DEPT. OB-GYN
ETSU COLLEGE OF MEDICINE
P. O. BOX 19,570A
JOHNSON CITY, TN 37614

ABDOMINAL ULTRASOUND

ABDOMINAL ULTRASOUND

Carol A. Mittelstaedt, M.D.

Associate Professor of Radiology
Associate Professor of Obstetrics and Gynecology
University of North Carolina at Chapel Hill
  School of Medicine
Chapel Hill, North Carolina

With a Contribution by

Lawrence M. Vincent, M.D.

Assistant Professor of Radiology
University of North Carolina at Chapel Hill
  School of Medicine
Chapel Hill, North Carolina

Churchill Livingstone
New York, Edinburgh, London, Melbourne   1987

Library of Congress Cataloging-in-Publication Data

Mittelstaedt, Carol A.
  Abdominal ultrasound.

  Includes bibliographies and index.
  1. Abdomen — Radiography. 2. Diagnosis, Ultrasonic.
3. Abdomen — Diseases — Diagnosis. I. Vincent, Lawrence M.
II. Title. [DNLM: 1. Abdomen — radiography. 2. Ultrasonic Diagnosis. WI 900 M6847a]
RC944.M58 1987   617′.5507′543   86-17143
ISBN 0-443-08341-X

© **Churchill Livingstone Inc. 1987**

Distributed in the United Kingdom by Churchill Livingstone, Robert Stevenson House,
1 – 3 Baxter's Place, Leith Walk, Edinburgh EH1 3AF, and by associated companies,
branches, and representatives throughout the world.

Accurate indications, adverse reactions, and dosage schedules for drugs are provided in this
book, but it is possible that they may change. The reader is urged to review the package
information data of the manufacturers of the medications mentioned.

Acquisitions Editor: *Robert A. Hurley*
Copy Editor: *Leslie Burgess*
Production Designer: *Jocelyn Eckstein*
Production Supervisor: *Jane Grochowski*

Printed in the United States of America

First published in 1987

Third printing in 1988

Fourth printing in 1989

To my parents,
Daisy and Stanley Mittelstaedt

Preface

I embarked on writing this text on abdominal ultrasound for three reasons. First, I love doing and teaching sonography and enjoy instilling my enthusiasm for this modality in medical students, residents, clinicians, and sonographers. Unfortunately, too many physicians do not "believe" in ultrasound because they do not understand what they are seeing in the images. It is a challenge to try to "convert" these "nonbelievers." Second, I wanted to fill a void in the ultrasound literature—having no comprehensive textbook on abdominal ultrasound had proven very frustrating. As a teacher, I was tired of always searching through my reprint file any time an interesting case came along in order to give a resident or student sonographer information about a particular entity. I wanted a convenient textbook for a reference. Third, I approached researching and writing this book as a tremendous intellectual exercise. Although it was a lot of work, I thoroughly enjoyed the project overall and gained immensely as a sonologist.

This text represents a culmination of the information published by sonographers and sonologists worldwide and from my personal experience. It is intended to be a comprehensive coverage of abdominal ultrasound. I organized each chapter with a preliminary discussion of sonographic technique and pertinent normal anatomy followed by a review of abnormalities. The areas covered include liver, biliary system, pancreas, urinary tract, retroperitoneum, vascular, peritoneal cavity and abdominal wall, spleen, gastrointestinal tract, interventional, and intraoperative. Obstetric, gynecologic, and small parts (thyroid, scrotum, and extremities) scanning are not covered, although there is a limited discussion of prostatic ultrasound. In each chapter, where appropriate, I include a discussion of ultrasound's diagnostic accuracy and a comparison between ultrasound and other imaging techniques. Many times, ultrasound texts present ultrasound as the modality of choice in all instances. I have made an attempt to place ultrasound in proper perspective, with regard to each area examined. I hope *Abdominal Ultrasound* will be useful as both a reference and a teaching text.

Carol A. Mittelstaedt, M.D.

Acknowledgments

This text represents the culmination of numerous individuals' efforts. Credit for photography goes to Robert Strain, for medical illustrations (except for Chapters 7 and 11) to Gwynne Moore, and for secretarial assistance to Joan Darnell. The UNC ultrasound images are the result of the technical expertise of staff and student sonographers over the years, but in particular Elizabeth ("Biffy") Daniel, R.D.M.S., and the student class of 1984–85: Linda Harris, R.D.M.S.; Carolyn Hedgepath, R.D.M.S.; Belinda Knight, R.D.M.S.; and Warwick Moss, R.D.M.S. I would like to thank William McCartney, M.D., the Director of the Imaging Division, and Lawrence Vincent, M.D., my ultrasound colleague, for their continued support (and contributions) in this endeavor. And, many thanks to the numerous individuals worldwide who kindly donated scans that made it possible to completely illustrate this text.

Contents

ABDOMINAL ULTRASOUND

1

The Liver

Even though the liver is the largest abdominal organ and the largest structure in the reticuloendothelial system, it is difficult to evaluate clinically because of its anatomic site. In addition, clinical detection of the liver 1 to 3 cm beneath the costal margin does not necessarily indicate hepatomegaly but, rather, may be due to a depressed diaphragm, as in emphysema, or may be a normal occurrence. As a result, ultrasound and other imaging techniques aid the clinician in the evaluation of liver disease.

TECHNIQUE

Preparation

No specific preparation is needed prior to an ultrasound of only the liver. If the gallbladder and pancreas are to be evaluated, it is preferable to have the patient fasting overnight. This allows for greater dilatation of the gallbladder and may be less likely to promote excessive bowel gas. In most cases, examination of the liver is not limited by bowel gas because the colon and the remainder of the bowel are usually inferior to the liver.

Real-Time Ultrasound

Some sonologists advocate real-time ultrasound as the sole method of examining the liver[1]; others feel it may be used in conjunction with static scanning.[2] The real-time scan has many advantages over the static scan. It is gen-

erally easier to perform, less sonographer-dependent, and more versatile. It is less hampered by bowel gas than static scans, perhaps because the bowel may be moved with the transducer and/or because there is greater maneuverability of the real-time sector transducer than the static fixed-arm transducer. The time required for a real-time examination is much less than that for the static examination, and the equipment is generally less expensive. Real-time ultrasound provides instant visualization of vascular landmarks, an advantage enhanced by the equipment's easy maneuverability.[1] Its disadvantages include the small field of view and the requirement of a more active role by the sonologist than that required with the static scan.

In one series, real-time scanning demonstrated an increased sensitivity over static scanning.[1] Real-time sonography was better able to examine the peripheral lateral portions of the liver, those portions near the junction of the diaphragm, and the anterior-posterior ribs.[1] The key to real-time examination of the liver is adherence to strict protocol.[1,2] One must examine all portions of the liver carefully, identifying certain anatomic landmarks. These include the various segments and fissures, the portal and hepatic venous structures and their branches, and the common hepatic artery and common bile duct.

Real-time ultrasound may be used as an adjunct to static ultrasound instead of the sole means of examination. Static scanning has certain problems that include nonvisualization of portions of the liver and kidney because of artifacts created by scanning over the lateral and anterior ribs and possible formation of "pseudolesions."[2] These problems can be overcome by use of sector real-time, which allows rapid access to alternate planes of view.[2] Many hepatic scans that would be suboptimal on static systems, due to "gas," can be "saved" by real-time systems, and more aggressively imaginative positioning.[2]

The technique for real-time examination of the liver is similar to that for static systems. The highest frequency transducer possible should be used to afford the best resolution. If adequate penetration to the posterior liver cannot be obtained with a high frequency transducer, a lower frequency transducer should be used. In most adults, the liver is examined using a 3 to 3.5 MHz transducer; in children and small adults, a 5 MHz transducer may be used. The near and far gain settings and the overall output (or system gain) should be adjusted in order to give a uniform representation of the hepatic parenchyma from the anterior to the posterior liver.[3,4] Many investigators have not found it helpful to vary the postprocessing settings.[5] The liver is generally examined during held inspiration in order to bring it beneath the costal margin. The liver is evaluated in both longitudinal and transverse planes, photographing sample scans at regular intervals and placing calibration marks on each scan. At times, one may need to scan in the left lateral decubitus position if the posterior liver is not adequately visualized.

Static Ultrasound

As with real-time ultrasound, the near and far gain on a static system, as well as the system gain, are set so that the liver parenchyma appears to have a uniform echopattern. The highest frequency transducer is used, which allows adequate penetration of the sound beam uniformly through to the posterior liver. Scans are usually performed at 1- to 2-cm intervals in the longitudinal and transverse planes during held inspiration. Because the transverse scan is a compound scan and takes longer to perform, the patient often is unable to hold his or her deep inspiration throughout the scan. These scans may have to be performed with quiet respiration. Other problems of static scanning include nonvisualization of portions of the liver and kidney because of the lateral and anterior ribs and possible formation of "pseudolesions."[2] At times, static scans of the liver may be hampered by bowel gas.

Future

Work is being done at the present time in evaluating ultrasound "contrast" agents. Perfluorochemicals such as perfluorodecalin, perfluorotripropylamine, and per-

fluoroctylbromide (PFOB) have been shown to produce increased liver echogenicity relative to kidney echogenicity in rabbits.[6,7] PFOB produces an echogenic rim around hepatic tumors in rabbits.[7] These compounds or others may sometime in the future serve as echogenic contrast materials that may facilitate the visualization of hepatic tumors.

NORMAL ANATOMY

Normally, the adult liver weighs from 1400 to 1600 g, with the right lobe six times larger than the left.[8] It is usually 15 to 17 cm in length with its upper border generally at the level of the nipples and its lower border at the level of the costal cartilage of the 8-9th rib. The hepatic flexure of the colon lies in immediate proximity to the free margin of the right lobe.[9] The left lobe is variable, with its inferior margin lying in close proximity to the body and antrum of the stomach; it frequently lies immediately adjacent to the body of the pancreas.[9] Clinical diagnosis of liver disease often rests on such nonspecific symptoms as anorexia, dyspepsia, malaise, and abdominal discomfort, while clinical signs of liver disease such as jaundice and hepatomegaly may not occur until liver failure is advanced.[10] Biochemical tests can be used to quantitate impaired liver function but are of limited use in the differential diagnosis in diffuse liver disease.

The liver is composed of three cell types: biliary epithelial cells, Kupffer cells, and hepatocytes.[3] In each liver lobule, hepatocytes radiate out to the periphery around a central vein.[8] These hepatocytes synthesize, metabolize, and excrete a variety of compounds.[3,8] The outer margins of the lobule are imcompletely demarcated by portal triads or tracts, which are connective tissue septa each containing branches of the hepatic artery, hepatic vein, and bile duct.[8] The vascular sinusoids are lined by endothelial cells and Kupffer cells. The Kupffer cells (portion of the reticuloendothelial system) phagocytize bacteria and foreign material.[3]

The liver function tests are estimates of deranged function. With cell necrosis, there is elevation of serum glutamic oxaloacetic transaminase (SGOT), and serum glutamic pyruvic transaminase (SGPT). With cholestasis or inhibition of bile secretion, there is an increased level of alkaline phosphatase. When there are defects in cell synthesis, there may be an elevation of serum bilirubin, serum albumin, and/or prothrombin time.

Ultrasound provides an excellent means of assessing internal structure of the liver and evaluating both diffuse and focal parenchymal abnormalities. Familiarity with the internal hepatic anatomy is important in order to diagnose disease. Knowledge of three-dimensional he-

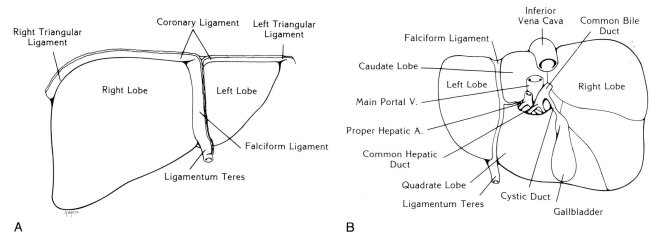

Fig. 1-1. Lobar anatomy. Anterior **(A)** and posterior **(B)** views. Using the traditional anatomic system for lobar division, the left lobe is considered that portion of the liver to the left of the falciform ligament with the remainder of the liver subdivided into the right, caudate, and quadrate lobes. Using the functional system for lobar division based on vessels, the "traditional" left lobe represents the lateral segment of the left lobe with the quadrate lobe representing the medial segment of the left lobe. With this system, the right and left lobes are divided with the plane of separation from the inferior vena cava to the gallbladder fossa.

patic anatomy results in greater ability to correlate the lesion location with various imaging methods. This is important in an era when ultrasound and computed tomography (CT) are used to confirm or add to the specificity of nuclear medicine findings. A knowledge of hepatic segmental anatomy is helpful in determining the extent of primary or secondary hepatic malignancy.[11]

Lobar Anatomy

The liver may be divided into lobes by certain anatomic landmarks visible at ultrasound (Fig. 1-1). The functional right lobe, by far the largest lobe, represents that portion of the liver located to the right of a line intersecting the gallbladder fossa and the sulcus for the inferior vena cava[9] (Fig. 1-2). The caudate lobe is located posterior to the porta hepatis, between the fissure for the ligamentum venosum and the inferior vena cava[9,12,13] (Fig. 1-3). It occasionally appears hypoechoic, possibly due to its position immediately posterior to the fissure of the ligamentum venosum and/or due to acoustic shadowing in a patient with more fat or fibrous tissue along the fissure of the ligamentum venosum.[12] It should not be confused with abnormalities, and if there is a question CT can be performed. The left margin of the caudate lobe forms the hepatic boundary of the superior recess of the lesser sac.[13] The right margin of the caudate extends in a tongue-like projection—caudate process—between the inferior vena cava, and adjacent to the main portal vein and the medial portion of the right hepatic lobe.[13,14]

The left lobe is always smaller than the right but varies in size.[14] The quadrate lobe (medial segment of the functional left lobe) lies between the fissure for the ligamentum teres and the gallbladder fossa, anterior to the porta hepatis[9] (Fig. 1-4). The lateral segment of the left lobe lies medial to the fissure of the ligamentum teres (Figs. 1-4 and 1-5). The degree of left lobe extension to the left is the key to visualization of the pancreas.[14] In rare instances, there may be a congenital absence of the left lobe of the liver; a failure to identify the falciform ligament or ligamentum teres supports evidence for this diagnosis.[15] Absence of liver tissue to the left of the gallbladder fossa further confirms the diagnosis.[15]

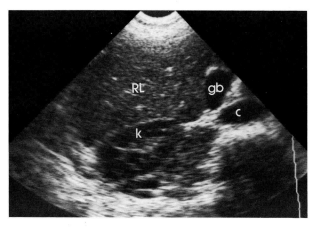

Fig. 1-2. Right lobe. Transverse scan. The right lobe *(RL)* represents that portion of the liver to the right of the gallbladder *(gb)* and the inferior vena cava *(c)*. (*k,* right kidney.)

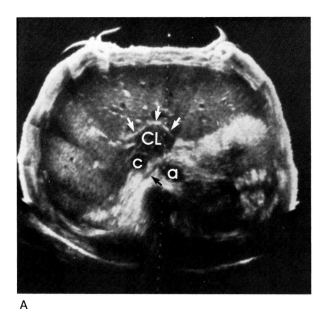

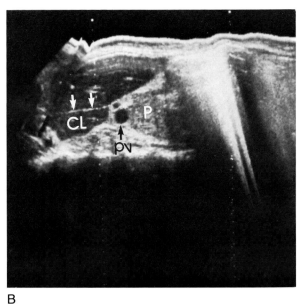

A   B

Fig. 1-3.   Caudate lobe. **(A)** Transverse static scan 12 cm above the umbilicus. The caudate lobe *(CL)* is seen posterior to the ligamentum venosum (white arrows). *(c,* inferior vena cava; *a,* aorta; black arrow, right renal artery.) **(B)** Longitudinal static scan. The caudate *(CL)* is again seen posterior to the ligamentum venosum (arrows) and superior to the portal vein *(pv).* *(P,* pancreas.)

Riedel's lobe, more common in women, is a tongue-like projection of the right lobe that may extend to the iliac crest.[14] It represents the enlarged anterior and posterior segments of this lobe[14] (Fig. 1-6).

The liver may also be visualized in terms of vascular planes (functional division).[9] The right and left lobes are divided by a line intersecting the gallbladder fossa and the inferior vena cava. The middle hepatic veins course within a plane of separation, the main lobar fissure, between the functional left and right lobes[14] (Fig. 1-7). The right functional lobe is divided into anterior and posterior segments based on the branching right hepatic vein in the right segmental fissure; the right portal vein (RPV) courses within this segment[11,14] (Fig. 1-8). The medial

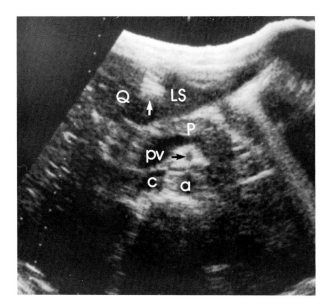

Fig. 1-4.   Quadrate lobe and ligamentum teres. Transverse static scan. The ligamentum teres (white arrow) is seen as a rounded echogenic area separating the medial *(Q,* quadrate lobe) and lateral *(LS)* segments of the left lobe. *(a,* aorta; *c,* inferior vena cava; *pv,* portal vein; *P,* pancreas; black arrow, superior mesenteric artery.)

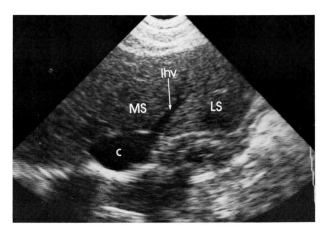

Fig. 1-5.   Left lobe. Lateral segment. Transverse real-time scan. The lateral segment *(LS)* is that portion of the left lobe medial to the left hepatic vein *(lhv),* which runs within the left segmental fissure. *(MS,* medial segment of left lobe; *c,* inferior vena cava.)

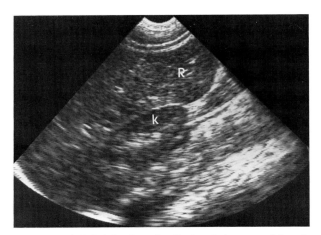

Fig. 1-6. Riedel's lobe. Longitudinal real-time scan. Note the inferior aspect of the liver extends inferior to the kidney *(k)*. This represents Riedel's lobe *(R)*.

Ligaments and Fissures

Ultrasound is capable of demonstrating the ligaments and fissures by virtue of the presence of collagen and fat within and around these structures, which make them highly reflective relative to hepatic parenchyma.[9] The falciform ligament travels over the anterior surface of the liver and runs in continuity with the ligamentum teres that courses within the liver (Figs. 1-1 and 1-9). It extends from the umbilicus to the diaphragm in a parasagittal plane; contained between its layers are the ligamentum teres and the umbilical vein remnant.[16] On the anterior-posterior axis, the falciform ligament extends from the right rectus muscle anterior to the bare area of the liver, where its reflections separate to contribute to the hepatic coronary ligaments.[16] On ultrasound, the ligamentum teres hepatis is seen as a round hyperechoic area just to the right of midline on a transverse scan[16-18] (Fig. 1-4). It is linear in longitudinal plane extending from the anterior surface posteriorly toward the porta hepatis. The ligamentum teres can sometimes be variable, so it is necessary to follow it in order to exclude metastasis.[19] The falciform ligament and the ligamentum teres mark the boundary of the lateral and medial (or quadrate) segments of the left lobe, both supplied by the left portal vein.[9] The major fissure of the liver dividing the left and right lobes is seen as a linear echo on longitudinal scans from the gallbladder to the porta hepatis (Fig. 1-7). The fissure for the ligamentum venosum contains the hepatogastric ligament, which is located between the caudate lobe and the lateral segment of the left lobe[9,13,18] (Fig. 1-3).

segment is the functional left lobe and the lateral segment is the traditional anatomic left lobe. The left segmental fissure divides the left lobe into medial and lateral segments; the portion of the falciform ligament that contains the ligamentum teres courses in the caudal aspect of the left intersegmental fissure[11,14] (Fig. 1-5). The functional lobar division has clinical relevance in assessing surgical resection of primary hepatic neoplasms, solitary metastatic lesions, and other nonmalignant hepatic abnormalities.[9] By employing each anatomic feature, it is possible to define the segmental anatomy.

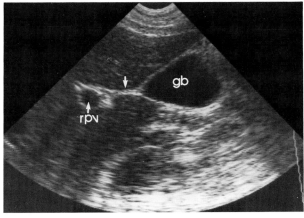

A

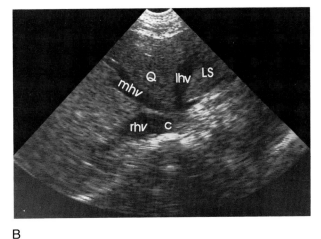

B

Fig. 1-7. Main lobar fissure. **(A)** Longitudinal real-time scan. The main lobar fissure is seen as a linear echodensity (arrow) extending from the gallbladder *(gb)* to the right portal vein *(rpv)*. It divides the functional left and right lobes. **(B)** High transverse real-time scan. The middle hepatic vein *(mhv)* is seen exiting from the inferior vena cava *(c)*. It courses within a plane of separation between the left and right lobes. (*lhv,* left hepatic vein; *rhv,* right hepatic vein; *Q,* quadrate lobe; *LS,* lateral segment of the left lobe.)

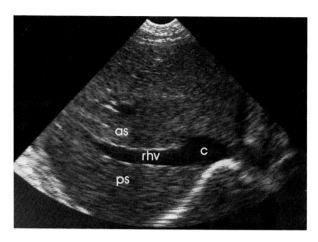

Fig. 1-8. Right segmental fissure. Transverse real-time scan. The right hepatic vein *(rhv)* is seen coursing in the right segmental fissure dividing the right functional lobe into anterior *(as)* and posterior *(ps)* segments. *(c,* inferior vena cava.)

Vessels

The liver receives its nutrients via the hepatic artery and the portal vein.[8] The portal vein is 80-percent saturated with oxygen and supplies 50 to 60 percent of the oxygen requirement of the hepatocytes.[8] With this dual blood supply, infarcts are rare. Because the distribution and branches of the hepatic veins and portal veins are used as a "road map" in localizing pathologic abnormalities and for orientation in follow-up studies, it is impor-

tant to be able to properly identify these vessels and their branches.[20]

At times, it may be difficult to differentiate portal and hepatic veins. Using real-time ultrasound, an hepatic vessel may be traced back to its origin—either portal or inferior vena cava.[9,14] Because portal veins are encased in collagenous sheaths running in common with the hepatic artery and bile duct, their margins tend to be echodense[9] (Fig. 1-10). This finding has been shown to be present in 99 percent of cases.[21] Hepatic veins have minimal collagen in their walls and are surrounded by hepatic parenchyma, and, as such, have imperceptible margins[9,21] (Fig. 1-10). In addition to the contrast in echodensity of the vessel walls, the portal and hepatic veins have different branching patterns. The apex of the angle of the portal vein has a horizontal orientation at the porta hepatis[9,21] (Fig. 1-11). The apex of the hepatic vein bifurcation is longitudinal toward the inferior vena cava[9,21] (Figs. 1-11B,C and 1-12A). The caliber of the hepatic veins increases as they course toward the diaphragm and inferior vena cava, while the caliber of the portal veins increases toward the porta hepatis.[9,21] In addition, as a general rule, hepatic veins course between lobes and segments (interlobar and intersegmental) while portal veins course within lobar segments (intrasegmental)[11] (Figs. 1-5, 1-7, 1-8, 1-11, and 1-12A).

The hepatic veins branch directly from the superior aspect of the inferior vena cava (Fig. 1-12A). They are best visualized on a high transverse scan through the liver. The right hepatic vein (RHV) is located in the right

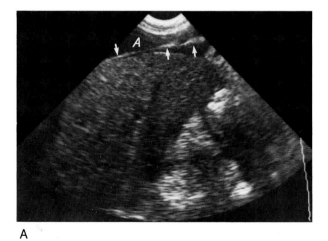

A

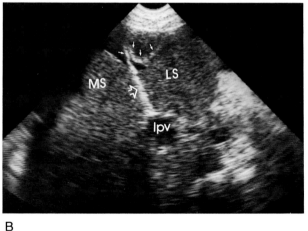

B

Fig. 1-9. Falciform ligament. **(A)** Longitudinal real-time scan through the liver. Ascites *(A)* is seen anteriorly. The linear echodensity (arrows) extending from the anterior aspect of the liver inferiorly is the falciform ligament. **(B)** Transverse scan in another patient demonstrates the falciform ligament (small arrows, open arrow) extending between the left portal vein *(lpv)* and the anterior abdominal wall, dividing the caudal portions of the medial *(MS)* and lateral *(LS)* left hepatic segments. The ligamentum teres runs in the inferior or free edge of the falciform ligament. It is the obliterated umbilical vein and is seen on transverse scans as a rounded echodense structure between the lateral and medial segments of the left lobe.

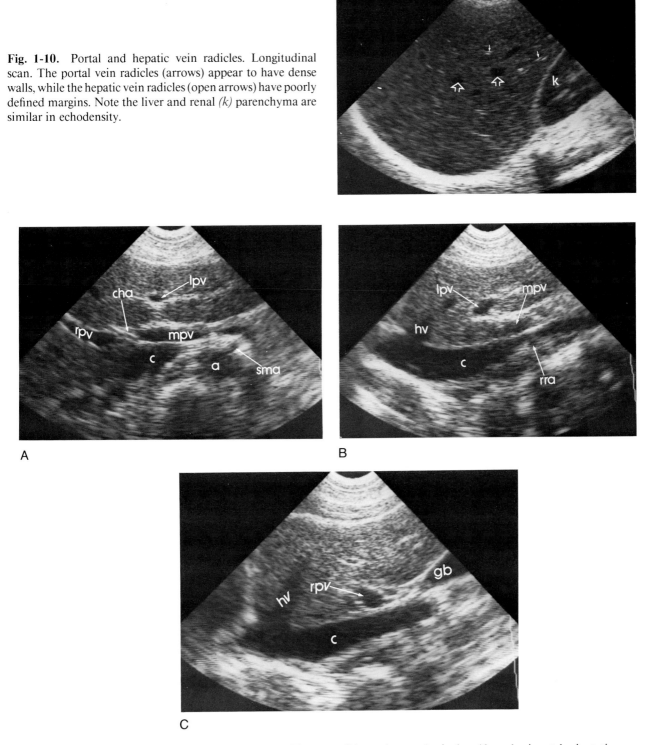

Fig. 1-10. Portal and hepatic vein radicles. Longitudinal scan. The portal vein radicles (arrows) appear to have dense walls, while the hepatic vein radicles (open arrows) have poorly defined margins. Note the liver and renal *(k)* parenchyma are similar in echodensity.

A

B

C

Fig. 1-11. Main portal vein. **(A)** Transverse scan. The apex of the main portal vein *(mpv)* has a horizontal orientation at the porta hepatis. The right portal vein *(rpv)* has a horizontal course from the main portal vein. (*lpv,* left portal vein; *c,* inferior vena cava; *a,* aorta; *sma,* superior mesenteric artery; *cha,* common hepatic artery.) **(B)** Longitudinal scan. The main portal vein *(mpv)* is round in this orientation with its left branch *(lpv).* (*hv,* hepatic vein; *c,* inferior vena cava; *rra,* right renal artery) **(C)** Longitudinal scan slightly to the right of midline. The right portal vein *(rpv)* is seen as the continuation of the main portal vein. (*c,* inferior vena cava; *gb,* gallbladder; *hv,* hepatic vein.)

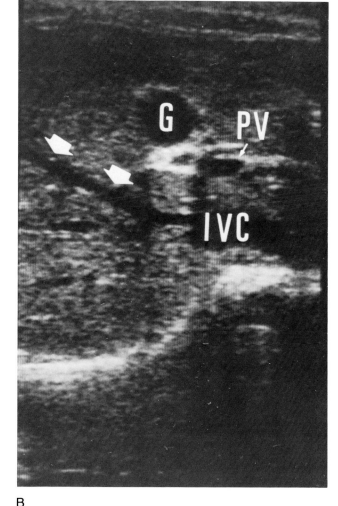

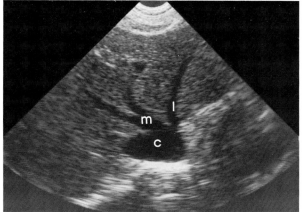

A   B

Fig. 1-12. Hepatic veins. **(A)** Transverse scan. The middle *(m)* and left *(l)* hepatic veins are seen extending from the inferior vena cava *(c)* on this high scan. There are two middle hepatic veins noted; the right hepatic vein is not seen in this view. The axis of the hepatic veins is superior. **(B)** Inferior right hepatic vein. Transverse linear real-time scan at a level lower in the abdomen than Fig. 1-12A. The inferior right hepatic vein (arrows) is seen extending from the inferior vena cava *(IVC)*. *(PV,* portal vein; *G,* gallbladder.) **(B** from Makunchi M, Hasegawa, H, Yamazaki S, et al: The inferior right hepatic vein: ultrasonic demonstration. Radiology 148:213, 1983.)

intersegmental fissure coursing between the anterior and posterior branches of the RPV[14,22] (Fig. 1-8). It divides the cephalic aspect of the anterior and posterior segments of the right hepatic lobe.[14] The middle hepatic vein (MHV) is located in the main lobar fissure separating the right and left lobes[14] (Figs. 1-7 and 1-12A). Located in the left intersegmental fissure, the left hepatic vein (LHV) divides the cephalic aspects of the medial and lateral segments of the left lobe[14,22] (Figs. 1-5, 1-7B, and 1-12A).

The main portal vein (MPV) emerges just to the right of midline at the junction of the superior mesenteric and splenic veins (Fig. 1-13). It courses cephalad to and to the

right of the porta hepatis and is anterior to the inferior vena cava; it is cephalad to the head of the pancreas with a normal measurement of 11 ± 2 mm.[23] It divides into a smaller, more anterior and more cranial left portal vein (LPV) and a larger, more posterior and more caudal RPV[14] (Figs. 1-11 and 1-14). The portal veins then branch into medial and lateral divisions on the left and into anterior and posterior divisions on the right, and become intrasegmental in their course.[14] Elongation of the MPV at the origin of the LPV represents the precise indication of the porta hepatis.[14] The LPV, which arises to the right of midline, proceeds cranially along the anterior surface of the caudate, and then arches back anteri-

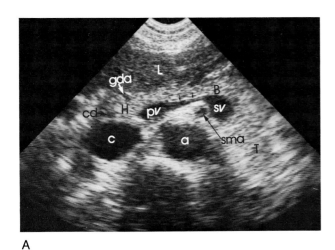

A

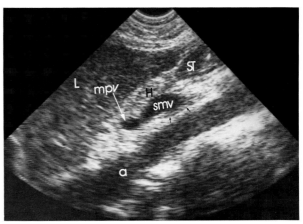

B

Fig. 1-13. Main portal vein. **(A)** Transverse scan. The main portal vein *(pv)* is formed by the junction of the superior mesenteric and splenic veins *(sv)* in the region of the neck (arrows) of the pancreas. *(c,* inferior vena cava; *a,* aorta; *sma,* superior mesenteric artery; *T,* pancreatic tail; *B,* pancreatic body; *H,* pancreatic head; *gda,* gastroduodenal artery; *cd,* common bile duct; *L,* liver.) **(B)** Longitudinal scan. The superior mesenteric vein *(smv)* is seen as a tubular structure paralleling the aorta *(a)* and draining into the main portal vein *(mpv).* The head *(H)* of the pancreas can be seen inferior to the main portal vein and anterior to the superior mesenteric vein. The uncinate process (arrows) is seen between the aorta and superior mesenteric vein. *(ST,* fluid-filled stomach; *L,* liver.)

orly and to the left (Fig. 1-14). It gives branches to the caudate lobe and divides into medial and lateral branches. The umbilical vein is also a branch of the LPV. At times, there are variations in the size of the LPV and the angle at which it travels from the MPV.[24] The LPV and its surrounding connective tissue frequently mimic the posterior margin of the lateral segment of the left lobe on the transverse scan.[25] The LPV has been found to be identifiable in 61 percent of patients.[25] The RPV is posterior and has a long, horizontal course (Fig. 1-11). Its appearance and course seem constant.[24]

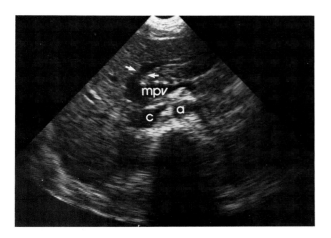

Fig. 1-14. Left portal vein. Transverse real-time scan. The left portal vein (arrows) is seen extending anteriorly from the main portal vein *(mpv).* *(c,* inferior vena cava; *a,* aorta.)

Both left and right portal triads give off portal venous and hepatic arterial branches to the caudate lobe.[13] The caudate is drained by a series of short venous channels that extend directly from the posterior aspect of the caudate into the inferior vena cava adjoining the posterior margin of the caudate.[13] Because the caudate has an independent vascular supply, there are important clinical implications.[13] The short intrahepatic course of the caudate lobe afferent vessels favors less attenuation of the caudate lobe vasculature by adjacent hepatic fibrosis. Discrepancy between perfusion of the caudate lobe and perfusion of the right hepatic lobe may be responsible for the caudate lobe enlargement and right hepatic lobe shrinkage seen in cirrhotic patients.[13] Caudate enlargement with compression of the underlying inferior vena cava is implicated in the development of various cirrhotic complications including inferior vena cava hypertension, ascites, portacaval shunt failure, and, possibly, hepatorenal syndrome.[13]

The common hepatic artery emerges from the celiac axis, crosses to the right, and runs adjacent to the portal vein and common bile duct at the porta hepatis[26,27] (Fig. 1-15). When the common hepatic artery arises from the superior mesenteric artery, it runs between the portal vein and common bile duct and joins the superior mesenteric artery.[26] As a branch of the common hepatic artery, the gastroduodenal artery curves caudally and runs along the right anterolateral surface of the head of the pancreas, posteromedial to the duodenum[27] (Figs. 1-13 and 1-16) The proper hepatic artery is the continua-

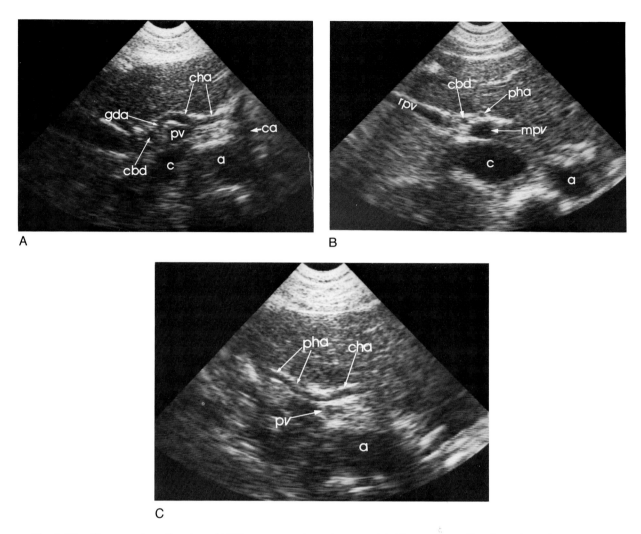

Fig. 1-15. Common hepatic artery. **(A)** The common hepatic artery *(cha)* is seen extending from the celiac artery *(ca)* running anterior to the main portal vein *(pv)*. The gastroduodenal artery *(gda)* is visualized branching from the common hepatic artery. *(cbd,* common bile duct; *c,* inferior vena cava; *a,* aorta.) **(B)** Transverse oblique scan. The common bile duct *(cbd)* is seen anterolateral to the main portal vein *(mpv)*, with the proper hepatic artery *(pha)* more anteromedial. *(a,* aorta; *c,* inferior vena cava; *rpv,* right portal vein.) **(C)** Transverse scan more oblique than **(A)**, following the course of the proper hepatic artery *(pha)*, the continuation of the common hepatic artery *(cha)*, after the gastroduodenal artery branch. *(a,* aorta; *pv,* main portal vein.)

tion of the common hepatic artery distal to the origin of the gastroduodenal artery. It turns anterior and cephalad and runs along the free edge of the lesser omentum (hepatoduodenal ligament) toward the porta hepatis. In the region of the porta, the proper hepatic artery divides into the right, middle, and left hepatic arteries (Fig. 1-16). The right hepatic artery runs in the right intersegmental fissure where it is posterior to the bile duct, between the duct and portal vein. Two thirds of the patients are noted to have a right hepatic artery that crosses behind the common bile duct or right hepatic duct, whereas the left hepatic artery crosses anterior to the left hepatic duct[26]

(Fig. 1-16). In most patients, the right hepatic artery is anterior to the right portal vein. The middle and left hepatic arteries are not usually imaged.

The parallel-channel has been described as a sign of dilated ducts.[26] It refers to simultaneous imaging of the RPV and right hepatic duct (RHD) and/or LPV and left hepatic duct (LHD) on transverse or longitudinal scan.[26] The common hepatic artery and duct are similar in size and may be difficult to distinguish. The following are helpful differentiating points: (1) intrinsic pulsations, (2) indentation or displacement of structures by arteries, (3) change in caliber of bile duct during real-time scanning,

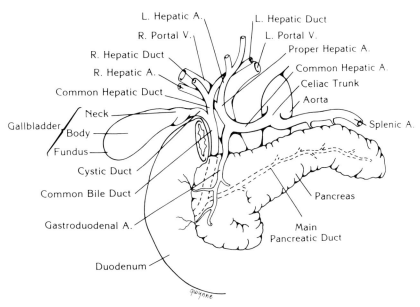

Fig. 1-16. Hepatic duct/hepatic artery/portal vein. Note the relationships of the hepatic ducts, hepatic arteries, and portal veins. On the right, the right hepatic artery is between the right portal vein and right hepatic duct, with the duct anterior. On the left, the left hepatic artery is anterior to the left hepatic duct and left portal vein. (Modified from Sauerbrei E: Ultrasound of the common bile duct. p. 1. In Sanders RC, Hill MC (eds): Ultrasound Annual 1983, Raven Press, New York, 1983.)

(4) orientation, (5) contour, (6) caliber, and (7) curvature of the tubular structure in the porta hepatis.[28] Doppler ultrasound also helps to distinguish duct from artery.[28]

Thus, there are three main structures of concern in the porta hepatis: hepatic artery, common bile duct, and portal vein. At the level of the porta hepatis, the common bile duct is lateral to the hepatic artery and both are anterior to the portal vein (Fig. 1-15B). Entering the liver, the common hepatic duct is anterior to the right hepatic artery, which in turn is anterior to the main portal vein (Fig. 1-16). The right and left hepatic ducts are located anterior to the right and left portal veins (Fig. 1-16).

In one series of 269 patients, 10 percent demonstrated an inferior RHV (an accessory RHV). The identification of this vessel is significant in patients undergoing hepatectomy with tumor thrombus in hepatocellular carcinoma, Budd-Chiari syndrome, and dilatation of the intrahepatic ducts.[29] The preoperative visualization of a hypertrophied inferior RHV would facilitate preservation of both it and the right posterior-inferior area of the liver during a resection of the RHV. In cases of Budd-Chiari syndrome, the main drainage vein of the right lobe of the liver may be the inferior RHV.[29] To identify the inferior RHV, it is necessary only to see the vessel posterior to the RPV and trace it back medially to the inferior vena cava (Fig. 1-12B). It should not be confused with the right posterior portal vein branch, which courses further caudad then the main right hepatic vein.

Echopattern

The parenchymal architecture is homogeneous, moderately echogenic, and interspersed with fluid-filled vessels. The liver may be isosonic (same relative echodensity) to the renal parenchyma or slightly more echogenic. It is usually isosonic to the pancreas or slightly less echogenic than the pancreas[9] (Fig. 1-10).

Size

One method for diagnosing hepatomegaly involves measuring the liver in two planes.[30] The liver is measured from the midspine to the outer surface of the liver on a transverse scan (Fig. 1-17A). On a longitudinal scan obtained at the midhepatic line, the liver is measured from its superior to inferior margins (Fig. 1-17B). This measurement has been found to be 87 percent accurate in determining the presence or absence of hepatomegaly.[30] If the liver is less than or equal to 13 cm in the midhepatic line, it is normal in 93 percent of cases. If the

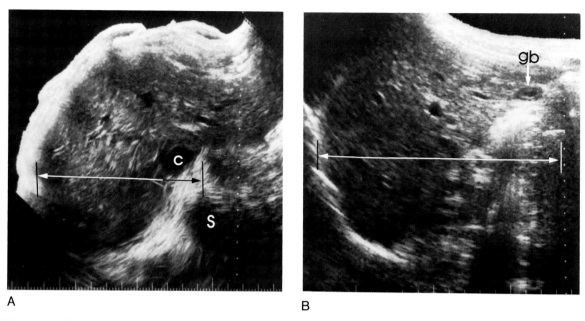

A   B

Fig. 1-17. Liver size. **(A)** The liver is measured on a transverse view from the midspine *(S)* to the outer surface of the liver. The measurement obtained transversely is halved and **(B)** a longitudinal scan is performed at that point (midhepatic line) to the right of midline. The liver is measured from its superior to inferior aspect (arrows). (*gb,* contracted gallbladder; *c,* inferior vena cava.)

liver is greater than or equal to 15.5 cm, it is enlarged in 75 percent of cases.[30]

Other investigators have evaluated the liver size relative to the midclavicular line.[31] The normal liver measures l0.5 ± 1.5 (standard deviation) cm in the longitudinal diameter in the midclavicular plane with a measurement of 8.1 ± 1.9 (standard deviation) cm in the anterior-posterior projection. The 95th percentile for these are 12.6 cm and 11.3 cm respectively.[31]

DIFFUSE DISEASE

Hepatocellular disease can be defined as a disease process that affects the hepatocytes and interferes with liver function. Such diseases may range from simple fatty change to hepatitis or cirrhosis depending on the severity and progression of the disease. There have been different sonographic patterns described with each.

Fatty Infiltration

With fatty infiltration, fat in the liver cells implies significant injury to the liver or some systemic disorder leading to either impaired metabolism of fat or excessive metabolism of depot fat.[8] This can be seen in diabetes mellitus, ethanol abuse, obesity, tuberculosis, ulcerative colitis, kwashiorkor, excessive overeating, starvation, corticosteroid therapy, hyperlipidemia, parenteral nutrition, Reye's syndrome, severe hepatitis, glycogen storage disease, cystic fibrosis, and jejunoileal bypass for obesity.[32] Fatty infiltration is particularly significant in chronic alcoholism.[8] If an echodense liver is demonstrated in a child who is not malnourished or receiving parenteral hyperalimentation or treatment with chemotherapy, metabolic disease should be suspected.[33]

The majority of patients with histologically moderate or severe fatty infiltration have brightly reflective echopatterns in their livers on ultrasound[34,35] (Figs. 1-18 and 1-19). The high-level echoes may be due to an increase in collagen content of the liver rather than to the fat.[35] One series was able to detect 60 percent of patients with fatty infiltration of the liver.[34] The sensitivity of detection by recognition of a bright liver echopattern was related to the degree of infiltration, and increased to 90 percent in moderate and severe cases.[34] The false-positive rate was very low.[34] Another study has correlated ultrasound and CT in the detection of fatty infiltration of the liver.[32] The overall accuracy of ultrasound was 85 percent with a 100-percent sensitivity and a 56-percent specificity.[32] Three grades were defined for fatty infiltration: grade 1 (mild)—slight diffuse increase in the fine echoes in the hepatic parenchyma with normal visualization of the diaphragm and intrahepatic vessel borders (Fig. 1-19A); grade 2 (moderate)—moderate diffuse increase in the

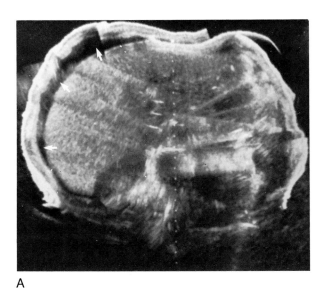

A

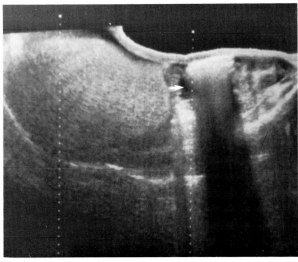

B

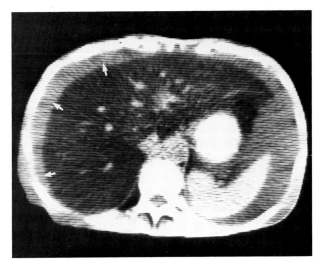

C

Fig. 1-18. Fatty infiltration. **(A)** Transverse static scan. There is a uniform echodense liver pattern. Ascites is seen as the anechoic area bordering the liver (arrows). **(B)** Longitudinal static scan 9 cm to right of midline. Fluid (arrow) is seen inferior to the liver. The liver echopattern is uniformly dense. **(C)** Enhanced CT revealing a uniformly low-density liver. Ascites (arrows) is seen.

fine echoes with slightly impaired visualization of the intrahepatic vessels and diaphragm (Fig. 1-19B); and grade 3 (severe)—marked increase in fine echoes with poor or nonvisualization of the intrahepatic vessel borders, diaphragm, and posterior portion of the right lobe of the liver[32] (Fig. 1-19C). A coarser, more scattered increase in echogenicity and an altered shape of the cirrhotic liver was sufficiently characteristic to permit differentiation from fatty infiltration, but there was some overlap.[32]

Fat infiltration of the liver is not uniform in all patients. Sometimes there is a patchy distribution of the fat throughout the liver. Cases of nonuniform distribution have been found to predominantly involve the right lobe; this nonuniformity may cause a problem in diagnosis[36] (Fig. 1-20). Nonuniform distribution of fat has been reported with alcohol abuse, administration of exogenous steroids, and malnutrition accompanying ma-

lignancy.[36,37] The reason for the nonuniformity is not known. Normally the time-gain-compensation (TGC) curve is set to provide relatively normal texture to the majority of the liver. In these cases, with most of the liver infiltrated by fat, there was an increased echogenicity.[36] When the fatty liver displayed normal texture, the true normal areas of the liver appeared as anechoic focal defects[36-38] (Fig. 1-20). The problem encountered in setting the correct TGC and gain factors for patients with liver disease just underlines the need for tissue phantoms for ultrasound.[36]

Hepatitis

Hepatitis is broadly defined as inflammation of the liver. In cases of viral hepatitis, the offending organism is generally hepatitis A, hepatitis B, or hepatitis non-A,

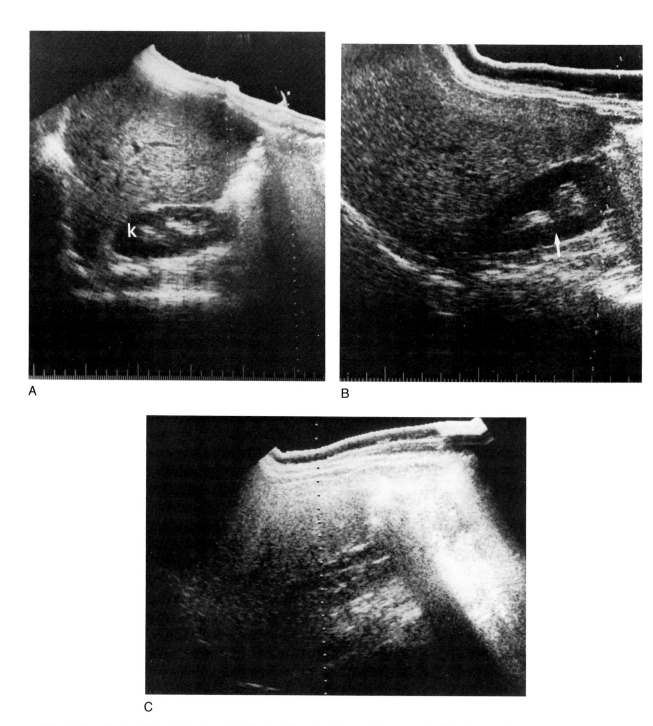

Fig. 1-19. Graded fatty infiltration. **(A)** Grade I. Longitudinal static scan with slight increase in the fine echoes in the liver compared to the right renal *(k)* cortex. **(B)** Grade 2. Longitudinal static scan with moderately increased fine echoes in the liver which impair visualization of the vessel walls and the right hemidiaphragm. (Arrow, right kidney). **(C)** Grade 3. Longitudinal static scan in which the echogenicity and sound attenuation are markedly increased. There is poor visualization of the diaphragm, vessels, and posterior right lobe. (From Scatarige JC, Scott WW, Donovan PJ, et al: Fatty infiltration of the liver: ultrasonographic and computed tomographic correlation. J Ultrasound Med 3:9, 1984.)

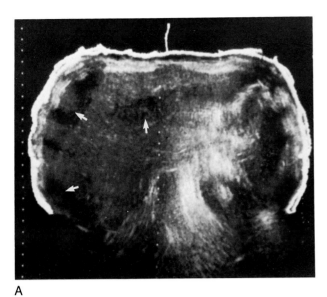
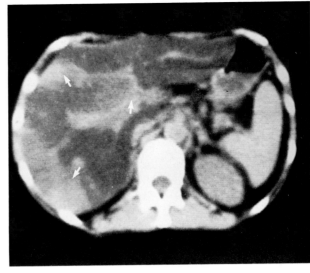

A   B

Fig. 1-20. Nonuniform fatty infiltration. **(A)** Transverse static scan at 12 cm above the umbilicus. There is an inhomogeneous echopattern. The normal parenchyma (arrows) appears lucent with the fat appearing dense. **(B)** CT scan demonstrating the inhomogeneous fatty infiltration. (Arrows, normal parenchyma.)

non-B virus. The incubation period for hepatitis A is 2 to 6 weeks; that of the B virus is 2 to 6 months. The A virus is transmitted from person to person via fecal-oral route, while the source of the B virus is a chronic carrier or patients with acute hepatitis B and is transmitted via parenteral inoculation (including toothbrushes and razor blades).[8] The extent of the liver injury in acute hepatitis may range from mild and subclinical cases to massive necrosis and liver failure. There is diffuse hepatocellular disarray and necrosis without portal or periportal abnormality.[39] The severity and extent of the necrosis appears to vary with the level of immune response evoked by the infected hepatocytes.[8] The pathologic changes seen include (1) liver cell injury — swelling of the hepatocytes and hepatocyte degeneration, which may lead to cell necrosis; (2) reticuloendothelial and lymphocytic response — Kupffer cells enlarge; and (3) regeneration — usual relationship of the liver cell to sinusoid disappears.[8] With chronic hepatitis, there is portal inflammatory infiltration without extension across the portal limiting plate and preservation of the lobular architecture.[39] In chronic active hepatitis, there is more extensive change than in chronic persistent hepatitis, with inflammation extending across the limiting plate, spreading out in a perilobular fashion, and causing piecemeal necrosis.[39] Fibrosis frequently accompanies this. The outcome may be complete recovery following an illness of 4 to 6 weeks in hepatitis A. The B infection tends to be more prolonged. If the hepatitis becomes

fulminant, massive necrosis may ensue, with the entire liver shrinking. While chronic persistent hepatitis is a benign, self-limiting process, chronic active hepatitis usually progresses to cirrhosis and liver failure.

Sonographic patterns associated with hepatitis have been described.[39] With acute hepatitis, the predominate findings are accentuated brightness, more extensive demonstration of the portal vein radicle walls, and overall decreased echogenicity of the liver[39] (Fig. 1-21). With chronic hepatitis, there is a decrease in brightness of the liver and the number of portal vein radicle walls and an overall increase in liver echogenicity[39] (Fig. 1-22). The liver exhibits a coarse echopattern. The patterns of acute and chronic hepatitis appear to be specific, with a confidence level of 95 percent (in a retrospective study).[39] The probability in detecting acute and chronic hepatitis patterns is thus 93 percent.

The ultrasound patterns are reported to be consistent with the histopathologic correlation.[39] In acute hepatitis, the major pathologic abnormality is in the intralobular portion of the liver; it is possible, therefore, that one sees portal walls better due to the fibrous walls of the portal vein radicles.[39] The swelling of the liver cells accounts for the decreased echoes. In chronic hepatitis, the pathologic findings of periportal, perilobular, and portal changes produce a coarse echopattern due to the increased amount of fibrous tissue and inflammatory cells surrounding hepatic lobules.[39] In more severe cases, since the abnormality abuts directly on the portal vein radi-

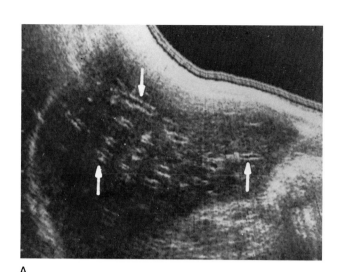
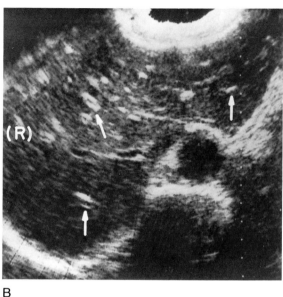

A   B

Fig. 1-21. Acute hepatitis. **(A)** Case 1. Longitudinal static scan showing overall decrease in the echopattern. The portal vein radial walls (arrows) are brighter than usual and are more clearly seen in the periphery, near, middle, and far fields. **(B)** Case 2. Transverse static scan showing the same findings as **(A).** (*R,* right.) (From Kurtz AB, Rubin CS, Cooper HS, et al: Ultrasound findings in hepatitis. Radiology 136:717, 1980.)

cals, there is decreased visualization of the portal vein radicle walls due to a similar brightness of adjacent portal and periportal echoes.[39]

The ultrasound technique is critical.[39] Because the predominant finding in acute hepatitis encompasses the portal vein radicles — the walls of which are large, specular, angle-dependent reflectors — the single sector scan is recommended particularly along the long axis of the

right lobe so that the transducer is perpendicular to the vein radicle walls. In chronic hepatitis, there is more effect produced by changes in the power (gain) and TGC curve. An inordinate increase in either produces a false overall brightness similar to true coarsening, as the compromised liver parenchyma contains small, diffuse, nonangle-dependent reflectors. In true coarsening, vessels remain echofree while vascular fill-in indicates in-

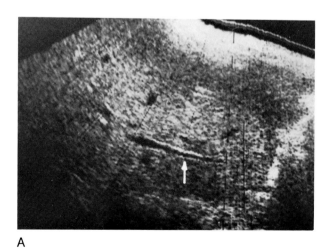
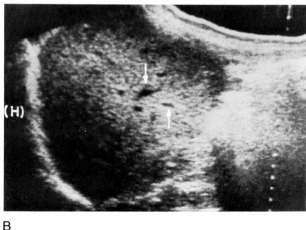

A   B

Fig. 1-22. Chronic hepatitis. **(A)** Case 1. Longitudinal static scan demonstrating marked coarsening. The brightness and number of portal vein radial walls (arrow) is decreased. **(B)** Case 2. Longitudinal static scan with marked coarsening of the liver pattern. There is increased brightness of the band through the midportion of the liver corresponding to the maximum zone of sensitivity. The portal vein radial walls within this bright band have no internal echoes (arrows). (From Kurtz AB, Rubin CS, Cooper HS, et al: Ultrasound findings in hepatitis. Radiology 136:717, 1980.)

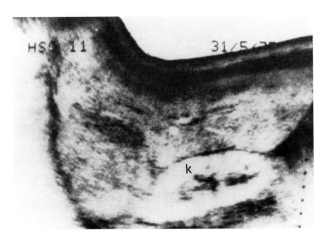

Fig. 1-23. Peliosis hepatitis. Longitudinal static scan 7 cm to the right of the midline. Numerous hypoechoic areas are seen throughout the liver. (*k*, right kidney.) (From Lloyd RL, Lyons EA, Levi CS, et al: The sonographic appearance of peliosis hepatis. J Ultrasound Med 1:293, 1982.)

correct TGC or power setting.[39] A normal ultrasound pattern may be seen in pathological minimal acute and chronic hepatitis.

Peliosis hepatitis is a rare disease process, usually found only postmortem.[40] The diagnosis is most often associated with wasting diseases such as tuberculosis, cancer, and androgenic steroid administration. It is characterized by blood-filled cystic spaces within the liver ranging from 1 to 5 mm in diameter. Each space is surrounded by a plate of normal appearing liver cells. Hepatomegaly is often present. There has been a report of a 2.4-percent incidence in renal transplants. The ultrasound pattern is not specific, but rather consists of a patchy pattern with echopoor and echogenic areas (Fig. 1-23). The value of ultrasound is in screening patients who are at high risk.[40]

Cirrhosis

The most common type of cirrhosis is associated with alcohol abuse. The alcohol itself may be a direct hepatotoxin or merely a caloric substitute predisposing to malnutrition. The earliest response to alcohol abuse is fatty change with accumulation of lipid in the liver cells.[8] The next response is pericentral venous sclerosis — sclerosis about the central veins or sclerosis with a necrotizing process; when advanced, it may obliterate the central veins and lead to portal hypertension. Alcoholic hepatitis is generally superimposed upon a fatty liver or previously developed cirrhotic lesion. In this instance, there is alcoholic hyalin found within the cytoplasm of the liver cells. In the early stages of cirrhosis, there is a fatty liver with little evidence of increased fibrous tissue or

scarring. As fibrosis evolves, the liver tends to decrease in size and progressively becomes finely nodular. Most patients with fatty livers are asymptomatic. In alcoholic hepatitis, there is tender hepatomegaly with pain, anorexia, nausea, jaundice, and ascites; in cirrhosis, the normal architecture of the liver is distorted by bands of connective tissue joining portal areas and central veins, forming pseudolobules.[8]

Cirrhosis is a diffuse process characterized by fibrosis and conversion of normal liver architecture into structurally abnormal nodules. The essential feature is generalized involvement of the liver by concurrent parenchyma necrosis, regeneration, and diffuse fibrosis resulting in disorganization of lobular architecture. As the process is chronic and progressive, liver cell failure and portal hypertension results. The scarring is irreversible and often progressive. In the United States, cirrhosis is the third most common cause of death in the 25-to 65-year age group and the fifth most common cause of death, overall[8] ; 30 to 60 percent of the cirrhosis is secondary to alcohol abuse (Laennec's, portal, and nutritional), with 2 to 5 percent representing pigment cirrhosis (cirrhosis associated with hemochromatosis and Wilson's disease), 10 to 30 percent postnecrotic cirrhosis, and 10 to 20 percent biliary cirrhosis.[8] In children, the causes of cirrhosis include infection (neonatal and viral hepatitis, ascending cholangitis), metabolic abnormalities, obstructive biliary disease, vascular disease, drugs, and toxins.[41]

Several investigators have evaluated the sonographic patterns associated with alcoholic liver disease and cirrhosis. Ultrasound has been found to be 95-percent sensitive, with a specificity of 94 percent when evaluating alcoholic liver disease.[42] Ultrasound is helpful in evaluating hepatomegaly, increased echo amplitude, ascites, and the biliary tract.[13] Though it is useful in detecting diffuse parenchymal disease of the liver, it is unable to give any quantitative estimate of the severity of the histologic change.[42] In this reported series, no difference was appreciated between fatty infiltration and cirrhosis.[42] In addition, the differentiation of fibrosis from primary biliary cirrhosis and chronic active hepatitis was not readily detected by ultrasound until late stages. Others also have noted no difference between fatty livers and cirrhosis on ultrasound, with hepatitis difficult to separate from normal livers.[43] As such, the diagnosis may simply be hepatocellular disease. The ultrasound findings include: (1) beam penetration — increased echoes anteriorly within the liver with echoes decreased posteriorly; (2) echogenicity — liver more echogenic than renal parenchyma; and (3) vascularity — small portal and venous vessels usually well seen but decreased in the peripheral liver[43] (Fig. 1-24). In the cases of fatty liver and hepatitis, the liver size does not aid in the diagnosis. Using these cri-

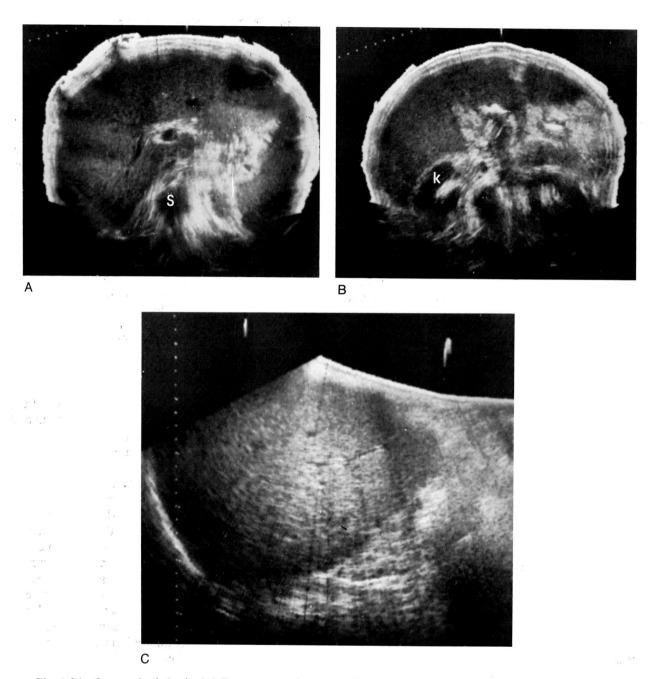

Fig. 1-24. Laennec's cirrhosis. **(A)** Transverse static scan at 12 cm above the umbilicus. There are course echoes within the liver and few internal vessels are seen. (*S,* spine.) **(B)** Transverse static scan 6 cm above the umbilicus. The liver is more dense than renal parenchyma *(k).* **(C)** Longitudinal static scan 8 cm to right of midline. The echopattern is coarse, with fewer echoes noted in the posterior liver.

teria to diagnose hepatocellular disease, 76 percent were correctly diagnosed as normal, with a 24-percent false-positive rate.[43] As such, ultrasound has a limited value in the diagnosis of diffuse liver abnormalities unless there is gross disruption of the normal echopattern.[39] Cirrhosis, the most frequent generalized liver disease, is most common. On ultrasound, there may be increased echogenicity of the parenchyma described as a coarsened echopattern or high amplitude echoes.[39] Decreased attenuation

and apparent vascularity are less constant findings and they can be seen with fatty infiltration, in cases of hemochromatosis, longstanding congestive heart failure, diffuse hepatomas, small multiple metastases, lymphoma, and lymphocytic infiltration and ascending cholangitis.[39]

Other investigators have studied the regional changes noted in hepatic morphology with cirrhosis.[44] There is right lobe shrinkage and caudate lobe enlargement (Fig.

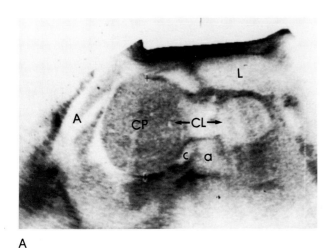
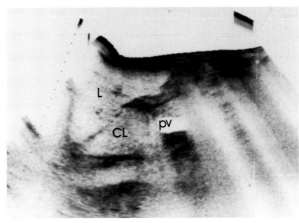

A   B

Fig. 1-25. Cirrhosis and caudate enlargement. **(A)** Transverse static view with enlarged caudate lobe (*CL*, arrows) and caudate process *(CP)* with little right lobe seen. Ascites **(A)** is present lateral to the caudate (*c*, inferior vena cava; *a*, aorta; *L*, left lobe of liver). **(B)** Longitudinal static scan 1 cm to the left of midline. The caudate lobe *(CL)* is even seen posterior to the left lobe of the liver *(L)*. (*pv*, portal vein.) (Courtesy of Dr. Charles A. Durrell III and Pinehurst Radiology, Moore Memorial Hospital, Pinehurst, N.C.)

1-25). Using a ratio of the transverse caudate lobe width to transverse right lobe width, cirrhotic livers can be separated from noncirrhotic livers. The caudate to right lobe ratio is determined as follows: (1) caudate—distance from the lateral margin of the main portal vein to the outside of the caudate; (2) right lobe—distance from the lateral margin to the lateral edge of the main portal vein; and (3) ratio—caudate measurement divided by right lobe measurement (C/RL) (Fig. 1-26). If the C/RL ratio is greater than 0.65, cirrhosis can be diagnosed with 96-percent confidence.[44] If the ratio is greater than 0.73, cirrhosis can be diagnosed with 99-percent confidence, and if less than 0.6, cirrhosis is unlikely.[44] When using the C/RL ratio of greater than 0.65 as posi-

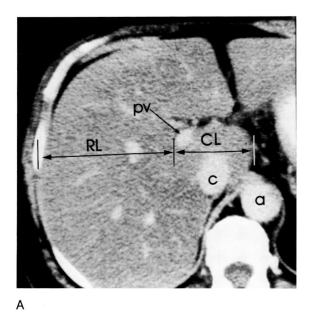
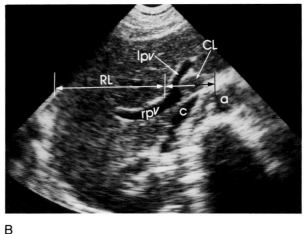

A   B

Fig. 1-26. Caudate/right lobe measurement. The caudate *(CL)* is measured from **(A)** the lateral margin of the main portal vein *(pv)* or **(B)** lateral margin of the portal bifurcation into left *(lpv)* and right *(rpv)* branches to the outside of the caudate. The right lobe *(RL)* is measured from the lateral margin of the main portal vein *(pv)* to the lateral margin of the right lobe. The first measurement (caudate lobe) is divided by the second (right lobe). If *C/RL* is greater than 0.65, cirrhosis can be diagnosed. (*c*, inferior vena cava; *a*, aorta.)

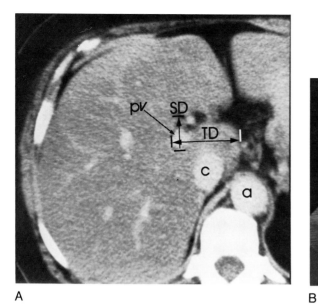

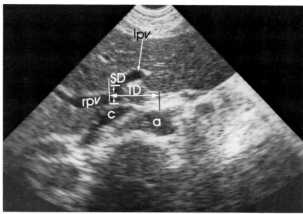

A   B

Fig. 1-27. Porta hepatis index. **(A,B)** Transverse *(TD)* and sagittal *(SD* —between small arrows) diameters of the porta hepatis may be obtained crossing the portal vein *(pv)*. When the margins of the porta hepatis are not clear-cut, the medial margin of the porta hepatis is taken as the most medial portion of the caudate lobe, while the lateral margin is taken as the bifurcation of the main portal vein into left *(lpv)* and right *(rpv)* branches. The product of the *SD* and *TD* divided by the right lobe measurement obtained in Figure 1-26 equals the portal hepatis index. Cirrhosis can be diagnosed if the measurement is greater than 1.15. *(c,* inferior vena cava; *a,* aorta.)

tive for cirrhosis, the diagnosis using this ratio alone has a sensitivity of 84 percent, a specificity of 100 percent, and an accuracy of 93 percent.[44] A ratio of 0.6 to 0.65 would be borderline. A widening of the porta hepatis is found in 84 percent of cirrhotic livers but is not specific for cirrhosis. The porta hepatis index represents the axis measurement traversing the main portal vein, with the greatest sagittal and transverse diameter of the porta hepatis recorded (Fig. 1-27). In some cases, the medial extent of the transverse diameter abuts the caudate lobe[44]; cirrhosis is then diagnosed when the C/RL ratio is equal to or greater than 0.65 and the porta hepatis index is greater than 1.15. This also constitutes a positive test for the diagnosis of cirrhosis with a 92-percent sensitivity, 100-percent specificity, and 96.6-percent accuracy.[44]

Enlargement of the caudate may exert pressure on the inferior vena cava leading to inferior vena caval hypertension, which may contribute to renal failure in patients with hepatorenal syndrome. The pathogenesis of right lobe fibrosis and caudate lobe enlargement in cirrhosis appears to be related to the caudate's separate blood supply. The vascular changes in cirrhosis play a major role in the reduction of hepatic parenchyma and may represent an irreparable stage of cirrhosis. In cirrhosis, hepatic fibrosis causes attenuation and irregular stenosis of the intrahepatic branches of the portal vein and hepatic artery and the overall hepatic vascular base is re-

duced. Because arteries and portal vein branches to the caudate lobe arise in or near the porta hepatis and have a shorter intrahepatic course than the vessels in the right lobe, and because the caudate veins have a shorter intrahepatic course than the other hepatic veins, it is believed that the caudate vessels are less attenuated and distorted by hepatic fibrosis; this results in a relatively greater blood supply to the caudate.[44]

Glycogen Storage Disease

Glycogen storage disease, or glycogenoses, is an autosomal recessive genetic disorder of carbohydrate metabolism characterized by a derangement of either the synthesis or degradation of glycogen and its subsequent utilization.[41,45,46] There are six categories of glycogen storage disease, divided on the basis of clinical symptoms and specific enzymatic defects. Type I glycogen storage disease (von Gierke's disease) is the most prevalent kind.[41] In this type, the activity of the enzyme glucose-6-phosphatase is impaired, preventing glycogenolysis and release of glucose. Excess glycogen accumulates in the hepatocytes and together with fatty metamorphosis accounts for hepatomegaly.[41,45] The livers are noted to be predominately echogenic[41,45] (Fig. 1-28). This disease is associated with hepatic adenomas, focal nodular hyper-

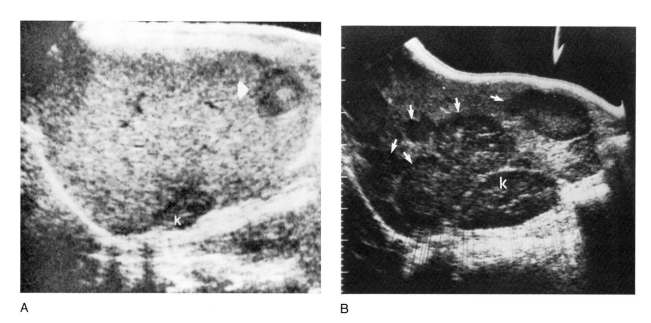

A   B

Fig. 1-28. Glycogen storage disease. **(A)** Longitudinal static scan. The liver has a dense echopattern. A single well-demarcated lesion containing echogenic and anechoic regions is seen (arrowhead). (k, right kidney.) **(B)** Longitudinal static scan. Multiple discrete, solid masses (both echogenic and anechoic) (arrows) are seen in an enlarged liver. (k, right kidney.) (From Grossman H, Ram PC, Coleman RA, et al: Hepatic ultrasonography in type I glycogen storage disease (von Gierke disease). Radiology 141:753, 1981.)

plasia, and hepatomegaly.[41] There is an 8-percent incidence of adenomas in glycogen storage disease with a frequency of 40 percent in Type I.[46]

Congenital Generalized Lipodystrophy

Congenital generalized lipodystrophy is a rare hereditary disease characterized by muscular hypertrophy and lack of adipose tissue throughout the body from birth. The characteristics of this disease include increased basal metabolic rate, hypertriglyceridemia, hepatomegaly with impaired liver function, and insulin-resistant diabetes without ketosis.[47] The enlargement of the liver is particularly marked during the child's first year of life. Investigators have described a hyperechoic pattern on ultrasound[47] (Fig. 1-29).

Schistosomiasis

Schistosomiasis, or bilharziasis, is a widespread disease in certain parts of the world. *Schistosoma haematobium* primarily involves the lower urinary tract and *S mansoni* and *S japonicum* mainly involve the colonic mucosa. The immature worm, or cercaria, exists in fresh water and the infection occurs when it punctures the skin of the human and migrates via the lymphatics or venous

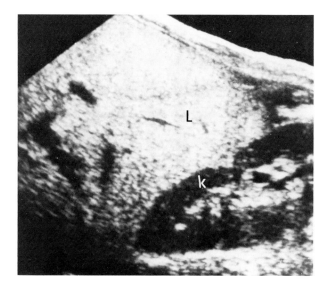

Fig. 1-29. Congenital generalized lipodystrophy. Longitudinal static scan. An echodense pattern compatible with fatty infiltration of the liver is noted. The liver *(L)* is much greater in density than the renal *(k)* cortex. (From Smevik B, Swensen T, Kolbenstvedt A, Trygstad O: Computed tomography and ultrasonography of the abdomen in congenital generalized lipodystrophy. Radiology 142:687, 1982.)

system to the general circulation. In the liver, it matures into adult form and lives in pairs. The female worm, once fertilized, migrates in a retrograde fashion into the terminal venous radicles of the bladder, ureters, and colon. The ova deposited by the female worm penetrate the mucosa and infect the urine and feces. The discharge of infected excreta into the water allows the cycle to continue.[48]

Some ova travel back to the liver via the portal venous system where they penetrate the walls of the smaller vessels and lodge in the periportal connective tissue. This causes an intense fibrotic response resulting in obstruction of the portal venous system with portal venous hypertension. This entire process occurs over a period of years. The presinusoidal portal hypertension that occurs results in splenomegaly and portosystemic venous collaterals. Ultrasound is often perfomed in the late stage of the disease and a large echogenic spleen is seen. The liver may be normal in size or small with foci of increased echoes secondary to diffuse fibrosis.[48] These dense echogenic bands are seen when scanning along the long axis of the intrahepatic portal vein radicles as well as along the central and peripheral bifurcation points of the portal vein.[49]

VASCULAR ABNORMALITIES

Portal Hypertension

Portal hypertension is due to cirrhosis in greater than 90 percent of cases.[8] It can also be caused by disorders obstructing the portal vein. It is sometimes, but uncommonly, caused by lesions such as neoplastic obstruction or thrombosis of hepatic veins or inferior vena cava or prolonged congestive heart failure. There are two types of portal hypertension: presinusoidal and intrahepatic.[8] The presinusoidal type includes sinusoidal obstruction by Kupffer and other cells and is generally associated with relatively normal hepatocellular function. The presinusoidal type can be further subdivided into extrahepatic presinusoidal and intrahepatic presinusoidal.[8] The extrahepatic presinusoidal is caused by obstruction of the portal vein. This type is more common in the child than the adult.[41] The causes of the portal vein obstruction can include neonatal sepsis, pyleophlebitis, tumor, and disease associated with intravascular clotting.[50] One-third of children with extrahepatic obstruction have a history of omphalitis, sepsis and dehydration, umbilical vein catheter, or no known cause.[41] The intrahepatic presinusoidal category of portal hypertension is due to lesions in the portal zone, including schistosomiasis, primary biliary cirrhosis, congenital hepatic fi-

brosis, sarcoidosis, and lesions within the sinusoids of liver such as reticuloendothelial disease.[8,22] The intrahepatic forms of portal hypertension are associated with hepatocellular disease and patients suffering from hemorrhage, who frequently develop liver failure. The most common and important cause of the intrahepatic type is cirrhosis; it accounts for greater than 90 percent of all cases of portal hypertension. In cirrhosis, obstruction to portal venous blood flow occurs at all levels of the liver. This results in (1) a decreased intrahepatic portal vascular bed; (2) compressed venous radicles and sinusoids due to regenerating nodules; and (3) obstruction to hepatic venous outflow at all levels of the portal zones through the sinusoids. Portal hypertension is followed by (1) ascites (46 percent), (2) formation of collateral venous channels, (3) splenomegaly, (4) gastrointestinal bleeding as a consequence of abnormal venous channels (23 percent), (5) signs and symptoms of hepatic failure (19 percent), and (6) jaundice (9 percent). Collateral venous channels develop as the portal vein is bypassed, and appear whenever systemic and portal circulation share a common capillary bed. Sixty-seven percent of patients with advanced cirrhosis have varices, 25 percent have hematemesis.[8]

There are many articles that deal with the sonographic findings in portal hypertension.[23,50-55] All discuss an evaluation of the portal venous system and identification of collateral vessels. Real-time ultrasound has made it possible to evaluate the portal vein rapidly, reliably, inexpensively, and noninvasively and provides a valid initial screening method. It is possible to identify portal vein hypertension before it has clinically manifested.[23] In most series, the normal portal vein has been found to measure 1.1 to 1.3 cm [23,54] and can be identified in as many as 97 percent of examinations[23] (Figs. 1-11 and 1-13). When determining portal hypertension on the basis of portal vein dilatation alone, a sensitivity of 41.8 percent is found.[54] The accuracy can be increased by an evaluation of the caliber variation of the splenic and superior mesenteric veins during respiration. Based on this, the sensitivity of ultrasound in the diagnosis of portal hypertension is 79.7 percent with a specificity of 100 percent.[54] The splanchnic venous outflow into hepatic veins is not steady; there is a variation resulting from a decrease or even an arrest of splanchnic outflow coinciding with a downstream inspiratory fall in intraluminal caval pressure and increased venous return in systemic circulation. The inspiratory interruption of splanchnic outflow would be determined by the compression of liver parenchmya with mechanical collapse of intrahepatic vasculature (with increased intrahepatic resistance) due to the descending diaphragm. On the contrary, increased splanchnic outflow is present during expiration. There is increased pressure and decreased outflow in the portal vein during inspiration and the reverse condition during expiration. With cirrhosis, there is a marked increase in the intrahepatic resistance leading to less variation due to respiration on the portal vein. Therefore, lack of normal caliber variation (i.e., increase during inspiration and decrease during expiration) in the superior mesenteric vein and splenic vein should lead one to the diagnosis of portal hypertension[54] (Fig. 1-30).

Though the portal vein caliber increases with portal vein hypertension secondary to chronic liver disease and cirrhosis, if shunts are present the portal vein may be small in caliber.[22] Portal hypertension develops when hepatopetal flow within the portal system is impeded. There may be spontaneous diversion of portal blood in the hepatofugal direction via various collateral venous

pathways with formation of multiple portosystemic anastomosis. The most common is the coronary-esophageal route, found in 80 to 90 percent of patients.[52] Documentation of portal hypertension and collaterals often require invasive, time-consuming, costly procedures, such as arteriography or direct portovenography, which can result in significant morbidity among patients with abnormal coagulation tests and other medical problems.[53]

The collaterals that develop represent closed or partially closed embryonic channels that reopen connecting portal and systemic venous systems. Portosystemic venous collaterals in portal hypertension have been evaluated with ultrasound.[52] There are several pathways to be evaluated: (1) patent umbilical vein, (2) splenorenal,

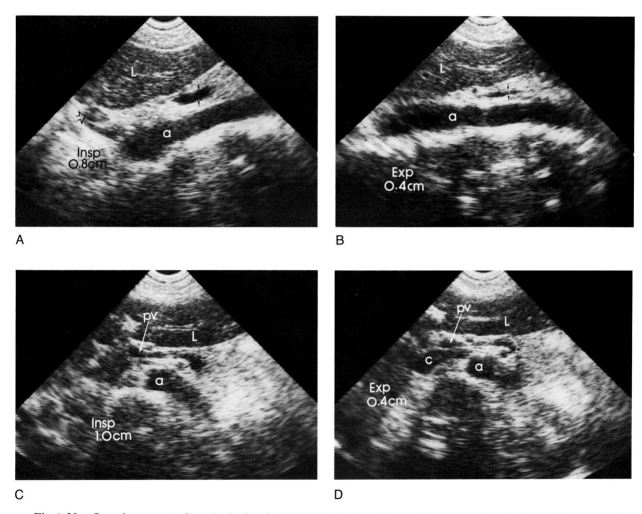

A

B

C

D

Fig. 1-30. Superior mesenteric and splenic veins. **(A)** In inspiration, the superior mesenteric vein (arrows) is measured on this longitudinal scan. (*a,* aorta; *L,* liver; open arrow, diaphragm level.) **(B)** With expiration, the superior mesenteric vein (arrows) is seen to decrease in size. (*a,* aorta; *L,* liver.) **(C)** In inspiration, the splenic vein (arrows) is measured on this transverse scan (*pv,* portal vein; *L,* liver, *a,* aorta). **(D)** With expiration, the splenic vein (arrows) is seen to decrease in size. (*pv,* portal vein; *L,* liver; *a,* aorta; *c,* inferior vena cava). With portal hypertension, there is lack of caliber variation in the superior mesenteric and splenic veins between expiration and inspiration.

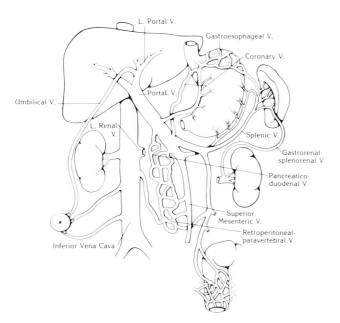

Fig. 1-31. Diagram of the common portosystemic collateral venous pathways in portal hypertension. (Modified from Subramanyam BR, Balthazar EJ, Madamba MR, et al: Sonography of portosystemic venous collaterals in portal hypertension. Radiology 146:161, 1983.)

(3) gastrorenal, (4) hemorrhoidal, and (5) intestinal[53] (Fig. 1-31). The patent umbilical vein extends from the left portal vein via the umbilical vein to the epigastric veins in the anterior abdominal wall at the level of the umbilicus; the umbilical vein opens to decompress the portal vein[51,56] (Figs. 1-31 and 1-32). The umbilical vein can be traced in the lower edge of the falciform ligament up from the LPV to the umbilicus.[51] There is further

potential for pulsed Doppler to demonstrate not only the presence of the umbilical vein but also the direction of flow.[51] The splenorenal collaterals extend from splenic hilar or capsular veins via the pancreatic and the retroperitoneal veins directly into the left renal vein[53] (Figs. 1-31 and 1-33). The pancreaticoduodenal veins drain the retroperitoneal structures such as the duodenum, pancreas, ascending and descending colon, and spleen.[52] These veins are seen in the region of the descending duodenum and the head of the pancreas, coexisting with the gastroesophageal varices[52] (Figs. 1-31 and 1-34). The retroperitoneal-paravertebral veins are below the level of the duodenum (Fig. 1-31). The gastrorenal collaterals connect the short gastric vein or coronary vein via gastric varices to the left adrenal vein, which empties into the left renal vein[53] (Figs. 1-31 and 1-35). The hemorrhoidal collaterals extend from the inferior mesenteric vein via the hemorrhoidal plexus into the systemic veins.[53] The intestinal collaterals extend from the superior mesenteric vein via collaterals to the inferior vena cava[53] (Figs. 1-31 and 1-36). An overall sensitivity of 80 percent for detection of the coronary collaterals and 64 percent for the gastroesophageal has been found.[52] The small size of the coronary-gastroesophageal varices in early portal hypertension seems to be the most important factor limiting detection.[52] The coronary vein runs between the two layers of the lesser omentum and cephalad toward the esophageal hiatus (Figs. 1-31, 1-37, and 1-38). At angiography, it is normally 1.3 to 3.8 mm in diameter; if it is greater than 5 mm it is abnormal.[22,52] The easiest portosystemic collateral to identify is the coronary vein with its associated gastroesophageal varices.[22] Examining the patient in the semierect, upright, or decubitus position can exaggerate the effect of hydrostatic pressure and en-

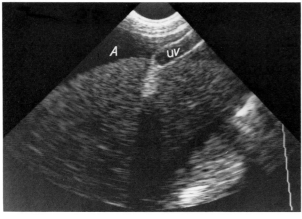

A

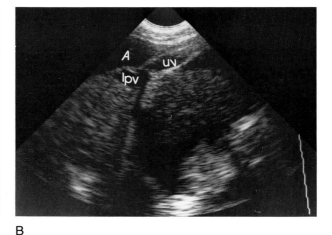

B

Fig. 1-32. Patent umbilical vein. **(A)** Transverse real-time image. A patent umbilical vein *(uv)* is seen extending anteriorly within the ligamentum teres hepatis. *(A,* ascites) **(B)** Transverse real-time image demonstrating the umbilical vein *(uv)* entering the liver to join the left portal vein *(lpv)*. *(A,* ascites.)

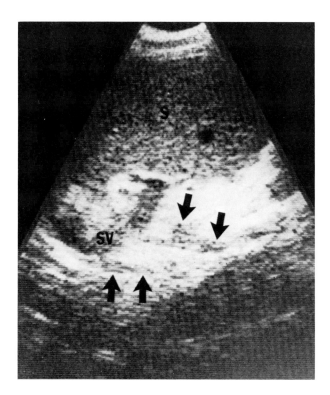

Fig. 1-33. Splenorenal collaterals. Longitudinal scan through the spleen *(S)* in the right lateral decubitus position. Splenorenal collaterals can be identified (arrows) running inferiorly from the splenic vein *(SV)* to the left renal vein. (From Hill MC, Sanders RC: Sonography of the upper abdominal venous system. p. 271. In Sanders RC, Hill MC (eds): Ultrasound Annual 1983. Raven Press, New York, 1983.)

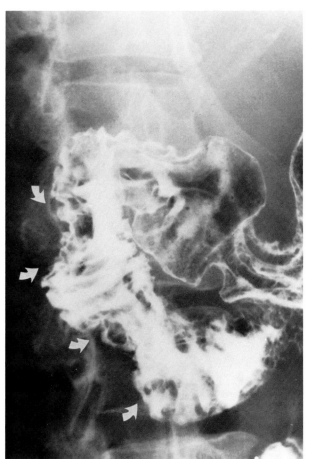

A

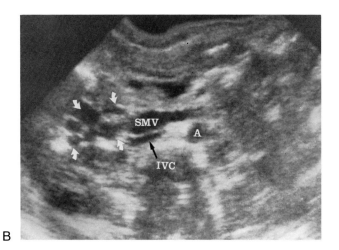

B

Fig. 1-34. Pancreaticoduodenal collaterals. **(A)** Radiograph of the upper gastrointestinal tract shows a nonspecific filling defect along the lateral aspect of the duodenum (arrows). **(B)** Transverse scan shows duodenal varices (arrows) corresponding to the descending duodenum. (*SMV*, superior mesenteric vein; *A*, aorta; *IVC*, inferior vena cava.) (From Subramanyam BR, Balthazar EJ, Madamba MR, et al: Sonography of portosystemic venous collaterals in portal hypertension. Radiology 146:161, 1983.)

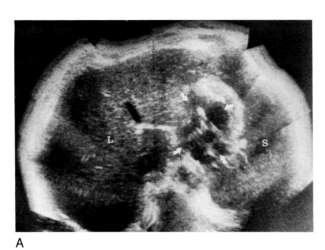

A

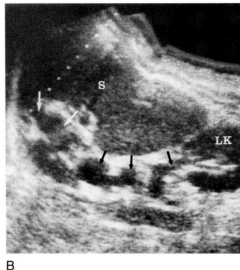

B

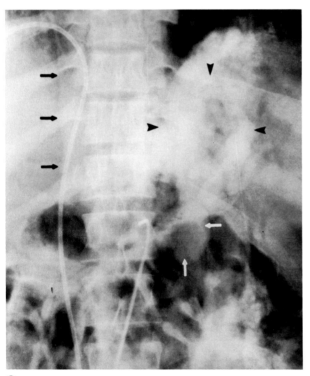

C

Fig. 1-35. Gastrorenal-splenorenal collaterals. **(A)** Transverse scan revealing large gastric varices (arrows). (*L*, liver; *S*, spleen.) **(B)** Longitudinal scan through the spleen *(S)* in the right lateral decubitus position demonstrating gastric varices (white arrows) and a large, tortuous vein (black arrows) connecting them to the left renal vein. (*LK*, left kidney.) **(C)** Venous phase of the superior mesenteric arteriogram. Gastric varices (arrowheads) are seen draining into the left renal vein (white arrows) with opacification of the inferior vena cava (black arrows). (From Subramanyam BR, Balthazar EJ, Madamba MR, et al: Sonography of portosystemic venous collaterals in portal hypertension. Radiology 146:161, 1983.)

hance detection; also the Valsalva maneuver increases portal pressure.[53] Ultrasound is a noninvasive way to screen patients.[23,52–54,56,57]

The sonographic evaluation for portal hypertension should include several steps. First, the maximum dimension of the main portal vein is measured (Figs. 1-11 and 1-13). Then, measurements of the superior mesenteric and splenic veins are made during held inspiration and expiration (Fig. 1-30). Next, evaluation for the presence of all the collaterals is done[52,53,56–58] (Figs. 1-32 to

1-38). To be significant, a patent umbilical vein must be at least 3 mm in diameter.[59] It can be identified at least throughout the course of the intrahepatic portion of the ligamentum teres.[58,59] When the umbilical vein does dilate, a "bull's-eye" pattern is seen in the area of the ligamentum teres due to the echodense fat surrounding the now dilated, fluid-filled vessel; this is seen in 11 percent of patients with cirrhosis.[22,60] When the coronary vein is involved, its internal diameter is greater than 4 to 5 mm.[22] The coronary vein is best seen on a longitudinal

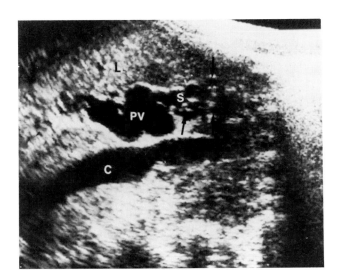

Fig. 1-36. Intestinal collaterals. Longitudinal scan along the dilated main portal vein *(PV)*. A large number of collateral vessels (arrows) can be identified around the superior mesenteric vein *(S)* in the area of the distal antrum of the stomach and proximal duodenum. *(C,* inferior vena cava; *L,* liver.) (From Hill MC, Sanders RC: Sonography of the upper abdominal venous system. p. 271. In Sanders RC, Hill MC (eds): Ultrasound Annual 1983. Raven Press, New York, 1983.)

scan lateral to where the splenic vein joins the superior mesenteric vein to form the main portal vein. Esophageal varices are seen on a transverse scan with the transducer angled cranially through the left lobe of the liver. The gastrorenal and splenorenal veins and the dilated short gastric branch are best seen on a longitudinal scan through the spleen with the patient in the right lateral decubitus position. The proximal splenic vein is formed by varying numbers of splenic branches in the splenic hilum. The short gastric vein is seen along the wall of the stomach above the splenic hilum, while the gastrorenal and splenorenal collaterals are seen longitudinally through the lower portion of the spleen and the upper pole of the left kidney.[22]

Ultrasound can be used to evaluate portosystemic shunts.[22] A portacaval shunt joins the end or side of the main portal vein to the adjoining portion of the inferior vena cava (Fig. 1-39). This type of shunt is the easiest to see with ultrasound.[22] With a mesocaval shunt, the end or side of the superior mesenteric vein is joined to the inferior vena cava. The splenic vein is joined to the side of the left renal vein in a splenorenal shunt. The size and site of the shunt can be determined by ultrasound and, with Doppler ultrasound, shunt patency can be determined.[22] Indirect evidence of shunt patency can be inferred by the absence of visualization of collaterals, which occurs when the shunt is occluded. If there is no

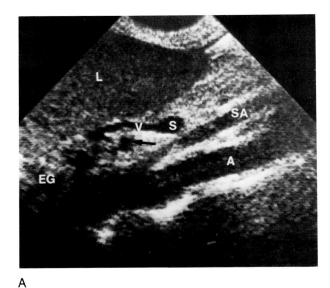

A

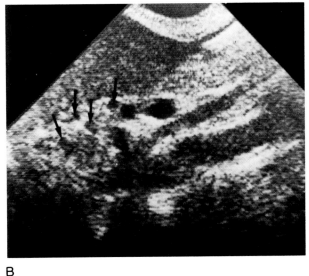

B

Fig. 1-37. Coronary veins. **(A)** Longitudinal midline scan demonstrating the coronary vein *(V)* arising from the superior aspect of the splenic vein *(S).* The coronary vein can be identified running toward the esophagogastric junction *(EG)* close to the under surface of the liver *(L).* *(A,* aorta; *arrow,* celiac axis; *SA,* superior mesenteric artery). **(B)** Longitudinal scan slightly to the left of that in **(A),** demonstrating varices (arrows) along the lesser curvature of the stomach at the level of and just below the esophagogastric junction. (From Hill MC, Sanders RC: Sonography of the upper abdominal venous system. p. 271. In Sanders RC, Hill MC (eds): Ultrasound Annual 1983. Raven Press, New York, 1983.)

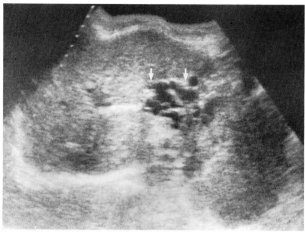

A   B

Fig. 1-38. Coronary-gastroesophageal collaterals. **(A)** Left longitudinal scan shows large, tortuous veins (arrows) within the lesser omentum, representing coronary-gastroesophageal varices. **(B)** Transverse scan reveals gastroesophageal varices posterior to the liver (arrows). (From Subramanyam BR, Balthazar EJ, Madamba MR, et al: Sonography of portosystemic venous collaterals in portal hypertension. Radiology 146:161, 1983.)

dilatation of the inferior vena cava just above the site of the portacaval anastomosis, then shunt occlusion should be suspected. Similarly, there should be dilatation of the superior mesenteric vein above the site of a functioning side to side mesocaval shunt. It is usually not possible to evaluate the patency of a splenorenal shunt, as the anastomotic site is often overlain by adipose and gas.[22]

Real-time ultrasound and pulsed Doppler may be used to evaluate splenorenal shunt patency.[61] With real-time ultrasound, a transplenic coronal approach is used

so that the proximal splenic vein and left renal vein are seen; the anastomotic site is not identified. The presence and direction of venous blood flow is determined by noting the presence of positive or negative frequency shifts of the Doppler signal from the baseline, obtained from a sample volume in the lumen of the vein.[61] Real-time and pulsed Doppler scans reliably demonstrate hepatopetal flow in the proximal splenic vein at the hilum, but proximal splenic vein flow is not indicative of shunt patency because flow may be through collaterals.[61] Difficulties arise in avoiding bowel gas, in identification of the vein, and with adipose.

Portal Vein Obstruction

Extrahepatic obstruction is most often related to thrombosis or direct invasion of the portal vein by cancer involving adjacent organs[8,62] (Fig. 1-40). The causes include (1) tumors—hepatocellular carcinoma, pancreatic or gastric carcinoma, and lymphoma; (2) inflammation—intraabdominal or pelvic infection, appendicitis, diverticulitis, inflammatory bowel disease, omphalitis, and sepsis; (3) cirrhosis; (4) trauma; (5) blood dyscrasia; and (6) idiopathic.[22] As high as 30 to 60 percent of patients have hepatocellular carcinoma with the obstruction due to intravascular tumor growth.[63,64] Ultrasound may demonstrate intraluminal tumor thrombus in 33 percent of hepatocellular carcinomas (sensitivity and specificity 100 percent) and in 1 percent of liver metastases.[65] In the absence of a known primary tumor and hepatic venous invasion, the presence of

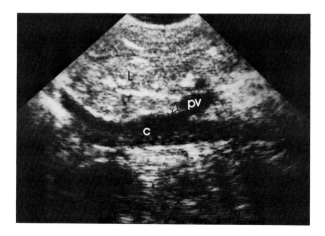

Fig. 1-39. Portacaval shunt. Longitudinal scan of the inferior vena cava *(c)* demonstrating an end-to-side portacaval shunt (arrow). (*pv,* main portal vein; *L,* liver.) (From Hill MC, Sanders RC: Sonography of the upper abdominal venous system. p. 271. In Sanders RC, Hill MC (eds): Ultrasound Annual 1983. Raven Press, New York, 1983.)

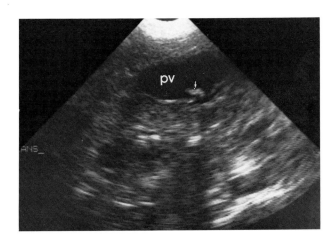

Fig. 1-40. Portal vein tumor. Retroperitoneal paraganglioma metastatic to the liver and portal vein. Transverse cone-down real-time scan of the dilated portal vein *(pv)* reveals an echodense area (arrow) within the vein lumen. This tumor-thrombus moved on real-time scan but was attached to the wall.

hepatocellular carcinoma is suggested. Ultrasound can suggest the histology and determine the feasibility of resection when evaluating venous extension. The intrahepatic position of the inferior vena cava, hepatic veins, and portal vein branches should be evaluated for tumor extension. The inferior vena cava, hepatic vein, and portal vein and its first order branches are seen in at least 90 percent of patients; the second order branches are seen in 85 percent.[62] Ultrasound reliably identifies these veins, detects hepatic or portal venous thrombosis, and suggests the origin of the thrombosis — neoplastic or nontumor — depending on the presence of a hepatic neoplasm.[62]

Thrombosis may be initiated by diffuse acute peritonitis or an abscess cavity lying with the peritoneal sac.[8] Portal vein thrombosis is the most significant cause of prehepatic portal hypertension.[66] Intrahepatic obstruction is frequently caused by primary carcinoma of the liver[8,67-69] and less frequently by metastatic disease.[8,63] Other predisposing factors include trauma, sepsis, and blood dyscrasia.[69] The liver of a patient with portal vein thrombosis is neither enlarged nor tender; in addition, no jaundice and little to no ascites is found.[8] All of this is in contrast to the Budd-Chiari syndrome. Congestive splenomegaly will eventually develop.[8] An inability to identify the portal vein on ultrasound is strong inferential evidence of portal vein occlusion, as the portal vein is seen in a high percentage of cases.[50,69] With nonvisualization of the portal vein or a diamond-shaped band of dense echoes in the place of the vein, thrombosis with recanalization producing irregular transonic channels is suggested.[69] As with portal hypertension, the umbilical

vein may become recanalized in cases of portal vein obstruction.[68] Real-time ultrasound is an excellent method of evaluating for portal vein obstruction.[63] The ultrasound findings of portal vein thrombosis, which is another cause of nonvisualization of the portal vein on ultrasound, include (1) presence of thrombi (echogenic material) within the portal vein; (2) dilatation of the splenic and superior mesenteric veins proximal to the point of the portal vein occlusion; and (3) loss of the normal portal venous landmarks with numerous periportal collaterals (cavernous transformation)[22,64,66] (Figs. 1-41 to 1-43). Intraluminal echoes are significant only if they can be shown to persist when major vessels (e.g., aorta and inferior vena cava) are clear of internal echoes.[64]

If portal occlusion occurs in infancy or the neonatal period, there is extensive collateral development in the porta hepatis, termed "cavernomatous transformation of the portal vein."[50,70,71] Clinically, the findings are various manifestations of Banti's syndrome, especially splenomegaly and gastrointestinal bleeding.[70] Pancreatitis is another well-known cause of portal vein thrombosis.[72] The ultrasound diagnosis is based on the associated findings of splenomegaly, normal liver, and a subhepatic sponge-like mass corresponding to the hepatopedal collaterals[70,71] (Figs. 1-42 and 1-43). Ultrasound demonstrates a characteristic diamond-shaped, densely echo-

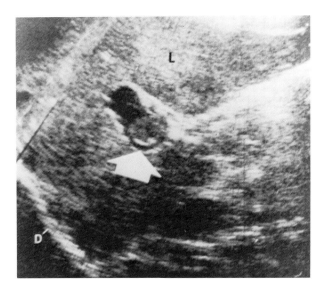

Fig. 1-41. Portal vein thrombosis. Longitudinal scan through the junction of the main portal vein with the left portal vein demonstrating a thrombus (arrow) almost completely occluding the vein lumen. The etiology of this thrombus is unknown. (*L*, liver; *D*, diaphragm.) (From Hill MC, Sanders RC: Sonography of the upper abdominal venous system. p. 271. In Sanders RC, Hill MC (eds): Ultrasound Annual 1983. Raven Press, New York, 1983.)

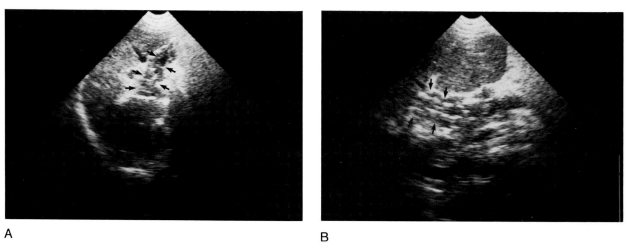

A   B

Fig. 1-42. Cavernous transformation of the portal vein. **(A)** Longitudinal real-time scan. In the porta hepatis area, there is a mass effect (arrows) with lucencies. **(B)** Oblique transverse real-time view through the porta hepatis. A main portal vein could not be found. Instead, several tubular lucencies (arrows) are seen.

genic band that replaces the portal vein and represents periportal fibrosis.[73] The ultrasound diagnosis in these cases is based on (1) failure to visualize the extrahepatic portal vein; (2) demonstration of high-level echoes seen in the porta hepatis ("diamond sign"); and (3) visualization of multiple serpiginous vascular channels around the thrombosed portal vein[73] (Figs. 1-42 and 1-43). With occlusion of the portal vein, adjacent collateral veins enlarge to span the obstruction and permit continued hepatofugal flow of blood.[71] Collateral channels represent cavernous transformation and recanalized channels within the portal vein often seen if occlusion is secondary to thrombosis.[71] The process of formation of collateral hepatopedal circulation involves organization and sub-

sequent recanalization of thrombus and development of venous periportal collateral circulation, and requires 1 to 12 months to occur.[73] Extrahepatic portal obstruction in children is usually due to occlusion of the portal vein by either a congenital anomaly or an extension to the portal system of the process responsible for obliteration of the fetal umbilical vein and ductus venosus.[70] Other causes for portal vein occlusion in infants include omphalitis, abdominal inflammation, sepsis, exchange transfusion, acute dehydration, and umbilical vein catherization.[41,70] Hepatofugal collaterals serve to shunt part of the blood into the inferior and superior vena cava in the vicinity of the distal esophagus, cardia, rectum, umbilicus, mesentery, and retroperitoneal spaces.[70] Calcified portal vein

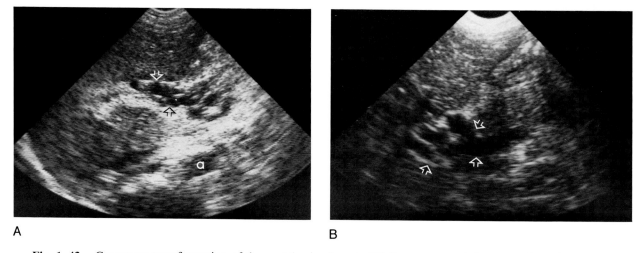

A   B

Fig. 1-43. Cavernous transformation of the portal vein. Case 1. **(A)** Transverse real-time scan through the porta hepatis. Serpiginous structures (open arrows) are seen. (*a,* aorta.) Case 2. **(B)** Transverse scan demonstrates dilated tubular structures (arrows) in the porta hepatis. Both of these children presented with varices and GI bleeding.

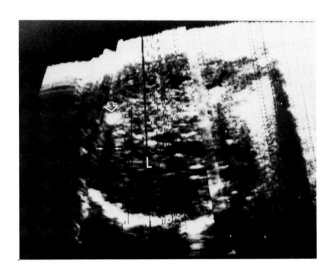

Fig. 1-44. Calcified portal vein thromboemboli. Longitudinal scan through the liver *(L)* reveals shadowing (small arrows) caused by the calcified portal vein thrombosis (open arrow). (From Friedman AP, Haller JO, Boyer B, Cooper R: Calcified portal vein thromboemboli in infants: Radiography and ultrasonography. Radiology 140:381, 1981.)

thromboemboli may also develop in infants. They are usually peripheral and associated with multiple anomalies in infants.[74] Calcified portal vein thromboemboli that were dense enough to cause shadowing on ultrasound have been shown[74] (Fig. 1-44). The etiology of

these are unknown, but the following mechanism is postulated: anemic shock in fetus leading to infarction and secondary venous thrombosis; placento-fetal embolization from chronic venous thrombi; and intravascular fibrin thrombus resulting from maternal or fetal release of thromboplastin.[74]

Portal Vein Aneurysm

Portal vein aneurysms occur either proximal at the junction of the superior mesenteric vein and splenic vein or more distal in the portal vein radicles[75] (Fig. 1-45). The etiologies are congenital or acquired secondary to portal hypertension. The portal venous system develops from the vitelline and umbilical veins that drain the primitive intestine. Various congenital abnormalities involving the portal vein may occur: (1) duplication of the portal vein; (2) the portal vein may receive anomalous pulmonary venous drainage; (3) atresia of the portal vein; and (4) the portal vein may assume an abnormal ventral position.[75] In addition, cavernous transformation may take place.[75]

Portal Vein Gas

Necrotizing enterocolitis (NEC) is an important diagnosis in the neonate and infant, which if not diagnosed and treated early in its course leads to sepsis and bowel

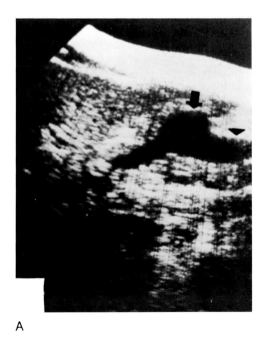

A

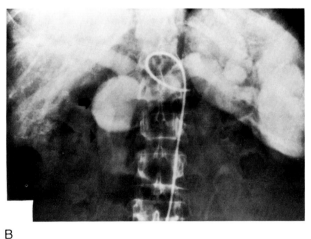

B

Fig. 1-45. Portal vein aneurysm. **(A)** Transverse scan through the porta hepatis. The splenic vein (arrowhead) drains into the enlarged portal vein (arrow). **(B)** Venous phase of celiac arteriogram. A large varix (arrow) of the portal vein is seen with reflux down the superior mesenteric vein (arrowhead). (From Vine HS, Sequeira JC, Widrich WC, Sacks BA: Portal vein aneurysm. AJR 132:557, © American Roentgen Ray Society, 1979.)

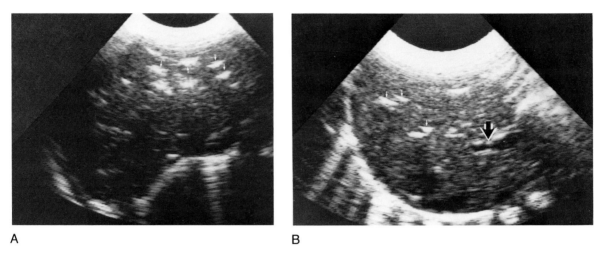

A   B

Fig. 1-46. Portal vein gas. Necrotizing enterocolitis (NEC). Transverse **(A)** and longitudinal **(B)** scans of an infant with NEC. Numerous echogenic patches (arrows) in the hepatic parenchyma tend to occupy the nondependent parts of the liver. In **(B)**, a microbubble is within the portal vein (large arrow). (From Merritt CRB, Goldsmith JP, Sharp MJ: Sonographic detection of portal venous gas in infants with necrotizing enterocolitis. AJR 143:1059, © Am Roent Ray Soc, 1984.)

perforation, and eventually death. These patients have abdominal distension, feeding intolerance, diarrhea (often bloody), and radiographic findings of dilated bowel loops, pneumatosis intestinalis, foamy bowel pattern, pneumoperitoneum, and portal vein gas. The gas results from diffusion of air from the smallest portal veins into the parenchyma.

The ultrasound findings are related to hepatic parenchymal and portal vein air. The most characteristic ultrasound pattern is that of highly echogenic particles believed to be microbubbles of gas flowing within the portal vein[76,77] (Figs. 1-46 and 1-47). This pattern is variable and intermittent and is not associated with acoustic shadowing. The second pattern seen consists of poorly defined, highly echogenic patches within the hepatic parenchyma[76,77] (Fig. 1-46). These hepatic echoes are seen to develop after the passage of microbubbles from the peripheral portal venous branches into the hepatic parenchyma. They are most apparent in the nondependent part of the liver and fade with time.[76,77] These findings have been reported in patients with necrotizing enterocolitis as well as those with ischemic bowel disease (Fig. 1-47). These findings are frequently observed before the characteristics of the disease process are noted on the radiograph. If they are seen, it allows early confirmation of the clinical impression, permitting earlier aggressive therapy with the potential of reducing mortality and complications of this serious illness.

Hepatoportal Fistula

Hepatic artery to portal vein fistula are relatively uncommon lesions with variable clinical presentation.[78] The causes include rupture of preexisting hepatic artery

aneurysm into the portal vein, trauma, cirrhosis, congenital arteriovenous malformation, and liver neoplasm eroding into the artery and portal vein.[78] A large majority of these cases arise from rupture of a preexisting aneurysm, with 75 percent of the aneurysms extrahepatic and 63 percent in the common hepatic artery. Real-time sonography is valuable in recognition of portal vein hypertension. With hepatoportal fistula, an enlarged hepatic artery is seen[78] (Fig. 1-48).

Budd-Chiari Syndrome

Budd-Chiari syndrome is a rare disorder caused by obstruction of the hepatic veins. The liver becomes enlarged and tender with intractable ascites.[8,22,79-83] The

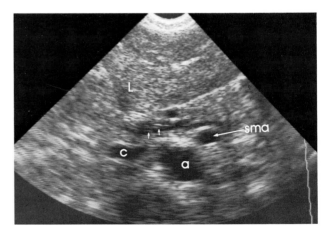

Fig. 1-47. Portal vein gas. Ischemic bowel. Transverse real-time scan. Microbubbles (arrows) were seen flowing in the portal vein at real-time scanning. (*a,* aorta; *c,* inferior vena cava; *sma,* superior mesenteric artery; *L,* liver.)

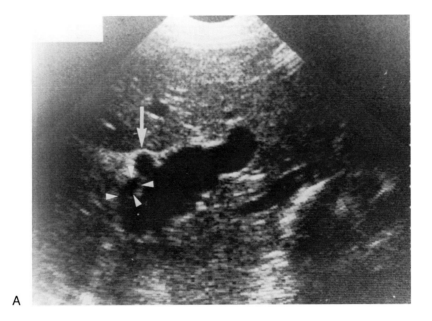

A

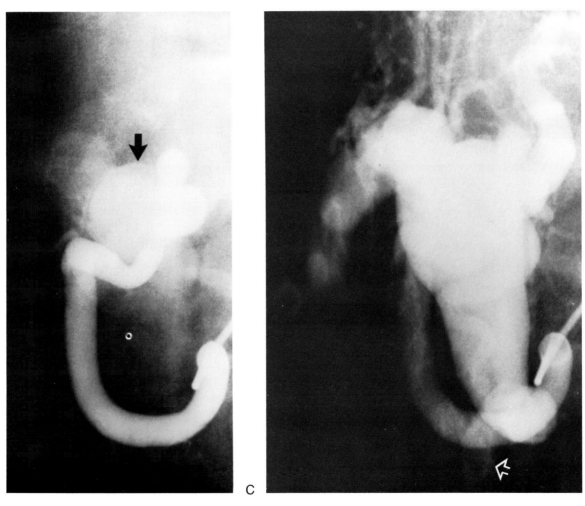

B   C

Fig. 1-48. Hepatoportal fistula. **(A)** Subcostal scan of the right upper quadrant. Main, right, and left portal veins are greatly enlarged. Hepatic artery (arrow) seen anterior to portal vein is markedly enlarged. There is fistulous communication between hepatic artery and portal vein (arrowheads); pulsations were seen in the region on real-time. **(B)** Early film of a selective hepatic arteriogram. There is an enlarged hepatic artery with a bilobed aneurysm in the region of the porta hepatis. Very early filling of portal vein (arrow) is noted. **(C)** Selective hepatic arteriogram 2 sec later than that in **(B)**. Bidirectional flow produces opacification of enlarged portal vein, its intrahepatic branches, and faint opacification of superior mesenteric vein (arrow). Poor filling of intrahepatic arterial branches is due to the large hepatoportal shunt. (From Ramchandani P, Goldenberg NJ, Soulen RL, White RI: Isobutyl 2-cyanoacrylate embolization of a hepataportal fistula. AJR 140:137, © American Roentgen Ray Society, 1983.)

single most common finding is unexplained partial or complete fibrous obliteration of the major hepatic veins.[8,79] In the majority of cases, the etiology of Budd-Chiari syndrome is never determined.[79] Thrombosis of the hepatic veins associated with hypercoagulable states, especially polycythemia vera or, rarely, paroxysmal nocturnal hemoglobinuria, may be responsible.[8,22,82,84] Hepatic vein thrombosis has been linked to oral contraceptives in some cases.[8,22,79,81,84] In addition, there can be invasion of the hepatic veins by tumors, in particular, hepatocellular carcinoma, renal carcinoma, and adrenal carcinoma; radiation to the liver with obliteration of the small hepatic veins is also associated with Budd-Chiari syndrome.[8,22,79,81,82] Chronic hepatic venous outflow obstruction may occur as a complication of polycythemia vera, paroxysmal nocturnal hemoglobinuria, hepatoma, trauma, renal tumor, liver abscess, and congenital webs of the inferior vena cava.[83] Pathologically, there is centrilobular congestion and necrosis first and central fibrosis and periportal regenerating nodules later.[4] There are three types of Budd-Chiari syndrome described: (1) occlusion of the inferior vena cava with or without secondary occlusion of the hepatic vein, (2) occlusion of the major hepatic veins, right and/or left, with or without occlusion of the inferior vena cava, and (3) veno-occlusive disease of the liver, a progressive thrombotic occlusion of small centrilobar veins.[79]

In cases of Budd-Chiari syndrome, the ultrasound findings depend on the stage of the disease. The caudate lobe hypertrophies because it has multiple small, direct connections to the patent portion of the inferior vena cava and this may be the only effective venous drainage of the liver.[13,79,81,83] As a result on ultrasound, not only

would a large caudate lobe be identified, but it should also be noted that the caudate is hypoechoic[22,82] (Fig. 1-49). In addition, there should be reduced or nonvisualization of hepatic veins, narrowing of the intrahepatic inferior vena cava, and ascites[22,80,82] (Fig. 1-50). With Doppler ultrasound, a lack of flow should be seen inside the suprahepatic inferior vena cava.[81] There is preferential flow from an obstructed segment of the liver to an unobstructed segment by one or more routes. These may be interlobular hepatic veins, subcapsular arcades, and retrograde flow (hepatofugal) through branches of the portal veins from obstructed segments to portal branches of unobstructed segments.[82] With primary Budd-Chiari syndrome, (primary membranous or segmental obstruction of the hepatic portion of the inferior vena cava) some investigators have defined certain ultrasound findings: (1) communicating vessels between the right and/or middle hepatic veins and the inferior right hepatic vein; (2) enlarged inferior right hepatic vein; (3) reversed flow in the hepatic veins; and (4) obstruction of the hepatic portion of the inferior vena cava.[85] A definitive diagnosis requires either hepatic venography or a liver biopsy demonstrating venous congestion with centrilobular necrosis, although ultrasound and CT can be helpful.[80,82]

Hereditary Hemorrhagic Telangiectasis

Hereditary hemorrhagic telangiectasia or Osler-Weber-Rendu disease is an autosomal dominant disorder that may involve every organ.[86] Liver involvement includes angiodysplasia, fibrosis, cirrhosis, portosys-

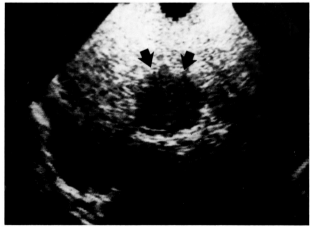
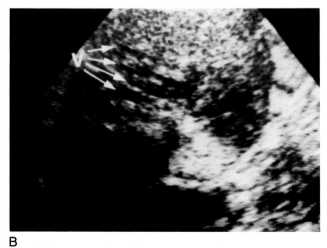

A
B

Fig. 1-49. Budd-Chiari syndrome. **(A)** Case 1. Transverse real-time scan of the liver demonstrating an enlarged, hypoechoic caudate lobe (arrows). (From Yang PJ, Glazer GM, Bowerman RA: Budd-Chiari syndrome: Computed tomographic and ultrasonographic findings. J Comput Assist Tomogr 7:148, 1983) **(B)** Case 2. Real-time scan. Multiple abnormal vessels *(V)* in the left lobe of the liver cannot be traced back to hepatic or portal veins. (From Harter LP, Gross BH, St. Hilaire J, et al: CT and sonographic appearance of hepatic vein obstruction. AJR 139:176, © Am Roent Ray Soc, 1982.)

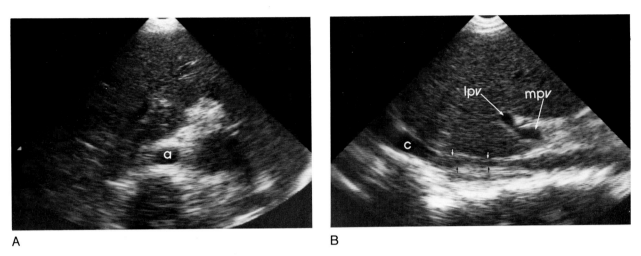

A   B

Fig. 1-50. Budd-Chiari syndrome. **(A)** High transverse scan. The inferior vena cava and hepatic veins are not seen. (*a,* aorta.) **(B)** Longitudinal scan. The hepatic portion (arrows) of the inferior vena cava *(c)* is compressed. No hepatic veins are seen. This patient had massive hepatomegaly and ascites. (*mpv,* main portal vein; *lpv,* left portal vein.)

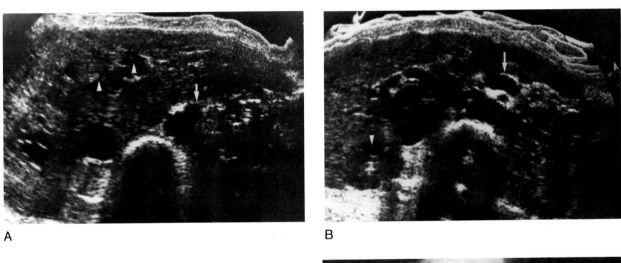

A   B

Fig. 1-51. Hereditary hemorrhagic telangiectasis. **(A)** Transverse scan of upper abdomen with a prominent celiac axis originating from the aorta (arrow). Multiple arteriovenous malformations (arrowheads) are seen in the liver. **(B)** This transverse scan through the porta hepatis demonstrates multiple prominent vascular structures mimicking dilated biliary ducts. The enlarged common hepatic artery (arrow) is present along with an incidental right renal cyst (arrowhead).**(C)** Arterial phase of an hepatic arteriogram. An enlarged hepatic artery (arrow), numerous arteriovenous malformations (arrowhead), and early draining hepatic veins *(v)* are confirmed. (From Cloogman HM, DiCapo RD: Hereditary hemorrhagic telangiectasia: Sonographic findings in the liver. Radiology 150:521, 1984.)

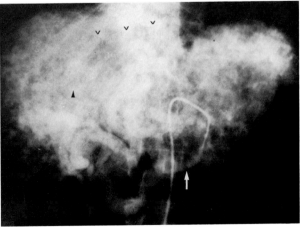

C

temic encephalopathy, and hepatocellular carcinoma. Classically, there is a familial incidence with multiple telangiectasias and recurrent episodes of bleeding; the most serious sequelae are the cardiovascular complications and gastrointestinal bleeding. On ultrasound, an abnormally dilated common hepatic artery with multiple arteriovenous malformations and an abnormal echogenicity of the liver are noted[86] (Fig. 1-51). Large feeding arteries, prominent pulsations, ectatic vascular structures, and large draining veins may be seen.

FOCAL ABNORMALITIES

At times it may be difficult to differentiate extra- and intrahepatic masses. The features most often observed of an extrahepatic mass include (1) internal invagination of the liver capsule, (2) discontinuity of the liver capsule, (3) formation of a triangular fat wedge, (4) anteromedial shift of the inferior vena cava, and (5) anterior displacement of the right kidney[87] (Fig. 1-52). With an intrahepatic mass, the features seen are (1) displacement of the hepatic vascular radicles, (2) external bulging of the liver capsule, and (3) posterior shift of the inferior vena cava[87] (Fig. 1-53). Using these criteria, accurate definition of the anatomic origin of many masses can be made. Masses exceeding 10 cm in diameter may present a diagnostic problem. The important contribution of ultrasound is its ability to create a multiplanal dynamic sectional image.

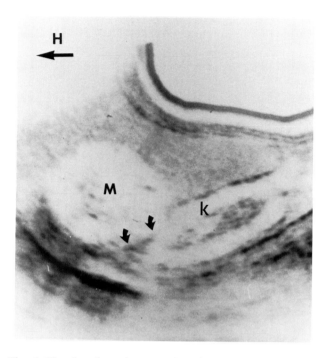

Fig. 1-53. Intrahepatic mass. Longitudinal scan. A large poorly echogenic mass *(M)* is seen surrounded by hepatic parenchyma and adjacent to the right kidney *(k).* This mass is hepatic in origin by virtue of the posterior-inferior displacement of the retroperitoneal fat (curved arrows). This was an echinococcal cyst of the liver. (*H,* head.) (From Gore RM, Callen PW, Filly RA: Displaced retroperitoneal fat: Sonographic guide to right upper quadrant mass localization. Radiology 142:701, 1982.)

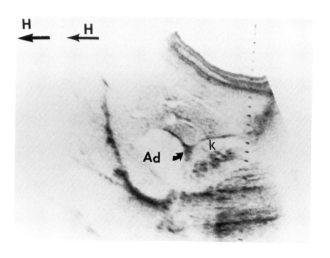

Fig. 1-52. Extrahepatic mass. Longitudinal scan. A large adrenal cyst *(Ad)* following a hemorrhage is seen to be causing wedging (curved arrow) of the retroperitoneal fat between the kidney *(k)* and adrenal mass. (*H,* head.) (From Gore RM, Callen PW, Filly RA: Displaced retroperitoneal fat: sonographic guide to right upper quadrant mass localization. Radiology 142:701, 1982.)

Cysts

NONPARASITIC CYSTS

Cysts may be congenital, traumatic, parasitic, or inflammatory in origin. Congenital cysts arise from developmental defects in the formation of bile ducts.[8,88] Cysts vary in diameter (3 cm to 13 liters), tend to be superficial, and are lined with cuboidal epithelium.[8,89] They usually do not cause liver enlargement and are rarely palpable.[8] The right lobe is affected twice as often as the left.[89] The incidence of hepatic cysts is said to be 17 in 10,000 at abdominal exploration[88,90] and 1 in 600 at laparotomy.[89] Polycystic kidney disease, which is a relatively common condition affecting 1 in 500 people and is autosomal dominant, is associated with liver cysts.[8] From 25 to 50 percent of patients with polycystic kidney disease have one to several cysts in the liver[8,89,91] (Fig. 1-54). On the other hand, 60 percent of patients with polycystic liver have renal cysts.[91]

Although patients with hepatic cysts are usually asymptomatic, these cysts occasionally cause epigastric

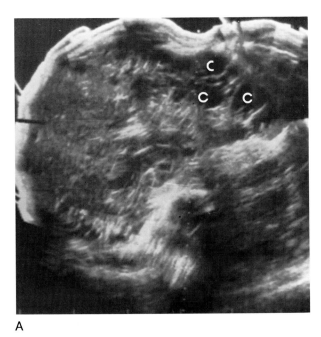

A

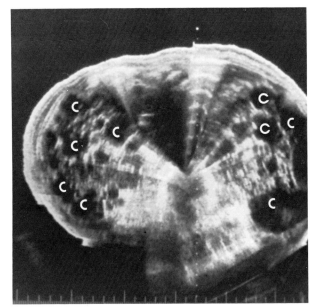

B

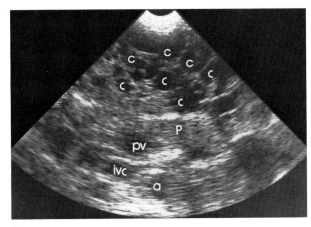

C

Fig. 1-54. Polycystic liver disease. (**A**) Transverse static scan at 18 cm above the umbilicus. Multiple anechoic areas *(c)* are seen within the left lobe. (**B**) Transverse static scan at 6 cm above the umbilicus. Multiple bilateral anechoic areas *(c)* are seen in each renal fossa. (**C**) Transverse real-time image of the left lobe. Multiple anechoic areas *(c)* are seen in the left lobe. (*a,* aorta; *pv,* portal vein; *ivc,* inferior vena cava; *P,* pancreas.)

pain or mass effect so that an infected cyst, abscess, or necrotic tumor may be suggested. Fifty-five percent of patients present with an abdominal mass, 40 percent with hepatomegaly, 33 percent with abdominal pain, and 9 percent with jaundice.[92] There is a slight female predominance (4 : 1)[89] and the clinical presentation is in the fifth to seventh decade. The average size is 3 cm. Besides being congenital, a cyst may be acquired (e.g. traumatic, parasitic, or inflammatory). These are most often symptomatic. On ultrasound, a cyst should be anechoic and well-defined, and should exhibit acoustic enhancement (increased through transmission)[88] (Figs. 1-55 and 1-56). The accuracy of ultrasound is 95 to 100 percent.[3,93] The differential diagnosis for such a lesion would have to include cyst, necrotic metastasis, echinococcal cyst, hematoma, hepatic cystadenocarcinoma, and abscess.[92] Fifty percent of the metastases of leio-

myosarcoma of the gastrointestinal tract are lucent but other primary tumors, including colon carcinoma, embryonal cell carcinoma, testicular carcinoma, carcinoid, and melanoma, have also been described.[92] If the diagnosis of a cyst is in doubt, an ultrasound-guided percutaneous cyst aspiration may be performed.[92] While still effective as a primary diagnostic maneuver, percutaneous aspiration seems to lack permanent therapeutic benefit.[94] In one series of 13 patients with cyst aspiration, all cysts recurred within 2 years. Definitive therapy requires surgical removal of the cyst lining or internal drainage by marsupialization.[94]

In a rare case, there may be a cyst of the falciform ligament.[95] The falciform ligament is composed of two mesothelial layers within which lies the ligamentum teres, paraumbilical vein, muscular fibers, and variable amounts of adipose. The cause of cysts in this location is

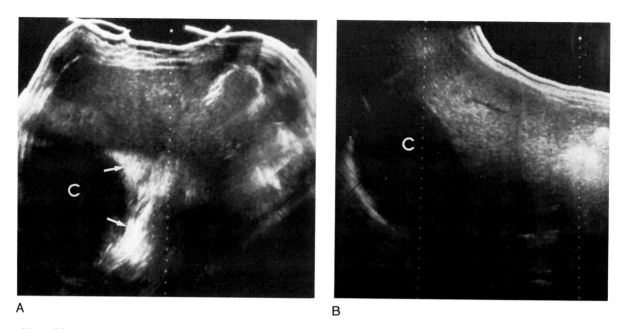

A   B

Fig. 1-55. Nonparasitic hepatic cyst. Solitary cyst. **(A)** Transverse static scan 11 cm above the umbilicus. An anechoic mass *(C)* is seen within the posterior liver. Acoustic enhancement is seen (arrows). **(B)** Longitudinal static scan 13 cm to the right of midline. An anechoic mass *(C)* is seen.

unclear. The diagnosis is based on the location of the cystic lesion.[95]

ECHINOCOCCAL CYST

Echinococcal cysts (hydatid disease) are common in the liver in regions of the world where the parasite is endemic, with the highest incidence in countries where sheep and cattle grazing is carried out with the help of

dogs.[96] Increased world-wide travel brought on by tourism and immigration has resulted in dissemination of many diseases formerly regarded as "tropical" and previously confined to large but localized endemic areas.[48] The eggs of the worm (*Echinococcus granulosis* and *E multilocularis*) are excreted in the feces of infected dogs; cattle, sheep, hogs, and humans serve as the intermediate host.[48] The eggs hatch in the intestine of the upper small bowel and the embryos permeate the intestinal mucosa

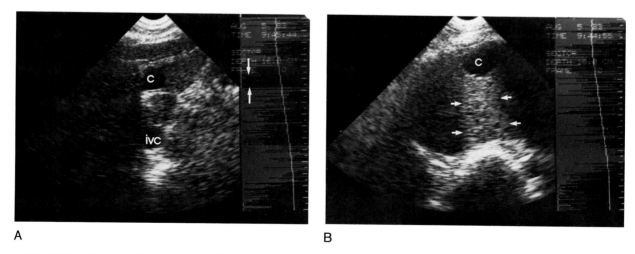

A   B

Fig. 1-56. Nonparasitic hepatic cyst. Multiple cysts in a patient with known carcinoma. **(A)** Transverse real-time scan. An anechoic area *(c)* is seen within the left lobe. Notice there are no echoes on the A-mode (arrows). *(ivc,* inferior vena cava.) **(B)** Transverse real-time scan in the left lateral decubitus position. An anechoic area *(c)* with acoustic enhancement (arrows) is seen in the lateral aspect of the right lobe.

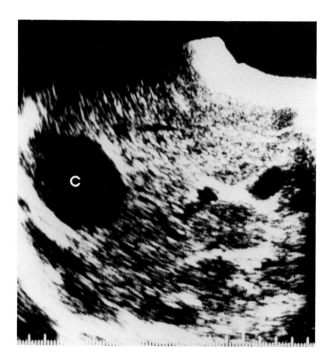

Fig. 1-57. Simple echinococcal cyst. Longitudinal scan. A simple liver cyst *(c)* is seen. (From Gharbi HA, Hassine W, Brauner MW, Dupuch K: Ultrasound examination of hydatic liver. Radiology 139:459, 1981.)

pancreatic involvement.[97] In these organs, the larvae lodge within capillaries and incite an inflammatory reaction composed principally of mononuclear leukocytes and esinophils.[8] Many such larvae are destroyed but the others encyst. The cyst begins at the microscopic level and progresses, taking 5 years or more to reach massive size.[8] Most grow at a rate of 0.25 to 1.00 cm per year and remain asymptomatic for 5 to 10 years.[96] Enclosing the fluid within the cyst is an inner, nucleated, germinative layer, which gives rise to the brood capsules, and an outer opaque non-nucleated layer.[8,98] The outer layer is quite distinctive with innumerable delicate laminations like fine tissue paper. Outside the opaque layer is an inflammatory reaction, which produces a layer of fibroblasts, giant cells, and mononuclear and eosinophilic infiltration.[8] When these cysts are present for about 6 months, daughter cysts develop within them arising from the germinal epithelium. Impingement upon blood vessels can lead to vascular thrombosis and infarction. The cyst may rupture and fluid may escape, evoking a massive anaphylactic reaction.[8,96]

There have been numerous articles that describe the sonographic findings associated with echinococcal cysts.[96,98-106] The patterns identified include (1) discrete simple cysts (with or without calcification) (Fig. 1-57); (2) multiple cysts (in multiple cysts the daughter cysts appear dense early on) (Fig. 1-58); (3) honeycomb cysts (fluid collection with septa) (Fig. 1-59); and (4) solid-appearing cysts (Fig. 1-60). An oval or spherical shape and regularity of the walls are common in most types of cysts.[98] The number and size of the cysts vary consider-

into the blood vessels traveling throughout the body. In man, greater than 50 percent of the cysts are in the liver.[8] Other sites, in decreasing order, include the lungs, the bones, and the brain. There also have been reports of

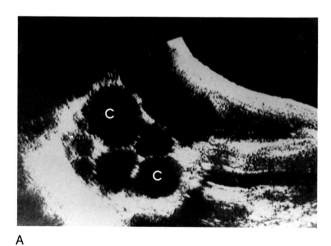

A

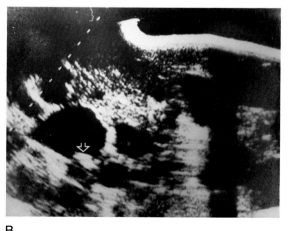

B

Fig. 1-58. Multiple echinococcal cysts. **(A)** Case 1. Scan through the left lobe of the liver showing a well-rounded cyst with multiple large daughter cysts *(C)* within it compressing each other to give a multilocular appearance. **(B)** Case 2. A small daughter cyst is developing within a parent cyst. Multiple fluid-filled hydated cysts are seen within the right lobe of the liver. In one of them, a small reflecting pole (open arrow) is seen attached to the wall of the parent cyst. This represents a developing daughter cyst. (From Itzchuk Y, Rubinstein Z, Shilo R: Ultrasound in tropical diseases. p. 69. In Sanders RC, Hill MC (eds): Ultrasound Annual 1983. Raven Press, New York, 1983.)

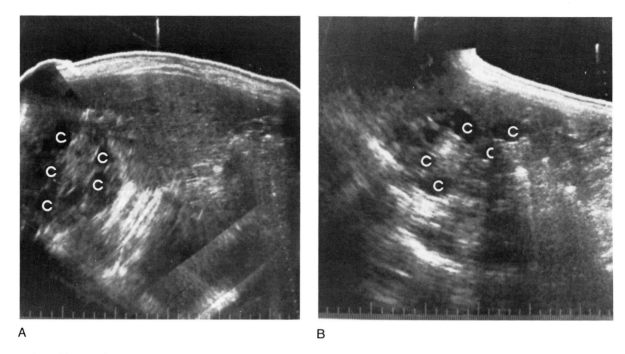

A   B

Fig. 1-59. Echinococcal cyst—Honeycomb pattern. **(A)** Transverse static scan 3 cm below the xyphoid. Multiple cystic areas *(c)* are seen within the right lobe. **(B)** Longitudinal static scan at 11 cm to the right of midline. Multiple cystic areas *(c)* are seen.

ably and calcification may occur in the wall many years after the initial infection.[48] Complete cyst wall calcification usually indicates an inactive lesion, but other viable noncalcified cysts may be present.[48] There usually is acoustic enhancement of the tissues immediately posterior to the lesion and identification of daughter cysts; the presence of these cysts is not indispensible to diagnosis but is highly pathognomonic of this disease.[98,102] An "ultrasound water lily sign" resulting from the detachment and collapse of the germinal layer has also been described and is analogous to the appearance seen on chest radiograph.[99] On ultrasound, the collapsed germinal layer is seen as an undulating linear collection of echoes either floating in the cyst fluid or lying in the most de-

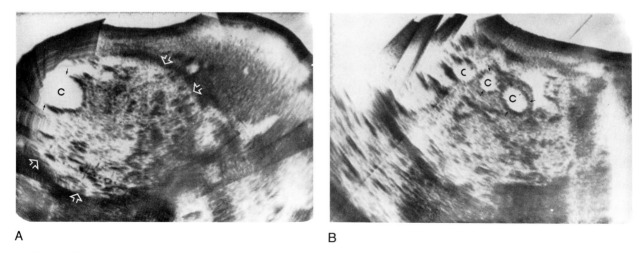

A   B

Fig. 1-60. Echinococcal cyst—Solid pattern. Transverse **(A)** and right longitudinal **(B)** scans of the abdomen. The giant mass (open arrows) is almost completely solid except for a few areas where some daughter cysts (*c*, arrows) can be identified, giving the clue to the diagnosis of echinococcal cyst. (From Barriga P, Cruz F, Lepe V, Lathrop R: An ultrasonographically solid tumor-like appearance of echinococcal cysts in the liver. J Ultrasound Med 2:123, 1983.)

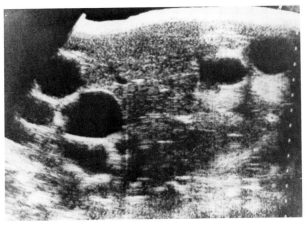
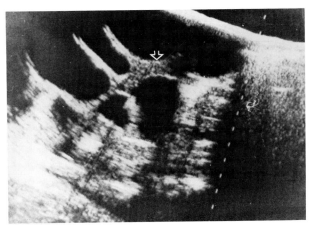

A   B

Fig. 1-61. Echinococcal cyst — Multiple parents. **(A)** Multiple well-defined separate fluid-filled cysts of various sizes are present within the liver. **(B)** Some cysts are compressed by others and lose their rounded appearance. There is liver tissue between the cysts (arrow), indicating that they are multiple parent cysts and not daughter cysts. (From Itzchuk Y, Rubinstein Z, Shilo R: Ultrasound in tropical diseases. p. 69. In Sanders RC, Hill MC, (eds): Ultrasound Annual 1983. Raven Press, New York, 1983.)

pendent portion of the cyst.[99] In addition, a "cyst within a cyst" pattern on ultrasound has been presented.[100]

In some instances, the liver may contain multiple parent cysts situated in both lobes, producing hepatomegaly.[48] To make this diagnosis, cysts with thick walls occupying different parts of the liver must be seen (Fig. 1-61). Tissue detected between the cysts indicates that each cyst is a separate parent cyst and not a daughter cyst.

A shell-like calcification in the thick wall around a cyst can indicate the true hydatid nature. If there are no daughter cells, the cyst may be inactive with disintegration of the daughter cysts.[49] Differentiation of hydatid cysts from other cystic masses is not difficult if a daughter cyst is found within the primary cyst.[102,103]

In contrast to previous reports, three cases with solid, well-defined masses that were rounded and clearly separated from normal parenchyma have been described[105] (Fig. 1-60). It is postulated that in cases in which the cysts appear solid, the germinative membranes of the cysts are very active, giving rise to many daughter cysts; pieces of the membrane may even detach, fall into such a cyst, and continue to proliferate.[105] The presence of daughter cells within hydatid cysts depends on many factors such as resistance of the organs where cysts grow and natural or acquired mechanisms of immunity of the host.[105]

When hydatid cysts become secondarily infected, a different pattern may be seen on ultrasound. With acute onset of secondary infection, the cyst may have a variable number of internal echoes that may give rise to an appearance of a solid mass (Fig. 1-62). The membrane may be in various shapes within the cyst, producing a

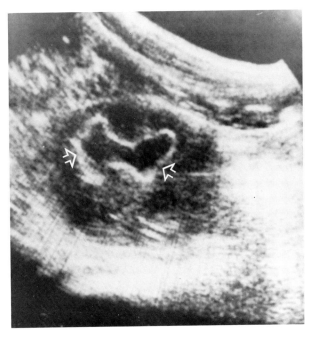

Fig. 1-62. Infected echinococcal cyst. Intermediate stage. Longitudinal scan. A 10-cm, well-defined mass with some internal echoes and with good through transmission is identified. An irregular membrane (arrows) is seen within the fluid-filled mass. (From Itzchuk Y, Rubinstein Z, Shilo R: Ultrasound in tropical diseases. p. 69. In Sanders RC, Hill MC, (eds): Ultrasound Annual 1983. Raven Press, New York, 1983.)

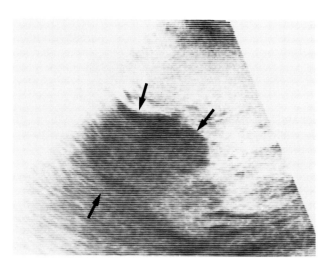

Fig. 1-63. Omenoplasty and hydatid cysts. Longitudinal scan. A sharply marginated echogenic focus in the area of resection of a cyst is seen representing the omentum used to pack the cavity. (From Papanicolaou N, Mueller PR, Simeone JF, Malt RA: The sonographic appearance of omentoplasty in the surgical treatment of large cystic lesions of the liver. J Ultrasound Med 3:181, 1984.)

bizarre appearance. These membranes usually indicate disintegration of the daughter cysts.[48]

Because world travel is so prevalent now, a hydatid cyst should be included in the differential diagnosis whenever a cystic liver lesion is identified on ultrasound. If after taking a careful history, hydatid disease is still considered, a serologic complement fixation test may be performed. It is generally not wise to puncture an hydatid cyst, as anaphylaxis is a known potential complica-

tion of spreading scolices into the peritoneal cavity.[92] Ultrasound is the modality of choice for screening relatives of affected patients with known hydatid disease; it can be used for planning therapy and for follow-up exams.[96]

Omentoplasy is used at times for the surgical treatment of cysts, particularly primary large hepatic hydatic cysts.[107] The cavity of the lesion is "unroofed" and a piece of omentum with its blood supply preserved is mobilized and spread into the cavity. It is fixed to the walls and edge. The use of "omental patching" of the space has dramatically decreased infection of the operative space and bile leaks and has shortened the hospital stay. On ultrasound, a well-circumscribed, sharply angulated echogenic focus is seen within the liver. The lesion's large size and sharply angulated margin should help to distinguish it from most naturally occurring abnormalities of the liver[107] (Fig. 1-63). When omentoplasty is not used, a large cystic cavity may be seen in the area of the previously resected echinococcal cyst (Fig. 1-64).

Infection

PYOGENIC ABSCESS

The routes for bacteria to gain access to the liver include the biliary tree, portal vein, hepatic artery, direct extension from contiguous infection, and, rarely, trauma.[8,88,108] The majority come from the biliary tree. Infection in the biliary tract, biliary obstruction, preexisting hepatic cyst, and biliary tumor are all conditions

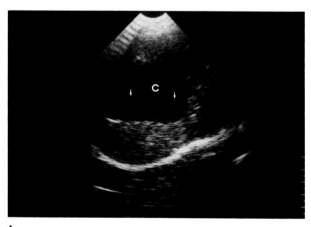

A

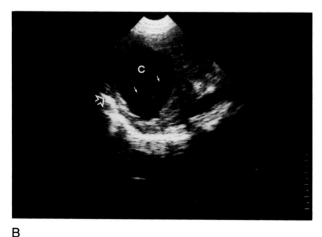

B

Fig. 1-64. Postoperative hydatid cyst. Transverse **(A)** and longitudinal **(B)** scans of the liver in a postoperative patient for hydatid cyst removal. A cystic (lucent) mass *(c)* is seen in the area of the previously resected cyst. It has a fluid-fluid level (arrows) within it. (Open arrow, diaphragm.) This was followed with ultrasound and serologic titers. By one year, it had disappeared.

that predispose to infection.[108-110] Not infrequently, the source of the infection is not found. The agent is usually *Escherichia coli* but anaerobic bacteria such as clostridia and bacteroides are also found.[8]

Rapid diagnosis and therapy are paramount since there is considerable morbidity and up to 100 percent mortality associated with untreated cases.[108] Ultrasound is an excellent modality for assessing the internal structure of the liver when looking for parenchymal abnormalities. It is superior to other radiologic modalities in detecting small, early hepatic lesions. Clinically, the presentation may be varied with fever, pain, pleuritic pain, nausea and vomiting, and diarrhea. There is usually leukocytosis, with elevated liver function tests and anemia. Real-time ultrasound requires careful scanning of the entire liver, identifying all landmarks. It allows a complete evaluation of the patient in a short period of time and can be done portably. The ultrasound features include (1) size—varying from 1 cm to extremely large; (2) location—right lobe most common (80 percent); (3) single or multiple (10 percent); (4) shape—variable but usually round or ovoid; (5) walls—usually irregular (90 percent) with poor definition; (6) pattern—anechoic to highly echogenic with the majority being less echogenic than liver; (7) acoustic enhancement (50 percent)— variable degree is prominent feature[108,110-113] (Figs. 1-65 to 1-68). Acoustic enhancement is the most diagnostic feature in a liver abscess when considering a differential diagnosis with other etiologies such as cyst, cyst with hemorrhage, necrotic tumor, echinococcal cysts, and primary or metastatic cystadencarcinoma.[108,110-113] The marked echogenicity in abscesses may be related to air or

actually to microbubbles that are not visible on radiographs[113,114] (Fig. 1-68). In the proper situation, acoustic shadowing is a reliable indicator of a gas-containing abscess.[115-117] In rare instances, an abscess can occur in the falciform ligament, as its layers represent a potential space providing communication between the gallbladder and falciform ligament.[118] Real-time ultrasound can be used to guide a puncture of an abscess for diagnosis and/or catheter drainage.[110,119,120]

AMEBIC ABSCESS

Although primarily an infection of the colon, amebiasis can spread to the liver, lungs, and brain. Hepatic abscesses are a common complication and one of the most widespread diseases of the world. The parasites (*Entamoeba histolytica*) reach the liver through the portal vein. They may burrow through the subdiaphragmatic space to enter the lung. The disease is contracted by ingesting the cysts in contaminated food and water. The wall of the cyst dissolves in the alkaline content of the small bowel and the trophozoite emerges to colonate and ulcerate the colon. The cecum and ascending colon are most commonly affected.[8] Most patients are asymptomatic and the organism is confined to the gastrointestinal tract. The amebas invade the colon mucosa and are carried to the liver via the portal venous system. The liver can be affected without overt colonic involvement.[48] Deposition in the capillaries of the portal vein presumably accounts for the peripheral location of the abscesses.[48,121] When the infestation has been established there is liquefaction necrosis of the hepatocytes with lit-

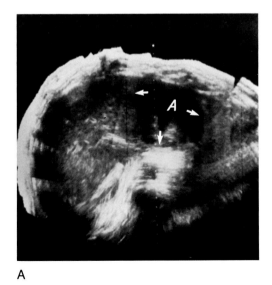

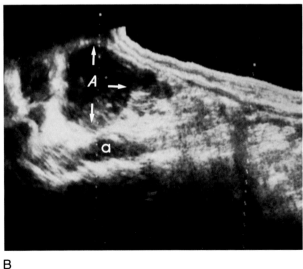

A   B

Fig. 1-65. Pyogenic abscess. **(A)** Transverse static scan at 16 cm above the umbilicus. A relatively cystic mass (*A*, arrows) is seen within the left lobe of the liver. **(B)** Longitudinal scan at 2 cm to the left of midline. The cystic mass (*A*, arrows) is seen within the left lobe. (*a*, aorta.)

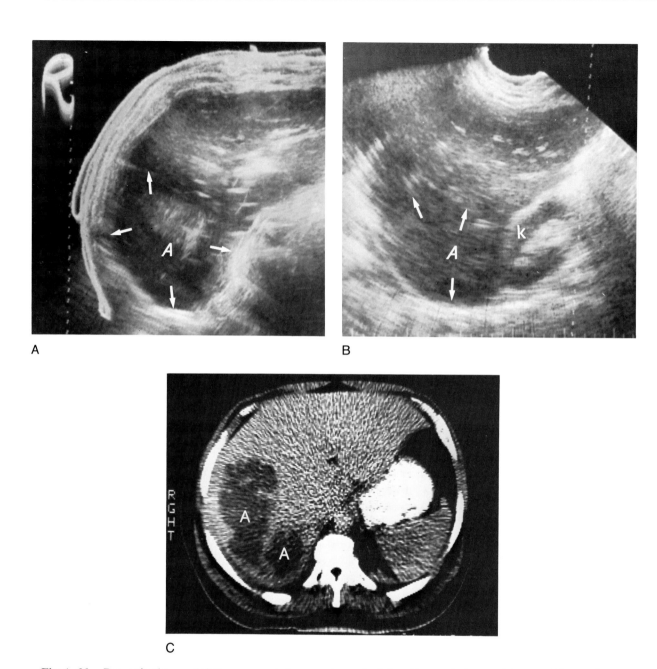

Fig. 1-66. Pyogenic abscess. **(A)** Transverse static scan. A poorly defined hypoechoic area (*A*, arrows) is seen in the posterior right lobe. **(B)** Longitudinal static scan. The poorly defined hypoechoic abscess (*A*, arrows) is seen. (*k*, right kidney.) **(C)** Unenhanced CT scan. The abscess appears as many low-density areas *(A).*

tle leukocytic response or fibrotic response resulting in the diagnostic "anchovy sauce" appearance.[48,121] The incidence of this infection is 5 percent and is increasing as a result of international travel and migration.[108]

Pathologically, the walls of this abscess have a shaggy fibrin lining surrounded by scant fibrovascular response. Because of hemorrhage into partially digested debris, abscess cavities are filled with chocolate-colored, pasty material. Patients may have clinical symptoms of ab-

dominal pain, diarrhea, and melena.[8] Complications include rupture into pleuropulmonary structures (15.8 percent), and rupture into the peritoneal cavity (6 percent).[108] The diagnosis is confirmed by direct hemaglutination titers with aspiration reserved for cases in which serologic tests are inconclusive.[8,108]

There are numerous descriptions of the ultrasound pattern of amebic abscesses of the liver.[48,92,108,121–126] Forty percent of patients exhibit findings suggestive of

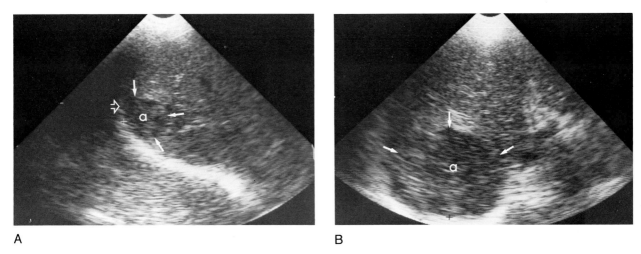

A   B

Fig. 1-67. Pyogenic abscess. Patient with Crohn's disease who was taking steroids and was not symptomatic for hepatic abscess. **(A)** Initial transverse scan. A poorly defined hypoechoic mass (*a*, arrows) is seen within the right lobe posteriorly and next to the diaphragm (open arrow). At the time of the scan, there was no clinical suspicion of an abscess. **(B)** Follow-up transverse scan one week after that of **(A)**, more magnified. The hypoechoic lesion (*a*, arrows) has tripled in size. The abscess was drained percutaneously.

the diagnosis: (1) lack of significant wall echoes; (2) round or oval configuration; (3) echogenicity less than normal liver parenchyma, with fine, homogeneous, low-level echoes at high gain; (4) location contiguous with liver capsule; and (5) distal sonic enhancement [48,124] (Figs. 1-69 and 1-70). Fifty percent over the above 40 percent were found to exhibit all but one or two charac-

teristics.[124] One series reported 7 of 74 amebic abscesses that appeared partly or predominately hyperechoic.[123] On follow-up exam, after a course of therapy, the appearance of four of six changed to a more typical hypoechoic form. After therapy, the healing process usually results in complete resolution of the ultrasound abnormality. This occurs in a period of 6 weeks to 23 months with a median

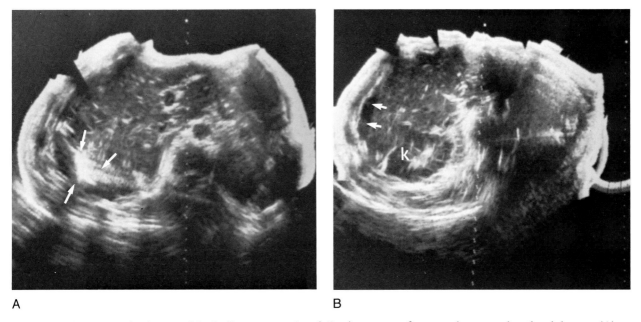

A   B

Fig. 1-68. Pyogenic abscess with air. Scans were taken following surgery for a gunshot wound to the abdomen. **(A)** Transverse static scan at 14 cm above the umbilicus. Air (arrows) is seen as an echogenic region within the posterior liver. The abscess as such is not defined. **(B)** Transverse static scan at 8 cm above the umbilicus. A subcapsular hematoma (arrows) is seen as a lucency bordering the liver. (*k*, right kidney.) *(Figure continues.)*

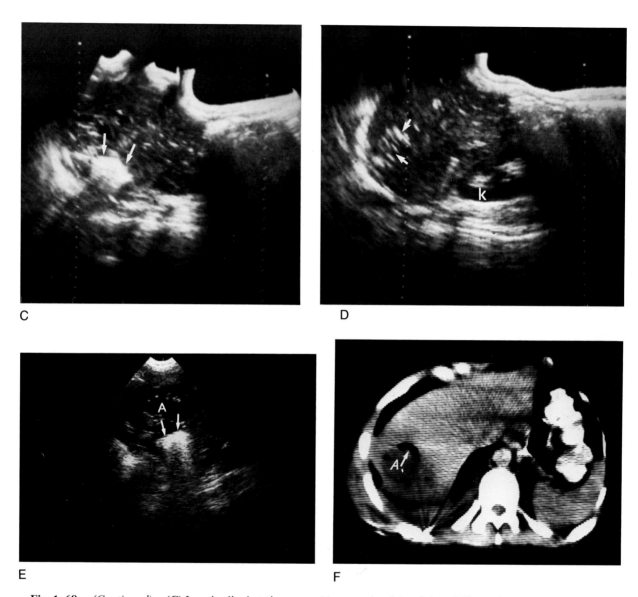

Fig. 1-68. *(Continued).* **(C)** Longitudinal static scan at 11 cm to the right of the midline. Air (arrows) is seen as an echogenic area within the posterior liver. **(D)** Longitudinal static scan at 9 cm to the right of midline. Air (arrows) is seen in the posterior liver. (*k*, kidney.) **(E)** Longitudinal real-time image through the abscess. The cystic cavity *(A)* is seen as well as the air (arrows). **(F)** CT scan similar to that of **(A)** with air (arrow) seen within a low density mass *(A)*.

period of 7 months.[106,124] Occasionally, a cystic residua remains[106,124,127] (Fig. 1-71). After therapy, ultrasound findings may vary; the cyst may enlarge, get smaller, or remain unchanged in echopattern.[48] It is important that a transient persistent abnormality seen after successful treatment not prompt reinstitution of therapy or further diagnostic testing in those patients.[106]

Aspiration rarely is indicated, as the diagnosis can be confirmed by hemagglutination titers and response to specific therapy.[121,124] Percutaneous aspiration is re-

served for use when the diagnosis is uncertain, superimposed pyogenic infection is suspected, response to drug therapy is inadequate, or impending rupture is considered likely.[48] Rupture is not infrequent and most commonly is into the peritoneal cavity or subhepatic space, or is through the diaphragm into the pleural cavity and may involve the lung and bronchial tree.[48] Untreated, the mortality is almost 100 percent and even treated the mortality is 10 percent. Early and accurate diagnosis followed by therapy is essential.[48]

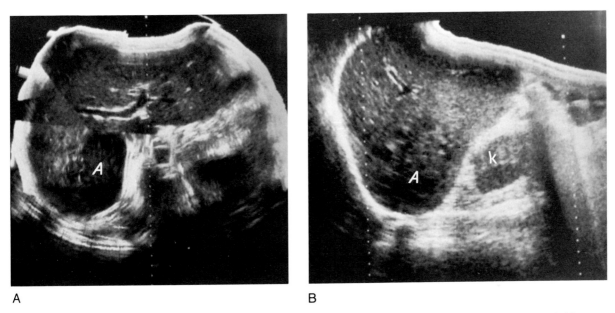

A   B

Fig. 1-69.   Amebic abscess. **(A)** Transverse static scan at 14 cm above the umbilicus. A hypoechoic area *(A)* is seen within the posterior aspect of the right lobe. **(B)** Longitudinal static scan at 6 cm to the right of midline. The abscess *(A)* is poorly defined. (*k,* right kidney.)

CANDIDIASIS

Noncutaneous candidiasis is uncommon and almost invariably is in immunologically compromised hosts. It occurs in patients with endogeneous immune deficiency, particularly T-cell function or underlying host defense mechanism defect. It is more common in patients undergoing therapy for neoplastic disorders (such as leukemia), renal transplants, or chronic granulomatous disease. With invasion of the bloodstream, the infection occurs in any organ with the kidneys, the heart, and the brain being the most commonly affected paren-

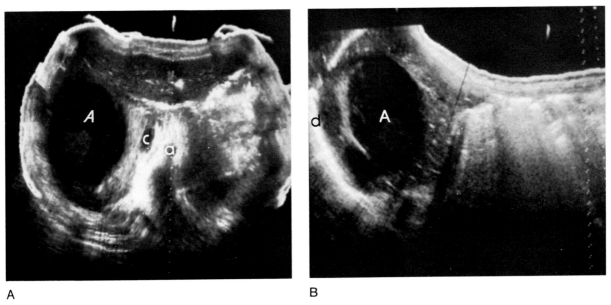

A   B

Fig. 1-70.   Amebic abscess. **(A)** Transverse static scan at 14 cm above the umbilicus. An almost anechoic mass *(A)* is seen within the posterior liver. (*a,* aorta; *c,* inferior vena cava.) **(B)** Longitudinal static scan at 7 cm to right of midline. The anechoic region *(A)* is seen. (*d,* diaphragm.)

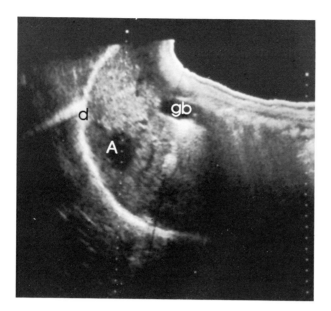

Fig. 1-71. Amebic abscess, follow-up. Patient in Figure 1.70 after Flagyl treatment. Longitudinal static scan similar to Figure 1.70B with only a small anechoic area *(A)* seen. (*d,* diaphram; *gb,* gallbladder.)

chymal organs; the pancreas, adrenal, liver, and spleen may also be affected.[128] The presenting symptoms are nonspecific with fever and pain referable to the area of involvement.[129] On ultrasound, the findings of the liver

are characteristic, that is, an hypoechoic area with a central area of increased echogenicity (bull's-eye or target)[128-130] (Fig. 1-72). A target lesion would be uncommon with lymphoma, but when it does occur, the central echodense focus is much larger.[128] A diagnosis of candidiasis is quickly made by percutaneous fine needle aspiration.

CHRONIC GRANULOMATOUS DISEASE

Chronic granulomatous disease is a familial disorder related to a congenital defect in the leukocyte, which is unable to inactivate catalase-positive, previously phagocytized bacteria.[131] It is an X-linked recessive trait. Clinically, when a child presents with recurrent infection of the lungs, paranasal sinuses, bone, lymph nodes, or liver, the diagnosis should be suggested. The catalase-positive bacteria involved is usually *Staphylococcus aureus* or *Escherichia coli,* but is rarely *Serratia marcescens* or *Aspergillus.* On ultrasound, hypoechoic, poorly marginated areas are seen with posterior enhancement[131] (Figs. 1-73 and 1-74). These lesions may be single or multiple. They are usually less defined than true abscesses. Early recognition of the disease is important, as antibiotics are especially effective at this stage. An aspiration biopsy may be needed for a definitive diagnosis. Ultrasound may be used to follow-up lesions after treatment.

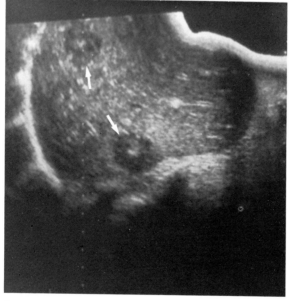

A

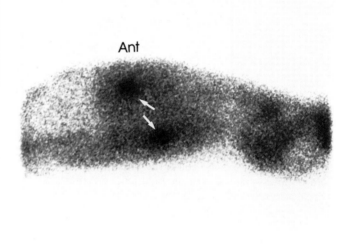

B

Fig. 1-72. Candidiasis. Acute myelogenous leukemia. **(A)** Longitudinal static scan. Two bull's-eye lesions (arrows) are seen within the liver. They have a small dense center and a hypoechoic rim. **(B)** Right lateral view of a gallium scan. The areas of increased activity (arrows) seen within the liver correspond to the areas seen on the ultrasound scan. (*Ant,* anterior.)

Benign Neoplasm

Primary liver tumors are less common than metastatic disease. They may originate from the hepatic parenchyma cells or bile duct epithelium, or represent a mixture of the two. Benign tumors are rare.[8]

MESENCHYMA HAMARTOMA

Mesenchyma hamartomas are rare and occur in children less than 2 years of age. They may enlarge such that they produce an abdominal mass. They are composed of well-differentiated ductal structures surrounded by loose mesenchymal connective tissue,[8] probably lymphangiomatous in origin.[132] On ultrasound, a mass is seen that is either well defined and predominantly anechoic with some evidence of trabeculation[133-135] or transonic with a reticular, lace-like configuration[132] (Fig. 1-75).

CAVERNOUS HEMANGIOMA

A cavernous hemangioma is the most common benign tumor of the liver. The incidence is 0.4 to 7.3 percent in an autopsy series.[136] It is composed of a large network of vascular endothelium-lined spaces filled with red blood cells.[8,137] They are more frequent in women and with increased age, and they may enlarge slowly with degeneration, fibrosis, and calcification.[88,138]

Most authors describe a homogeneous echodense (94 percent) pattern that is sharply marginated with this tumor[136-144] (Fig. 1-76). The echogenicity of the hemangioma may be due to the multiple interfaces between the

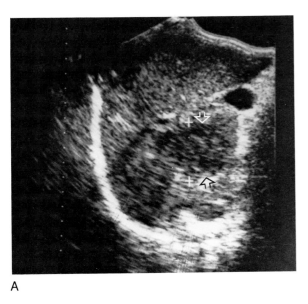

A

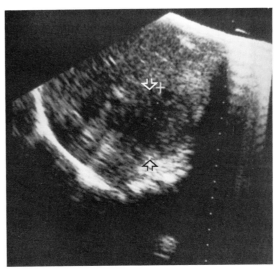

B

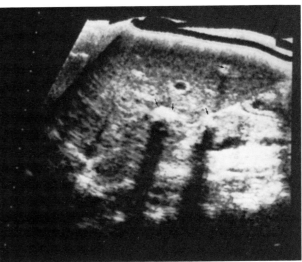

C

Fig. 1-73. Chronic granulomatous disease. Longitudinal scans (**A–E**) of the liver. Two poorly marginated, hypoechoic areas (open arrows) are seen in the right lobe. Calcifications with distal acoustic shadowing (arrows) are visible in (**C**) suggesting previous chronic granulomatous disease of the left lobe. *(Figure continues.)*

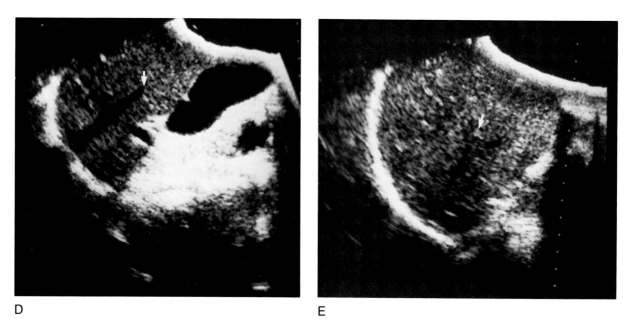

D   E

Fig. 1-73. *(Continued).* **(D,E)** Two months later after treatment with antibiotics, the hypoechoic areas have subsided. Scars are still visible (arrows) with a single calcification which remained unchanged 2 years later. (From Garel LA, Pariente DM, Nezelop C, et al: Liver involvement in chronic granulomatous disease: the role of ultrasound in diagnosis and treatment. Radiology 153:117, 1984.)

walls of the cavernous sinuses and blood within them.[142] As the hemangioma undergoes degeneration and fibrous replacement, the echopattern becomes more heterogeneous.[142] Some lesions have been complex or anechoic with acoustic enhancement.[138,140] One series described a

76.5-percent incidence of posterior acoustic enhancement in hemangiomas, with all lesions greater than 25 mm diameter demonstrating enhancement[143] (Fig. 1-77). No acoustic enhancement was found in 87.5 percent of the hemangiomas less than 25 mm diameter.[143]

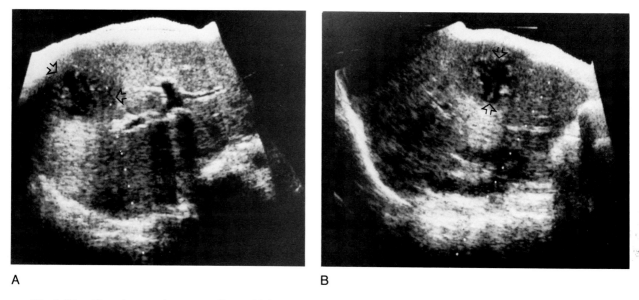

A   B

Fig. 1-74. Chronic granulomatous disease (CGD). This patient with known CGD had fever, right upper quadrant pain, and liver enlargement. Oblique **(A)** and longitudinal **(B)** scans demonstrate a transonic mass (arrows) with distal enhancement suggestive of abscess. An abscess was found at surgery. (From Garel LA, Pariente DM, Nezelop C, et al: Liver involvement in chronic granulomatous disease: the role of ultrasound in diagnosis and treatment. Radiology 153:117, 1984.)

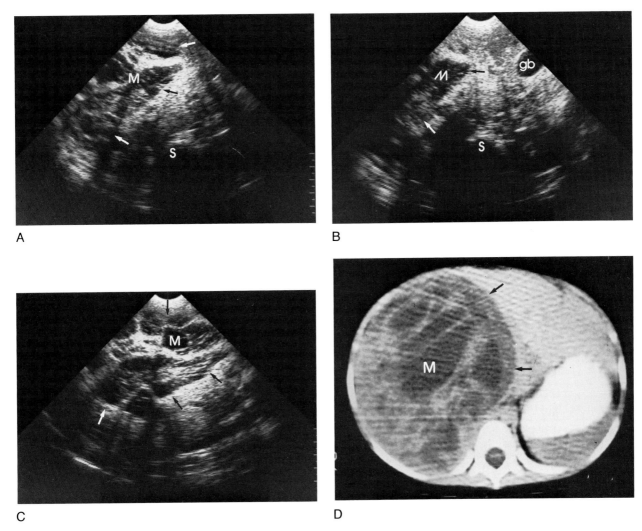

Fig. 1-75. Mesenchymal hamartoma. **(A,B)** Transverse real-time images demonstrating a mass (*M*, arrows) containing hypoechoic to anechoic areas within the liver. The gallbladder *(gb)* is seen in **(B)** and is displaced to the left of midline. The mass appears to only involve the right lobe. (*S,* spine.) **(C)** Longitudinal real-time scan. The mass (*M*, arrows) contains multiple lucent areas. **(D)** Enhanced CT scan. A large low-density mass (*M*, arrows) is seen filling the right lobe of the liver. The mass contains many septations.

The posterior enhancement correlated with hypervascularity on angiography. The zone of distal enhancement results from better sound penetration in the mass than in the liver and is an indicator of lower attenuation coefficient.

Most hemangiomas are in the posterior right lobe of the liver[142,144]; 73 percent are in the right lobe, with 27 percent in the left lobe.[143] These lesions are (1) subcapsular in location (70 percent), (2) less than 2 cm in size (32 percent), (3) multiple (35 percent), and (4) greater than 3 cm with a polylobular contour (90 percent).[139] They have been described as round (75.5 percent), oval (13.5 percent), or lobulated (11 percent).[143] The contours were well defined in 92 percent, with poorly defined margins in 8 percent.[143]

In one study, ultrasound was found to be more reliable than CT in detecting cavernous hemangiomas less than 1.5 cm in size.[145] Although the CT enhancement pattern with this lesion is characteristic, it is difficult to evaluate in lesions smaller than 1.5 cm. Those lesions smaller than 3 cm were universally found to be strongly echogenic on ultrasound.[145] If a lesion has a characteristic ultrasound pattern and is too small to evaluate with CT enhancement, the use of an angiogram might be questioned, especially if the patient has no history of malignancy or liver dysfunction nor is at high risk for hepatocellular carcinoma. The differential diagnosis would include hepatocellular carcinoma, liver cell adenoma, focal nodular hyperplasia, and solitary metastasis.[142] A definitive diagnosis cannot be made with ultrasound

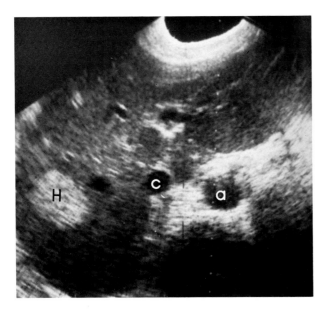

Fig. 1-76. Cavernous hemangioma. Transverse scan at 9 cm below the xyphoid. A well-defined echogenic area *(H)* is seen within the right lobe. (*c,* inferior vena cava; *a,* aorta.)

alone, but can be when ultrasound is combined with dynamic CT, angiogram, and/or biopsy. In a patient with no known primary tumor, dynamic CT could be done after ultrasound. If CT is not characteristic, an angiogram or biopsy might follow. The CT patterns of a hemangioma include (1) low-density area before bolus of contrast, followed by irregular enhancement of the mass with the mass becoming isodense to surrounding liver; (2) low-density area followed by irregular periph-

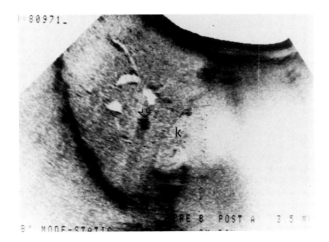

Fig. 1-77. Cavernous hemangioma. Longitudinal static scan with a hyperechoic mass (open arrow) with slight distal acoustic enhancement (small arrows). (*k,* right kidney.) (Courtesy of Dr. Charles A. Durrell III, and Pinehurst Radiology, Moore Memorial Hospital, Pinehurst, North Carolina.)

eral enhancement of the mass, with the mass becoming predominately isodense but with a central low density area; (3) low-density area followed by irregular peripheral enhancement of the mass, with the mass becoming hyperdense compared to surrounding liver[142] (Fig. 1-78). If the lesion is characteristic of the findings on CT, a follow-up ultrasound may be performed in 6 to 12 months.[142]

INFANTILE HEMANGIOENDOTHELIOMA

Infantile hemangioendothelioma is the most common symptomatic vascular liver tumor in infancy.[146] Eighty-five percent occur before 6 months of age, more commonly in females with a 2:1 ratio.[146,147] A normal α-fetoprotein (AFP) level would exclude a diagnosis of hepatoblastoma.[146] The tumor usually grows rapidly after presentation and then regresses gradually.[146] The spontaneous regression of an infantile hemangioendotheliomatosis of the liver has been reported.[148] The child presents with an abdominal mass and high cardiac output failure secondary to arteriovenous shunting throughout the tumor.[132,147,149] Congestive heart failure associated with this mass is not as common as once thought.[146] Complications of this lesion include thrombocytopenia, angiopathic anemia, gastrointestinal bleeding, and intraabdominal rupture with hemorrhage.[132,148]

Pathologically, the mass is round, smooth, multilobular or irregular, and tends to be well demarcated. There are central areas in large lesions of infarction, hemorrhage, fibrosis, and foci of dysmorphic calcification.[146] There are two types described. The first is seen to contain variable-sized vascular spaces lined by relatively immature, plump endothelial cells with supporting fibrous stroma with some foci of less well-differentiated myxomatous tissue. Between the vascular spaces are scattered bile ducts, which may contain hematopoietic cells. The second type consists of more immature, bigger pleomorphic cells, which reflect the more aggressive end of the spectrum and may mimic hemangioendothelial sarcoma (generally seen in older adults) with poorly formed vascular spaces and branching structures.[146,148]

Plain film shows hepatomegaly, and, rarely, calcification, which may be numerous and sponge-like or in the form of spicules radiating from a central core.[148] On ultrasound, the lesion has been described as hyperechoic, hypoechoic, and diffuse[146,150] (Fig. 1-79). Multiple lucent lesions varying from 1 to 3 cm with few low-level echoes and hyperechoic margins may also be seen.[148] Large draining veins and a dilated proximal abdominal aorta may be seen in the lesion, with arteriovenous shunting.[135]

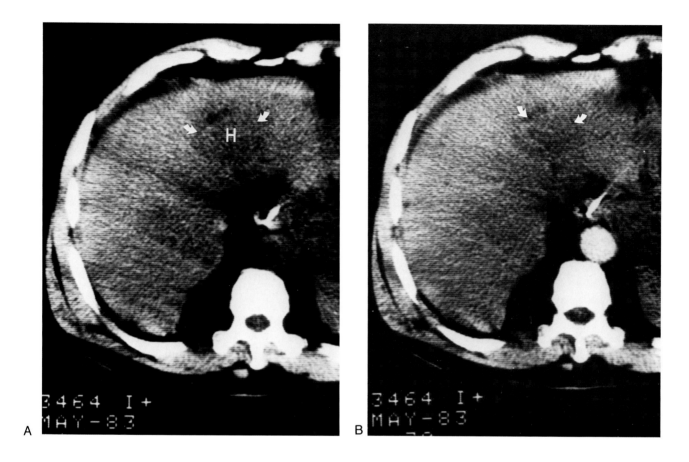

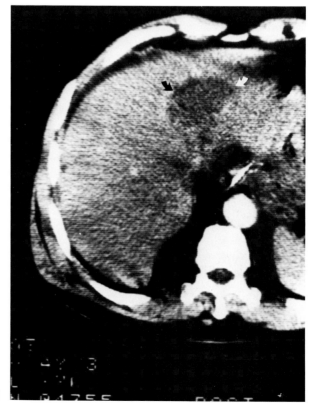

Fig. 1-78. Cavernous hemangioma. (A) Unenhanced CT scan. A poorly defined low-density area *(H)* is seen. (B,C) Dynamically enhanced CT scans. The low-density area (arrows) on (A) is seen to become more lucent on (C) with peripheral enhancement. *(Figure continues.)*

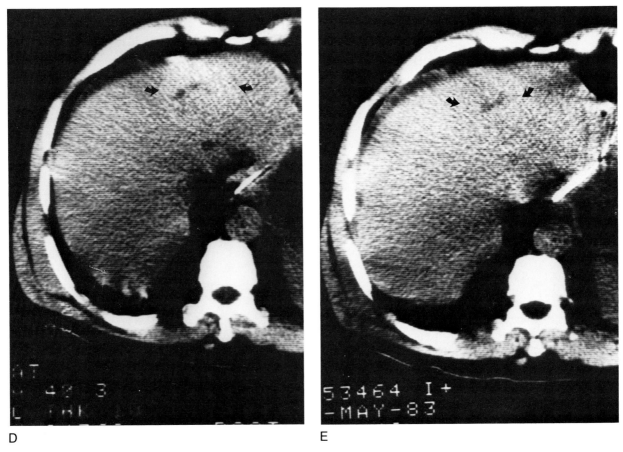

D   E

Fig. 1-78. *(Continued).* **(D)** Seven minutes after a bolus of contrast the lesion (arrows) is almost isodense. **(E)** By 20 minutes, the lesion (arrows) is even more isodense.

FOCAL NODULAR HYPERPLASIA

Focal nodular hyperplasia is a rare benign tumor that is usually discovered serendipitously by imaging procedures. It is most common in females less than 40 years of age, and an increased incidence with the use of oral contraceptives has been shown. It is usually asymptomatic and is most frequently located near the free edge of the liver (subcapsular).[8] It is usually a solitary, well-circumscribed, nonencapsulated multinodular mass. The mass is composed of normal hepatocytes, Kupffer cells, bile duct elements, and fibrous connective tissue.[151,152] Multiple nodules are separated by bands of fibrous tissue often radiating from a large central scar.[8] Others describe a well-circumscribed nodular cirrhotic-like mass within normal tissue.[153] The characteristic depressed central or eccentric stellate scar is composed of dense fibrous connective tissue, proliferating bile ducts, and thin-walled blood vessels.[152,153] The typical features include (1) a size of 0.5 to 20 cm; (2) a central scar from which fibrous septa extend radially, which divides the mass into nodules; (3) usually in right lobe, or lateral segment of the left lobe (13 percent multiple); (4) an unknown natural

history—rarity of complications led to conservative management; and (5) no malignant transformation.[151,152] The only known complication is intraperitoneal bleeding, and this is rare.[151,152]

On ultrasound, the mass may be slightly less echogenic than the liver,[151] hyperechoic, or may appear as a mass isosonic to normal liver[152–155] (Figs. 1-80 to 1-82). Most of these tumors have similar acoustic characteristics to surrounding liver.[155] A dense nonshadowing linear or stellate group of echoes in a solitary hepatic mass may also be seen[152,153] (Fig. 1-82). A 100-percent sensitivity for ultrasound in detecting focal nodular hyperplasia has been reported while CT has a 78-percent sensitivity, angiography, an 82-percent and nuclear medicine, a 55-percent.[152] Normal colloid uptake by a focal hepatic mass is virtually diagnostic of this entity.[152]

LIVER CELL ADENOMA

Liver cell adenoma represents normal or slightly atypical hepatocytes frequently containing areas of bile stasis and focal hemorrhage or necrosis, but not containing

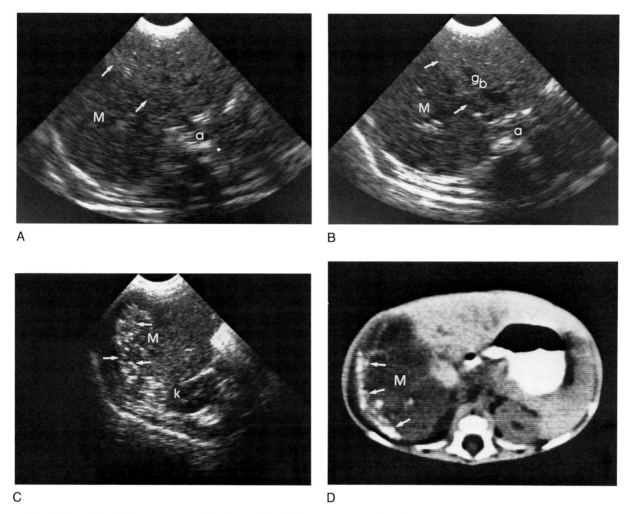

Fig. 1-79. Infantile hemangioendothelioma. **(A,B)** Transverse real-time images. A hypoechoic mass (*M*, arrows) is seen within the posterior liver. The gallbladder *(gb)* is seen in **(B)** and it appears to be displaced to the left. The mass *(M)* involves only the right lobe. (*a,* aorta.) **(C)** Transverse real-time scan through the lower part of the mass *(M)*. Note the dense areas (arrows) within the lateral aspect of the mass, representing the calcification. (*k,* kidney.) **(D)** Unenhanced CT scan, which corresponds to the level of that of **(C)** with the lateral calcification (arrows). The mass *(M)* is of low density and is well defined.

bile ducts or Kupffer cells.[87,156] It is usually a solitary, marginated, encapsulated mass.[132] It is more common in females and oral contraceptives have been linked to it.[8,88] The mass is usually symptomatic with presentations that may include a palpable mass or severe right upper quadrant pain (due to rupture lesion with hemoperitoneum or bleeding into tumor), or both.[88] The ultrasound pattern is variable; if bleeding has occurred, the mass may be lucent or a greater density than the surrounding liver[88,132,156,157] (Fig. 1-83). Adenomas and focal nodular hyperplasia often look similar on ultrasound.[156]

These lesions have been reported in Type I glycogen storage disease.[46,158] In glycogen storage disease, there is an 8-percent incidence of adenomas, with a frequency of 40 percent in Type I.[46] Since the liver in von Gierke's disease is abnormally echogenic, the adenomas in these patients appear as solitary or multiple hyperechoic solid lesions (Fig. 1-28). The larger adenomas are heterogeneous with hypoechoic foci secondary to necrosis or hemorrhage, or both.[158] Marked acoustic enhancement deep to the adenoma was noted; this was postulated to be related to relative paucity of lipid and glycogen within the adenoma.[158] This acoustic enhancement is not seen deep to adenomas not associated with glycogen storage disease.[158]

LIPOMAS

Lipomas are rare, benign primary solid tumors of the liver, derived from mesenchymal elements.[159] They are nonencapsulated and in continuity with the normal liver parenchyma. These fatty masses are invariably hyper-

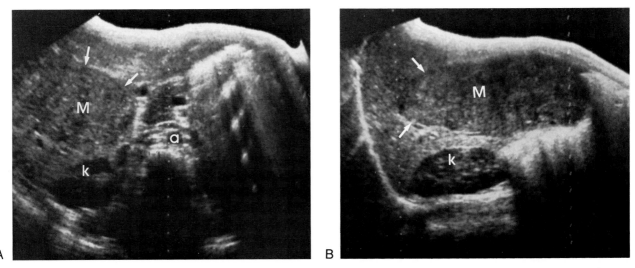

A B

Fig. 1-80. Focal nodular hyperplasia. **(A)** Transverse static image at 3.5 cm below the xyphoid. A mass (*M*, arrows) is seen with a similar density to liver. The borders are poorly defined. (*k*, kidney; *a*, aorta.) **(B)** Longitudinal static scan 4 cm to right of midline. The mass (*M*, arrows) is more easily seen. (*k*, kidney.) On a sulfur colloid liver/spleen scan, the mass was found to contain less activity than the remainder of the liver.

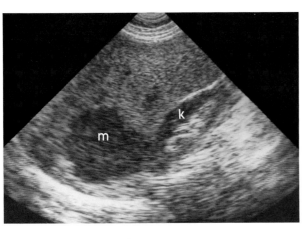

Fig. 1-81. Focal nodular hyperplasia. Right longitudinal scan. A hypoechoic mass *(m)* is seen in the posterior right lobe. (*k*, right kidney.) On a sulfur colloid liver/spleen scan, the mass contained less activity than the remainder of the liver. (From Parker LA, Banning B: Focal nodular hyperplasia of the liver: Scintigraphic demonstration with Tc-99m sulfur colloid emission computed tomography. Clinical Nuc Med, 10:601, 1985.)

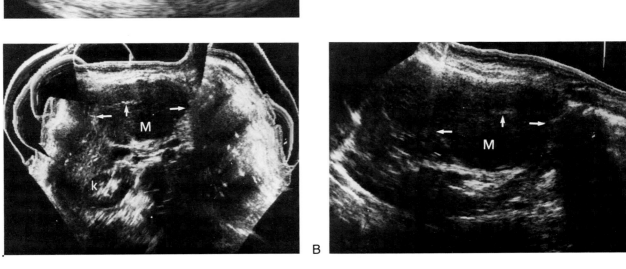

A B

Fig. 1-82. Focal nodular hyperplasia. **(A)** Transverse and **(B)** longitudinal static scans of a mass (*M*, long arrows) occupying most of the left lobe. The echopattern of the mass is slightly less than that of the remainder of the liver. A short linear horizontal cluster of bright echoes (short arrow) is seen within the mass on both projections. This represented a prominent central fibrous scar with radiating septa. (*k*, kidney.) (From Scatarige JC, Fishman EK, Sanders RC: The sonographic "scar sign" in focal nodular hyperplasia of the liver. J Ultrasound Med 1:275, 1982.)

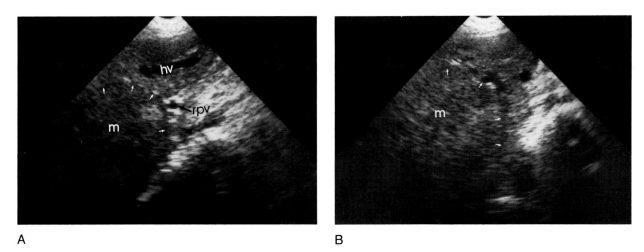

A   B

Fig. 1-83.   Liver cell adenoma. **(A,B)** Right longitudinal scans. The mass (*m*, arrows) is barely perceived on these scans. It is very similar in echodensity to the remainder of the liver. A dilated hepatic vein *(hv)* is seen in **(A)**. (*rpv,* right portal vein.)

echoic, which is explained by the presence of multiple fat/nonfat interfaces[159] (Fig. 1-84). A posterior "shadow conus" is seen due to the diminished penetration of the sound beam to the posterior liver.

Malignant Tumors

HEPATOBLASTOMA

Hepatoblastoma is a rare malignant tumor that is seen in infancy and childhood. The patient presents with abdominal enlargement with hepatomegaly. Calcification may be seen on radiographs and the α-fetoprotein (AFP)

level is increased. There are two types of hepatoblastoma: (1) epithelial—sheets of cells resembling fetal liver cells or undifferentiated "embryonal" cells and (2) mixed—epithelial, mesenchymal connective tissue and other elements, particularly osteoid tissue.[8,132] On ultrasound, these lesions have been found to be echogenic[134] or cystic with internal septations[160] (Fig. 1-85).

HEPATOCELLULAR CARCINOMA

The pathogenesis of hepatocellular carcinoma (HCC) appears to be related to hepatocarcinogens in food, cirrhosis, and chronic hepatitis B virus infection.[8] Eighty

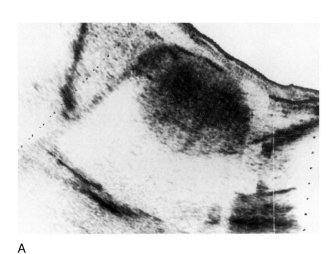

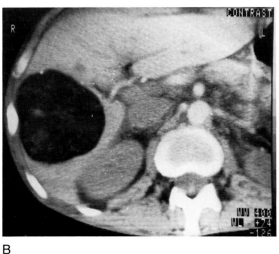

A   B

Fig. 1-84.   Hepatic adenolipoma. **(A)** Longitudinal scan of the liver. A hyperechogenic mass with a reflective pattern and a posterior shadow conus is seen. **(B)** CT scan through the mass. There is a specific fat attenuation valve (−65HU), clear delineation, and network enhancement at angio CT. (From Kurdziel JC, Stines J, Parache RM, Chaulieu C: Adenolipoma of the liver: An unique case with ultrasound and CT patterns. Europ J Radiol 4:45, 1984.)

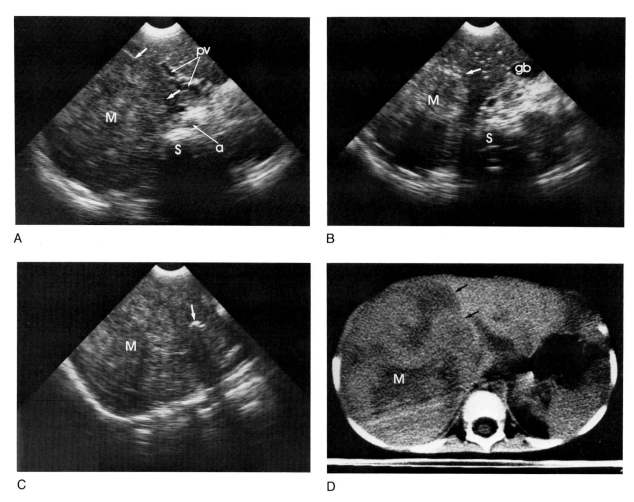

Fig. 1-85. Hepatoblastoma. **(A)** Transverse real-time scan with a mass *(M)* filling the posterior right lobe. It has an inhomogeneous echogenic pattern — more dense than normal liver parenchyma. The borders of the mass (arrows) are poorly defined. Note that the axis of the portal vein *(pv)* has assumed an almost vertical axis due to the mass. (*S,* spine; *a,* aorta.) **(B)** Somewhat similar scan to that of **(A)** but reveals the gallbladder *(gb)*. The gallbladder is displaced to the left of midline. The mass appears to only involve the right lobe since it is to the right of the gallbladder and major fissure. (*S,* spine.) **(C)** Longitudinal real-time through the mass. Calcification (arrow) is seen within the mass *(M)*. **(D)** Unenhanced CT scan. The mass (*M,* arrows) has an inhomogeneous appearance.

percent of HCCs occur in livers with preexisting cirrhosis, most frequently in those with postnecrotic or macronodular cirrhosis (13 to 24 percent) and alcoholic cirrhosis (3.2 percent).[8] The overall incidence of HCC with cirrhosis in the United States is 5 percent. Morphologically, there are several patterns: (1) solitary massive tumor, (2) multiple nodules throughout the liver, and (3) diffuse infiltrative types.[8] All of these cause hepatic enlargement.[8] HCC tends to invade the hepatic veins, producing Budd-Chiari syndrome.[8] Thrombosis or tumor invasion of the portal system is seen in 30 to 68 percent of hepatocellular carcinomas; in 13 percent of cases the tumor invades the hepatic veins and can invade the biliary tree.[63] Hepatocellular carcinoma has a distinct tendency to destroy the portal venous radicle wall with inva-

sion into the vessel lumen. The tumor then grows within the vessel with its blood supply from the capillary bed, surrounding vein, and/or adjacent bile duct.[63] Vascular invasion can be an early event and does not indicate inoperability.[63]

Clinically, patients present with a palpable mass in the liver, rapid liver enlargement, an unexplained mild fever, and a complex of signs and symptoms associated with underlying cirrhosis. One should suspect HCC when the condition of a patient with cirrhosis suddenly worsens or there is a sudden progressive enlargement of the liver with bloody ascites. Liver function tests often disclose surprisingly little abnormality and cirrhosis may explain any abnormality found. An AFP level is sometimes helpful in determining the diagnosis; 70 percent of

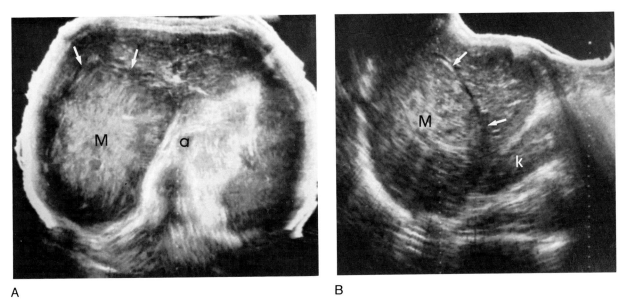

Fig. 1-86. Hepatocellular carcinoma. Dense pattern. **(A)** Transverse static scan at 12 cm above the umbilicus. The posterior aspect *(M)* of the right lobe appears echogenic and inhomogeneous. (*a*, aorta.) **(B)** Longitudinal static scan 7 cm to right of midline. The anteroinferior outline (arrows) of the mass *(M)* is seen. (*k*, kidney.)

patients with HCC have an elevated AFP level. Some investigators recommend screening patients for hepatocellular carcinoma, with AFP followed by ultrasound and CT.[161] AFP is synthesized by HCC; elevation can be seen in severe liver necrosis as well.[8]

In one series, 90 percent of patients with HCC had clinical hepatomegaly.[162,163] There are various ultrasound patterns described in patients with HCC: discrete echogenic, discrete echofree, mixed, isoechoic, and diffuse infiltrative[162-165] (Figs. 1-86 to 1-88). A 90-percent sensitivity for ultrasound in detecting HCC has been reported with a specificity of 93 percent.[166] One study suggests a close relationship between the echopattern and the histologic findings.[167] The hypoechoic tumors

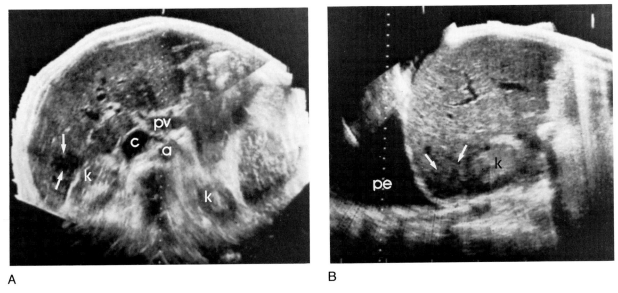

Fig. 1-87. Hepatocellular carcinoma. Lucent pattern. **(A)** Transverse static scan 12 cm above the umbilicus. A poorly defined hypoechoic area (arrows) is seen in the posterior liver. (*k*, kidney; *c*, inferior vena cava; *a*, aorta; *pv*, portal vein.) **(B)** Longitudinal static scan 7 cm to the right of midline. A poorly defined hypoechoic area (arrows) is seen. (*pe*, pleural effusion; *k*, kidney.)

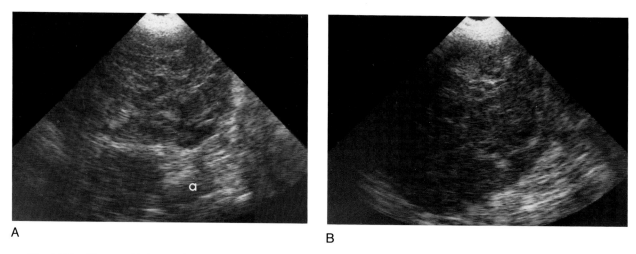

A   B

Fig. 1-88.   Hepatocellular carcinoma. Diffuse pattern. Transverse **(A)** and longitudinal **(B)** images demonstrate a liver with a diffusely inhomogeneous pattern. This patient had chronic hepatitis with rapidly worsening liver function. At autopsy, the liver exhibited a diffuse hepatocellular carcinoma. (*a,* aorta.)

were without necrosis and were hypoechoic presumably because of a lack of any structure within the tumor to serve as a reflective source. The hyperechoic lesion was the site of nonliquefactive necrosis. The anechoic lesion was the site of extensive liquifactive necrosis. Fatty metamorphosis, as well as severe sinusoidal dilatation, was visualized as hyperechoic.[167]

In one series, ultrasound was found to be the most sensitive method for the detection of small tumors.[168] Real-time ultrasound was felt to play a prominent role in the early detection and diagnosis of small hepatocellular carcinomas. In their series of 36 tumors of less than 3 cm, real-time scans revealed 93.9 percent of the small tumors, CT revealed 84.3 percent (those missed were < 2 cm), angiography revealed 75.7 percent, and nuclear medicine revealed 12.1 percent.[168] Most of these small tumors were noted to be hypoechoic (77.4 percent); as the tumor grows, it becomes larger and more dense, so larger ones are hyperechoic. In correlating the echopattern with the histology, the hypoechoic tumor contained only carcinoma cells; the hyperechoic tumor exhibited a mixture of hemorrhage, fibrous tissue, and necrosis.[168]

METASTASES

Metastases are the most common form of neoplastic involvement of the liver.[8] The usual primary sites are the gastrointestinal tract (particularly colon), the breast, and

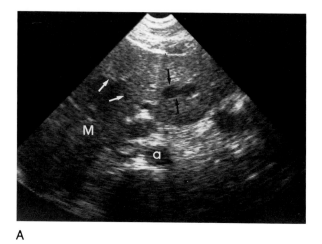

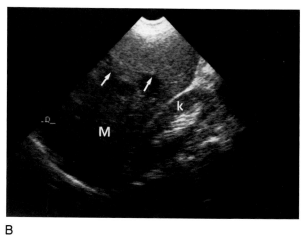

A   B

Fig. 1-89.   Hypoechoic hepatic metastases. Papillary cystadenocarcinoma of the ovary. **(A)** Transverse real-time scan with poorly defined hypoechoic areas (*M,* arrows). (*a,* aorta.) **(B)** Longitudinal real-time scan with a hypoechoic area (*M,* arrows). (*k,* kidney.)

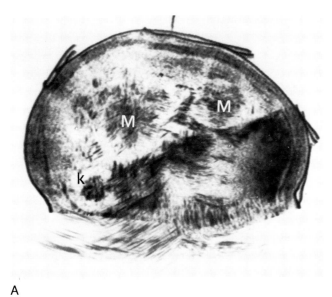

A

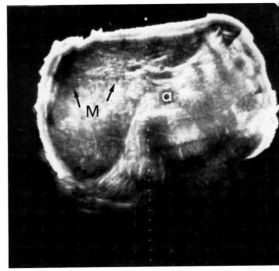

B

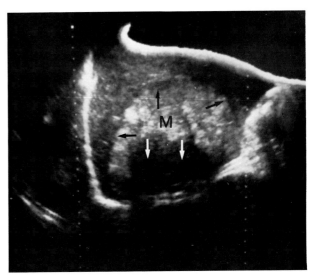

C

Fig. 1-90. Echogenic hepatic metastases. Case 1. Carcinoma of the colon. **(A)** Transverse static scan 8 cm above the umbilicus. Two large echogenic areas *(M)* are seen within the liver. (*k*, right kidney.) Case 2. Carcinoma of the colon. **(B)** Transverse static scan 10 cm above the umbilicus. A poorly defined echodense mass (*M*, arrows) is seen within the posterior liver. (*a*, aorta) **(C)** Longitudinal static scan 9 cm to right of midline. A large echodense mass (*M*, black arrows) is seen. There is absorption of the sound beam by the mass such that there is poor penetration of the sound beam (white arrows).

the lung. Dissemination of the tumor to the liver occurs via portal vein, lymphatics, hepatic artery, and, less frequently, by direct extension (e.g., from the gallbladder or stomach).[8] Metastatic disease usually causes liver enlargement. Multiple nodules throughout both lobes are typical.[8]

The following patterns have been described with ultrasound: (1) discrete hypoechoic (Fig. 1-89), (2) discrete echogenic (Figs. 1-90 and 1-91), (3) anechoic (Fig. 1-92), and (4) diffuse inhomogeneity[169-172] (Fig. 1-93). The majority of echogenic metastasis are from a colon primary (54 percent) and hepatoma (25 percent).[171] The ultrasound appearance of hepatic metastases seem to lack specificity in defining the organ of origin,[146,170,173] although there does appear to be a high correlation between the hyperechoic metastases and colon carcinoma.

Besides identifying the lesions, ultrasound can be employed to follow the progress of the lesions in assessing chemotherapeutic response. The following parameters should be assessed: (1) no change, (2) progression in size or extent, (3) decrease in size or extent, and (4) pattern change.[169] Ultrasound cannot be used to assess a change in echopattern, but can evaluate improvement, worsening, or no change based on number and size of lesions.[174]

A series of lucent metastasis has been reported, with the lucency felt to be due to extensive necrosis[175] (Fig. 1-94). A fluid-fluid level in some supported the concept of necrosis as the causative agent; this presumably demarcated layering of various components of the cavity was secondary to gravity.[175,176] As metastatic nodules increase rapidly in size and outgrow their blood supply, central necrosis and hemorrhage may result. By identi-

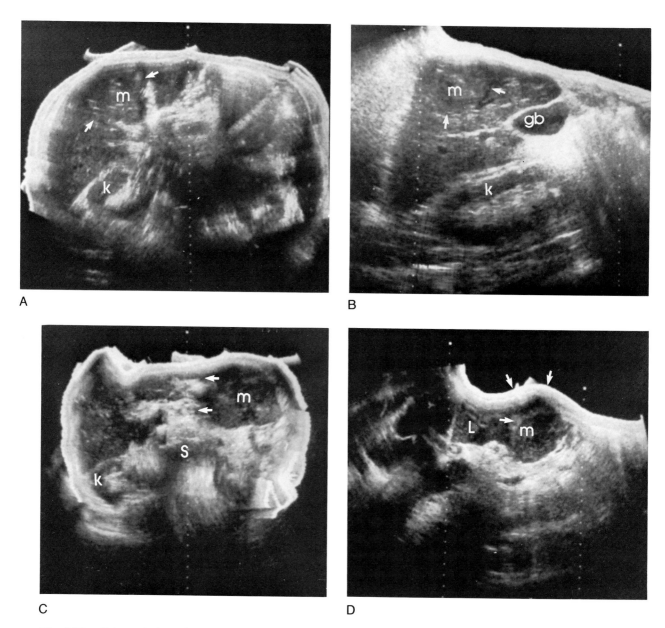

Fig. 1-91. Echogenic hepatic metastases. Case 1. Very subtle echogenic metastasis, squamous cell carcinoma. **(A)** Transverse static scan 12 cm above the umbilicus. The mass (*m*, arrows) is barely identifiable. (*k*, right kidney.) **(B)** Longitudinal scan 10 cm to right of midline. The same mass (*m*, arrows) is seen. (*k*, kidney; *gb*, gallbladder.) Case 2. Metastasis from carcinoma of the lung presenting as a left upper quadrant mass. **(C)** Transverse static scan 6 cm above the umbilicus. A mass (*m*, arrows) is seen in the left upper quadrant. (*S*, spine; *k*, right kidney.) **(D)** Longitudinal scan at 4 cm to the left of midline. The mass *(m)* is seen to be extending from the inferior aspect of the left lobe of the liver *(L)*. Note the mass produces a bulge (arrows) in the anterior abdominal wall.

fying wall thickness, mural nodules, septations, and fluid-fluid levels, ultrasound determines the morphology of cystic lesions and helps differentiate them from uncomplicated hepatic cysts.[177] In identifying irregular margins or presence of internal echoes, it helps distinguish a tumor from a cyst. Metastatic sarcomas tend to undergo degenerative changes more frequently than

metastatic carcinoma. Half of the cases in one series were leiomyosarcomas. It was difficult to differentiate cysts, abscesses, and tumors.[175]

Another feature described is calcification of metastases (Fig. 1-95). One ultrasound series revealed 13 cases of calcified metastases; in only 9, had the calcification been identified on radiographs.[178] The calcification of

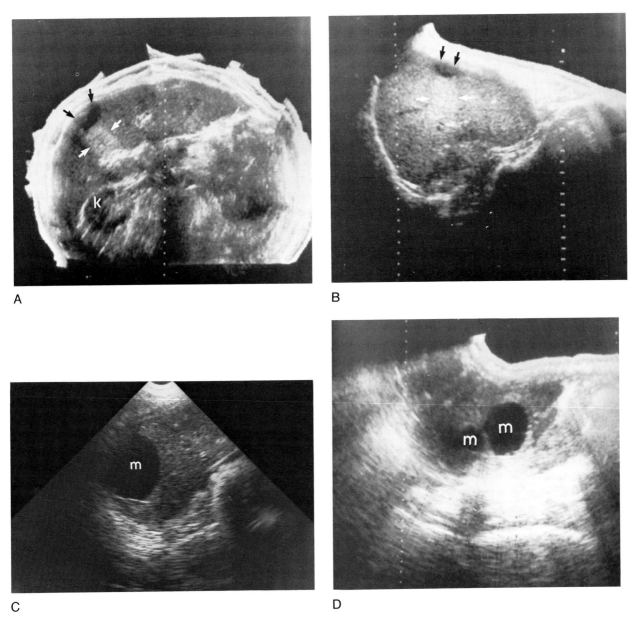

Fig. 1-92. Anechoic hepatic metastases. Case 1. Adenocarcinoma of the stomach. **(A)** Transverse scan 11 cm above the umbilicus. A well-defined anechoic area (black arrows) is seen within the liver. Note the acoustic enhancement (white arrows). (*k,* right kidney.) **(B)** Longitudinal scan 12 cm to the right of midline. A well-defined anechoic area (black arrows) with acoustic enhancement (white arrows) is seen within the anterior portion of the liver. Case 2. Carcinoma of the ovary. Longitudinal real-time **(C)** and static **(D)** images with well-defined anechoic *(m)* metastases.

metastases corresponds to at least partial involution; it is always associated with a polymetastatic hepatic condition and does not affect prognosis. It is noted as an echo-density with acoustical shadowing (Fig. 1-95). The shadowing is partial or total obliteration of echoes behind the echogenic area due to the high acoustic impedance and attenuation by the calcium-containing structure.[179] Cancer of the colon is the cancer most frequently associated with calcification.[171,178,179] Less frequent are en-

docrine tumors of the pancreas, leiomyosarcoma, malignant melanoma, cystadenocarcinoma of the ovary, adenocarcinoma of the stomach, lymphoma, osteosarcoma, pleural mesothelioma, neuroblastoma, and breast cancer.[178,179]

The relationship of the vascularization of the lesions to the echographic pattern has been evaluated.[180] Most cases of hypervascular lesions corresponded to hyperechoic patterns, while hypovascular lesions furnished

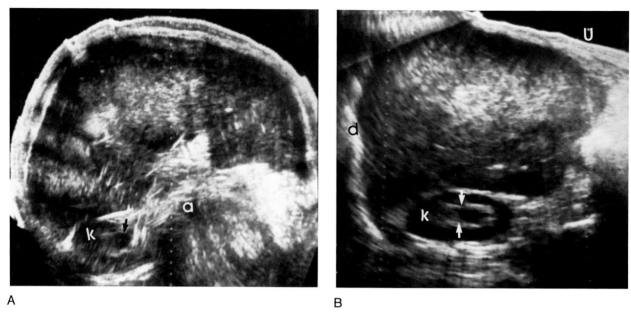

A   B

Fig. 1-93. Diffuse inhomogeneity with hepatic metastases. Carcinoma of the prostate. Transverse static scan at 12 cm above the umbilicus **(A)** and longitudinal static scan 4 cm to the right of midline **(B)** demonstrate an inhomogeneous liver echopattern. Note the dilated right collecting system (arrows). (*k,* right kidney; *U,* level of the umbilicus; *d,* diaphragm; *a,* aorta.)

hypoechoic lesions. Although the nature of the vascular substrate seem to be the predominate factor in formation of the echographic image of the metastatic lesion, the tissue component may not be excluded. In hypoechoic lesions, along with necrosis and hypovascularity, there are ischemic areas resulting from neoplastic thrombosis.[180] The most common hypervascular metastases are

renal cell carcinoma, carcinoid, choriocarcinoma, transitional cell carcinoma, islet cell carcinoma, papillary cell carcinoma of the pancreas, and hepatocellular carcinoma.[143]

The ultrasound patterns in hepatic lymphoma have been studied, with the most common pattern identified as hypoechoic[181,182] (Fig. 1-96). Hypoechic and diffuse

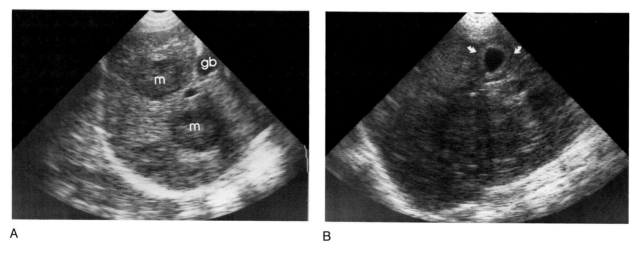

A   B

Fig. 1-94. Lucent hepatic metastases with necrosis. Malignant melanoma. **(A)** Longitudinal scan. Multiple echodense masses *(m)* are seen. (*gb,* gallbladder.) After therapy, one lesion (*m,* arrows) has developed a necrotic (lucent) center as seen on **(B)** longitudinal scan.

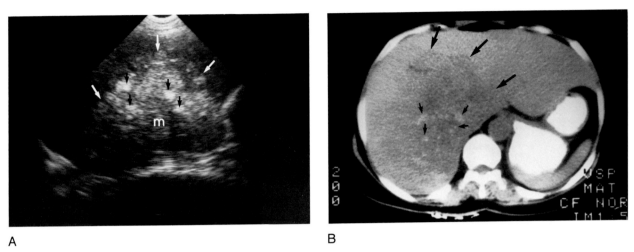

A   B

Fig. 1-95. Calcification within hepatic metastases. Colon carcinoma metastatic to the liver. **(A)** Longitudinal real-time scan of the liver. The liver mass (*m*, white arrows) is more dense than the surrounding liver parenchyma. It contains focal echodense areas (black arrows) with acoustic shadowing representing calcification. **(B)** Unenhanced CT scan. Speckled calcification (small arrows) is seen within the posterior liver. The borders of the mass are barely seen (large arrows). The mass is less dense than the surrounding liver parenchyma.

patterns have been found in both Hodgkin's and non-Hodgkin's lymphoma while target and echogenic patterns have been found only in non-Hodgkin's lymphoma[181,182] (Fig. 1-97). Similarly, intrahepatic lucent areas with Burkitt's lymphoma have been described[183] (Fig. 1-98). There is no correlation between the type of Hodgkin's lymphoma and the ultrasound appearance.[181] In Hodgkin's disease, the liver is the second most commonly involved extranodal site.[181] In an autopsy series, the liver was found to be invaded in 51 percent of non-Hodgkin's and 50 to 80 percent of Hodgkin's lymphoma.[182]

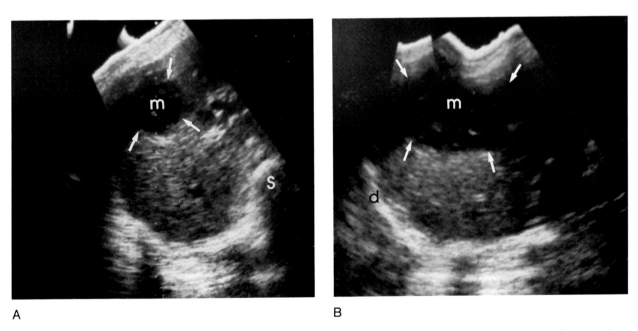

A   B

Fig. 1-96. Nodular poorly differentiated lymphoma. Hypoechoic pattern. **(A)** Transverse real-time scan with a poorly defined hypoechoic area (*m*, arrows) within the anterior aspect of the liver. (*S*, spine.) **(B)** Longitudinal real-time scan. The poorly defined hypoechoic mass (*m*, arrows) is more difficult to see. (*d*, diaphragm.)

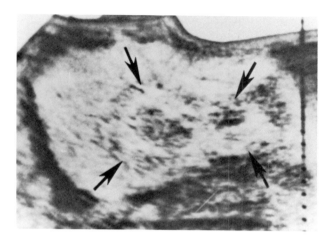

Fig. 1-97. Non-Hodgkin's lymphoma. Target pattern. Longitudinal scan through the right hepatic lobe. Multiple areas of increased echogenicity surrounded by hypoechoic rings (arrows) are seen. (From Ginaldi S, Bernardino ME, Jing BS, Green B: Ultrasonographic patterns of hepatic lymphoma. Radiology 136:427, 1980.)

In leukemia, there may be multiple discrete hepatic masses. These lesions have been observed to be solid anechoic masses with no acoustic enhancement[184] (Fig. 1-99). Many may exhibit a "bull's-eye" appearance with a dense center resulting from necrosis. Liver involvement with leukemia is uncommon. Acute myelogeneous or lymphocytic leukemia may have microscopic involvement and, as such, the ultrasound appearance may be normal.[184]

In children, the most common metastatic disease is produced by neuroblastoma, Wilms' tumor, and leukemia.[132,149,185] Neuroblastoma, which is a malignant neoplasm of the sympathetic nerve cell origin, produces a

densely reflective pattern with liver involvement similar to hepatoma, hepatoblastoma, and Wilms'[132] (Fig. 1-100). The liver is commonly involved, as compared to Wilms', in which the lungs are the most frequent site of involvement.[132] Wilms' tumor produces a densely reflective pattern often with lucencies resulting from necrosis or hypoechoic lesions[132,185] (Fig. 1-101). Metastatic adenocarcinoma is unusual in a child.

Ultrasound is an accurate method for monitoring a patient's disease and determining whether there is improvement or progression. It is an excellent way to determine the exact lobar location and resectability of a lesion prior to surgery, utilizing hepatic and portal veins for localizing purpose; this is particularly true in aggressive management of the oncologic patient in which segmentectomy or lobectomy of the liver is considered.[20]

Biopsy/Aspiration

Ultrasound is excellent for biopsy localization of lesions larger than 3 cm; CT should be used for lesions smaller than 3 cm.[2] A series of 23 tumors biopsied has been reported in which there were no false-positive findings and only one complication—a pneumothorax was found.[186] The risk of serious complication increases with caliber of canula.[186] The yield of a single pass was 75 percent with greater than 90-percent accuracy in diagnosing malignancy or benignancy.[186] Some report an 83-percent yield in obtaining enough cytologic material to correctly make a diagnosis without significant complication.[187] Others report an accuracy in cytohistologic evaluation of 91.6 percent with a sensitivity of 92.2 percent, a specificity of 88.9 percent, and a high predictive value of positive results.[188] Still others report a rate of

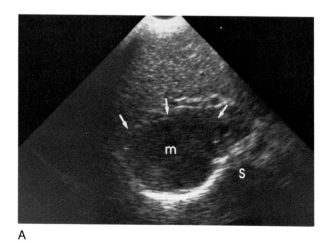

A

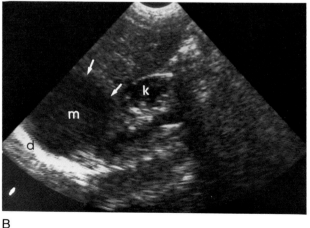

B

Fig. 1-98. Burkitt's lymphoma. Hypoechoic pattern. Transverse **(A)** and longitudinal **(B)** scans demonstrate a well-defined hypoechoic mass *(m)* in the posterior right lobe. (*S,* spine; *d,* diaphragm, *k,* right kidney.)

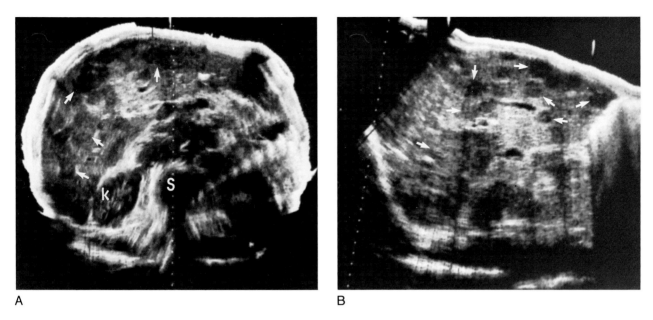

A   B

Fig. 1-99. Hairy-cell leukemia (B-cell lymphoma). Hypoechoic pattern. **(A)** Transverse static scan at 8 cm above the umbilicus with multiple poorly defined hypoechoic areas (arrows) within the liver. (*k,* right kidney; *S,* spine.) **(B)** Longitudinal scan at 2 cm to right of midline. Multiple hypoechoic areas (arrows) are seen within the liver.

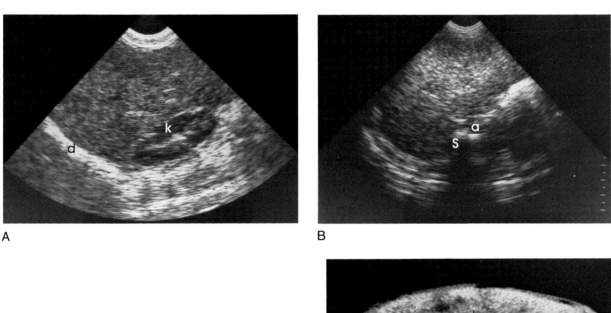

A   B

Fig. 1-100. Metastatic neuroblastoma. Fairly normal appearing parenchymal pattern on longitudinal **(A)** and transverse **(B)** real-time scans. The pattern is somewhat inhomogeneous. (*S,* spine; *a,* aorta; *k,* kidney; *d,* diaphragm.) **(C)** CT scan demonstrating multiple focal low-density areas (arrows) within the liver. The patient had diffuse metastatic disease involving the liver from neuroblastoma.

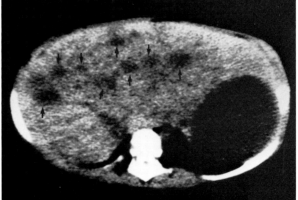

C

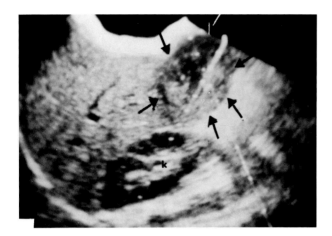

Fig. 1-101. Metastatic Wilms' tumor. Longitudinal scan. A large (5 × 6 cm) hypoechoic mass (arrows) is seen in the inferior aspect of the liver (k, kidney). (From Filiatrault D, Garel L, Tournade MF, Zucker JM: Echographic aspects of hepatic metastases of nephroblastomas. Pediatr Radiol 12:72, 1982.)

positive diagnosis in guided liver biopsy of 96.5 percent with a 9.5-percent false-negative for malignant lesion.[189] When comparing liver biopsy with 18-and 22-gauge needles, the overall accuracy of the 18 gauge was 98 percent while the accuracy of the 22 gauge was 84 percent.[190] In that particular series, there were no complications with either needle. The major advantage of the 18-gauge needle was a more consistent retrieval of adequate cellular material.

Percutaneous aspiration with ultrasound is a safe, useful, highly accurate method. Compared to CT, real-time ultrasound has a higher level of practicality and requires no ionizing radiation and is widely applicable. Guided fine-needle aspiration is the procedure of choice in cases of malignant metastases because of its simplicity and safety and because it can be performed on an outpatient basis.[189]

Besides assisting in the biopsy of tumors, ultrasound can guide successful aspiration and localization for catheter drainage of abscesses.[110,119] Real-time ultrasound allows dynamic visualization of the procedure.[120] Some surgeons use the catheter location in an abscess to define the surgical approach.[119]

TRAUMA

The etiology of a liver hematoma may be due to trauma or rupture of a neoplasm such as an adenoma, metastatic choriocarcinoma, or cavernous hemangioma.[191] In children, blunt abdominal trauma accounts for 94 percent of all abdominal injuries.[183] There are three categories of liver trauma: (1) rupture of the liver

and its capsule, (2) separation of the capsule and the subcapsular hematoma, and (3) central rupture of the liver.[192] In the past, aggressive treatment was advocated. The newer imaging modalities have allowed a more conservative approach. If the patient's clinical status is stable, the liver may be evaluated with CT initially and followed serially with ultrasound.[192]

Generally, a hepatic hematoma has been described as hypoechoic with poorly defined margins[191,193] (Fig. 1-102). With an acute bleed, the pattern tends to be echogenic due to fibrin and erythrocytes in layered linkage, so in initial blunt trauma, the hematoma appears echodense.[193] If subcapsular, the fluid borders the liver; if it ruptures, it is difficult to identify (Figs. 1-103 and 1-104). The progression of the hematoma varies in relation to the site of injury.[192] When following these hematomas on a serial basis, there may be a significant increase in the cystic component before there is reduction in size and complete resolution.[192]

OTHER

Besides tumors, there are other causes of focal lesions in the liver. Echodensities with strong posterior reverberation echoes can be seen with metallic foreign bodies in the liver[194] (Fig. 1-105). Calcified granulomas seen with tuberculosis, syphilis, parasitic diseases, and bacterial diseases can produce echodensities within the liver[195] (Fig. 1-106). With biliary tract air, linear echodensities may be seen in the anterior liver[17,113,195] (Fig. 1-107). This air may produce a reverberation artifact. The air in the biliary system may be secondary to passage of a stone through the duct, a spontaneous or surgically created choledochoenteric fistula, or biliary tract infection.[195] Portal venous gas is also seen as linear echodensities within the hepatic parenchyma (Fig. 1-46). A transient flow pattern is seen within the portal vein with real-time ultrasound but this disappears with time[113] (Figs. 1-46 and 1-47). Portal venous air is seen in a more peripheral location than is biliary air[113] (Fig. 1-46).

CORRELATIVE IMAGING

Although there are those who advocate the use of the sulfur colloid radionuclide scan as the initial diagnostic procedure in the patient suspected of hepatic neoplasm, others feel ultrasound should supercede nuclear medicine.[2] Some feel that ultrasound is the most sensitive and specific of the available noninvasive techniques.[196] The sensitivity and accuracy of ultrasound when compared to CT and nuclear medicine vary, as there have been

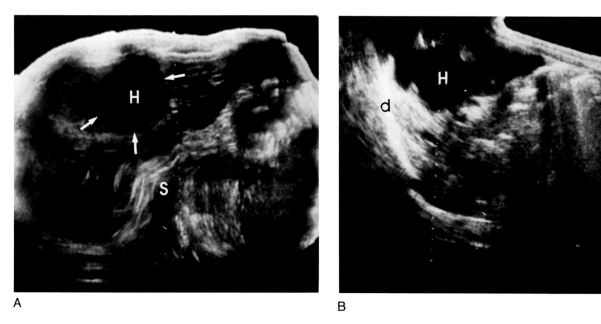

A   B

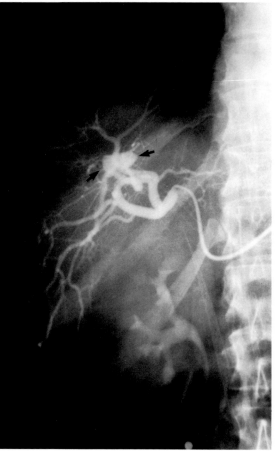

Fig. 1-102. Intrahepatic hematoma. **(A)** Transverse static scan at 18 cm above the iliac crest. An anechoic area (*H,* arrows) is seen within the anterior aspect of the liver. (*S,* spine.) **(B)** Longitudinal static scan at 5 cm to the right of midline. The anechoic area *(H)* is seen with some acoustic enhancement. (*d,* diaphragm.) **(C)** Angiogram demonstrating a false aneurysm (arrows) of the distal hepatic artery. This had bled into the liver.

C

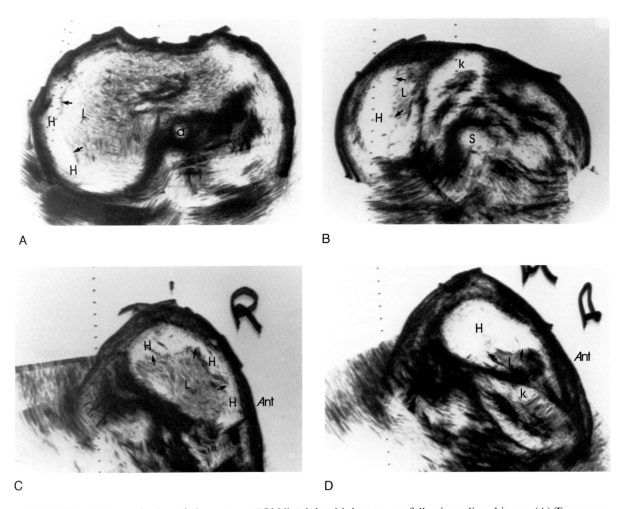

Fig. 1-103. Subcapsular hepatic hematoma. "Old." Adult with hematoma following a liver biopsy. **(A)** Transverse scan at 16 cm above the umbilicus. Fluid (*H*, arrows) is seen as a lucency bordering the liver (*L*; *a*, aorta). **(B)** Transverse scan at 4 cm above the umbilicus. Fluid (*H*, arrows) is visualized as a lucency around the liver tip *(L)*. Note the right kidney *(k)* is displaced anteriorly. (*S*, spine.) To verify that the fluid was subcapsular, left lateral decubitus scans **(C,D)** were performed. The fluid (*H*, arrows) continues to border the liver *(L)* and, as such, is not mobile. (*Ant,* anterior; *k* kidney.)

changes in CT and ultrasound.[2] Past claims no longer are valid. Ultrasound is believed to be as effective as nuclear medicine but less effective than CT.[2] Nuclear medicine reveals only the liver, while ultrasound and CT reveal other structures. Ultrasound diagnostic accuracy depends almost entirely on the quality of the image, which is a direct result of a close interplay between physician, technologist, and machine.[3]

There have been many studies comparing the imaging modalities of CT, ultrasound, and nuclear medicine in the evaluation of the liver. In general, the better resolution of ultrasound detected smaller and deeper focal lesions than did nuclear medicine, but nuclear medicine was more informative concerning hepatocellular disease.[197] Many believe nuclear medicine to be the best

initial screening exam providing anatomic and physiologic information.[197,198]

Others believe CT should be the first choice for examination of the patient with suspected liver disease.[199] This opinion was based on (1) the greater sensitivity and specificity of contrast-enhanced CT for focal lesions, as compared to ultrasound and nuclear medicine; (2) the ability of CT to detect diffuse liver abnormalities; (3) the greater ease in standardization and interpretation of CT exams; (4) the ability of CT to predict accurately the histology of many focal and diffuse diseases; and (5) the superiority of CT accuracy in detection and characterization of extrahepatic abnormalities.[199] They felt that ultrasound should be done (1) when CT scanning was not available, (2) when intravenous contrast could not be given, (3)

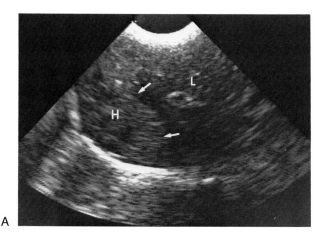

A

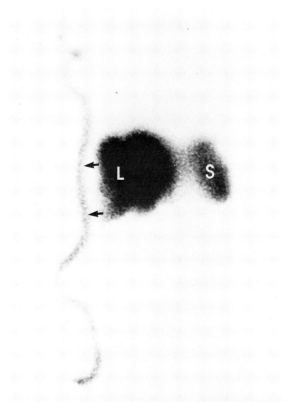

B

Fig. 1-104. Subcapsular hepatic hematoma. "Fresh." Neonate with a traumatic delivery and decreased hematocrit. **(A)** Transverse view of the liver demonstrating the subtle difference between the liver *(L)* parenchyma and the "fresh" subcapsular hematoma (*H*, arrows). **(B)** Anterior view of a sulfur colloid liver-spleen scan verifying the separation between the liver *(L)* and the skin (arrows; *S*, spleen).

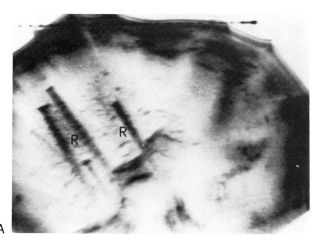

A

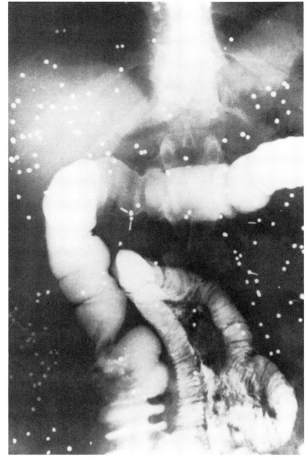

B

Fig. 1-105. Metallic foreign body. **(A)** Transverse scan of the upper portion of the abdomen demonstrates numerous intrahepatic echodensities with posterior reverberations *(R)*. **(B)** Selected film from a barium enema examination shows several lead shot pellets. (From Wendell BA, Athey PA: Ultrasonic appearance of metallic foreign bodies in parenchymal organs. J Clin Ultrasound 9:133, 1981.)

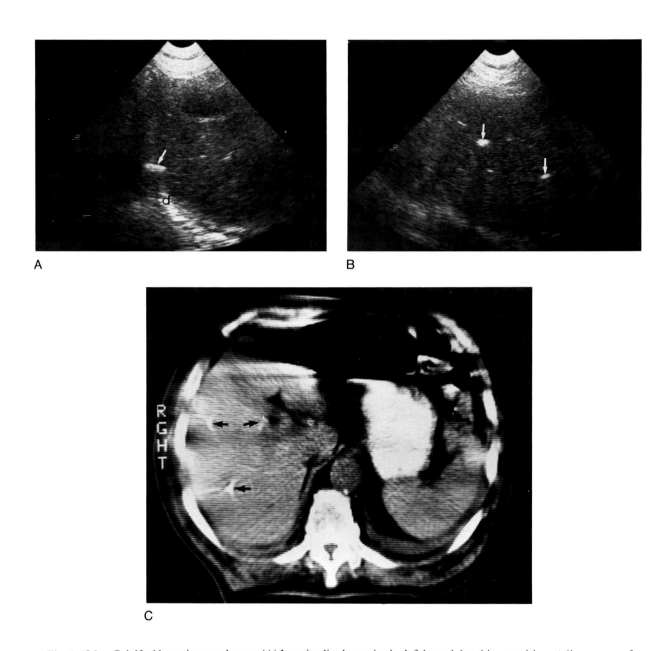

Fig. 1-106. Calcified hepatic granulomas. **(A)** Longitudinal scan in the left lateral decubitus position. A linear area of calcification (arrow) is noted in the area of the right hemidiaphragm *(d)*. **(B)** Longitudinal scan to the right of midline with multiple echogenic foci (arrows) in the liver. **(C)** CT image demonstrating the hepatic calcifications (arrows).

when there were other problems with technique, (4) for patients requiring ultrasound for other reasons, and (5) when the delay in scheduling CT was too long. Nuclear medicine should play a very limited role in early evaluation of liver disease; it should be reserved for occasional classifications of previous diffuse disease or for patients who are difficult to study on either CT or ultrasound.

Ultrasound plays a complementary role by further differentiating and characterizing an abnormality on nuclear medicine.[147,197,200] With an equivocal nuclear medicine scan, ultrasound is helpful in differentiating

normal variant from disease state.[147,201] Ultrasound has a reported accuracy of 94 percent in differentiating normal from abnormal on an "indeterminate" nuclear medicine scan.[20]

When evaluating a liver mass, many favor nuclear medicine as the method of choice for the initial evaluation.[202] Others feel ultrasound should replace nuclear medicine liver scanning as the initial diagnostic procedure in patients with liver neoplasm because of the versatility of ultrasound.[2] When the nuclear medicine scan is abnormal, CT or ultrasound can be used for anatomic definition. The accuracies of the various modalities have been reported as follows: CT 85 to 98 percent, ultrasound 75 to 93 percent, and nuclear medicine 73 to 94 percent.[20,199,201,203–207] The false-positive rates for these techniques have been reported as 12 percent, 17 percent, and 26 percent, respectively.[205] In contrast, others report nuclear medicine as having the lowest false-positive rate.[207]

When evaluating diffuse hepatocellular disease, nuclear medicine is usually the preferred modality.[198,204] Ultrasound scans may be normal and by the time they are abnormal, late disease is usually present. In addition, it is difficult to assess increases and decreases in echogenicity — this is technically dependent.[2] As far as fatty infiltration is concerned, ultrasound detected 85 percent with a 100-percent sensitivity and a 56-percent

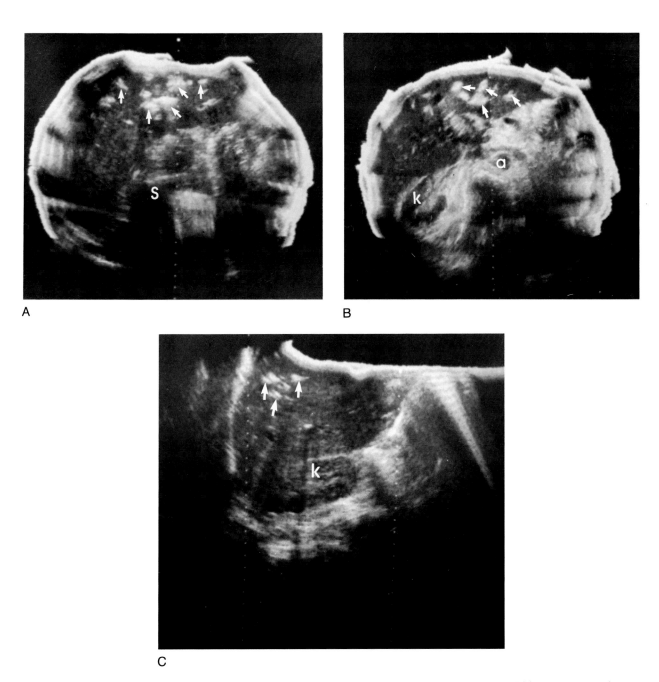

A

B

C

Fig. 1-107. Biliary tract air. **(A,B)** Transverse scans at 12 cm **(A)** and 8 cm **(B)** above the umbilicus demonstrating biliary tract air as linear echodensities (arrows) in the anterior aspect of the liver. (*k*, kidney; *S*, spine; *a*, aorta.) **(C,D)** Longitudinal scans at 8 cm **(C)** to the right of midline. *(Figure continues.)*

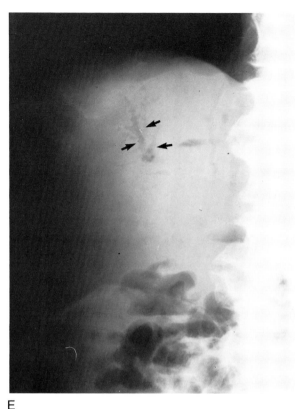

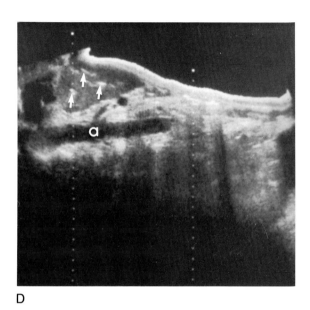

D   E

Fig. 1-107 *(Continued).*   **(D)** and midline with air (arrows, linear echodensities) in the anterior aspect of the liver (*a,* aorta). **(E)** Plain radiograph of right upper quadrant with air in the biliary tract (arrows). This patient developed a hepaticocholedochoduodenal fistula due to a gallstone perforation.

specificity.[32] With regard to diffuse disease, including cirrhosis, chronic hepatitis, diffuse type of hepatoma, lymphoma, and diffuse microscopic metastatic disease, ultrasound has been reported to detect abnormalities with a sensitivity of 80 percent.[20] All can produce similar ultrasound appearances, so a biopsy is needed for a definitive diagnosis.[20]

In the evaluation of cystic lesions, ultrasound is generally better because the wall thickness, mural nodule septation, and fluid-fluid levels can be identified.[177] It has been reported to have an accuracy of 100 percent in cyst identification.[93] There is a potential danger in overreliance on CT attenuation values, and complementary roles of ultrasound and CT should be stressed.[177] Again, ultrasound is superior to CT in determining the morphology of the cystic lesion and differentiating uncomplicated cysts from cystic neoplasms.[177]

The traumatized patient poses still another dilemma. Some physicians prefer nuclear medicine for screening[72], others recommend CT or ultrasound so that multiple organs can be examined. The decision of using CT or ultrasound might depend on the tenderness and mobility of the patient, the time of the trauma, and the availability of the CT scanner.

In the case of abscesses, there are also mixed preferences. One series reported 50 percent of abscesses missed with sulfur colloid nuclear medicine scans.[208] Nuclear medicine has an 85-percent sensitivity for focal intrahepatic lesions smaller than 2 cm.[208] The accuracy of gallium in detecting abscess is greater than 90 percent.[208] Again, the modality of choice depends on many factors including patient's portability and patient's condition. Generally, CT or ultrasound is preferred, especially in the immunosuppressed patient.[208]

When very specific lesions are questioned, one modality may be more accurate than another. With focal nodular hyperplasia, the sensitivity rate of ultrasound is 100 percent; of CT, is 78 percent; of angiography, is 82 percent; and of nuclear medicine is 55 percent.[152] A normal sulfur colloid scan makes the diagnosis when combined with the ultrasound scan. In hepatocellular carcinoma, one series reported CT to be 79-percent accurate.[209] Another described the following sensitivities for detecting lesions smaller than 5 cm: nuclear medicine — 39 percent, ultrasound — 50 percent, CT — 56 percent, and angiography — 94 percent.[161] When detecting small hepatocellular carcinomas (under 3 cm), one investigator found ultrasound to be most accurate, with a 93.9-percent detection rate; CT demonstrated an 84.3-percent rate, angiography, a 75.7-percent rate, and nuclear medicine, a 12.1-percent rate.[168] When evaluating the detection of liver metastases from colon and breast carcinoma, CT was found to have the highest true-positive ratio, with a sensitivity of 93 percent and a specificity of 88 percent.[210] Ultrasound had a sensitivity of 86 percent with a specificity of 83 percent, while nuclear medicine had a sensitivity of 82 percent with a specificity of 85 percent.[210]

Increased technologic developments including the development of larger digital memories and the development of tissue signaturing (or characterization by measuring B-scan echo amplitude by the degree of acoustic attenuation or spectral analysis) may present several interesting new possibilities.[20,211] Once tissue characterization is developed in a clinical setting, the diagnostic potential of ultrasound may be further increased.[20]

REFERENCES

1. Eftekhari F, Barnes PA, Thomas JL, Bernardino ME: Real-time scanning as an adjunct to conventional hepatic sonography. Texas Medicine 78:61, 1982
2. Bernardino ME, Thomas JL, Maklad N: Hepatic sonography: Technical considerations, present applications, and possible future. Radiology 142:249, 1982
3. Pertcheck L, Mack L, Johnson ML: Ultrasound evaluation of the liver. Applied Radiology 7:139, 1978
4. Kane RA, Lavery M: Techniques of liver examination. p. 198. In Raymond HW, Zwiebel WJ (eds): Seminars in Ultrasound. Grune and Stratton, Vol II, New York, 1981
5. Bernardino ME, Thomas JL, Mayes GB: An initial experience with post-data processing in hepatic sonography. AJR 136:521, 1981
6. Mattrey RF, Leopold GR, VanSonnenberg E, et al: Perfluorochemicals as liver and spleen-seeking ultrasound contrast agents. J Ultrasound Med 2:173, 1983
7. Mattrey RF, Scheible FW, Gosink BB, et al: Perfluoroctylbromide: a liver/spleen-specific and tumor-imaging ultrasound contrast material. Radiology 145:759, 1982
8. O'Brien MJ, Gottlieb LS: The Liver and Biliary Tract. p. 1009. In Robbins SL, Cotran RS (eds): Pathologic basis of disease. W.B. Saunders Co, Philadelphia, 1979
9. Kane RA: Sonographic Anatomy of the liver. p. 190. In Raymond HW, Zwiebel WJ (eds): Seminars in Ultrasound. Grune and Stratton, Vol II, New York, 1981
10. Taylor KJW, Carpenter DA, Hill CR, McCready VR: Gray scale ultrasound imaging. Radiology 119:415, 1976
11. Sexton CC, Zeman RK: Correlation of computed tomography, sonography and gross anatomy of liver. AJR 141:711, 1983
12. Mitchell SE, Gross BH, Spitz HB: The hypoechoic caudate lobe: An ultrasonic pseudolesion. Radiology 144:569, 1982
13. Brown BM, Filly RA, Callen PW: Ultrasonographic anatomy of the caudate lobe. J Ultrasound Med 1:189, 1982
14. Marks WM, Filly RA, Callen PW: Ultrasonic anatomy of the liver: A review with new applications. J Clin Ultrasound 7:137, 1979
15. Belton RL, VanZandt TF: Congenital absence of the left lobe of the liver: a radiologic diagnosis. Radiology 147:184, 1983
16. Hillman BJ, D'Orsi CJ, Smith EH, Bartrum RJ: Ultrasonic appearance of the falciform ligament. AJR 132:205, 1979
17. Prando A, Goldstein HM, Bernardino ME, Green B: Ultrasonic pseudolesions of the liver. Radiology 130:403, 1979
18. Parulekar SG: Ligaments and fissures of the liver: Sonographic anatomy. Radiology 130:409, 1977
19. Sones PJ, Torres WE: Normal ultrasonic appearance of the ligamentum teres and falciform ligament. J Clin Ultrasound 6:392, 1978
20. Lewis E: Screening for diffuse and focal liver disease: The case for hepatic sonography. J Clin Ultrasound 12:67, 1984
21. Chafetz N, Filly RA: Portal and hepatic veins: accuracy of margin echoes for distinguishing intrahepatic vessels. Radiology 130:725, 1979
22. Hill MC, Sanders RC: Sonography of the upper abdominal venous system. p. 289. In Sanders RC, Hill MC (eds): Ultrasound Annual 1983. Raven Press, New York, 1983
23. Weinreb J, Kumari S, Phillips G, Pochaczevsky R: Portal vein measurements by real-time sonography. AJR 139:497, 1982
24. Filly RA, Laing FC: Anatomic variation of portal venous anatomy in the porta hepatis: ultrasonographic evaluation. J Clin Ultrasound 6:83, 1978
25. Callen PW, Filly RA, DeMartini WJ: The left portal vein: A possible source of confusion on ultrasonograms. Radiology 130:205, 1979
26. Willi UV, Teele RL: Hepatic arteries and the parallel-channel sign. J Clin Ultrasound 7:125, 1979
27. Ralls PW, Quinn MF, Rogers W, Halls J: Sonographic anatomy of hepatic artery. AJR 136:1059, 1981
28. Berland LL, Lawson TL, Foley WD: Porta hepatis: sonographic discrimination of bile ducts from arteries with pulsed Doppler with new anatomic criteria. AJR 138:833, 1982
29. Makunchi M, Hasegawa H, Yamazaki S, et al: The inferior right hepatic vein: ultrasonic demonstration. Radiology 148:213, 1983
30. Gosink BB, Leymaster CE: Ultrasonic determination of hepatomegaly. J Clin Ultrasound 9:37, 1981
31. Niederau C, Sonnenberg A, Muller JE, et al: Sonographic measurements of the normal liver, spleen, pancreas and portal vein. Radiology 149:537, 1983
32. Scatarige JC, Scott WW, Donovan PJ, et al: Fatty infiltration of the liver: ultrasonographic and computed tomographic correlation. J Ultrasound Med 3:9, 1984
33. Henschke CI, Goldman H, Teele RL: The hyperechogenic liver in children: cause and sonographic appearance. AJR 138:841, 1982

34. Foster KJ, Dewbury KC, Griffin AH, Wright R: The accuracy of ultrasound in the detection of fatty infiltration of the liver. Brit J Radiol 53:440, 1980

35. Behan M, Kazam E: The echographic characteristics of fatty tissues and tumors. Radiology 129:143, 1978

36. Scott WW, Sanders RC, Siegelman SS: Irregular fatty infiltration of the liver: diagnostic dilemmas. AJR 135:67, 1980

37. Wilson SR, Rosen IE, Chin-Sang HB, Arenson AM: Fatty infiltration of the liver—an imaging challenge. J Can Assoc Radiol 33:227, 1982

38. Scott WW, Donovan PJ, Sanders RC: The sonography of diffuse liver disease. p. 219. In Raymond HW, Zwiebel WJ (eds): Seminars in Ultrasound, Vol II, Grune and Stratton, New York, 1981

39. Kurtz AB, Rubin CS, Cooper HS, et al: Ultrasound findings in hepatitis. Radiology 136:717, 1980

40. Lloyd RL, Lyons EA, Levi CS, et al: The sonographic appearance of peliosis hepatis. J Ultrasound Med 1:293, 1982

41. Gates GF: The liver, gallbladder and biliary tree. p. 56. In Haller JO, Shkolnik A (eds): Clinics in Diagnostic Ultrasound: Ultrasound in Pediatrics. Churchill Livingstone, New York, 1981

42. Taylor KJW, Gorelick FS, Rosenfield AT, Riely CA: Ultrasonography of alcoholic liver disease with histological correlation. Radiology 141:157, 1981

43. Gosink BB, Lemon SK, Scheible W, Leopold GR: Accuracy of ultrasonography in diagnosis of hepatocellular disease. AJR 133:19, 1979

44. Harbin WP, Robert NJ, Ferrucci JT: Diagnosis of cirrhosis based on regional changes in hepatic morphology. Radiology 135:273, 1980

45. Grossman H, Ram PC, Coleman RA, et al: Hepatic ultrasonography in type I glycogen storage disease (von Gierke disease). Radiology 141:753, 1981

46. Brunelle F, Tammam S, Odievre M, Chaumont P: Liver adenomas in glycogen storage disease of children: ultrasound and argiographic study. Pediatr Radiol 14:94, 1984

47. Smevik B, Swensen T, Kolbenstvedt A, Trygstad O: Computed tomography and ultrasonography of the abdomen in congenital generalized lipodystrophy. Radiology 142:687, 1982

48. Itzchuk Y, Rubinstein Z, Shilo R: Ultrasound in tropical diseases. p. 69. In Sanders RC, Hill MC, (eds): Ultrasound Annual 1983. Raven Press, New York, 1983

49. Fataar S, Bassiony H, Satyanath S, et al: Characteristic sonographic features of Schistosomal periportal fibrosis. AJR 143:69, 1984

50. Kane RA, Katz SG: The spectrum of sonographic findings in portal hypertension: a subject review and new observations. Radiology 142:453, 1982

51. Funston MR, Goudie E, Richter IA, et al: Ultrasound diagnosis of the recanalized umbilical vein in portal hypertension. J Clin Ultrasound 8:244, 1980

52. Subramanyam BR, Balthazar EJ, Madamba MR, et al: Sonography of portosystemic venous collaterals in portal hypertension. Radiology 146:161, 1983

53. Juttner H-V, Jeeney JM, Ralls PW, et al: Ultrasound demonstration of portosystemic collaterals in cirrhosis and portal hypertension. Radiology 142:459, 1982

54. Bolondi L, Gandolfi L, Arienti V, et al: Ultrasonography in the diagnosis of portal hypertension: diminished response of portal vessels to respiration. Radiology 142:167, 1982

55. Abel-Latif Z, Abdel-Wahab F, El-Kady NM: Evaluation of portal hypertension in cases of hepatosplenic schistosomiasis using ultrasound. J Clin Ultrasound 9:409, 1981

56. Dach JL, Hill MC, Pelaez JC, et al: Sonography of hypertensive portal venous system: correlation with arterial portography. AJR 137:511, 1981

57. Dokmeci AK, Kimura K, Matsutani S, et al: Collateral veins in portal hypertension: demonstration by sonography. AJR 137:1173, 1981

58. Glazer GM, Laing FC, Brown TW, Gooding GAW: Sonographic demonstration of portal hypertension: the patent umbilical vein. Radiology 136:161, 1980

59. Saddekni S, Hutchinson DE, Cooperberg PL: The sonographically patent umbilical vein in portal hypertension. Radiology 145:441, 1982

60. Schabel SI, Rittenberg GM, Javid LH, et al: The "bull's-eye" falciform ligament: a sonographic finding of portal hypertension. Radiology 136:157, 1980

61. Foley WD, Gleysteen JJ, Lawson TL, et al: Dynamic computed tomography and pulsed Doppler ultrasonography in the evaluation of splenorenal shunt patency. J Comput Assist Tomogr 7:106, 1983

62. Subramanyam BR, Balthazar EJ, Hilton S, et al: Sonography in neoplastic and non-tumorous portal and hepatic venous thrombosis. Proceedings from 28th American Institute of Ultrasound in Medicine, J Ultrasound Med 2:31, 1983

63. Jackson VP, Martin-Simmerman P, Becker GJ, Holden RW: Real-time ultrasonographic demonstration of vascular invasion by hepatocellular carcinoma. J Ultrasound Med 2:277, 1983

64. Pauls CH: Ultrasound and computed tomographic demonstration of portal vein thrombosis in hepatocellular carcinoma. Gastrointest Radiol 6:281, 1981

65. Subramanyam BR, Balthazar EJ, Hilton S, et al: Hepatocellular carcinoma with venous invasion: sonographic-angiographic correlation. Radiology 150:793, 1984

66. Merritt CRB: Ultrasonographic demonstration of portal vein thrombosis. Radiology 133:425, 1979

67. Miller EI, Thomas RH: Portal vein invasion demonstrated by ultrasound. J Clin Ultrasound 7:57, 1979

68. Fakhry J, Gosink BB, Leopold GR: Recanalized umbilical vein due to portal vein occlusion: documented by sonography. AJR 137:410, 1981

69. Miller EI, Thomas RH: Portal vein invasion demonstrated by ultrasound. J Clin Ultrasound 7:57, 1979

70. Grand MP, Remy J: Ultrasound diagnosis of extrahepatic portal vein obstruction in childhood. Pediatr Radiol 8:155, 1979

71. Marx M, Scheible W: Cavernous transformation of the portal vein. J Ultrasound Med 1:167, 1982

72. Froelich JW, Simeone JF, McKusick KA, et al: Radionu-

clide imaging and ultrasound in liver/spleen trauma: a prospective comparison. Radiology 145:457, 1982

73. Kauzlaric D, Petrovic M, Barmeir E: Sonography of cavernous transformation portal vein. AJR 142:383, 1984

74. Friedman AP, Haller JO, Boyer B, Cooper R: Calcified portal vein thromboemboli in infants: radiography and ultrasonography. Radiology 140:381, 1981

75. Vine HS, Sequeira JC, Widrich WC, Sacks BA: Portal vein aneurysm. AJR 132:557, 1979

76. Merritt CRB, Sharp MJ, Goldsmith JP: Ultrasound findings in infants with necrotizing enterocolitis. Proceedings from the 28th American Institute of Ultrasound in Medicine, J Ultrasound Med 2:136, 1983

77. Merritt CRB, Goldsmith JP, Sharp MJ: Sonographic detection of portal venous gas in infants with necrotizing enterocolitis. AJR 143:1059, 1984

78. Ramchandani P, Goldenberg NJ, Soulen RL, White RI: Isobutyl 2-cyanoacrylate embolization of a hepatoportal fistula. AJR 140:137, 1983

79. Tisnado J, Cho S-R, Carithers RL, et al: The Budd-Chiari syndrome: Angiographic-pathologic correlation. Radiographics 3:155, 1983

80. Baert AL, Fevery J, Marchal G, et al: Early diagnosis of Budd-Chiari syndrome by computed tomography and ultrasonography: Report of five cases. Gastroenterology 84:587, 1983

81. Redel D, Fehske W, Kirchhoff PG: Budd-Chiari syndrome in child with post-traumatic obstruction of inferior vena cava. Radiology 139:151, 1981

82. Yang PJ, Glazer GM, Bowerman RA: Budd-Chiari syndrome: Computed tomographic and ultrasonographic findings. J Comput Assist Tomogr 7:148, 1983

83. Cooper RA, Picker RH, Fulton AJ, Lonzer MR: The ultrasonic appearance of the liver in hepatic venous outflow obstruction (Budd-Chiari syndrome). J Clin Ultrasound 10:35, 1982

84. Harter LP, Gross BH, St. Hilaire J, et al: CT and sonographic appearance of hepatic vein obstruction. AJR 139:176, 1982

85. Makuuchi M, Hasegawa S, Yamazaki S, et al: Primary Budd-Chiari syndrome: Ultrasonic demonstration. Radiology 152:775, 1984

86. Cloogman HM, DiCapo RD: Hereditary hemorrhagic telangiectasia: Sonographic findings in the liver. Radiology 150:521, 1984

87. Graif M, Manor A, Itzchak Y: Sonographic differentiation of extra- and intrahepatic masses. AJR 141:553, 1983

88. Sandler MA, Marks DS, Hricak H, et al: Benign focal diseases of the liver. p. 202. In Raymond HW, Zwiebel WJ (eds): Seminars in Ultrasound. Vol II, No. 3. Grune and Stratton, New York 1981

89. Taylor KJW, Viscomi GN: Ultrasound diagnosis of cystic disease of the liver. J Clin Gastroenterol 2:197, 1980

90. Weaver RM, Goldstein HM, Green B, Perkins C: Gray scale ultrasonographic evaluation of hepatic cystic disease. AJR 130:849, 1978

91. Kuni CC, Johnson ML, Holmes JH: Polycystic liver disease. J Clin Ultrasound 6:332, 1978

92. Roemer CE, Ferrucci JT, Mueller PR, et al: Hepatic cysts: Diagnosis and therapy by sonographic needle aspiration. AJR 136:1065, 1981

93. Spiegel RM, King DL, Green WM: Ultrasonography of primary cysts of liver. AJR 131:235, 1978

94. Saini S, Mueller PR, Ferrucci JT Jr., et al: Percutaneous aspiration of hepatic cysts does not provide definitive therapy. AJR 141:559, 1983

95. Enterline DS, Rauch PE, Silverman PM, et al: Cyst of the falciform ligament of the liver. AJR 142:327, 1984

96. Fulton AJ, Picker RH, Cooper RA: Ultrasonic appearance of hydatid cysts of the liver. Australas Radiol 26:64, 1982

97. Andrew WK, Thomas RG: Hydatid cyst of the pancreatic tail: Ultrasonic features including application of the Escudero-Nemenow sign. SA Med J 59:235, 1981

98. Hadidi A: Sonography of hepatic echinococcal cysts. Gastrointest Radiol 7:349, 1982

99. Niron EA, Ozer H: Ultrasound appearances of liver hydatid disease. Br J Radiol 54:335, 1981

100. Babcock DS, Kaufman L, Cosnow I: Ultrasound diagnosis of hydatid disease (echinococcosis) in two cases. AJR 131:895, 1978

101. Calder JF, Okelo GBA, Chemtai A, Stass B: Ultrasonic diagnosis of abdominal hydatid disease in Kenya. Diagnostic Imaging 50:107, 1981

102. Itzchak Y, Rubinstein Z, Heyman Z, Gerzof S: Role of ultrasound in the diagnosis of abdominal hydatid disease. J Clin Ultrasound 8:341, 1980

103. Hadidi A: Ultrasound findings in liver hydatid cysts. J Clin Ultrasound 7:365, 1979

104. Gharbi HA, Hassine W, Brauner MW, Dupuch K: Ultrasound examination of hydatic liver. Radiology 139:459, 1981

105. Barriga P, Cruz F, Lepe V, Lathrop R: An ultrasonographically solid tumor-like appearance of echinococcal cysts in the liver. J Ultrasound Med 2:123, 1983

106. Ralls PW, Quinn MF, Bowswell WD Jr., Colletti PM, et al: Patterns of resolution in successfully treated hepatic amebic abscess: sonographic evaluation. Radiology 149:541, 1983

107. Papanicolaou N, Mueller PR, Simeone JF, Malt RA: The sonographic appearance of omentoplasty in the surgical treatment of large cystic lesions of the liver. J Ultrasound Med 3:181, 1984

108. Kuligowska E, Noble J: Sonography of hepatic abscesses. p. 102. In Raymond HW, Zwiebel WJ, (eds): Seminars in Ultrasound Vol IV, No. 2. Grune and Stratton, New York, 1983

109. Weed TE, Merritt CRB, Bowen JC: Surgical management of multiple hepatic abscesses using ultrasonography for sequential evaluation. So Med J 75:1270, 1982

110. Kuligowska E, Conners SK, Shapiro JH: Liver abscess: Sonography in diagnosis and treatment. AJR 138:253, 1982

111. Dewbury KC, Joseph AEA, Sadler M, Birch SJ: Ultrasound in the diagnosis of the early liver abscess. Brit J Radiol 53:1160, 1980

112. Newlin N, Silver TM, Stuck KJ, Sandler MA: Ultrasonic

features of pyogenic liver abscesses. Radiology 139:155, 1981

113. Gosink BB: Intrahepatic Gas: Differential Diagnosis. AJR 137:763, 1981

114. Powers TA, Jones TB, Karl JH: Echogenic hepatic abscess without radiographic evidence of gas. AJR 137:159, 1981

115. Jones M, Kovac A, Geshner J: Acoustic shadowing by gas-producing abscesses. So Med J 74:247, 1981

116. Burt TB, Knochel JQ, Lee TG: Gas as a contrast agent and diagnostic aid in abdominal sonography. J Ultrasound Med 1:179, 1982

117. Conrad MR, Bregman R, Kilman WJ: Ultrasonic recognition of parenchymal gas. AJR 132:395, 1979

118. Sones PJ, Thomas BM, Masand PP: Falciform ligament abscess: appearance on computed tomography and sonography. AJR 137:161, 1981

119. Yaremchuk MJ, Kane R, Cady B: Ultrasound-guided catheter localization of intrahepatic abscesses—an aid in open surgical drainage. Surgery 91:482, 1982

120. Kimura M, Tsuchiya Y, Ohto M, et al: Ultrasonically guided percutaneous drainage of solitary liver abscess: Successful treatment in four cases. J Clin Gastroenterol 3:61, 1981

121. Ralls PW, Colletti PM, Quinn MF, Halls J: Sonographic findings in hepatic amebic abscess. Radiology 145:123, 1982

122. Boultbee JE, Simjee AE, Rooknoodeen F, Engelbrecht HE: Experiences with grey scale ultrasonography in hepatic amoebiasis. Clin Radiol 30:683, 1979

123. Dalrymple RB, Fataar S, Goodman A, et al: Hyperechoic amoebic liver abscesses: an unusual ultrasonic appearance. Clin Radiol 33:541, 1982

124. Ralls PW, Mikity VG, Colletti P, et al: Sonography in the diagnosis and management of hepatic abscesses in children. Pediatr Radiol 12:239, 1982

125. Sukov RJ, Cohen LJ, Sample WF: Sonography of hepatic amebic abscesses. AJR 134:911, 1980

126. Abul-Khair MH, Kenawi MM, Korasky EE, Arafa NM: Ultrasonography and amoebic liver abscesses. Ann Surg 193:221, 1981

127. Gooding GAW: Amebic abscess: Sonographic follow-up of persistent hepatic defects in two patients one year after successful treatment for amebiasis of the liver. J Clin Ultrasound 9:451, 1981

128. Ho B, Cooperberg PL, Li DKB, et al: Ultrasonography and computed tomography of hepatic candidiasis in immunosuppressed patients. J Ultrasound Med 1:157, 1982

129. Miller JH, Greenfield LD, Wald BR: Candidiasis of the liver and spleen in childhood. Radiology 142:375, 1982

130. Callen PW, Filly RA, Marcus FS: Ultrasonography and computed tomography in the evaluation of hepatic microabscesses in the immunosuppressed patient. Radiology 136:433, 1980

131. Garel LA, Pariente DM, Nezelop C, et al: Liver involvement in chronic granulomatous disease: the role of ultrasound in diagnosis and treatment. Radiology 153:117, 1984

132. Gates GF: Liver and Spleen. p. 16. In Atlas of Abdominal Ultrasonography in Children. Churchill Livingstone, New York, 1978

133. Rosenbaum DM, Mindell HJ: Ultrasonographic findings in mesenchymal hamartoma of the liver. Radiology 138:425, 1981

134. Donovan AT, Wolverson MK, deMello D, et al: Multicystic hepatic mesenchynal hamartoma of childhood. Pediatr Radiol 11:163, 1981

135. Abramson SJ, Lack EE, Teele RL: Benign vascular tumors of the liver in infants: Sonographic appearance. AJR 138:629, 1982

136. Onodera H, Ohta K, Oikawa M, et al: Correlation of the real-time ultrasonographic appearance of hepatic hemangiomas with angiography. J Clin Ultrasound 11:421, 1983

137. McArdle CR: Ultrasonic appearances of a hepatic hemangioma. J Clin Ultrasound 6:124, 1978

138. Mirk P, Rubaltelli L, Bazzocchi M, et al: Ultrasonographic patterns in hepatic hemangiomas. J Clin Ultrasound 10:373, 1982

139. Marchal G, Baert AL, Fevery J, et al: Ultrasonography of liver haemangioma. Fortschr Rontgenstr 138:201, 1983

140. Wiener SN, Parulekar SG: Scintigraphy and ultrasonography of hepatic hemangioma. Radiology 132:149, 1979

141. Freeny PC, Vimont TR, Barnett DC: Cavernous hemangioma of the liver: ultrasonography, arteriography, and computed tomography. Radiology 132:143, 1979

142. Bree RL, Schuab RE, Neiman HL: Solitary echogenic spot in the liver: is it diagnostic of a hemangioma? AJR 140:41, 1983

143. Taboury J, Porcel A, Tubiana J-M, Monnier J-P: Cavernous hemangiomas of the liver studied by ultrasound: enhancement posterior to a hyperechoic mass as a sign of hypervascularity. Radiology 149:781, 1983

144. Bruneton JN, Drouillard J, Fenart D, et al: Ultrasonography of hepatic cavernous haemangiomas. Brit J Radiol 56:791, 1983

145. Itai Y, Ohtomo K, Araki T, et al: Computed tomography and sonography of cavernous hemangiomas of the liver. AJR 141:315, 1983

146. Dachman AH, Lichtenstein JE, Friedman AC, Hartman DS: Infantile hemangioendothelioma of the liver: a radiologic-pathologic-clinical correlation. AJR 140:1091, 1983

147. Taylor KJW, Sullivan D, Rosenfield AT, Gottschalk A: Gray scale ultrasound and isotope scanning: complementary techniques for imaging the liver. AJR 128:277, 1977

148. Pardes JG, Bryan PJ, Gauderer MWL: Spontaneous regression of infantile hemangioendotheliomatosis of the liver: demonstration by ultrasound. J Ultrasound Med 1:349, 1982

149. Kassner EG, Friedman AP: Liver masses. p. 80. In Haller JO, Shkolnik A (eds): Clinics in Diagnostic Ultrasound: ultrasound in Pediatrics, Churchill Livingstone, New York, 1981

150. Kaude JV, Felman AH, Hawkins IF: Ultrasonography in

primary hepatic tumors in early childhood. Pediatr Radiol 9:77, 1980

151. Atkinson GO, Kodroff M, Sones PJ, Gay BB: Focal nodular hyperplasia of the liver in children: a report of three new cases. Radiology 137:171, 1980

152. Rogers JV, Mack LA, Freeny PC, et al: Hepatic focal nodular hyperplasia: angiography, CT, sonography, and scintigraphy. AJR 137:983, 1981

153. Scatarige JC, Fishman EK, Sanders RC: The sonographic "scar sign" in focal nodular hyperplasia of the liver. J Ultrasound Med 1: 275, 1982

154. Whitley NO, Cunningham JJ: Angiographic and echographic findings in avascular focal nodular hyperplasia of the liver. AJR 130:777, 1978

155. Majaewski A, Gratz KF, Brolsch C, Gebel M: Sonographic pattern of focal nodular hyperplasia of the liver. Europ J Radiol 4:52, 1984

156. Sandler MA, Petrocelli RD, Marks DS, Lopez R: Ultrasonic features and radionuclide correlation in liver cell adenoma and focal nodular hyperplasia. Radiology 135:393, 1980

157. Cimmino CV, Scott DW: Case report: benign liver tumor with central necrosis. J Clin Ultrasound 6:119, 1978

158. Bowerman RA, Samuels BI, Silver TM: Ultrasonographic features of hepatic adenomas in type I glycogen storage disease. J Ultrasound Med 2:51, 1983

159. Kurdziel JC, Stines J, Parache RM, Chaulieu C: Adenolipoma of the liver: an unique case with ultrasound and CT patterns. Europ J Radiol 4:45, 1984

160. Miller JH: The ultrasonographic appearance of cystic hepatoblastoma. Radiology 138:141, 1981

161. Takashima T, Matsui O, Suzuki M, Ida M: Diagnosis and screening of small hepatocellular carcinomas. Radiology 145:635, 1982

162. Kamin PD, Bernardino ME, Green B: Ultrasound manifestations of hepatocellular carcinoma. Radiology 131:459, 1979

163. Boultbee JE: Grey scale ultrasound appearances in hepatocellular carcinoma. Clin Radiol 30:547, 1979

164. Dubbins PA, O'Riordan D, Melia WM: Ultrasound in hepatoma—can specific diagnosis be made? Br J Radiol 54:307, 1981

165. Broderick TW, Gosink B, Menuck L, et al: Echographic and radionuclide detection of hepatoma. Radiology 135:149, 1980

166. Cottone M, Marceno MP, Maringhini A, et al: Ultrasound in the diagnosis of hepatocellular carcinoma associated with cirrhosis. Radiology 147:517, 1983

167. Tanaka S, Kitamura T, Imaoka S, et al: Hepatocellular carcinoma: sonographic and histologic correlation. AJR 140:701, 1983

168. Sheu J-C, Sung J-L, Chen D-S, et al: Ultrasonography of small hepatic tumors using high resolution linear-array real-time instruments. Radiology 150:797, 1984

169. Mayes GB, Bernardino ME: The role of ultrasound in the evaluation of hepatic neoplasms. p. 212. In Raymond HW, Zwiebel WJ (eds): Seminars in Ultrasound. Vol. 2. Grune and Stratton, New York, 1981

170. Green B, Bree RL, Goldstein HM, Stanley C: Gray scale ultrasound evaluation of hepatic neoplasms: Patterns and correlations. Radiology 124:203, 1977

171. Viscomi GN, Gonzalez R, Taylor KJW: Histopathological correlation of ultrasound appearances of liver metastases. J Clin Gastroenterol 3:395, 1981

172. Scheible W, Gosink BB, Leopold GR: Gray scale echographic patterns of hepatic metastatic disease. Am J Roentgenol 129:983, 1977

173. Hillman BJ, Smith EH, Gammelgaard J, Holm HH: Ultrasonographic-pathologic correlation of malignant hepatic masses. Gastrointest Radiol 4:361, 1979

174. Bernardino ME, Green B: Ultrasonographic evaluation of chemotherapeutic response in hepatic metastases. Radiology 133:437, 1979

175. Wooten WB, Green B, Goldstein HM: Ultrasonography of necrotic hepatic metastases. Radiology 128:447, 1978

176. Baker DA, Morin ME: Gravity dependent layering in necrotic metastatic carcinoma to the liver. J Clin Ultrasound 5:282, 1977

177. Federle MP, Filly RA, Moss AA: Cystic hepatic neoplasms: Complementary roles of CT and sonography. AJR 136:345, 1981

178. Bruneton JN, Ladree D, Caramella E, et al: Ultrasonographic study of calcified hepatic metastases: a report of 13 cases. Gastrointest Radiol 7:61, 1982

179. Katrugadda CS, Goldstein HM, Green B: Gray scale ultrasonography of calcified liver metastases. Am J Roentgenol 129:591, 1977

180. Rubaltelli L, Del Mashio A, Candiani F, Miotto D: The role of vascularization in the formation of echographic patterns of hepatic metastases: microangiographic and echographic study. Brit J Radiol 53:1166, 1980

181. Sekiya T, Meller ST, Cosgrove DO, McCready VR: Ultrasonography of Hodgkin's disease in the liver and spleen. Clin Radiol 33:635, 1982

182. Ginaldi S, Bernardino ME, Jing BS, Green B: Ultrasonographic patterns of hepatic lymphoma. Radiology 136:427, 1980

183. Siegal MJ, Melson GL: Sonographic demonstration of hepatic Burkitt's lymphoma. Pediatr Radiol 11:166, 1981

184. Lepke R, Pagani JJ: Sonography of hepatic chloromas. AJR 138:1176, 1982

185. Filiatrault D, Garel L, Tournade MF, Zucker JM: Echographic aspects of hepatic metastases of nephroblastomas. Pediatr Radiol 12:72, 1982

186. Nosher JL, Plafker J: Fine-needle aspiration of the liver with ultrasound guidance. Radiology 136:177, 1980

187. Zornoza J, Wallace S, Ordonez N, Lukeman J: Fine-needle aspiration biopsy of the liver. AJR 134:331, 1980

188. Schwerk WB, Schmitz-Moormann P: Ultrasonically guided fine-needle biopsies in neoplastic liver disease: cytohistologic diagnoses and echopattern of lesions. Cancer 48:1469, 1981

189. Elyaderani MK: Ultrasonic guidance of liver biopsy and fine-needle aspiration in difficult cases. So Med J 76:850, 1983

190. Pagani JJ: Biopsy of focal hepatic lesions: comparison of 18 and 22 gauge needles. Radiology 147:673, 1983

191. Green B, Goldstein HM: Hepatic ultrasonography. p. 62. In Sarti DA, Sample WF (eds): Diagnostic Ultrasound Text and Cases, G. K. Hall, Boston, 1980

192. Lam AH, Shulman L: Ultrasonography in the management of liver trauma in children. J Ultrasound Med 3:199, 1984

193. VanSonnenberg E, Simeone JF, Mueller PR, et al: Sonographic appearance of hematomas in the liver, spleen, and kidney: A clinical, pathologic, and animal study. Radiology 147:507, 1983

194. Wendell BA, Athey PA: Ultrasonic appearance of metallic foreign bodies in parenchymal organs. J Clin Ultrasound 9:133, 1981

195. Weeks LE, McCune BR, Martin JF, O'Brien TF: Differential diagnosis of intrahepatic shadowing on ultrasound examination. J Clin Ultrasound 6:399, 1978

196. Cosgrove DO: Liver. p. 1. In Goldberg BB (ed): Clinics in Diagnostic Ultrasound: Ultrasound in Cancer. Churchill Livingstone, New York, 1981

197. Elyaderani MK, Gabrielle OF: Comparison of radionuclide imaging and ultrasonography of the liver. So Med J 76:37, 1983

198. McClees EC, Gedgaudas-McClees RK: Screening for diffuse and focal liver disease: the case for hepatic scintigraphy. J Clin Ultrasound 12:75, 1984

199. Berlard LL: Screening for diffuse and focal liver disease: The case for hepatic computed tomography. J Clin Ultrasound 12:83, 1984

200. Sample WF, Gray RK, Poe ND, et al: Nuclear Imaging, tomographic nuclear imaging and gray scale ultrasound in the evaluation of the porta hepatis. Radiology 122:773, 1977

201. Sullivan DC, Taylor KJW, Gottschalk A: The use of ultrasound to enhance the diagnostic utility of the equivocal liver scintigraph. Radiology 128:727, 1978

202. Petasnick JP, Ram P, Turner DA, Fordham EW: The relationship of computed tomography, gray-scale ultrasonography and radionuclide imaging in the evaluation of hepatic masses. Sem Nuc Med 9:8, 1979

203. Knopf DR, Torres WE, Fajman WJ, Sones PJ: Liver lesions: Comparative accuracy of scintigraphy and computed tomography. AJR 138:623, 1982

204. Frick MP, Knight LC, Feinberg SB, et al: Computer tomography, radionuclide imaging and ultrasonography in hepatic mass lesions. Comput Tomogr 3:49, 1979

205. Snow JH, Goldstein HM, Wallace S: Comparison of scintigraphy, sonography and CT in evaluation of hepatic neoplasams. AJR 132:915, 1979

206. Bondestam S, Liahde S, Annala R, et al: Scintigraphy and sonography in the investigation of liver metastases. Diagn Imaging 49:339, 1980

207. Bryan PJ, Dinn WM, Grossman ZD, et al: Correlation of computed tomography, gray scale ultrasonography, and radionuclide imaging of the liver in detecting space-occupying processes. Radiology 124:387, 1977

208. Sty JR, Starshak RJ: Comparative imaging in the evaluation of hepatic abscesses in immunocompromised children. J Clin Ultrasound 11:11, 1983

209. Itai Y, Nishikawa J, Tasaka A: Computed tomography in the evaluation of hepatocellular carcinoma. Radiology 131:166, 1979

210. Alderson PO, Adams DF, McNeil BJ, et al: Computed tomography, ultrasound, and scintigraphy of the liver in patients with colon or breast carcinoma: a prospective comparison. Radiology 149:225, 1983

211. Shawker TH, Moran B, Linzer M, et al: B-scan echo-amplitude measurement in patients with diffuse infiltrative liver disease. J Clin Ultrasound 9:293, 1981

2

The Biliary System

The biliary system has become one of the primary areas for evaluation with ultrasound in the 1980s. With the use of the newer high-resolution sector real-time ultrasound systems, the gallbladder and extrahepatic ducts can be identified in the majority of patients despite body habitus or clinical condition. Unlike radiographic evaluation, ultrasound may be performed rapidly, repeatedly (if necessary), without radiation or contrast administration, and at the bedside in critically ill patients. As a result, ultrasound has become the primary tool in evaluation of the gallbladder and the jaundiced patient. It is also an accurate and reliable technique for evaluating the common bile duct and intrahepatic ducts, and is effective for evaluation of neighboring structures (e.g., the liver and pancreas).

TECHNIQUE

Preparation

In order to perform an optimal examination of the gallbladder, the patient should fast for at least 6 hours prior to the ultrasound study. It is desirable to perform the gallbladder ultrasound after an overnight fast whenever possible. This fasting allows for maximum distention of the gallbladder, which promotes better visualization not only of the gallbladder but also of intraluminal abnormalities and/or wall abnormalities. In the case of an emergency study or a critically ill patient, a satisfactory gallbladder examination can still usually be per-

formed, as many of these patients have eaten little to nothing anyway.

It is also helpful for the patient to have been fasting when the extrahepatic ducts are studied. As one study is rarely performed without the other, this fasting is needed mainly for gallbladder distention.

Ultrasound Technique

ULTRASOUND SYSTEM

There is no comparison between the effectiveness of real-time and static systems for studying the biliary system. Static systems, as a rule, just do not have the capability and, ultimately, the resolution of real-time systems. With real-time ultrasound, evaluation of the biliary system can average 10 to 15 minutes in trained hands. The gallbladder can be quickly identified and meticulously scanned in various scan planes and body positions. In addition, with sector real-time systems, one can quickly identify the extrahepatic ducts because the real-time system has the advantage of easy maneuverability of the scanhead. A similar examination using a static system would take 30 to 45 minutes, at least.

EXAMINATION TECHNIQUE

Examination of the gallbladder begins with the patient in the supine position. In the longitudinal plane, the gallbladder is located by identifying the major fissure of the liver (Fig. 2-1). Once located, the gallbladder is

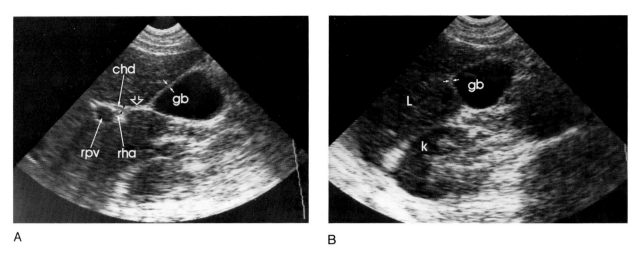

A   B

Fig. 2-1. Normal gallbladder. **(A)** Longitudinal supine real-time scan. The gallbladder *(gb)* is seen as an oval-shaped anechoic structure with a thin wall (small arrows). It is located by identifying the major fissure (open arrow) of the liver. The internal diameter (arrowheads) of the common hepatic duct *(chd)* is measured anterior to the right portal vein *(rpv)*. *(rha,* right hepatic artery.) **(B)** Transverse supine scan. The gallbladder *(gb)* is seen as a thin-walled (arrows) anechoic structure in the area of the major fissure. The gallbladder *(gb)* wall is most easily measured next to the liver *(L)*. *(k,* right kidney.)

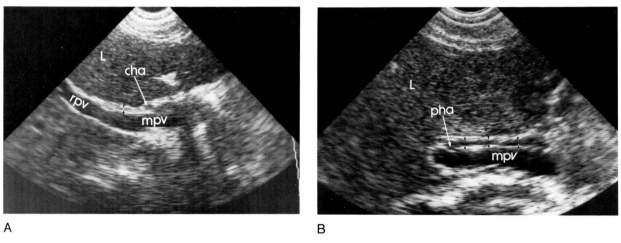

A   B

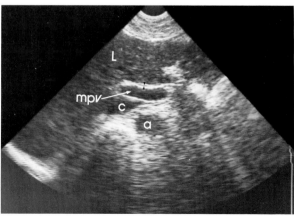

Fig. 2-2. Common bile duct. Transverse, oblique real-time scans **(A–C)** paralleling the costal margin with two different patients in the left lateral decubitus position. The long axis view of the main portal vein *(mpv)* is depicted with the common bile duct (arrowheads) seen as a tubular lucency paralleling the portal vein in this plane. These ducts varied from 3 to 5 mm in internal diameter (arrowheads). **(A)** is more lateral to the porta hepatis with **(C)** most medial. **(B)** is more magnified than **(A)** or **(C)** with the duct measuring 4 mm. *(rpv,* right portal vein; *cha,* common hepatic artery; *pha,* proper hepatic artery; *L,* liver; *a,* aorta; *c,* inferior vena cava.) *(Figure continues.)*

C

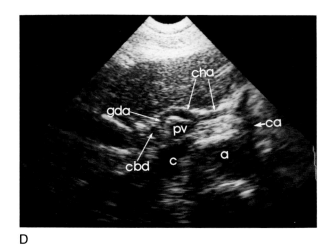

D

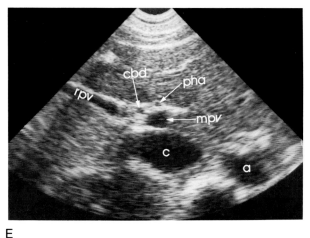

E

Fig. 2-2. *(Continued).* Transverse scans of common hepatic artery and duct. **(D)** The common hepatic artery (*cha*) is seen extending from the celiac artery (*ca*) running anterior to the main portal vein (*pv*). The gastroduodenal artery (*gda*) is visualized branching from the common hepatic artery. (*cbd,* common bile duct; *c,* inferior vena cava; *a,* aorta.) **(E)** Transverse oblique scan. The common bile duct (*cbd*) is seen anterolateral to the main portal vein (*mpv*) with the proper hepatic artery (*pha*) more anteromedial. (*a,* aorta; *c,* inferior vena cava; *rpv,* right portal vein.)

scanned very slowly from its medial to lateral borders taking at least three freeze-frame images. It is then scanned transversely from its inferior to superior extent (Fig. 2-1). The transducer frequency used for the examination depends on the patient's body habitus. The highest frequency transducer possible should be used, as this affords better resolution. The depth of the gallbladder should be matched to the focal zone of the transducer.

When examining the gallbladder, the extrahepatic ducts are always evaluated. With the patient in the same supine position as above, several longitudinal scans of the common hepatic duct are obtained following longitudinal scans of the gallbladder. The common hepatic duct can be seen as a small anechoic tubular structure anterior to the right portal vein on this projection (Fig. 2-1). While it is impossible to say exactly where the common hepatic duct ends and the common bile duct begins (the cystic duct is not generally identified), there is a general rule that the common hepatic duct is that portion of the common duct located above the level of the gallbladder on longitudinal scan and the common bile duct is that portion located inferiorly. When examining in the transverse plane, the common bile duct can be quickly identified by finding the long axes of the main and right portal veins. The duct can be seen anterior to the portal vein (Fig. 2-2). This plane parallels the costal margin in most patients. The transducer is thus placed in an oblique position. In a straight transverse plane, the bile duct can be seen anterior and lateral to the portal vein with the common hepatic artery anterior and medial to the portal vein (Fig. 2-2D,E). The bile duct and hepatic artery should not be confused. If there is a ques-

tion, the common hepatic artery can be followed back to its origin in the celiac artery by using the real-time system.

Once supine views are obtained, the patient is positioned in the left lateral decubitus position, which often affords improved clarity and visualization of abnormalities.[1] No gallbladder examination should be done in only one position unless the patient is simply not clinically able to be moved. Longitudinal and transverse views of the gallbladder are also obtained in the decubitus position. If stones were questioned in the supine views, one needs to evaluate for movement of the stones (Fig. 2-3). As with examination of the gallbladder, views of the extrahepatic ducts are again obtained in this position with the technique described above. Sometimes the ducts are poorly imaged in the supine position and can be seen only in the decubitus position. Some investigators report an accuracy of 96 percent in identifying the common bile duct in the decubitus view.[2]

If the gallbladder is quite high or there is still a question after the decubitus examination, the gallbladder may be examined in the erect position (Fig. 2-3C). Once again, the longitudinal and transverse views are obtained. This change in position may demonstrate a shifting position of stones, confirming their presence.[3] It may also allow a different view of the extrahepatic ducts.

If the examiner is specifically interested in evaluating the cystic duct, the patient may be placed in the Trendelenburg position (with the head lower than the feet). Since most ultrasound tables don't tilt, this position may be obtained by placing a pillow and/or rolled sheets under the patient's hips. Once the position is obtained,

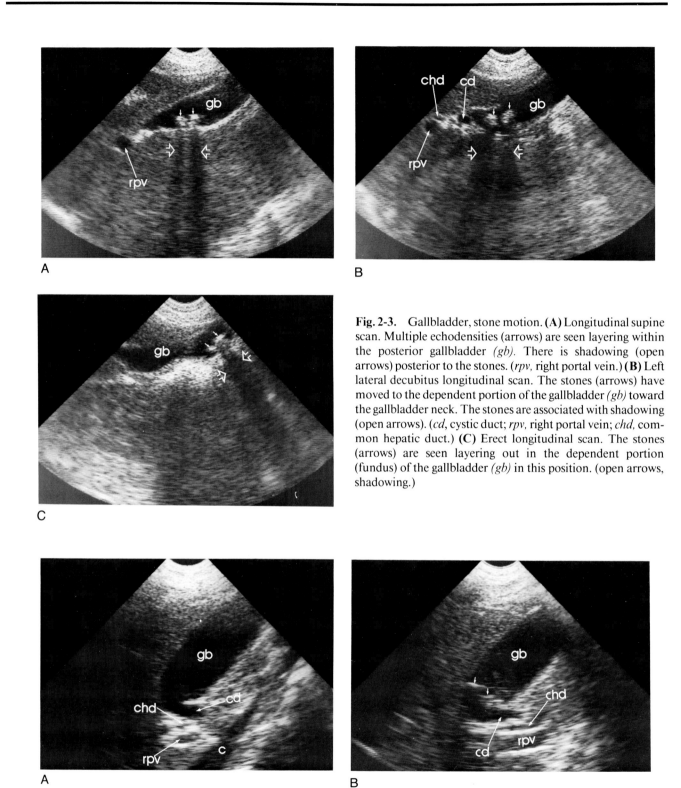

Fig. 2-3. Gallbladder, stone motion. **(A)** Longitudinal supine scan. Multiple echodensities (arrows) are seen layering within the posterior gallbladder *(gb)*. There is shadowing (open arrows) posterior to the stones. (*rpv,* right portal vein.) **(B)** Left lateral decubitus longitudinal scan. The stones (arrows) have moved to the dependent portion of the gallbladder *(gb)* toward the gallbladder neck. The stones are associated with shadowing (open arrows). (*cd,* cystic duct; *rpv,* right portal vein; *chd,* common hepatic duct.) **(C)** Erect longitudinal scan. The stones (arrows) are seen layering out in the dependent portion (fundus) of the gallbladder *(gb)* in this position. (open arrows, shadowing.)

Fig. 2-4. Gallbladder and cystic duct, Trendelenberg position. **(A)** Longitudinal scan supine. The cystic duct *(cd)* is clearly identified medial to the gallbladder *(gb)*. (*chd,* common hepatic duct; *rpv,* right portal vein; *c,* inferior vena cava.) **(B)** Longitudinal scan slightly right lateral decubitus. The cystic duct *(cd)* is seen anterior to the common hepatic duct *(chd)* and right portal vein *(rpv)*. There were stones in the gallbladder; the interface with the lateral edge of the stones (arrows) is noted. (*gb,* gallbladder.)

the gallbladder and cystic duct may be scanned in the longitudinal and transverse planes. In addition, it may be helpful to scan the cystic duct with the patient in the left and/or right lateral decubitus position (with patient still in the Trendelenburg position). These positions appear to open up the long axis of the cystic duct for maximum visualization (Fig. 2-4). Still, in many patients, a complete evaluation of the cystic duct cannot be obtained.

At times, it may be desirable to measure the contraction of the gallbladder in response to cholecystokinin (CCK) when cystic duct obstruction is questioned.[4] While the demonstration of significant contraction after CCK is strong evidence of cystic duct patency, the converse does not always hold true. Failure of contraction is not specific.[4,5]

If stones are identified in the gallbladder, careful evaluation of the extrahepatic ducts, as well as that of the pancreas, must be obtained. The bile duct is scrutinized for stones in the supine and left and right lateral decubitus positions (Fig. 2-1–2-4). Some investigators recommend the 45° or 90° right anterior oblique position to better demonstrate the duct.[6] Visualization of the distal common duct is improved by placing the patient in the erect or semi-erect position[7] (Fig. 2-5). At times, the patient may be given 32 oz (4 glasses) of water to drink in order to better evaluate the distal common duct (the retroduodenal and intrapancreatic parts). The scans may then be performed transversely in the erect and/or

right lateral decubitus position (Fig. 2-6). (The right lateral decubitus position allows the air in the stomach to float to the fundus and the second portion of the duodenum tends to fill with fluid, nicely outlining the head of the pancreas.) Because stones in the gallbladder and/or duct may be associated with pancreatitis, the pancreas should be evaluated for its parenchymal echopattern, mass effect, and ductal size and configuration. With careful scanning, the main pancreatic duct can be identified in the body of the pancreas on a transverse scan (Fig. 2-7). The parenchymal pattern of the pancreas should be similar to or denser than the liver. If the pancreas is lucent or a mass effect is identified, pancreatitis should be questioned.

If no gallstones are identified but dilated intra- or extrahepatic ducts are seen, a careful search for the etiology should be undertaken. One should identify the level of obstruction (e.g., distal common bile duct or common hepatic duct — intrahepatic dilatation without common bile duct dilatation) and then search for the etiology. The pancreas should always be evaluated for mass effect. Unfortunately, not all pancreases can be visualized due to overlying bowel gas and/or body habitus. (Evaluation of the pancreas is thoroughly discussed in Chapter 3). The examination is not complete until an evaluation for lymphadenopathy in the porta hepatis and metastatic liver disease has been undertaken.

If the patient is referred to ultrasound for right upper quadrant pain and the biliary exam is negative, careful

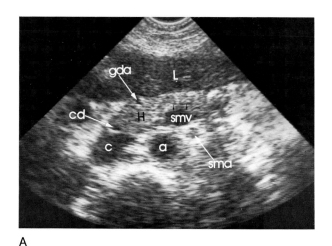
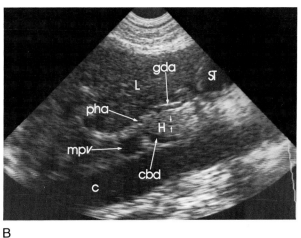

A   B

Fig. 2-5. Distal common bile duct. Erect. **(A)** Transverse scan. The distal common bile duct *(cd)* can be seen within the inferolateral portion of the pancreatic head *(H)*. (*smv,* superior mesenteric vein; *sma,* superior mesenteric artery; *gda,* gastroduodenal artery; *a,* aorta; *c,* inferior vena cava; *L,* liver; arrows, pancreatic neck.) **(B)** Longitudinal scan. The distal common bile duct *(cbd)* is noted to be running posterior to the pancreatic head *(H)* with the gastroduodenal artery *(gda)* running anteriorly. The proper hepatic artery *(pha)* is at the superior margin of the pancreas with the main portal vein *(mpv).* The pancreatic duct (arrows) can be seen in the center of the pancreatic head. (*ST,* fluid-filled stomach; *L,* liver; *c,* inferior vena cava.)

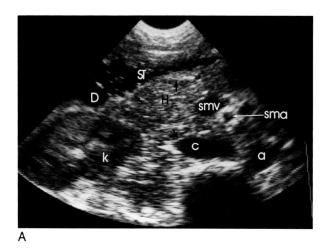
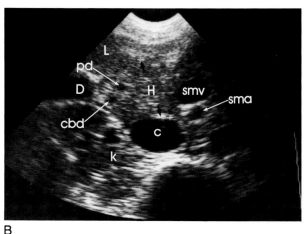

Fig. 2-6. Distal common bile duct, Water Technique. Magnified right lateral decubitus views. (**A**) The pancreatic head (*H*, arrows) is seen outlined by the fluid-filled stomach *(ST)* and duodenum *(D)* with the right kidney *(k)* and inferior vena cava *(c)* posterior and the superior mesenteric vein *(smv)* medial. (*sma,* superior mesenteric artery; *a,* aorta.) (**B**) On this view, the fluid-filled stomach is not seen anteriorly. The border (arrows) of the pancreatic head *(H)* blends with the liver *(L);* the pancreas is isoechoic to liver. The common bile duct *(cbd)* and pancreatic duct *(pd)* are seen within the pancreatic head. (*smv,* superior mesenteric vein; *c,* inferior vena cava; *k,* right kidney; *sma,* superior mesenteric artery; *D,* fluid-filled duodenum.)

examination of other structures (e.g., right kidney, diaphragm, liver, and vessels) should be obtained. Liver or kidney abnormalities may then be identified.

NORMAL ANATOMY

Gallbladder

The gallbladder is a conical musculomembranous sac lying in a fossa under the liver.[8] Its segments include (1) the fundus—a hemispheric blind end, (2) the body—

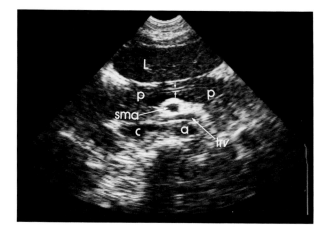

Fig. 2-7. Normal pancreas. Transverse scan. The normal pancreas *(p)* is seen. The pancreatic duct (arrows) is seen as a tubular lucency within the body of the pancreas. (*L,* liver; *c,* inferior vena cava; *a,* aorta; *sma,* superior mesenteric artery; *lrv,* left renal vein.)

portion between the fundus and neck, and (3) the neck —narrow tube-like structure that tapers to the cystic duct[8] (Fig. 2-8). The fundus is usually close to the hepatic flexure of the colon and duodenum.[9] The neck of the gallbladder is oriented posteromedially toward the porta hepatis, with the fundus situated lateral, caudad, and anterior to the neck.[9] The size and shape of the gallbladder are variable. When relaxed, the gallbladder is 7 to 10 cm in length and 2 to 3 cm in width.[8] It has a capacity of 30 to 50 ml.[8] The Rokitansky-Aschoff sinuses of the gallbladder are small outpouchings of the mucosa of the gallbladder that extend into the underlying connective tissue and sometimes into the muscular layer.[8] They communicate directly with the lumen of the gallbladder.[8]

Bile secreted by the liver contains water, cholesterol, bile salts, bile acids, bilirubin, lecithin in micellar complexes, inorganic ions, and mucoproteins secreted by epithelium. Bile salts (sodium salts of taurocholic and glycocholic acids) aid in maintaining cholesterol in solution. The gallbladder concentrates bile by selective absorption of water, inorganic ions, and small amounts of bile salts. Contraction and partial emptying of the gallbladder occurs when foods, especially fatty ones, or other stimulants enter the duodenum. The gallbladder activity is mediated through cholecystokinin, a hormone that is released from the duodenum into the blood.[8]

On ultrasound, the gallbladder is seen as an anechoic fluid-filled ellipsoid structure adjacent to and indenting the inferior-medial aspect of the right lobe of the liver (Fig. 2-1). It is situated along the junction of the medial

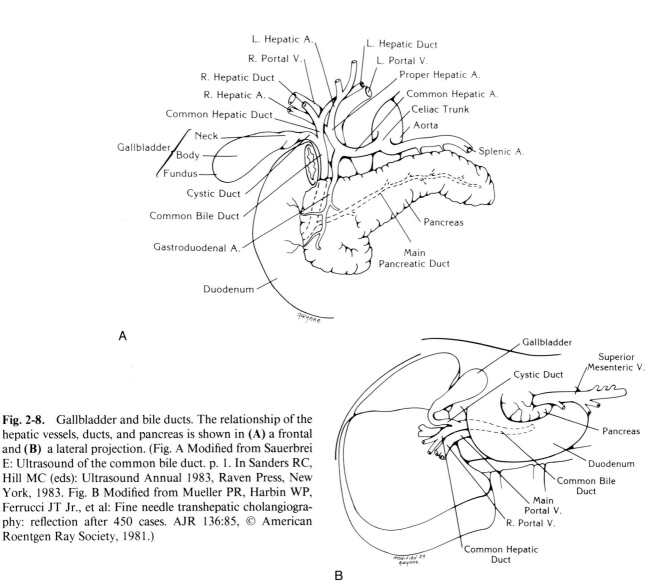

A

Fig. 2-8. Gallbladder and bile ducts. The relationship of the hepatic vessels, ducts, and pancreas is shown in **(A)** a frontal and **(B)** a lateral projection. (Fig. A Modified from Sauerbrei E: Ultrasound of the common bile duct. p. 1. In Sanders RC, Hill MC (eds): Ultrasound Annual 1983, Raven Press, New York, 1983. Fig. B Modified from Mueller PR, Harbin WP, Ferrucci JT Jr., et al: Fine needle transhepatic cholangiography: reflection after 450 cases. AJR 136:85, © American Roentgen Ray Society, 1981.)

B

segment of the left lobe and the right lobe.[10] A linear echodensity connecting the gallbladder to the right or main portal vein is seen on ultrasound in a high percentage of cases (68 percent)[11] (Fig. 2-1A). This linear echodensity is the main lobar fissure of the liver and appears to be a reliable anatomic indicator of gallbladder location.[11] The gallbladder lies in the posterior and caudal aspect of this fissure with the right portal vein under the medial segment of the left hepatic lobe before it bifurcates and enters the parenchyma of the right lobe.[11] The neck of the gallbladder usually is in contact with the main segment of the right portal vein or the main portal vein near the origin of the left portal vein.[11] A redundant or folded neck of the gallbladder should not be confused with a dilated common bile duct[12] (Fig. 2-9). Ninety-eight percent of gallbladders can be visualized with ultrasound.[13]

The gallbladder, in its distended state, has a smooth wall that is usually not measurable. The anterior wall is normally seen as a thin, strongly reflective structure, while the posterior wall may be difficult to evaluate because of transmission of sound and its contact with bowel[14] (Fig. 2-1A). The wall thickness is never more than 3 mm, even in the child.[15] The gallbladder wall measurement is most accurate if it is obtained along that portion of the gallbladder wall that is perpendicular to the sound beam[16] (Fig. 2-1). In addition, it is best to measure the anterior wall adjacent to the liver.

The gallbladder may vary in size and shape. It is usually 8 cm in length and less than 3.5 cm in diameter in the adult and child.[9,15] In the neonate, the mean gallbladder width to length ratio is 0.37.[17] It may be dilated in diabetics, bedridden patients with protracted illness or pancreatitis, and patients taking anticholinergics.[9]

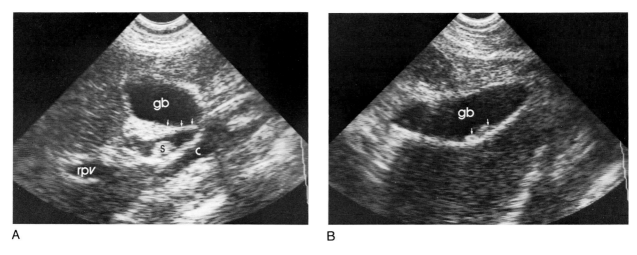

A   B

Fig. 2-9. Gallbladder, folded neck. (**A**) Longitudinal left lateral decubitus scan. There is a stone *(s)* in the neck of the gallbladder *(gb)*. The gallbladder is folded (arrows) upon itself in region of the neck. (*rpv,* right portal vein; *c,* inferior vena cava.) (**B**) Transverse long axis view of the gallbladder *(gb)* in the right lateral decubitus position. In this view, the gallbladder is unfolded and the stones (arrows) are clearly within the gallbladder.

A variety of folds and kinks in the body are noted in 14.5 percent of gallbladders[18] (Figs. 2-9 to 2-11); the most common is at the incisura between the body and infundibulum analogous to the junctional fold[18] (Fig. 2-10). Care should be taken not to mistake septations or a phrygian cap for stones.[19] The phrygian cap is a fold toward the fundus of the gallbladder in the distal segment[10] (Fig. 2-11). It may be caused by angulation, kinking, or circumferential constriction of the body of the gallbladder, producing an apparently expanded bulbous end to the fundus.[8]

A well-contracted gallbladder has a striking appearance on ultrasound.[14] It changes from a single to a double concentric structure with three components: (1) a strongly reflective outer contour, (2) a poorly reflective inner contour, and (3) an anechoic area between both contours[14] (Fig. 2-12). After a fatty meal, 69 percent of gallbladders are seen to completely contract, while 31 percent incompletely contract.[14]

Developmental anomalies of the gallbladder take many forms and are of varied clinical significance. There may be agenesis, hypoplasia, hyperplasia, total reduplication to form a double gallbladder, or subtotal division of the fundus and body to create a bilobed structure.[8] The incidence of gallbladder duplication is 1 in 4000 individuals with a 2:1 female-to-male ratio.[20] With a

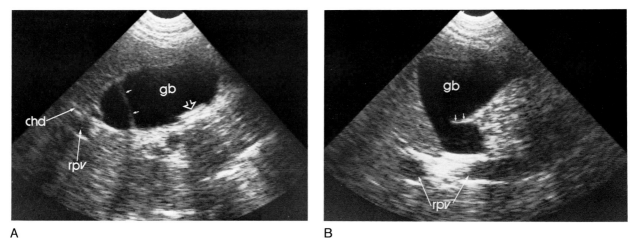

A   B

Fig. 2-10. Gallbladder, junctional fold. (**A**) Longitudinal scan. A fold (arrows) or kink is seen at the incisura between the body and infundibulum of the gallbladder *(gb)*. On this view, it appears more like a septum. (*rpv,* right portal vein; *chd,* common hepatic duct; open arrow, stones.) (**B**) Transverse oblique scan. The fold (arrows) in the gallbladder *(gb)* is more clearly defined in this view. (*rpv,* right portal vein.)

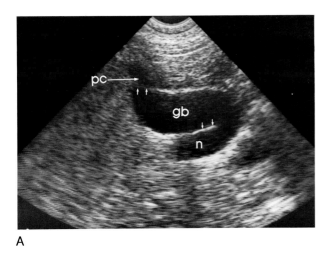

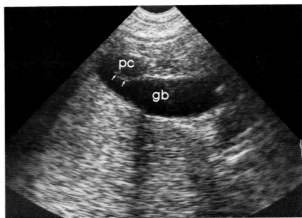

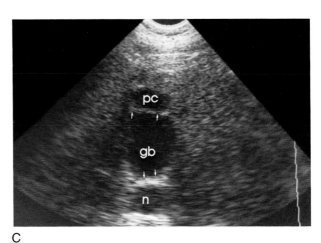

Fig. 2-11. Phrygian cap. In this case, there are multiple folds including a phrygian cap and a junctional fold. **(A)** Left lateral decubitus longitudinal scan. Folds (arrows) are demonstrated in the fundic and neck *(n)* ends of the gallbladder *(gb)*. A phrygian cap *(pc)* is a fold in the distal segment toward the fundus. **(B)** Oblique longitudinal view performed to open the folds demonstrate the phrygian cap *(pc)*. (*gb*, gallbladder.) **(C)** Erect longitudinal view. With the folds (arrows), there is the appearance of three cystic structures. The more anterior one is the phrygian cap *(pc)* and the more posterior one is the neck *(n)*, the middle section being the body of the gallbladder *(gb)*.

Fig. 2-12. Contracted gallbladder. Longitudinal scan. The contracted gallbladder is seen as a double concentric structure with a strongly reflective outer contour (arrows), a poorly reflective inner contour and an anechoic area between both.

double gallbladder, two parallel pear-shaped cystic structures are seen in the gallbladder fossa.[16] The gallbladder may be abnormally located in the left lobe of the liver; sometimes it is intrahepatic or floating on a long pendulous mesentery. An intrahepatic gallbladder may be difficult to diagnose; its diagnosis may be inferred if the cystic intrahepatic area has a pear-shape and contracts after a fatty meal. There is a congenital absence of the gallbladder in 0.03 percent of cases.[21]

Bile Ducts

The extrahepatic biliary system (gallbladder and extrahepatic ducts) maintains direct connection between the liver and the gastrointestinal tract and serves as an essential link in the enterohepatic circulation.[8] The ducts passively transfer bile from the liver to the duodenum, directly or via the gallbladder.[8] The extrahepatic duct system has two functions: the storage and concentration of bile and the delivery of bile to the duodenum.[8] Bile flows if intraductal pressure is less than hepatic secretary pressure. Pressure differences are affected by (1) activity of the sphincter at the distal end of the common bile duct, (2) gallbladder filling and resorption of bile in the gallbladder, and (3) bile flow from the liver.[22] Contractility at the distal sphincter is probably the most important dynamic factor in affecting intraductal pressure. Normally, there is a regular cycle of contractions and relaxations causing flow of bile into the duodenum. The common duct has no motor role in bile flow.

The right and left hepatic ducts emerge from the liver parenchyma in the porta hepatis and unite to form the common hepatic duct, which passes caudad and medial (Fig. 2-8). It is joined by the cystic duct to form the common bile duct, which descends along the free border of the lesser omentum for a variable distance, crossing behind the first portion of the duodenum and entering the parenchyma of the head of the pancreas. It then turns somewhat toward the right and enters the second portion of the duodenum where it ends at the ampulla of Vater (Fig. 2-8). In its supraduodenal segment, the common bile duct is situated lateral to the hepatic artery and anterior to the portal vein (Fig. 2-2D,E). As it descends behind the duodenal bulb and enters the pancreas, the duct becomes more posterior, lying close to the anterior margin of the inferior vena cava (Fig. 2-5). Within the liver parenchyma, the bile ducts follow the same course as the portal venous and hepatic arterial branches. All are encased in a common collagenous sheath, forming the so-called portal triad. The common duct is tethered superiorly to the liver, where the left and right hepatic ducts converge, and inferiorly, where it enters the posterior portion of the head of the pancreas. The rest of the common bile duct is relatively unfixed as it passes along the lateral edge of the hepatoduodenal ligament, with the main portal vein and proper hepatic artery superior to the pancreas.[22] The main right and left bile ducts nearly always lie anterior to the corresponding portal vein trunk. The hepatic artery may lie anterior to the portal vein, although the left hepatic artery is often posterior to the left portal vein. In the periphery of the liver, the orientation of ducts and vessels is variable.[9]

On a section at the level of the hepatoduodenal ligament (just below the porta hepatis and just above the head of the pancreas) the portal vein lies immediately anterior to the inferior vena cava and the common bile duct is situated anterolateral to the portal vein (Fig. 2-2D,E). Slightly more inferior, the common bile duct is more posterior as it courses through the head of the pancreas. This distal duct is best seen on a transverse scan inferior to the level of the superior mesenteric vein in the region of the uncinate process[7] (Figs. 2-5 and 2-6). An anterior-to-posterior course to the common bile duct is seen on a longitudinal scan, which allows differentiation of the common bile duct from the superior mesenteric vein (Fig. 2-5B). The superior mesenteric vein is

slightly to the left and pursues a relatively horizontal course. The cystic duct itself is seldom visualized because of its small size.

Many studies have been performed with high-resolution real-time equipment to evaluate the normal size of the extrahepatic ducts. In 98 percent of normals, the common hepatic duct has been found to measure 4 mm or less as it passes anterior to the right portal vein[23] (Fig. 2-1A). This and all measurements reflect the internal dimension of the duct or a measurement of the lucency and not an external measurement, which could be affected by technique. The upper limits of normal size for the common bile and hepatic ducts are thus 4 to 8 mm. In the child, the lumen of the common hepatic duct increases with age but never exceeds 4 mm.[15] In the neonate, the common bile duct is less than or equal to 1 mm.[17] A measurement of 6 to 8 mm in the adult is equivocal.

Some feel that if the common hepatic duct is greater than 4 mm, biliary obstruction is probably present; thus, a measurement of 5 mm is considered borderline, while a measurement of 6 mm is consistent with obstruction.[24] Using these measurements, a sensitivity of 99 percent and a specificity of 87 percent is achieved.[24] The range of size considered normal is greater if the patient has had prior biliary surgery, with an upper limit of 10 mm.

There is a discrepancy between the radiographic and sonographic bile duct measurements.[25] The ultrasound measurement is smaller than the radiographic (11 mm) one due to several factors: (1) radiographic magnification, (2) ultrasound underestimation—wall reverberation causing underestimation of lumen size, (3) possible choleretic effect of radiographic contrast material, and (4) the fact that different regions of the duct are measured with different techniques.[25] The choleretic effect of contrast has been shown to significantly increase ductal size in a small percentage of cases. The radiographic magnification factor is usually 1.3. The ultrasound diameter measurement is generally 1.5 to 2.0 mm smaller than true size. The most important cause of the discrepancy between the ultrasound and radiographic values is the measurement of different regions of the duct with different techniques. Some recommend always measuring the common hepatic duct anterior to the right portal vein.[25] Although the ultrasound measurements are generally assumed to be accurate, reverberation and other artifacts can cause a slight increase or decrease in size. The artifactual thickening of the duct wall encroaches upon the lumen of fluid-filled duct, which makes the duct smaller.[25]

At times it may be difficult to differentiate bile ducts from vessels. Some investigators have offered suggestions in making this distinction. The "parallel-channel sign" is used to describe the image of a dilated duct. It refers to the simultaneous visualization on a transverse or longitudinal scan of the right portal vein and the right hepatic duct and/or the left portal vein and the left hepatic duct. The common hepatic artery normally emerges from the celiac axis and crosses to the right to run adjacent to the portal vein and common bile duct at the porta hepatis (Figs. 2-2D,E and 2-8A). There it branches into the right and left hepatic arteries. In two thirds of patients, the right hepatic artery crosses behind the common bile duct or right hepatic duct, whereas the left hepatic artery crosses anterior to the left hepatic duct (Fig. 2-8A). In most patients, on cross-section, the right hepatic artery is anterior to the right portal vein (Fig. 2-1A). When the common hepatic artery arises from the superior mesenteric artery, it runs between the portal vein and common bile duct to join the superior mesenteric artery.[26] Duplex scanning of the porta hepatis may be performed to help in the identification of the common bile duct and common hepatic artery. In 59 percent of patients, the hepatic artery is as large or larger than the duct. Ultrasound signs that help differentiate the two structures include (1) intrinsic pulsations of the arteries; (2) indentation or displacement of structures by arteries; (3) change in caliber of the duct during real-time ultrasound; and (4) orientation, contour, caliber, and curvature of the tubular structures in the porta hepatis.[27]

Differentiation of the umbilical portion of the left portal vein and intrahepatic bile ducts may also be difficult. The left branch of the portal vein courses horizontally as a transverse portion then veers anteriorly at an acute angle, to form the umbilical portion. This can be demonstrated in normal and 95 percent of jaundiced patients (see Figs. 1-11A, 1-11B, and 1-14). The left hepatic duct does not curve anteriorly at an acute angle, but branches off to the lateral segment running superior to the umbilical portion. This anatomic relationship and characteristic form of the umbilical portion is useful in differentiating the portal vein and bile duct.[28]

The common bile duct may take on various contours. The normal duct courses dorsally as it goes inferiorly, making a sharp dorsal bend as it passes over the portal vein (Fig. 2-2). Most dilated common bile ducts display a convex ventral configuration that allows easy differentiation from the portal vein (Fig. 2-13). The common duct courses caudally, medially, and dorsally in the hepatoduodenal ligament, ventral and lateral to the portal vein. At the termination of the hepatoduodenal ligament, the duct runs dorsally and continues through the dorsal part of the pancreatic head until it empties into the duodenum. As described above, the proximal end of the common bile duct is tethered by its intrahepatic tributary ducts as it merges from the porta and the distal end is fixed by surrounding pancreatic tissue. In patients with a dilated duct, the ventral convex configuration of the prepancreatic segment (hepatoduodenal ligament) occurs in most cases. Since the duct is tethered both inferiorly and superiorly and is constrained dorsally by the portal vein, the dilated duct bows ventrally. Thus, when a ventrally convex large tubular structure is noted in the hepatoduodenal ligament region, it may be confidently identified as a dilated duct, even when other anatomic landmarks are not imaged.[29]

In reviewing intraoperative cholangiograms, investi-

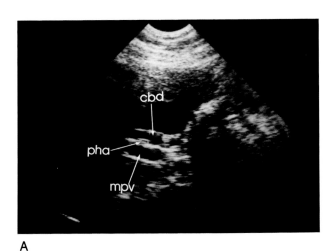

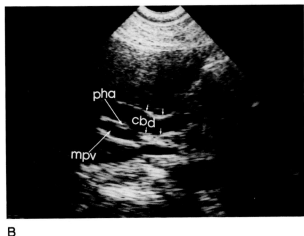

A   B

Fig. 2-13. Dilated common bile duct. Postcholecystectomy patient with biliary colic. **(A)** Long axis view in the left lateral decubitus position. The proximal common bile duct *(cbd)* seen anterior to the main portal vein *(mpv)* measures 6 mm. (*pha,* proper hepatic artery.) **(B)** Long axis left lateral decubitus scan (same location and magnification as **A).** Ten minutes after a fatty meal, the duct is rescanned; it has dilated to 10 mm. This represents an abnormal response. Note the convex ventral configuration (arrows) is more pronounced on this view. At ERCP, the patient was found to have ampullary stenosis. (*mpv,* main portal vein; *pha,* proper hepatic artery.)

gators have found that the transverse segment of the common duct is longer than 35 mm in 18 percent of dilated extrahepatic ducts and 6 percent of normal caliber ducts. When dilated, the transverse segment may be confused with the portal and splenic veins on ultrasound. The course of the extrahepatic duct is largely dependent on positions of the porta hepatis, the head of the pancreas, and the site of insertion of the duct into the duodenum. In 6 percent of normal patients, the extrahepatic duct has a long transverse segment that may reach or extend beyond the midline.[30]

Some authors have studied the distensibility of the common bile duct.[31] Initially, the grossly dilated common hepatic duct returns to normal size within minutes. This rapid size change probably occurs only in patients without a normally functioning gallbladder. The wall of the duct is composed largely of fibroelastic tissue and the stretch potential of the elastic fibers permits duct dilatation; the elastic recoil of the fibers is responsible for the return of the duct to normal size after relief of the obstruction.[31] In humans, the size of the common bile duct is largely determined by intraductal pressure. With increase in intraductal pressure, the common bile duct progressively dilates to a limit governed by the elastic properties of the ductal wall.[32] Some obstructive lesions affect elastic tone of the duct, creating irreversible damage and effectively converting the duct to a passive, or "floppy tube." On ultrasound, this duct may appear normal. On direct cholangiogram, the duct quickly dilates to abnormal size. It is postulated that in these, the elastic network is damaged or distorted and an actual "floppy duct" phenomenon develops. The discrepancies between individual static measurements of duct caliber underscore the need of assessment by other techniques.[31]

As with the gallbladder, there are congenital anomalies associated with the ducts. The bile ducts may have a variety of anomalous connections. There may be agenesis of all or a portion of the hepatic or common bile duct. Agenesis, or severe stenosis, is usually discovered shortly after birth and is incompatible with life.[8]

GALLBLADDER ABNORMALITIES

Normally, the gallbladder is an elongated, smoothly marginated, anechoic structure in the right upper quadrant. Its anterior wall is a single thin, strongly reflective structure. Its posterior wall is difficult to evaluate because of sound transmission and the fact that it is in contact with the bowel. After a fatty meal, 69 percent of gallbladders demonstrate complete contraction, with 31 percent demonstrating incomplete contraction. The most striking finding of a well-contracted gallbladder is its appearance, which changes from a single to a double

concentric structure with three components: (1) a strongly reflective outer contour, (2) a poorly reflective inner contour, and (3) an anechoic area between both[14] (Fig. 2-12).

The gallbladder, as a fluid-filled structure, is an ideal sonographic subject. The ultrasound evaluation of the gallbladder has become more sophisticated with the advances in technology and an increased understanding of sonographic appearances of various gallbladder disease processes. In evaluating the gallbladder for abnormalities, one must search for more than just gallstones; the gallbladder should be evaluated for size, wall thickness, intraluminal echopattern, and pericholecystic area. In addition, one must recognize the limitations of the nonspecific ultrasound findings; often ultrasound may be used as an adjunct with other imaging modalities, specifically hepatobiliary nuclear medicine.[33]

Gallstones

There is a 10 to 20 percent incidence of gallstones in adults. The occurrence increases progressively and reaches a peak in the sixth and seventh decade. It is more common in females than males with a 4:1 ratio. It has been said that the perfect candidate for gallstones is "fat, fertile, female, and forty." There is a predisposition for the formation of pigment stones in biliary infection, alcoholic cirrhosis, and anemias characterized by abnormal hemolysis and increased production of bilirubin pigment.[8]

The pathogenesis for gallstones is varied depending on the type. There is an increased risk of cholesterol stones in patients with ileal disease or ileal resection, females receiving estrogens, intestinal bypass for morbid obesity, and type IV hyperlipidemia, as well as obesity, pregnancy, diabetes, and clofibrate therapy. The three most important factors affecting gallstone formation are abnormal bile composition, stasis, and infection. The abnormalities of composition of the bile appear to be the most important.[8]

Gallstone formation occurs in three stages: (1) formation of saturated bile, (2) nucleation (initiation of stone formation), and (3) growth of the gallstone to a detectable size. Inflammation can be caused by chemical irritation secondary to alteration in bile caused by invasion of bacteria. Stasis may result from obstruction to outflow, which predisposes to infection.[8]

Gallstone composition is variable. They may be composed of cholesterol, calcium bilirubinate (pigment stones), and calcium carbonate. Most are either bilirubin or cholesterol. Pure calcium carbonate stones are very rare. Cholesterol stones are usually mixtures of cholesterol with pigment and carbonate.[8] Pure cholesterol stones represent 10 percent of all stones. Calcium bilirubinate stones (pigment stones) are less common than pure cholesterol in the Western countries but are more common in the Asiatic ones. Pure calcium carbonate stones are the rarest of stones. Ninety percent of all gallstones are mixed or combined. Mixed stones are those having varying proportions of the three stone-forming constituents. Combined stones have a central core or external layer that is pure, with the remainder being mixed.[8]

The clinical implications of gallstones are varied. In 80 percent of cases, the gallbladder stones evoke no clinical manifestations. The most serious consequence of calculous disease is obstruction of the cystic duct or common bile duct. With complete blockage of the cystic duct, hydrops of the gallbladder results. In calculous obstruction, the gallbladder is often not distended and may be small (gallbladder fibrotic); in neoplastic obstruction of the common bile duct, an association with chronic cholecystitis is less likely and so continual formation of bile results in a distended gallbladder (Courvoisier's law). Calculous obstruction of the cystic or common bile duct predisposes to bacterial infection, which may lead to cholangitis and ascending cholangitis. Presumably, stasis, distention of the biliary system, impaired lymphatic drainage and vascular supply, and chemical irritation are operative factors. Rarely, in patients with gallstones and acute inflammatory disease, a stone erodes through the gallbladder wall and adherent intestinal loop to create a cholecystointestinal fistula. Most stones pass unnoticed through the gastrointestinal tract. Large ones, however, may impact at the ileocecal valve, resulting in gallstone ileus. There is a high incidence (65 to 95 percent) of stones associated with a cancerous gallbladder.[8]

ULTRASOUND PROPERTIES

Several studies have been performed with ultrasound to evaluate the sonographic characteristics of gallstones. Stones have been shown to be echodense on ultrasound with a posterior acoustic shadow[34–37] (Fig. 2-14). It has been shown that all stones larger than 3 mm demonstrate a shadow.[38,39] This acoustic shadow does not relate to the calcium content of the stone, shape, surface characteristics, or specific gravity of the stone.[38,39] The shadow is due to the high reflectivity of the near surface of the gallstone and absorption by the stone of the remainder of the sound that is reflected.[10] Further, it has been shown that stones containing greater than 88 percent cholesterol float and produce a shadow.[39] If, however, nonshadowing echogenic foci that are smaller than 5 mm are seen in the gallbladder, 81 percent of these will represent stones[40] (Fig. 2-15). In addition, any echogenic structure within the gallbladder lumen that causes a posterior shadow and moves with gravity will be a gallstone in 100 percent of cases.[40,41]

The ability to demonstrate the acoustic shadow is highly dependent on the relationship between the stone and the acoustic beam.[10,35,42–45] If the transducer is situated such that the peripheral edge of the acoustic beam encounters the stone, no shadow is demonstrated. If sound waves at or near the center or focal zone of the beam strike the same stone, and the stone is large in comparison to the beam width or wavelength employed, an acoustic shadow will be easily perceived[42,44] (Fig. 2-16).

Using in vivo and in vitro techniques, stones with higher attenuation have been shown to show the most

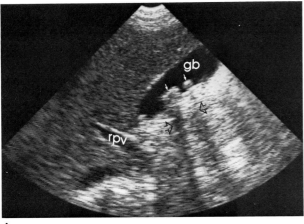

A

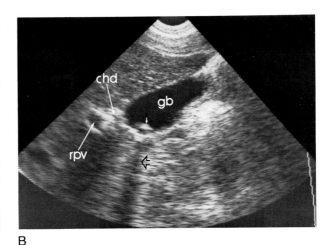

B

Fig. 2-14. Gallstones, typical. Longitudinal left lateral decubitus scans in two different patients **(A,B)**. Echodense stones (arrows) are seen in the dependent portion of the gallbladder *(gb)* with associated posterior acoustic shadowing (open arrows). (*rpv,* right portal vein; *chd,* common hepatic duct.)

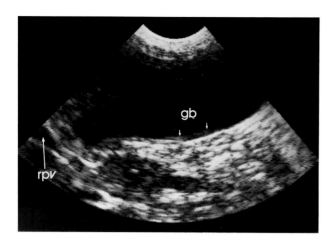

Fig. 2-15. Gallstones, nonshadowing. Longitudinal left lateral decubitus scan. Multiple small echodensities (arrows) are seen within the dependent portion of the gallbladder *(gb)*. There is no associated shadow. At surgery, small stones (2 to 4 mm) were found. *(rpv,* right portal vein.) (From Durrell CA III, Vincent LM, Mittelstaedt CA: Gallbladder ultrasonography in clinical context. p. 315. In Mueller PR (ed): Seminars in Ultrasound, CT and MR. Vol. 5 Grune and Stratton, Orlando, 1984.)

shadowing.[46] Attenuation is correlated with physical structure; more highly attenuating stones tend to have the largest percentage of crystalline material, a larger average crystal size, and more rigid structure. Use of a higher frequency transducer is recommended if no shadow is demonstrated (Fig. 2-17). A shadow occurs when the attenuation of the stone is greater than that of an equivalent amount of tissue. The difference increases

with frequency; so a greater shadow is seen with a higher frequency.[46] The high attenuation of the gallstone results in the formation of a shadow at ultrasound. The shadow is best seen when the stone lies within the focal zone of the transducer and is large in comparison to the beam width or wavelength employed.[44]

Some investigators have evaluated the characteristics of the acoustic shadow associated with gallstones.[47] The shadow is described as a "clean shadow" if there are distinct margins and a lack of reverberation echoes (Fig. 2-18). Because calcification in stones reflects a much larger percent of the incident sound beam, reverberation echoes are seen within this shadow. The heavier the calcification, the stronger the reverberations are within this shadow (Fig. 2-19). The lack of reverberation echoes does not exclude calcification because its production is dependent on the size and shape of the stone and its orientation to the sound beam. The in vitro ultrasound compositional analysis of stones for detection of calcification might influence the therapeutic decision regarding selection of patients for chemodexycholic acid therapy for stone dissolution.[47]

At times it may be difficult to differentiate the acoustic shadow due to calculi from that due to gas collections. In vitro, the acoustic shadows distal to calculi contain significantly fewer echoes and are more sharply defined than those distal to gas collection (Figs. 2-14, 2-18, and 2-19). Artifactual reverberation echoes within the acoustic shadows distal to gas collection result from virtually total sound reflection at tissue-air interfaces, whereas shadows distal to calculi are primarily due to sound absorption[48] (Fig. 2-20).

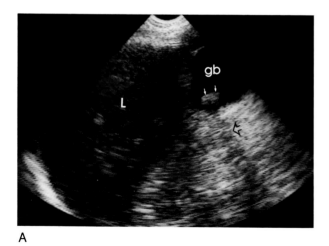 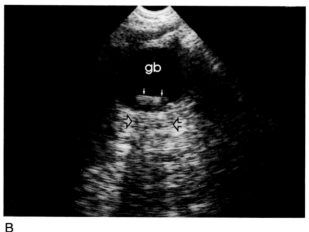

A   B

Fig. 2-16. Gallstone, shadow. **(A)** Longitudinal scan. An echodense gallstone (arrows) is seen within the dependent portion of the gallbladder *(gb).* A shadow (open arrow) is barely visible. The transducer is situated such that the peripheral edge of the acoustic beam encounters the stone and little shadowing is demonstrated. (*L*, liver.) **(B)** Longitudinal scan, same case as **(A).** The stone (arrows) is near the center or focal zone of the sound beam, so a well-defined shadow (open arrows) is produced. (*gb*, gallbladder.)

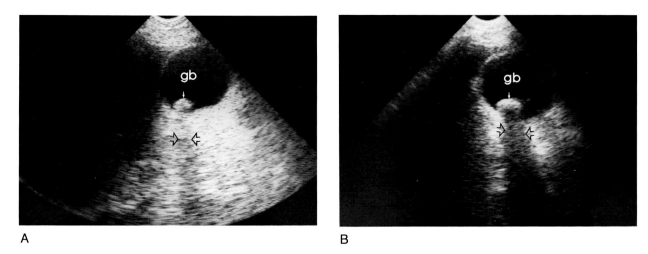

A B

Fig. 2-17. Gallstone, shadow. In both of these longitudinal scans **(A,B)** of the gallbladder *(gb)*, the stone (arrows) is within the focal zone of the transducer. The shadowing (open arrows) is not as well defined in **(A)** as in **(B)**. The scan **(A)** was performed with a 3 MHz transducer and scan **(B)** with the well-defined shadow was performed with a 5 MHz scanhead.

There are several criteria that must be met to diagnose gallstones clinically on an ultrasound scan. The gallbladder must be well visualized in at least two body positions and two scan planes. Intraluminal gallbladder densities that move with change in body position should be seen. These densities must shadow and/or move rapidly with change in body position.[33,49,50] (Figs. 2-14 to 2-19).

At times, these intraluminal densities may be seen to float. If a patient has had a recent oral cholecystogram, the contrast raises the specific gravity of the bile and causes this phenomenon (Figs. 2-21 and 2-22). The stones seek a level where their specific gravity equals that of the mixture of bile and contrast.[51,52] These "floating" gallstones may be difficult to see, as they will be quite superficial. Some investigators suggest the use of an oral cholecystogram agent in conjunction with ultrasound in cases where the ultrasound scans are equivocal; this combination facilitates the demonstration of small cholesterol stones by inducing the phenomenon of layering.[52] The identification of floating gallstones is a favorable indicator for dissolution therapy.[52] Floating stones may also be seen with gas-containing stones.[53] Fissuring preferentially takes place in rapidly formed stones and can proceed eventually to complete rupture of a stone

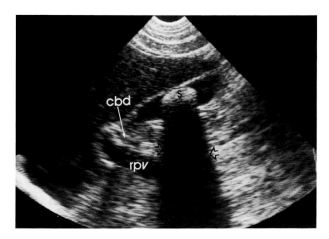

Fig. 2-18. Gallstone, "clean shadow". Slightly oblique longitudinal left lateral decubitus scan. The shadow associated with this gallstone *(s)* has distinct margins (open arrows) and lacks reverberation echoes. *(rpv,* right portal vein; *cbd,* common bile duct.)

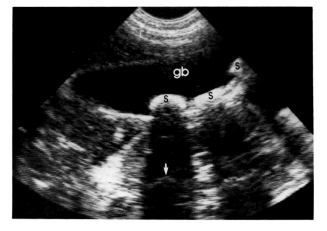

Fig. 2-19. Gallstone, reverberations in shadow. Longitudinal scan. With the central gallstone *(s),* there are reverberations (arrow) within the acoustic shadow. The heavier the calcification, the stronger the reverberations are within the shadow. There are many other stones *(s)* that are not in the center of the sound beam. *(gb,* gallbladder.)

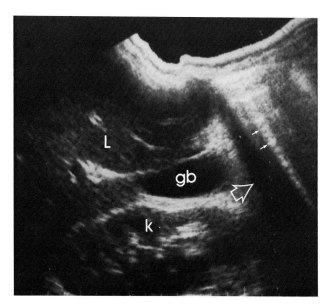

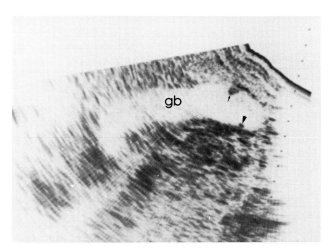

Fig. 2-20. Gas shadow. Longitudinal scan. The shadow (open arrow) distal to this gas collection results from a virtually total sound reflection at the tissue-air interface, whereas shadows distal to calculi are primarily due to sound absorption. As such, there are artifactual reverberation echoes (small arrows) within the gas shadow. (*gb,* gallbladder; *L,* liver; *k,* right kidney.)

into smaller fragments. Gas may be generated by low pressure in the stone due to fissuring, out of the small amount of fluid that is present in the stone. At ultrasound, the gas produces floating stones in a nonopacified gallbladder[53] (Fig. 2-23). In addition, there has been a report of food particles in the gallbladder mimicking cholelithiasis in a patient with a cholecystojejunostomy.[54]

Fig. 2-22. Floating gallstone. Longitudinal supine scan demonstrates an echodense stone (arrow) that is seen floating in the gallbladder *(gb)* fundus. It moved at real-time scan. There is also a nonfloating stone (arrowhead).

GALLBLADDER NECK/CYSTIC DUCT STONE

Ultrasound is uniformly successful in the diagnosis of impacted stones within the gallbladder neck.[54] A typical appearance is seen: curved, highly reflective intraluminal echoes with a prominent acoustic shadow[55] (Fig. 2-24). To document that the stone is indeed impacted, the patient is rescanned in the upright position and then in the supine and/or decubitus position. If the stone is impacted, there will be no apparent change in its position (Figs. 2-24 and 2-25).

In contrast to scanning for gallbladder neck stones, ultrasound is uniformly unsuccessful in the diagnosis of

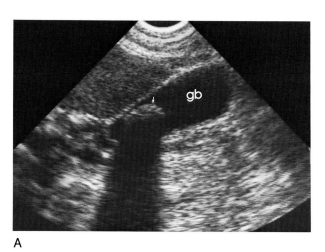

A

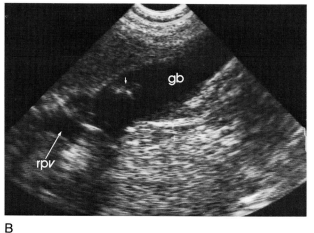

B

Fig. 2-21. Floating gallstone. Left lateral decubitus longitudinal scans **(A,B).** An echodense gallstone (arrow) is noted to be floating. This patient had taken an oral cholecystographic agent. The contrast is thought to raise the specific gravity of the bile causing the stone to float. The associated acoustic shadowing is "clean" in **(A)** but not well seen in **(B)**; on **(B)**, the sound beam is only visualizing the edge of the stone. (*rpv,* right portal vein; *gb,* gallbladder.)

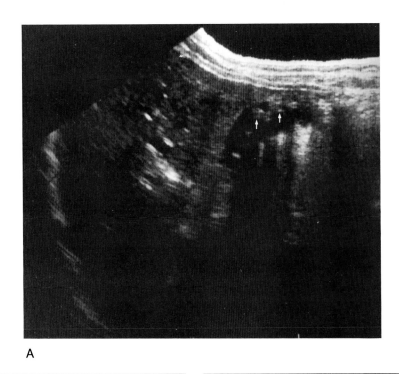

A

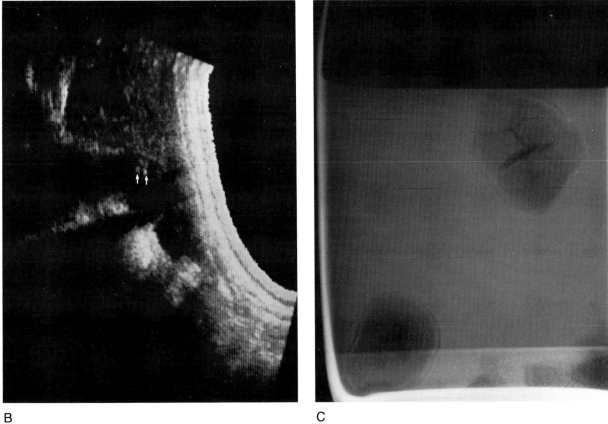

B   C

Fig. 2-23. Fissured gallstones. (**A**) Longitudinal supine scan. Multiple floating stones (arrows) are present. (**B**) Longitudinal erect scan. Multiple floating and sedimentary stones (arrows) are seen. (**C**) Radiograph with horizontal beam of the gallstones in a container filled with saline (specific gravity is 1.006). One stone is floating under the surface and one is lying on the bottom. (From Strijk SP, Boetes C, Rosenbusch G: Floating stones in a nonopacified gallbladder: Ultrasonographic sign of gas-containing gallstones. Gastrointest Radiol 6:261, 1981.)

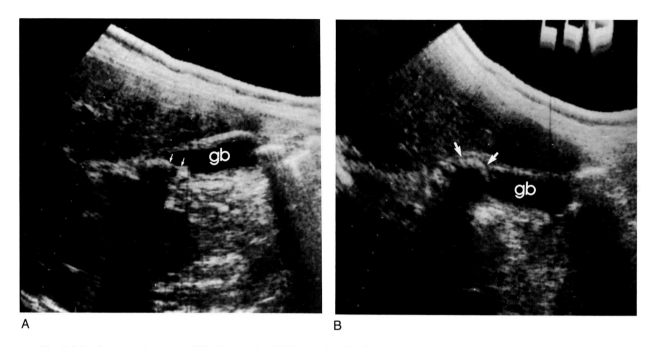

A   B

Fig. 2-24.   Impacted stone, gallbladder neck. **(A)** Supine longitudinal scan. A gallstone (arrows) is seen in the area of the gallbladder *(gb)* neck. **(B)** Left lateral decubitus longitudinal scan. The stone (arrows) has not moved, which is consistent with an impacted stone. On hepatobiliary nuclear medicine scan at 45 minutes following injection, isotope was seen in the common bile duct, gut, and duodenum, but not in the gallbladder (*gb*). This is consistent with cystic duct obstruction.

impacted stones in the cystic duct.[55] The normal cystic duct is not usually seen at ultrasound. Even when enlarged and containing an impacted stone, the cystic duct does not contain enough bile surrounding the stone to create the acoustic contrast necessary for definitive visualization.[55] There are a number of nonbiliary structures that can mimic a cystic duct stone: echogenic fat in the porta hepatis, duodenal gas, refractive shadow from the valves of Heister, and calcification in masses in the porta hepatis.[55] If a cystic duct stone is suspected, hepatobiliary nuclear medicine is recommended.

Mirizzi syndrome is an uncommon, surgically correc-

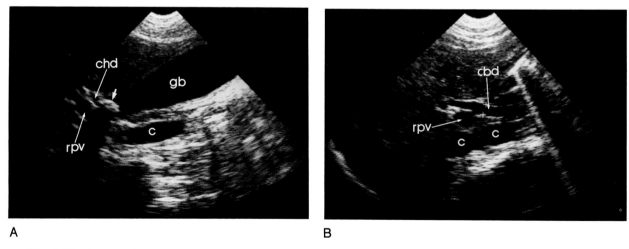

A   B

Fig. 2-25.   Impacted stone, gallbladder neck. **(A)** Longitudinal supine scan. A stone (arrow) is seen in the area of the gallbladder *(gb)* neck. It does not move with change in position. (*chd,* common hepatic duct; *rpv,* right portal vein; *c,* inferior vena cava.) **(B)** Oblique long axis view of the common bile duct *(cbd)*. It was noted to be dilated. (*c,* inferior vena cava; *rpv,* right portal vein.)

table cause of extrahepatic obstruction.[56-58] The features of this syndrome include (1) presence of an impacted stone in the cystic duct, cystic duct remnant, or gallbladder neck; (2) partial mechanical obstruction of the common hepatic duct by compression or by resulting inflammatory reaction around the impacted stone; and (3) sequelae of jaundice, recurrent cholangitis, formation of biliobiliary fistulas, or cholangitic cirrhosis.[56-58] The typical signs include dilatation of the common hepatic duct above the level of the gallstone impacted in the cystic duct, with a normal duct width below the stone.[57] In most cases, there is an anomalous insertion of the cystic duct or gallbladder neck allowing a parallel arrangement of the cystic duct adjacent to the common hepatic duct.[56,58] When ultrasound demonstrates two parallel tubular structures in the position of the common bile duct, the diagnosis should be suggested.[58] The differential diagnosis based on visualization of a smooth, generally curved segmental stenosis of the common hepatic duct would include metastatic adenopathy in the porta, gallbladder carcinoma, focal sclerosing cholangitis, primary liver tumor, or tumor of the duct. In the proper situation, the ultrasound appearance of dilated intrahepatic ducts, normal caliber common bile duct, and stone in the neck of the gallbladder or cystic duct should suggest the diagnosis[56-58] (Figure 2-26). It is important to exclude the presence of a mass in the porta hepatis or secondary signs of malignancy as possibilities. Direct cholangiography is often necessary because cholecystobiliary fistula secondary to stone penetration into the common bile duct can be demonstrated by only cholangiography.[57] The main features of Mirizzi syndrome at direct cholangiography include partial common hepatic duct obstruction due to either external compression at the level of the cystic duct or to the partly or completely

eroded calculus.[57] The findings may mimic cholangiocarcinoma.

CONTRACTED OR NONVISUALIZED GALLBLADDER

In some instances, gallstones may prevent ultrasound visualization of the gallbladder. In 15 to 25 percent of patients with stones, there is gallbladder nonvisualization.[59] If many strong echoes that cast a large shadow are seen in the gallbladder area, the possibility of gallbladder stones is great (Fig. 2-27). This may represent a gallbladder that is contracted or simply packed with stones; the anterior layer of stones casts a shadow that prevents the visualization of the gallbladder.[60] A specific image may also be observed — that of two parallel arcuate echogenic lines separated by a thin anechoic space with distal acoustic shadowing[59,61] (Fig. 2-28). The proximal arc represents the near wall of the gallbladder, the anechoic space is bile, and the distal arc is secondary to gallstones. This "double arc" sign or "WES triad" (W, the wall; E, the stone; and S, the shadow) can increase the confidence of the examiner. These findings help to differentiate the gallbladder from a bowel loop.[61] Care must be taken in such cases to examine the gallbladder in various body positions, particularly the left lateral decubitus position. An echogenic focus and an associated shadow that persist in the same location are more evidence suggestive of gallstones.[62] In addition, the patient may be examined on a subsequent day. If the findings persist, a diagnosis of cholelithiasis may be made.

There are numerous causes of nonvisualization of a gallbladder on ultrasound. Gallbladder disease may obliterate the lumen; the patient may not be truly fasting; there may be obstruction of the biliary tree proximal to

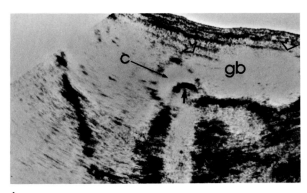

A

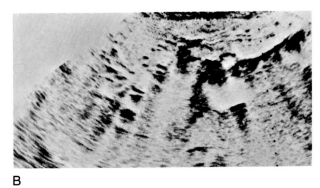

B

Fig. 2-26. Mirizzi syndrome. (A) Longitudinal scan. A distended gallbladder (gb, open arrows) is seen, as well as a large stone (arrow) within the dilated cystic duct (c). (B) Transverse scan of the liver demonstrating intrahepatic biliary dilatation. The common bile duct was of normal caliber. (From Jackson VP, Lappas JC: Sonography of the Mirizzi syndrome. J Ultrasound Med 3:281, 1984.)

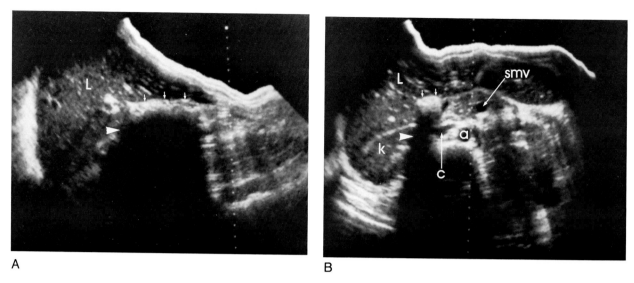

Fig. 2-27. Contracted gallbladder. Longitudinal **(A)** and transverse **(B)** views of the right upper quadrant demonstrate a strongly echogenic structure (arrows) in the gallbladder fossa. No gallbladder lumen is seen. There is posterior acoustic shadowing (arrowhead). (*k*, right kidney; *L*, liver; *c*, inferior vena cava; *a*, aorta; *smv*, superior mesenteric vein.)

the cystic duct; and, rarely, there may be congenital absence of the gallbladder. The nonvisualization may also be due to a small gallbladder, a technical error, or floating stones containing gas.[63] Fissuring preferentially takes place in rapidly formed stones and can proceed eventually to complete rupture of the stone into smaller fragments that can pass. The gas in the stones causes them to float. The gas is generated by low pressure in the stone due to fissuring, out of the small amount of fluid that is present in the stone.[53]

PORCELAIN GALLBLADDER

The incidence of calcification in the gallbladder wall is 0.6 to 0.8 percent of cholecystectomy specimens.[64] It is associated with stones in 95 percent of cases and is more common in females, with a 5:1 female-to-male ratio. The pathogenesis is controversial. Some speculate that obstruction of the cystic duct leads to mucosal precipitation of calcium carbonate salts, which in turn causes bile to stagnate in the gallbladder. Others feel the calcium is a

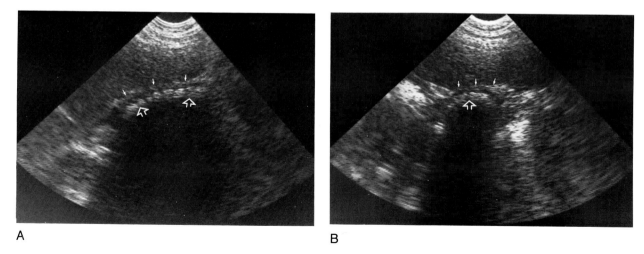

Fig. 2-28. Double arc sign or WES triad. Longitudinal **(A)** and transverse **(B)** scans. The echogenic anterior line (small arrows) represents the anterior wall of the gallbladder with the second echogenic arc (open arrows) representing stones. A distal shadow is seen. (Fig. A from Durrell CA III, Vincent LM, Mittelstaedt CA: Gallbladder ultrasonography in clinical context. p. 315. In Mueller PR (ed): Seminars in Ultrasound, CT and MR. Vol. 5, Grune and Stratton, Orlando, 1984.)

dystrophic process resulting from chronic low-grade infection and/or compromised circulation due to the impacted cystic duct stone resulting in hemorrhage, scarring, and hyalinization of the wall, which in turn provide the matrix for deposition of lime salts. The third theory is that chronic irritation of the wall by a stone or other foreign body produces the calcification.[64]

Histologically, there are two types of calcification.[64] In one type, there is a continuous broad band of calcification within the muscularis, which is seen on radiographs as a large plaque-like area. The second type includes numerous calcified microliths scattered diffusely throughout the mucosa and submucosa, localized within the glandular spaces and in the Rokitansky-Aschoff sinuses. On radiographs, this type appears as granular and plaque-like calcifications. Between 11 and 33 percent of carcinomas of the gallbladder have calcification in the wall.

There are several patterns of the porcelain gallbladder seen on ultrasound.[64] A hyperechoic semilunar structure with a posterior acoustic shadow may be seen (Fig. 2-29). This may simulate a stone-filled gallbladder devoid of bile. Instead, a biconvex curvilinear echogenic structure with variable acoustic shadowing may be seen (Fig. 2-30), or irregular clumps of echoes with posterior acoustic shadowing may be demonstrated.[64]

CHOLELITHIASIS IN CHILDREN

When children develop cholelithiasis, there is usually a prior predisposing disease or underlying circumstance. Possible predisposing diseases are hemolytic anemia,

thalassemia, cystic fibrosis, metabolic disease, liver disease, neonatal septicemia, Crohn's disease, and cardiac disease. Possible underlying circumstances are prior orthopedic surgery, chemotherapy, postpartum state, and prior bowel resection or malabsorption.[49,65,66] Two mechanisms are involved in cholelithiasis in children: interruption of the enterohepatic circulation of bile salts and bile stasis.[49] Bile is a supersaturated solution of bilirubin and cholesterol held in balance by the presence of bile salts and phospholipids. Factors such as increased secretion of cholesterol and bilirubin, decreased secretion of bile salts and phospholipids, and damage to biliary mucosa by inflammation, stasis, or abnormal pH level can alter this balance and initiate the formation of calculi. Developing gallstones require a period in which incipient microliths increase in size without being discharged from the biliary tree, implying impairment of gallbladder contractility.[66] In one series, cholesterol stones were found most commonly; pigmented stones were found less commonly.[66]

One study done to evaluate the incidence of gallstones in children found an apparent increase. In 55 percent of these cases, there was an underlying predisposing disease or circumstance. The rest did not have predisposing factors. It is felt that if a child is at high risk for gallstones, ultrasound is mandatory in order to prevent complications of unrecognized gallstones.[49]

Although cholelithiasis is rare in the newborn, it has been associated with total parenteral nutrition, septicemia, and furosemide therapy.[49,67,68] These patients have respiratory distress syndrome complicated by bronchopulmonary dysplasia and are treated with assisted venti-

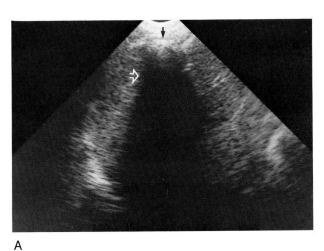

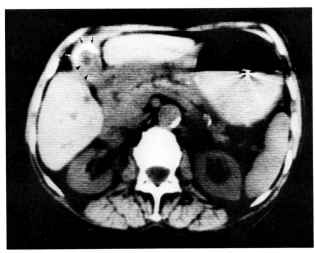

A
B

Fig. 2-29. Porcelain gallbladder. **(A)** Longitudinal real-time scan. A dense line (black arrow) is seen in the gallbladder fossa with acoustic shadowing (open arrow). This finding persisted in various body positions. **(B)** CT scan. The calcification (small arrows) within the gallbladder wall is seen, as well as stones (arrowheads).

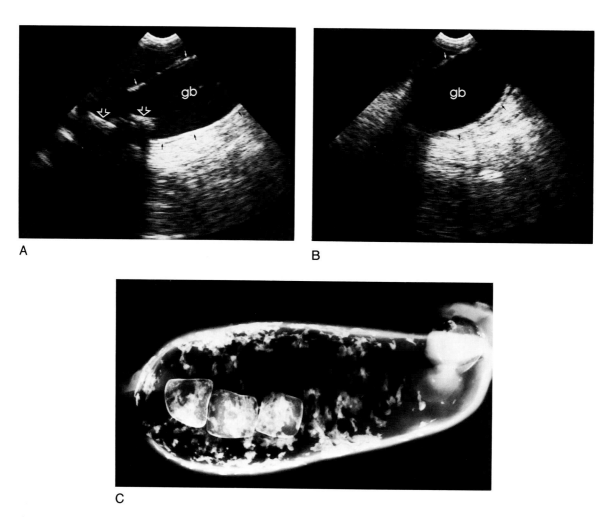

Fig. 2-30. Porcelain gallbladder. Longitudinal real-time scans of a patient with a palpable pelvic mass **(A,B)**. The gallbladder *(gb)* wall (small arrows) appears denser than usual. There are gallstones (open arrows) associated. The palpated mass was the gallbladder. **(C)** Specimen radiograph. Note the stones and the dense wall to the gallbladder. (Figs. A&C from Durrell CA III, Vincent LM, Mittelstaedt CA: Gallbladder ultrasonography in clinical context. p. 315. In Mueller PR (ed): Seminars in Ultrasound, CT and MR. Vol. 5, Grune and Stratton, Orlando, 1984.)

lation, total parenteral nutrition, and furosemide. In these cases, it is theorized that the patients on total parenteral nutrition are deprived of the normal stimulatory effect, which leads to stasis within the biliary system. In addition, there is immaturity of the hepatocellular enzyme system with disturbance in the transport of conjugated bilirubin, which impairs bile secretion. Furosemide enhances the excretion of calcium into the urine. It is not known whether it has similar actions on bile.[67]

In sickle cell anemia, there is a 27 to 30 percent incidence of gallstones.[69,70] This is in contrast to the range of 0.1 to 0.28 percent in the average child population.[71] The incidence of gallstones appears to increase significantly with age. In addition, these patients appear to have a significantly higher mean bilirubin level.[70] In one series, it was found that one third of the patients had stones,

with one fifth demonstrating sludge.[72] Patients with thalassemia major also have an increased incidence of gallstones. One series reported an incidence of 23 percent in these patients.[71]

Sludge

Echogenic bile or sludge is identified in many cases. The source of the echoes in the biliary sludge particles is predominantly pigment granules with lesser amounts of cholesterol crystals.[73] The sludge consists mainly of calcium bilirubinate.[73] Echogenic bile is most often found in patients with extrahepatic biliary obstruction and acute and chronic cholecystitis, and patients undergoing a fast or hyperalimentation.[73,74] The common factor in all instances is stasis of bile in the gallbladder.

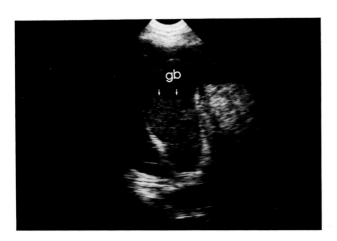

Fig. 2-31. Gallbladder sludge. Transverse left lateral decubitus scan. There is a fluid-fluid level (arrows) within the gallbladder *(gb)* with the denser layer located posteriorly. (From Durrell CA III, Vincent LM, Mittelstaedt CA: Gallbladder ultrasonography in clinical context. p. 315. In Mueller PR (ed): Seminars in Ultrasound, CT and MR. Vol. 5, Grune and Stratton, Orlando, 1984.)

Sludge is visualized as nonshadowing low-amplitude echoes that layer in the dependent part of the gallbladder.[75] Because of its high-specific gravity, sludge forms a fluid-fluid level that moves slowly with change in patient position[74] (Fig. 2-31). The straight horizontal line's nondependence on receiver gain and lack of change in height of debris between transverse and longitudinal scans are important clues that help differentiate true sludge from debris due to slice-thickness artifact.[74]

The clinical implications of sludge are difficult to assess. When the gallbladder bile contains cholesterol crystals or calcium bilirubinate granules in moderate to large amounts, there is a strong correlation with the presence of gallstones or other abnormalities such as cholesterolosis.[73] It can, however, be seen in normal individuals.[73] Sludge is an indicator of abnormal biliary dynamics and a possible precursor to cholecystitis.[76] One cannot distinguish thick bile from multiple nonshadowing calculi, pus, cholesteral crystals, and possibly abnormal mucous in the gallbladder.[75]

"Pseudosludge" is indistinguishable from true sludge and is seen as low-amplitude echoes in the posterior portion of the gallbladder.[76] Its appearance is created by a beam averaging effect or "partial-volume phenomenon" at the diverging portion of the ultrasound beam. The overall appearance is due to an averaging of echoes from the liver adjacent to the gallbladder, containing normally anechoic bile. It must be differentiated from sedimented calcium bilirubinate granules and cholesterol crystals. On the decubitus view, the location of the sludge changes to the dependent portion of the gallbladder. The interface of the sludge and the bile is oblique to the beam while the interface of the pseudosludge remains perpendicular to the beam.[76]

Many entities may simulate sludge. Blood seen with hematobilia may cause echogenic bile[77] (Fig. 2-32). Hemobilia or bleeding into the biliary tree is associated with a variety of disorders among which are rupture of a hepatic artery aneurysm, blunt abdominal trauma, and, rarely, percutaneous liver biopsy.[78] As with any echogenic foci in the gallbladder lumen, the differential diagnosis includes stone, tumor, polyp, and sludge. Early diagnosis of hemobilia may be lifesaving, as bleeding may be intermittent and massive hemorrhage may not

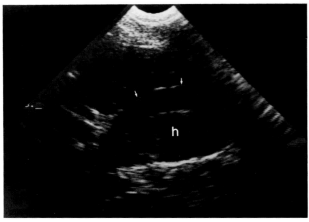

A

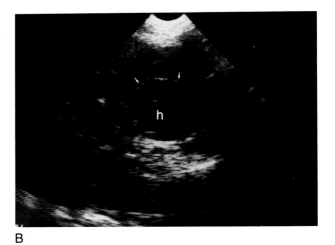

B

Fig. 2-32. Hematobilia. Longitudinal **(A)** and transverse **(B)** real-time scans demonstrate a smooth, ovoid, relatively hypoechoic mass within the gallbladder lumen, representing a hematoma *(h)*. The gallbladder wall (arrows) is of normal caliber and the remaining portion of the gallbladder lumen is echofree. (From Grant EG, Smirniotopoulos JG: Intraluminal gallbladder hematoma: Sonographic evidence of hemobilila. J Clin Ultrasound 11:507, 1983.)

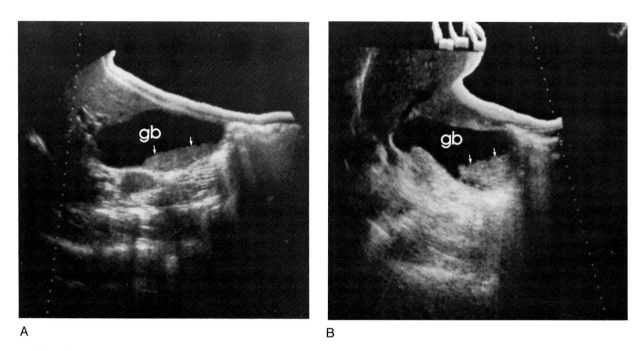

A   B

Fig. 2-33. Gallbladder mass, sludge. **(A)** Longitudinal supine static scan. A layer of sludge (arrows) is seen posteriorly within the gallbladder *(gb)*. **(B)** Left lateral decubitus longitudinal scan. A mass effect (arrows) is produced by the sludge, which has not as yet layered out after the change in body position *(gb,* gallbladder.)

occur until weeks following biopsy. Parasitic infestation, blood clot, and aggregate material containing pus or sludge may be seen.[79] These may produce mobile intraluminal gallbladder masses.

At times biliary sludge may simulate tumor. Sludge

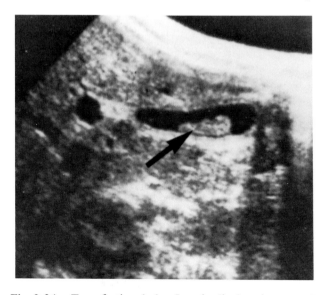

Fig. 2-34. Tumefactive sludge. Longitudinal supine scan. A polypoid mass (arrow) is seen within the lumen of the gallbladder. Repeat examination one day later demonstrated that the mass was no longer present. (From Fakhry J: Sonography of tumefactive biliary sludge. AJR 139:717, © Am Roent Ray Soc, 1982.)

layers within the gallbladder, due to thick or inspissated bile, multiple tiny nonshadowing calculi, pigment granules, or cholesterol crystal formation, hemobilia, or purulent bile. A mass effect may be seen due to temporary clumping of highly viscous material resulting from bile stasis[74,80] (Fig. 2-33). Upon reexamination, the "mass" is seen to disappear further confirming the "pseudotumor" nature.[74] At times, the gallbladder full of sludge may simulate a solid mass.[81] This has been described in a Courvoisier gallbladder with a long duration of obstruction. "Tumefactive biliary sludge" and "sludge balls" are echogenic masses that more closely resemble masses or stones than sludge[82] (Figs. 2-34 and 2-35). These nonshadowing sludge balls eventually attenuate enough sound to cause a distal shadow and prove to be calculi.

The sonographic appearance of milk of calcium bile has been described by several authors.[83,84] Pathologically, the gallbladder appears chronically inflammed, functionless, and contains thickened bile with a high calcium content (usually as calcium carbonate). The calcium carbonate can be deposited on already existing stones that are commonly associated with this condition, or can settle out as semifluid or a putty-like mass.[84] There is cystic duct obstruction in most cases. Clinically, this entity is indistinguishable from chronic cholecystitis. Stratification of bile creates a layering effect on ultrasound with two zones separated by a fluid-fluid level. The less dependent fraction has a lower specific gravity and appears lucent, simulating normal bile (Fig.

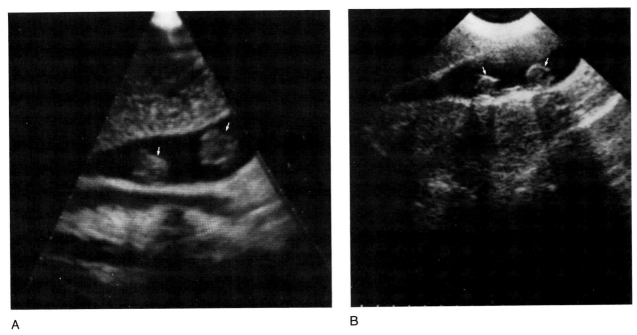

A   B

Fig. 2-35. Tumefactive sludge. **(A)** Longitudinal real-time scan with two nonshadowing "sludge balls" (arrows). **(B)** Longitudinal real-time scan 2 years after **(A)**, showing clear-cut shadowing deep to the masses (arrows). At surgery, these were found to be gallstones, largely aggregrations of calcium bilirubinate crystals with a much smaller component of cholesterol crystals. The sludge ball matrix was composed of approximately 5-percent calcium. (From Britten JS, Golding RH, Cooperberg PL: Sludge balls to gallstones. J Ultrasound Med 3:81, 1984.)

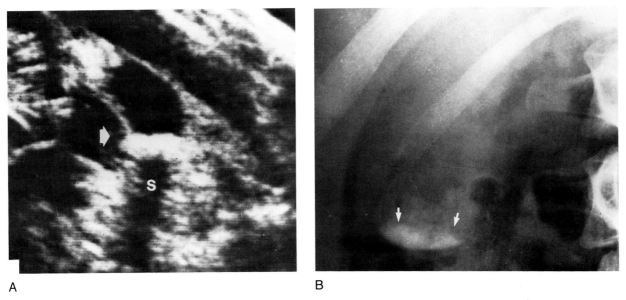

A   B

Fig. 2-36. Milk of calcium bile. **(A)** Transverse scan in the left lateral decubitus position. High-amplitude reflections (arrow) are demonstrated within the dependent portion of the gallbladder. Prominent posterior acoustic shadowing **(S)** is noted. **(B)** Upright radiograph of the right upper quadrant demonstrating the characteristic appearance of milk of calcium layering (arrows) within the dependent portion of the gallbladder. (From Chun GH, Deutsch AL, Scheible W: Sonographic findings in milk of calcium bile. Gastrointest Radiol 7:371, 1982.)

2-36). The dependent layer is dense, dissolved calcium and absorbs and reflects the sound causing a shadow. On ultrasound, the findings are similar to the floating gallstone.[83,84]

Distended Gallbladder

Occasionally in an adult or child, a distended gallbladder may cause the patient to present with a palpable mass.[85-87] This is seen while fasting and receiving parenteral hyperalimentation.[85,86] Ultrasound can quickly distinguish the gallbladder origin from other masses (Fig. 2-37).

Bile flow is controlled by the sphincter of Oddi. Under basal conditions and interdigestive periods, the sphincter of Oddi is closed and bile is diverted into the gallbladder. Neural and hormonal stimuli triggered by eating cause gallbladder emptying by simultaneously stimulating gallbladder contraction and relaxation of the sphincter of Oddi. During fasting, the lack of neural and hormonal stimuli on the biliary system results in the accumulation of large amounts of bile in the gallbladder.[85] Bile viscosity and the bile salt concentration are increased by water resorption and mucin secretion in the gallbladder.[86] The inspissated bile may not pass readily through the biliary tract and can cause either functional obstruction or dilatation secondary to stasis.[86]

Cholecystitis

Cholecystitis represents inflammation of the gallbladder, which may be acute or chronic. The acute stage is subdivided on the basis of the severity of the inflammatory response into acute supportive and gangrenous cholecystitis. There is a 70-percent incidence of cholecystitis in adults, but it does not occur in significant numbers until the midthirties and reaches a peak in the fifth and sixth decades. There is a female-to-male ratio of 3 : 1 with the typical clinical pattern being "female, fat, forty, and fertile."[8]

There are several factors that affect the pathogenesis of cholecystitis. These include chemical irritation by concentrated bile, bacterial infection, and pancreatic reflux.[8,88] Stones obstructing the cystic duct are implicated in 80 to 95 percent of cases of acute cholecystitis.[8,88] Venous or lymphatic stasis may play a contributory role in the chemical irritation; an impacted stone or extrinsic pressure may interfere with the blood supply of the gall-

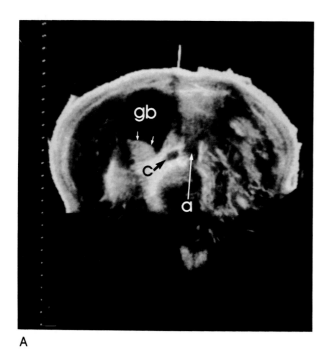

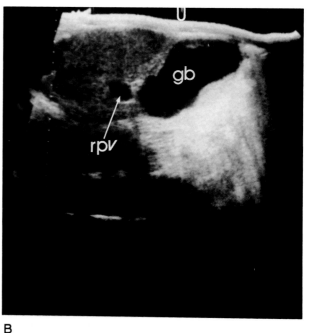

A   B

Fig. 2-37.   Distended gallbladder. Transverse (**A**) and longitudinal (**B**) scans of a patient with known hepatocellular disease and a palpable right abdominal mass. The "mass" was noted to be gallbladder *(gb)*, which was distended (note cm marks) and extended well below the level of the umbilicus *(U)*. There is sludge (arrows) present on the transverse scan at the level of the umbilicus. (*rpv*, right portal vein; *c*, inferior vena cava; *a*, aorta.) (Fig. A from Durrell CA III, Vincent LM, Mittelstaedt CA: Gallbladder ultrasound in clinical context. p. 315. In Mueller PR (ed): Seminars in Ultrasound, CT, and MR. Vol. 5, Grune and Stratton, Orlando, 1984.)

bladder and predispose to an acute inflammatory reaction. Such patients are prone to develop secondary bacterial infection. As such, there is a strong association (75 percent of acute cholecystitis) with bacterial infection.[88] Most commonly, the offending microorganisms are staphylococci, enterococci and gram-negative rods. Evidence for bacterial infection as the initiating etiologic factor is seen in a minority (5 to 10 percent) of patients, and there is usually concomitant septicemia or severe infection elsewhere in the body.[8] Pancreatic reflux also creates an inflammatory response. The evolution of chronic cholecystitis is very obscure but only rarely is it preceded by a well-defined bout of acute cholecystitis.[8]

Several distinct changes are seen pathologically in cholecystitis. In acute cholecystitis, the gallbladder is enlarged and tense with serosal hemorrhages and a serosal covering layered by fibrin, and at times a definite suppurative coagulated exudate.[8] There is increased vascular permeability with edema, extravasation of blood in the wall, and initially monocytic and later polymorphonuclear infiltration.[88] With acute inflammation, there is edema, leukocytic infiltration, vascular congestion, frank abscess formation, or gangrenous necrosis when vascular stasis complicates the edematous inflammatory response. In more severe cases, the mucous membrane is completely destroyed.[88] The pathologic changes depend on the severity of involvement and the length of the time process. The lumen may be filled with cloudy or turbid bile containing large amounts of fibrin and pus. If there is deposition of calcium within the gallbladder wall, a calcified gallbladder or porcelain gallbladder results.

With empyema of the gallbladder, there is pure pus in the lumen and gallstones are present in up to 80 percent of cases. The gallbladder wall is up to 10 times its normal thickness and has a rubbery consistency with edema fluid, exudate, and hemorrhage.

In gangrenous cholecystitis, the mucosa of the gallbladder is patchily or totally hyperemic with a necrotic surface, small ulcerations, or desquamation.[8,88] These ulcerations may penetrate the wall to give rise to a pericholecystic abscess or generalized peritonitis.

In chronic cholecystitis, the gallbladder is contracted, normal, or enlarged. The size depends on the balance between the development of fibrosis in the wall and the element of obstruction in the genesis of inflammation. Ninety percent of these patients have associated gallstones. The wall is variably thickened but rarely more than five times its normal size. In extreme cases, the wall is permeated by fibrosis seen with a considerable obliteration of the smooth musculature. Rokitansky-Aschoff sinuses are seen in 90 percent of chronically inflamed gallbladders. This is presumably because inflammatory damage to the wall predisposes to herniation of the lining epithelium.[8]

The clinical course associated with cholecystitis can be variable. Acute right upper quadrant pain may be referred to the shoulder when inflammatory exudate tracks up beneath the diaphragm causing irritation of the phrenic nerve. Fever, nausea, vomiting, leukocytosis, and a rigid abdominal wall may be seen. Jaundice is found in 25 percent of cases. Complications of an acute attack include pericholecystic abscess due to permeative infection or perforation of the gallbladder, generalized peritonitis, ascending cholangitis, liver abscess, subdiaphragmatic abscess and septicemia. In chronic cholecystitis, there is a vague insidious disorder with intolerance to fatty food, belching, postcibal epigastric distress, nausea, and vomiting. Complications of chronic cholecystitis and gallstones are a development of carcinoma of the gallbladder and passage of gallstones into the common bile duct.[8]

GALLBLADDER WALL THICKENING

One of the sonographic findings described with cholecystitis is an increase in the thickness of the gallbladder wall[16,89,90] (Figs. 2-38 to 2-41). A wall thickness of greater than 3.5 mm is said to be highly accurate in predicting disease.[91-95] If the wall is less than 3 mm, cholecystitis cannot be excluded.[95] However, no patients with acute cholecystitis have had a wall less than 5 mm thick.[96] The average gallbladder wall thickness has been reported to be less than or equal to 2 mm in 97 percent of asymptomatic patients without gallstones[97,98] (Fig. 2-1). It was noted to be 3 mm or greater in 45 percent of patients with stones in that same series.[98] Though increased wall thickness is a hallmark in chronic cholecystitis, only 55 percent of these patients were found to exhibit this at surgery in one series.[98]

It should be noted that wall thickness varies with transducer placement and angulation.[16,99] It is necessary to locate the true central long axis of the gallbladder for an accurate wall measurement. The wall measurement is most accurate if the region of the gallbladder wall perpendicular to the sound beam is measured[16] (Fig. 2-1). Measuring the anterior wall adjacent to the liver is most accurate, correlating within a millimeter to that found at surgery in 90 percent of cases.[16] Real-time ultrasound is the most accurate method of measuring the gallbladder wall.[99] Minor angulation or decentering of the sound beam with respect to the gallbladder's true central long axis can cause pseudothickening of the gallbladder wall.[99]

Though increased gallbladder wall thickness has been associated with cholecystitis, it has also been found to be associated with other abnormalities.[93,97] A thickened wall may be seen with hepatitis, ascites, alcoholic liver disease, hypoproteinemia, hypoalbuminemia, heart fail-

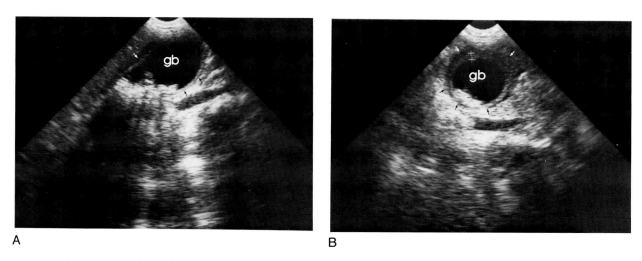

A   B

Fig. 2-38. Gallbladder wall thickening. Longitudinal (**A**) and transverse (**B**) scans of the gallbladder *(gb)* demonstrate wall thickening (arrows) as well as cholelithiasis. Note that it is easier to define the gallbladder wall laterally, medially, and superiorly.

ure, systemic venous hypertension, renal disease, multiple myeloma, and with physiologic thickening resulting from partial wall contraction.[92,97,100] Increased gallbladder wall thickness has also been seen with adenomyomatosis, gallbladder tumor, pericholecystic abscess, and, possibly, varices resulting from portal hypertension.[93] In hepatitis, the virus excreted into the biliary system may produce a mild pericholecystic inflammation.[92,100] There is a strong correlation between gallbladder wall thickening and hypoalbuminemia.[99] In one series, all patients with ascites demonstrated gallbladder wall thickening.[101] (Fig. 2-41). With ascites formation, the

plasma colloid oncotic pressure and portal venous pressure seem to influence the thickness.[102] Hypoproteinemic states probably produce this by a decreased intravascular osmotic effect just as in the bowel wall. With congestive heart failure, there is increased systemic and portal venous engorgement, which may produce edema of the wall. A thickened gallbladder wall may also be secondary to focal obstruction of the gallbladder lymphatic drainage by malignant lymphoma in portal lymph nodes.[103] Obstruction of the lymphatic drainage of an organ results in increased interstitial fluid and thickening of the tissues. This ultrasound appearance is

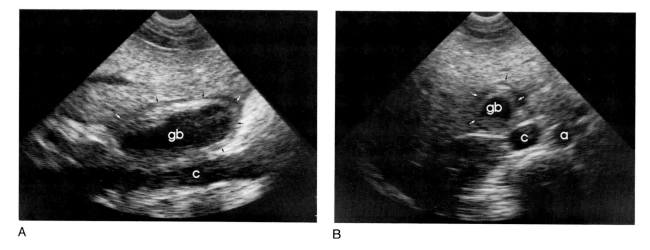

A   B

Fig. 2-39. Gallbladder "halo". Longitudinal (**A**) and transverse (**B**) scans of a patient with acute cholecystitis. A thickened gallbladder wall (arrows) is seen. There is an inner hyperreflective layer representing the lamina propria and muscularis with the outer poorly defined hypoechoic layer representing edema and cellular infiltration in the subserosa and adjacent liver. (*c*, inferior vena cava; *a*, aorta.) (From Durrell CA III, Vincent LM, Mittelstaedt CA: Gallbladder ultrasonography in clinical context. p. 315. In Mueller PR (ed): Seminars in Ultrasound, CT and MR. Vol. 5, Grune and Stratton, Orlando, 1984.)

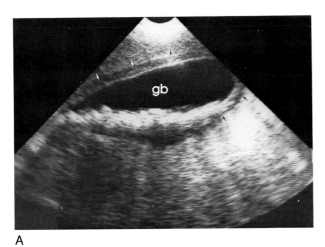
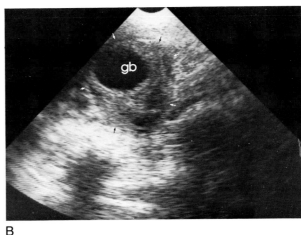

A   B

Fig. 2-40. Gallbladder wall thickening. Longitudinal (**A**) and transverse (**B**) left lateral decubitus scans of the gallbladder *(gb)* demonstrate echodense gallstones on (**A**) with wall thickening (arrows). The gallbladder wall is thickest in the fundic area as seen on (**B**). At surgery, there were changes of both acute and chronic cholecystitis with a hematoma in the wall of the fundus.

similar to that of hemorrhagic cholecystitis, a severe inflammatory process involving the gallbladder wall, and pericholecystic fluid collections including bilomas, pancreatic pseudocyst, and abscess.[103]

Besides gallbladder wall thickening in cholecystitis, a "halo" around the gallbladder has been described[91] (Fig. 2-39). In acute cholecystitis, there is diffuse hyperreflective wall thickening, hazy wall delineation, and gallbladder distention. Additionally, there is a hyporeflective or lucent layer, which is continuous or interrupted within the hyperreflective, thickened gallbladder wall. On follow-up, this lucency represents subserosal edema and necrosis. The inner, hyperreflective contour coincides with the lamina propria and muscularis, with the thick-

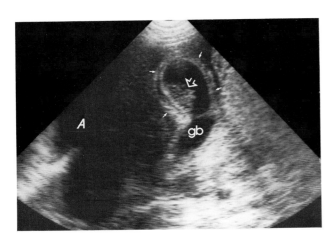

Fig. 2-41. Gallbladder wall thickening, ascites. Transverse scan demonstrates a gallbladder *(gb)* with a thickened wall (arrows). Ascites *(A)* is seen. There is thick sludge (open arrow) that has not reached the dependent portion of the gallbladder.

ness and irregularity of the outer contour probably related to the degree of edema and cellular infiltration in the subserosa and adjacent liver parenchyma.[104] This halo has been demonstrated in 26 percent of patients with acute cholecystitis.[91]

ULTRASOUND SIGNS OF CHOLECYSTITIS

In order to make an accurate diagnosis of cholecystitis on ultrasound, it is necessary to adhere to specific criteria (Fig. 2-42). The major criteria are visualization or nonvisualization of a fluid-filled gallbladder in the right upper quadrant and presence or absence of stones. The minor criteria are (1) a gallbladder wall thickness, measured at a point perpendicular to the beam, of greater than 4 mm, (2) a round or oval gallbladder, and (3) a greatest transverse diameter of the gallbladder of greater than 5 cm. The most common minor criterion identified with acute cholecystitis is increased wall thickness.[91,105] In one study of patients with acute cholecystitis, 70 percent met all of the following ultrasound criteria: (1) gallbladder wall thickening of 5 mm or greater, (2) gallbladder wall anechocity, (3) gallbladder distension as determined by external anteroposterior width of 5 cm or greater, and (4) cholelithiasis.[96] Gallbladder distension (> 4 cm) was seen in 87 percent of patients with cholecystitis.[96]

RIGHT UPPER QUADRANT PAIN

Several groups have evaluated the role of ultrasound in evaluating acute right upper quadrant pain.[91,106,107] The diagnosis of acute cholecystitis is based on the highly

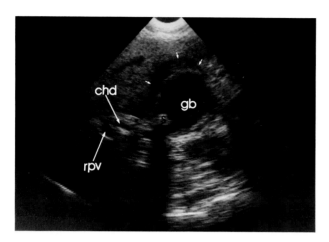

Fig. 2-42. Acute cholecystitis. Longitudinal scan is a patient with pain over the gallbladder *(gb)* when scanning. Gallstones *(s)* are present in a gallbladder that has a thickened wall (arrows), an oval shape, and a transverse diameter of 5 cm. *(rpv,* right portal vein; *chd,* common hepatic duct.) (From Durrell CA III, Vincent LM, Mittelstaedt CA: Gallbladder ultrasonography in clinical context. p. 315. In Mueller PR (ed): Seminars in Ultrasound, CT, and MR. Vol. 5, Grune and Stratton, Orlando, 1984.)

significant observations of focal gallbladder tenderness and calculi; sludge and wall thickness are statistically significant, but to a lesser degree.[107] In one study, maximum tenderness was found over the gallbladder in 85 percent of patients with acute cholecystitis.[91] The accuracy of the sonographic Murphy's sign is 87.2 percent with a sensitivity of 63 percent, a specificity of 93.6 percent, a predictive value for a positive test of 72.5 percent and a predictive value for a negative test of 90.5 percent.[108]

In patients with normal appearing, nontender gallbladders, ultrasound may be able to localize the site of pathology or may direct the patient's workup. When screening patients with right upper quadrant pain, ultrasound was able to detect nonbiliary pathology in 21 percent.[106] The limiting feature of ultrasound is that it requires substantial technical expertise to obtain satisfactory images. With the introduction of high-resolution real-time equipment, it is possible to perform accurate exams with considerably less operator dependence. Because of ultrasound's multiorgan imaging capability and its ability to localize areas of maximum tenderness, it is recommended as the imaging technique of choice in evaluation of patients with right upper quadrant pain.[107] The diagnosis of acute cholecystitis is confirmed if calculi are visualized in a tender gallbladder. The diagnosis is further supported if the gallbladder contains sludge and a thickened wall. If the gallbladder is nontender and stones are present, a diagnosis of chronic cholecystitis is

made. If the gallbladder is normal and not tender, gallbladder disease is unlikely and clinical attention should be directed away from the gallbladder and biliary system.[107]

GALLBLADDER CONTRACTION

At times, it may be desirable to measure the contraction of the gallbladder in response to cholecystokinin (CCK) when cystic duct obstruction is questioned.[4] While the demonstration of significant contraction after CCK is strong evidence of cystic duct patency, the converse does not always hold true. Failure of contraction is not specific.[4,5]

ACALCULOUS CHOLECYSTITIS

Acalculous cholecystitis is difficult to diagnose by clinical means or contrast radiograph. The sensitivity of ultrasound in detecting it is 67 percent and that of nuclear medicine is 68 percent, which is not as high as in calculous cholecystitis.[109] Acalculous cholecystitis represents acute or chronic gallbladder inflammation in the absence of biliary stones. It is seen in 5 to 15 percent of cases of cholecystitis and 47 percent of postoperative cholecystitis.[109] The incidence of acute acalculous cholecystitis in patients with acute cholecystitis is 5 to 10 percent.[110] It may be associated with previous unrelated surgery, trauma, hyperalimentation, burns, cardiac arrest, diabetes, and pancreatitis. Fifty-two percent of untreated cases progress to gangrene and gallbladder rupture.

There are numerous pathophysiologic mechanisms postulated to be the basis for acalculous cholecystitis.[109] It may be caused by substances directly toxic to the gallbladder wall such as pancreatic enzymes and hyperconcentrated bile. Pancreatitis, and/or surgery for biliary tract revision may predispose to the reflux of pancreatic juices into the gallbladder. When organisms in the gallbladder invade the mucosa and wall, inflammation results. Infarction of the gallbladder wall or mucosa may be due to decreased perfusion pressure or gallbladder vessel damage.[109]

The ultrasound findings with acalculous cholecystitis include (1) enlarged gallbladder, (2) diffuse or focal wall thickening, (3) focal hypoechoic regions in the wall, (4) pericholecystic fluid, (5) diffuse homogeneous echogenicity within the gallbladder lumen, and (6) a positive Murphy's sign[109] (Fig. 2-43). Using these ultrasound criteria, the sensitivity is 63 to 67 percent.[109] After a patient fasts for at least 5 hours, a positive ultrasound diagnosis may be made if one or all of the following signs is seen: (1) gallbladder wall thickening of greater than 6 mm,

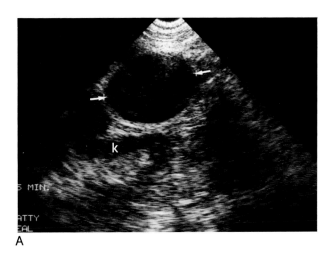

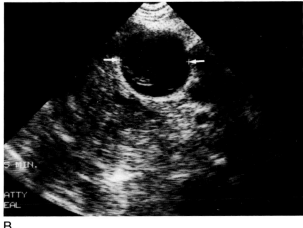

A   B

Fig. 2-43. Acalculous cholecystitis. Longitudinal (**A**) and transverse (**B**) scans in a patient with a postive Murphy's sign and a palpable mass. The gallbladder (arrows) is enlarged, tense, and filled with diffuse internal echoes that do not layer. (*k*, right kidney.)

diffuse or focal; (2) enlarged gallbladder with a positive Murphy's sign; and (3) diffuse, homogeneous nonshadowing median level echogenicity within the gallbladder lumen, suggestive of pus in combination with a Murphy's sign.[109]

GANGRENOUS CHOLECYSTITIS

Acute emphysematous cholecystitis is a complication or uncommon variant of acute cholecystitis and is associated with a significant increase in morbidity and mortality. With this entity, ischemia is followed by invasion of the gallbladder wall by gas-forming microorganisms. Cholelithiasis is not a major pathologic factor and 38 percent of patients are diabetic.[111,112] Gangrene is common and the incidence of perforation is five times greater than with acute cholecystitis.[16,112] Gangrenous cholecystitis occurs in 2 to 38 percent of patients with acute cholecystitis, and perforation occurs in 10 percent of patients with acute cholecystitis.[113] Patients with gangrenous cholecystitis present with right upper quadrant pain, tenderness, fever, leukocytosis and often a palpable gallbladder.[114] Pathologically, it differs from acute cholecystitis by the observation of intramural hemorrhage, necrosis, and microabscesses.[113] The gallbladder wall is thickened and edematous with focal areas of exudate, hemorrhage, and even abscess.[114] Stones or fine gravel are seen in 80 to 95 percent of cases.[114]

Gangrenous cholecystitis and empyema of the gallbladder have been described with ultrasound.[114,115] The typical pattern is that of diffuse, medium-to-coarse intraluminal echoes within the gallbladder, which do not show layering or acoustic shadowing[91,113-115] (Fig. 2-44). Other findings include thickening of the gallbladder wall

and localized peritoneal fluid collections. The echogenic debris described probably represents purulent and fibrinous debris within the gallbladder, perhaps contributed from the focal exudative and ulcerative changes in

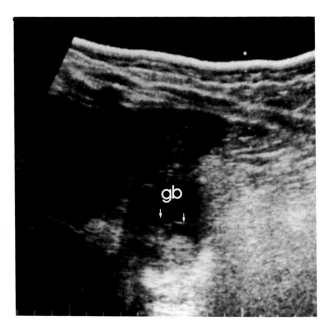

Fig. 2-44. Gangrenous cholecystitis. Typical pattern. Longitudinal static scan in a burn patient with right upper quadrant pain. A poorly defined mass *(gb)* is seen in the area of the gallbladder fossa. There are layering echoes (arrows) within the mass. On hepatobiliary nuclear medicine scan at 60 minutes, there was isotope within the gut but the gallbladder was not visualized. (From Durrell CA III, Vincent LM, Mittelstaedt CA: Gallbladder ultrasonography in clinical context. p. 315. In Mueller PR (ed): Seminars in Ultrasound, CT, and MR. Vol. 5, Grune and Stratton, Orlando, 1984.)

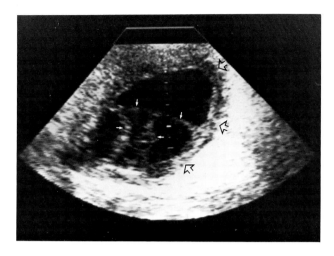

Fig. 2-45. Gangrenous cholecystitis. Membranes. A distended gallbladder with a thickened wall (open arrows) is seen longitudinally with intraluminal linear densities (arrows).

the gallbladder wall. The lack of layering effect is attributed to the markedly increased viscosity of the bile.[114] In one series, 42 percent of patients with gangrenous cholecystitis had no specific features different from acute cholecystitis.[113]

There have been atypical findings seen with gangrenous cholecystitis. In one study, 58 percent of patients had atypical findings present including intraluminal membranes and/or marked irregularities of the gallbladder wall, which is unusual in acute cholecystitis and should prompt close clinical observation for possible gangrenous cholecystitis[113] (Fig. 2-45). These linear, nonshadowing densities producing gallbladder septation seen within the gallbladder lumen represent desquamated necrotic mucosa reflecting separation of the inflammed necrotic mucosa, which is rare in cholecystitis.[88] At times high-density echoes are seen within the gallbladder fossa with posterior shadowing in cases of gangrenous cholecystitis[111,112] (Fig. 2-46). Gas in the gallbladder wall may cause it to be hyperechoic with or without acoustic shadowing, depending upon the amount of the gas. In most, there are large amounts of

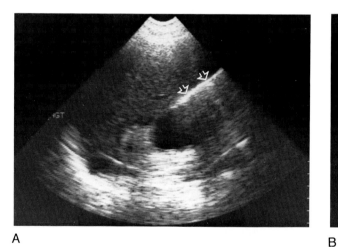

A

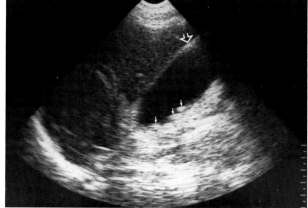

B

C

Fig. 2-46. Emphysematous gangrenous cholecystitis. Longitudinal (A,B) and transverse (C) real-time scans. Gallstones (small arrows) are seen on (B,C), as well as a hyperreflective layer (air, open arrows) in the superificial portion of the gallbladder. (Figs. A&C from Durrell CA III, Vincent LM, Mittelstaedt CA: Gallbladder ultrasonography in clinical context. p. 315. In Mueller PR (ed): Seminars in Ultrasound, CT and MR. Vol. 5, Grune and Stratton, Orlando, 1984.)

gas in the lumen of the gallbladder. The key on ultrasound is to see reverberations within the acoustic shadow, which is produced by gas in the gallbladder (Fig. 2-46). Since reverberations are rarely seen within the shadows produced by gallstones, a "reverberation shadow" arising from the gallbladder (in absence of biliary-enteric anastomosis or fistula) should be confirmed by abdominal radiograph.[111]

GALLBLADDER PERFORATION

Perforation of the gallbladder occurs in 8 to 12 percent of patients with acute cholecystitis and typically occurs 3 to 7 days after the onset of symptoms.[116,117] Predisposing factors include not only cholelithiasis but also infection, malignancy, trauma, drugs (corticosteroids), and impaired vascular supply.[118] Perforation occurs due to calculi obstructing the cystic duct, producing mucosal injury, edema, congestion, and eventual circulatory compromise of the gallbladder wall, which leads to gangrene and perforation.[117] The time interval between the onset of symptoms and gangrene/perforation may be as short as 24 hours or as long as 24 days.[96] The associated mortality has been reported to be 19 to 24 percent.[117]

An accepted mechanism for perforation includes (1) impaction of a calculus in the cystic duct; (2) gallbladder distension due to secretion into its lumen by the mucous glands located in the walls of the gallbladder; (3) vascular impairment of the gallbladder due to distension of the viscus; and (4) ischemia, necrosis and perforation of the gallbladder wall.[118] The risk of gallbladder perforation decreases the earlier cholecystectomy is performed after

the onset of acute cholecystitis. Distension of the gallbladder and edema of its walls may be the earliest signs of impending gallbladder perforation detectable on ultrasound (Figs. 2-40 and 2-42). The gallbladder is considered dilated on ultrasound if it is greater than 3.5 to 4 cm in its anterior-posterior width. Once perforation occurs, pericholecystic collections that are easily detectable on ultrasound will develop.

The various types of perforation are: (1) acute — free perforation causing bile peritonitis; (2) subacute (most common) — walled-off perforation causing a pericholecystic abscess; and (3) chronic — perforation resulting in internal biliary fistula (cholecystoenteric or cholecystocutaneous).[117-119] Pericholecystic abscess is a serious complication of cholecystitis, which develops after gallbladder perforation and usually is associated with acute inflammatory signs and symptoms. The perforation occurs in an area of gangrene or infarction in the wall. The most common site of perforation is in the fundus of the gallbladder. The extraluminal fluid collection is located contiguous to a thick-walled gallbladder in the fundic region and is usually constant in location.[116] Pericholecystic fluid collections can also occur when there is inflammation in adjacent organs in such diseases as peptic ulcer disease, pancreatitis, ascites, and peritonitis.[118,120]

The ultrasound findings in perforation of the gallbladder range from a well-defined band of low-level echoes around the gallbladder (well-encapsulated abscess) to multiple poorly defined hypoechoic masses surrounding an irregular indistinct gallbladder (extensive abscess)[118,119,121] (Figs. 2-47 and 2-48). The ultrasound

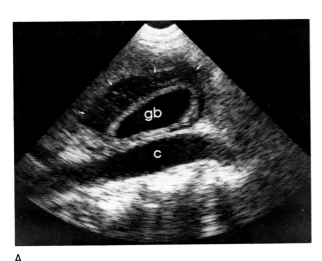

A

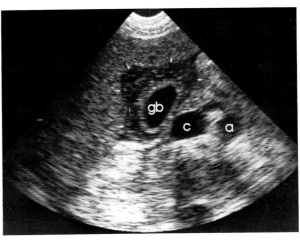

B

Fig. 2-47. Gallbladder perforation. Longitudinal **(A)** and transverse **(B)** real-time scans. A well-defined hypoechoic layer (arrows) is seen encircling the gallbladder *(gb)* wall. This is consistent with pericholecystic fluid. (*c*, inferior vena cava; *a*, aorta.) (From Durrell CA III, Vincent LM, Mittelstaedt CA: Gallbladder ultrasonography in clinical context. p. 315. In Mueller PR (ed): Seminars in Ultrasound, CT and MR. Vol. 5, Grune and Stratton, Orlando, 1984.)

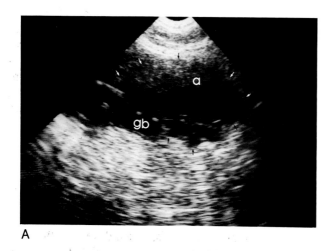

A

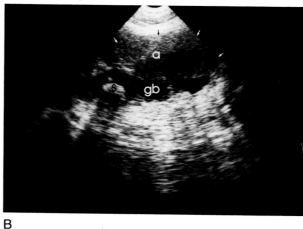

B

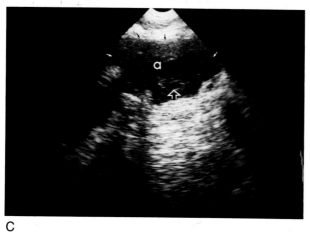

C

Fig. 2-48. Gallbladder perforation. Longitudinal **(A,B)** and transverse **(C)** left lateral decubitus scans. An echodense stone **(s)** is seen within the neck of the gallbladder *(gb)* on **(B)** with a poorly defined mass effect (*a* with arrows) in the fundic region mainly anterior. The mass has a mixed echopattern. This proved to be a pericholecystic abscess. (open arrow, gb lumen.)

findings depend on the presence or absence of inflammation or gangrene of the gallbladder wall, size and location of the perforation, and extent and location of the bile leakage.[117] Pericholecystic collections develop after gallbladder perforation; they range from anechoic to complex collections and their internal characteristics are dependent on the duration of the pericholecystic process.[118] The residual gallbladder lumen or calculi can be identified within or peripheral to the pericholecystic process.

XANTHOGRANULOMATOUS CHOLECYSTITIS

The etiology of xanthogranulomatous cholecystitis must be similar to xanthogranulomatous pyelonephritis, which is a chronic infection in which the formation of calculi play a role. The pathologic pattern is that of lipid-containing histiocytes infiltrating the outer layer of the muscularis of the gallbladder wall. On ultrasound, one sees a complex right upper quadrant mass with poorly marginated, intense reflections within it[122] (Fig. 2-49).

HEMORRHAGIC CHOLECYSTITIS

Hemorrhagic cholecystitis is a rare complication of biliary tract disease and is usually associated with cholelithiasis. Other causes include anticoagulation, biliary neoplasms, and trauma, including liver biopsy and vascular disease. On ultrasound, the gallbladder bile is dense, similar to what is seen with pus or thick sludge. (Fig. 2-50). Blood clots appear as clumps of echogenic material[123] (Fig. 2-32).

HYDROPS OF THE GALLBLADDER

In hydrops of the gallbladder, there is distention of the gallbladder invariably due to total obstruction of the cystic duct. The trapped bile is resorbed and the gallbladder is filled with a clear mucinous secretion derived from the gallbladder wall. The gallbladder is tense and enlarged, and the wall is thin (Fig. 2-51). This condition is usually asymptomatic, but some have epigastric pain, discomfort, nausea, and vomiting.[8]

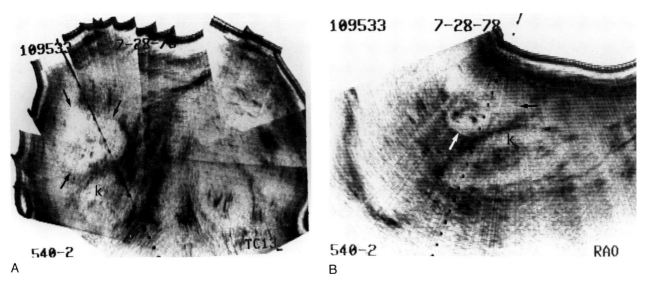

Fig. 2-49. Xanthogranulomatous cholecystitis. Transverse (**A**) and right anterior oblique (**B**) views of the abdomen 16 cm above the iliac crest. A complex mass (arrows) with internal reflections is seen just superior to the right kidney *(k)*. (From Bluth EI, Katz MM, Merritt CRB, et al: Echographic findings in xanthogranulomatous cholecystitis. J Clin Ultrasound 7:213, 1979.)

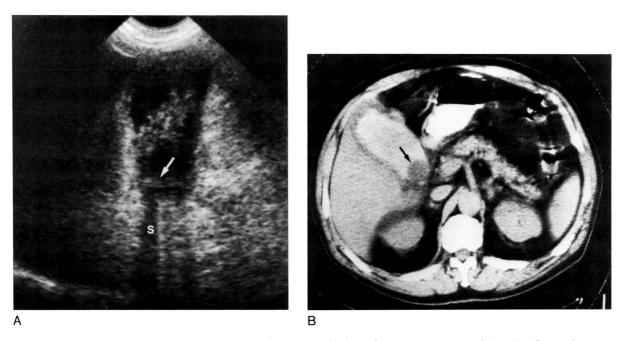

Fig. 2-50. Hemorrhagic cholecystitis. (**A**) Real-time long axis view of the gallbladder. A thick-walled fundus is seen with an echo (arrow) and acoustic shadow *(S)* of a calculus, along with clumps of echogenic material within the gallbladder. (**B**) CT scan. A thick-walled fundus is seen with a negative filling defect (arrow) of the calculus with increased density of blood in bile (80 CT units). (From Jenkins M, Golding RH, Cooperberg PL: Sonography and computed tomography of hemorrhagic cholecystitis. AJR 140:1197, © Am Roentgen Ray Soc, 1983.)

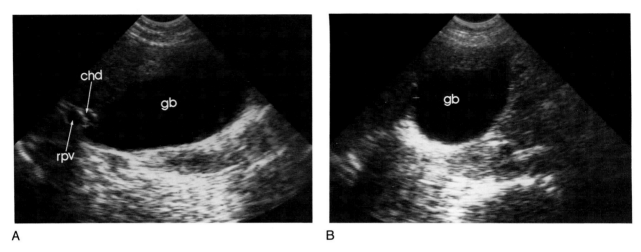

Fig. 2-51. Gallbladder hydrops. Palpable mass in the right upper quadrant. Longitudinal (**A**) and transverse (**B**) scans display a tremendously dilated gallbladder *(gb)* with a thin wall. (*rpv,* right portal vein; *chd,* common hepatic duct.)

There have been reports of children presenting with an abdominal mass that turns out to be gallbladder. Hydrops is a rare cause of right upper quadrant pain in the child. It is not a form of cholecystitis because the gallbladder is not acutely inflamed. Acute distention occurs secondary to preceding illness and a focus of infection elsewhere in the body.[124] Ultrasound can certainly identify the mass as gallbladder in these cases.[85]

In the neonate, hydrops may be associated with numerous diseases including salmonellosis, pseudomonas, and group B-β streptococcal sepsis, prolonged biliary obstruction, shock, congestive heart failure, and hyperalimentation.[17] In a series of three premature neonates, the gallbladder distension was felt to be due to lack of enteric feeding, as it disappeared with feeding. The normal contraction of the gallbladder and simultaneous relaxation of the sphincter of Oddi is stimulated by the enteric hormone cholecystokinin with little influence from the autonomic nervous system.[87] The gallbladder has also been noted to be enlarged in the neonate with extrahepatic biliary atresia, choledochal cyst, and inspissated bile syndrome. Fasting patients receiving total parenteral hyperalimentation develop biliary stasis, and they, too, develop gallbladder distension.[86] If a follow-up ultrasound is done after initiation of oral feedings, the gallbladder size is seen to diminish.

CHOLECYSTITIS IN CHILDREN

The ultrasound signs of cholecystitis in the child are the same as those in the adult. These include gallbladder wall thickening, biliary sludge, gallbladder stones, Murphy's sign, increased gallbladder size, and nonvisualization of the gallbladder.[15] Acalculous cholecystitis is more common in the child than the adult so one must carefully examine the gallbladder wall; 50 percent of childhood cases are not associated with stones.[15,125] In the adolescent group, there is a higher association with stones. In addition, 25 to 45 percent of children present with jaundice and only 6 percent with common bile duct stones.[125] Many cases are associated with congenital malformations of the biliary tract.[124]

MUCOCUTANEOUS LYMPH NODE SYNDROME

Mucocutaneous lymph node syndrome (MLNS) is an acute febrile illness associated with cervical lymphoadenopathy and involvement of the oral cavity, lips, and skin. The etiology of MLNS is unknown. Its features include (1) persistent high fever for more than 1 week; (2) bilateral conjunctival infection; (3) abnormal mucous membranes, including erythema of the oral cavity and dry fissured lips; (4) changes on the extremities, including indurative edema, erythema of the palms and soles, and desquamation; (5) erythematous rash; and (6) cervical lymphadenopathy.[126] Most patients are less than 5 years of age, and greater than 50 percent are less than 2 years of age.

One of the complications of MLNS is acute hydrops of the gallbladder; this can be a major component of abdominal crisis.[126,127] The pathophysiology of hydrops in MLNS is uncertain. No organism is identified. Patients with MLNS are known to have adenopathy and vasculitis in other areas of the body, which could be the cause of the obstruction.[128] If a patient with MLNS presents with pain, distension, and/or palpable right upper quadrant mass, hydrops of the gallbladder, which can be identified on ultrasound, should be considered.[126,128] (similar to Fig. 2-51). The condition is usually self-limiting and transient; the patients respond to conservative medical management.[126] Ultrasound is useful in evaluating complications of acute hydrops of the gallbladder, such as perforation, where a fluid collection is demonstrated surrounding the distended gallbladder.[128]

Gallbladder Disease in Pregnancy

Pregnancy is thought to be one possible cause of gallbladder disease.[129,130] It may be related to an alteration in the composition of the bile with a decrease in concentration of bile salts and an increase in cholesterol. The gallbladder volume increases during gestation probably as a predominant effect of progesterone or a consequence of a combined progesterone-estrogen influence, or the hormones may act directly on the gallbladder musculature. In one series of pregnant patients, 4.2 percent had abnor-

malities.[129] In another, 11.3 percent of obstetrical patients were found to have gallstones.[130]

Biliary Ascariasis

In 1967, there was a report that estimated that the ascaris roundworm *(Ascaris lumbricoides)* infests one quarter of the world's population due to heavy endemicity in the Far East, USSR, Latin America, and Africa. It has a lower endemicity in many other areas including the southeastern United States and Europe. The adult worm is 15 to 49 cm long, 3 to 6 mm thick, and lives mainly in the jejunum. The most common clinical presentation apart from passage per rectum or vomiting worms, is small bowel obstruction by a bolus of worms.[131] In a small number of patients, one or more ascarides migrate through the biliary tract reaching the ducts and gallblad-

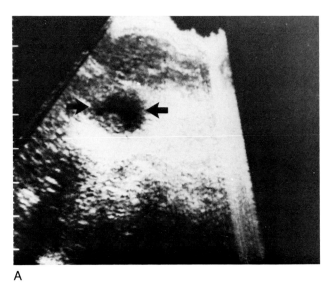

A

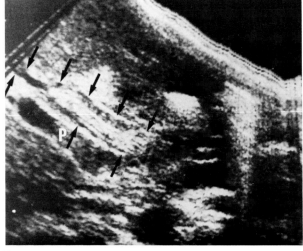

B

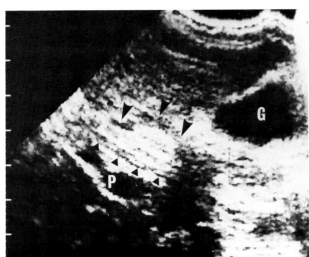

C

Fig. 2-52. Biliary ascariasis Case 1. **(A)** Transverse scan of the gallbladder (arrows) containing coiled-up worms. Case 2. **(B)** Spaghetti appearance of the main bile duct worms. The main bile duct (arrows) expands to contain numerous longitudinal interfaces. (*P*, portal vein). Case 3. **(C)** Spaghetti appearance of main bile duct worms. The lumen of the main bile duct is entirely replaced by the longitudinally disposed bundle of echogenic interfaces. (large arrowheads, anterior margin; small arrowheads, posterior margins; *P*, portal vein; *G*, gallbladder.) *(Figure continues.)*

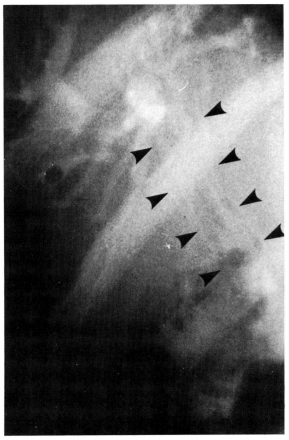

D

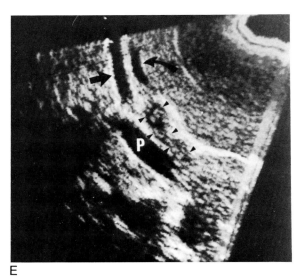

E

Fig. 2-52. *(Continued).* **(D)** Intravenous cholangiogram. The distended main bile duct (arrowheads) contains worms throughout its length. The intrahepatic bile ducts are also dilated. **(E)** Improved appearance 9 days later. The lumen of the main bile duct is now seen (arrowheads), but still contains echogenic fragments of worms. (curved arrow, left hepatic bile duct; straight arrow, left portal vein.) (From Shulman A, Loxton AJ, Heydenrych JJ, Abdurahman KE: Sonographic diagnosis of biliary ascariasis. AJR 139:485, © Am Roentgen Ray Soc, 1982.)

der, causing cholecystitis, cholangitis, biliary obstruction, and hepatic abscess.[131,132] The clinical manifestations are seen mainly in children.[131]

On ultrasound, these worms are seen as (1) echogenic, nonshadowing images in the main bile duct and/or gallbladder; (2) single strips (on occasion, with its digestive tract seen as an anechoic "inner tube"); (3) multiple strips giving a spaghetti-like appearance; (4) coils; or (5) more amorphous fragments[131,133] (Fig. 2-52). On real-time ultrasound, one may even see a moving image of a worm in duct.[132]

Benign Neoplasms

PAPILLOMA AND ADENOMA OF THE GALLBLADDER

Papillomas and adenomas of the gallbladder are infrequent benign epithelial tumors. They represent localized overgrowths of the lining epithelium. Papillomas grow as a pedunculated complex branching structure and adenomas as a flat sessile thickening. Papillomas may occur singly or multiply as small branching, pedunculated

masses less than 1 cm in diameter that project into the lumen of the gallbladder. They are connected to the wall by a slender stalk. Adenomas are broad-based hemispheric elevations, less than 1 cm in diameter and firmly attached to the underlying wall[8] (Fig. 2-53). Adenomas represent the most frequent (28 percent) of benign gallbladder neoplasms with nearly half (43 percent) having a papillary configuration.[134]

ADENOMYOMATOSIS OF THE GALLBLADDER

Adenomyomatosis of the gallbladder represents proliferation of the surface epithelium of the gallbladder with gland-like formation and out-pouchings of mucosa into or through a thickened muscular layer (Rokitansky-Aschoff sinuses).[135,136] Adenomyomatous hyperplasia belongs to a group of diseases known as "hyperplastic cholecystoses." There are various forms of adenomyomatosis: (1) diffuse—entire gallbladder involved; (2) segmental—proximal, middle, or distal third of the gallbladder involved in a circular fashion; and (3) localized—confined almost exclusively to the fundus (occurs in the majority of cases). The ability to diagnose adenoma-

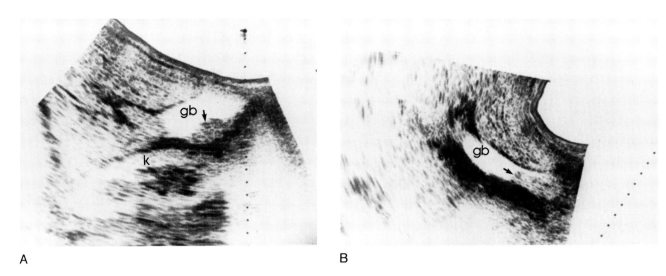

A   B

Fig. 2-53. Gallbladder adenoma. **(A)** Longitudinal supine view of the gallbladder *(gb)* containing a polyp (arrow). (*k*, right kidney.) **(B)** Erect longitudinal view. The polyp (arrow) moved slightly with change in body position.

tosis with ultrasound is dependent upon the degree and nature of the gallbladder wall thickening and identification of the intramural diverticula.[136,137]

Adenomyomatosis of the gallbladder should be suspected on ultrasound when there is diffuse or segmental thickening of the gallbladder wall and intramural diverticula are seen as anechoic or echogenic foci with or without associated acoustic shadowing or reverberation artifacts[136-138] (Figs. 2-54 to 2-56). The ultrasound appearance of the intramural diverticula varies depending on the size and content and whether papillary projections are present. When the intramural diverticula contain bile, they appear as anechoic spaces. Those diverticula that are small or contain biliary sludge, stones, or papillary projections appear as echogenic foci at varying intervals within the gallbladder wall with or without acoustic shadowing or reverberation artifacts.[136,137] Diffuse adenomyomatosis has been described as a hyperechoic mass arising from the fundus of the gallbladder with a diffusely thickened wall (Fig. 2-54). The mass, in such a case, represents the effect of circumferential thickening of the wall.[135]

CHOLESTEROLOSIS

Cholesterolosis results from the accumulation of triglycerides and esterified sterols in macrophages in the lamina propria of the gallbladder wall.[139] It represents a local disturbance in cholesterol metabolism and is not associated with any derangement in blood levels of cholesterol. Histologically, there is enlargement and distention of the mucosal folds into club shapes with aggregation of round to polyhedral histiocytes within these clubbed ends.[8] The polypoid type of cholesterolosis is

associated with cholesterol polyps that are attached to the mucosa by a fragile pedicle composed of an epithelium covering a core of lipid-filled macrophages.[136] The polyps may break off (contain no glandular elements) and form a nidus for stones. On ultrasound, one looks for nonshadowing single or multiple fixed echodense masses that project into the lumen of the gallbladder[136,139] (Fig. 2-57). Some investigators describe shadowing associated with cholesterol polyps.[140]

Malignant Neoplasms

PRIMARY CARCINOMA

Carcinoma of the gallbladder is the fifth most frequent gastrointestinal malignancy and represents 1 to 3 percent of all malignancies.[131-145] It is more frequent than the aggregate of all other types of malignancies and a much more common lesion than benign adenomas and papillomas. It is the most frequent cancer of the biliary system. It is more common in the sixth and seventh decades, in whites, and in females (4:1).[141-143] Gallbladder stones are present in 65 to 95 percent of cases, which strongly suggests an etiologic role for inflammation.[16,141-145] In 70 to 80 percent of cases, the neoplasm is adenocarcinoma (most, well differentiated), with 15 percent of these fungating papillary carcinoma and 65 percent infiltrating parietal carcinoma.[146] In up to 25 percent of cases, there is calcification in the gallbladder wall.[145] The most common site is in the fundus and neck.

There are several principal forms of gallbladder carcinoma, including localized infiltrating or fungating tumors.[146] The infiltrating type is more common and is

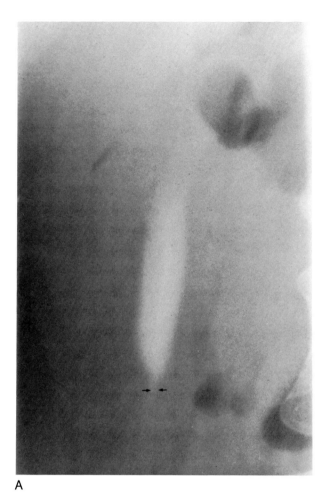

A

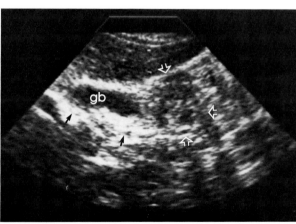

B

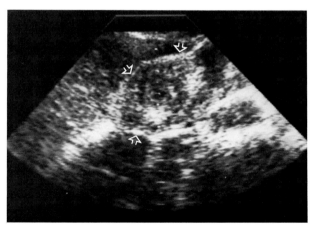

C

Fig. 2-54. Gallbladder adenomyomatosis. Diffuse disease. **(A)** Oral cholecystogram. The gallbladder appears narrow with a peculiar tapering at its fundus (arrows). **(B)** Longitudinal real-time scan revealing a diffusely thickened gallbladder wall (arrows) measuring 0.5 cm to 1 cm with a mass (open arrows) in the area of the fundus. (*gb*, gallbladder lumen.) **(C)** Transverse scan of the hyperechoic "mass" (open arrows) 3 cm in diameter. The less echogenic central part represents gallbladder lumen. (From Detweiler DG, Biddinger P, Staab EV, et al: The appearance of adenomyomatosis with the newer imaging modalities: a case with pathologic correlation. J Ultrasound Med 1:295, 1982.)

usually a poorly defined area of diffuse thickening and induration in the gallbladder wall. The fungating type grows into the lumen as an irregular cauliflower mass invading the wall. Most invade the liver centrifugally and many have extended to the cystic duct and adjacent bile ducts. There is direct liver invasion in 69 percent of cases.[147]

The clinical course is extremely insidious, and frequently the patient is asymptomatic over long periods of time. The symptoms include loss of appetite, nausea and vomiting, intolerance to fatty foods, and belching, all of which are suggestive of some form of gallbladder involvement. Jaundice is usually not seen until there is infiltration of the major biliary ducts and extension into

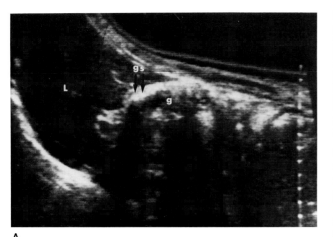

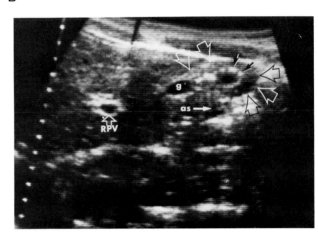

A   B

Fig. 2-55. Gallbladder adenomyomatosis. Case 1. Longitudinal **(A)** and transverse **(B)** scans of the gallbladder *(g),* with intramurally located gallstones *(gs)* and Rokitansky sinuses *(ra).* There was mucosal hypertrophy and intramural diverticula on gross specimen. *(L,* liver; *RK,* right kidney.) Case 2. **(C)** Longitudinal scan of the gallbladder *(g)* with wall thickening (open arrows) confined to the body and fundus of the gallbladder. Note echogenic dots (closed arrows) paralleling the luminal surface in the fundus. On gross specimen, there was marked thickening of the gallbladder wall with intramural diverticula. *(as,* acoustic shadow from gallstone; *RPV,* right portal vein.) (From Raghavendra BN, Subramanyam BR, Balthazar EJ, et al: Sonography of adenomyomatosis of the gallbladder: radiologic-pathologic correlation. Radiology 146:747, 1983.)

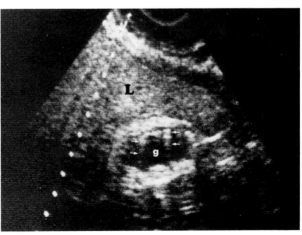

C

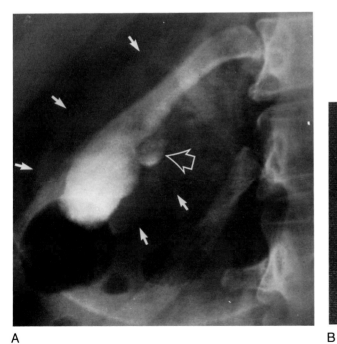

A   B

Fig. 2-56. Gallbladder adenomyomatosis. Case 1. **(A)** Oral cholecystogram (OCG) shows markedly thickened gallbladder wall (arrows) and contrast-filled intramural diverticulum (open arrow). **(B)** Longitudinal scan of the gallbladder *(g)* shows reverberation artifacts (small arrows) emanating from the thickened gallbladder wall. *(L,* liver.) There was mucosal hypertrophy and intramural diverticula. Frond-like projections within the diverticulum might have been responsible for the reverberation artifact. *(Figure continues.)*

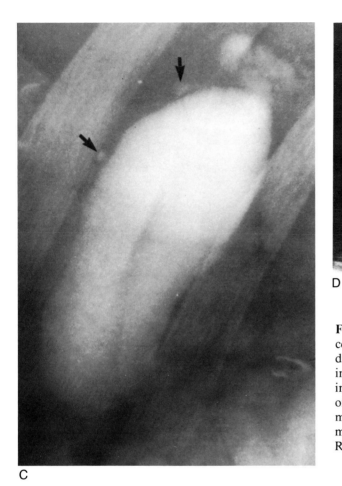

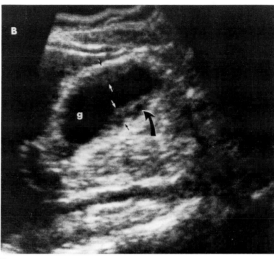

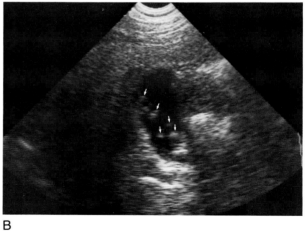

Fig. 2-56. *(Continued.)* Case 2. **(C)** OCG shows at least two contrast-filled intramural diverticula (arrows). **(D)** Longitudinal scan of the gallbladder *(g)* shows segmented wall thickening (straight arrows). A rounded anechoic area representing an intramural diverticulum is seen within the thickened portion of the wall (curved arrow). (From Raghavendra BN, Subramanyam BR, Balthazar EJ, et al: Sonography of adenomyomatosis of the gallbladder: Radiologic-pathologic correlation. Radiology 146:747, 1983.)

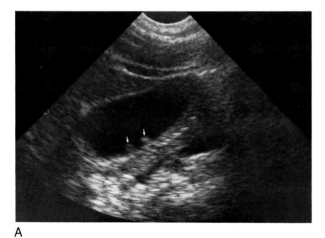

Fig. 2-57. Gallbladder cholesterolosis. Longitudinal **(A)** and transverse **(B)** scans of the gallbladder. Multiple polypoid masses (arrows) are seen and with change in body position, they remain attached to the wall.

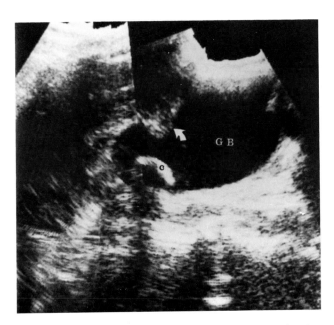

Fig. 2-58. Gallbladder carcinoma. Tumor protruding into gallbladder lumen. Longitudinal scan shows well-defined mass (arrow) protruding into fluid-filled gallbladder *(GB)*. Calculi *(c)* with acoustic shadowing are also noted. (From Weiner SN, Koenigsberg M, Morehouse H, Hoffman J: Sonography and computed tomography in the diagnosis of carcinoma of the gallbladder. AJR 142:735, © Am Roent Ray Soc, 1984.)

the liver bed. In half the cases, there is a mass and in half there is right upper quadrant pain. The diagnosis of gallbladder carcinoma is difficult. An early diagnosis is rare, as clinical signs appear late and are due to extension to contiguous structures. The average duration of life after diagnosis is 1 to 1 ½ years and rarely does survival reach 5 years.[8] The 5-year survival rate has been reported to be 4 to 12 percent.[145]

The findings of gallbladder carcinoma on ultrasound represent a spectrum that is dependent upon the size of the tumor, its morphologic character, and the extent of secondary spread.[141] The early findings include (1) localized area of thickening of the gallbladder wall, (2) polypoid lesion with irregular borders, and/or (3) loss of the usual smooth outline of the gallbladder with replacement by an undulated configuration.[141] Other patterns described with gallbladder carcinoma include (1) a solid mass (with diffuse weak or strong echoes) filling the gallbladder (most common type in 42 percent of cases); (2) infiltrating mass with gallbladder wall markedly thickened due to infiltration by carcinoma (15 percent); (3) fungating mass on the wall producing an intraluminal mass with an irregular contour (23 percent); and (4) a fungating or polypoid mass with a markedly thickened posterior wall[141,142,144,145,148,149] (Figs. 2-58 to 2-61). With localized lesions, one may see a thickened hypoechoic gallbladder wall, gradual or abrupt junction with normal

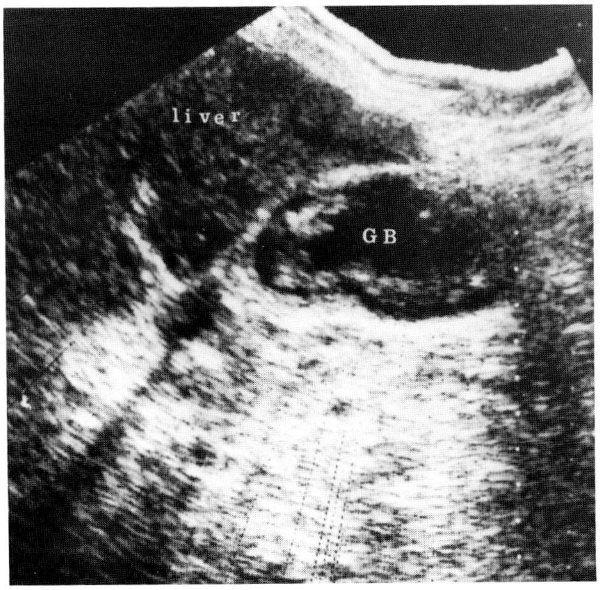

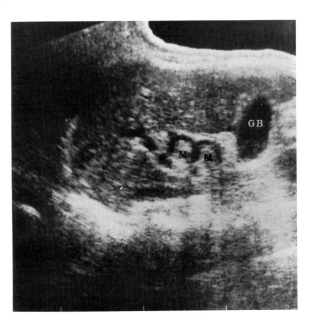

Fig. 2-59. Gallbladder carcinoma. Carcinoma infiltrating the gallbladder wall. Longitudinal left lateral decubitus scan shows a fluid-filled gallbladder *(GB)* with an asymmetrically thickened, irregular wall. (From Weiner SN, Koenigsberg M, Morehouse H, Hoffman J: Sonography and computed tomography in the diagnosis of carcinoma of the gallbladder. AJR 142:735, © Am Roent Ray Soc, 1984.)

Fig. 2-60. Gallbladder carcinoma. Intraductal extension of gallbladder tumor. Longitudinal scan shows a lobulated mass *(M)* in the common bile duct. The gallbladder *(GB)* contains sludge. (From Weiner SN, Koenigsberg M, Morehouse H, Hoffman J: Sonography and computed tomography in the diagnosis of carcinoma of the gallbladder. AJR 142:735, © Am Roent Ray Soc, 1984.)

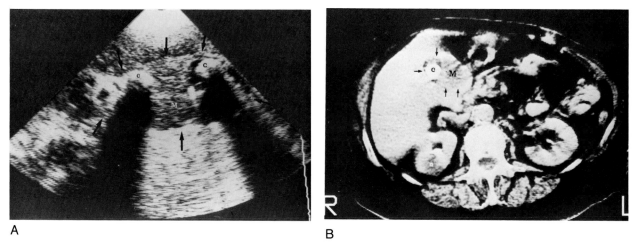

A   B

Fig. 2-61. Gallbladder carcinoma. Carcinoma replacing the gallbladder. Longitudinal scan of the right upper quadrant **(A)** and CT scan **(B)** show a large soft-tissue mass *(M)* in the gallbladder (arrows) and calculi *(c)* with acoustic shadowing. (From Weiner SN, Koenigsberg M, Morehouse H, Hoffman J: Sonography and computed tomography in the diagnosis of carcinoma of the gallbladder. AJR 142:735, © Am Roentgen Ray Soc, 1984.)

wall tissue, and, later, a bilobed appearance to the gallbladder lumen[146] (Figs. 2-58 and 2-59). Localized tumors are usually located in the infundibular or fundal region and rarely involve the body of the gallbladder.[146] When such tumors are localized in the neck, they are often associated with hydrops and porta hepatis invasion (Fig. 2-60). The gallbladder wall may be poorly distinguished from the liver. In some instances, the gallbladder wall may be hyperechoic with irregular limits and a large

base of implantation. When the lesions extend into the liver, the masses may lie in contact with the gallbladder or numerous tumor masses may be seen within the liver from hematogenous spread.[146] With diffuse tumor, the wall may be totally infiltrated with a hypoechoic thickened wall (Figs. 2-59 and 2-61), or the gallbladder wall may be collapsed.[146] With advanced neoplasm, a complex echogenic mass may be present, obliterating the gallbladder lumen.[150] Seeing a stone encased within a

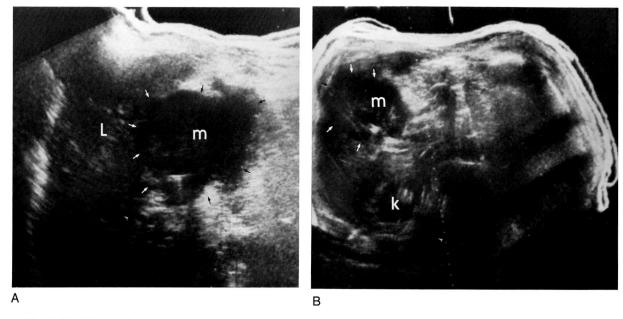

A   B

Fig. 2-62. Metastatic gallbladder disease. Squamous cell carcinoma metastatic to the gallbladder. Longitudinal **(A)** and transverse **(B)** scans demonstrate a poorly defined hypoechoic mass *(m,* arrows) in the gallbladder fossa. *(k,* right kidney; *L,* liver.)

gallbladder mass (constrained stone sign) is almost pathognomonic for carcinoma[16] (Fig. 2-61). Other lesions such as cholesterol polyp, mucosal hyperplasia, inflammatory polyp, granulomatas, and blood clot may simulate gallbladder carcinoma.[142]

Awareness of the subtle ultrasound findings in this condition will permit its early detection. A diagnosis of gallbladder carcinoma can be made by ultrasound in 84.6 percent of patients.[142] A clear-cut solid tumor of the gallbladder, which infiltrates the liver, is highly suggestive of carcinoma.[147]

METASTATIC DISEASE TO THE GALLBLADDER

Metastatic tumor to the gallbladder should be suspected in the presence of focal gallbladder wall thickening in association with nonshadowing intraluminal soft tissue masses. Unlike primary carcinoma of the gallbladder, cholelithiasis is usually absent. Several patterns have been described: (1) focal thickening of the gallbladder wall due to localized metastatic deposit; (2) intraluminal mass without shadowing, with sonographically normal gallbladder wall; (3) combination of these two with polypoid or irregular intraluminal mass based on an area of focal thickening of the gallbladder wall; and (4) indistinct walls that contain low-level, irregular echoes with decreased through transmission (Figs. 2-62 and 2-63). The tumors that metastasize to the gallbladder are from stomach, pancreas, and bile ducts; they reach the gallbladder by direct invasion while metastatic disease from organs such as lung, kidneys, esophagus, and malignant melanoma reach the gallbladder via blood-borne embolic phenomenon.[151,152]

Postcholecystectomy Patients

Postoperative complications are infrequent. They include wound, common duct injury, retained cystic duct, drainage tube problems, retained stones, hepatic artery injury, and fluid collections. These fluid collections represent the most frequent complications (5 to 6 percent of cases).[153] The fluid may be blood, bile, lymph, or peritoneal fluid. Most are in the area of the falciform ligament in either the right subhepatic or right subphrenic space. These areas are vulnerable to infection because the medium provided by pooling blood, lymph, bile, and a denuded liver bed is right for bacterial growth.[153]

One should be cautious in making a diagnosis of retained duct calculi in a postcholecystectomy patient.[154] A strong echo with distal acoustic shadowing may be seen in patients without stones (Fig. 2-64). This is assumed to be caused by a postoperative scar in the gallbladder bed.[154] If an echodense structure with an associated shadow is seen in the area of the gallbladder fossa, and is surrounded by a lucency, a diagnosis of cystic duct remnant stone should be entertained (Fig. 2-65).

Percutaneous Cholecystostomy

Percutaneous ultrasound-guided puncture of the gallbladder is a new method for antegrade study of the gallbladder and common bile duct. The following represent

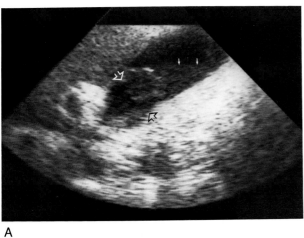

A

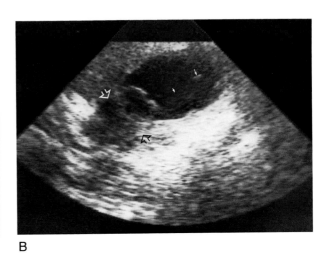

B

Fig. 2-63. Metastatic gallbladder disease. **(A)** Supine long axis view of the gallbladder. Apparent debris (small arrows) is lying dependent in the gallbladder. A mass within the gallbladder is suspected (open arrows) because of the abnormal configuration of the gallbladder neck. **(B)** Erect long axis view. A lobulated mass (open arrows) remains in the neck of the gallbladder and debris (small arrows) layers out dependently. At surgery, there was metastatic melanoma with acute or chronic cholecystitis. (From Bundy AL, Ritchie WGM: Ultrasonic diagnosis of metastatic melanoma of the gallbladder presenting as acute cholecystitis. J Clin Ultrasound 10:285, 1982.)

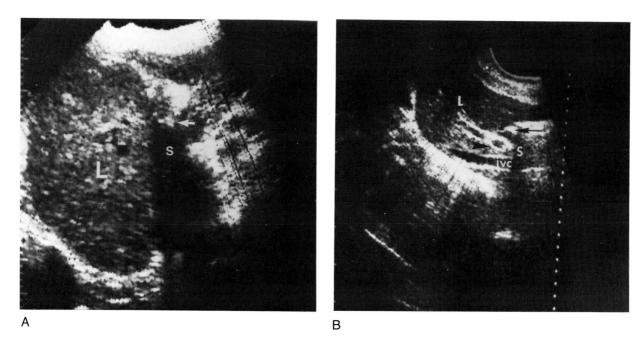

Fig. 2-64. Postcholecystectomy shadow. Pseudocalculus pattern. Longitudinal scans after cholecystectomy without **(A)** and with **(B)** surgical clips in the right upper abdomen. **(A)** Oblique scan parallel to costal margin. **(B)** Slight oblique right parasagital scan. (arrow, strong echoes; arrowhead, portal vein; *S*, acoustic shadow; *L*, liver; *ivc,* inferior vena cava.) (From Raptopoulos V: Ultrasonic pseudocalculus effect in post-cholecystectomy patients. AJR 134:145, © Am Roentgen Ray Soc, 1980.)

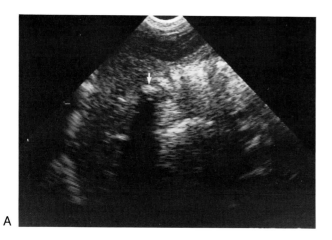

Fig. 2-65. Postcholecystectomy shadow. Retained stone. Longitudinal scan **(A)** of the gallbladder fossa. An echodense structure *(arrow)* with associated shadowing is seen. **(B)** Percutaneous transhepatic cholangiogram. A stone (arrow) is seen within the cystic duct remnant.

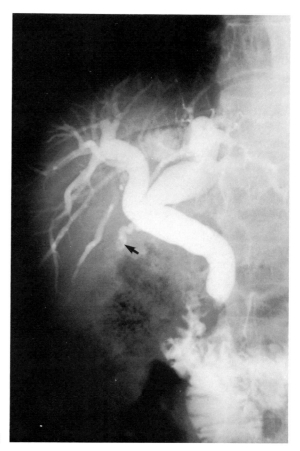

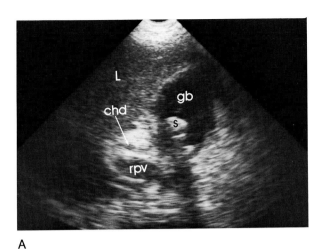
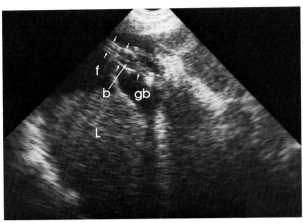

A   B

Fig. 2-66.   Cholecystostomy. Cholelithiasis. **(A)** Longitudinal scan in the left lateral decubitus position demonstrating echodense stones *(s)* within the gallbladder *(gb)* with shadowing. The patient was acutely ill with a positive Murphy's sign. Since the patient was not an operative candidate, a cholecystostomy tube was placed. *(rpv,* right portal vein; *chd,* common hepatic duct; *L,* liver.) **(B)** Transverse scan of the gallbladder *(gb)* with a catheter (arrows) inserted. The catheter balloon *(b)* is seen within the lumen of the gallbladder. The tip is the bright echo. Peritoneal fluid *(f)* has developed. *(L,* liver.)

the indications for the procedure: (1) evaluation of the common bile duct for calculi and/or obstruction; (2) aspiration of bile for Gram stain, crystal analysis, and cytology; (3) evaluation of the gallbladder lumen for intraluminal mass; and (4) to establish the anatomic site for occult abscess.[155] This technique can be successfully used to treat severely ill patients—those at considerable surgical risk. It may be indicated as a preoperative measure in patients with known cholelithiasis or acute cholecystitis in whom prolonged anesthesia or surgery may be hazardous[155-157] (Fig. 2-66).

This percutaneous approach can be used for biliary drainage when a transhepatic approach is not possible.[158] Once the gallbladder is localized with ultrasound, a 22-gauge sheathed needle is placed into the gallbladder (using an anterior abdominal wall approach, right axillary line) and dilute (25 to 30 percent) diatriozoate meglumine (Hypaque) can be injected into the gallbladder. Needling the gallbladder without catheterization will frequently lead to bile peritonitis.[159] Thus, it is important to introduce a pigtail catheter, which keeps the gallbladder collapsed, preventing the catheter from being pulled out.[159] Although complications with this procedure are few, they include peritonitis, fatal septic shock, and severe vasovagal reaction.[157]

BILIARY ABNORMALITIES

Biliary Dilatation

Common bile duct measurement is a sensitive indicator of biliary obstruction and its demonstration by noninvasive or invasive means is mandatory even when in-

trahepatic ducts appear normal.[160] The physical law of Laplace applies to the biliary system, accounting for the preferential dilatation of the extrahepatic ducts.[160] For a given pressure, the bursting force in a cylinder is directly proportional to the diameter of the cylinder. The gallbladder may also act as a reservoir and prevent dilatation of the biliary system and elevation of the bilirubin level early in the course of obstruction. The total transmural pressure applied to the intrahepatic bile ducts by adjacent hepatic parenchyma or fibrosis (as in cirrhosis) may account for the lack of ease with which they dilate. Extrahepatic duct measurement is a more sensitive measurement of biliary obstruction than intrahepatic duct dilatation, particularly if the duration of the jaundice is less than 4 weeks.[160]

Experimental studies have been performed to evaluate biliary tract obstruction. Within 24 hours after occlusion of the distal common bile duct, there is dilatation of the common bile duct and gallbladder before elevation of the bilirubin. After a brief interval of several hours following acute biliary obstruction, the ultrasound appearance of the ducts may be normal when nuclear medicine studies document total obstruction.[161] The ducts expand centrifugally from the obstructive point with dilatation of the intrahepatic ducts occurring days after the onset of the obstruction. After release of the obstruction, the biliary ducts contract centripetally with the common bile duct requiring 30 to 50 days to return to normal.[162] Others describe decompression within 43 hours after relief of acute obstruction.[163]

Some investigators have shown that a dilated common hepatic duct may return to normal size within minutes.[32] It is postulated that the rapid size change probably

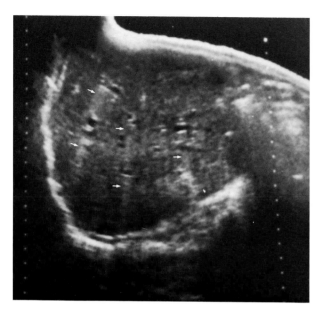

Fig. 2-67. Dilated intrahepatic ducts. Right lobe. Longitudinal scan to the right of midline. Tubular lucencies are seen within the right lobe of the liver. These are associated with acoustic enhancement (arrows) characteristic of ducts.

occurs only in patients without a normally functioning gallbladder. The wall of the duct is composed of largely fibroelastic tissue, with the stretch potential of the elastic fibers permitting duct dilatation, while the elastic recoil of the fibers is responsible for return of the duct to nor-

mal size after relief of obstruction. In humans, the size of the common bile duct is largely determined by intraductal pressure. With an increase in intraductal pressure, the common bile duct progressively dilates to a limit governed by the elastic properties of the duct wall.[32] Ductal dilatation may be followed by inflammation and fibrosis and may preclude further dilatation or reduction in ductal size.[164]

Dynamic changes have been demonstrated with biliary dilatation. The common hepatic duct can be evaluated before and after fat ingestion.[165] In normal patients, the common hepatic duct remains the same or decreases in caliber after a fatty meal. A response is abnormal if a normal-sized duct increases in size or a slightly dilated duct remains the same or increases in size. Evaluation before and after a fatty meal may aid in evaluation of a common hepatic duct that is equivocally or mildly dilated and can indicate the need for further invasive studies. After the fat enters the duodenum, cholecystokinin is released by the intestinal mucosa. The release of bile into the duodenum is mediated by cholecystokinin. It produces gallbladder contraction, relaxation of the sphincter of Oddi, and increased bile flow from the liver.[165] This test can also be used on the postoperative cholecystectomy patient. In these patients, the common hepatic duct is 5 mm or less; a fatty meal is helpful in those whose common hepatic duct is 5 mm or greater.[165] With the gallbladder removed, the response of the normal duct should remain the same. Even if the common duct

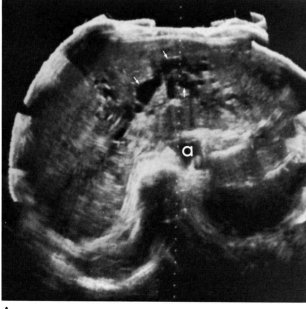

A

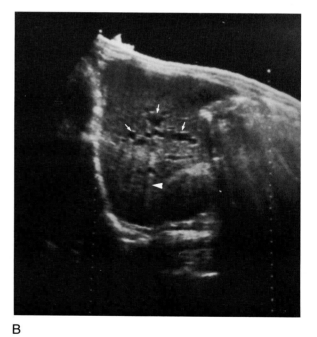

B

Fig. 2-68. Dilated intrahepatic ducts. Antler branching pattern. There are tubular lucencies (arrows) within the right lobe of the liver, which appears to exhibit an antler branching pattern on transverse (**A**) and longitudinal (**B**) scans. Note the acoustic enhancement (arrowhead) on (**B**). (*a*, aorta.)

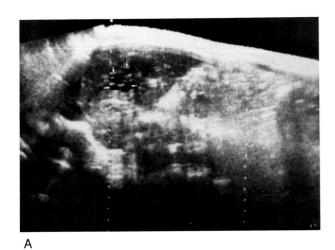

A

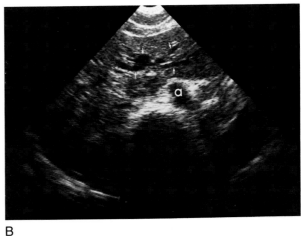

B

Fig. 2-69. Dilated intrahepatic ducts. Left lobe. There are lucencies (arrows) within the left lobe on these longitudinal **(A)** and transverse **(B)** scans of two different patients. There is subtle acoustic enhancement. As a rule vessels are not seen in the left lobe. (*a,* aorta.)

is mildly dilated (6 to 10 mm) before a fatty meal, a decrease of 5 mm or less seems to indicate normal bile duct dynamics and excludes the possibility of obstruction.[165] If the duct is of normal caliber or slightly dilated before fat and increases in caliber after fat, this is a strong indicator of bile duct pathology.[165]

There have been several ultrasound signs described for dilatation of the biliary system. These include (1) periph-

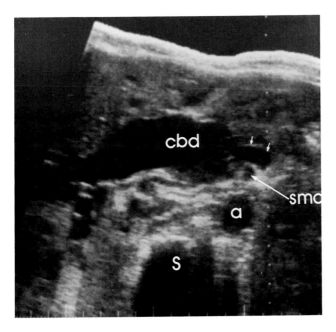

Fig. 2-70. Dilated common bile duct. Long axis view of the common bile duct *(cbd)* with narrowing of the distal end (arrows). (*a,* aorta; *sma,* superior mesenteric artery; *S,* spine.) On transverse scan at a lower level, a hypoechoic mass was seen. This mass represented adenocarcinoma of the pancreatic head.

eral lucencies within the liver, which demonstrate acoustic enhancement; (2) tubular lucencies within the liver, which have an antler or stellate branching pattern; (3) lucencies within the left lobe of the liver; (4) dilated common bile duct identified as a tubular lucency anterior to the portal vein on a long axis view of the portal vein; (5) dilated common hepatic duct identified as a tubular lucency anterior to the right portal vein; and (6) more than two tubular lucencies seen on a longitudinal scan in the porta hepatis region[166] (Figs. 2-67 to 2-72). While there are often lucencies seen within the right lobe of the liver on a longitudinal scan, these are usually vessels and there is no acoustic enhancement. Bile, being less dense than blood, exhibits increased through transmission (Figs. 2-67 and 2-68). This sign of intrahepatic duct dilatation may be subtle at times. Normally, no intrahepatic vessels are seen on a longitudinal scan through the left lobe of the liver (Fig. 2-69). If lucencies are seen, one should suspect dilated intrahepatic ducts. The abnormal common hepatic duct has an internal dimension of greater than 4 mm[24] (Fig. 2-71). A measurement of 5 mm would be borderline, with one of 6 mm required to diagnose dilatation of the common hepatic duct.[24] The abnormal common bile duct has an internal dimension of greater than 6 mm, with a dimension of 7 mm definitely abnormal (Figs. 2-70 and 2-71).

Another finding with dilatation is the "parallel channel" sign. This refers to the simultaneous imaging of the dilated right or left hepatic duct and adjacent contiguous main portal vein branch. It is highly reliable in minimal duct dilatation.[167] The "shotgun" sign is similar to the "parallel-channel" sign. It describes the presence of two parallel ducts as pathologic.[168] As dilatation of the biliary tree progresses, the portal system becomes flattened, thus reversing the initial proportion between the diameter of the biliary junction and that of the biliary tree. With appropriate positioning, the junction of the right and left ducts can be demonstrated.[168]

Ultrasound has proved to be a more sensitive indicator of obstructive jaundice than the serum bilirubin level or biochemical profile.[169-171] Since peripheral biliary dilatation may be diagnosed as early as 4 hours after biliary obstruction and before elevation of the serum bilirubin, it is suggested that obstruction may be diagnosed with ultrasound before the onset of icterus.[172] However, obstruction has been demonstrated in the absence of biliary dilatation.[173]

How does ultrasound fare in a prospective evaluation of the site and cause of obstructive jaundice? In one series, the site of obstruction could be identified in 27 percent, with 73 percent indeterminate because of the inability to visualize the complete biliary tract.[174] The cause of obstruction was determined in 23 percent, with 76 percent indeterminate.[174] The determination of the anatomic site of obstruction and its cause is critical in the management of jaundiced patients. While ultrasound is an excellent screen for distinguishing dilated from non-dilated ducts, direct cholangiography or possibly CT is necessary if stringent criteria are applied to determine the site and cause of biliary obstruction.[174]

POSTOPERATIVE CHOLECYSTECTOMY PATIENTS

There have been many reports that indicate that there is dilatation of the extrahepatic ductal system following a cholecystectomy. However, one study found no evidence of common bile duct dilatation in 95 percent of patients; all of their postoperative cholecystectomy patients had common bile ducts that measured 6 mm or less.[175] In most instances (84 percent), the common hepatic duct measured 4 mm or less.[176,177] If the common hepatic duct measures 6 mm or larger and the common bile duct measures 8 mm or larger, further studies are indicated.[176] These may include ultrasound evaluation of the biliary system before and after a fatty meal, as has been discussed, or a hepatobiliary nuclear medicine study (Fig. 2-13).

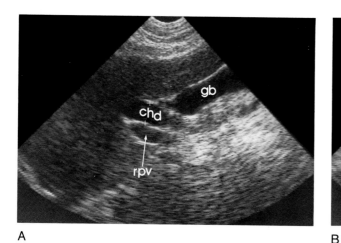

A

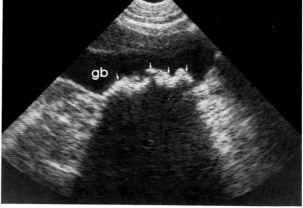

B

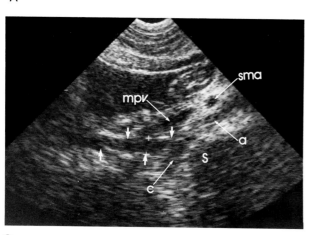

C

Fig. 2-71. Dilated common hepatic and bile duct. **(A)** Left lateral decubitus longitudinal scan. The dilated common hepatic duct *(chd)* (1.3 cm) is seen anterior to the right portal vein *(rpv)* and superior to the gallbladder neck. *(gb)*. **(B)** Longitudinal view of the gallbladder *(gb)* demonstrating multiple stones (arrows) with shadowing. **(C)** Oblique transverse scan of the proximal common bile duct (arrows) (9 mm) in the porta hepatis. *(mpv,* main portal vein; *a,* aorta; *sma,* superior mesenteric artery; *c,* inferior vena cava; *S,* spine.) *(Figure continues.)*

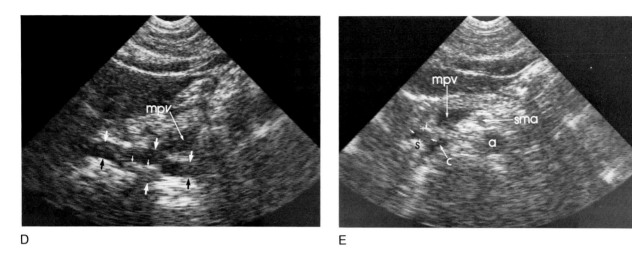

D   E

Fig. 2-71 *(Continued).* **(D)** Similar scan to **(C)** but in the right lateral decubitus position. Now the ductal stones (small arrows) are visible within the proximal common bile duct (larger arrows). (*mpv,* main portal vein.) **(E)** Transverse supine view of the pancreatic head taken before **(D)**. The distal common bile duct (small arrow) is seen to be dilated within the pancreatic head. It contains echodensities *(s)* representing stones. (*a,* aorta; *c,* inferior vena cava; *sma,* superior mesenteric artery; *mpv,* main portal vein.)

BILIARY DILATATION IN CHILDREN

Neonate. Jaundice in the neonate may develop for various reasons.[178] These include overproduction of bilirubin due to fetomaternal blood incompatibility, hemoglobinopathies, enzymatic and structural red blood cell defects, and polycythemia. It can also occur with

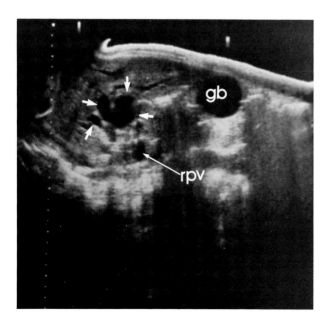

Fig. 2-72. "Too-many tubes" sign. Longitudinal scan to the right of midline. Multiple tubular lucencies are seen in the porta hepatis (arrows). Only one, the right portal vein *(rpv),* is a vessel. (*gb,* gallbladder.)

hemorrhage anywhere in the body. It is seen with Hirschsprung's disease, intestinal atresia or stenoses, or meconium ileus or meconium plug syndrome. With mixed hyperbilirubinemia, there may be metabolic abnormalities, storage disease, alpha$_1$-antitrypsin deficiency, prenatal infection (toxoplasmosis, cytomegalovirus, herpes, syphilis), neonatal sepsis, and neonatal hepatitis. The leading diagnoses to be considered when all of the above have been excluded are neonatal hepatitis and biliary atresia. These entities are difficult to differentiate on ultrasound and are further discussed later in this chapter. In biliary atresia, the atretic segment may involve any or all parts of the biliary tree. The noninvolved part may be normal in caliber but there may be normal-sized extrahepatic ducts with atresia.[178]

Older Child. In the older child, the etiologies to be considered include choledochal cyst, Caroli's disease, cholelithiasis, cholecystitis, and hepatic and obstructive extrahepatic masses. Not only does ultrasound permit rapid detection of bile duct dilatation, but it also can permit localization for percutaneous cholangiography, which aids in the choice of surgical procedure by locating the site of obstruction.[179] Cholelithiasis and cholecystitis have already been discussed. Choledochal cyst and Caroli's disease will be discussed in subsequent sections in this chapter. The major hepatic masses in infants and children are not associated with jaundice, but present with a palpable mass and are discussed in Chapter 1. Abdominal lymphoma or metastatic nodes can obstruct the biliary tree. Hepatic hemangiomas may also present with jaundice. These hemangiomas are capillary he-

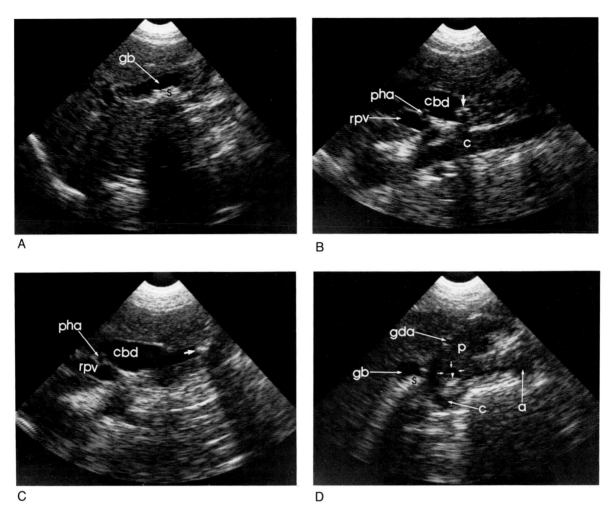

Fig. 2-73. Choledocholithiasis. **(A)** Longitudinal scan of the gallbladder *(gb)* with gallstones *(s).* **(B)** Longitudinal view of the common bile duct *(cbd)* with a stone (small arrow) with shadowing. (*pha,* proper hepatic artery; *rpv,* right portal vein; *c,* inferior vena cava.) **(C)** Oblique longitudinal view of the common bile duct *(cbd)* in the left lateral decubitus position. The echodense stone (arrow) has moved. (*rpv,* right portal vein; *pha,* proper hepatic artery.) **(D)** Transverse scan of the pancreatic head *(p).* A dilated distal common bile duct (arrows) is seen with calculi (arrowhead). (*gb,* gallbladder; *c,* inferior vena cava; *a,* aorta; *gda,* gastroduodenal artery; *s,* gallbladder stone.)

mangiomas or hemangioendotheliomas. The jaundice is due to a low-grade hemolysis. As discussed in Chapter 1, these masses are seen on ultrasound with multiple lucent and hypoechoic areas within the liver parenchyma. Most of these patients present by 6 months of age.[178]

Choledocholithiasis

While ultrasound is the method of choice in diagnosing cholelithiasis and for evaluation of intra-and extra-hepatic biliary ductal dilatation in jaundiced patients, its role in the diagnosis of choledocholithiasis is uncertain. Ductal stones are identified by the presence of echogenic material within the duct (Figs. 2-71, 2-73 to 2-74). The

absence of surrounding bile makes the diagnosis difficult. Also, a high percentage of common bile duct stones do not shadow (probably due to size).[180] The echogenic nature of the calculus in the ampulla is difficult to distinguish from pancreas and mucus in the duodenum.[55] While the proximal common bile duct can usually be reliably identified in its long axis, the distal duct is difficult to see due to bowel gas. The administration of small amounts of water containing microbubbles, while simultaneously scanning the ampulla and pancreatic head, frequently defines the duodenum more clearly and allows better delineation of the medial aspect of the pancreas. The distal duct is best visualized in the transverse plane with the patient in the erect and/or right lateral decubitus position[7] (Figs. 2-71E, 2-73D, and 2-74E).

Occasionally, by placing the patient in the Trendelenberg position, the stone may be seen migrating cephalically into the more visible part of the duct.[55] The stones in the proximal common bile duct are best demonstrated by sagittal sections with the patient in the right anterior oblique position[181] (Figs. 2-71D and 2-74D). This evaluation is best with high-resolution real-time sector ultrasound. It is especially helpful to reevaluate a dilated common duct on a subsequent day if no stones are seen.[181]

The reasons for difficulties with this diagnosis of choledocholithiasis rest on these factors: (1) deeper position of the common bile duct as compared to the gallbladder; (2) difficulty in continuously observing a stone secondary to interference from changing pockets of gas within overlying bowel; (3) reflection and refraction of the beam by the curved wall of the duct; (4) position of the common bile duct such that it may lie out of the optimal focal zone of the transducer; and (5) very small amount of fluid surrounding the stone, especially in the minimally dilated or normal-sized duct.[181] Structures that create confusion include (1) air or residue in adjacent bowel, mimicking stone; (2) right hepatic artery crossing the common bile duct and indenting it; (3) postoperative cholecystectomy clips; (4) impression on the common bile duct by the cystic duct; (5) air in the biliary tree; (6) mucous plug; and (7) calcification in the head of the pancreas[181] (Fig. 2-75). As such, one needs to be familiar with the artifacts created by such things as clips, catheters, and air, which can lead to a false-positive diag-

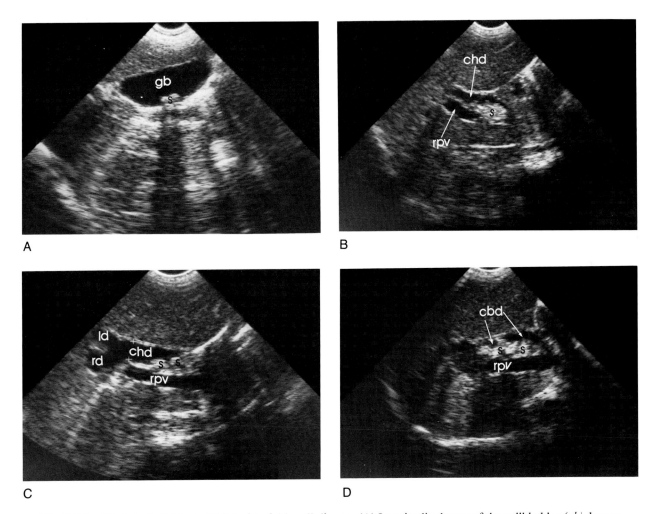

Fig. 2-74. Choledocholithiasis. Child with sickle cell disease. **(A)** Longitudinal scan of the gallbladder *(gb)* demonstrating cholelithiasis. Echodense stones *(s)* are seen. **(B)** Longitudinal view of the common hepatic duct *(chd),* which contains small echodense stones *(s)*. *(rpv,* right portal vein.) **(C)** Longitudinal view of the dilated common hepatic duct *(chd)* more superior on the duct than **(B).** Echodense stones *(s)* are seen as well as the dilated right *(rd)* and left *(ld)* hepatic ducts. *(rpv,* right portal vein.) **(D)** Right lateral decubitus longitudinal scan of the dilated proximal common bile duct *(cbd).* Multiple echodense stones *(s)* are seen. *(rpv,* right portal vein.) *(Figure continues.)*

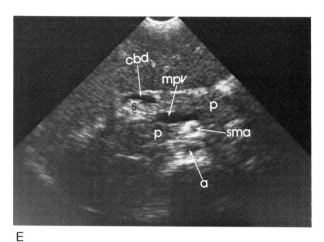

E

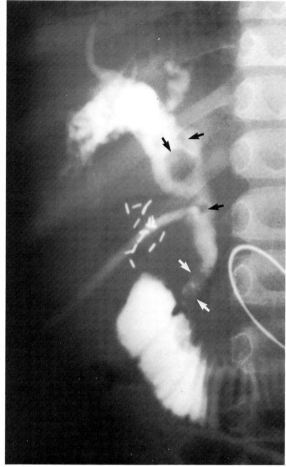

F

Fig. 2-74 *(Continued).* **(E)** Transverse view of the pancreatic head. The dilated distal common bile duct *(cbd)* is seen within the pancreatic head. It is dilated and contains stones *(s).* (*a,* aorta; *mpv,* main portal vein; *p,* pancreas; *sma,* superior mesenteric artery.) **(F)** Intraoperative cholangiogram demonstrating multiple stones (arrows) within the extrahepatic ducts. The common hepatic duct is more dilated than the common bile duct.

nosis.[182] A history of previous surgery and a plain radiograph are important in such cases, as well. A positive diagnosis of choledocholithiasis can only be made if ultrasound demonstrates hyperechoic structures within the common bile duct with an associated shadow; it is especially helpful to diagnosis if the echodense structures are seen to change position within the common bile duct as the patient changes position.[181]

Primary Biliary Neoplasm

ADENOCARCINOMA AND SQUAMOUS CELL CARCINOMA

The predisposing influences of inflammation and cholelithiasis are less established for carcinoma of the bile ducts than for carcinoma of the gallbladder.[8] Stones are found in one third of cases. With chronic ulcerative colitis, there is also an increased incidence of this type of carcinoma. These tumors occur in the same age range as carcinoma of the gallbladder with a greater frequency in

males than females. Most are adenocarcinoma with some squamous cell carcinoma. There are three types: nodular, infiltrating, and papillary.[183] Most are annular infiltrating scirrhous carcinomas, which are slow growing and usually extend along the length of the ducts, resulting in longer lesions.[184] In the minority of cases, the tumor may be papillary or polypoid.[184] The relatively inaccessible location of this carcinoma and frequent local invasion of the liver, portal vein, and hepatic artery make en bloc resection difficult.[183] The sites of location of the tumor in descending frequency include common bile duct (especially lower end); junction of cystic duct, hepatic and common bile duct; hepatic ducts; cystic duct; and duodenal portion of the common bile duct.[8] Cholangiocarcinoma is intrahepatic in 13 percent of patients, common hepatic duct and bifurcation in 37 percent, junction of the cystic duct and common bile duct in 15 percent, cystic duct in 6 percent, and common bile duct in 33 percent.[184] These lesions are insidious in their development, with most presenting with right upper quadrant pain of acute onset, biliary colic, jaundice, weight loss, and nonspecific digestive disturbances.

High-resolution real-time ultrasound can evaluate the extrahepatic biliary system in multiple planes, so if abrupt termination of the duct is seen on long axis views, malignancy should be considered.[185] The ultrasound features of cholangiocarcinoma may include (1) marked biliary obstruction in the presence of a normal pancreas; (2) focal biliary tract stricture or abrupt termination; (3) delineation of a mass involving the bile duct; (4) irregu-larly defined coarse acoustic shadowing arising from the obstructive mass; (5) contained intraluminal soft-tissue echoes; and (6) echogenic bands across the lumen[183–187] (Fig. 2-76). In most cases, a mass itself will not be identi-fied.[186,187] When dilated ducts and a main pancreatic duct are demonstrated, a primary bile duct carcinoma should be suspected in the presence of a normal pancre-atic head, although a small pancreatic or ampullary car-

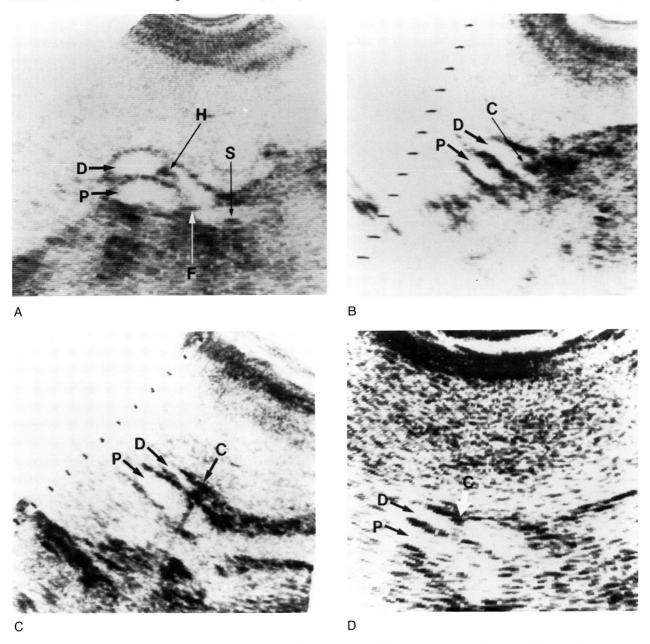

Fig. 2-75. Artifacts mimicking choledocholithiasis. **(A)** Longitudinal scan. A large (9 mm) right hepatic artery identation echo *(H)* mimics a stone in the common bile duct. A fold *(F)* caused by tortuosity of the common bile duct also mimics a stone. (*D*, common bile duct; *P*, portal vein; *S*, stone.) **(B)** A large (8 mm) echo *(C)* from a surgical clip close to the common bile duct, mimics stone. (*D*, common bile duct; *P*, portal vein) **(C,D)** Longitudinal scans. Surgical clip echoes *(C)* are associated with "comet tail" reverberation artifact. (*D*, common bile duct; *P*, portal vein.) *(Figure continues.)*

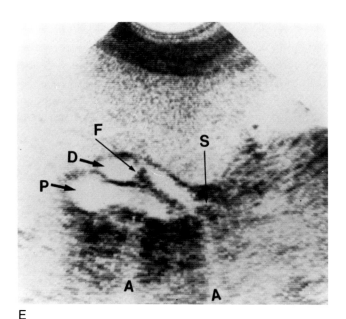

E

Fig. 2-75 *(Continued).* **(E)** Longitudinal scan. A fold *(F)* resulting from tortuosity of the common bile duct creates an echo with an acoustic shadow *(A).* (*S*, stone with acoustic shadow; *D*, common bile duct; *P*, portal vein.) (From Parulekar SG, McNamara MP: Ultrasonography of choledocholithiasis. J Ultrasound Med 2:395, 1983.)

cinoma cannot be excluded.[183,186] An intraductal neoplasm should be suggested by finding an intraluminal focus of low-level echoes within the biliary tree, without a shadow.[187] The accuracy of ultrasound detection depends on the location of the tumor. It is more accurate for lesions involving the bifurcation and common hepatic duct than for the common bile duct.[184] Cholangiography is superior to ultrasound in determining the length of the involved segment, but ultrasound is superior in detecting hepatic invasion and lymphadenopathy.[184] At times, it is difficult to distinguish cholangiocarcinoma from hepatocellular carcinoma or hepatic metastases.[184]

Klatskin is the name given to the bile duct carcinomas arising at the hepatic duct bifurcation. It has the worst prognosis. The ultrasound features include (1) dilatation of the intrahepatic ducts but not extrahepatic ducts; (2) nonunion of the right and left hepatic ducts; and (3) small, solid masses of the hepatic hilum[183] (Fig. 2-77). In the face of intrahepatic duct dilatation without extrahepatic duct dilatation, a primary tumor should be suspected. The location of the tumor allows significant obstruction to occur before the primary tumor attains considerable size.[183] It may not be possible to distinguish the tumor from lymphadenopathy as a source of obstruction. Tumors of the gastrointestinal tract, breast, pancreas, and gallbladder show a propensity for spread to the porta hepatis.

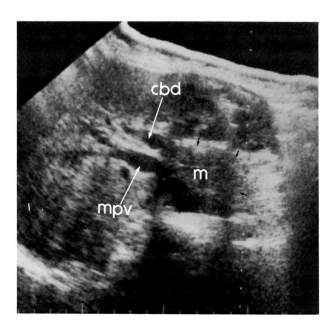

Fig. 2-76. Cholangiocarcinoma. Long axis view of the dilated common bile duct *(cbd).* A solid mass (*m*, arrows) is seen at the distal end of the duct. (*mpv,* main portal vein.)

CYSTADENOMA AND CYSTADENOCARCINOMA

Biliary cystadenoma and cystadenocarcinoma are rare hepatic neoplasms constituting 4.6 percent of the total intrahepatic cysts of bile duct origin.[188] The incidence is greater in females, with a peak in the fifth decade; 80 percent are older than 30 years of age.[188,189] The right lobe is more commonly involved with a size that ranges from 1.5 to 30 cm with most greater than 10 cm in diameter.[188] They may present as a painful epigastric mass, occasionally with intermittent jaundice.[190] They

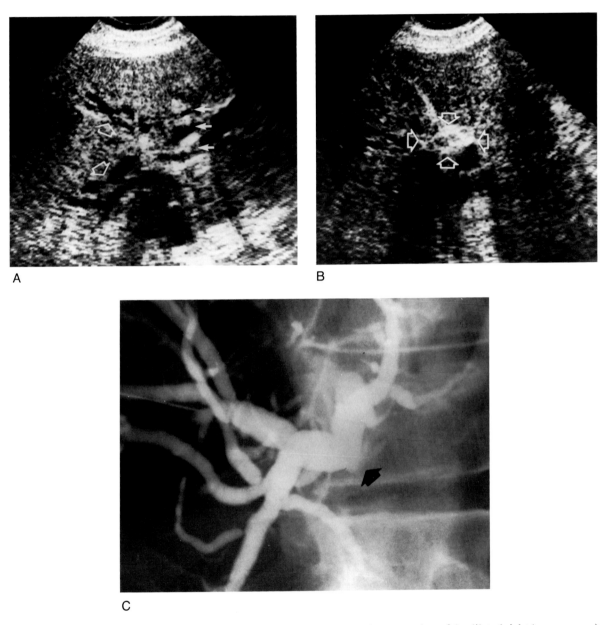

A

B

C

Fig. 2-77. Klatskin tumor. **(A)** Transverse scan of the liver demonstrating nonunion of the dilated right (open arrows) and left hepatic ducts (solid arrows) at the hilum. **(B)** Transverse scan at a slightly lower level, showing several small, solid masses in the region of the bifurcation (arrows). **(C)** Percutaneous transhepatic cholangiogram demonstrating that filling is limited to the right hepatic ducts, which terminate abruptly at the hilum (arrowhead). (From Meyer DG, Weinstein BJ: Klatskin tumors of the bile ducts: sonographic appearance. Radiology 148:803, 1983.)

grow slowly but a rapid increase in tumor size may result from fluid accumulation.[190]

The cystadenomas appear well encapsulated, and are composed of numerous cystic spaces lined by cuboidal or columnar epithelium of biliary tract origin.[190] The cyst wall contains biliary-type epithelium with a capsule of connective tissue, with mural cysts and polypoid cystic spaces that may communicate with the ducts.[190] The cysts contain mucinous material, serous fluid, hemosid-

erin, cholesterol crystals, and necrotic or purulent material.

Biliary cystadenoma and cystadenocarcinomas are characteristically cystic multiloculated intrahepatic masses with thick, highly echogenic internal septations and papillary projections[188-190] (Figs. 2-78 and 2-79). These findings are similar to those in the pancreas and ovary. The differential diagnosis of such a lesion would include a complicated cyst, echinococcal cyst, abscess,

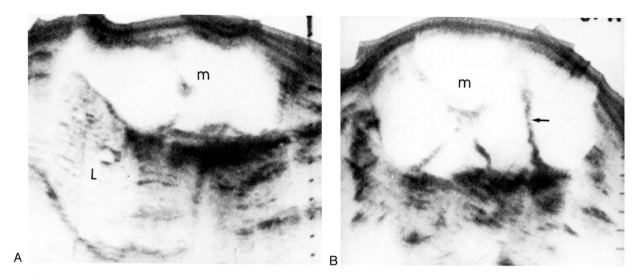

Fig. 2-78. Biliary cystadenoma. **(A)** Longitudinal scan 3 cm to the right of midline with an ovoid septated cystic mass *(m)* demonstrated with an irregular posterior margin, and increased sound transmission. The mass is partly surrounded by hepatic parenchyma. *(L,* liver.) **(B)** Transverse scan at 8 cm above the umbilicus. Septa of variable thickness (arrow) form multiple locules. Thick irregular echoes in the center of the lesion *(m)* form papillary projections. (From Forrest ME, Cho KJ, Shields JJ, et al: Biliary cystadenomas: Sonographic-angiographic pathologic correlations. AJR 135:723, © American Roentgen Ray Society, 1980.)

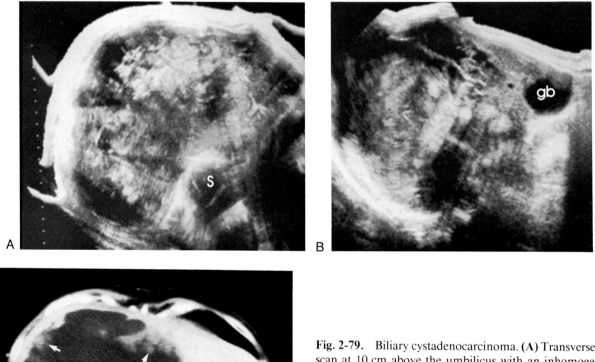

Fig. 2-79. Biliary cystadenocarcinoma. **(A)** Transverse static scan at 10 cm above the umbilicus with an inhomogeneous pattern throughout the liver. There are echodense and anechoic areas. *(S,* spine.) **(B)** Longitudinal static scan at 1 cm to the right of midline. A mixed echopattern is seen. *(gb,* gallbladder.) **(C)** Enhanced CT scan. A large low-density mass is seen, which contains multiple septations. There are small soft-tissue density masses (arrows) within the mass.

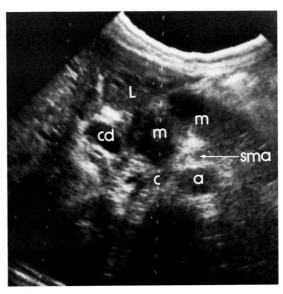

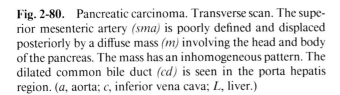

Fig. 2-80. Pancreatic carcinoma. Transverse scan. The superior mesenteric artery *(sma)* is poorly defined and displaced posteriorly by a diffuse mass *(m)* involving the head and body of the pancreas. The mass has an inhomogeneous pattern. The dilated common bile duct *(cd)* is seen in the porta hepatis region. (*a*, aorta; *c*, inferior vena cava; *L*, liver.)

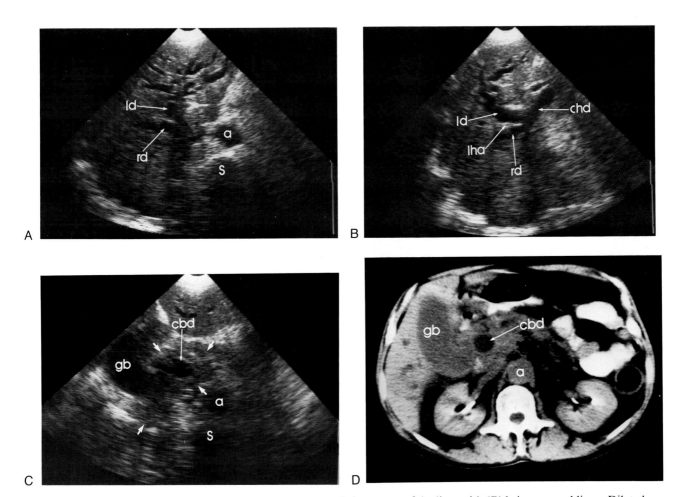

Fig. 2-81. Pancreatic carcinoma. **(A,B)** Transverse real-time scans of the liver with **(B)** being more oblique. Dilated intrahepatic ducts are seen in the left lobe. On **(B)**, the dilated left *(ld)*, right *(rd)* and common *(chd)* hepatic ducts are demonstrated. (*a*, aorta; *S*, spine; *lha*, left hepatic artery.) **(C)** Transverse view of a pancreatic head mass (arrows) and dilated distal common bile duct *(cbd)*. Dilated intrahepatic ducts are seen as well. (*gb*, gallbladder; *a*, aorta; *S*, spine.) **(D)** Enhanced CT scan that is similar to **(C)**. The gallbladder *(gb)* and dilated distal common bile duct *(cbd)* are seen. The pancreatic head is enlarged. Dilated intrahepatic ducts are seen as low-density areas within the liver. (*a*, aorta.)

hematoma, and cystic metastases.[190] Aspiration may be performed in indeterminate cases with mucinous bile-tinged or brownish cloudy fluid obtained.

Metastatic Disease to the Biliary System

Pancreatic carcinoma is the most common cause of malignant obstruction of the biliary ductal system (Figs. 2-80 to 2-82). Less common causes are carcinoma of the ampulla of Vater, nodal masses due to either lymphoma (usually histiocytic) or other metastatic disease involving the liver hilum or peripancreatic lymph nodes, and primary biliary and gallbladder carcinoma. (Fig. 2-83)[191] Lymphomatous involvement of the pancreas with ex-trahepatic bile duct obstruction is rare and represents an uncommon cause of obstructive jaundice.[192] The majority develop jaundice due to nodes in the porta hepatis. With pancreatic involvement, the mass is a relatively hypoechoic lobulated area in the pancreatic head.[192] Ultrasound of an intrinsic bile duct lesion can help in the differential diagnosis by demonstrating the presence or absence of shadowing.[193]

Hepatocellular carcinoma has also been shown to produce biliary obstruction. Hepatoma should be included in the differential diagnosis of filling defects in the proximal extrahepatic ducts.[194] The characteristic features include bulky obstructing intraluminal masses in the proximal extrahepatic ducts (Fig. 2-84). The location of

the hepatoma is suggested to be intraductal rather than extraductal by the fact that a thin anechoic rim representing the lumen nearly circumscribes the mass.[195] The distal common bile duct defects usually signify hematobilia and clots.

Other Causes of Biliary Dilatation

Mirizzi syndrome is an uncommon, surgically correctable cause of extrahepatic obstruction.[56-58] This entity was discussed previously in this chapter. In the proper situation, the ultrasound appearance of dilated intrahepatic ducts, normal caliber common bile ducts and stones in the neck of the gallbladder or cystic duct should suggest the diagnosis[56-58] (Fig. 2-26).

Unusual causes of biliary dilatation have been reported. These include obstruction due to compression by an aortic aneurysm.[196]

Cholangitis

ORIENTAL CHOLANGIOHEPATITIS

With the recent influx of immigrants from Southeast Asia into the United States, there is an increased likelihood of encountering oriental cholangiohepatitis or pyogenic cholangitis in this country. The symptoms in-

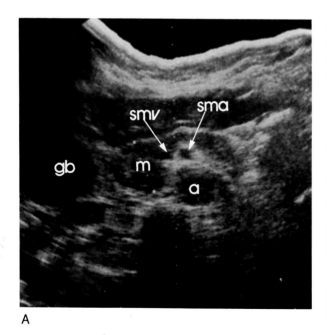

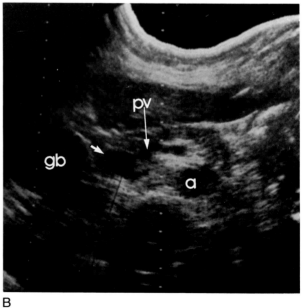

A   B

Fig. 2-82. Pancreatic carcinoma. Transverse static scans with **(A)** 1 cm below **(B)**. The dilated common bile duct (arrow) is seen on **(B)**. The pancreatic head mass *(m)* is seen on **(A)**. (*a*, aorta; *sma*, superior mesenteric artery; *smv*, superior mesenteric vein; *pv*, main portal vein; *gb*, gallbladder.)

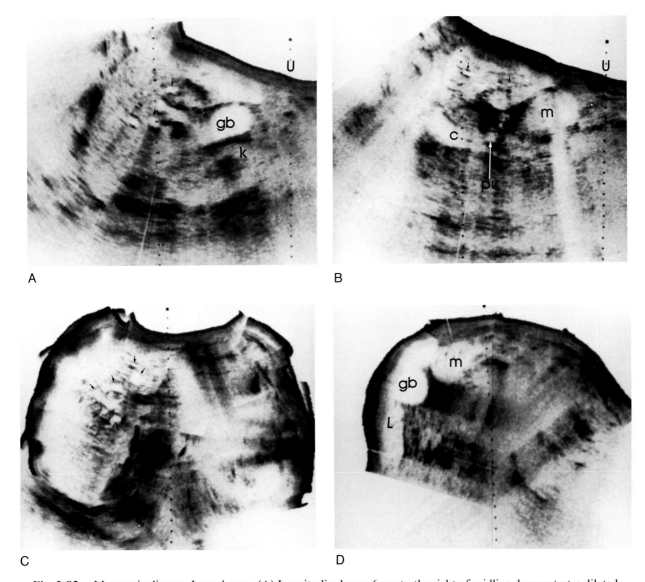

Fig. 2-83. Metastatic disease. Lymphoma. **(A)** Longitudinal scan 6 cm to the right of midline demonstrates dilated intrahepatic ducts (arrows) with increased through transmission. (*gb*, gallbladder; *k*, right kidney; *U*, level of the umbilicus.) **(B)** Longitudinal scan 2 cm to the right of midline demonstrates a hypoechoic lymphomatous mass *(m)* inferior to the liver. Dilated ducts (arrows) are seen as lucencies within the left lobe. (*c*, inferior vena cava; *pv*, portal vein; *U*, level of the umbilicus.) **(C)** Transverse scan at 12 cm above the umbilicus. The dilated intrahepatic ducts (arrows) are seen. **(D)** Transverse scan 4 cm above the umbilicus with a lymphomatous hypoechoic mass *(m)* in the porta hepatis. (*gb*, gallbladder; *L*, liver.)

clude repetitive attacks of cholangitis with fever, chills, epigastric or right upper quadrant pain, and jaundice.[197,198] The male to female ratio is equal with a 20- to 49-year age of incidence.[197,199] This process is histologically characterized by peribiliary fibrosis and grossly characterized by bile duct stricture with marked ductal dilatation, ductal stones, local hepatic necrosis, and hepatic abscess. Many possible etiologies have been cited; a combination of causes is probable.[199] These may include

(1) congenital or acquired stricture; (2) coliform bacterial infection of bile; and (3) parasitic infestation (commonly found), particularly *Clonorchis sinensis.*[198,199] If untreated, cholangitis leads to intrahepatic bile stasis and ultimately to death from liver failure. The treatment is surgical decompression of the biliary tree with a permanent drainage procedure.[198]

On ultrasound, massively dilated ducts are demonstrated frequently as large as 3 to 4 cm in diameter (Figs.

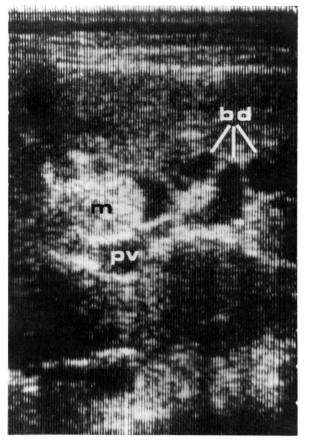

A

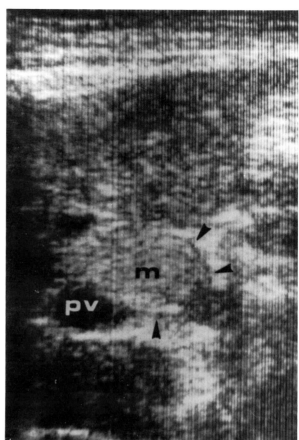

B

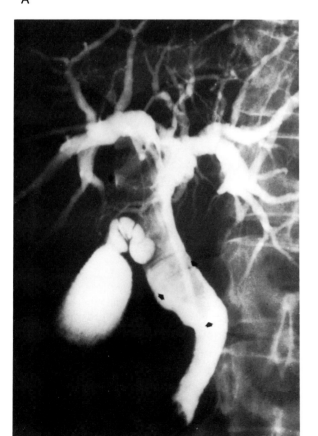

C

Fig. 2-84. Hepatoma. **(A)** Subcostal scan. There is a small echogenic mass *(m)* anterior to the portal vein *(pv)*. The intrahepatic biliary ducts *(bd)* are dilated. **(B)** Longitudinal scan. A thin anechoic rim (arrowheads) is visible around the mass *(m)*. *(pv,* portal vein.) **(C)** Transhepatic cholangiogram after placement of a catheter for drainage and injection of more contrast material. A bulky filling defect (arrows) is evident within an enlarged common duct. (From Maffessanti MM, Bazzochi M, Melato M: Sonographic diagnosis of intraductal hepatoma. J Clin Ultrasound 10:397, 1982.)

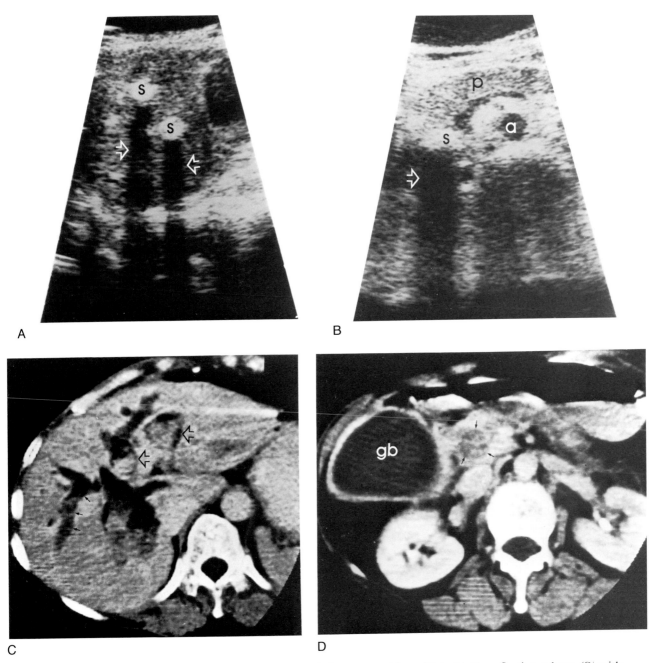

Fig. 2-85. Oriental cholangitis. **(A)** Longitudinal real-time scan with multiple highly reflective echoes *(S)* with acoustic shadowing (arrows) representing intrahepatic calculi. **(B)** Transverse scan demonstrates similar marked echoes *(S)* with posterior shadowing (arrow) in the distal common duct within the head of the pancreas *(p).* (*a*, aorta.) **(C)** CT scan shows massive dilatation of the intrahepatic ducts with some discrete calculi (open arrows) and other intraductal debris, which forms a cast of the dependent ducts (small arrows). **(D)** CT scan caudad to **(C)** with a dilated common bile duct (arrows) within the pancreatic head. The duct is filled by a calculus that is higher in attenuation than the bile in the gallbladder *(gb).* At surgery, numerous pigmented stones were present in the intra- and extrahepatic ducts, along with biliary "mud" and pus. (From Federle MP, Cello JP, Laing FC, Jeffrey RB: Recurrent pyogenic cholangitis in Asian immigrants: use of ultrasonography, computed tomography and cholangiography. Radiology 143:151, 1982.)

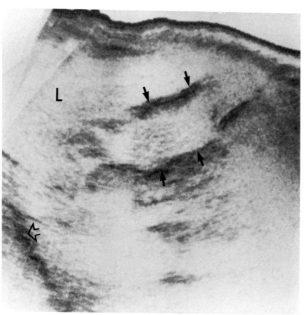

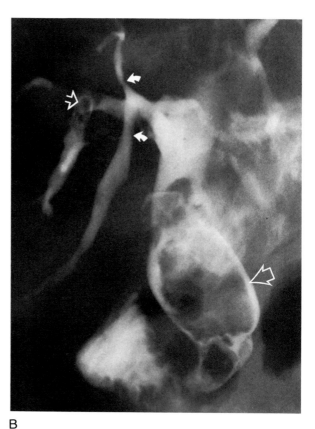

A   B

Fig. 2-86. Oriental cholangitis. **(A)** Longitudinal scan with a large lesion (arrows) extending from the porta hepatis to the pancreatic head and containing diffuse low-level echoes interpreted as a complex solid mass. Good definition of the backwall and through-transmission of sound suggests a tubular fluid-filled containing structure. No dilated intrahepatic ducts are seen. (*L*, liver; open arrow, diaphragm.) **(B)** Transhepatic cholangiogram demonstrates gross dilatation of the common bile duct and less striking dilatation of the hepatic ducts, with irregular areas of stenosis (curved arrows) and rapid tapering characteristic of recurrent pyogenic cholangitis. The left ductal system is incompletely filled. Large, amorphous filling defects form a virtual cast of the common bile duct (large open arrow) and are present in the intrahepatic ducts as well (small open arrow). At surgery, the ducts were filled with soft, pigmental calculi, sludge and mud-like pus. (From Federle MP, Cello JP, Laing FC, Jeffrey RB: Recurrent pyogenic cholangitis in Asian immigrants: Use of ultrasonography, computed tomography and cholangiography. Radiology 143:151, 1982.)

2-85 and 2-86). Striking dilatation of the extrahepatic ducts is seen with the ducts packed with huge pigmented stones. The common bile duct is the most frequently involved structure, followed by the left and right hepatic ducts. In 81.1 percent of cases there are bilirubinate stones.[197] In 60 percent, there are ductal stones, with cholelithiasis seen in 15 to 20 percent.[199] The gallbladder is large and palpable in 30 percent. Ultrasound may fail to demonstrate the ductal calculi and extrahepatic dilatation due to the soft-mudlike consistency of the stones.[199] The differential diagnosis on ultrasound would have to include biliary obstruction and Caroli's disease.[197]

SCLEROSING CHOLANGITIS

The etiology of sclerosing cholangitis is unknown but may be secondary to either bacterial or metabolic alteration of bile acids. It is seen in less than 1 percent of patients with ulcerative colitis. It is also associated with Riedel's struma, Crohn's disease, retroperitoneal fibrosis, and, possibly, mediastinal fibrosis.[200] It is more common in young men with jaundice, pruritis, fever, pain, weight loss, and hepatomegaly. Histologically, sclerosing cholangitis demonstrates nonspecific inflammation characterized by lymphocytic and plasma cells, bile duct proliferation, periportal fibrosis, cholestasis, and copper accumulation in the hepatic tissue.[200] Secondary cholangitis can be caused by tumors, previous surgery or trauma, and passage of large gallstones with resultant strictures.[200] On ultrasound, one sees evidence of biliary obstruction associated with marked concentric thickening of the intra- and extrahepatic biliary tree[200] (Fig. 2-87).

Congenital Abnormalities of the Biliary System

BILIARY ATRESIA

The differentiation of biliary atresia from neonatal hepatitis is critical and a difficult problem even with ultrasound and nuclear medicine. Biliary atresia exists

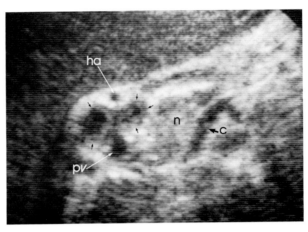

A

B

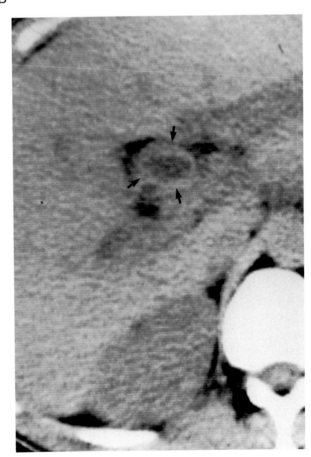

C

Fig. 2-87. Sclerosing cholangitis. **(A)** Longitudinal left decubitus scan through the porta hepatis. There is concentric thickening of the walls of the common hepatic and common bile duct to 1.5 cm (arrows). The lumen of the common duct (open arrow) is less than 5 mm in diameter. (*L*, liver; *pv*, portal vein; *n*, portal adenopathy; *c*, inferior vena cava; *ha*, hepatic artery.) **(B)** Oblique scan through the porta hepatis. There is concentric thickening of the walls of the right and left hepatic ducts (arrows). (*ha*, hepatic artery; *pv*, portal vein; *n*, node; *c*, inferior vena cava.) **(C)** CT scan at the level of the porta hepatis. There is concentric thickening of the dilated common bile duct (arrows). (From Carroll BA, Oppenheimer DA: Sclerosing cholangitis: sonographic demonstration of bile duct thickening. AJR 139:1016, © Am Roentgen Ray Soc, 1982.)

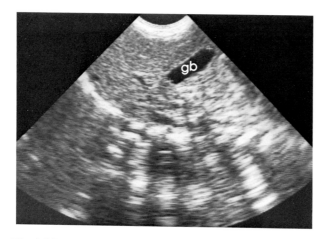

Fig. 2-88. Neonatal hepatitis. Longitudinal scan in a fasting newborn. A gallbladder *(gb)* is seen, which is 2.1 cm in length.

when the ducts from the hilum of the liver to the duodenum (including the gallbladder) are shown at surgery to be obliterated.[201] If a normal gallbladder (≥ 1.5 cm) is seen on ultrasound, the diagnosis of neonatal hepatitis is supported[201,202] (Fig. 2-88). However, gallbladders are present in 20 percent of patients with extrahepatic biliary atresia.[203] The liver may be echogenic or normal.[202] If there is nonvisualization of the gallbladder or the gallbladder is small (< 1.5 cm) on ultrasound without evidence of excretion of the radionuclide into the gastrointestinal tract and an indeterminate hepatic biopsy, surgical exploration is indicated.[201] It is most helpful to combine ultrasound and hepatobiliary nuclear medicine in these cases. Nuclear medicine has a sensitivity of 97 to 100 percent in the evaluation of neonatal jaundice with a specificity of 83 to 87 percent depending on phenobarbitol stimulation.[202,203] If there is passage of the radionu-

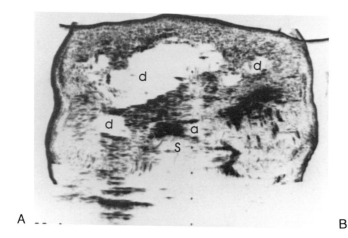

A

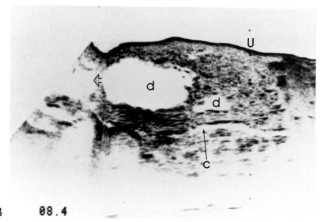

B   08.4

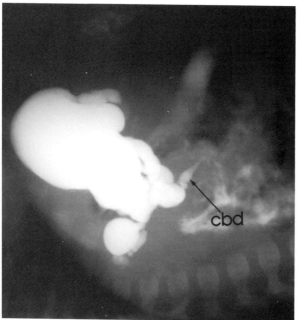

C

Fig. 2-89. Caroli's disease. **(A)** Transverse scan 3 cm below the xyphoid. Dilated ducts *(d)* are seen as anechoic spaces within the liver. (*a*, aorta; *S*, spine.) **(B)** Longitudinal scan 1 cm to the right of midline. (*c*, inferior vena cava; *U*, level of the umbilicus; open arrow, level of the diaphragm.) **(C)** Transhepatic cholangiogram, lateral view. The intrahepatic ducts are dilated but the common bile duct *(cbd)* is not dilated. (From Mittelstaedt CA, Volberg FM, Fischer GJ, McCartney WH: Caroli's disease: Sonographic findings. AJR 134:585, © American Roentgen Ray Society, 1980.)

clide from the liver to the gastrointestinal tract, patency of the biliary tree is noted.

CAROLI'S DISEASE

Caroli's disease is an entity characterized by (1) segmental saccular dilatation of the intrahepatic ducts; (2) marked predisposition for biliary calculous disease, cholangitis, and liver abscesses; (3) absence of portal hypertension and cirrhosis; and (4) association with renal tubular ectasia or other forms of cystic disease of the kidney.[204] Most coexist with hepatic fibrosis. Characteristically, there is a segmental, saccular, or beaded appearance to the intrahepatic ducts, which contain bile and communicate with the biliary tree. This condition leads to bile stasis, predisposes to bacterial growth, and, by compression of parenchymal cells, impairment of liver function. It is probably a Mendelian recessive trait. Patients present with crampy pain secondary to stone formation, which in turn is felt to be secondary to bile stasis within the cyst and to cholangitis. Pain, fever, and intermittent jaundice are the most common symptoms and usually develop during childhood or young adulthood.[205] Ultrasound enables the early diagnosis and can be used for follow-up examinations.[204] On ultrasound, one sees multiple cystic structures within the liver, which communicate with the biliary tree (Fig. 2-89). Stones, echogenic structures, may be seen with the ducts.

CHOLEDOCHAL CYST

A choledochal cyst is an uncommon abnormality with greater incidence in females and orientals.[206] It occurs four times more often in females than males.[207] The favored etiology is that of an anomalous insertion of the common bile duct into the pancreatic duct, permitting reflux of pancreatic juice into the bile duct leading to cholangitis and dilatation.[206,208,209] The theory of primary weakness in the wall with a distal obstructing lesion is now less favored.[208] Patients present in the first decade of life with pain, intermittent jaundice, and a palpable mass (in 20 to 25 percent).[178,208-211] Jaundice occurs in 70 percent of patients.[206] The incidence of carcinoma in a choledochal cyst is 20 times greater than bile duct carcinoma in the general population.[212]

There are four basic types of choledochal cysts: (1) cystic dilatation of the common bile duct (most common); (2) diverticulum of the common bile duct; (3) choledochocele; and (4) multiple intrahepatic and extrahepatic cysts.[206,208-210] In 50 percent of cases, there are associated dilated ducts.[213] The common hepatic duct is usually normal with variable portions of the extrahepatic ductal system involved.[178] The preoperative diagnosis is important, as the surgical morbidity and mortality is significantly diminished in cases in which the diagnosis is made correctly prior to surgery.[211] Prompt surgery is indicated to arrest possible complications of portal hypertension, cirrhosis, cholangitis, perforation, sepsis, and stone formation.[211]

On ultrasound, one finds a large cystic mass in the porta hepatis separate from the gallbladder with a dilated common hepatic duct or common bile duct entering directly into the cyst[206] (Fig. 2-90). Calculi may be seen within the cyst.[207] These lesions have even been observed antenatally.[208] The differential diagnosis would include hepatic cyst, pancreatic pseudocyst, enteric duplication, hepatic artery aneurysm, and spontaneous perforation of the extrahepatic ducts.[206] An accurate ultrasound diagnosis may lead to early corrective surgery, which may prevent irreversible biliary cirrhosis.[209]

Hydatid Disease of the Biliary System

Hydatid cysts may rupture into the biliary tree, with hydatid debris and daughter cysts entering the ducts and giving rise to jaundice and biliary colic.[214,215] The site and incidence of intrabiliary rupture is the right hepatic duct in 55 percent of cases, left hepatic duct in 29 percent, bifurcation in 9 percent, gallbladder in 6 percent, and common bile duct in 1 percent.[215] The development of jaundice is caused by the accumulation of hydatid sand in the extrahepatic ducts.[215] The diagnosis should be suggested on ultrasound if a complex mass is noted to be communicating with the biliary ducts[214] (Fig. 2-91). The lesion may be cystic with or without septation or it may exhibit a heterogeneous pattern with a hypo- or hyperechoic pattern.[215]

Biliary Drainage Procedures

Percutaneous biliary drainage and transhepatic cholangiography may be performed with the guidance of real-time ultrasound. The merits of the procedure include (1) single-step procedure, (2) no contrast, (3) left-sided approach permitting longer intubation, and (4) no use of irradiation.[216] Ultrasound can detect catheters used for decompression of the biliary tree and is an appropriate method for determining the success of biliary decompression without instilling contrast[217] (Fig. 2-92).

Ultrasound is indispensible as an aid in delineation of the left duct anatomy for directing needle puncture (Fig. 2-93). Accurate documentation and successful catheter drainage of the left duct obstruction are important contributions to total management of patients with high biliary obstruction.[218] A left hepatic duct approach is

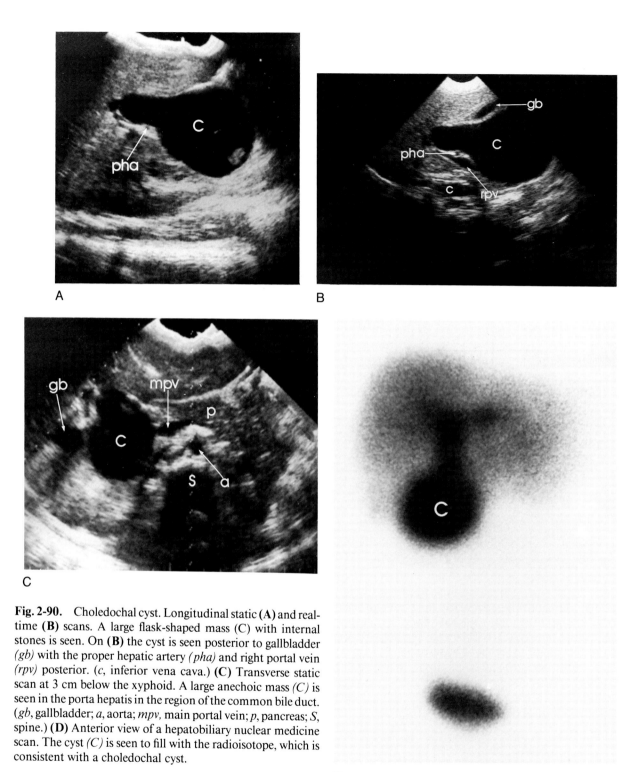

Fig. 2-90. Choledochal cyst. Longitudinal static **(A)** and real-time **(B)** scans. A large flask-shaped mass (C) with internal stones is seen. On **(B)** the cyst is seen posterior to gallbladder *(gb)* with the proper hepatic artery *(pha)* and right portal vein *(rpv)* posterior. (c, inferior vena cava.) **(C)** Transverse static scan at 3 cm below the xyphoid. A large anechoic mass *(C)* is seen in the porta hepatis in the region of the common bile duct. (*gb*, gallbladder; *a*, aorta; *mpv*, main portal vein; *p*, pancreas; *S*, spine.) **(D)** Anterior view of a hepatobiliary nuclear medicine scan. The cyst *(C)* is seen to fill with the radioisotope, which is consistent with a choledochal cyst.

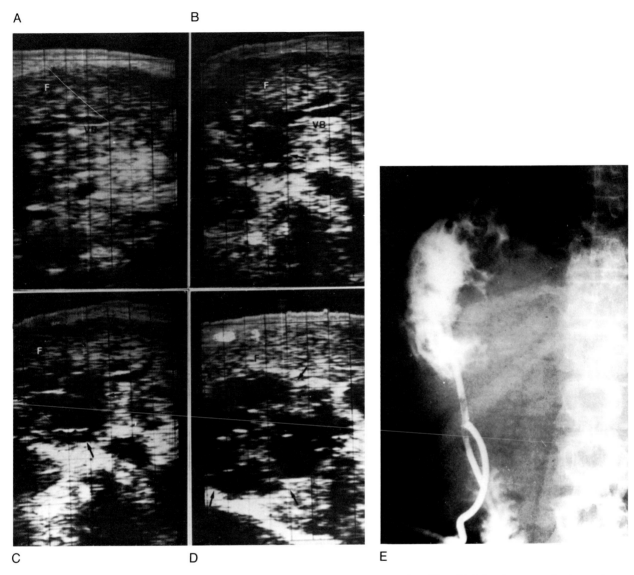

Fig. 2-91. Hydatid disease. **(A)** Transverse scan. An enlarged liver is seen with diffuse high-level structural echoes; the biliary ducts are dilated. **(B)** Transverse scan. The right biliary ducts are seen to communicate with a rounded irregular complex mass (arrow). **(C,D)** Oblique subcostal scans. A mass seen with many rounded cystic spaces divided by thick septa of solid tissue. The mass measured 18 × 12 cm with an oval shape with polycyclic margins (arrow) clearly separated from surrounding liver. (*F*, liver; *VB*, biliary ducts.) **(E)** T-tube cholangiogram. The mass is clearly demonstrated communicating with the biliary ducts. Within the tube, hydatid debris and/or small daughter cysts can be seen. (From Biggi E, Derchi L, Cicio GR, Valente M: Sonographic findings of hydatid cyst of the liver ruptured into the biliary duct. J Clin Ultrasound 7:381, 1979.)

often selected for the following reasons: (1) it is the largest hepatic duct in most patients and is nearest to the body surface; and (2) the entire biliary system can be opacified because contrast is heavier than bile and the left duct is located more anteriorly than the junction of the main hepatic duct.[219]

Bilomas

Bilomas are localized collections of bile within the peritoneal cavity, which may occur after surgery or after blunt or penetrating trauma; they are readily detected with ultrasound or CT.[220-223] The symptoms occur as

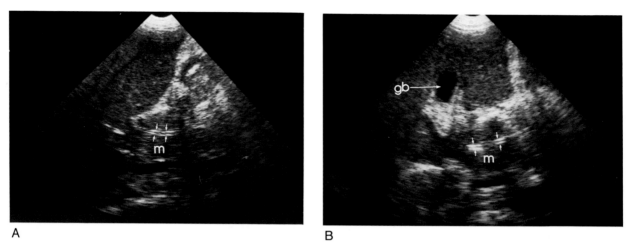

Fig. 2-92. Biliary decompression. The patient with pancreatic carcinoma in Figure 2.81 underwent percutaneous biliary decompression. The catheter (arrows) is seen within the common duct as two parallel echogenic lines on longitudinal (**A**) and transverse (**B**) scans. (*gb*, gallbladder; *m*, pancreatic head mass.)

the biloma, formed by a bile leak, grows. As such, they are manifested at a variable delayed interval after the initial injury. Some patients are asymptomatic. Many bilomas present with unexpected clinical features such as pyogenic subhepatic abscess, localized biloma in the left upper quadrant despite surgery on the right side, and presence of an active bile fistula.

The ultrasound features of bilomas include (1) a sharply defined echofree mass; (2) acoustic enhancement; (3) loculation; (4) location in the right, mid-upper or left upper quadrant; and (5) contiguity with the liver or biliary structures[222-224] (Fig. 2-94). The loculation

and size of the collection may be explained by the inflammatory reaction of the bile. Bile generates an intense inflammatory response that produces the sharply defined pseudocapsule.[222] The differential diagnosis would include hematoma and abscess, neither of which have pronounced acoustic enhancement.[224]

A percutaneous aspiration may be guided with ultrasound to evaluate a gallbladder fossa fluid collection following biliary tract surgery.[225] Bile can be identified by visual inspection and an initial rapid dip-stick (Multistix) technique as well as formal chemical analysis.[223] To confirm the diagnosis further and for drainage purposes,

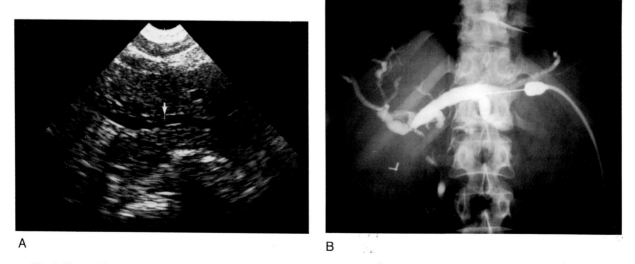

Fig. 2-93. Biliary decompression. Left duct approach. (**A**) Transverse scan localizing the depth (arrow) of a dilated left hepatic duct. (**B**) Transhepatic cholangiogram. There are dilated intrahepatic ducts with an area of stricture immediately distal to the right and left hepatic ducts. The common duct was normal in size.

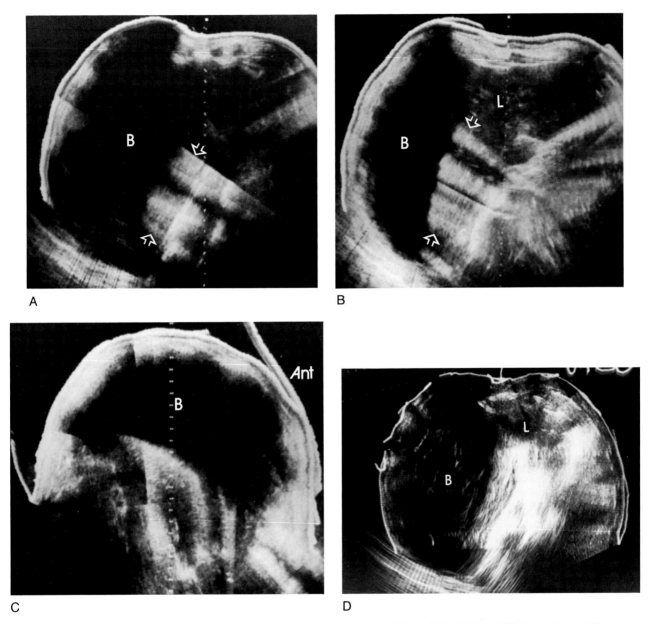

Fig. 2-94. Biloma. Postoperative cholecystectomy. Transverse scans at 22 cm **(A)** and 16 cm **(B)** above the umbilicus. A large fluid collection *(B)* is seen lateral to the liver *(L)*. It exhibits acoustic enhancement (open arrows). **(C)** Left lateral decubitus transverse scan at 15 cm above the iliac crest. The fluid *(B)* does not move. (*Ant,* anterior.) Follow-up transverse scan **(D)** at 20 cm above the umbilicus 1 month after **(A–C)**. The fluid collection *(B)* has developed internal septations. The fluid was aspirated and found to be bile. (*L,* liver.)

a catheter may be placed into the biloma. Percutaneous radiologic catheter drainage provides adequate therapeutic drainage in most patients, except for those with continuing active bile leak that eventually requires surgical correction.[223]

The diagnosis of biloma may be confirmed by hepatobiliary nuclear medicine study.[224,226] Delayed views usually confirm the diagnosis.[224] Evidence for continued free bile leak includes a positive hepatobiliary nuclear

medicine scan and copious amounts of bilious catheter drainage over a prolonged period.

Biliary Enteric Anastomoses

Cholecystocolic fistula may occur infrequently as a complication of long-standing cholelithiasis and cholecystitis in the elderly patient. The importance in making the diagnosis lies in the fact that the patient is at an increased risk for the development of cholangitis, gastrointestinal tract bleeding, malabsorption syndrome, and other medical problems—leading many physicians to advocate surgical intervention. Cholecystocolic fistulous tract formation constitutes 15 percent of the enterobiliary communications. It is second in frequency to the cholecystoduodenal fistula, which constitutes 70 percent of enterobiliary communications. The incidence in the general population of all enterobiliary fistula is 0.1 to 0.5 percent. Ninety percent occur in patients with cholelithiasis and chronic cholecystitis. Fibrous adhesions develop between the gallbladder and adjacent tissue with necrosis of the gallbladder wall and perforation. The site for communication is usually the hepatic flexure or proximal transverse colon. In the absence of a stone, the fistula usually communicates with the common bile duct. Symptoms disappear after the gallbladder decompresses into the colon. The failure to demonstrate, on ultrasound, a previously revealed gallstone indicates passage. The fistula itself is usually obscured by biliary air[227] (Fig. 1-107).

For evaluation of the surgically established biliary-enteric anastomoses, hepatobiliary nuclear medicine is the preferred technique. Ultrasound is limited because of the gas within the anastomosis obscuring the bile ducts, and gas within the biliary tree producing confusing echoes that mimic intrahepatic biliary calculi. Ultrasound may be useful regarding bile duct caliber, but refluxed biliary air and persistent postoperative biliary dilatation are significant obstacles. Nuclear medicine is the best technique for this evaluation.[228]

CORRELATIVE IMAGING

Gallbladder Disease

When evaluating for gallbladder disease in general (e.g., stones or cholecystitis), ultrasound is the preferred modality.[229] It has been shown to have an overall accuracy of 98.9 percent with a false-negative rate of 7.2 percent and a false-positive rate of 7.8 percent.[229] Because of its high accuracy, minimal preparation, speed, and cost-effectiveness, ultrasound is recommended for screening for gallbladder disease.[229]

Cholelithiasis

Studies have been undertaken to answer the question of how real-time and static ultrasound compare in the accuracy of diagnosing stones. In one study, the gallbladder was seen with real-time sonography in 97.6 percent

of cases and 94.5 percent of the gallstones were identified in those patients with cholelithiasis. With static ultrasound, the gallbladder was visualized in only 89.5 percent of cases and 78.8 percent of the gallstones were identified in the patients with cholelithiasis. Another study reported an accuracy of 86.3 percent for static scans and 96 percent for real-time scans.[59] One study reported no nonvisualized gallbladders with real-time ultrasound, with a 12- to 16-percent nonvisualization rate with static ultrasound.[230] This demonstrates that real-time ultrasound is more accurate because it can show the contracted, stone-filled gallbladder faster; it is also more convenient to both patient and examiner, making it the procedure of choice in the primary evaluation of the gallbladder.[231] The apparent improvement in spatial resolution observed with real-time ultrasound is probably due to the highly flexible cable of the transducer, which permits optimal positioning and selection of an infinite variety of oblique scanning planes.[59]

The accuracy of ultrasound in diagnosing cholelithiasis has also been compared to that of other gallbladder imaging techniques. The accuracy of the various ultrasound criteria for gallstones have been reported to be (1) shadowing moving intraluminal densities—100 percent; (2) nonvisualization of the gallbladder lumen—96 percent; and (3) nonshadowing opacities within the gallbladder—61 percent.[41,229,232] An accuracy of 98.6 percent for diagnosing cholelithiasis with ultrasound has been reported when using the following criteria: (1) gallbladder well visualized in at least two projections; (2) intraluminal gallbladder densities well defined; and (3) densities either shadow and/or move rapidly with change in patient position.[50] Early studies with static and real-time ultrasound reported accuracies of 89 to 93 percent.[233-237] Later studies have demonstrated an overall accuracy of 96 to 98.9 percent, with a sensitivity of 98 percent, a specificity of 93.5 to 97.7 percent, a false-negative rate of 2.2 to 4 percent and a false-positive rate of 2.8 percent.[229,232,238] The accuracy of the oral cholecystogram has been reported to be 93 to 93.2 percent.[232,239]

There is thus much evidence suggesting that ultrasound is the modality of choice for an accurate evaluation of many pathologic states of the gallbladder, as it is an ideal organ for ultrasound evaluation. While the oral cholecystogram is one of the most trusted radiographic procedures, various protocols proposed for film and pill taking probably reflect dissatisfaction with the procedure. Ultrasound allows a rapid examination to obtain a definitive diagnosis. Also, many studies have shown stones with ultrasound that were not demonstrated on oral cholecystograms.[240] In addition, ultrasound is more sensitive than CT for detecting the presence of gallstones because of the partial volume averaging errors that occur with CT.[241] Because of its high accuracy, minimal preparation, speed of diagnosis, and cost-effectiveness, real-time ultrasound is recommended for screening in patients with suspected gallbladder disease.[50,229]

With regard to gallbladder neck/cystic duct area, ultrasound has been reported to have a sensitivity of 30 percent, a specificity of 100 percent, and an accuracy of 74 percent.[55] Ultrasound is generally not a good method for diagnosis of cystic duct obstruction.

Cholecystitis

Which diagnostic modality is the method of choice for evaluation of cholecystitis is a much more controversial topic than that of cholelithiasis. Some favor ultrasound because of its capabilities to view the entire right upper quadrant and to assess for pinpoint gallbladder tenderness.[107] Others favor hepatobiliary nuclear medicine because it is a better test for evaluating gallbladder function.[242,243] Most institutions do not use intravenous cholangiography because of the morbidity and mortality associated with it.[244]

Much data support the use of ultrasound as the initial imaging procedure for patients with suspected acute cholecystitis, but a comparison between ultrasound and nuclear medicine studies should be made. The rapid assessment of the patient with suspected acute cholecystitis poses a difficult and important problem. Hepatobiliary nuclear medicine is useful in those cases without stones, which exhibit minor criteria for gallbladder abnormality. The major diagnostic feature is the presence (cystic duct patency) or absence (cystic duct obstruction) of gallbladder visualization.[245] While visualization of the gallbladder with hepatobiliary nuclear medicine usually precludes the possibility of acute cholecystitis, nonvisualization does not, and delayed views would have to be obtained. One study reported the visualization of a gallbladder on nuclear medicine with acute cholecystitis and a patent cystic duct.[246] Another reports visualization of an obstructed gallbladder via an accessory hepatic duct.[247] The visualization of two gallbladders involved with acute cholecystitis has been described with nuclear medicine.[248]

How do the accuracies of ultrasound and nuclear medicine compare with regard to acute cholecystitis? Numerous studies have reported the following statistics for nuclear medicine: accuracy of 84.7 to 88 percent, specificity of 90.2 to 100 percent, sensitivity of 95 to 98.3 percent, and false-negative rate of 5 percent.[105,249–252] The comparative values for ultrasound are: accuracy of 88.1 percent, specificity of 60.2 to 100 percent, and sensitivity of 76 to 97 percent.[105,249–252] The ultrasound criteria of gallbladder roundness or a diameter of greater than 5 cm was less sensitive and less specific. When dif-

ferentiating normality from all types of gallbladder disease, nuclear medicine had a sensitivity of 80 percent with a specificity of 100 percent[105]; ultrasound had a sensitivity of 100 percent with a specificity of 96 percent, using the major and minor criteria for gallbladder disease.[105] The most common minor criterion seen in acute cholecystitis was increased wall thickness.[105] Some believe the choice of the examination—nuclear medicine or ultrasound—should depend on (1) quality of available equipment, (2) capability of technologist to perform the exam, (3) relative experience of the physician, and (4) willingness of the surgeon to accept a positive result as an indication to perform emergency surgery.[249]

The reliability of the elicitation of pin-point right upper quadrant pain in making the diagnosis of cholecystitis has also been studied. Investigators have examined the role of ultrasound in evaluating acute right upper quadrant pain, with a clinical suspicion of acute cholecystitis. The diagnosis of acute cholecystitis is based on the highly significant observations of focal gallbladder tenderness and calculi. Sludge and wall thickness are statistically significant but to a lesser degree. Cholelithiasis allows differentiation of patients with chronic cholecystitis from patients with normal gallbladders; these latter patients do not have significant focal gallbladder tenderness, sludge, or a thickened wall. Ultrasound has a sensitivity of 94 percent, a specificity of 85 percent, and an overall accuracy of 88 percent with regard to acute cholecystitis.[107] Maximum tenderness is demonstrated over the gallbladder in 85 to 87.2 percent of cases of acute cholecystitis.[91,108] The sensitivity of focal tenderness is 63 to 94 percent with a specificity of 93.6 percent, a predictive value for a positive sign of 72.5 percent, and a predictive value for a negative sign of 90.5 percent.[107,108] Focal tenderness distinguishes acute from chronic cholecystitis. With chronic cholecystitis, the sensitivity is 71 percent with a specificity of 97 percent and an overall accuracy of 88 percent.[107] Of the patients with symptoms of acute cholecystitis in this study, only 34.6 percent truly had it.[107] In addition, when the gallbladder wall is thicker than 3.5 mm in the absence of ascites in patients suspected of acute acalculous cholecystitis, ultrasound can make a diagnosis with a specificity of 98 percent.[110]

While ultrasound's accuracy is not as high as that of nuclear medicine, there are several factors that lend support to the proposition that ultrasound be performed as the initial exam in the patient with acute right upper quadrant pain. Inclusive are that (1) two out of three patients do not have acute cholecystitis; (2) ultrasound is an extremely accurate method in determining whether or not the gallbladder is abnormal—either acute or chronically (sensitivity 94 percent, specificity 97 percent, accuracy 96 percent); and (3) in patients with normal appearing nontender gallbladders, ultrasound may be able to localize the site of pathology or may direct the patient's work-up such that extrabiliary site of disease will be evaluated more directly.[107] If ultrasound is normal and the pain is localized to the gallbladder fossa, a nuclear medicine scan may be performed to exclude the possibility of a stone impacted in the duct. Because of ultrasound's multiorgan imaging capabilities and its ability to localize areas of maximum tenderness, it is felt that it is the imaging technique of choice in evaluation of patients with right upper quadrant pain. The diagnosis of acute cholecystitis can be confirmed if calculi are visualized in a tender gallbladder; the diagnosis is further supported if the gallbladder contains sludge and has a thickened wall. If the gallbladder is not tender and stones are present, the diagnosis of chronic cholecystitis is made. If the gallbladder is not tender and normal, gallbladder disease is unlikely and clinical attention should be directed away from the gallbladder and biliary system. In conclusion, because acute cholecystitis is only found in a minority of patients with acute right upper quadrant pain, and because ultrasound is a rapid, accurate, and noninvasive test, it should be the initial modality used to evaluate these patients.[107,253]

Biliary Dilatation

The method of choice for evaluation of biliary tract dilatation is once again ultrasound.[254] Ultrasound is the preferred initial screening procedure for biliary tract dilatation in the jaundiced patient in whom obstruction must be differentiated from hepatocellular disease; this is because of the accuracy and sensitivity of ultrasound, although CT more precisely displays the level and cause of obstruction.[254,255] When evaluating the accuracy of ultrasound in identifying dilatation of the common hepatic duct, the sensitivity is reported to be 99 percent, with a specificity of 87 percent if the common hepatic duct is greater than 4 mm.[24] Ultrasound studies describe an accuracy of 86 to 97 percent for ultrasound in differentiating obstructive from nonobstructive jaundice, with a predictive value of 97 percent in obstruction and 84 percent in nonobstruction.[256-260] The level of obstruction is demonstrated in 95 percent and the cause of obstruction in 68 percent.[257] When comparing ultrasound and CT, ultrasound has been reported to identify the precise level of obstruction in 60 percent and CT in 88 percent.[261] The cause of obstruction can be accurately predicted in 38 percent with ultrasound and 70 percent with CT.[261] While ultrasound can be used as a screen for obstructive jaundice, it is not as helpful in identifying the level of the obstruction and the cause; CT is more accurate in this respect.[261] If the ultrasound scan is normal,

no further studies are needed. If there is evidence of obstruction, CT and/or percutaneous transhepatic cholangiography is performed. The markedly obese patient or the patient with a biliary-enteric anastomosis is better suited to CT.[261]

Other investigators have compared ultrasound and nuclear medicine in the evaluation of biliary tract obstruction.[262] They found nuclear medicine to have a sensitivity of 18 percent with a specificity of 100 percent for large duct obstruction, while ultrasound had a sensitivity of 82 percent and specificity of 86 percent, with a predictive value for a negative interpretation of 97 percent.[262]

Choledocholithiasis

The method of choice in evaluating a patient for choledocholithiasis is less clear-cut. While ultrasound is the method of choice in the diagnosis of cholelithiasis and for evaluation of biliary tract obstruction, its role in the diagnosis of choledocholithiasis is uncertain. It is not accurate in the diagnosis (sensitivity 22 to 25 percent) or exclusion (value-negative study 73 percent) of choledocholithiasis.[180,263] The overall accuracy of ultrasound is reported to be 15 to 60 percent.[182] There are several explanations for this low accuracy.[264] In both dilated and nondilated ducts, the distal area of the common bile duct, where impacted stones usually lie, often is obscured by bowel gas from the duodenum or colon. Occasionally in dilated ducts, a stone can be visualized by placing the patient in the Trendelenberg position and observe the stone floating cephalad. Lack of a bile pool in the dilated and nondilated duct preclude detection of the obstructing stone.[264]

Several studies have demonstrated an improved accuracy in the diagnosis of choledocholithiasis with the new high resolution real-time systems.[7,55] In one study, the earlier results demonstrated a sensitivity of 29 percent, a specificity of 91 percent, and an accuracy of 55 percent.[55] In the last part of their study using high-resolution real-time ultrasound, the sensitivity increased to 55 percent, specificity to 90 percent, and accuracy to 71 percent.[55] The improved results were felt to be secondary to several factors: (1) the high-resolution real-time ultrasound with flexibility and ability to display rapidly many planes of sections; and (2) improved skills to image the common bile duct.[55] By adding an evaluation of the distal common bile duct in another study, the overall sensitivity of ultrasound for the diagnosis of choledocholithiasis was 75 percent.[7] Eighty-nine percent of proximal and 70 percent of distal common bile duct calculi were identified.[7]

CT and ultrasound have been compared with regard to choledocholithiasis.[265] Ultrasound demonstrated a sensitivity of 18 percent with an accuracy of 19 per-

cent.[265] CT had a sensitivity of 87 percent with an accuracy of 84 percent.[265] CT is felt to be effective in imaging for common bile duct stones and is superior to ultrasound in diagnosing the cause of obstruction. While ultrasound is an excellent initial procedure to detect biliary dilatation, CT is effective in the definition of the level and cause of obstruction. Ultrasound is limited in its ability to image a calculus in the distal common bile duct. Percutaneous cholangiography is reserved for cases in which (1) further confirmation is required preoperatively; (2) cause is not determined by CT; (3) ducts are not dilated on ultrasound or CT but there is clinical suspicion of obstruction; (4) percutaneous biliary decompression is indicated; and (5) endoscopic retrograde cholangiopancreatography (ERCP) sphinecterotomy is the treatment of choice.[265]

Postoperative Cholecystectomy Patients

Finally, the method of choice in examining the postoperative cholecystectomy patient must be discussed. In these patients, ERCP is recommended as the initial diagnostic modality.[263] Ultrasound demonstrates a specificity of 87 percent in these cases; the value of a positive diagnosis is 60 percent and that of a negative diagnosis is 64 percent.[263] When comparing ultrasound to ERCP, ultrasound is 88-percent sensitive with a specificity of 93 percent.[263] The sensitivity of the sonographic measurement of the common hepatic duct as an indicator of biliary obstruction is 88 percent with a specificity of 57 percent.[176] ERCP is thus recommended for evaluation of the postoperative gallbladder patient even though the complication rate of the procedure is 3 percent, the mortality is 0.2 percent, and the failure rate is 12 percent.[263]

REFERENCES

1. Foster SC, McLaughlin SM: Improvement in the ultrasonic evaluation of the gallbladder by using the left lateral decubitus position. J Clin Ultrasound 5:253, 1977
2. Behan M, Kazam E: Sonography of the common bile duct: Value of the right anterior oblique view. AJR 130:701, 1978
3. Albarelli JN: Erect cholecystosonography. J Clin Ultrasound 3:309, 1975
4. Okulski TA, Eikman EA, Williams JW: Ultrasound measurement of contraction response of the gallbladder: Comparison with the radionuclide test for cystic duct patency. Clin Nuclear Med 3:117, 1982
5. Davis GB, Berk RN, Scheible FW, et al: Cholecystokinin cholecystography, sonography and scintigraphy: detection of chronic acalculous cholecystitis. AJR 139:1117, 1982
6. Parulekar SG: Ultrasound evaluation of common bile duct size. Radiology 133:703, 1979
7. Laing FC, Jeffrey RB, Wing VW: Improved visualization of choledocholithiasis by sonography. AJR 143:949, 1984
8. O'Brien MJ, Gottlieb LS: The Liver and Biliary Tract p. 1071. In Robbins SL, Cotran RS (eds): Pathologic Basis of Disease. W.B. Saunders, Philadelphia, 1979
9. Kane RA: Ultrasonographic anatomy of the liver and biliary tree. p. 87. In Raymond HW, Zwiebel WJ (eds): Seminars in Ultrasound. Vol. 1. Grune and Stratton, New York, 1980
10. Cooperberg PL: Real-time ultrasonography of the gallbladder. p. 49. In Winsberg F, Cooperberg PL (eds): Clinics in Diagnostic Ultrasound:Real-time Ultrasonography. Churchill Livingstone, New York, 1982
11. Callen PW, Filly RA: Ultrasonographic localization of the gallbladder. Radiology 133:687, 1979
12. Laing FC, Jeffrey RB: The pseudo-dilated common bile duct: Ultrasonographic appearance created by the gallbladder neck. Radiology 135:405, 1980
13. Birnholz JC: Population survey: ultrasonic cholecystography. Gastrointest Radiol 7:165, 1982
14. Marchal G, deVoorde V, Dooren MV, et al: Ultrasonic appearance of the filled and contracted normal gallbladder. J Clin Ultrasound 8:439, 1980
15. McGahan JP, Phillips HE, Cox KL: Sonography of the normal pediatric gallbladder and biliary tree. Radiology 144:873, 1982
16. Yeh H-C: Update on the gallbladder. p. 135. In Sanders RL (ed): Ultrasound Annual 1982. Raven Press, New York, 1982
17. Carroll BA, Oppenheimer DA, Muller HH: High-frequency real-time ultrasound of the neonatal biliary system. Radiology 145:437, 1982
18. Sukov RJ, Sample WF, Sarti DA, Whitcomb MJ: Cholecystosonography — the junctional fold. Radiology 133:435, 1979
19. Bova JG: Gallstone simulated by gallbladder septation. AJR 140:287, 1983
20. Cunningham JJ: Empyema of a duplicated gallbladder: echographic findings. J Clin Ultrasound 8:511, 1980
21. Taylor KJW, Rosenfield AT, DeGraaff CS: Anatomy and pathology of the biliary tree as demonstrated on ultrasound. p. 103. In Taylor KJW (ed): Clinics in Diagnostic Ultrasound: Diagnostic Ultrasound in Gastrointestinal Disease. Churchill Livingstone, New York, 1979
22. Sauerbrei E: Ultrasound of the Common Bile Duct. p. 1. In Sanders RC, Hill MC (eds): Ultrasound Annual 1983. Raven Press, New York, 1983
23. Cooperberg P: High-resolution real-time ultrasound in the evaluation of the normal and obstructed biliary tract. Radiology 129:477, 1978
24. Cooperberg PL, Li D, Wong P, Cohen MM, Burhenne HJ: Accuracy of common hepatic duct size in the evaluation of extrahapatic biliary obstruction. Radiology 135:141, 1980
25. Sauerbrei EE, Cooperberg PL, Gordon P, et al: The dis-

crepancy between radiographic and sonographic bile-duct measurements. Radiology 137:751, 1980

26. Willi UV, Teele RL: Hepatic arteries and the parallel-channel sign. J Clin Ultrasound 7:125, 1979

27. Berland LL, Lawson TL, Foley WD: Porta hepatis: Sonographic discrimination of bile ducts from arteries with pulsed doppler with new anatomic criteria. AJR 138:833, 1982

28. Bandai Y, Masatoshi M, Watanabe G, et al: Sonographic differentiation between umbilical portion of the left portal vein and intrahepatic bile ducts. J Clin Ultrasound 8:207, 1980

29. Ralls PW, Quinn MF, Halls J: Biliary sonography: Ventral bowing of the dilated common duct. AJR 137:1127, 1981

30. Jacobson JB, Brodey PA: The transverse common duct. AJR 136:91, 1981

31. Mueller PR, Ferrucci JT, Simeone JF, et al: Observations on the distensibility of the common bile duct. Radiology 142:467, 1982

32. Glazer GM, Filly RA, Laing FC: Rapid change in the caliber of the nonobstructed common duct. Radiology 140:161, 1981

33. Durrell CA, Vincent LM, Mittelstaedt CA: Gallbladder ultrasound in clinical context. p. 315. In Mueller PR (ed): Seminars in Ultrasound, CT and MR. Vol. 5. Grune & Stratton, Orlando, 1984

34. Lawson TL: Gray scale cholecystosonography: Diagnostic criteria and accuracy. Radiology 122:247, 1977

35. Grossman M: Cholelithiasis and acoustic shadowing. J Clin Ultrasound 6:182, 1978

36. Simeone JF, Ferrucci JT: New trends in gallbladder imaging. JAMA 246:380, 1981

37. Crow HC, Bartrum RJ, Foote SR: Expanded criteria for the ultrasonic diagnosis of gallstones. J Clin Ultrasound 4:289, 1976

38. Carroll BA: Gallstones: In vitro comparison of physical radiographic and ultrasonic characteristics. AJR 131:223, 1978

39. Good LI, Edell SL, Soloway RD, et al: Ultrasonic properties of gallstones—effect of stone size and composition. Gastroenterology 77:258, 1979

40. Simeone JF, Mueller PR, Ferrucci JT, et al: Significance of nonshadowing focal opacities at cholecystosonography. Radiology 137:181, 1980

41. Philbrick TH, Kaude JK, McInnis AN, Wright PG: Abdominal ultrasound in patients with acute right upper quadrant pain. Gastrointest Radiol 6:251, 1981

42. Filly RA, Moss AA, Way LW: In vitro investigation of gallstone shadowing with ultrasound tomography. J Clin Ultrasound 7:255, 1979

43. Gonzalez L, MacIntyre WJ: Acoustic shadow formation by gallstones. Radiology 135:217, 1980

44. Taylor KJW, Jacobson P, Jaffee CC: Lack of an acoustic shadow on scans of gallstones: a possible artifact. Radiology 131:463, 1979

45. Bartrum RJ Jr, Crow HC: Inflammation diseases of the biliary system. p. 102. In Raymond HW, Zwiebel WJ (eds): Seminars in Ultrasound. Vol. 1. Grune and Stratton, New York, 1980

46. Purdom RC, Thomas SR, Kereiakes JG, et al: Ultrasonic properties of biliary calculi. Radiology 136:729, 1980

47. Parulekar SG: Ultrasonic detection of calcification in gallstones: "the reverberation shadow". J Ultrasound Med 3:123, 1984

48. Sommer FG, Taylor KJW: Differentiation of acoustic shadowing due to calculi and gas collections. Radiology 135:399, 1980

49. Garel L, Lallemand D, Montagne JP, Forel F, Sauve-grain J: The changing aspects of cholelithiasis in children through a sonographic study. Pediatr Radiol 11:75, 1981

50. Hessler PC, Hill DS, Detorie FM, Rocco AF: High accuracy sonographic recognition of gallstones. AJR 136:517, 1981

51. Scheske GA, Cooperberg PL, Cohen MM, Burhenne HJ: Floating gallstones: The role of contrast material. J Clin Ultrasound 8:227, 1980

52. Lebensart PD, Bloom RA, Meretyk S, et al: Oral cholecystosonography: A method of facilitating the diagnosis of cholesterol gallstones. Radiology 153:255, 1984

53. Strijk SP, Boetes C, Rosenbusch G: Floating stones in nonopacified gallbladder: Ultrasonographic sign gas-containing gallstones. Gastrointest Radiol 6:261, 1981

54. Gooding GAW: Food particles in the gallbladder mimic cholelithiasis in a patient with a cholecystojejunostomy. J Clin Ultrasound 9:346, 1981

55. Laing FC, Jeffrey RB: Choledocholithiasis and cystic duct obstruction: difficult ultrasonographic diagnosis. Radiology 146:475, 1983

56. Jackson VP, Lappas JC: Sonography of the Mirizzi syndrome. J Ultrasound Med 3:281, 1984

57. Becker CD, Hassler H, Terrier F: Preoperative diagnosis of the Mirizzi syndrome: limitations of sonography and computed tomography. AJR 143:591, 1984

58. Koehler RE, Melson GL, Lee JKT, Long J: Common hepatic duct obstruction by cystic duct stone: Mirizzi syndrome. AJR 132:1007, 1979

59. Raptopoulos V, D'Orsi C, Smith E, et al: Dynamic cholecystosonography of the contracted gallbladder: the double-arc-shadow sign. AJR 138:275, 1982

60. Laing FC, Gooding GAW, Herzog KA: Gallstones preventing ultrasonographic visualization of the gallbladder. Gastrointest Radiol 1:301, 1977

61. MacDonald FR, Cooperberg PL, Cohen MM: The WES triad—a specific sonographic sign of gallstones in the contracted gallbladder. Gastrointest Radiol 6:39, 1981

62. Conrad MR, Leonard J, Landay MJ: Left lateral decubitus sonography of gallstones in the contracted gallbladder. AJR 134:141, 1980

63. Harbin WP, Ferrucci JT, Wittenberg J, Kirkpatrick RH: Nonvisualized gallbladder by cholecystosonograph. AJR 132:127, 1979

64. Kane RA, Jacobs R, Katz J, Costello P: Porcelain gallbladder: ultrasound and CT appearance. Radiology 152:137, 1984

65. Buschi AJ, Brenbridge NAG: Sonographic diagnosis of cholelithiasis in childhood. Am J Dis Child 134:575, 1980

66. Henschke CI, Teele RL: Cholelithiasis in children: recent observations. J Ultrasound Med 2:481, 1983

67. Callahan J, Haller JO, Cacciarelli AA, et al: Cholelithiasis in infants: association with total parenteral nutrition and furosemide. Radiology 143:437, 1982

68. Brill PW, Winchester P, Rosen MS: Neonatal cholelithiasis. Pediatr Radiol 12:285, 1982

69. Cunningham JJ: Sonographic diameter of the common hepatic duct in sickle cell anemia. AJR 141:321, 1983

70. Sarnaik S, Slovis TL, Corbett DP, et al: Incidence of cholelithiasis in sickle cell anemia using the ultrasonic gray-scale equipment. J Pediatr 96:1005, 1980

71. Borgna-Pignatti C, De Stefano P, Pajno D, et al: Cholelithiasis in children with thalassemia major: an ultrasonographic study. J Pediatr 99:243, 1981

72. Cunningham JJ, Houlihan SM, Altay C: Cholecystosonography in children with sickle cell disease: technical approach and clinical results. J Clin Ultrasound 9:231, 1981

73. Filly RA, Allen B, Minton MJ, et al: In vitro investigation of the origin of echoes within biliary sludge. J Clin Ultrasound 8:193, 1980

74. Fakhry J: Sonography of tumefactive biliary sludge. AJR 139:717, 1982

75. Conrad MR, Janes JO, Dietchy J: Significance of low level echoes within the gallbladder. AJR 132:967, 1979

76. Fiske CE, Filly RA: Pseudo-sludge. A spurious ultrasound appearance within the gallbladder. Radiology 144:631, 1982

77. Buschi AJ, Brenbridge NAG, Cochrane JA, Teates CD: A further observation on gallbladder debris. J Clin Ultrasound 7:152, 1979

78. Grant EG, Smirniotopoulos JC: Intraluminal gallbladder hematoma: Sonographic evidence of hemobilia. J Clin Ultrasound 11:507, 1983

79. Jeanty P, Ammann W, Cooperberg PL, et al: Mobile intraluminal masses of the gallbladder. J Ultrasound Med 2:65, 1983

80. Anastasi B, Sutherland GR: Biliary sludge — ultrasonic appearance simulating neoplasm. Br J Radiol 54:679, 1981

81. Weeks LE, McCune BR, Martin JF, O'Brien TF: Unusual echographic appearance of a courvoisier gallbladder. J Clin Ultrasound 5:341, 1977

82. Britten JS, Golding RH, Cooperberg PL: Sludge balls to gallstones. J Ultrasound Med 3:81, 1984

83. Love MB: Sonographic features of milk of calcium bile. J Ultrasound Med 1:325, 1982

84. Chun GH, Deutsch AL, Scheible W: Sonographic findings in milk of calcium bile. Gastrointest Radiol 7:371, 1982

85. Burth RA, Brasch RC, Filly RA: Abdominal pseudotumor in childhood: distended gallbladder with parenteral hyperalimentation. AJR 136:341, 1981

86. Oppenheimer DA, Carroll BA: Spontaneous resolution of hyperalimentation-induced biliary dilatation: ultrasonic description. J Ultrasound Med 1:213, 1982

87. Liechty EA, Cohen MD, Lemons JA, et al: Normal gallbladder appearing as abdominal mass in neonates. Am J Dis Child 136:468, 1982

88. Wales LR: Desquamated gallbladder mucosa: unusual sign of cholecystitis. AJR 139:810, 1982

89. Mindell HJ, Ring BA: Gallbladder wall thickening: ultrasonic finding. Radiology 133:699, 1979

90. Marchal G, Crolla D, Baert AL, et al: Gallbladder wall thickening: a new sign of gallbladder disease visualized by gray-scale cholecystosonography. J Clin Ultrasound 6:177, 1978

91. Elyaderani MK, Gabriele OF: Cholecystosonography in detection of acute cholecystitis: the halo sign — A significant sonographic finding. So Med J 76:174, 1983

92. Juttner H-U, Ralls PW, Quinn MF, Jenney JM: Thickening of the gallbladder wall in acute hepatitis: ultrasound demonstration. Radiology 142:465, 1982

93. Fiske CE, Laing FC, Brown TW: Ultrasonographic evidence of gallbladder wall thickening in association with hypoalbuminemia. Radiology 135:713, 1980

94. Handler SJ: Ultrasound of gallbladder wall thickening and its relation to cholecystitis. AJR 132:581, 1979

95. Engel JM, Deitch EA, Sikkema W: Gallbladder wall thickness: sonographic accuracy and relation to disease. AJR 134:907, 1980

96. Raghavendka BN, Feiner HD, Subramanyam BR, et al: Acute cholecystitis: sonographic-pathologic analysis. AJR 137:327, 1981

97. Patriquin HB, DiPietro M, Barber FE, Teele RL: Sonography of thickened gallbladder wall: causes in children. AJR 141:57, 1983

98. Finberg JH, Birnholtz JC: Ultrasound evaluation of the gallbladder wall. Radiology 133:693, 1979

99. Lewandowski B, Winsberg F: Gallbladder wall thickness distortion by ascites. AJR 137:519, 1981

100. Shlaer WJ, Leopold GR, Scheible FW: Sonography of the thickened gallbladder wall: a nonspecific finding. AJR 136:337, 1981

101. Sanders RC: The significance of sonographic gallbladder wall thickening. J Clin Ultrasound 8:143, 1980

102. Ralls PW, Quinn MF, Juttner HU, et al: Gallbladder wall thickening: patients without intrinsic gallbladder disease. AJR 137:65, 1981

103. Carroll BA: Gallbladder wall thickening secondary to focal lymphatic obstruction. J Untrasound Med 2:89, 1983

104. Marchal GJF, Casaer M, Baert AL, et al: Gallbladder wall sonolucency in acute cholecystitis. Radiology 133:429, 1979

105. Worthen NJ, Uszler JM, Funamura JL: Cholecystitis: prospective evaluation of sonography and 99mTc-HIDA cholescintigraphy. AJR 137:973, 1981

106. Shuman WP, Mack LA, Rudd TG, et al: Evaluation of acute right upper quadrant pain: sonography and 99mTc-PIPIDA cholescintigraphy. AJR 139:61, 1982

107. Laing FC, Federle MP, Jeffrey RB, Brown TW: Ultra-

sonic evaluation of patients with acute right upper quadrant pain. Radiology 140:449, 1981

108. Ralls PW, Halls J, Lapin SA, et al: Prospective evaluation of the sonographic Murphy sign in suspected acute cholecystitis. J Clin Ultrasound 10:113, 1982

109. Shuman WP, Rogers JV, Rudd TG, et al: Low sensitivity of sonography and cholescintigraphy in acalculous cholecystitis. AJR 124: 541, 1984

110. Deitch EA, Engel JM: Acute acalculous cholecystitis — Ultrasonic diagnosis. Am J Surg 142:290, 1981

111. Parulekar SG: Sonographic findings in acute emphysematous cholecystitis. Radiology 145:117, 1982

112. Hunter ND, Macintosh PK: Acute emphysematous cholecystitis: an ultrasonic diagnosis. AJR 134:592, 1980

113. Jeffrey RB, Laing FC, Wong W, Callen PW: Gangrenous cholecystitis: diagnosis by ultrasound. Radiology 148: 219, 1983

114. Kane RA: Ultrasonographic diagnosis of gangrenous cholecystitis and empyema of the gallbladder. Radiology 134:191, 1980

115. Garcia OM, Kovac A, Plauche WE: Empyema of the gallbladder detected by gallium scan and abdominal ultrasonography. So Med J 74:1020, 1981

116. Deitch EA, Engel JM: Ultrasonic detection of acute cholecystitis with pericholecystic abscesses. Am Surg 47:211, 1981

117. Fleischer AC, Muhletaler CA, Jones TB: Sonographic detection of gallbladder perforation. So Med J 75:606, 1982

118. Madrazo BL, Francis I, Hricak H, et al: Sonographic findings in perforation of the gallbladder. AJR 139:491, 1982

119. Bergman AB, Neiman HL, Kraut B: Ultrasonographic evaluation of pericholecystic abscesses. AJR 132:201, 1979

120. Nyberg DA, Laing FC: Ultrasonographic findings in peptic ulcer disease and pancreatitis that simulate primary gallbladder disease. J Ultrasound Med 2:303, 1983

121. Crade M, Taylor KJW, Rosenfield AT, Walsh JW: Ultrasonic imaging of pericholecystic inflammation. JAMA 244:708, 1980

122. Bluth EI, Katz MM, Merritt CRB, et al: Echographic findings in xanthogranulomatous cholecystitis. J Clin Ultrasound 7:213, 1979

123. Jenkins M, Golding RH, Cooperberg PL: Sonography and computed tomography of hemorrhagic cholecystitis. AJR 140:1197, 1983

124. Kumari S, Lee WJ, Baron MG: Hydrops of the gallbladder in a child: Diagnosis by ultrasonography. Pediatrics 63:295, 1979

125. Greenberg M, Kangarloo H, Cochran ST, Sample WF: The ultrasonographic diagnosis of cholecystitis and cholelithiasis in children. Radiology 137:745, 1980

126. Bradford BF, Reid BS, Weinstein BJ, et al: Ultrasonographic evaluation of the gallbladder in mucocutaneous lymph node syndrome. Radiology 142:381, 1982

127. Koss JC, Coleman BG, Mulhern CB, et al: Mucocutaneous lymph node syndrome with hydrops of the gallbladder diagnosed by ultrasound. J Clin Ultrasound 9:477, 1981

128. Sty JR, Starshak RJ, Gorenstein L: Gallbladder perforation in a case of Kawasaki disease: image correlation. J Clin Ultrasound 11:381, 1983

129. Stauffer RA, Adams A, Wygal J, Lavery JP: Gallbladder disease in pregnancy. Am J Obstet Gynecol 144:661, 1982

130. Williamson SL, Williamson MR: Cholecystosonography in pregnancy. J Ultrasound Med 3:329, 1984

131. Schulman A, Loxton AJ, Heydenrych JJ, Abdurahman KE: Sonographic diagnosis of biliary ascariasis. AJR 139:485, 1982

132. Cerri GG, Leite GJ, Simoes JB, et al: Ultrasonographic evaluation of ascaris in the biliary tract. Radiology 146:753, 1983

133. Schulman A, Roman T, Dalrymple R, et al: Sonography of biliary worms (ascariasis). J Clin Ultrasound 10:77, 1982

134. Carter SJ, Rutledge J, Hirsch JH, et al: Papillary adenoma of the gallbladder: ultrasonic demonstration. J Clin Ultrasound 6:433, 1978

135. Detweiler DG, Biddinger P, Staab EV, et al: The appearance of adenomyomatosis with the newer imaging modalities: a case with pathologic correlation. J Ultrasound Med 1:295, 1982

136. Berk RN, van der Vegt JH, Lichtenstein JE: The hyperplastic cholecysterolosis: cholesterolosis and adenomyomatosis. Radiology 146:593, 1983

137. Raghavendra BN, Subramanyam BR, Balthazar EJ, et al: Sonography of adenomyomatosis of the gallbladder: radiologic-pathologic correlation. Radiology 146:747, 1983

138. Rice J, Sauerbrei EE, Semogas P, et al: Sonographic appearance of adenomyomatosis of gallbladder. J Clin Ultrasound 9:336, 1981

139. Price RJ, Stewart ET, Foley WD, Dodds WJ: Sonography of polypoid cholesterolosis. AJR 139:1197, 1982

140. Ruhe AH, Zachman JP, Mulder BD, Rime AE: Cholesterol polyps of the gallbladder: ultrasound demonstration. J Clin Ultrasound 7:386, 1979

141. Allibone GW, Fagan CJ, Porter SC: Sonographic features of carcinoma of the gallbladder. Gastrointest Radiol 6:169, 1981

142. Yeh H-C: Ultrasonography and computed tomography of carcinoma of gallbladder. Radiology 133:167, 1979

143. Oken SM, Bledsoe R, Newmark H: The ultrasonic diagnosis of primary carcinoma of the gallbladder. Radiology 129:481, 1978

144. Raghavendra BN: Ultrasonographic features of primary carcinoma of the gallbladder: Report of five cases. Gastrointest Radiol 5:239, 1980

145. Weiner SN, Koenigsberg M, Morehouse H, Hoffman J: Sonography and computed tomography in the diagnosis of carcinoma of the gallbladder. AJR 142:735, 1984

146. Ruiz R, Teyssou H, Fernandez N, et al: Ultrasonic diagnosis of primary carcinoma of the gallbladder: a review of 16 cases. J Clin Ultrasound 8:489, 1980

147. Bondestam S: Sonographic diagnosis of primary carcinoma of the gallbladder. Diagnostic Imaging 50:197, 1981
148. Yum HY, Fink AH: Sonographic findings in primary carcinoma of the gallbladder. Radiology 134:693, 1980
149. Harolds JA, Dennehy DC: Preoperative diagnosis of gallbladder carcinoma by ultrasonography. So Med J 74:1024, 1981
150. Crade M, Taylor KJW, Rosenfield AT, et al: The varied ultrasonic character of gallbladder tumor. JAMA 241:2195, 1979
151. Phillips G, Pochaczevsky R, Goodman J, Kumari S: Ultrasound patterns of metastatic tumors in the gallbladder. J Clin Ultrasound 10:379, 1982
152. Bundy AL, Ritchie WGM: Ultrasonic diagnosis of metastatic melanoma of the gallbladder presenting as acute cholecystitis. J Clin Ultrasound 10:285, 1982
153. Love L, Kucharski P, Pickleman J: Radiology of cholecystectomy complications. Gastrointest Radiol 4:33, 1979
154. Raptopoulos V: Ultrasonic pseudocalculus effect in post cholecystectomy patients. AJR 134:145, 1980
155. Phillips G, Bank S, Kumari-Subaiya S, Kurtz LM: Percutaneous ultrasound-guided puncture of the gallbladder (PUPG). Radiology 145:769, 1982
156. Salerno NR: Percutaneous aspiration and drainage of gallbladder. J Ultrasound Med 1:129, 1982
157. Shaver RW, Hawkins IF, Soong J: Percutaneous cholecystostomy. AJR 138:1133, 1982
158. Elyaderani MK, McDowel DE, Gabriele OF: A preliminary report of percutaneous cholecystostomy under ultrasonography and fluoroscopy guidance. J Clin Gastroenterol 5:277, 1983
159. Radder RW: Ultrasonically guided percutaneous catheter drainage for gallbladder empyema. Diagnostic Imaging 49:330, 1980
160. Zeman RK, Dorfman GS, Burrell MI, et al: Disparate dilatation of the intrahepatic and extrahepatic bile ducts in surgical jaundice. Radiology 138:129, 1981
161. Floyd JL, Collins TL: Discordance of sonography and cholescintigraphy in acute biliary obstruction. AJR 140:501, 1983
162. Shawker TH, Jones BL, Girton ME: Distal common bile duct obstruction: an experimental study in monkeys. J Clin Ultrasound 9:77, 1981
163. Gooding GAW: Acute bile duct dilatation with resolution in 43 hours: an ultrasonic demonstration. J Clin Ultrasound 9:201, 1981
164. Scheske GA, Cooperberg PL, Cohen MM, Burhenne JH: Dynamic changes in the caliber of the major bile ducts, related to obstruction. Radiology 135:215, 1980
165. Simeone JF, Mueller PR, Ferrucci JT, et al: Sonography of the bile ducts after a fatty meal: an aid in detection of obstruction. Radiology 143:211, 1982
166. Laing FC, London LA, Filly RA: Ultrasonographic identification of dilated intrahepatic bile ducts and their differentiation from portal venous structures. J Clin Ultrasound 6:90, 1978
167. Conrad MR, Landay MJ, Janes JO: Sonographic "parallel channel" sign of biliary tree enlargement in mild to moderate obstructive jaundice. AJR 130:279, 1978
168. Weill F, Eisencher A, Zeltner F: Ultrasonic study of the normal and dilated biliary tree: the "shotgun" sign. Radiology 127:221, 1978
169. Weinstein BJ, Weinstein DP: Biliary tract dilatation in the nonjaundiced patient. AJR 134:899, 1980
170. Zeman R, Taylor KJW, Burrell MI, Gold J: Ultrasound demonstration of anicteric dilatation of biliary tree. Radiology 134:689, 1980
171. Weinstein DP, Weinstein BJ, Brodmerkel GJ: Ultrasonography of biliary tract dilatation without jaundice. AJR 132:729, 1979
172. Zeman RK, Taylor KJW, Rosenfield AT, et al: Acute experimental biliary obstruction in the dog: sonographic findings and clinical implications. AJR 136:965, 1981
173. Thomas JL, Zornoza J: Obstructive jaundice in the absence of sonographic biliary dilatation. Gastrointest Radiol 5:357, 1980
174. Honickman SP, Mueller PR, Wittenberg J, et al: Ultrasound in obstructive jaundice—prospective evaluation of site and cause. Radiology 147:511, 1983
175. Mueller PR, Ferrucci JT, Simeone JF, et al: Postcholecystectomy bile duct dilatation: myth or reality. AJR 136:355, 1981
176. Graham MF, Cooperberg PL, Cohen MM, Burhenne HJ: Ultrasonographic screening of the common hepatic duct in symptomatic patients after cholecystectomy. Radiology 138:137, 1981
177. Graham MF, Cooperberg PL, Cohen MM, Burhenne HJ: The size of the normal common hepatic duct following cholecystectomy: an ultrasonographic study. Radiology 135:137, 1980
178. Markle BM, Potter BM, Majd M: The jaundiced infant and child. p. 123. In Raymond HW, Zwiebel WJ (eds): Seminars in Ultrasound. Vol. 1. Grune and Stratton, New York, 1980
179. Douillet P, Brunelle F, Chaumont P, et al: Ultrasonography and percutaneous cholangiography in children with dilated bile ducts. Am J Dis Child 135:131, 1981
180. Einstein DM, Lapin SA, Ralls PW, Halls JM: The insensitivity of sonography in the detection of choledocholithiasis. AJR 142:725, 1984
181. Parulekar SG, McNamara MP: Ultrasonography of choledocholithiasis. J Ultrasound Med 2:395, 1983
182. Mueller PR, Cronan JJ, Simeone JF, et al: Choledocholithiasis: Ultrasonographic caveats. J Ultrasound Med 2:13, 1983
183. Meyer DG, Weinstein BJ: Klatskin tumors of the bile ducts: Sonographic appearance. Radiology 148:803, 1983
184. Subramanyam BR, Raghavendra BN, Balthazar EJ, et al: Ultrasonic features of cholangiocarcinoma. J Ultrasound Med 3:405, 1984
185. Jones TB, Dubrisson RL, Hughes JJ, Robinson AE: Abrupt termination of the common bile duct: a sign of

malignancy identified by high-resolution real-time sonography. J Ultrasound Med 2:345, 1983

186. Levine E, Maklad NF, Wright CH, Lee KR: Computed tomographic and ultrasonic appearances of primary carcinoma of the common bile duct. Gastrointest Radiol 4:147, 1979

187. Schnur MJ, Hoffman JC, Koenigsberg M: Ultrasonic demonstration of intraductal biliary neoplasms. J Clin Ultrasound 10:246, 1982

188. Forrest ME, Cho KJ, Shields JJ, et al: Biliary cystadenomas: sonographic-angiographic pathologic correlations. AJR 135:723, 1980

189. Carroll BA: Biliary cystadenoma and cystadenocarcinoma: Gray-scale ultrasound appearance. J Clin Ultrasound 6:337, 1978

190. Frick MP, Feinberg SB: Biliary cystadenoma. AJR 139:393, 1982

191. Arger PH: Obstructive jaundice of malignant origin. p. 113. In Raymond HW, Zwiebel WJ (eds): Seminars in Ultrasound. Vol. 1. Grune and Stratton, New York, 1980

192. Swartz TR, Ritchie WGM: Bile duct obstruction secondary to lymphomatous involvement of the pancreas. J Clin Ultrasound 11:391, 1983

193. Belta KS, Donnelly PB, Wexler JS: Sonographic demonstration of the intraluminal bile duct metastasis: a case report. Connecticut Med 46:636, 1982

194. vanSonnenberg E, Ferrucci JT: Bile duct obstruction in hepatocellular carcinoma (hepatoma)—clinical and cholangiographic characteristics: report of 6 cases and review of the literature. Radiology 130:7, 1979

195. Maffessanti MM, Bazzochi M, Melato M: Sonographic diagnosis of intraductal hepatoma. J Clin Ultrasound 10:397, 1982

196. Spinelli GD, Kleinclaus DH, Wenger JJ, et al. Obstructive jaundice and abdominal aortic aneurysm: an ultrasonographic study. Radiology 144:872, 1982

197. Ralls PW, Colletti PM, Quinn MF, et al: Sonography in recurrent oriental pyogenic cholangitis. AJR 136:1010, 1981

198. Scheible FW, David GB: Oriental cholangiohepatitis: preoperative radiographic and ultrasonographic diagnosis. Gastrointest Radiol 6:269, 1981

199. Federle MP, Cello JP, Laing FC, Jeffrey RB: Recurrent pyogenic cholangitis in Asian immigrants: use of ultrasonography, computed tomography and cholangiography. Radiology 143:151, 1982

200. Carroll BA, Oppenheimer DA: Sclerosing cholangitis: Sonographic demonstration of bile duct wall thickening. AJR 139:1016, 1982

201. Abramson SJ, Treves S, Teele RL: The infant with possible biliary atresia: evaluation by ultrasound and nuclear medicine. Pediatr Radiol 12:1, 1982

202. Kirks DR, Coleman RE, Filston HC, et al: An imaging approach to persistent neonatal jaundice. AJR 142:461, 1984

203. Majd M: 99mTc-IDA scintigraphy in the evaluation of neonatal jaundice. Radiographics 3:88, 1983

204. Mittelstaedt CA, Volberg FM, Fischer GJ, McCartney

205. Lucaya J, Gomez JL, Molino C, Atienza JG: Congenital dilatation of the intrahepatic bile ducts (Caroli's disease). Radiology 127:746, 1978

206. Han BK, Babcock DS, Gelfand MH: Choledochal cyst with bile duct dilatation: sonography and 99mTc IDA cholescintigraphy. AJR 136:1075, 1981

207. Reuter K, Raptopoulous VD, Cantelmo N, et al: The diagnosis of choledochal cyst by ultrasound. Radiology 136:437, 1980

208. Frank JL, Hill MC, Chirathivat S, et al: Antenatal observation of a choledochal cyst by sonography. AJR 137:166, 1981

209. Kangarloo H, Sarti DA, Sample WF, Amundson G: Ultrasonographic spectrum of choledochal cysts in children. Pediatr Radiol 9:15, 1980

210. Glass TA, Buschi AJ, Brenbridge NAG, Shaffer H: Choledochal cyst: sonographic evaluation of an unusual case. So Med J 73:1391, 1980

211. Richardson JD, Grant EG, Barth KH, et al: Type II choledochal cyst: diagnosis using real-time sonography. J Ultrasound Med 3:37, 1984

212. Filly RA, Carlsen EN: Choledochal cyst: report of a case with specific ultrasonographic findings. J Clin Ultrasound 4:7, 1976

213. Mettler FA, Wicks JD, Requard CK, Christie JH: Diagnostic imaging of choledochal cyst. Clin Nuclear Med 6:513, 1981

214. Biggi E, Derchi L, Cicio GR, Valente M: Sonographic findings of hydatid cyst of the liver ruptured into the biliary duct. J Clin Ultrasound 7:381, 1979

215. Subramanyam BR, Balthazar EJ, Naidich DP: Ruptured hydatid cyst with biliary obstruction: diagnosis by sonography and computed tomography. Gastrointest Radiol 8:341, 1983

216. Makuuchi M, Bandai Y, Ito T, et al: Ultrasonically guided percutaneous transhepatic bile drainage. Radiology 136:165, 1980

217. Gooding GAW, Munyer TP: Ultrasonic localization of biliary decompression catheters. J Ultrasound Med 2:325, 1983

218. Mueller PR, Ferrucci JT, vanSonnenberg E, et al: Obstruction of the left hepatic duct: diagnosis and treatment by selective fine-needle cholangiography and percutaneous biliary drainage. Radiology 145:297, 1982

219. Makuuchi M, Bandai Y, Ito T, et al: Ultrasonically guided percutaneous transhepatic cholangiography and percutaneous pancreatography. Radiology 134:767, 1980

220. Gould L, Patel A: Ultrasound detection of extrahepatic encapsulated bile: "biloma". AJR 132:1014, 1979

221. Ralls PW, Eto R, Quinn M, Boger D: Gray-scale ultrasonography of a traumatic biliary cyst. J Trauma 21:176, 1981

222. Zegal HG, Kurtz AB, Perlmutter GS, Goldberg BB: Ultrasonic characteristics of bilomas. J Clin Ultrasound 9:21, 1981

WH: Caroli's disease: sonographic findings. AJR 134:585, 1980

223. Mueller PR, Ferrucci JT, Simeone JF, et al: Detection and drainage of bilomas: special considerations. AJR 140:715, 1983

224. Esensten M, Ralls PW, Colletti P, Halls J: Posttraumatic intrahepatic biloma: sonographic diagnosis. AJR 140: 303, 1983

225. Hillman BJ, Smith EH, Holm HH: Ultrasound diagnosis and treatment of gallbladder fossa collections following biliary tract surgery. Br J Radiol 52:390, 1979

226. Weissman HS, Chun KJ, Frank M, et al: Demonstration of traumatic bile leakage with cholescintigraphy and ultrasonography. AJR 133:843, 1979

227. White M, Simeone JF, Muller PR: Imaging of cholecystocolic fistulas. J Ultrasound Med 2:181, 1983

228. Zeman RK, Lee C, Stahl RS, et al: Ultrasonography and hepatobiliary scintigraphy in the assessment of biliary-enteric anastomoses. Radiology 145:109, 1982

229. McIntosh DMF, Penney HF: Gray-scale ultrasonography as screening procedure in detection of gallbladder disease. Radiology 136:725, 1980

230. Clair MR, Rosenberg ER, Ram PC, Bowie JD: Comparison of real-time and static-mode gray-scale ultrasonography in the diagnosis of cholelithiasis. J Ultrasound Med 1:201, 1982

231. Raptopoulos V, Moss L, Reuter K, Kleinman P: Comparison of real-time and gray-scale static ultrasonic cholecystography. Radiology 140:153, 1981

232. Crade M, Taylor KJW, Rosenfield AT, et al: Surgical and pathologic correlation of cholecystosonography and cholecystography. AJR 131:227, 1978

233. Bartrum RJ, Crow HC, Foote SR: Ultrasonic and radiographic cholecystography. N Engl J Med 296:538, 1977

234. Arson S, Rosenquist CJ: Gray-scale cholecystosonography: an evaluation of accuracy. Am J Roentgenol 127:817, 1976

235. Anderson JC, Harned RK: Gray-scale ultrasound of the gallbladder: an evaluation of accuracy and report of additional ultrasound signs. Am J Roentgenol 129:975, 1977

236. Bartrum RJ, Crow HC, Foote SR: Ultrasound examination of the gallbladder—an alternate to "double-dose" oral cholecystography. JAMA 236:1147, 1979

237. Leopold GR, Amberg J, Gosink BB, Mittelstaedt CA: Gray-scale ultrasonic cholecystography: A comparison with conventional radiographic techniques. Radiology 121:445, 1976

238. Cooperberg PL, Burhenne HJ: Real-time ultrasonography: diagnostic technique of choice in calculous gallbladder disease. N Engl J Med 302:1277, 1980

239. Crade M: Comparison of ultrasound and oral cholecystogram in the diagnosis of gallstones. p. 123. In Taylor KJW (ed): Clinics in Diagnostic Ultrasound: Diagnostic Ultrasound in Gastrointestinal Disease. Churchill Livingstone, New York, 1979

240. McCluskey PL, Prinz RA, Guico R, Greenlee HB: Use of ultrasound to demonstrate gallstones in symptomatic patients with normal oral cholecystograms. Am J Surg 138:655, 1979

241. Raskin MM: Hepatobiliary disease: A comparative evaluation by ultrasound and computed tomography. Gastrointest Radiol 3:267, 1978

242. Zeman RK, Burrell MI, Cahow CE, Caride V: Diagnostic utility of cholescintigraphy and ultrasonography in acute cholecystitis. Am J Surg 141:446, 1981

243. Weissman HS, Frank M, Rosenblatt R, et al: Cholescintigraphy, ultrasonography and computerized tomography in the evaluation of biliary tract disorders. Semin Nuc Med 9:22, 1979

244. Sherman M, Ralls PW, Quinn M, et al: Intravenous cholangiography and sonography in acute cholecystitis: prospective evaluation. AJR 135:311, 1980

245. Weissman HS, Badin J, Sugarman LA, et al: Spectrum of 99m-Tc-IDA cholescintigraphic patterns in acute cholecystitis. Radiology 138:167, 1981

246. Massie JD, Moinuddin M, Phillips JC: Acute calculous cholecystitis in patient with patent cystic duct. AJR 141:39, 1983

247. Reimer DE, Donald JW: Technetium-99-m-HIDA visualization of an obstructed gallbladder via an accessory hepatic duct. AJR 137:610, 1981

248. Echevarria RA, Gleason JL: False-negative gallbladder scintigram in acute cholecystitis. J Nuclear Med 21:841, 1980

249. Ralls PW, Colletti PM, Halls JM, Siemsen JK: Prospective evaluation of 99mTc-IDA cholescintigraphy and gray-scale ultrasound in the diagnosis of acute cholecystitis. Radiology 144:369, 1982

250. Freitas JE, Mirkes SH, Fink-Bennett DM, Bree RL: Suspected acute cholecystitis: comparison of hepatobiliary scintigraph versus ultrasonography. Clin Nuclear Med 7:364, 1982

251. Weissman HS, Frank MS, Bernstein LH, Freeman LM: Rapid and accurate diagnosis of acute cholecystitis with 99mTc-HIDA cholescintigraphy. AJR 132:523, 1979

252. Samuels BI, Freitas JE, Bree RL, et al: A comparison of radionuclide hepatobiliary imaging and real-time ultrasound for the detection of acute cholecystitis. Radiology 147:207, 1983

253. Dillon E, Parkin GJS: The role of upper abdominal ultrasonography in suspected acute cholecystitis. Clin Radiol 31:175, 1980

254. Ferrucci JT, Adson MA, Mueller PR, et al: Advances in the radiology of jaundice: a symposium and review. AJR 141:1, 1983

255. Berk RN, Cooperberg PL, Gold RP, et al: Radiology of the bile ducts: a symposium on the use of new modalities for diagnosis and treatment. Radiology 145:1, 1982

256. Koenigsberg M, Weiner SN, Walzer A: The accuracy of sonography in the differential diagnosis of obstructive jaundice: a comparison with cholangiography. Radiology 133:157, 1979

257. Haubek A, Pedersen JH, Burcharth F, et al: Dynamic sonography in the evaluation of jaundice. AJR 136:1071, 1981

258. Malini S, Sabel J: Ultrasonography in obstructive jaundice. Radiology 123:429, 1977

259. Taylor KJW, Rosenfield AT, Spiro HM: Diagnostic ac-

curacy of gray-scale ultrasonography for the jaundiced patient: a report of 275 cases. Arch Intern Med 139:60, 1979

260. Hadidi A: Distinction between obstructive and non-obstructive jaundice by sonography. Clin Radiol 31:181, 1980

261. Baron RL, Stanley RJ, Lee JKT, et al: A prospective comparison of the evaluation of biliary obstruction using computed tomography and ultrasonography. Radiology 145:91, 1982

262. Klingensmith WC, Johnson ML, Kuni CC, et al: Complimentary role of Tc-99m-Diethyl-IDA and ultrasound

in large and small duct biliary tract obstruction. Radiology 138:177, 1981

263. Gross BH, Harter LP, Gore RM, et al: Ultrasonic evaluation of common duct stones: prospective comparison with endoscopic retrograde cholangiopancreatography. Radiology 146:471, 1983

264. Crohan JJ, Mueller PR, Simeone JF, et al: Prospective diagnosis of choledocholithiasis. Radiology 146:467, 1983

265. Mitchell SE, Clark RA: A comparison of computed tomography and sonography in choledocholithiasis. AJR 142:729, 1984

3

The Pancreas

It has only been in recent years that the radiologist has been able to offer direct evaluation of the pancreas with computerized tomography (CT) or ultrasound. Prior to that time, pancreatic disease was diagnosed by indirect changes seen on plain radiograph or upper gastrointestinal series. Now disease processes can be detected at an early stage, and follow-up studies provide greater insight into correlation between clinical findings and morphologic changes in the gland. Pancreatic carcinoma is detected at an earlier stage, but it appears that long-term survival in these patients is not at present altered significantly. With the development of gray-scale imaging, the role of ultrasound in pancreatic disease has improved significantly. However, as abdominal organs go, the pancreas is the most difficult to adequately visualize with ultrasound. To evaluate the pancreas successfully with ultrasound, the examiner must be meticulous with technique as well as knowledgeable of the normal and abnormal.

TECHNIQUE

Patient Preparation

It is best to perform an ultrasound examination of the pancreas after an overnight fast whenever possible. If this is not possible, then the patient should have been fasting for at least 6 to 8 hours. The purpose of the fasting is threefold. First, because the biliary system and pancreas are intimately related, they are usually examined to-gether. If gallstones are seen, and/or dilated ducts and/or choledocholithiasis, an examination of the pancreas is performed. If the pancreas is abnormal, the gallbladder and ducts are always evaluated. Fasting promotes greater dilatation of the gallbladder, thereby giving better evaluation of that structure. The second reason for fasting is to ensure an empty stomach. Because the stomach is directly anterior to the pancreas, its contents affect the sound beam transmission to the pancreas. Thirdly, by fasting there tends to be less bowel gas as a whole; this also improves the visualization of the pancreas.

Ultrasound System

Although most of the early work performed to evaluate the pancreas was done with the static ultrasound system, the equipment of choice today for the most successful examination of the pancreas is a real-time system, preferably a sector, because it requires a smaller contact surface. With this system, there is greater success in adequate visualization of the pancreas in more cases. This is due to the flexibility of the scanhead, which can be manuevered easily, and the ability to displace bowel gas by moving the scanhead. Also, the patient can be examined in almost any position and, very importantly, at the bedside or portably. Besides being able to visualize the pancreas with the real-time system, bowel loops and the stomach may be easily identified by their peristalsis; whereas, with the static system, these structures may appear as masses.

Transducers

As with any other ultrasound study, one should use the highest frequency transducer possible to be able to adequately visualize the structure being examined.[1] The focal zone of the transducer should be matched to the depth of the pancreas, by measuring from the skin to the pancreas.[2-4] In adults, this may vary from a 3 MHz long-focused transducer to a 5 MHz medium-focused transducer. In children, a 5 or 7.5 MHz transducer may be used routinely. Again, one must check the focal zones for each transducer. The time gain compensation (TGC) must be adjusted to optimize visualization of the entire gland.[5]

Scan Technique

In order to perform a complete examination of the pancreas, the examiner must identify and measure all portions of the pancreas — head, neck, body, and tail — in longitudinal and transverse planes. The pancreatic contour, shape, and texture should be evaluated. The following structures must also be identified: superior mesenteric artery (SMA), superior mesenteric vein (SMV), portal vein, splenic vein, aorta, inferior vena cava (IVC), and common bile duct (CBD). In each study, the examiner should attempt to identify the following: gastroduodenal artery (GDA), common hepatic artery (CHA), pancreatic duct, left renal vein, duodenal bulb, and posterior wall of the stomach. Often, however, the examiner is frustrated by bowel gas artifact and the technical inability to see the pancreas. He or she must be prepared to improvise as needed and alter the standard routine in order to see the most pancreases. It is easier to say the pancreas cannot be visualized and refer the patient to CT. All possible innovative techniques should be tried before concluding that the pancreas is impossible to visualize. The success of visualization of the pancreas is directly linked to the persistence of the examiner.

The routine pancreatic examination begins with the patient in the supine position. The lie and elevation of the pancreas must be identified for each patient to establish the correct scan plane and setting.[5] Scans should be taken along the long axis of the gland, as well as perpendicular to the long axis.[5] Longitudinal and transverse scans of the head, neck, and body of the pancreas are taken. Measurements of the various portions of the pancreas are also noted. The echopattern of the pancreas is compared to that of the liver. Prone scans are taken through the left kidney to evaluate the remainder of the tail of the pancreas. The prone position is particularly helpful when ascites interferes with pancreatic visualization.[6] Care should be taken to not mistake splenic flexure

and distal transverse colon for tail because they cross anterior to the left kidney.[7] The colon is caudal to the tail of the pancreas. Coronal scans also improve the visibility of the pancreas and provide an additional view of the pancreas and peripancreatic region.[8]

As indicated, the goal of every pancreatic ultrasound is to successfully visualize the gland in its entirety. To do this in many cases, the examiner must find or produce a suitable acoustic window through which the pancreas can be visualized.[1] The stomach or colon are situated between the anterior abdominal wall and the pancreas. Many times, the left lobe of the liver overlies the area of the pancreas. These structures then can be used for possible acoustic windows in better visualizing the pancreas.

To improve the evaluation of the pancreas, especially if it is poorly seen supinely, the water technique is added.[9-11] To successfully apply this technique, the examiner must have an accurate conception of the positional changes of the stomach in various examining positions, and of relative movements of air and fluid within the stomach.[1,10] The patient is asked to drink approximately 32 to 300 cc of water through a straw in the erect or the left lateral decubitus position.[9] By using a straw, air swallowing is kept to a minimum. Also, if the water is drawn up (tap water) and allowed to sit overnight, there will be fewer microbubbles within it.[1]

Once the patient has completed the fluid intake, the examination can begin either erect or in the left lateral decubitus position. In the erect position, the pancreas is localized and scanned (air in the gastric fundus) (Fig. 3-1). The examiner may need to maneuver the patient and/or transducer positioning in order to maximize the stomach as an acoustic window. Once the stomach is positioned over the pancreas, the evaluation can begin. Again, by moving the patient and/or transducer, all portions of the pancreas can be identified.

At times, the examiner may be more successful in examining the patient in the decubitus position, especially if the patient is unable to sit up. By moving the patient progressively from the left lateral decubitus to the right lateral decubitus positions, portions of the pancreas may be selectively visualized as water distends the gut lumen[9] (Figs. 3-2 and 3-3; see Fig. 2-6). In the right lateral decubitus position, fluid in the gastric antrum and duodenum can be seen, nicely outlining the pancreas (Fig. 3-3; see Fig. 2-6). The air in the stomach has moved to the fundus in this position. The pancreas may even be visualized well in the straight supine position. In the left decubitus position, by scanning far to the patient's left one may see portions of the tail of the pancreas (Fig. 3-2).

What if the patient cannot drink fluid or is not allowed fluid orally? Many times, there can be significant improvement in the visualization of the pancreas by just changing to the erect position.[1,10]

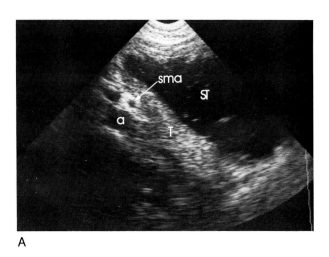

A

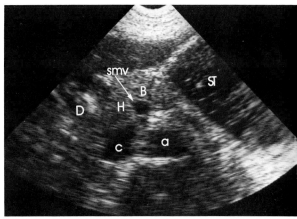

B

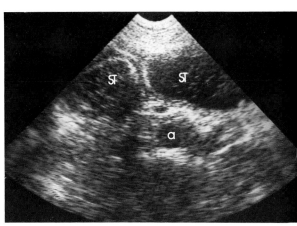

C

Fig. 3-1. Water technique. Erect position. **(A)** Transverse real-time scan with the transducer angled upward. The fluid-filled stomach *(ST)* is seen anterior to the pancreatic tail *(T)*. (*a*, aorta; *sma*, superior mesenteric artery.) **(B)** Transverse real-time scan at a lower level then **(A)**. The fluid-filled stomach *(ST)* is seen to the left with the duodenum *(D)* to the right. The pancreatic head *(H)* and a portion of the body *(B)* are seen. (*a*, aorta; *c*, inferior vena cava; *smv*, superior mesenteric vein.) **(C)** Transverse real-time scan lower than **(B)**. The distended stomach *(ST)* is seen anterior to the aorta *(a)*. The pancreas is not visualized at this level. In the erect position with the stomach distended with fluid, the gastric antrum and body may project inferior to the level of the pancreas.

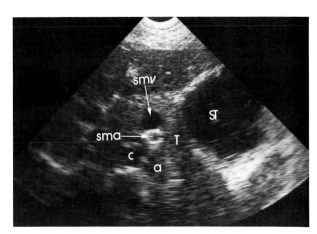

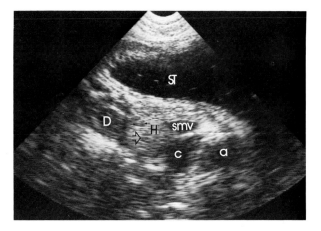

Fig. 3-2. Water technique. Left lateral decubitus position. Transverse real-time scan. Fluid is seen within the gastric fundus *(ST)*, which allows visualization of a portion of the pancreatic tail *(T)*. (*a*, aorta; *sma*, superior mesenteric artery; *smv*, superior mesenteric vein; *c*, inferior vena cava.)

Fig. 3-3. Water technique. Right lateral decubitus position. Transverse slightly oblique real-time scan. Fluid is seen in the duodenum *(D)* as well as gastric antrum *(ST)*. This position is particularly useful in visualizing the head *(H)* of the pancreas and distal common bile duct (open arrow).(*a*, aorta; *c*, inferior vena cava; small arrows, pancreatic duct; *smv*, superior mesenteric vein.)

Some authors in the past have advocated the use of glucagon to inhibit peristalsis. Because real-time ultrasound is used in the majority of cases, peristalsis is not a problem. If there is a case in which the water flows too quickly from the stomach to the small bowel to get an adequate examination of the pancreas, then 0.5 to 1 U of glucagon may be given subcutaneously, followed by more oral fluids.[1] The use of glucagon produces gastric fundal dilatation, which provides a "sonic window" for the examination of the pancreas.[12]

Another technique to inhibit peristalsis is to give a fatty meal prior to the oral water.[1] Two to three ounces of fluid fat (Lipomul-oral) may be given, which not only decreases peristalsis but is a potent inhibitor of gastric emptying.[1,10] One would not give a fatty meal to a patient with pancreatitis, or gallbladder disease.

Still other investigators promote the use of methylcellulose solution prior to fluids.[13] This is an aqueous suspension that fills the stomach, allowing increased through transmission and contains inert, viscid mucilages. There is little air swallowing associated with it. After administering intravenous glucagon, the patient may be examined prone.

How often is the pancreas visualized on an ultrasound examination? This depends on the patient as well as the persistence and thoroughness of the examiner. The head and body should be visualized 90 percent of the time.[14] For obvious reasons, ultrasound has its greatest success in thin patients.[15] When the water technique is not used, there has been a reported nonvisualization rate of 19 percent.[10] By using the water technique, this can be decreased to 1 percent.[10] As such 93 percent of pancreases (head, neck, body, and tail) can be visualized using all available techniques.[10] The erect position alone without water may improve the visualization in 48 percent.[10]

Future

Conventional ultrasound is often compromised by intervening bowel gas. Endoscopic ultrasound represents a new method for visualization of the pancreas. A small transducer (10 MHz linear array or 7 to 7.5 MHz sector) is coupled to an endoscope.[16,17] Because the endoscopic visualization of the gastrointestinal (GI) mucosa and the ultrasound examination of the extraluminal organs is obtained during a single procedure, rapid differentiation among mucosal and intramural disease of hollow gut and disease of extraluminal organs is possible. The examiner is able to visualize the heart, aorta, spleen, pancreas, liver, gallbladder, kidney, and GI mucosa, detect moderate size pancreatic tumors and hepatic metastases less than 1 cm in diameter.[16] However, the topographic anatomic orientation is difficult because the scan plane is strictly determined by the endoscope and the pancreas cannot be examined in two planes.[17] However, this technique holds promise for better visualization of pancreatic lesions in the future.

NORMAL ANATOMY

The pancreas arises from two duodenal buds, dorsal and ventral, which fuse.[18] The ventral bud grows slowly and swings around the gut to join the dorsal bud. The entire body and tail are the dorsal anlage and the remainder are from the ventral bud. The duct drainage system anatomose with the major duct, the dorsal one, being the duct of Wirsung that drains into the duodenum. The ventral duct usually disappears; if it persists, it represents an accessory duct, the duct of Santorini. In 60 percent of adults, the main pancreatic duct does not empty directly into the duodenum but into the common bile duct just proximal to the ampulla of Vater.[18]

The normal pancreas in the adult is 15 cm in length and weighs 60 to 100 gm.[18] Although the position of the gland may be variable, most are located at the level of the first or second lumbar vertebra.[5] The pancreas is a nonencapsulated multilobular gland located in the retroperitoneal space extending from the second portion of the duodenum to the splenic hilum. Histologically, the pancreas is composed of two components—exocrine and endocrine. The exocrine portion is composed of numerous small glands (acini) aggregated into lobular acini separated by connective tissue. The ductal system begins with extremely fine radicles in secretor acini and by progressive anastomosis eventually drain into the duct of Wirsung. The endocrine portion of the pancreas is represented by the islets of Langerhans, which are groups of cells scattered throughout the pancreas.[4]

The regulation of pancreatic secretion is complex; it is related to humoral, vagal, and local neurogenic reflexes.[18] The most important humoral agent is secretin, which is produced in the duodenum. Fats and alcohol are particularly active stimulators of secretin. Pancreatic secretory activity is also correlated with the ingestion of food. The proteolytic enzymes—trypsin and chymotrypsin—are secreted as inactive precursors. They are most important in protein digesting ferments. In addition to the proteases, amylase, lipase, phospholipase, and elastases are all elaborated by the pancreas and activated in the duodenum.[18] The main hormones produced by the endocrine portion of the gland include insulin (in beta cells), and glucagon (in alpha cells).

Examination of the pancreas not only takes persistence and compulsiveness, but also an understanding of the normal anatomy of the pancreas and its anatomic landmarks (Fig. 3-4). When evaluating the pancreas, one

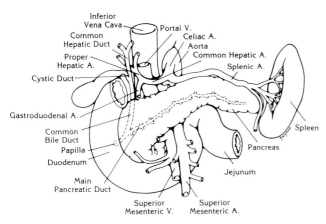

Fig. 3-4. Vascular and ductal landmarks. The relationship of the pancreas to associated vessels and ducts can be seen.

must look at the parenchymal texture, contour, shape, and echopattern as well as the size of the various portions of the gland and the pancreatic duct. Its blood supply is from the splenic artery, gastroduodenal artery, and superior mesenteric artery.[5] Its venous drainage is through tributaries of the splenic and superior mesenteric veins.

Vascular and Ductal Landmarks

PORTAL VEIN AND TRIBUTARIES

The portal vein is formed behind the neck of the pancreas by the junction of the superior mesenteric vein and the splenic vein (Fig. 3-5A,B). The splenic vein runs from the splenic hilum along the posterior superior aspect of the pancreas (Fig. 3-5C). The superior mesenteric vein runs posterior to the lower neck of the pancreas and anterior to the uncinate (Fig. 3-6). The portal vein courses superiorly at various obliquity.[4]

SPLENIC ARTERY

The splenic artery arises from the celiac artery and runs along the superior margin of the gland, slightly anterior and superior, to follow its vein (Fig. 3-7). As it approaches the lateral portion of the tail, it may run anterior to the pancreatic parenchyma[19] (Figs. 3-7D and 3-7F).

COMMON HEPATIC ARTERY

The common hepatic artery arises from the celiac artery in 92 percent of patients (Fig. 3-7A). It courses along the superior margin of the first portion of the duodenum and divides into the proper hepatic artery and GDA,

usually when it crosses onto the front of the portal vein (Fig. 3-8). The proper hepatic artery is seen in 75 percent as it proceeds superiorly along the anterior aspect of the portal vein with the common bile duct lateral to it (Fig. 3-8C). The GDA is less frequently seen (30 percent) (Figs. 3-6A, 3-6C, and 3-8B) as it travels a short distance along the anterior aspect of the head just to the right of the neck before it divides into the superior pancreaticoduodenal branches (anterior and posterior). They join with their counterparts (inferior pancreaticoduodenal), which arise from the SMA. In some (14 percent), the right hepatic artery arises from the SMA and courses posterior to the medial portions of the splenic vein and runs along the aspect of the portal vein.

SUPERIOR MESENTERIC ARTERY

The superior mesenteric artery arises from the aorta behind the lower portion of the body and courses anterior to the third portion of the duodenum to enter the small bowel mesentery (Fig. 3-9). The SMA runs directly anterior to the aorta but may be tortuous (Figs. 3-1A, 3-2, 3-5, 3-6A, and 3-7B).

COMMON BILE DUCT

The common bile duct crosses the anterior aspect of the portal vein to the right of the proper hepatic artery (Fig. 3-8C). As the portal vein crosses anterior to the IVC, the duct passes off the front of the portal vein and goes behind the first portion of the duodenum to course inferior and somewhat posterior in the parenchyma of the head of the pancreas where it is close to the second portion of the duodenum (Figs. 3-5A and 3-6). It joins the pancreatic duct close to the ampulla. In the head of the pancreas, the internal diameter is not more than 4 mm (Figs. 3-5A and 3-6).

Portions of the Pancreas

HEAD

The head of the pancreas is that portion of the pancreas that is to the right of the superior mesenteric vein (Fig. 3-6). Its right lateral border is the second portion of the duodenum, which can often be identified by its air and/or shadow or fluid within it (Fig. 3-3). The inferior vena cava is posterior to the head of the pancreas.[5] Often, anteriorly the gastroduodenal artery (first branch of the common hepatic artery) can be identified (Fig. 3-6). The common bile duct can be seen anterior and lateral to the gastroduodenal artery (Fig. 3-6A). The portal vein is cranial to the head[5] (Figs. 3-5B and 3-6). The uncinate pro-

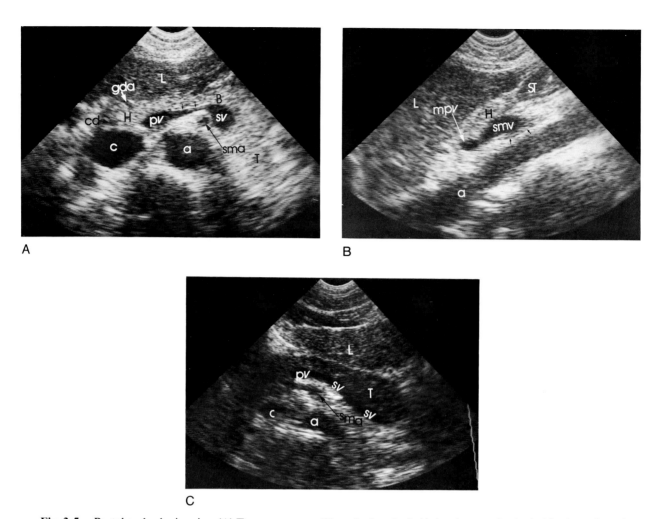

A

B

C

Fig. 3-5.   Portal and splenic veins. **(A)** Transverse scan. The splenic vein *(sv)* joins the portal vein *(pv)* in the region of the neck (arrows) of the pancreas. The body *(B)* is measured anterior to the aorta *(a)* and splenic vein. The pancreas is more echodense or hyperechoic compared to the liver *(L)*. (*sma,* superior mesenteric artery; *c,* inferior vena cava; *T,* pancreatic tail; *H,* pancreatic head; *gda,* gastroduodenal artery; *cd,* common bile duct). **(B)** Longitudinal scan. The superior mesenteric vein *(smv)* is seen as a tubular structure paralleling the aorta *(a)* and draining into the main portal vein *(mpv)*. The head *(H)* of the pancreas, can be seen inferior to the main portal vein and anterior to the superior mesenteric vein. The uncinate process (arrows) is seen between the aorta and the superior mesenteric vein. The anteroposterior and craniocaudal measurements of the head can be made on this scan (*ST,* fluid-filled stomach; *L,* liver). **(C)** Splenic vein. Slightly oblique transverse scan. The splenic vein *(sv)* is seen extending from the area of the spleen along the posterior superior aspect of the pancreas. The tail of the pancreas *(T)* can be measured diagonally at the left lateral border of the aorta *(a)* and splenic vein (*pv,* main portal vein; *sma,* superior mesenteric artery; *L,* liver).

cess is usually included as that portion of the pancreatic head that is directly posterior to the superior mesenteric vein (Fig. 3-6). The head of the pancreas is measured in the anteroposterior axis in the transverse plane, taking the maximum dimension (Fig. 3-6A). It is also measured in the longitudinal plane, again taking the maximum anteroposterior axis (Figs. 3-5B and 3-6). Normally, the head should measure 2.08 ± 0.40 cm transversely and 2.0l ± 0.39 cm in the longitudinal plane.[4,20,21]

NECK

The neck of the pancreas is that portion of the gland that is directly anterior to the superior mesenteric vein on longitudinal or transverse scan[5] (Figs. 3-5 and 3-6). The portal vein is formed behind the neck of the pancreas by the junction of the superior mesenteric vein and the splenic vein[4] (Fig. 3-5). It separates the body from the head of the pancreas. The neck is measured over the

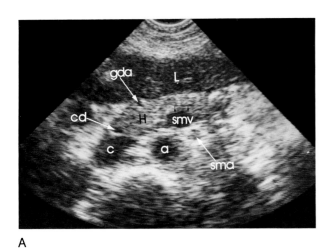

A

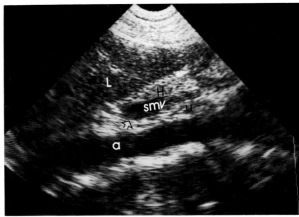

B

Fig. 3-6. Superior mesenteric vein and pancreatic head. **(A)** Transverse scan. The superior mesenteric vein *(smv)* is seen as a circular lucency to the right of the superior mesenteric artery *(sma)*. The pancreatic head *(H)* includes that portion of the pancreas to the right of the *smv*. The gastroduodenal artery *(gda)* is along the anterolateral border of the pancreatic head with the common duct *(cd)* inferior and lateral. The head can be measured in its anteroposterior axis on this view. The neck (arrows) of the pancreas, directly anterior to the superior mesenteric vein, can be measured anterior to the *smv* (*a*, aorta; *c*, inferior vena cava; *L*, liver). **(B)** Longitudinal scan. The uncinate process *(u)* is seen between the superior mesenteric vein *(smv)* and aorta *(a)*. (*H*, pancreatic head; open arrow, main portal vein; *L*, liver.) **(C)** Longitudinal scan to the right of **(B)**. The pancreatic head *(H)* can be seen bordered by the gastroduodenal artery *(gda)* anteriorly, and the common bile duct *(cbd)* posteriorly. The proper hepatic artery *(pha)* is at its superior margin as is the main portal vein *(mpv)*. The pancreatic duct (arrows) can be seen in the center of the pancreatic head (*ST*, fluid-filled stomach; *c*, inferior vena cava).

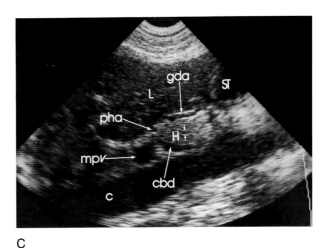

C

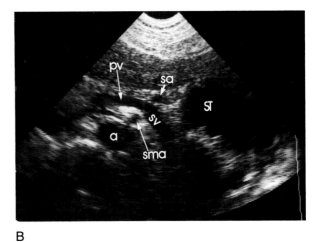

A

B

Fig. 3-7. Splenic artery and pancreatic tail. **(A)** High transverse scan. The splenic artery *(sa)* is seen arising from the celiac artery (arrows). The common hepatic artery *(cha)* is seen as the right branch of the celiac artery. (*a*, aorta; *L*, liver) **(B)** Slightly oblique transverse scan lower than **(A)**. The splenic artery *(sa)* is seen anterior to the splenic vein *(sv)*. (*pv*, main portal vein; *a*, aorta; *sma*, superior mesenteric artery; *ST*, fluid-filled stomach) *(Figure continues.)*

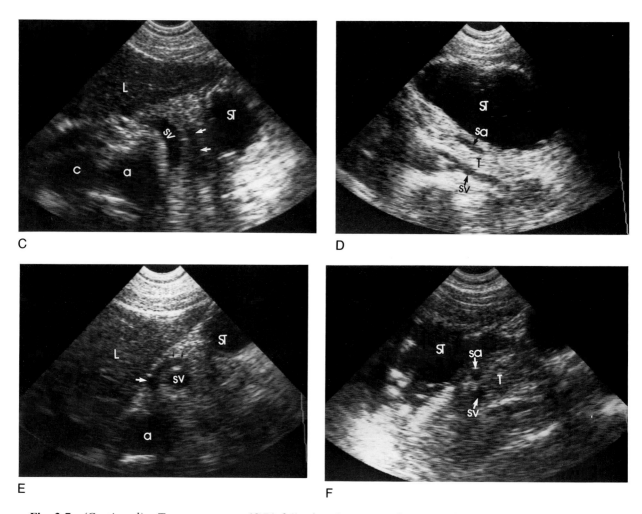

Fig. 3-7 *(Continued).* Transverse scans **(C,D)** following the course of the splenic artery (*sa*, arrows) along the anterior margin of the pancreatic tail *(T)*. (*ST*, fluid-filled stomach; *sv*, splenic vein; *a*, aorta; *c*, inferior vena cava; *L*, liver.) **(E,F)** Longitudinal scans with **(F)** more lateral. In **(E)**, the splenic artery (black arrows) is seen extending inferiorly from the celiac artery (white arrow) anterior to the splenic vein *(sv)*. (*a*, aorta; *ST*, fluid-filled stomach; *L*, liver.) In **(F)**, the pancreatic tail *(T)* is visualized with the splenic artery *(sa)* seen anterior to the splenic vein *(sv)* and posterior to the fluid-filled stomach *(ST)*.

superior mesenteric vein. Its anteroposterior measurement in the longitudinal plane is 1.00 ± 0.30 cm and 0.95 ± 0.26 cm in the transverse plane.[4,20]

BODY

Although the anteroposterior dimensions of the body are small, it still represents the largest section of the pancreas. It can be seen anterior to the superior mesenteric artery (Fig. 3-5A). Its anterior border is the posterior wall of the antrum of the stomach. Its right lateral border is the neck of the gland that is anterior to the superior mesenteric vein. Its left lateral border is not definite. The splenic vein courses along the posterior surface of the body[5] (Fig. 3-5C). The tail of the pancreas begins to the

left lateral margin of the vertebral body. The body measures 1.18 ± 0.36 cm in the longitudinal plane and 1.16 ± 0.29 cm in the transverse plane when measured over the superior mesenteric artery in the anteroposterior projection.[4,20]

TAIL

The tail of the pancreas is the most difficult to visualize. It begins just to the left of the left lateral border of the vertebral body and extends to the splenic hilum[4] (Fig. 3-5). The tail may be at a higher level (41 percent) or at the same level (51 percent) as the body and is infrequently (2 percent) at a lower level.[4] The splenic vein courses along the posterior surface of the body and tail

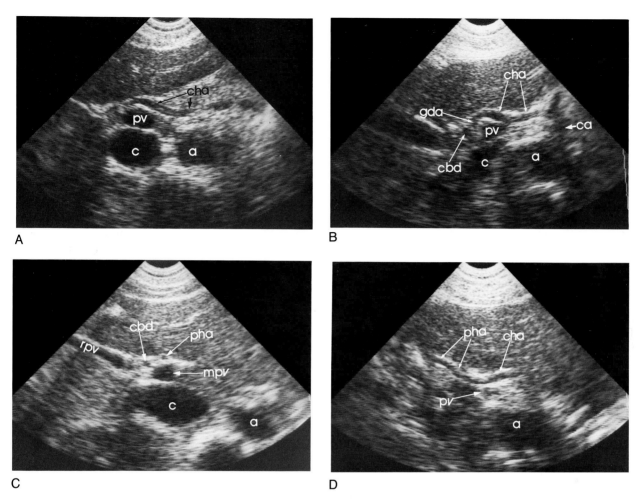

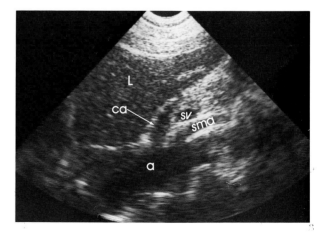

Fig. 3-8. Common hepatic artery. **(A)** Transverse slightly oblique scan. The common hepatic artery *(cha)* is seen extending anterior to the main portal vein *(pv)*. (*a*, aorta; *c*, inferior vena cava.) **(B)** The common hepatic artery *(cha)* is seen extending from the celiac artery *(ca)* running anterior to the main portal vein *(pv)*. The gastroduodenal artery *(gda)* is visualized branching from the common hepatic artery. (*cbd*, common bile duct; *c*, inferior vena cava; *a*, aorta). **(C)** Transverse oblique scan. The common bile duct *(cbd)* is seen anterolateral to the main portal vein *(mpv)* with the proper hepatic artery *(pha)* more anteromedial (*rpv*, right portal vein; *a*, aorta; *c*, inferior vena cava). **(D)** Transverse scan more oblique than **(B)**, following the course of the proper hepatic artery *(pha)*, the continuation of the common hepatic artery after the gastroduodenal artery branch (*pv*, main portal vein; *a*, aorta).

Fig. 3-9. Superior mesenteric artery. Longitudinal scan. The superior mesenteric artery *(sma)* is seen to be the second branch of the abdominal aorta *(a)* with the celiac artery *(ca)* being the first branch. (*sv*, splenic vein; *L*, liver.)

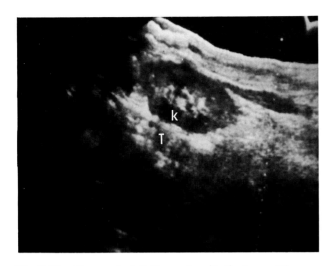

Fig. 3-10. Pancreatic tail. Prone, longitudinal scan. The pancreatic tail *(T)* is seen anterior to the left kidney *(k)*.

(Fig. 3-5C). The tail is seen anterior to the left kidney, posterior to the stomach and medial to the spleen (Figs. 3-5C, 3-7, and 3-10). It appears ovoid or elliptical and has the same echogenicity as on the supine view.[6] It should not be confused with the empty stomach; oral fluid may be given if there is a question.[22]

Size

ADULT

A number of investigators have evaluated pancreatic size.[20,21,23] As expected, size is noted to normally decrease with age. All of the following measurements are made in the anteroposterior projection obtained at a right angle to the true axis of the gland. They include head: 2.01 ± 0.39 cm longitudinal, 2.08 ± 0.40 cm transversely; body: 1.18 ± 0.36 cm longitudinally, 1.16 ± 0.29 cm transversely; neck: 1.00 ± 0.30 cm longitudinally, 0.95 ± 0.26 cm transversely; and tail: 0.7 ± 2.8 cm.[4,20,21] The craniocaudal measurements include head: 2.4 to 4.8 cm; body: 2.4 to 3.6 cm; and tail: 1.6 to 2.4 cm.[4] Taking a maximum dimension of 2.8 cm will embrace 96 percent of the normal population but normal measurements do not exclude pathology.[20] Absolute measurements of pancreatic size may be misleading; symmetry and contour may be more important.[4]

CHILD

As expected, the pancreatic size is smaller in the child and increases with age.[24] With advanced age, the gland again becomes smaller.[4] The head of the pancreas is

TABLE 3-1. Measurements of Pancreatic Size in the Child.*

Age	Head (cm)	Body (cm)	Tail (cm)
0–6 yr	1.6 (1.0–1.9)	0.7 (0.4–1.0)	1.2 (0.8–1.6)
7–12 yr	1.9 (1.7–2.0)	0.9 (0.6–1.0)	1.4 (1.3–1.6)
13–18 yr	2.0 (1.8–2.2)	1.0 (0.7–1.0)	1.6 (1.3–1.8)

(Coleman BG, Arger PH, Rosenberg HK et al: Gray-scale sonographic assessment of pancreatitis in children. Radiology 146:145, 1983.)
* Measurements made in anteroposterior axis on a transverse scan.

measured in an anteroposterior projection including the uncinate process. The body measurement is in an anteroposterior projection anterior to the aorta and splenic vein. The tail is measured in an anteroposterior projection diagonally at the left lateral border of the aorta, and splenic vein. The measurements are given in Table 3-1.

Other investigators have correlated pancreatic size to the transverse lumbar vertebral body measurement.[25] The ratio of the greatest anteroposterior dimension of the body of the pancreas relative to the transverse vertebral body measurement (P/V ratio) was noted to be greater than 0.3 when associated with a hypoechoic parenchyma indicative of acute pancreatitis. The measurements are given in Table 3-2.

Shape

Various shapes have been ascribed to the pancreas. They include sausage, dumbbell, and tadpole.[5,26] More commonly, the pancreas is comma-shaped with the larger portion being the head of the pancreas (see Figs. 3-5 and 3-6).

Texture

A number of investigators have evaluated the normal echopattern or texture of the pancreas. The degree of echogenicity is determined to a greater extent on the amount of fat between the lobules and to a lesser extent on interlobular fibrous tissue.[4] The internal echoes of the

TABLE 3-2. Correlation of Pancreatic Size to the Transverse Lumbar Vertebral Body Measurement.

Group	Range	Average	Standard Deviation
Control	0.24–0.41	0.3	0.06
Acute Pancreatitis	0.21–1.0	0.58	0.24
Chronic Pancreatitis	0.28–0.30	0.3	0.12

(Fleischer AC, Parker P, Kirchner SG, James AE Jr.: Sonographic findings of pancreatitis in children. Radiology 146:151, 1983.)

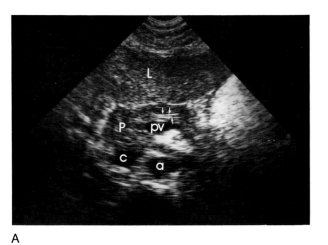 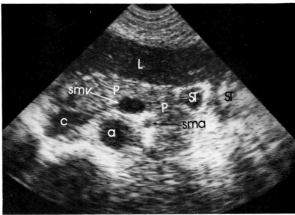

A   B

Fig. 3-11. Normal pancreatic texture. Transverse scans. (**A**) Note the pancreas *(P)* and liver *(L)* are isosonic (equal in echodensity). The pancreatic duct (arrows) is seen as a tubular lucency bordered by two echogenic lines. (*a*, aorta; *c*, inferior vena cava; *pv*, main portal vein.) (**B**) In this case, the pancreas *(P)* is more dense than the liver *(L)*. (*c*, inferior vena cava; *a*, aorta; *smv*, superior mesenteric vein; *sma*, superior mesenteric artery; *ST*, fluid-filled stomach.)

pancreas consist of regularly and closely spaced elements of uniform intensity with uniformly distributed variation throughout the gland.[2]

Normally, when comparing the echopattern of the pancreas to the liver, the pancreas is either isosonic (equal to the liver) (Fig. 3-11A; see Fig. 2-6) or hyperechoic (more dense than liver)[5,15,27–29] (Figs. 3-5A, 3-6A, and 3-11B; see Fig. 2-5A). Several studies have shown that the isosonic pattern represents 46 to 48 percent of normals with the hyperechoic pattern 49 to 52 percent of

normals.[4,30] All agree that the normal pancreas is not less echodense than liver.[30] This entire assignment of pattern is based on the assumption the liver is normal, using it as an internal standard. If there is significant hepatocellular disease and the liver is abnormally dense, it is possible that the normal pancreas may appear less dense than liver (Fig. 3-12).

It is known that with increasing age and body fat deposition, there are increased amounts of fat in the pancreas accounting for an increased echodensity and these function independently.[31] The echopattern of the pancreas in adults is greater than that in children because there is less fat in children.[4] In a histologic study, it was shown that after age 60, there is moderate to severe fat accumulation in the acinar cells of the pancreas.[31] This may account for some of the problems in visualizing the pancreas. As the pancreas becomes more echodense, it tends to become less distinguishable from surrounding retroperitoneal fat (Fig. 3-13). The pancreas should normally be less echogenic than retroperitoneal fat.[5] But, the pancreatic echogenicity may not be entirely due to fat; fibrous tissue may account for a portion of the increased echogenicity not attributed to fat.[27] When the pancreas is quite dense so it cannot be distinguished, it can be identified by the vascular anatomy.[4]

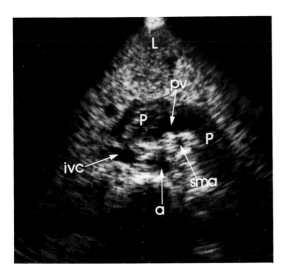

Fig. 3-12. Pancreatic texture. Transverse scan. This patient is known to have severe hepatocellular disease. The normal pancreas *(P)* appears less dense than the liver *(L)*. (*ivc*, inferior vena cava; *a*, aorta; *sma*, superior mesenteric artery; *pv*, main portal vein.)

Pancreatic Duct

Although it was once thought there was a high incidence of pancreatic disease associated with the visualization of the pancreatic duct, the normal pancreatic duct is commonly seen with the high resolution real-time ultra-

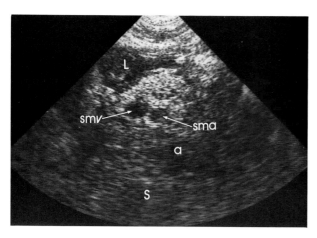

Fig. 3-13. Echodense pancreatic texture. Transverse slightly oblique scan. The pancreatic outline cannot be identified in this elderly obese patient. The pancreas is similar in density to retroperitoneal fat. Many of the normal vascular landmarks for the pancreas are seen. (*a*, aorta; *sma*, superior mesenteric artery; *smv*, superior mesenteric vein; *L*, liver; *S*, spine.)

sound systems currently available.[32-34] It is seen more frequently in the body (straightest portion) (82 to 86 percent) of the pancreas and least frequently in the tail.[4,5,32,35] The duct appears as an echogenic line (Fig. 3-14) or a lucency bordered by two echogenic lines[5,36,37] (Fig. 3-11A). This duct is the duct of Wirsung or the main pancreatic duct and originates at the junction of the small ducts in the lobules of the tail as the conduit for pancreatic juice.[5] The accessary duct of Santorini runs transversely in the upper anterior portion of the pancreatic head at a higher level than the main pancreatic duct.[4]

The main duct passes steeply cephalad from the pa-

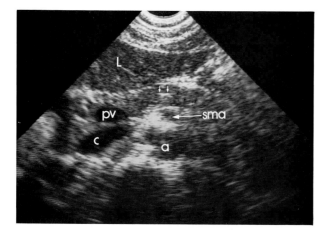

Fig. 3-14. Pancreatic duct, body. Transverse scans. The duct (arrows) is seen as an echogenic line within the body of the pancreas. (*a*, aorta; *c*, inferior vena cava; *sma*, superior mesenteric artery; *pv*, main portal vein; *L*, liver.)

pilla of Vater obliquely to the left, then transversely and upwards across the midline to the left of the spine; then upwards more steeply in the tail.[38] The duct can be easily seen in the standard ventral abdominal wall approach and axial plane.[33] The scanhead may need to be tilted or in an off-axis plane frequently for optimal visualization. To see the duct in the tail is more difficult; it is aided by changes in patient position or oral ingestion of fluid. Failure to see the duct in the tail is presumed to be secondary to the small caliber as well as technical difficulty. In the head, the duct has a dorsal-ventral course and is parallel to the ultrasound beam so the right coronal view is usually needed for optimal visualization[33] (Figs. 3-3, 3-6C, and 3-15; see Fig. 2-6).

The mean diameter (measured in anteroposterior projection on a transverse scan) of the main duct in the area of the head/neck is 3 mm, in the body proximal to neck it is 2.1 mm, and in the body distal to neck it is 1.6 mm.[39] The duct caliber then decreases toward the tail.[5,39] Normally, the duct should not measure more than 2 mm in its internal diameter.[32,33,35,37] It is considered abnormal if it is greater than 2 mm or has walls nonparallel or convex outward (focal dilatation or beading).[32,33] Analysis of the pancreatic duct size and wall contour changes are not helpful in arriving at a specific histologic diagnosis.[33,37,40] In one series, 50 percent of patients with pancreatitis had a dilated duct.[33]

There is noted to be a discrepancy between ultrasound and ERCP in the normal duct measurements.[36] The discrepancy may be due to the contrast injection in the duct under pressure. The ultrasound measurement may be underestimated because the echoes of the wall of the duct are strong, causing apparent thickening of the walls, resulting in underestimation of the inner diameter. There may also be difficulty in visualizing the duct in the head and tail, which is thought to be caused by a variable course of the duct and interfering echoes from neighboring organs, particularly bowel gas.[36]

Real-time ultrasound may be used to guide a thin needle puncture of the duct. Percutaneous pancreatic ductography and percutaneous biopsy can be successfully performed as a single procedure without major complications.[36]

When identifying the pancreatic duct, the examiner should take care not to mistake the splenic vein, splenic artery, or the posterior wall of the stomach for the duct.[32,41,42] The splenic vein can be followed by real-time scanning to its portal vein junction if there is a question (Fig. 3-5). The splenic artery is superior to the body and tail of the pancreas (Fig. 3-7). It can be followed back to its origin in the celiac axis with real-time ultrasound.[41] The posterior wall of the antrum is directly anterior to the body of the pancreas (Fig. 3-16). It appears as an anechoic structure surrounded on both sides by an echogenic rim with the lumen of the stomach appearing

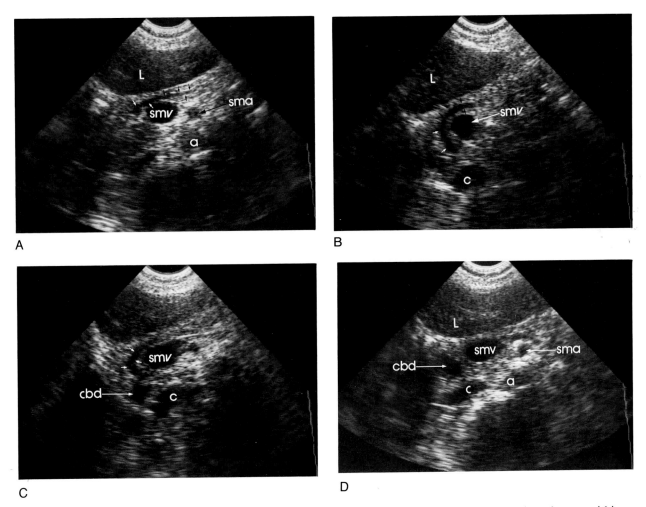

Fig. 3-15. Pancreatic duct, head. Oblique transverse views. **(A)** The pancreatic duct (small arrows) can be seen within the pancreatic body and neck. (*sma*, superior mesenteric artery; *smv*, superior mesenteric vein; *a*, aorta; *L*, liver.) **(B)** Scan slightly lower and more oblique than **(A)**. The pancreatic duct (small arrows) can be seen within the pancreatic head. (*c*, inferior vena cava; *smv*, superior mesenteric vein; *L*, liver.) **(C)** At a slightly lower level than **(B)**, the dilated distal end of the common bile duct *(cbd)* is seen as well as the pancreatic duct (arrows). (*smv*, superior mesenteric vein; *c*, inferior vena cava) **(D)** Lower scan than **(C)**. The dilated distal common bile duct *(cbd)* is seen. This asymptomatic patient was status postcholecystectomy in the distant past, with an incidental finding of a dilated distal common bile duct and a pancreatic duct (3 mm) at upper limits for normal. The patient was not obstructed. (*L*, liver; *smv*, superior mesenteric vein; *c*, inferior vena cava; *a*, aorta; *sma*, superior mesenteric artery.)

Fig. 3-16. Posterior wall of the stomach. Transverse scan. The anterior and posterior walls (arrows, lucency) of the stomach *(ST)* are outlined anterior to the pancreatic body *(B)*. To differentiate posterior gastric wall from the pancreatic duct, the patient may be given water to drink while observing for peristalsis with real-time. (*pv*, main portal vein; *sv*, splenic vein; *L*, liver)

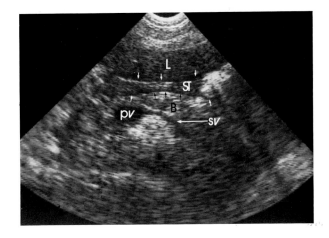

dense.[5,42] It can easily be identified by having the patient drink fluid and by identifying the vascular landmarks.

CONGENITAL ABNORMALITIES

General

Congenital abnormalities other than cystic fibrosis are uncommon.[18] There can be agenesis or hypoplasia of the pancreas; neither can be diagnosed with ultrasound. An annular pancreas represents persistence of the dorsal and ventral pancreas with the head encircling the duodenum.[18] Ultrasound may be able to identify a mass associated with the duodenal obstruction; there have been no case reports. Aberrant or ectopic pancreas is present in 2 percent of routine postmortem examinations.[18] The most favored sites are the stomach and duodenum with jejunum, a Meckel's diverticulum and ileum less common. The mass is usually 3 to 4 cm. There have been no ultrasound reports of this entity either.

Cysts

Congenital cysts result from anomalous development of the pancreatic ducts.[18] There are usually multiple ranging from microscopic to 3 to 5 cm in size.[18] They appear as well-defined anechoic areas with acoustic enhancement (Fig. 3-17).

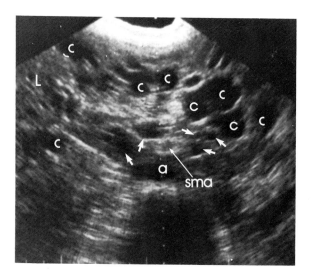

Fig. 3-17. Pancreatic cyst. Transverse scan. Several pancreatic cysts (arrows) are seen as well-defined anechoic areas within the pancreatic area in this patient with polycystic liver and kidney disease. (*c*, liver cysts; *sma*, superior mesenteric artery; *a*, aorta; *L*, liver.)

Cystic Fibrosis

Cystic fibrosis is the single most lethal genetic disease in the white population with a conservative estimation of an incidence of 1 in 2000; 1 in 20 individuals are genetic carriers.[43] Because of improvements in antimicrobial therapy, physical therapy and general medical care, patients with cystic fibrosis are living longer and the disease is becoming recognized as a disease of adolescents and adults.[43,44] The incidence of abdominal problems specifically related to the liver, biliary tract and pancreas increase with age.[44] Now greater than 50 percent of newly diagnosed patients with cystic fibrosis survive to be 20 years old or older.[43]

In cystic fibrosis, the complications are related to the increased secretion of abnormal mucus by the exocrine glands.[4,44] As such the disease is variable. In the pancreas, there is precipitation or coagulation of secretions in the small pancreatic ducts that form obstructing eosinophilic concretions.[44] The proximal distention of the ductules and acini leads to their degeneration and replacement by small cysts. Atrophy of glandular elements and replacement of the altered architecture by fibrosis or fat are late changes. Pancreatic achylia (in 80 percent of patients) results with attendant malabsorption.[44]

The identification of the pancreas in cystic fibrosis is hampered by distention and redundancy of the gastrointestinal tract related to malabsorption and a lack of a scan window through the left lobe of the liver. The anteroposterior diameter of the abdomen is increased due to emphysema. In most, the pancreas will appear echogenic but often the pancreas is not appreciated as a defined homogeneous organ[43-45] (Fig. 3-18). The increased echoes are felt to be due to fibrosis and fat infiltration.[4] The echopattern of the pancreas and the liver cannot be compared because the liver is often abnormal. Up to the stage where there is total or near total fat replacement of the pancreas, there is no correlation between histologic findings and pancreatic function as judged by pancreatic function tests. The availability of ultrasound and CT to monitor the progression of the disease is helpful in assessing the prognosis of a patient with cystic fibrosis.[45]

The hepatic disease in cystic fibrosis is an enigma. There is focal biliary cirrhosis (or fibrosis) with increasing frequency as patients age. This may be due to mechanical obstruction of the bile ductules due to inspissated secretions. Progressive multinodular biliary cirrhosis occurs. The incidence of complications (specifically portal hypertension and sequelae) related to chronic hepatic disease occurs in 2 percent of patients.[44] The liver is enlarged with an increased echogenicity.[4] The spleen is noted to be enlarged with increased echogenicity assumed to be due to hemosiderin and/or fibrosis.[44]

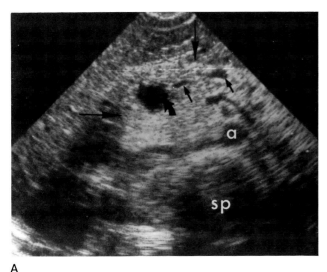

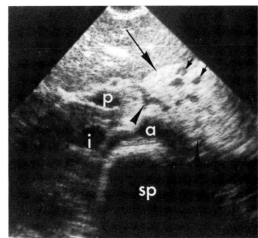

A   B

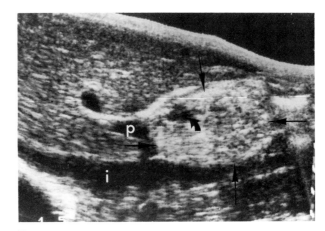

C

Fig. 3-18. Cystic fibrosis. Transverse scans show head and body **(A)** and tail **(B)**. The pancreas (large arrows) is markedly enlarged and has increased echogenicity. The small hypoechoic areas probably represent small cysts (small arrows). The dilated common bile duct (curved arrow) is seen in transverse and longitudinal **(C)** scans. (*sp*, spine; *a*, aorta; *i*, inferior vena cava; *p*, portal vein; arrowhead, celiac bifurcation.) (From Daneman A, Gaskin K, Martin DJ, Cutz E: Pancreatic changes in cystic fibrosis: CT and sonographic appearances. AJR 141:653, © American Roentgen Ray Society, 1983.)

In the gastrointestinal tract, there are thickened irregular folds in cystic fibrosis. Hyperplasia of Brunner's glands may account for the "donut" sign often seen in these patients.[44]

As far as the biliary tract is concerned, there is nonvisualization of the gallbladder in many. There may be obstruction of the cystic duct from mucosal hyperplasia, inspissated mucus or actual atresia of the duct. The lumen is filled with thick bile, sludge, or defined concretions. The wall of the gallbladder is thickened or normal.[44]

ACUTE PANCREATITIS

The etiology and pathogenesis of acute pancreatitis is not clearly understood. The attack is related to biliary tract disease and alcoholism.[4,46] Gallstones are present in 40 to 60 percent of patients with 5 percent of patients with gallstones presenting with acute pancreatitis.[18] Other rare causes include trauma, extension of inflam-

mation from adjacent peptic ulcer disease or abdominal infection, blood borne bacterial infection, viral infection (mumps), vascular thrombosis and embolism, polyarteritis nodosa, hypothermia, drugs (corticosteroids, sulfonamides, oral contraceptives), and is associated with hyperlipoproteinemia and hyperparathroidism. It is idiopathic in 9 to 50 percent of patients.[18] The majority of cases occur in middle age.

The mechanism for acute pancreatitis is not firmly established. The anatomic changes in the pancreas are caused by the destructive lytic effects of the pancreatic enzymes—proteases, lipase, and elastase—which are the keys to pancreatic destruction. There are several proposals to explain the production of acute pancreatitis: (1) bile reflux—important mechanism for activation of pancreatic enzymes; (2) hypersecretion and obstruction —rupture of ducts by pancreatic hypersecretion possibly potentiated by partial duct obstruction; (3) alcohol induced changes—precise manner of its production of pancreatitis is unknown but it is a potent stimulator of pancreatic secretions; and (4) duodenal reflux—favored as initiating mechanism by many.[18,47]

The morphologic changes in acute pancreatitis are many and varied.[46] The basic alterations include (1) proteolytic destruction of the pancreatic substance; (2) necrosis of blood vessels with subsequent hemorrhage; (3) necrosis of fat by lipolytic enzymes; and (4) accompanying inflammatory reaction.[18] The extent and predominance of each of these changes depends on the duration and severity of the process. It may be mild and self-limiting with transient edema. There may be interstitial edema that eventually leads to focal and frank necrosis. Leukocyte reaction between areas of hemorrhage and necrosis and secondary bacterial invasion convert the areas into foci of suppurative necrosis or abscess. With time, the gland is replaced by diffuse or focal parenchymal or stromal fibrosis, calcifications, and irregular duct dilatation.[18]

The process may be severe with damage to the acinar tissue and duct system producing damage by the exudation of pancreatic juice into the interstitium of the gland, leakage of secretions into the peripancreatic tissues, or both. After the acini or duct disrupt, the pancreatic secretions migrate to the surface of the gland. There are several pathways these secretions may take. The most common course is for the fluid to break through the pancreatic connective tissue layer and thin posterior layer of the peritoneum and enter the lesser sac. The pancreatic juice enters the anterior pararenal space by breaking through the thin layer of the fibrous connective tissue; or the fluid might migrate to the surface of the gland and remain within the confines of the fibrous connective tissue layer.[47]

The collections of fluid in the peripancreatic area generally retain communication with the pancreas. A dynamic equilibrium is established so that fluid is continuously absorbed from the collection and replaced by additional pancreatic secretions. Centrifugal drainage of the pancreatic juices may cease as the pancreatic inflammatory response subsides and the rate of pancreatic secretion returns to normal. Collections of extrapancreatic fluid should be reabsorbed or, if drained, should not recur with recovery of proper drainage through the duct.[47]

Because acute pancreatitis produces a combination of unfavorable and favorable consequences, the phenomenon of escape and pooling of pancreatic secretions occurs. The symptoms of patients with this complication are prolonged with persistent abdominal pain, fever, and leukocytosis beyond the five days of the usual attack of acute pancreatitis. These patients are at risk for abscess and hemorrhage. With expulsion of the pancreatic secretions, the pancreas itself appears to be spared, serving to decompress the gland. In complicated pancreatitis, there is an inverse relationship between the degree of autodigestion of the gland and the volume of peripancreatic fluid.[47]

The clinical course of the patient with acute pancreatitis usually begins with severe pain that usually occurs after a large meal or alcoholic binge. The pain is constant and intense. The serum amylase increases within 24 hours and the serum lipase increases within 72 to 94 hours.[18] Five percent of these patients will die from the acute effects of the peripheral vascular collapse and shock during the first week of the clinical course.[18] Acute adult respiratory distress syndrome and acute tubular necrosis frequently accompany pancreatitis and are particularly ominous. Other complications include pseudocyst formation (10 percent), phlegmon (18 percent), abscess (1 to 9 percent), hemorrhage (5 percent), and duodenal obstruction.[18,48,49]

On ultrasound, there are several characteristic findings associated with acute pancreatitis.[4,24,47,50-54] The pancreas may appear normal on ultrasound in 29 percent of cases.[4] There is a diffuse (52 percent) increase in size to the gland with loss of the normal sonographic texture or focal (28 percent) enlargement.[4] The gland is hypoechoic to anechoic and is less echogenic than liver (Figs. 3-19 to 3-21). The borders of the pancreas may be smooth, but they are usually indistinct. In addition, there may be loss of distinction of the splenic vein.[50] The textural changes in acute pancreatitis with the development of edema without overall enlargement of the pancreas may be seen at an earlier stage with ultrasound than with CT. Patients have been seen to demonstrate an abnormal pancreatic ultrasound before an abnormal serum amylase. Ultrasound usually does not reveal the peripancreatic thickening of the surrounding fascial planes as is seen on CT.[47]

Hemorrhagic Pancreatitis

In acute hemorrhagic pancreatic necrosis or acute hemorrhagic pancreatitis, there is the sudden more or less diffuse enzymatic destruction of the pancreatic substance caused presumably by sudden escape of the active lytic pancreatic enzymes into the glandular parenchyma. The enzymes cause focal areas of fat necrosis in and about the pancreas, which lead to rupture of pancreatic vessels and hemorrhage. Forty-five percent of patients have a sudden necrotizing destruction of the pancreas following an alcoholic debauch or excessively large meal.[18] Patients with acute hemorrhagic pancreatitis represent the severe form of the disease with decreased hemocrit and serum calcium, hypotension despite volume replacement, metabolic acidosis, and adult respiratory distress syndrome.[18]

Hemorrhagic complications of pancreatitis include hemorrhagic necrosis of the pancreatic parenchyma, deposition of hemorrhagic fluid into the retroperitoneal tissue or peritoneal cavity, and hemorrhage into a pan-

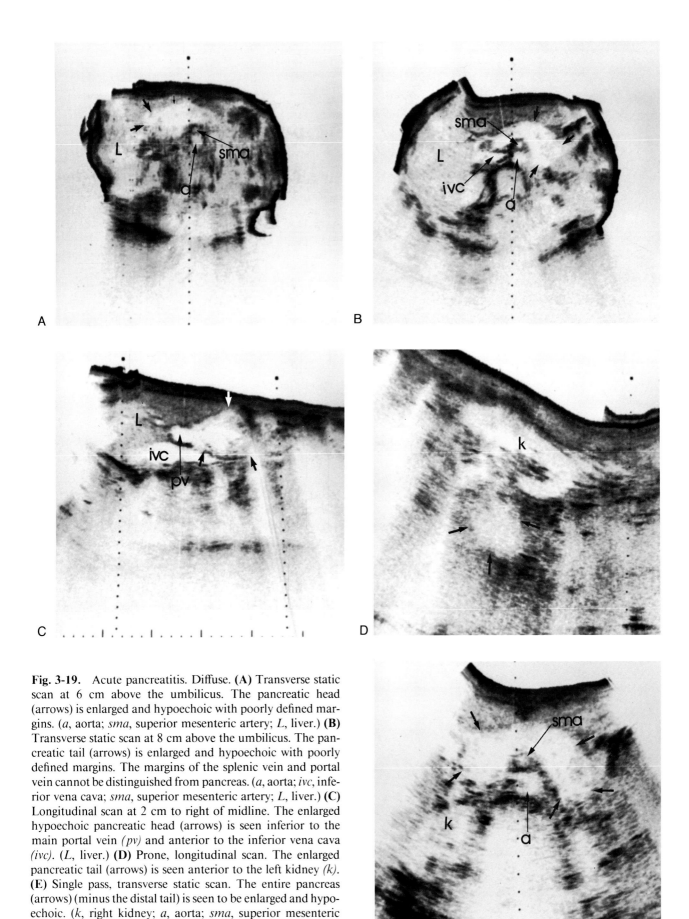

Fig. 3-19. Acute pancreatitis. Diffuse. **(A)** Transverse static scan at 6 cm above the umbilicus. The pancreatic head (arrows) is enlarged and hypoechoic with poorly defined margins. (*a*, aorta; *sma*, superior mesenteric artery; *L*, liver.) **(B)** Transverse static scan at 8 cm above the umbilicus. The pancreatic tail (arrows) is enlarged and hypoechoic with poorly defined margins. The margins of the splenic vein and portal vein cannot be distinguished from pancreas. (*a*, aorta; *ivc*, inferior vena cava; *sma*, superior mesenteric artery; *L*, liver.) **(C)** Longitudinal scan at 2 cm to right of midline. The enlarged hypoechoic pancreatic head (arrows) is seen inferior to the main portal vein *(pv)* and anterior to the inferior vena cava *(ivc)*. (*L*, liver.) **(D)** Prone, longitudinal scan. The enlarged pancreatic tail (arrows) is seen anterior to the left kidney *(k)*. **(E)** Single pass, transverse static scan. The entire pancreas (arrows) (minus the distal tail) is seen to be enlarged and hypoechoic. (*k*, right kidney; *a*, aorta; *sma*, superior mesenteric artery.)

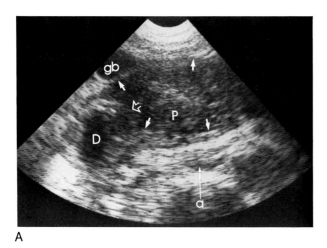 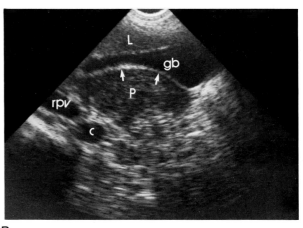

A   B

Fig. 3-20. Acute pancreatitis. Diffuse. **(A)** Transverse scan. The pancreas *(P)* is markedly enlarged with poorly defined margins (arrows) and is relatively hypoechoic. It is difficult to define the medial border (open arrow) of the fluid-filled duodenum *(D)*. (*gb*, gallbladder; *a*, aorta.) **(B)** Longitudinal left lateral decubitus scan. The enlarged pancreas *(P)* produces a mass effect (arrows) on the posterior wall of the gallbladder *(gb)* in this projection. (*rpv*, right portal vein; *c*, inferior vena cava; *L*, liver.)

creatic pseudocyst. The incidence of hemorrhage is 2 to 33 percent.[55] The hemorrhagic complication of pancreatitis is reported to have a poor prognosis with a mortality of 25 to 100 percent.[55] With increasing awareness of the spectrum of the appearance of hemorrhagic pancreatic fluid collections, more clinically benign hemorrhagic

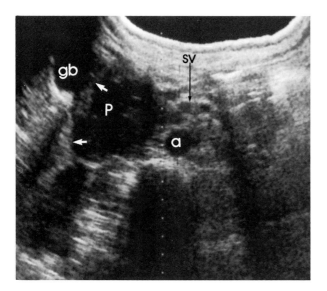

Fig. 3-21. Acute pancreatitis and phlegmonous extension. Focal. Transverse scan demonstrates focal enlargement of the pancreatic head *(P)*. The "mass effect" has poorly defined margins and is hypoechoic relative to the remainder of the gland. The inferior vena cava is not identified. There is phlegmonous extension into the area of the lesser sac (arrows). (*a*, aorta; *gb*, gallbladder; *sv*, splenic vein.)

events may be diagnosed. The presence of hemorrhagic fluid collections does not necessarily warrant drastic measures. The overall clinical setting should be a major factor in determining whether therapeutic intervention is warranted.[55]

The appearance of hemorrhagic pancreatic fluid collections on ultrasound depends on the age of the hemorrhage.[4,55] Acutely, a well-defined homogeneous mass (on CT 45 to 65 HU) is seen (Figs. 3-22 to 3-24). At one week of age, the mass may appear cystic (on CT 14 to 25 HU) with solid elements or septation. At several weeks of age, the hemorrhage may appear cystic. In vitro studies have shown that hemorrhage and clotted blood appear either echogenic or lucent, depending on the age of the hemorrhage and the transducer used. So, in the appropriate clinical setting, ultrasound may demonstrate an echogenic well-defined pancreatic mass that suggests an acute hemorrhage (Figs. 3-22, 3-23). Abscess or pseudocyst appear similar but are not as homogeneous or as strongly echogenic.

Phlegmonous Pancreatitis

A phlegmon is spreading diffuse inflammatory edema of soft tissues that may proceed to necrosis, and even suppuration. Extension outside the gland occurs in only 18 to 20 percent of patients with acute pancreatitis. A phlegmon appears hypoechoic with good through transmission. It does not represent extrapancreatic fluid. It usually involves the lesser sac, the left anterior pararenal

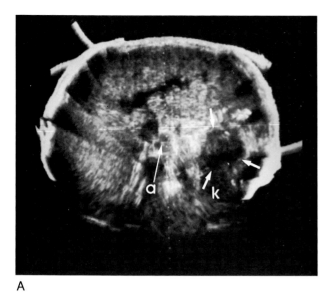

A

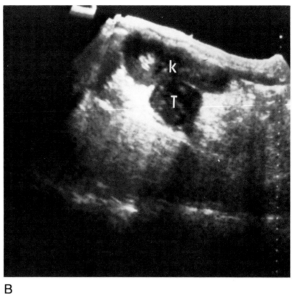

B

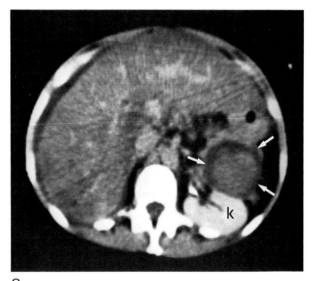

C

Fig. 3-22. Hemorrhagic pancreatitis. Focal. **(A)** Transverse static scan at 12 cm above the umbilicus. This patient had known hepatocellular disease with a dense echopattern. A poorly defined mass (arrows) is seen in the region of the pancreatic tail. The mass is similar in density to liver. (*a*, aorta; *k*, left kidney.) **(B)** Prone longitudinal scan. The pancreatic tail *(T)* mass is seen anterior to the left kidney *(k)*. It is similar in density to kidney. **(C)** CT scan. The focal pancreatic enlargement is seen as a mass (arrows) anterior to the left kidney *(k)*. The mass exhibited an increased density both on enhanced **(C)** and unenhanced views. This represented focal hemorrhagic pancreatitis.

Fig. 3-23. Hemorrhagic pancreatitis. Focal. Transverse scan through the pancreas *(P)*. A poorly defined mass (arrows), seen in the area of the pancreatic tail, has a similar echodensity to the liver *(L)*. The remainder of the pancreas was enlarged with a mass effect. On a CT scan this mass was shown to be very dense consistent with hemorrhage. (*sma*, superior mesenteric artery; *a*, aorta.)

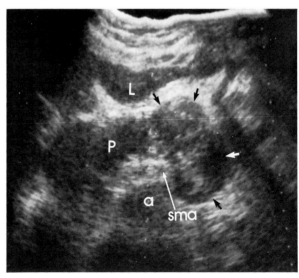

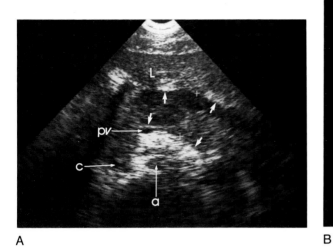
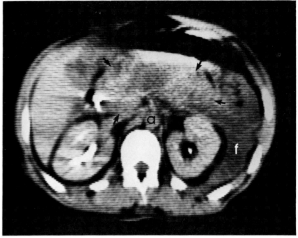

A   B

Fig. 3-24. Hemorrhagic pancreatitis. Diffuse. **(A)** Transverse scan through the pancreatic body (arrows). The pancreas is inhomogeneously echodense and diffusely enlarged. (*pv*, main portal vein; *L*, liver; *a*, aorta; *c*, inferior vena cava.) **(B)** CT scan. There is fluid *(f)* in the left anterior pararenal space and the pancreas is enlarged with increased density (arrows) consistent with hemorrhage. (*a*, aorta.)

space, and transverse mesocolon (Fig. 3-21). Less commonly, it involves the small bowel mesentery, lower retroperitoneum, and pelvis.[4]

Liquefactive Necrosis

In unusual cases, a necrotic pancreas may become an excavated necrotic sac surrounded by a shell of tissue forming a sac that conforms to the axis and contour of the pancreas.[4,47] This debris-containing sac could be misinterpreted on ultrasound and CT and is often best defined by direct injection into the pancreatic duct.[48] On ultrasound, a debris containing cystic structure is seen in the region of the pancreas without a definite extrapancreatic pseudocyst. It appears hypoechoic and resembles a diffusely edematous gland or cyst (Fig. 3-25). On ERCP, a ductal stricture and communication with the pancreatic sac is seen.[48] The lesion is usually treated with drainage like a pseudocyst.

Acute Pancreatitis in Children

The pancreas can be more reliably seen in children than adults because they tend to be smaller with less body fat.[24] In the young child, the liver normally lies lower in the abdomen and the left lobe is more prominent, which provides an excellent sonic window for improved visualization. As with adults, the normal pancreas is generally isosonic or hyperechoic with respect to the liver.[56] In children, the gland tends to be more often isosonic then hyperechoic.[25] The size, echogenicity, and contour must be assessed in evaluation for acute pancreatitis. The gland will be seen increased in size (generally in a diffuse fashion), hypoechoic (less dense than liver), and indistinct in outline.[24]

Ultrasound is valuable in children with unexplained acute and chronic abdominal pain. In one series, the serum amylase and/or amylase clearance ratio correlated poorly with the ultrasound and clinical evidence of pancreatitis.[56]

In the child, there are diverse causes for acute pancreatitis. These include trauma, drugs (steroids, L-asparaginase, hydrochlorothiazide, azothioprine, salicylazosulfapyridine), infection (viral, measles, mumps, and rubella), congenital anomalies, and familial or idiopathic.[24]

Aspiration/Biopsy

As a rule, there would not be a need to perform a biopsy or aspiration in cases of acute pancreatitis unless complications occurred.

Clinical Considerations

A patient with acute edematous pancreatitis may have a normal appearance on ultrasound in 28 percent of cases but there is usually focal or diffuse enlargement (61 percent) or phlegmonous changes (11 percent). Patients with a diagnosis of acute necrotizing pancreatitis never

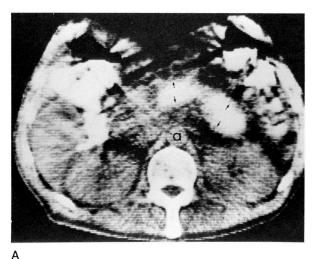
A

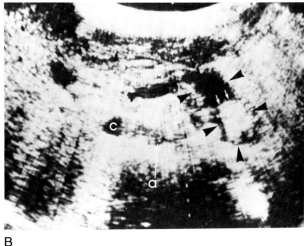
B

Fig. 3-25. Liquefactive necrosis. **(A)** CT scan performed immediately following an ERCP, demonstrating a central contrast-filled area (arrows), surrounded by a shell of pancreatic tissue, completely replacing the core and occupying the normal pancreatic axis. (*a*, aorta.) **(B)** Transverse scan showing a localized collection of solid material (necrotic tissue) layering out (white arrows) in the sac-like fluid collection (arrowheads) in the area of the pancreatic tail. (*a*, aorta; *c*, inferior vena cava.) (From Burrell M, Gold JA, Simeone J et al: Liquefactive necrosis of the pancreas: The pancreatic sac. Radiology 135:157, 1980.)

have a normal pancreas on ultrasound and most (89 percent) have evidence of phlegmonous pancreatitis. The ultrasound appearance persists in phlegmonous pancreatitis for weeks to months after the patient has made a full clinical recovery.

In patients with an acute pancreatitis diagnosis, the pancreas is visualized 62 percent of the time by ultrasound and 98 percent of the time by CT.[4] Ultrasound is useful in pancreatitis to evaluate for biliary tract disease because biliary disease is often associated with stones and dilatation. A CT is performed for those who fail to visualize on ultrasound and when complications of acute pancreatitis are suspected.

COMPLICATIONS OF PANCREATITIS

Aneurysms Secondary to Pancreatitis

Aneurysms secondary to acute pancreatitis are an uncommon complication.[57] The splenic artery is the most often involved, but other splanchnic vessels can be involved including celiac, common hepatic artery, gastric artery, and gastroduodenal artery. The pancreatic arteries that are subject to aneurysm are the pancreaticoduodenal arcades and dorsal and transverse pancreatic arteries. A superior mesenteric artery aneurysm is an uncommon complication.

Because of the risk of aneurysm formation, the patient should be scanned carefully with real-time ultrasound

(Fig. 3-26); not all lucent masses are pseudocysts.[57] Most will demonstrate intrinsic pulsations of the arterial wall with real-time scanning. However, a splanchnic aneurysm need not show pulsation. If a massive gastrointestinal hemorrhage has occurred in association with acute pancreatitis, the examiner should look carefully for an aneurysm.[57] Some may be too small to identify. Ten percent of patients with chronic pancreatitis have pseudoaneurysms. Aneurysms occasionally do occur in the pancreatic bed secondary to pancreatitis.[57]

Abscess

The incidence of pancreatic abscess is 1 to 9 percent and is related to the severity of acute pancreatitis.[49] The likelihood of abscess development appears to be directly related to the degree of tissue necrosis.[47] Forty percent are associated with postoperative pancreatitis, 4 percent with an alcoholic binge and 7 percent with biliary disease.[49] There is an associated high mortality (32 to 65 percent) even with surgical drainage with an untreated mortality of 100 percent.[25]

An abscess develops due to the superinfection of the necrotic pancreatic and retroperitoneal tissues and less commonly due to superinfection of a pseudocyst. The infection occurs due to hematogenous, lymphatic, or transmural spread of enteric organisms from the adjacent gastrointestinal tract. The abscess may be unilocular or multilocular and can spread superiorly into the

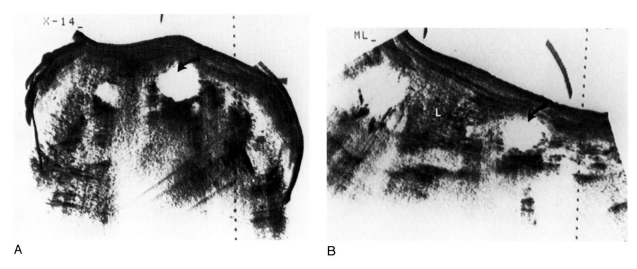

Fig. 3-26. Superior mesenteric artery aneurysm. **(A)** Transverse scan. A superior mesenteric artery aneurysm (arrow) is seen mimicking the appearance of a pancreatic pseudocyst. **(B)** Longitudinal scan of the same aneurysm (arrow). (*L*, liver.) (From Gooding GAW: Ultrasound of superior mesenteric artery aneurysm secondary to pancreatitis: A plea for real-time ultrasound of sonolucent masses in pancreatitis. J Clin Ultrasound 9:255, 1981. By permission, John Wiley & Sons, New York.)

mediastinum, inferiorly into the transverse mesocolon or down the retroperitoneum into the pelvis.

The clinical patterns are variable. The clinical diagnosis is difficult as a patient with acute necrotizing pancreatitis can have the signs and symptoms of an acute supportive process. If the patient with acute necrotic pancreatitis has a persistent fever and leukocytosis, an abscess should be considered.[4] With acute necrotizing pancreatitis, an abscess may develop 7 to 14 days after the onset of symptoms.[49] Most patients improve with acute pancreatitis in 1 to 10 days with conservative therapy with 2 to 9 percent developing abscesses.[4,58,59] With acute interstitial pancreatitis, the patient may suffer a relapse within 2 to 3 weeks complicated by abscess.[49] The cardinal signs of abscess include fever, chills, hypotension, and a tender abdomen with a growing mass. A leukocytosis and bacteremia strengthen the diagnosis.[49]

The ultrasound appearance of an abscess may be very similar to acute pancreatitis or a pseudocyst. A hypoechoic mass will be seen that may have smooth walls with little to no internal echoes; some have irregular walls with increased internal echoes (Figs. 3-27 and 3-28). The mass may range from completely echofree to echodense.[4] Hidden by bowel gas, a gas-containing abscess can be missed with ultrasound. The only suggestive sign of an abscess on CT is gas, but the air may be present in the absence of abscess with sterile necrosis, phlegmon, or a pseudocyst that has ruptured into the gastrointestinal tract.[4,47,49] A positive diagnosis of an abscess cannot be made by ultrasound alone. If an abscess is clinically suspected, then an aspiration of the pancreatic/peripancreatic fluid should be performed.[4,47,49]

ASPIRATION/BIOPSY

As has been described, the ultrasound findings with a pancreatic abscess are not greatly different than those with acute pancreatitis or at times pseudocyst. Because a patient with a pancreatic abscess is at significant risk, if an abscess is suspected, an ultrasound guided needle aspiration should be performed.[49] An immediate gram-stain should be performed in order to determine if the fluid is sterile or not making an immediate diagnosis. With an immediate diagnosis of a pancreatic abscess, appropriate therapy may be instituted. With the addition of percutaneous aspiration, perhaps the high mortality rate associated with a pancreatic abscess may be reduced while surgery may be avoided in those patients with sterile fluid collections.[49]

Pseudocyst

Pseudocysts represent collections of fluid that arise from a loculation of inflammatory processes, necrosis, or hemorrhage. The overwhelming majority are clinically important cysts and are almost always associated with pancreatitis. In 9 out of 10 cases, they are due to acute pancreatitis or trauma.[18] Pseudocysts are said to occur in 10 to 50 percent of patients with acute pancrea-

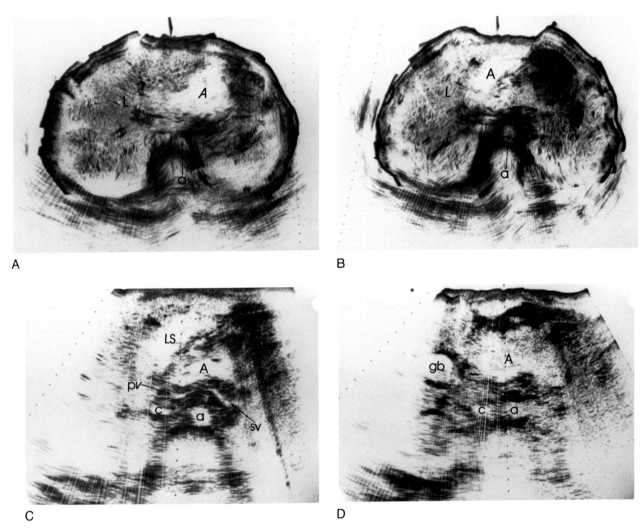

A

B

C

D

Fig. 3-27. Pancreatic abscess. **(A)** Transverse scan at 16 cm above the umbilicus. A hypoechoic mass *(A)*, seen in the area of the lesser sac, is poorly defined and contains internal echoes. It represents extension of a pancreatic abscess. (*L*, liver; *a*, aorta.) **(B)** Transverse scan at 12 cm above the umbilicus. The poorly defined hypoechoic abscess *(A)* is seen in the midabdomen at this level. A portion of this mass is in the pancreatic area with the anterior component in the lesser sac. (*L*, liver; *a*, aorta.) **(C)** Transverse cone-down scan at 5 cm below the xyphoid. The lesser sac *(LS)* component is seen anterior to the pancreatic component *(A)*. (*pv*, main portal vein; *c*, inferior vena cava; *sv*, splenic vein; *a*, aorta.) **(D)** Transverse cone-down scan at 6.5 cm below the xyphoid. The hypoechoic pancreatic abscess *(A)* is seen in the area of the pancreatic body. (*gb*, gallbladder; *c*, inferior vena cava; *a*, aorta.)

titis.[4,48,60] They are usually single, oval to round in shape, and vary in size; they arise in any portion of the pancreas and can cause dilatation of the pancreatic duct. They are situated within the pancreas or adjacent to the pancreas particularly in the region of the tail. The wall may be thin or quite thick and fibrotic. There is no epithelial lining, no communication with the duct, and marked inflammatory reaction associated.[18] They are said to occur because of obstruction followed by rupture of the pancreatic duct, which allows pancreatic juice to escape into the interstitium of the gland. Because there is absence of a

capsule, the fluid may rupture into and accumulate in the lesser sac or extend down into the retroperitoneal soft tissue planes in any direction.[4]

On ultrasound, a pseudocyst has a typical appearance. It usually has sharply defined smooth walls and demonstrates acoustic enhancement[2,47,54,61,62] (Fig. 3-29). At times the lesion may demonstrate multiple septations, multiple internal echoes, and even fail to exhibit acoustic enhancement[61] (Fig. 3-30). The ultrasound success rate in detecting pseudocysts varies from 50 to 92 percent.[4] Those in the head and body are usually seen while those

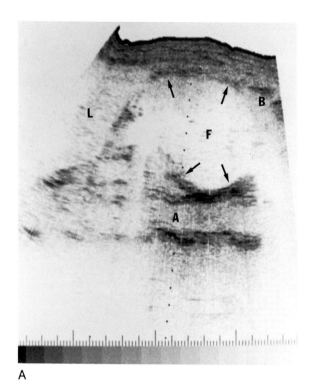

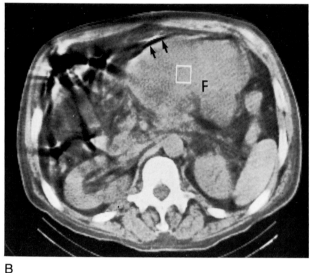

A   B

Fig. 3-28.   Pancreatic abscess. Lesser sac abscess. **(A)** Longitudinal midline scan with a well-defined fluid collection *(F)* with smooth walls (arrows) and some internal echoes. (*L,* liver; *A,* aorta; *B,* bowel gas.) **(B)** CT scan. Well-defined, loculated lesser sac collection *(F)* is seen. (Arrows, stomach.) (From Hill MC, Dach JL, Barkin J et al: The role of percutaneous aspiration in the diagnosis of pancreatic abscess. AJR 141:1035, © Am Roent Ray Soc, 1983.)

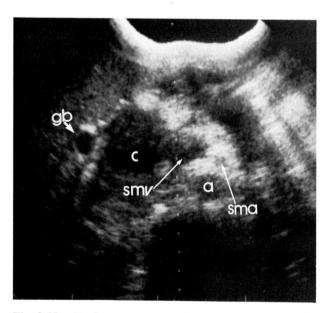

Fig. 3-29.   Typical pseudocyst. Transverse scan. A well-defined, round anechoic mass *(c)* is seen in the area of the head of the pancreas. The pancreatic head is enlarged (*a,* aorta; *gb,* gallbladder; *smv,* superior mesenteric vein; *sma,* superior mesenteric artery.)

in the tail are often "hidden" by the stomach. The wall of the cyst is usually smooth although some are irregular. The fluid is often echofree with some filled with internal echoes; if a fluid-debris level is superimposed, abscess or hemorrhage should be considered. This lesion can mimic cystadenoma or cystadenocarcinoma by its ultrasound appearance.

There are various locations for these pseudocysts.[33,47,48,58] The most common site is the lesser sac as it is directly anterior to the pancreas and posterior to the body of the stomach[47,54] (Figs. 3-30 and 3-31). The second most common location of the extrapancreatic fluid collection is the anterior pararenal space[47] (Figs. 3-32 and 3-33). This is directly posterior to the lesser sac and bounded by the anterior layer of Gerota's fascia. The spleen represents the lateral border of the anterior pararenal space on the left. Fluid occurs more commonly in the left pararenal space than the right. Sometimes the posterior pararenal space is also fluid-filled as fluid spreads from the anterior pararenal space to the posterior pararenal space on the same side. In addition, fluid may enter the peritoneal cavity either via the foramen of Winslow or by disrupting the peritoneum in the anterior surface of the lesser sac.[47]

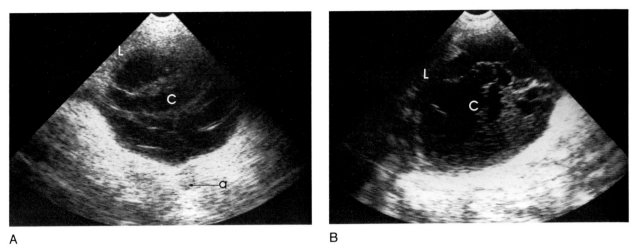

A   B

Fig. 3-30. Pseudocyst, septations. Case 1: **(A)** Transverse scan through the midline. A large cystic mass *(C)* is seen anterior to the aorta *(a)*. It contains many internal septations. (*L*, liver) Case 2: **(B)** Transverse scan through a multiseptated pancreatic pseudocyst *(C)*. (*L*, liver.)

At times, the location of a pseudocyst may be confusing. One can be located in the mediastinum by extending through the esophageal (T10) or aortic (T12) hiatus[63,64] (Figs. 3-34 and 3-35). A mediastinal pseudocyst may be commonly associated with a pleural effusion rich in protein and amylase.[63] It is important to identify the location of the pseudocyst and identify it as such because the operative procedure entails internal drainage below the xyphoid.[63] Besides extending into the mediastinum, a pseudocyst may extend into the small bowel mesentery or down into the retroperitoneum into the pelvis and even the groin.[4] A pseudocyst may also be located in the transverse mesocolon or anterior pararenal space adjacent to the left kidney and be confused with renal pathology[65] (Figs. 3-32 and 3-33). Since at times, the diagnosis of a renal cyst versus a pseudocyst cannot be made by imaging alone, a fine needle aspiration may be performed obtaining fluid for amylase evaluation.[66]

At times, the pseudocyst may be in the region of the spleen[67,68] (Fig. 3-36). There may be release of proteolytic active enzymes with erosion of the splenic hilum and further extension into the splenic parenchyma as a known complication of pancreatitis.[67,69] If an intrasplenic pseudocyst is suspected, this must be confirmed.

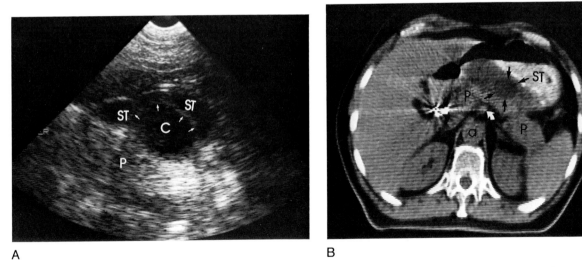

A   B

Fig. 3-31. Pseudocyst, lesser sac. **(A)** Slightly oblique transverse scan with fluid in the stomach *(ST)*. A cystic mass *(C,* arrows) is seen posterior to the stomach. Many of the usual pancreatic *(P)* landmarks are not identified. **(B)** CT similar to **(A)** demonstrating a pancreatic pseudocyst (arrows) as a well-defined low-density area between the stomach *(ST)* and the pancreas *(P)*. (*a*, aorta; curved arrow, superior mesenteric artery.)

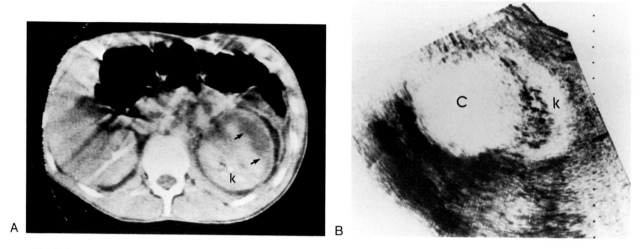

Fig. 3-32. Pseudocyst, pararenal. **(A)** Contrast CT through the upper pole of the kidneys. An intrarenal-appearing mass (arrows) is seen involving the anterior aspect of the left kidney *(k)*. **(B)** Prone, longitudinal scan. An anechoic mass *(C)* is seen at the anterior, superior aspect of the left kidney *(k)*. (From Baker MK, Kopecky KK, Wass JL: Perirenal pancreatic pseudocysts: Diagnostic management. AJR 140:729, © American Roentgen Ray Society, 1983.)

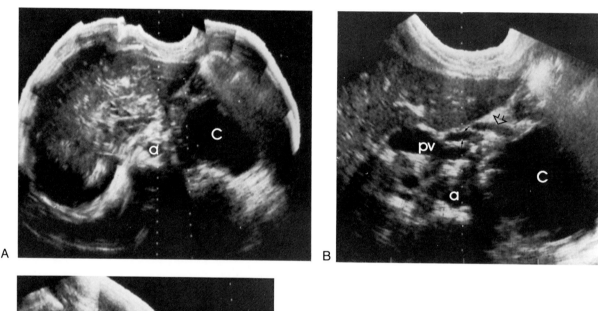

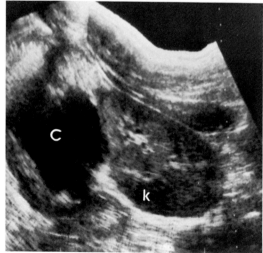

Fig. 3-33. Pseudocyst, pararenal. Transverse scan at 14 cm above the umbilicus **(A)** and transverse cone-down scan 1 cm below the xyphoid **(B)**. A cystic mass *(C)* is seen in the left upper quadrant. (*a*, aorta; *pv*, main portal vein; solid arrows, pancreatic duct; open arrow, splenic artery.) **(C)** Longitudinal prone scan. A cystic mass *(C)* that appears to involve the left kidney is seen *(k)*. By using the vascular landmarks, the pancreatic origin of the mass could be established.

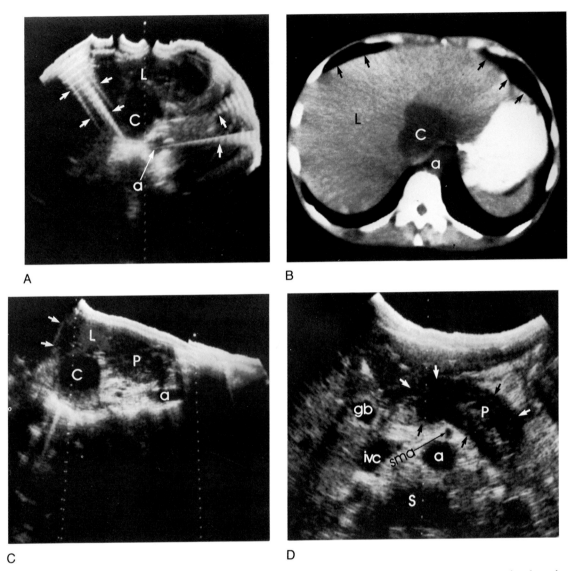

Fig. 3-34. Pseudocyst, mediastinal. Patient with acute pancreatitis and a pseudocyst extending up to the chest through the lesser sac. **(A)** High transverse scan. The pseudocyst *(C)* is seen in the midline extending up from the lesser sac. (*a,* aorta; *L,* liver; arrows, relective pattern due to air from the lung.). **(B)** CT scan at a slightly lower level than **(A)** demonstrating a low density area *(C)* in the lesser sac region. (*a,* aorta; *L,* liver; arrows, lung producing reflective pattern in **(A)**) **(C)** Longitudinal midline scan. The pseudocyst *(C)* is seen next to the diaphragm (arrows) extending upward. The pancreas *(P)* itself is enlarged and hypoechoic. (*a,* aorta; *L,* liver.) **(D)** Transverse cone-down scan through the pancreas *(P).* The body and tail are seen to be enlarged (arrows) and hypoechoic consistent with acute pancreatitis. (*a,* aorta; *ivc,* inferior vena cava; *sma,* superior mesenteric artery; *gb,* gallbladder; *S,* spine.)

Once confirmed, surgical intervention is mandatory because of the danger of secondary hemorrhage.[68] Nuclear medicine and angiography may be used in conjunction with ultrasound to verify the diagnosis.[68]

Besides stimulating splenic, renal, and mediastinal pathology, a pseudocyst may also involve the duodenum.[70] Duodenal involvement may occur because the nonperitonealized posterior surface of the duodenum is in direct contact with the head of the pancreas with no effective barrier to the anatomically disruptive effect of the secretions. Whether these appear intramural or as severe extrinsic compressive lesions depend on the variable interplay between the depth of penetration and extent of infiltration. With accumulation of secretions and increased pressure, extension may occur within the wall of the duodenum or it may rupture from the cyst cavity into the bowel lumen. The second portion of the duodenum is the most frequently involved with the site of

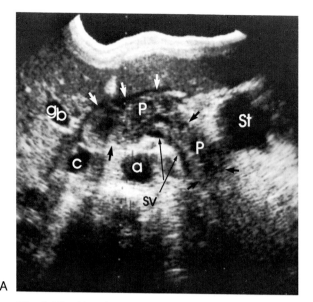 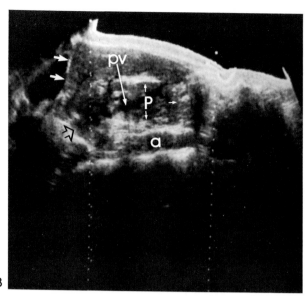

Fig. 3-35. Pseudocyst, mediastinal - followup. These scans were performed 2 weeks after those in Figure 3-34. (A) Transverse scan, similar to Figure 3-34D. The pancreas (*P*, arrows) is smaller and more echogenic. Now the splenic vein *(sv)* can be identified. (*St*, fluid-filled stomach; *c*, inferior vena cava; *a*, aorta; *gb*, gallbladder.) (B) Longitudinal midline scan similar to Figure 3-34C. No pseudocyst is seen where the previous lesion was seen (open arrow.) (*P*, small arrows, pancreas; large solid arrows, diaphragm; *pv*, portal vein; *a*, aorta.)

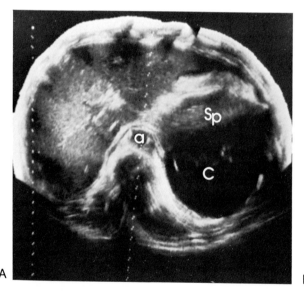 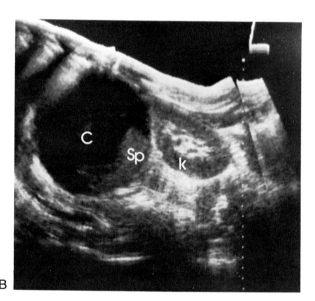

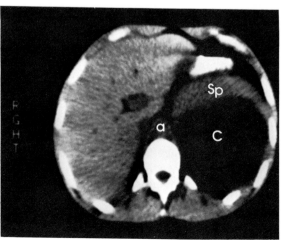

Fig. 3-36. Pseudocyst, splenic. (A) Transverse static scan. An anechoic mass *(C)* is seen posterior to the spleen *(Sp)*. (*a*, aorta.) (B) Prone longitudinal static scan. The same pseudocyst *(C)* is seen superior and posterior to the spleen *(Sp)*. (*k*, left kidney.) (C) CT scan similar to (A). (*C*, pseudocyst; *Sp*, spleen; *a*, aorta.) (Figs. A and C from Mittelstaedt CA, McCartney WH, Mauro M et al: Spleen. p. 235. In Simeone J (ed): Clinics in Diagnostic Ultrasound: Coordinated Diagnostic Imaging. Churchill Livingstone, New York, 1984. Fig. B from Mittelstaedt CA: Ultrasound of the spleen. p. 233. In Raymond HW, Zwiebel WJ (eds): Seminars in Ultrasound,CT and MR. Vol. 2. Grune and Stratton, New York, 1981.)

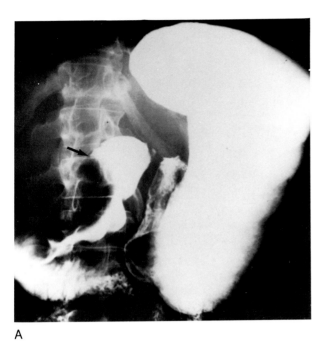

A

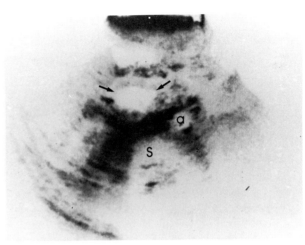

B

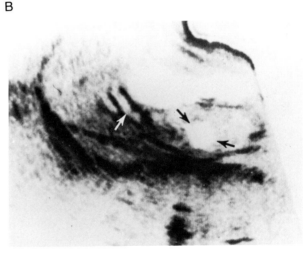

C

Fig. 3-37. Pseudocyst, duodenual. **(A)** Upper gastrointestinal series, right anterior oblique view. A smooth lobulated filling defect is seen within the lumen of the distal first and second parts of the duodenum. The lumen is severely narrowed. An acute angle is formed at the junction of the filling defect and the duodenal wall (arrow). Transverse **(B)** and longitudinal **(C)** static scans at the level of the pancreas. A 5 cm mass is seen in the region of the head of the pancreas. It has an anechoic center (black arrows). The common bile duct (white arrow) measures 7 mm. (*a*, aorta; *S*, spine.) (From Bellon EM, George CR, Schreiber H, Marshall JB: Pancreatic pseudocysts of the duodenum. AJR 133:827, © Am Roent Ray Soc, 1979.)

involvement usually on its lateral or posterolateral surface[70] (Fig. 3-37).

Many pseudocysts regress with a 20 percent rate of spontaneous regression reported.[4,60] Some decompress into the pancreatic duct, others into the GI tract.[4] Five to 15 percent of the cysts rupture.[61,71,72] Fifty percent of those that resolve rupture into the gastrointestinal tract and 50 percent rupture into the peritoneal cavity.[61] The stomach is most commonly involved with drainage into the duodenum rare.[73] These cysts rupture from the tryptic digestion of the wall; in those cases whose erosion into an adjacent hollow viscus occurs, digestion of the visceral wall and pressure necrosis is produced by the expanded cyst.[72] There is a 70 percent mortality associated with rupture into the peritoneal cavity.[71] There is an operative mortality of 25 percent for surgical excision with a 6 percent mortality for external drainage of an acute immature pseudocyst.[74] There is a 7 percent mortality for internal drainage.[74]

The introduction of CT and ultrasound have enhanced the rational management of patients with fluid.[47] The availability of ultrasound monitoring has led the surgeon to advocate a more conservative approach. If the patient is stable or improving, he is treated conservatively for 3 to 4 weeks. This delay eliminates surgery on those who resolve and provides time for formation of a firm fibrous wall that holds suture for internal anatomosis.[47] It generally takes 4 to 6 weeks for cyst wall maturation.[71]

In the past, a persistent pseudocyst was an indication

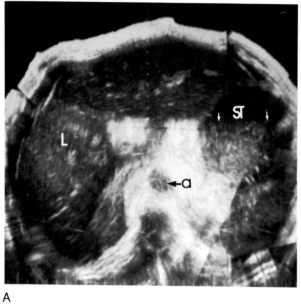

A

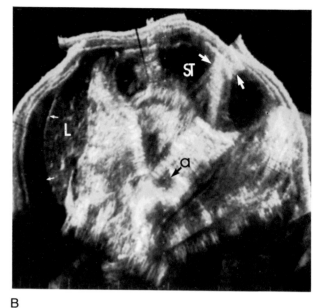

B

C

Fig. 3-38. Pseudocyst versus fluid-filled stomach. Case 1: Fluid-filled stomach. **(A)** Transverse scan at 17 cm above the umbilicus. A large cystic mass *(ST)* seen in the region of the tail of the pancreas contains a fluid-fluid level (arrows). (*a*, aorta; *L*, liver) **(B)** Transverse scan at 11 cm above the umbilicus. The fluid-filled mass *(ST)* seen within the mid-abdomen contains a reflective pattern (large arrows) anteriorly. (*L*, liver; small arrows, ascites; *a*, aorta) **(C)** Longitudinal scan to the left of midline. A cystic mass *(ST)* is seen posterior to the left lobe of the liver *(L)*. It is anterior to the spleen *(Sp)* and left kidney *(k)*. A reflective pattern (arrow) is seen within the most anterior aspect of the mass. (*U*, level of the umbilicus.) On real-time ultrasound, peristalsis confirmed that the mass was a fluid-filled stomach. The patient presented with an abdominal mass that was a distended stomach, secondary to involvement with amyloidosis. *(Figure continues.)*

for surgery. Now these lesions can be successfully drained percutaneously. The success rate with no recurrence is 16 to 18 percent.[4] Pseudocysts in the lesser sac tend to reaccumulate so aspiration is more successful in those not contiguous with the pancreas. The amylase of the fluid on those successfully treated with drainage is lower than those unsuccessfully treated. Successful drainage is more likely if the cyst is mature although it can be used to relieve symptoms.[4]

There are several structures that may be confused with a pseudocyst. One might be a fluid filled stomach (Fig. 3-38). This diagnosis should be made using real-time ultrasound and by identifying the characteristic appear-

ance of the stomach with peristalsis. A pancreatic pseudocyst may also mimic a dilated pancreatic duct, which may have an unusual configuration at times[69,75] (Fig. 3-39). Because there is no capsule, the cyst's unusual configuration conforms to the borders of the surrounding tissue.[75] With careful scanning, the examiner should try to identify whether the cystic structure in question is in the middle of the gland and whether it connects with the duct on real-time scanning. Several transverse sections along the pancreatic axis with various degrees of angulation may be necessary to show the interconnection between the cystic structure and duct.[69] Lastly, a left renal vein varix has been reported to simulate a pseudo-

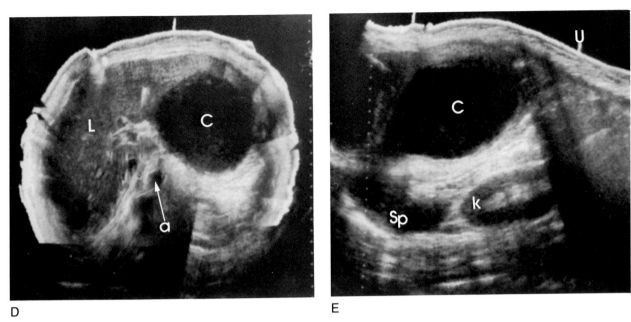

D   E

Fig. 3-38 *(Continued).* Case 2: Pseudocyst. **(D)** Transverse scan similar to **(A)** at 12 cm above the umbilicus. A large anechoic mass *(C)* is seen in the left upper quadrant. Stomach with peristalsis was seen to be separate from the mass at real-time. *(a,* aorta; *L,* liver.) **(E)** Longitudinal scan 4 cm to the left. Similarly to **(C)**, a cystic mass *(C)* is seen anterior to the spleen *(Sp)* and left kidney *(k).* *(U,* level of the umbilicus.)

cyst.[76] It can appear as a hypoechoic, well-circumscribed mass anterior to the left kidney (Fig. 3-40). Venous dilatation should be considered in a patient with known portal hypertension because it is in a location where portosystemic shunting is known to occur.[76]

In the child, blunt trauma to the abdomen is the main cause of pseudocysts.[77-79] Child abuse is one of the most common causes of this injury.[77] Pancreatitis, cyst, and loculated peripancreatic effusion are sequelae of trauma.[77] The patients present with pain, fullness, nausea, and vomiting, anorexia, and weight loss.[79] The cyst may occur rapidly and is seen as an echofree, unilocular ellipsoid mass.[77] A significant number of the cysts will resolve spontaneously and as such should be followed with ultrasound. Size alone should not be an absolute criterion in determining surgical intervention.[78] Ultrasound can be used to establish the diagnosis of cyst and for followup evaluation.[80]

ASPIRATION/BIOPSY

Some investigators advocate the percutaneous drainage of pancreatic pseudocysts to verify the diagnosis and as treatment in patients where surgery is contraindicated.[81,82] Ultrasound can be used to guide the percutaneous puncture of a pseudocyst; it is an easy and simple procedure with little risk and discomfort to the patient. It can be used for verification of the diagnosis, for defini-

tive therapy, for decompression in case of threatening rupture and for allowance of time for maturation of the cyst membrane before surgical intervention.[81,83] In one series, 4 cysts were treated this way without any recurrence or surgical intervention by 6 to 12 months.[84] The surgery for acute pseudocysts may be postponed or eliminated with this technique.[84] Relief of pain and obstructive symptoms and time gained when necessary for maturation of the cyst wall is achieved by this technique. Surgical management of pseudocysts consist of internal drainage into an adjacent viscus. This is a safe reliable procedure once the cyst wall has thickened to facilitate satisfactory anastomosis. Ten percent of cysts resolve while waiting for maturation.[84]

CHRONIC PANCREATITIS

Chronic relapsing pancreatitis is a better term for this disease process. It often represents progressive destruction of the pancreas by repeated flare-ups of a mild or subclinical type of acute pancreatitis. The same type of patient gets chronic pancreatitis as acute pancreatitis but most commonly it is alcoholics and, less frequently, patients with biliary tract disease. Hypercalcemia and hyperlipidemia predispose to chronic pancreatitis. Chronic pancreatitis is not usually preceded by an attack of classic hemorrhagic pancreatitis. This disease is much more

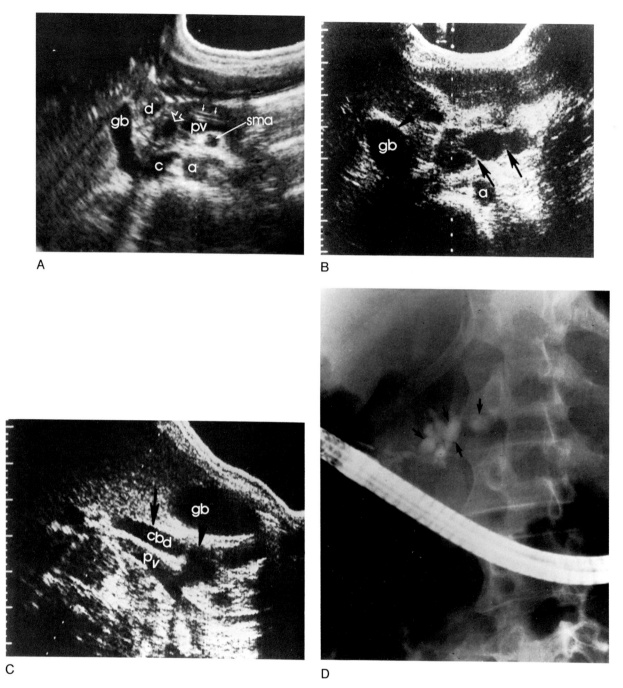

Fig. 3-39. Dilated duct versus pseudocyst. Case 1: Pseudocyst. **(A)** Transverse scan. A round cystic area (open arrow) representing a pseudocyst is seen in the region of the head of the pancreas. With careful real-time scanning, the pancreatic duct (small arrows) was seen as a separate structure. (*gb*, gallbladder; *a*, aorta; *d*, duodenum; *c*, inferior vena cava; *pv*, portal vein; *sma*, superior mesenteric artery) Case 2: Dilated pancreatic duct. *(B)* Transverse scan showing interconnecting cystic structures (arrows). (*gb*, gallbladder; *a*, aorta.) **(C)** Longitudinal decubitus scan. A dilated 1 cm common bile duct (*cbd*, arrow) terminates in a lobulated cystic structure at the head of the pancreas (arrowhead). (*pv*, portal vein; *gb*, gallbladder.) **(D)** ERCP with contrast media. An irregular lobulated cystic structure (arrows) is seen within the head of the pancreas. (Figs. **B–D** from Kuligowska E, Miller K, Birkett D, Burakoff R: Cystic dilatation of the pancreatic duct simulating pseudocysts on sonography. AJR 136:409, © American Roentgen Ray Society, 1981.)

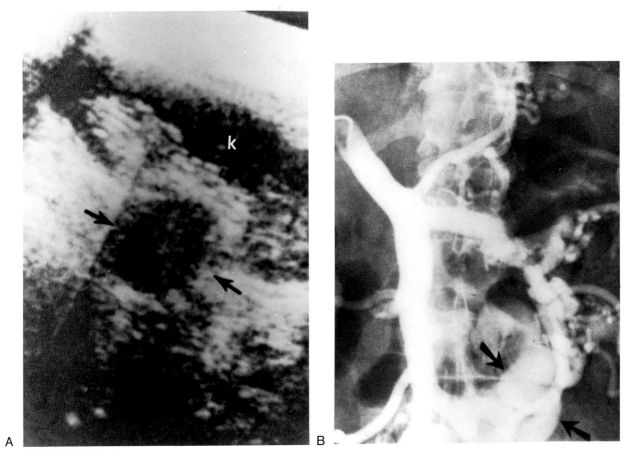

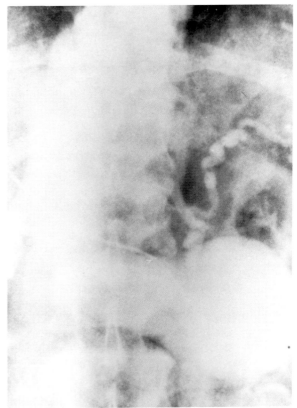

Fig. 3-40. Renal vein varix. **(A)** Longitudinal prone scan. A 5 cm hypoechoic mass (arrows) is seen anterior to the left kidney *(k)*. **(B)** Transhepatic portal venogram. There is retrograde flow in the portal, splenic, and superior mesenteric veins. Collaterals (arrows) from the splenic vein and enlarged branch of superior mesenteric vein form spontaneous portosystemic shunts. **(C)** Late film of the selective splenic venogram. A markedly enlarged left renal vein is seen with a localized 5 cm dilatation ("varix") accounting for the mass on **(A)**. (From Spira R, Kwan E, Gerzof SG, Widrich WC: Left renal vein varix simulating a pancreatic pseudocyst by sonography. AJR 138:149, © American Roentgen Ray Society, 1982.)

common in males than females. Forty percent or less of patients have no recognizable predisposing factors. The pathogenesis of chronic pancreatitis is obscure.[18]

The morphologic changes associated with chronic pancreatitis are many. Most commonly, there are chronic calcifying changes. With this there is atrophy of the acini, increase in the interlobular fibrous tissue and chronic inflammatory infiltration. Stones of calcium carbonate are located inside the ductal system. And pseudocysts are common occurrences. The second type of chronic pancreatitis is a chronic obstructive pancreatitis. The lesions are in the lobules and the ductal epithelium is less involved. The most common cause of this type is stenosis of the sphincter of Oddi with associated cholelithiasis.[18]

The patients with chronic pancreatitis experience recurrent bouts of pain at intervals of months to years. As time goes on, the intervals between bouts decrease. The precipitating factor appears to be alcohol, overeating, or the use of opiates. Diabetes, steatorrhea, and pancreatic pseudocysts occur frequently. Frank diabetes occurs in 14 to 90 percent with steatorrhea in 25 to 35 percent. Duodenal obstruction and jaundice occur in one-third of patients.[18]

With chronic pancreatitis, there are several changes one sees on ultrasound.[37,40,47,54] There is increased echogenicity of the pancreas beyond the normal amount due to fibrotic changes, fatty changes, or both.[4,85] Calcification, ductal dilatation and an irregular outline to the gland are seen[40,47,49] (Figs. 3-41 to 3-44). There may be strictures, stenoses, irregularities, and dilatation of the duct.[37] Focal or diffuse enlargement (27 percent) of the gland may be associated with an irregular outline (45 percent) of the gland (Fig. 3-44). Pancreatic duct dilatation is present in 41 percent and is most likely present when there is pancreatic calcification (92 percent)[4] (Fig. 3-43). At times, it may be difficult to even identify the pancreas on ultrasound if its density blends in with the surrounding retroperitoneal fat.[54] Also, in some instances, chronic pancreatitis appears as a focal enlargement of the gland[54] (Fig. 3-45). In such instances, it is difficult to distinguish it from neoplasm with ultrasound or CT alone.

Pancreatic lithiasis is associated with alcoholic pancreatitis. Pancreatic ductal calculi result from preexisting chronic pancreatic disease rather than the cause and have no significance over and above that of ordinary pancreatic calculi.[86] Twenty to 40 percent of patients with chronic pancreatitis develop lithiasis.[87] The incidence is greater in males than females and there is a high association with alcoholic pancreatitis. In chronic pancreatitis, the calcifications seen are almost always true stones lying free in the pancreatic duct rather than the parenchyma.[36] The stones consist of a protein matrix

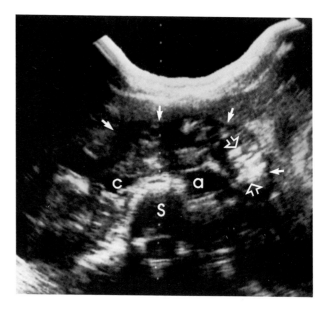

Fig. 3-41. Chronic pancreatitis. Calcifications. Transverse static scan. The entire pancreas is enlarged (arrows) with a mixed echopattern. There are multiple calcifications (open arrows) seen within the tail as echodense areas. (*a*, aorta; *c*, inferior vena cava; *S*, spine.)

and varying amounts of calcium carbonate. Initially the lesion probably consists of a protein plug that precipitates into the small ducts, causing obstruction with secondary dilatation.[87] Calcium carbonate salts are subsequently deposited onto the protein matrix forming the stone. The stone extrudes into the duct as the disease progresses and obstructs the main pancreatic duct or even the ampulla of Vater. The progression of the disease can be seen on subsequent follow-up examinations. In 92 percent of patients there is ductal dilatation and in 54 percent there is lithiasis involving the main pancreatic duct.[87]

Although a radiograph may be sufficient to establish the presence of pancreatic calcifications, in many, ultrasound provides additional information concerning the duct dilatation and lithiasis in the main duct. The duct may be dilated secondary to stricture or as a result of an extrinsic stone from a smaller pancreatic duct into a major duct.[4] Ultrasound can be employed to determine the distribution of the calculi and the characteristics of the calculi — peripheral or ductal. They may have a focal or diffuse distribution. The calcifications on ultrasound appear as small highly reflective particles that give the gland a stippled appearance[87] (Figs. 3-41, 3-42, and 3-46). Shadowing is sometimes associated with the stones. The intraductal location for the stones can be determined accurately by ultrasound. Stones in the duct are identified by the fact that they are surrounded by the echo-free structure of the duct[87] (Fig. 3-46). The signifi-

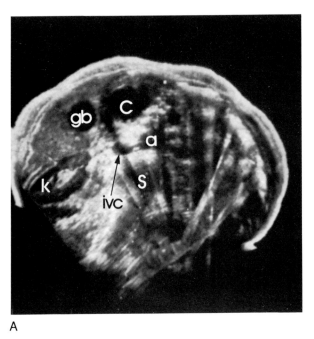

A

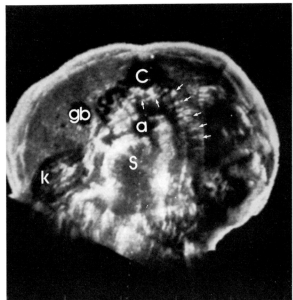

B

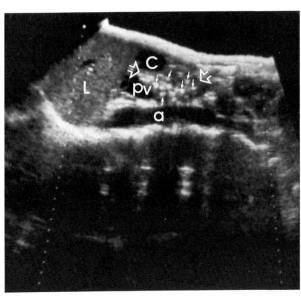

C

Fig. 3-42. Chronic pancreatitis. Calcifications and pseudo-cysts. **(A)** Transverse static scan at 3 cm above the umbilicus. A pseudocyst *(C)* is seen in the area of the head of the pancreas. (*gb*, gallbladder; *ivc*, inferior vena cava; *a*, aorta; *k*, right kidney; *S*, spine.) **(B)** Transverse static scan at 7 cm above the umbilicus. Another pseudocyst **(C)** is seen extending from the anterior aspect of the enlarged pancreas. The pancreas is stippled with multiple echodensities (arrows) representing calculi. (*a*, aorta; *gb*, gallbladder; *S*, spine; *k*, right kidney) **(C)** Midline static longitudinal scan. The anterior pseudocyst *(C)* seen on **(B)** is demonstrated as is the pancreatic enlargement (open arrows) with multiple calcifications (arrows.) (*a*, aorta; *pv*, portal vein; *L*, liver.) *(Figure continues.)*

cance of ductal stones is unclear.[86] The exact site and cause of an obstruction cannot be seen as well on ultrasound as endoscopic retrograde cholangiopancreatography (ERCP).[86] ERCP is the most accurate method to investigate duct dilatation and intraductal lithiasis.[87] The most common site of obstruction is at the papilla and the site of origin of the main duct.[37] The ultrasound finding of ductal dilatation and calculi can forewarn the endoscopist to expect difficulty. Lastly, the incidence of carcinoma with pancreatic calcification is 25 percent so tumor must be searched for carefully.[87]

There are several complications of chronic pancreatitis. Psuedocysts develop in 20 percent of patients.[4] Thrombosis of the splenic vein and/or portal vein can be seen. When a focal mass is seen with chronic pancreatitis, carcinoma should be considered because it occurs in 4 to 25 percent of such patients.[4] The symptoms of both carcinoma and chronic pancreatitis are so similar that they are not helpful in differentiating between the two conditions. Ultrasound cannot distinguish a benign or malignant mass unless secondary signs of carcinoma are present: adjacent nodes or liver metastases. The ac-

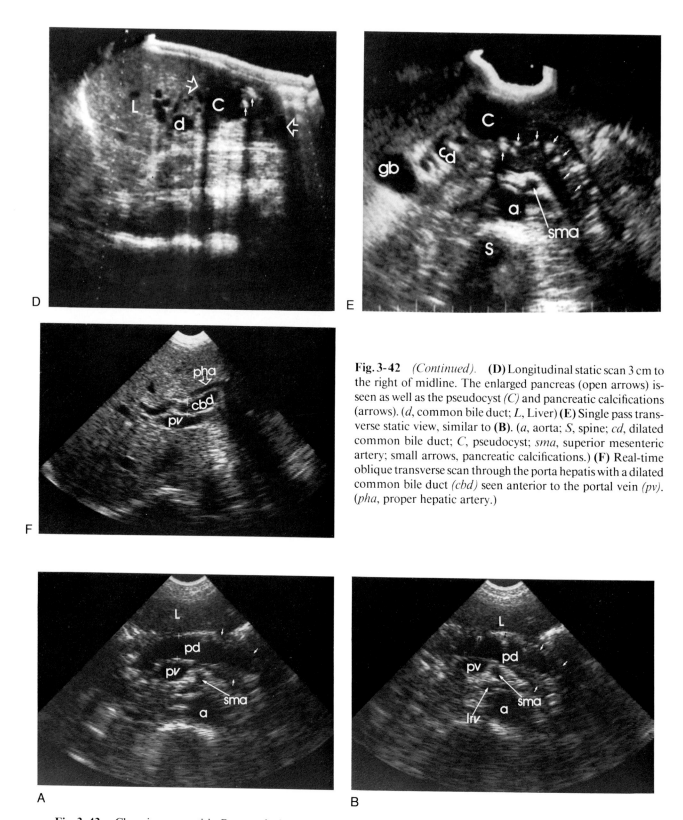

Fig. 3-42 *(Continued).* **(D)** Longitudinal static scan 3 cm to the right of midline. The enlarged pancreas (open arrows) is seen as well as the pseudocyst *(C)* and pancreatic calcifications (arrows). (*d,* common bile duct; *L,* Liver) **(E)** Single pass transverse static view, similar to **(B).** (*a,* aorta; *S,* spine; *cd,* dilated common bile duct; *C,* pseudocyst; *sma,* superior mesenteric artery; small arrows, pancreatic calcifications.) **(F)** Real-time oblique transverse scan through the porta hepatis with a dilated common bile duct *(cbd)* seen anterior to the portal vein *(pv).* (*pha,* proper hepatic artery.)

Fig. 3-43. Chronic pancreatitis. Pancreatic ductal dilatation. Transverse scans **(A,B)** demonstrate a markedly dilated pancreatic duct *(pd).* There is very little pancreatic tissue (arrows) surrounding the duct. There are pancreatic calcifications (black arrows) bordering the duct anteriorly on **(B).** (*sma,* superior mesenteric artery; *a,* aorta; *pv,* main portal vein; *L,* liver; *lrv,* left renal vein.)

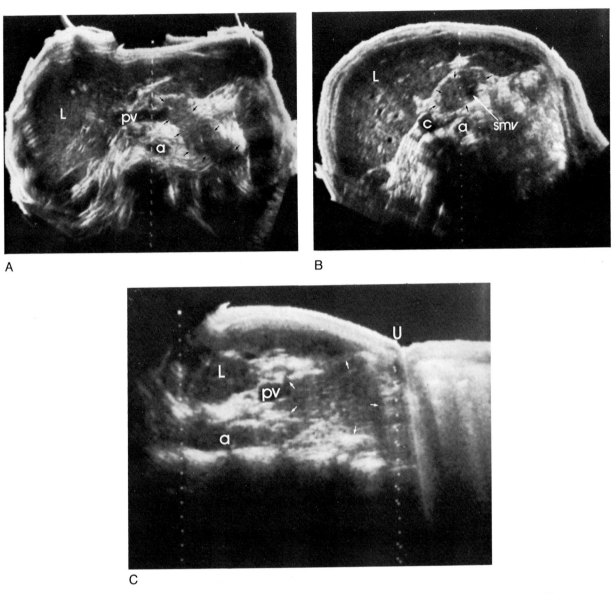

Fig. 3-44. Chronic pancreatitis. Diffuse enlargement. **(A)** Transverse scan at 10 cm above the umbilicus. The pancreatic tail (arrows) is enlarged and isoechoic to the liver *(L)*. (*pv*, main portal vein; *a*, aorta.) **(B)** Transverse scan at 6 cm above the umbilicus. The enlarged pancreatic head (arrows) is seen. (*L*, liver; *c*, inferior vena cava; *a*, aorta; *smv*; superior mesenteric vein.) **(C)** Longitudinal midline scan. The pancreas (arrows) is markedly enlarged in its craniocaudad axis. (*L*, liver; *pv*, portal vein; *a*, aorta; *U*, level of the umbilicus) *(Figure continues.)*

curacy rate in the absence of metastases varies and can be as high as 100 percent.[4] The presence of calcification in the mass makes tumor unlikely. CT has the same difficulty as ultrasound in the diagnosis of pancreatic carcinoma in the presence of chronic pancreatitis and in such patients, ERCP or percutaneous biopsy may be necessary. Still false negatives may be obtained.

Chronic pancreatitis may require palliative surgery, generally pancreatojejunostomy with or without pancreatic resection, to relieve pain. Recurrence of symptoms postoperatively may lead to an attempt at retrograde opacification of the anstomosis by endoscopy to establish patency. With real-time guidance, a 22-gauge needle can be inserted with injection of 5 cc of water soluble iodinated contrast diluted with genomycin into the pancreatojejunostomy, jejunal loop, and biliary tree.[88] Per-

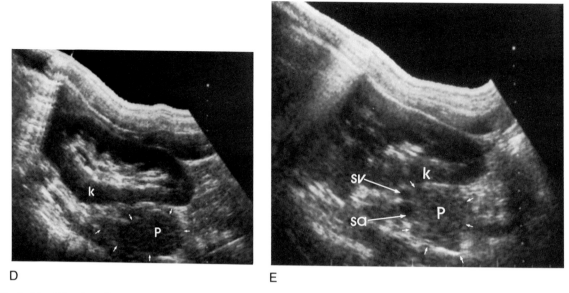

D   E

Fig. 3-44 *(Continued).* **(D,E)** Longitudinal prone scans with **(D)** more medial. The enlarged pancreatic tail (arrows) is seen anterior to the left kidney *(k)*. (*sa*, splenic artery; *sv*, splenic vein.)

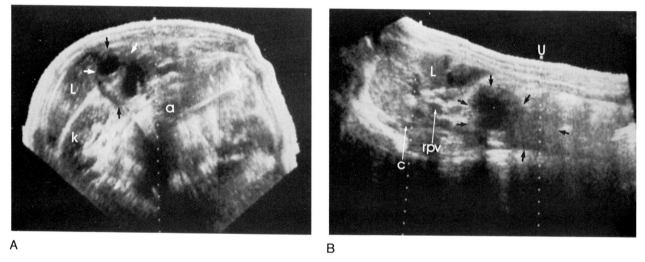

A   B

Fig. 3-45. Chronic pancreatitis. Focal enlargement. **(A)** Transverse scan at 4 cm above the umbilicus. The pancreatic head (arrows) is enlarged with a mixed echopattern; there are several anechoic areas. (*L*, liver; *k*, right kidney; *a*, aorta.) **(B)** Longitudinal scan at 3 cm to the right of midline. The pancreatic head is enlarged (arrows) and contains a poorly defined anechoic area. A percutaneous biopsy revealed a diagnosis of chronic pancreatitis. (*L*, liver; *c*, inferior vena cava; *rpv*, right portal vein; *U*, level of the umbilicus.)

cutaneous pancreatography can be used in selected cases of pancreatic duct dilatation not opacified by endoscopy.

Pancreatography

A good pancreatogram provides valuable information for planning surgery.[89] Although a preoperative pancreatogram may be obtained by endoscopic retrograde cannulation of the duct, it can also be obtained percutaneously. A needle placed in the obstructed duct may cause pancreatitis, and as in transhepatic cholangiography, in the obstructed biliary tree, it should be followed by surgical decompression within 24 to 48 hours.[89] The pancreatic duct can be demonstrated in 84 percent of normals with this technique.[36]

Using real-time guidance, a percutaneous pancreatic ductogram and a percutaneous aspiration biopsy can be

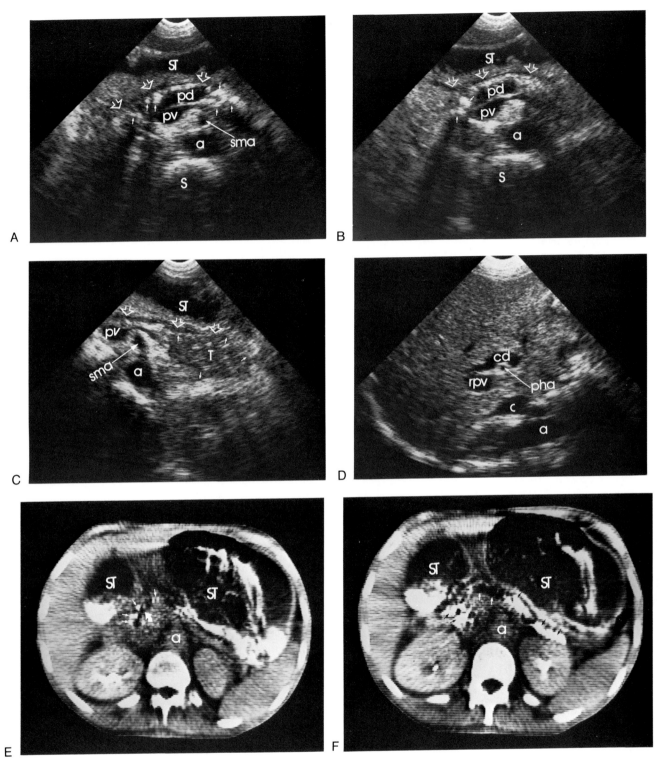

Fig. 3-46. Pancreatic lithiasis. **(A)** Transverse real-time scan. A dilated pancreatic duct *(pd)* is seen which is bordered by echodensities (solid arrows) representing calcifications. (*pv*, main portal vein; *a*, aorta; *sma*, superior mesenteric artery; open arrows, posterior wall of stomach; *ST*, fluid-filled stomach; *S*, spine.) **(B)** Transverse real-time scan at a slightly lower level than **(A)**. A calculus (arrows) is seen within the pancreatic duct *(pd)*. (*a*, aorta; *pv*, main portal vein; *S*, spine; *ST*, stomach; open arrows, posterior wall of the stomach.) **(C)** Transverse real-time scan through the fluid-filled stomach *(ST)*. The enlarged pancreatic tail (*T*, arrows) is seen. (*a*, aorta; *pv*, portal vein; *sma*, superior mesenteric artery; open arrows, posterior wall of the stomach) **(D)** Longitudinal oblique real-time scan in the left lateral decubitus position. The dilated common duct *(cd)* is seen anterior to the proper hepatic artery *(pha)* and right portal vein *(rpv)*. (*a*, aorta; *c*, inferior vena cava) **(E)** CT scan further demonstrating the dilated fluid-filled stomach *(ST)*, dilated pancreatic duct (low density area, curved arrow) and dense calcifications (arrows). (*a*, aorta) **(F)** CT scan at a higher level than **(E)**. The dilated pancreatic duct (white arrows) is seen as well as the pancreatic calcifications (black arrows) posterior to the fluid-filled stomach *(ST)*. (*a*, aorta.)

successfully performed as a single procedure without major complication.[36] Because the distinction between chronic pancreatitis and carcinoma is not always feasible with ultrasound alone, this combination technique is especially helpful.[36] When there is abrupt obstruction of the pancreatic duct with extensive dilatation proximal to the obstruction, a carcinoma should be suspected.[36]

Hereditary Pancreatitis

Hereditary pancreatitis is a recurrent inflammation of the pancreas from childhood with an unusual prevalence among blood relatives in accordance with Mendel's law —autosomal dominant. The sex distribution is equal and it occurs exclusively in whites. The patients present with recurrent attacks of severe pain in childhood. There are pancreatic calcifications in 30 to 50 percent and a dilated pancreatic duct. Pseudocysts develop in 10 percent of patients.[90]

TRAUMA

Pancreatic injury from nonpenetrating abdominal trauma is uncommon and the diagnosis is made difficult by the absence of specific signs during physical examination. In the child, blunt trauma is a common cause of

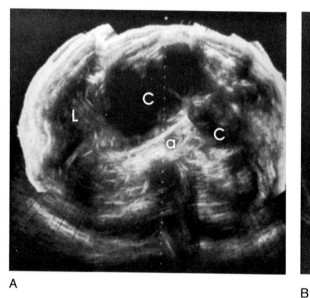

A

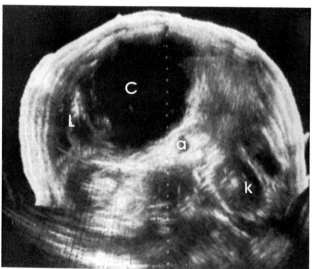

B

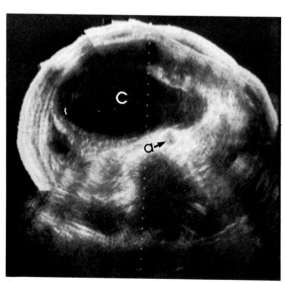

C

Fig. 3-47. Trauma, pseudocyst. This patient experienced abdominal trauma in an automobile accident. Transverse static scan at 10 cm (**A**), and 6 cm (**B**) above and at the level (**C**) of the umbilicus. A large traumatic pseudocyst (**C**) is seen. (*L*, liver; *a*, aorta; *k*, left kidney.) (*Figure continues.*)

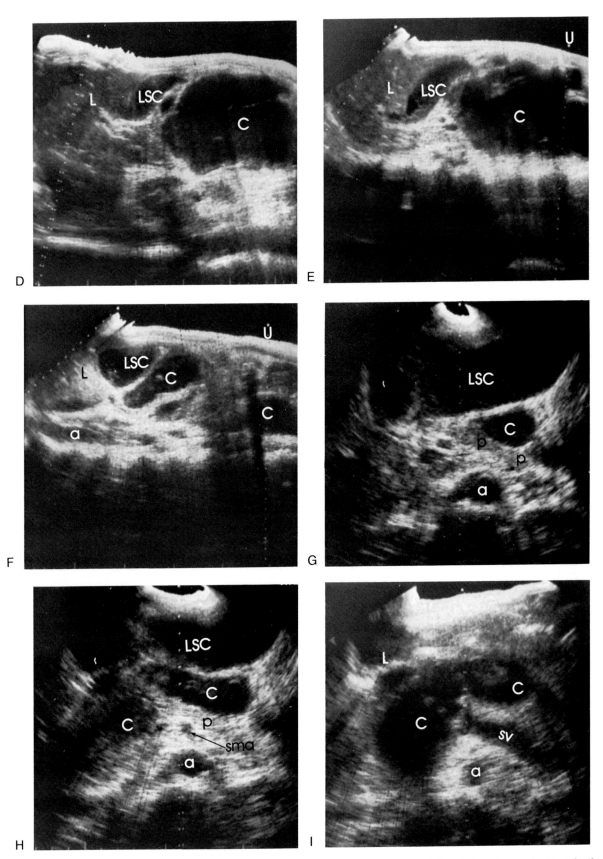

Fig. 3-47 *(Continued).* Longitudinal scans at 3 cm to the right of midline **(D)**, midline **(E)**, and 3 cm to the left of midline **(F)**. There is extension of the pseudocyst *(C)* into the lesser sac *(LSC)* and below the level of the umbilicus *(U)* (*L*, liver; *a*, aorta). Transverse cone-down scans of the pancreatic area at 0.5 cm **(G)**, 2 cm **(H)**, and 3 cm **(I)** below the xyphoid demonstrate the pancreatic pseudocyst *(C)* with the lesser sac extension *(LSC)* anterosuperiorly. (*p*, pancreas; *a*, aorta; *sma*, superior mesenteric artery; *L*, liver; *sv*, splenic vein.)

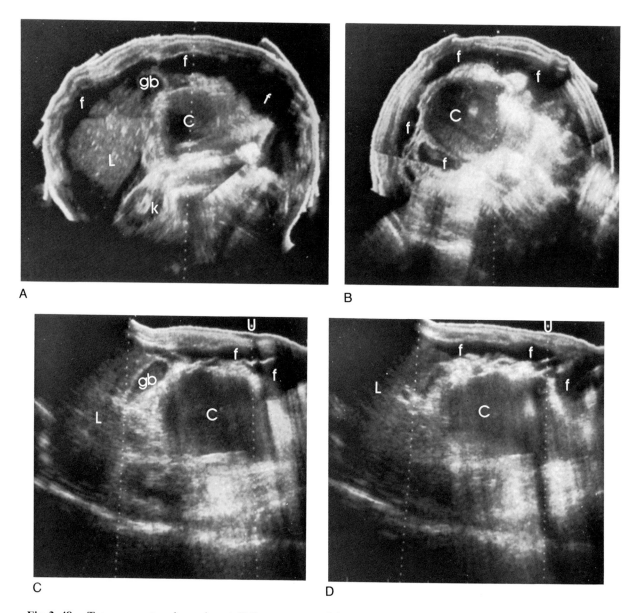

Fig. 3-48. Trauma, ruptured pseudocyst. Follow-up scans of the patient in Figure 3-47. Transverse scans at 12 cm **(A)** and 2 cm **(B)** above the umbilicus demonstrate that the traumatic pancreatic pseudocyst *(C)* has decreased in size by rupturing into the peritoneum. Free peritoneal fluid *(f)* is seen bordering the liver *(L)* and extending into the flanks. (*k*, right kidney; *gb*, gallbladder.) Longitudinal scans at 2 cm **(C)** to the right of midline and midline **(D)**. The cyst *(C)* is smaller than in Figure 3-47 and peritoneal fluid *(f)* is seen. (*L*, liver; *U*, level of the umbilicus; *gb*, gallbladder.)

pseudocyst. Acute traumatic injury to the pancreas includes contusion with edema, laceration, hemorrhage, and transection, which almost always occurs in the body of the pancreas since it is compressed against the spine.[91,92] The pancreas and duodenum are fixed in position so they absorb the total force of the abdominal blow. The relation of these structures to the spine and ribs make them damaged in such situations.[92] Clinically, these patients present with epigastric pain with or without radiation and nausea and vomiting. In one series in

children, there were 3 percent isolated pancreatic injuries and 8 percent isolated duodenal injuries.[92]

The ultrasound findings with pancreatic trauma depend on the extent of the trauma. With contusion, a focal hypoechoic mass or a diffuse hypoechoic enlargement of the gland may be seen. A well-defined anechoic mass with associated acoustic enhancement may be seen with a traumatic pseudocyst (Fig. 3-47). With rupture, fluid may be demonstrated in the retroperitoneum and/ or peritoneum (Fig. 3-48).

PANCREATIC NEOPLASM

Pancreatic Cyst

True cysts are lined by a mucous epithelium and may be congenital or acquired.[18] The congenital ones are believed to be the result of anomalous development of the pancreatic duct.[4,18] They may be single but are usually multiple and without septation. They vary in size from microscopic to 3 to 5 cm.[18] The acquired cysts are retention cysts (cystic dilatation of the pancreatic duct due to any cause), parasitic cysts, and neoplastic cysts. Besides true cysts, there are pseudocysts that are not lined by epithelium but have a fibrous wall when mature. They are postinflammatory or posttraumatic in origin.[4]

Cystadenoma and Cystadenocarcinoma

Some authors have classified these as macrocystic (premalignant) adenomas and carcinoma (classic cystadenoma and cystadenocarcinoma) and microcystic (no malignant potential) adenomas.[93] The macrocystic adenoma is an uncommon, slow growing tumor that is thought to arise as a cystic neoplasm from the ducts.[18] It is composed primarily of a large cyst (2 to 20 cm), with or without septations, that is lined by mucin producing cells.[4,18] There is significant malignant potential. The patients generally present with epigastric pain and/or a palpable mass. Several concurrent diseases are reported with this neoplasm including diabetes, calculous disease

of the biliary tract, and arterial hypertension.[4,99] The macrocystic adenomas occur more frequently in middle age females with 60 percent in the tail and 5 percent in the head of the pancreas.[93] The body and tail are the most frequent sites.[4,94,95] There are frequently foci of calcification. The therapy of choice is surgical excision.

The microcystic adenoma is comprised of tiny cysts (less then 2 cm) lined by flattened or cuboidal cells that contain glycogen and little to no mucin. These lesions are totally benign. Microcystic adenomas also occur more frequently in females and involve the body and tail (60 percent) but may arise in the head (30 percent) or may be diffuse (10 percent).[4,93]

On ultrasound, these cystic neoplasms look similar to pseudocysts.[4,47,93–99] The macrocystic adenomas contain cysts greater than 2 cm. They are classic anechoic cysts with acoustic enhancement and internal septations[4,93,95,97,98] (Figs. 3-49 to 3-51). The internal septations usually are thin and as the gain is increased the cystic areas fill in with echoes.[4] In 10 to 18 percent, calcification may be present within the wall seen as focal echogenic areas with shadowing; these cannot be distinguished as benign or malignant.[4] Other investigators have identified four ultrasound patterns associated with cystadenocarcinoma: (1) anechoic mass with posterior enhancement and irregular margins; (2) anechoic mass with internal homogeneous echoes stratified supine and mobile decubitus; (3) anechoic mass with irregular internal vegetations protruding into the lumen and showing no movement; and (4) completely echogenic mass with nonhomogeneous pattern.[96] The microcystic adenomas

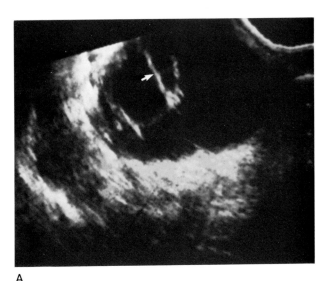
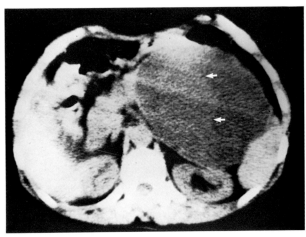

A   B

Fig. 3-49. Macrocystic adenoma. **(A)** Longitudinal static scan. A large cystic lesion in the tail of the pancreas is seen with thin septations (arrow) in the superior part of the mass. **(B)** CT scan. The septations (arrows) are only faintly visualized within the large cystic mass in the tail of the pancreas. (From Wolfman NT, Ramquist NA, Karstaedt N, Hopkins MB: Cystic neoplasms of the pancreas: CT and sonography. AJR 138:37, © Am Roent Ray Soc, 1982.)

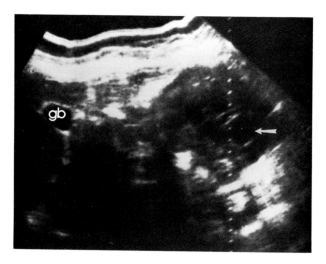

Fig. 3-50. Macrocystic adenocarcinoma. Transverse static scan. A mass is seen in the tail of the pancreas containing cysts (arrow) that are larger than 2 cm. Acoustic enhancement is seen. (*gb*, gallbladder.) (From Wolfman NT, Ramquist NA, Karstaedt N, Hopkins MB: Cystic neoplasms of the pancreas: CT and sonography. AJR 138:37, © Am Roent Ray Soc, 1982.)

contain cysts less than 2 cm with a central, stellate scar that may be calcified with radiating bands of connective tissue[4] (Fig. 3-52). This tumor is usually well circumscribed and oval. The scan occasionally contains calcification; these are seen as focal echogenic areas with shadowing.[4] On ultrasound, there are small cysts with central calcification.[93] When the cysts are small, the tumor appears echogenic.[4] A preoperative biopsy with pathology aids in making a definitive diagnosis and directs appropriate therapy.

Adenocarcinoma

Carcinoma of the pancreas is a highly fatal tumor involving the exocrine portion of the gland, with its beginning in the ductal epithelium. It represents 6 percent of all neoplastic deaths in the United States and it represents 95 percent of all malignant pancreatic tumors.[4] Cures by surgical resection are rare. There is an increased risk of carcinoma of the pancreas in patients who smoke. There is an unexplained correlation between cancer of the pancreas mortality and per capita consumption of fats and possibly calories. It occurs in the sixth, seventh, and eighth decades of life with a male preponderance. There have been rare reports of this lesion in children.[100] In 60 to 70 percent of cases, it is in the head of the pancreas with 20 to 30 percent in the body and 5 to 10 percent in the tail; 21 percent are diffuse.[4,18] The tumors in the head present earlier than the others in the body or tail.[4,18] The detection rate depends on an adequately visualized gland, which varies from 81 to 94 percent.[4] When there is adequate visualization of the pancreas, the

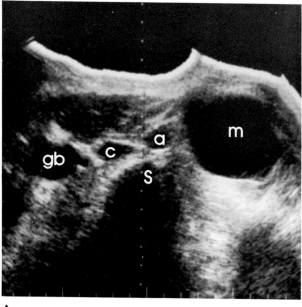

A

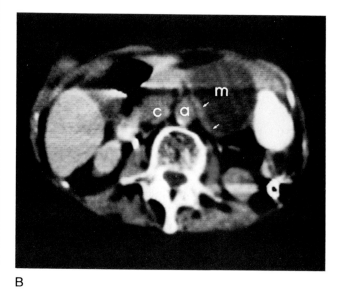

B

Fig. 3-51. Cystadenocarcinoma. **(A)** Transverse static scan at a level inferior to the tail of the pancreas. An anechoic mass *(m)* is seen. (*a*, aorta; *c*, inferior vena cava; *gb*, gallbladder; *S*, spine.) **(B)** CT scan. A low-density mass *(m)* is seen anterior to the pancreatic tail (arrows). (*a*, aorta; *c*, inferior vena cava.)

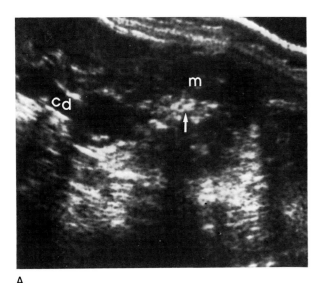

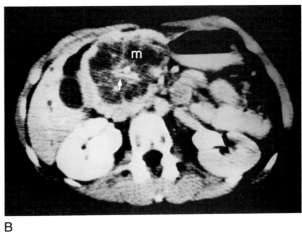

A   B

Fig. 3-52. Microcystic adenoma. **(A)** Longitudinal static scan to the right of midline. A dilated common bile duct *(cd)* is seen obstructed by a large mass *(m)* in the head of the pancreas. Centrally located calcifications are seen within the mass (arrow). Tiny cysts are barely visible. **(B)** Enhanced CT scan. A mass *(m)* is seen in the head of the pancreas with central calcification (arrow) and numerous cysts are separated by radiating bands of fibrosis. (From Wolfman NT, Ramquist NA, Karstaedt N, Hopkins MB: Cystic neoplasms of the pancreas: CT and sonography. AJR 138:37, © Am Roent Ray Soc, 1982.)

likelihood of missing a pancreatic neoplasm is extremely low with a negative predictive value of 99 percent.[4,14]

The clinical course of carcinoma of the pancreas is insidious. Some of the symptoms include weight loss (70 percent of cases), abdominal pain (50 percent), back pain (25 percent), anorexia, nausea and vomiting, generalized malaise and weakness.[4,18] The average time from symptoms until diagnosis is 4 months and that between symptoms until death is 8.3 months to 1.6 years.[4,18,101] The 5-year survival is only 0.9 to 2 percent.[4,18,100,101] Poor survival is a reflection that 80 to 85 percent of patients with carcinoma of the pancreas have local spread or distant metastases at the time seen clinically.[101]

There have been various signs described that are consistent with carcinoma of the pancreas on ultrasound.[2,15,18,19,52,53,103,104] As a rule, these lesions represent a localized change in echodensity of the pancreas. The echopattern is hypoechoic—less dense than normal pancreas and liver (Figs. 3-53 and 3-54; see Figs. 2-80 to 2-82). One series reported 95 percent of these tumors to be hypoechoic.[19] In another series, 3 percent were reported to be echogenic.[4] The borders of the mass are irregular and the mass is usually quite distinct from the rest of the gland.[4,62] There may or may not be pancreatic enlargement. Masses in the head tend to be smaller than those seen in the tail due to compression of the common bile duct[4] (Figs. 3-55 and 3-56). Other associated changes include dilatation of the pancreatic duct (18 percent), biliary dilatation, liver metastases, nodal metastases, portal venous system involvement, splenic vein enlarge-

ment, superior mesenteric artery displacement, and ascites.[19,40,103,105] The pancreatic ductal dilatation shows either a smooth pattern or irregular duct dilatation that closely corresponds to the dilatation patterns on ERCP.[36] Abrupt obstruction of the pancreatic duct and

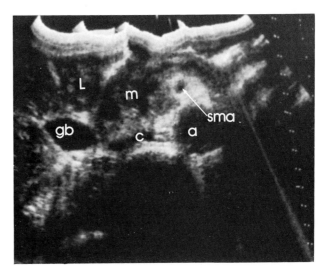

Fig. 3-53. Adenocarcinoma, head. Transverse scan. A large inhomogeneous mass *(m)* is seen within the head of the pancreas. The borders of the mass are irregular and the mass compresses the inferior vena cava *(c)*. The superior mesenteric artery *(sma)* is displaced anteriorly and to the right. *(a,* aorta; *gb,* gallbladder; *L,* liver.)

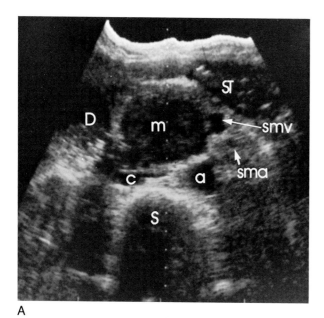

A

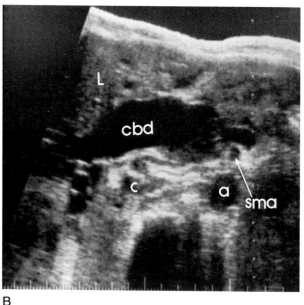

B

Fig. 3-54. Adenocarcinoma, head. Common bile duct obstruction. **(A)** Transverse scan demonstrating a hypoechoic mass *(m)* compressing the inferior vena cava *(c)* and displacing the superior mesenteric artery *(sma)* and vein *(smv)* to the left. (*a*, aorta; *ST*, fluid-filled stomach; *D*, fluid-filled duodenum; *S*, spine.) **(B)** Oblique transverse scan higher than **(A)** demonstrating a dilated common bile duct *(cbd)*. (*a*, aorta; *c*, inferior vena cava; *sma*, superior mesenteric artery; *L*, liver.)

extensive dilatation proximal to the dilatation suggests carcinoma.

The superior mesenteric vessels may be displaced posteriorly by a pancreatic mass.[19] The amount of the displacement depends on the site of the tumor.[4] They are displaced anteriorly when carcinoma is in the uncinate

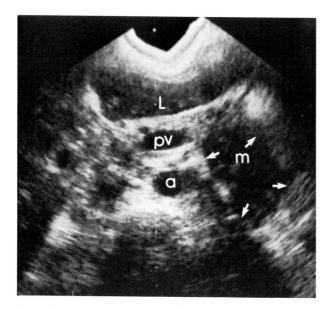

Fig. 3-55. Adenocarcinoma, tail. Transverse static scan. A poorly defined hypoechoic mass *(m)* is seen in the region of the pancreatic tail. (*a*, aorta; *pv*, portal vein; *L*, liver.)

process and posteriorly to the left and often to the right with tumor in the head or body (Figs. 3-53 and 3-54; see Fig. 2-80). Soft tissue thickening caused by neoplastic infiltration of the perivascular lymphatics may be seen surrounding the celiac axis or superior mesenteric artery (see Fig. 2-80). This occurs more commonly with carcinoma of the body and tail (52 percent) than with carcinoma of the head (25 percent). In some (11 percent), this may be the only sign of carcinoma.

Since most of the patients with carcinoma of the head of the pancreas also have obstructive jaundice, one should search for a mass anytime an obstructive biliary tree is noted. Obstruction of the common bile duct can be produced by the direct effect of the mass in the head or adenopathy in the porta hepatis[4] (see Figs. 2-80 to 2-82 and 3-54). The pancreatic duct may also be dilated (Fig. 3-57). In some cases ductal dilatation is the only sign of carcinoma. This can be seen with carcinoma of the ampulla, cholangiocarcinoma near the ampulla, Crohn's disease of the duodenum, and stenosis of the ampulla. ERCP may be needed for the diagnosis. If the mass is very hypoechoic with extensive adenopathy, lymphoma should be considered.

The pancreatic mass can compress the splenic vein producing secondary splenic enlargement. Tumor may displace or invade the splenic or portal vein or produce thrombosis (12 to 48 percent)[4] (Fig. 3-58). Collateral venous channels may develop and be visualized in the periportal area and along the wall of the stomach. In

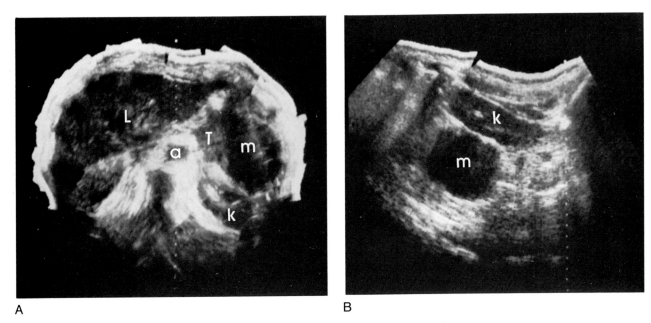

A   B

Fig. 3-56. Adenocarcinoma, tail. **(A)** Transverse static scan. A hypoechoic mass *(m)* is seen in the pancreatic tail *(T)*. (*k*, left kidney; *a*, aorta; *L*, liver.) **(B)** Prone longitudinal static scan. A hypoechoic mass *(m)* is seen anterior to the left kidney *(k)*.

addition, a mass in the head may compress the anterior wall of the inferior vena cava (50 percent)[4,106] (Figs. 3-53 and 3-54).

Focal masses of the pancreas can be seen with chronic or acute pancreatitis as well as tumor. In acute pancreatitis, the mass is usually uniformly hypoechoic with good through transmission unless there is hemorrhage or gas caused by necrosis and/or suppuration. A focal mass confined to the pancreas directly anterior to the aorta is not likely to be inflammation. The presence of adenopathy silhouetting the wall of the aorta by a contiguous

pancreas process is most likely tumor. The differentiation from chronic pancreatitis is difficult.[4]

Islet Cell Tumor

There are several types of islet cell tumors; some are functional (85 percent) and others are nonfunctional (15 percent).[4] They represent either benign adenomas or malignant tumors. The nonfunctioning islet cell tumors constitute one third of all the islet cell tumors.[107] While

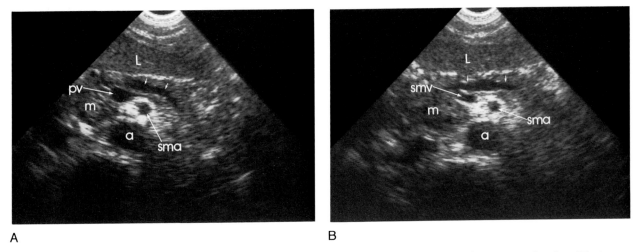

A   B

Fig. 3-57. Adenocarcinoma, head. Pancreatic duct obstruction. Transverse scans with **(A)** more superior than **(B)**. An inhomogeneous mass *(m)* is seen in the pancreatic head. The pancreatic duct (arrows) is dilated within the pancreatic body. (*sma*, superior mesenteric artery; *smv*, superior mesenteric vein; *pv*, portal vein; *a*, aorta; *L*, liver.)

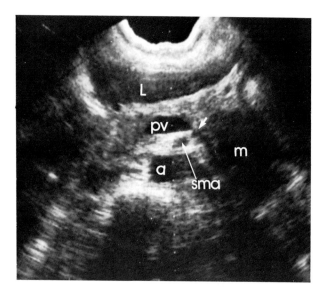

Fig. 3-58. Adenocarcinoma, tail. Splenic vein compression. Transverse scan. The splenic vein (arrow) is compressed by the hypoechoic pancreatic tail mass *(m)*. (*a*, aorta; *L*, liver; *sma*, superior mesenteric artery; *pv*, main portal vein.)

these tumors may be malignant or benign, 92 percent of the nonfunctional tumors are malignant.[4] The diagnosis is based on clinical and endocrinology features. Ultrasound can detect 51 percent of the tumors. The presence of malignancy is difficult to determine at the cellular

level and can be diagnosed when there is invasion of surrounding structures or liver metastases.[4] These tumors are slow-growing with a 5 year survival of 44 percent.[4] There is a 1.6 percent incidence of these tumors in an autopsy series.[108]

The most common functioning islet cell tumor is the insulinoma (60 percent) followed by the gastrinoma (18 percent), and the tumors producing watery diarrhea, hypokalemia, and achlorhydria (WDHA).[4,109] Functioning tumors are more difficult to detect than nonfunctional ones as functioning tumors present when small as a consequence of their hormonal activity. They occur most frequently in the body and tail where there is the greatest concentration of Langerhans islets.[108] The rate of malignancy is higher in gastrinomas (25 to 60 percent) than with insulinomas (10 percent).[4] The diabetes producing tumors—glucagonoma and somatostatinoma—are usually malignant and several centimeters in size. Of the nonbeta islet cell tumors responsible for WDHA syndrome, 50 percent are malignant. Clinically, these patients with insulinomas experience hypoglycemia and fasting hypoglycemia and inappropriate elevated plasma insulin levels.[109] In 70 percent of cases there is a solitary adenoma, in 10 percent there are multiple adenomas, and in 10 percent there are metastases. The lesions may be minute to 1500 gm. In Zollinger-Ellison syndrome, the lesions are gastrinomas. These pancreatic lesions are associated with gastric hypersecretion and peptic ulcer

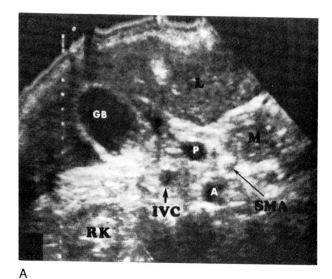

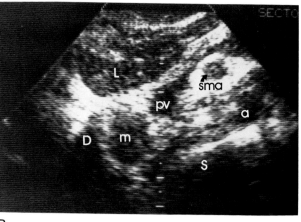

A   B

Fig. 3-59. Islet cell tumors. Case 1: **(A)** Transverse static scan, 1 cm caudad to the xyphoid process. A solid mass *(M)* is seen in the tail of the pancreas. (*A*, aorta; *IVC*, inferior vena cava; *GB*, gallbladder; *RK*, right kidney; *L*, liver.) (From Raghavendra BN, Glickstein ML: Sonography of islet cell tumor of the pancreas: Report of two cases. J Clin Ultrasound 9:331, 1981.) Case 2: Insulinoma. **(B)** Real-time transverse scan demonstrates a 2 cm solid mass *(m)* in the head of the pancreas. (*D*, fluid-filled duodenum; *L*, liver; *S*, spine; *pv*, portal vein; *sma* superior mesenteric artery; *a*, aorta.) (From Shawker TH, Doppman JL, Dunnick NR, McCarthy DM: Ultrasonic investigation of pancreatic islet cell tumors. J Ultrasound Med 1:193, 1982. By permission, John Wiley & Sons, New York.)

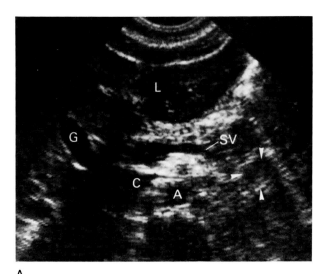
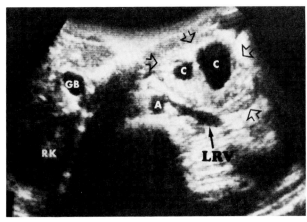

A   B

Fig. 3-60. Islet cell tumors. Case 1: Insulinoma 10 × 20 mm. **(A)** Transverse scan with hypoechoic tumor (arrowheads) in the tail of the pancreas. (*G*, gallbladder; *SV*, splenic vein; *C*, inferior vena cava; *A*, aorta; *L*, liver.) (From Gunther RW, Klose KJ, Ruckert K et al: Islet-cell tumors: Detection of small lesions with computed tomography and ultrasound. Radiology 148:485, 1983.) Case 2: Cystic degeneration. **(B)** Transverse scan 3 cm caudad to the xyphoid. A mass in the tail of the pancreas (open arrows) is seen containing two cystic cavities *(C)*. (*A*, aorta; *LRV*, left renal vein; *GB*, gallbladder; *RK*, right kidney.) (From Raghavendra BN, Glickstein ML: Sonography of islet cell tumor of the pancreas: Report of two cases. J Clin Ultrasound 9:331, 1981. By permission, John Wiley & Sons, New York.)

disease. Most of the lesions are in the pancreas with 13 percent in the duodenum and over 60 percent are malignant. Each functioning tumor with the exception of somatostatinoma is described in association with multiple endocrine neoplasia (MEN) type I syndrome. In MEN syndrome, there are adenomas in the pituitary, pancreas, and parathyroid. With MEN I (autosomal dominant, multiglandular), there are tumors or hyperplasia of the parathyroid, pituitary, adrenal cortex, and pancreas with peptic ulcer disease and gastric hypersecretion. In MEN II (Sipple syndrome) there are multiple pheochromocytomas, medullary carcinoma of the thyroid, parathyroid hyperplasia or adenoma and no pancreatic islet cell tumor.[4] The nonfunctioning tumors are easier to detect as they reach a larger size before they cause symptoms. They are usually solitary and present with pain (36 percent), jaundice (28 percent), or a palpable mass (8 percent).[4]

Ultrasound is very effective in evaluating the nonbeta cell tumors looking for a primary pancreatic mass, hepatic metastases in patients with glucagonomas, somatostinoma, nonfunctioning tumors, and WDHA syndrome.[109] In detection of Zollinger-Ellison syndrome, ultrasound compares favorable with gastrinomas detection by angiography and CT. On ultrasound, these lesions are homogeneously hypoechoic.[109] Ultrasound has been reported to identify lesions less than 1 cm.[110] Insulinomas are homogeneously solid with no cavitation or

calcification.[109] In general, the islet cell tumors appear homogeneous and solid, frequently hypoechoic while some larger ones are moderately echogenic[108,109,111] (Figs. 3-59 and 3-60). Calcification and fluid spaces may be seen in the larger lesions (Fig. 3-60). The tumors are

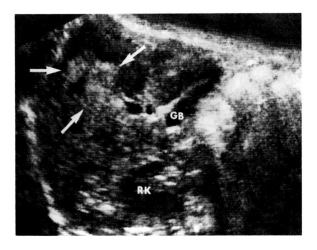

Fig. 3-61. Islet cell tumor, metastases. Longitudinal scan of the patient in Figure 3-59A, 7 cm to the right of midline. Poorly defined echogenic lesions (arrows) are seen within the liver. (*GB*, gallbladder; *RK*, right kidney.) (From Raghavendra BN, Glickstein ML: Sonography of islet cell tumor of the pancreas: Report of two cases. J Clin Ultrasound 9:331, 1981. By permission, John Wiley & Sons, New York.)

spherical, well-marginated homogeneous, and slow-growing. The solid masses are more likely functional with those containing necrotic cystic areas more likely nonfunctional.[107] The overall detection rate is 51 percent with the lowest in the insulinomas (30 percent) because of their small size and the patient's obesity. In 31 percent of patients there are liver metastases. Those from functioning tumors tend to be echogenic,[4] (Fig. 3-61); whereas those from the nonfunctioning tumors run the gamet from high-level to low-level echoes with target lesions being present.[4,109] Others describe the liver me-

tastases in functioning islet cell tumors to be characteristically isodense.[109] The role of ultrasound varies with the type of pancreatic islet cell tumor.

Metastatic Disease to the Pancreas

Extramedullary plasmacytomas of the gastrointestinal tract are rare (10 to 13 percent) and are found in 71 percent of multiple myelomas at autopsy with the vast majority involving the head and neck.[112] Pancreatic in-

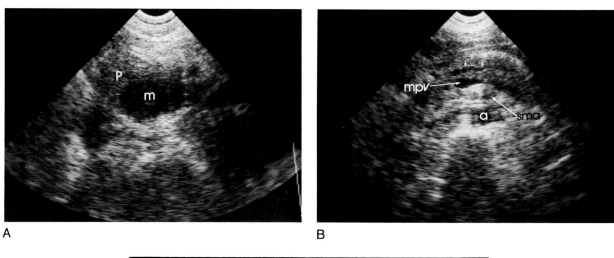

A   B

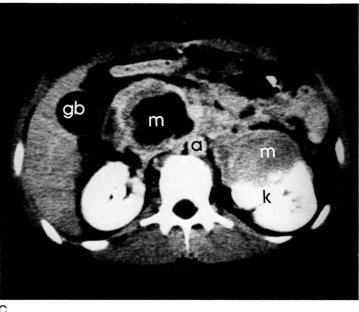

C

Fig. 3-62. Pancreatic lymphoma. Histiocytic lymphoma. **(A)** Transverse scan through the pancreatic head *(P)*. A hypoechoic mass *(m)* is seen. The usual vascular landmarks are not identified. **(B)** Transverse scan at a higher level than **(A)**. The pancreatic duct (arrows) is noted to be dilated within the pancreatic body. *(mpv,* main portal vein; *a,* aorta; *sma,* superior mesenteric artery.) **(C)** Enhanced CT scan. The pancreatic head lymphomatous mass *(m)* appears to be low-density. There is also a similar mass *(m)* in the left kidney *(k)*. *(a,* aorta; *gb,* gallbladder.)

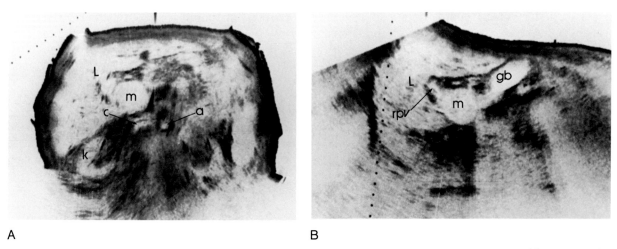

A   B

Fig. 3-63. Pancreatic lymphoma. Histiocytic lymphoma. **(A)** Transverse scan at 11 cm above the umbilicus. A round hypoechoic mass *(m)* is seen in the area of the pancreatic head. *(c,* inferior vena cava; *L,* liver; *k,* right kidney; *a,* aorta.) **(B)** Longitudinal scan to the right of midline. The hypoechoic lymphomatous mass *(m)* is seen inferior to the right portal vein *(rpv)* and posterosuperior to the gallbladder *(gb)*. *(L,* liver.)

volvement is usually microscopic. There has been a report of a plasmacytoma involving the pancreas appearing as a multilobular mass with fine low-level echoes and moderate acoustic enhancement that suggest lymphoma. The definitive diagnosis would have to be made with a percutaneous needle biopsy.[112]

Intraabdominal lymphomas may also involve the pancreas producing a large lumpy mass that is hypoechoic (Figs. 3-62 to 3-64). The superior mesenteric vessels should be displaced anteriorly instead of the posterior displacement seen with a primary pancreatic mass

(Fig. 3-65 and 3-66). Again, the definitive diagnosis would be made on percutaneous needle biopsy.[19]

The pancreatic head and body are ringed along their lateral and posterior margins by anterior and posterior pancreaticoduodenal, anterior paracaval, and superior mesenteric lymph nodes.[113] These nodes can be involved with metastatic disease and can be a source of a false positive diagnosis for pancreatic carcinoma. These nodes may appear as well-defined, echo-poor, ovoid or rounded masses in the retropancreatic location or may surround and silhouette the region of the pancreatic

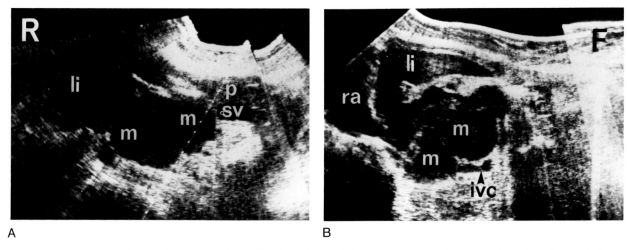

A   B

Fig. 3-64. Pancreatic lymphoma. Non-Hodgkins lymphoma. **(A)** Transverse scan demonstrating a large hypoechoic mass *(m)* engulfing the pancreatic head. The mass is slightly lobulated. *(p,* pancreas; *SV,* splenic vein; *li,* liver.) **(B)** Longitudinal scan through the confluent mass *(m)* in the region of the pancreatic head. The mass is more distinctly lobulated on this view. *(ivc,* inferior vena cava; *li,* liver; *ra,* right atrium; *F,* toward patient's feet.) (From Schnur MJ, Hoffman JC, Koenigsberg M: Gray-scale ultrasonic demonstration of peripancreatic adenopathy. J Ultrasound Med 1:139, 1982.)

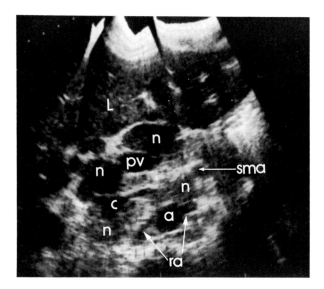

Fig. 3-65. Peripancreatic nodes. Lymphocytic leukemia. Transverse scan demonstrating multiple nodes *(n)* compressing and displacing the inferior vena cava *(c)* and the superior mesenteric artery *(sma)* anteriorly. (*a*, aorta; *pv*, main portal vein; *ra*, renal arteries; *L*, liver.)

head and body[113] (Fig. 3-65). With a confluent mass of peripancreatic nodes, they may be impossible to distinguish from pancreatic disease. The nodes are usually retropancreatic, lying posterior to the splenic vein and splenic-portal confluence, anterior to the inferior vena

cava, and lateral to the superior mesenteric artery (Figs. 3-66 and 3-67).

Direct invasion by tumors from surrounding organs may also appear as a primary pancreatic mass with a hypoechoic echopattern[114] (Fig. 3-68). This can occur with gastric, colonic, duodenal, and biliary tumors. Because the mass cannot be distinguished from a primary carcinoma, the diagnosis would be made with a percutaneous needle biopsy. The pancreas is rarely involved by metastatic disease from other primary malignancies[4]; when secondarily involved, most often it is from direct extension.

Aspiration Biopsy

The diagnosis of pancreatic carcinoma is difficult to make and in the majority of patients the diagnosis is made only at the stage of the disease in which the lesion is not resectable. Several investigators have described the aspiration/biopsy procedure in evaluating for pancreatic carcinoma.[101,115-125] The indications for a fine needle biopsy would include the following: (1) avoid surgery by obtaining histologic diagnosis; (2) determine staging of neoplastic disease process; and (3) facilitate treatment planning.[115] The essential indication is to obtain pathologic evidence of malignancy without exploratory laparotomy. With the recent improvements in localizing methods, the availability of thin needles for aspiration and the increased sophistication of cytologic techniques,

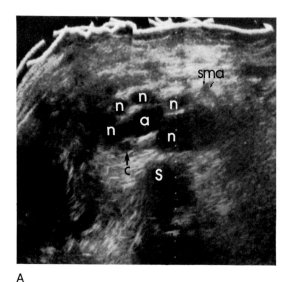

A

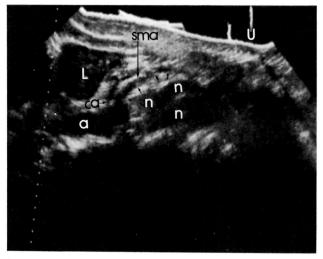

B

Fig. 3-66. Peripancreatic nodes. Histiocytic lymphoma. **(A)** Transverse scan at 9 cm above the umbilicus. Multiple hypoechoic nodes *(n)* are seen surrounding and displacing the aorta *(a)* to the right. The inferior vena cava *(c)* is compressed anteriorly and the superior mesenteric artery *(sma)* is displaced anteriorly and to the left. (*S*, spine.) **(B)** Longitudinal scan 0.5 cm to the left of midline. The superior mesenteric artery *(sma)* is displaced anteriorly *(arrows)* by the nodes *(n)*. The inferior aspect of the aorta *(a)* is not seen on this scan since it is displaced to the right. (*ca*, celiac artery; *L*, liver; *U*, level of the umbilicus.)

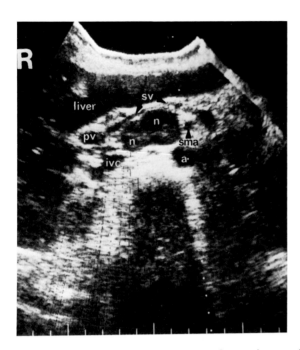

Fig. 3-67. Peripancreatic nodes. Metastatic ovarian carcinoma. Transverse oblique static scan with nodes *(n)* behind the splenic vein *(sv)*, and anterior to the inferior vena cava *(ivc)* and aorta *(a)* displacing the superior mesenteric artery *(sma)* to the left. *(pv,* portal vein; *R,* right.) (From Schnur MJ, Hoffman JC, Koenigsberg M: Gray-scale ultrasonic demonstration of peripancreatic adenopathy. J Ultrasound Med 1:139, 1982.)

the use of aspiration-biopsy has extended to that of the mass lesions of the pancreas and other abdominal structures. With fine needle biopsy, a diagnosis can be made in 78 to 88.7 percent of pancreatic carcinomas.[101,115,118,123,125] The positive cytology diagnosis is not influenced by the location of the tumor, but positive results are more frequent in patients with distant metastases than in those with localized tumor or locally invasive carcinoma.[118] The sensitivity of the procedure has been reported to be 86 percent with a specificity of 100 percent.[101] The rate of over 75 percent correct results with percutaneous aspiration biopsy of the pancreas.[115] There are no false positive diagnoses. Negative cytology does not exclude malignancy. By combining cytology with carcinoembryonic antigen (CEA) assay, the specimen obtained by percutaneous biopsy has increased the diagnostic rate to 100 percent.[118] Success with the fine needle aspiration biopsy technique requires experienced and skilled cytopathologists.[115]

CORRELATIVE IMAGING

Acute Pancreatitis

What is the accuracy of ultrasound with regards to acute pancreatitis and how does it compare to other imaging modalities? The role of an imaging study in

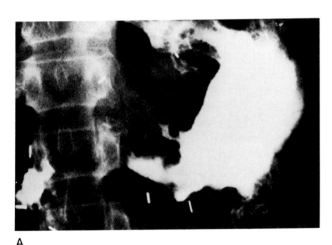

A

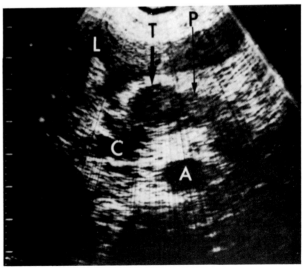

B

Fig. 3-68. Pancreas, direct metastatic invasion. Gastric carcinoma. **(A)** UGI series demonstrating numerous surgical clips from a prior operative procedure. There is poor filling of the distal stomach caused by an irregular mass involving the distal antrum consistent with a malignant lesion. **(B)** Transverse scan demonstrates the normal pancreatic tissue *(P)* to be approximately as echogenic as the adjacent liver *(L)* in the body and tail. In the region of the head and neck, a well-defined focal area of decreased echogenicity *(T)* is seen bulging the anterior border of the pancreas. *(A,* aorta; *C,* inferior vena cava.) (From Simeone JF, Dembner AG, Mueller PR: Invasion of the pancreas by gastric carcinoma: Ultrasonic appearance. J Clin Ultrasound 8:501, 1980. By permission, John Wiley & Sons, New York.)

evaluation of acute pancreatitis is to make a diagnosis of complications.[126] Some studies would indicate that CT is most sensitive in patients with acute pancreatitis.[51,126] CT can better visualize the fascial thickening and more accurately identify the locations and true extent of associated fluid collections. These patients on the whole tend to have more bowel gas due to ileus and the pancreas is not visualized as often with ultrasound as with other patients. In one study, there was good to excellent visualization on CT in 64 percent with only 20 percent visualized on ultrasound.[126] In 27 percent of patients with a normal CT, there was pancreatitis.[126]

In patients with pancreatitis, ultrasound is recommended as the initial examination to document the pancreatitis, check the gallbladder for stones, and evaluate for chronic pancreatitis, collections of fluid or other conditions predisposing to recurrent attacks.[47] If the technique is satisfactory, CT is not necessary if ultrasound is normal or shows mild changes. Pancreatic abscess or hemorrhage never develops in an intact pancreas. If ultrasound shows signs of a pancreatic mass or collections of fluid, a baseline CT is obtained. With ultrasound and CT available to monitor the stasis of the pancreas, the clinical condition of the patient becomes the pivotal item in the management of the progress of the patient.

Abscess

With pancreatic abscess, which modality is best? In one series, CT was able to detect gas in 50 percent of cases thus making a positive diagnosis.[58] Ultrasound suggested the diagnosis in 31 percent of these same cases.[58] But, as has been previously discussed, the presence of gas does not necessarily mean the lesion is an abscess. If an abscess is clinically suspected, then a percutaneous needle biopsy should be performed in order to make an immediate diagnosis.

Pseudocyst

Several series have been reported in comparing CT and ultrasound and their detection of pseudocysts.[127,128] In one, CT was correct in identifying 75 percent of uncomplicated pseudocysts, and 100 percent of infected pseudocysts. Ultrasound was correct in identifying 87.5 percent of the uncomplicated pseudocysts, and 50 percent of the infected ones.[128] In still another series, CT was correct in 95 percent of cysts with one false negative and two false positives; ultrasound was correct in 75 percent of cysts with one false negative and three false positives.[127] Some authors report an accuracy of 96 percent in the ultrasound detection of cyst.[104] All comparison

studies depend on having state of the art CT and ultrasound. As far as the ultrasound is concerned, the examiner must be persistent and meticulous in obtaining the images. Ultrasound is recommended as the best method to screen a patient for a cyst. CT may be used to plan the surgical approach or confirm the nature of the lesion, prior to surgery particularly in difficult cases. CT also may be used when the ultrasound results in a poor examination.

Tumor

There have been various reports as to the accuracy of ultrasound with regards to pancreatic cancer. One study reports a positive predictive value of 84 percent with a negative predictive value of 99 percent and a sensitivity of 94 percent with a specificity of 96 percent.[129] Others report a 94 percent sensitivity with a specificity of 99 percent.[14] In comparing CT and ultrasound, one investigation reports an accuracy for CT of 96 percent and for ultrasound 84 percent.[102] Still another study reports a CT sensitivity of 87 percent with a specificity of 90 percent; the sensitivity of ultrasound was 69 percent with a specificity of 82 percent.[130] In detecting a lesion and identifying it as malignant or inflammatory, CT was 84 percent sensitive with ultrasound 56 percent sensitive.[130] Because symptoms of this disease are common in the elderly, ultrasound allows reliable exclusion of this disease in a noninvasive way.[14,129] Others would recommend CT as the initial diagnostic imaging modality for evaluation for pancreatic carcinoma.[102,130] Both CT and ultrasound lack the ability to identify small lesions particularly in the head.[102] By combining CT/ultrasound with ERCP the accuracy rate increases to greater than 90 percent.[130]

CT and ultrasound have broadened the diagnostic spectrum in the diagnosis of islet cell tumors. Ultrasound is recommended as the first examination in evaluation for these tumors followed by CT, angiography, and transhepatic venous sampling.[109,111] The ultrasound detection rate is 57 percent overall.[109] The CT scan requires rapid sequential scanning with a bolus of contrast; there is marked contrast enhancement with dynamic CT. If CT/ultrasound are negative or inconclusive, then an angiogram is recommended.

CONCLUSION

Some investigators recommend ultrasound as the method of choice in evaluating patients for pancreatic pathology.[15] It is a rapid and economical tool allowing a scan in 15 to 30 minutes as opposed to CT, which takes 30 to 60 minutes, with equipment that costs 1/15th as much as CT. Ultrasound is able to define pancreatic anatomy in detail and has a high degree of accuracy in evaluating for gallstones, biliary dilatation, and helping to identify patients with gallstone pancreatitis. It is reported to have an accuracy of 90 percent in detecting pancreatic disease.[131] Small defects in the parenchyma may be seen with ultrasound before there are any changes in size or contour of the gland.[14] By performing a physical examination at the time of the ultrasound, a tender mass can be correlated with the examination. In addition, ultrasound is mobile and as such can be performed in conjunction with special procedures or in the intensive care unit. An initial ultrasound does not preclude other studies.

Both ultrasound and ERCP provide accurate information in evaluation of pancreatic disease.[132] A combination of ultrasound and ERCP constitute a comprehensive complementary diagnostic approach to the patient with upper abdominal problems. Ultrasound shows the size, outline, and consistency of the gland and ERCP outlines the duct. Both techniques require considerable expertise and results depend on the individual expertise in obtaining and interpreting the images. ERCP is an invasive procedure and carries the possibility of complication. Each technique fails to provide information in less than 10 percent of cases and each has a sensitivity and specificity in excess of 90 percent. Together they provide a powerful diagnostic combination.[132]

Despite the fact that overall CT is a little more accurate than ultrasound, ultrasound because of its noninvasive nature, lack of ionizing radiation, and lower cost per examination has not been replaced by CT for the pancreatic examination as predicted by some years ago. In considering the modality of choice, the body habitus is one of the most important factors. Thin patients do better with ultrasound; obese patients do better with CT.[4] Patients may be screened with ultrasound except those suspected of having complications of acute pancreatitis, i.e. phlegmon, abscess, and hemorrhage. If the ultrasound screening test is normal, CT is performed only if there is a high index of suspicion of pancreatic disease or the ultrasound was a suboptimal examination.[4]

REFERENCES

1. Bowie JD, MacMahon H: Improved techniques in pancreatic sonography. p.170. In Raymond HW, Zwiebel WJ (eds): Seminars in Ultrasound. Vol. 1. Grune and Stratton, New York, 1980

2. Kunzman A, Bowie JD, Rochester D: Texture patterns in pancreatic sonograms. Gastrointest Radiol 4:353, 1979

3. Kwa A, Bowie JD: Transducer selection for pancreatic ultrasound based on skin to pancreas distance in the supine and upright position. Radiology 134:541, 1980

4. Hill MC: Pancreatic sonography: An update. p.1. In Sanders RC (ed): Ultrasound Annual 1982. Raven Press, New York, 1982

5. Weinstein BJ, Weinstein DP: Sonographic anatomy of the pancreas. P.156. In Raymond HW, Zwiebel WJ (eds): Seminars in Ultrasound. Vol. 1. Grune and Stratton, New York, 1980

6. Goldstein HM, Katragadda CS: Prone view ultrasonography for pancreatic tail neoplasm. AJR 131:231, 1978

7. Berger M, Smith EH, Bartrum RJ Jr. et al: False-positive diagnosis of pancreatic tail lesions caused by colon. J Clin Ultrasound 5:343, 1977

8. Lawson TL, Berland LL, Foley WD: Coronal upper abdominal anatomy: Technique and gastrointestinal applications. Gastrointest Radiol 6:115, 1981

9. Crade M, Taylor KJW, Rosenfield AT: Water distention of the gut in the evaluation of the pancreas by ultrasound. AJR 131:348, 1978

10. MacMahon H, Bowie JD, Beezhold C: Erect scanning of pancreas using a gastric window. AJR 132:587, 1979

11. Jacobson P, Crade M, Taylor KJW: The upright position while giving water for the evaluation of the pancreas. J Clin Ultrasound 6:353, 1978

12. Weighall SL, Wolfman NT, Watson N: The fluid-filled stomach: A new sonic window. J Clin Ultrasound 7:353, 1979

13. Warren PS, Garrett WJ, Kossoff G: The liquid-filled stomach: An ultrasonic window to the upper abdomen. J Clin Ultrasound 6:315, 1979

14. Taylor KJW, Buchin PJ, Viscomi GN, Rosenfield AT: Ultrasonographic scanning of the pancreas: Prospective study of clinical results. Radiology 138:211, 1981

15. Crade M, Taylor KJW: Ultrasound diagnosis of pancreatic pathology. J Clin Gastroenterol 1:171, 1979

16. Dimagno EP, Regan PT, Clain JE et al: Human endoscopic ultrasonography. Gastroenterology 83:824, 1982

17. Lutz H, Lux G, Heyder N: Transgastric ultrasonography of the pancreas. Ultrasound in Med and Biol 9:503, 1983

18. Robbins SL, Cotran RS: The Pancreas. p.1092. In Pathologic basis of disease. WB Saunders Co, Philadelphia, 1979

19. Weinstein DP, Weinstein BJ: Pancreas. p.35. In Goldberg BB (ed): Clinics in Diagnostic Ultrasound: Ultrasound in Cancer. Churchill Livingstone, New York, 1981

20. deGraaff CS, Taylor KJW, Simonds BD, Rosenfield AJ: Gray-scale echography of the pancreas. Radiology 129:157, 1978

21. Niederau C, Sonnenberg A, Muller JE et al: Sonographic measurements of the normal liver, spleen, pancreas and portal vein. Radiology 149: 537, 1983

22. Gooding GAW, Laing FC: Rapid water infusion: A technique in the ultrasonic discrimination of gas-free stom-

ach from a mass in pancreatic tail. Gastrointest Radiol 4:139, 1979

23. Haber K, Freimanis AK, Asher WM: Demonstration and dimensional analysis of the normal pancreas with gray-scale echography. Am J Roentgenol 126:624, 1976

24. Coleman BG, Arger PH, Rosenberg HK et al: Gray-scale sonographic assessment of pancreatitis in children. Radiology 146:145, 1983

25. Fleischer AC, Parker P, Kirchner SG, James AE Jr.: Sonographic findings of pancreatitis in children. Radiology 146:151, 1983

26. Weill F, Schraub A, Eisenscher A, Bourgoin A: Ultrasonography of the normal pancreas: Success rate and criteria for normality. Radiology 123:417, 1977

27. Marks WM, Filly RA, Callen PW: Ultrasonic evaluation of normal pancreatic echogenicity and its relationship to fat deposition. Radiology 137:475, 1980

28. Ghorashi B, Rector WR: Gray scale sonographic anatomy of the pancreas. J Clin Ultrasound 5:25, 1977

29. Taylor KJW: Anatomy of pancreas by gray-scale ultrasonography. J Clin Gastroenterol 1:67, 1979

30. Filly RA, London SS: The normal pancreas: Acoustic characteristics and frequency of imaging. J Clin Ultrasound 7:121, 1979

31. Worthen NJ, Beabeau D: Normal pancreatic echogenicity: Relation to age and body fat. AJR 139:1095, 1982

32. Parulekar SG: Ultrasonic evaluation of the pancreatic duct. J Clin Ultrasound 8:457, 1980

33. Lawson TL, Berland L, Foley WD et al: Ultrasonic visualization of the pancreatic duct. Radiology 144:865, 1982

34. Eisenscher A, Weill F: Ultrasonic visualization of Wirsung's duct: Dream or Reality? J Clin Ultrasound 7:41, 1979

35. Bryan PJ: Appearance of normal pancreatic duct: A study using real-time ultrasound. J Clin Ultrasound 10:63, 1982

36. Ohto M, Saotome N, Saisho H et al: Real-time sonography of the pancreatic duct: Application to percutaneous pancreatic ductography. AJR 134:647, 1980

37. Weinstein DP, Weinstein BJ: Ultrasonic demonstration of the pancreatic duct: An analysis of 41 cases. Radiology 130:729, 1979

38. Porter A, Warren G: The morphology of the main pancreatic duct at E.R.C.P. as a guide to its demonstration by ultrasound. Australas Radiol 26:149, 1982

39. Hadidi A: Pancreatic duct diameter: Sonographic measurement in normal subjects. J Clin Ultrasound 11:17, 1983

40. Kaude JV, Wood MB, Cerda JJ, Nelson EW: Ultrasonographic demonstration of the pancreatic duct. Gastrointest Radiol 4:239, 1979

41. Sanders RC, Chang R: A variant position of splenic artery mimicking the pancreatic duct. J Clin Ultrasound 10:391, 1982

42. McGahan JP: The posterior gastric wall: A possible source of confusion in the identification of the pancreatic duct. J Clin Ultrasound 12:366, 1984

43. Phillips HE, Cox KL, Reid MH, McGahan JP: Pancreatic sonography in cystic fibrosis. AJR 137:69, 1981

44. Willi UV, Reddish JM, Teele RL: Cystic fibrosis: Its characteristic appearance on abdominal sonography. AJR 134:1005, 1980

45. Daneman A, Gaskin K, Martin DJ, Cutz E: Pancreatic changes in cystic fibrosis: CT and sonographic appearances. AJR 141:653, 1983

46. Mack E: Clinical aspects of pancreatic disease. p.166. In Raymond HW, Zwiebel WJ (eds): Seminars in Ultrasound. Vol. 1. Grune and Stratton, New York, 1980

47. Donovan PJ, Sanders RC, Siegelman SS: Collections of fluid after pancreatitis: Evaluation of computed tomography and ultrasonography. Radiol Clin North Am 20:653, 1982

48. Burrell M, Gold JA, Simeone J et al: Liquefactive necrosis of the pancreas: The pancreatic sac. Radiology 135:157, 1980

49. Hill MC, Dach JL, Barkin J et al: The role of percutaneous aspiration in the diagnosis of pancreatic abscess. AJR 141:1035, 1983

50. Doust BD, Pearce JD: Gray-scale ultrasonic properties of normal and inflamed pancreas. Radiology 120:653, 1976

51. Foley WD, Stewart ET, Lawson TL et al: Computed tomography, ultrasonography and endoscopic retrograde cholangiopancreatography in the diagnosis of pancreatic disease: A comparative study. Gastrointest Radiol 5:29, 1980

52. Johnson ML, Mack LA: Ultrasonic evaluation of the pancreas. Gastrointest Radiol 3:257, 1978

53. Lee JKT, Stanley RJ, Melson GL, Sagel SS: Pancreatic imaging by ultrasound and computed tomography: A general review. Radiol Clin North Am 14:105, 1979

54. Sarti DA, King W: The ultrasonic findings in inflammatory pancreatic disease. p.178. In Raymond HW, Zwiebel WJ (eds): Seminars in Ultrasound. Vol 1. Grune and Stratton, New York, 1980

55. Hashimoto BE, Laing FC, Jeffrey RB Jr., Federle MP: Hemorrhagic pancreatic fluid collections examined by ultrasound. Radiology 150:803, 1984

56. Cox KL, Ament ME, Sample WF et al: The ultrasonic and biochemical diagnosis of pancreatitis in children. J Pediatr 96:407, 1980

57. Gooding GAW: Ultrasound of superior mesenteric artery aneurysm secondary to pancreatitis: A plea for real-time ultrasound of sonolucent masses in pancreatitis. J Clin Ultrasound 9:255, 1981

58. Woodard S, Kelvin FM, Rice RP, Thompson WM: Pancreatic abscess: Importance of conventional radiology. AJR 136:871, 1981

59. Ranson JHC, Spencer FC: Prevention, diagnosis and treatment of pancreatic abscess. Surgery 82:99, 1977

60. Gonzalez AC, Bradley EL, Clements JL Jr.: Pseudocyst formation in acute pancreatitis: Ultrasonographic evaluation of 99 cases. Am J Roentgenol 127:315, 1976

61. Laing FC, Gooding GAW, Brown T, Leopold GR: Atypical pseudocysts of the pancreas: An ultrasonographic evaluation. J Clin Ultrasound 7:27, 1979

62. Stuber JL, Templeton AW, Bishop K: Sonographic diagnosis of pancreatic lesion. Am J Roentgenol 11:406, 1972

63. Gooding GAW: Pseudocyst of the pancreas with medias-

tinal extension: An ultrasonographic demonstration. J Clin Ultrasound 2:121, 1977

64. Asokan S, Alagratnam D, Eftaha M et al: Ultrasonography of a mediastinal pseudocyst. Am J Roentgenol 129:923, 1977

65. deGraff CS, Taylor KJW, Rosenfield AT, Kinder B: Gray-scale ultrasonography in the diagnosis of pseudocyst of pancreas simulating renal pathology. J Urol 120:751, 1978

66. Baker MK, Kopecky KK, Wass JL: Perirenal pancreatic pseudocysts: Diagnostic management. AJR 140:729, 1983

67. Conrad MR, Landay MJ, Khoury M: Pancreatic pseudocysts: Unusual ultrasound features. AJR 130:265, 1978

68. Farman J, Dallemand S, Schneider M et al: Pancreatic pseudocysts involving the spleen. Gastrointest Radiol 1:339, 1977

69. Kuligowska E, Miller K, Birkett D, Burakoff R: Cystic dilatation of the pancreatic duct simulating pseudocyst on sonography. AJR 136:409, 1981

70. Bellon EM, George CR, Schreiber H, Marshall JB: Pancreatic pseudocysts of the duodenum. AJR 133:827, 1979

71. Sarti DA: Rapid development and spontaneous regression of pancreatic pseudocysts documented by ultrasound. Radiology 125:789, 1977

72. Clements JL Jr., Bradley EL III, Eaton SB Jr.: Spontaneous internal drainage of pancreatic pseudocysts. Am J Roentgenol 236:985, 1976

73. Leopold GR, Berk RN, Reinke RT: Echographic radiological documentation of spontaneous rupture of a pancreatic pseudocyst into the duodenum. Radiology 120:699, 1972

74. Czaja AJ, Fisher M, Marin GA: Spontaneous resolution of pancreatic masses (pseudocysts?): Development and disappearance after acute alcoholic pancreatitis. Arch Intern Med 135:558, 1975

75. Semogas P, Cooperberg PL: Atypical pseudocyst of pancreas mimicking a diluted pancreatic duct. J De L'Association Canadienne Des Radiologists 31:258, 1980

76. Spira R, Kwan E, Gerzof SG, Widrich WC: Left renal vein varix simulating a pancreatic pseudocyst by sonography. AJR 138:149, 1982

77. Slovis TL, VonBerg VJ, Mikelic V: Sonography in the diagnosis and management of pancreatic pseudocysts and effusion in children. Radiology 135:153, 1980

78. Bloom RA, Abu-Dalu K, Pollak D: Spontaneous resolution of a large pancreatic pseudocyst in a child. J Clin Ultrasound 11:37, 1983

79. Kagan RJ, Reyes HM, Asokan S: Pseudocyst of the pancreas in childhood. Arch Surg 116:1200, 1981

80. Harkanyi Z, Vegh M, Hittner I, Popik E: Gray-scale echography of traumatic pancreatic cysts in children. Pediatr Radiol 11:81, 1981

81. Hancke S, Pedersen JF: Percutaneous puncture of pancreatic cysts guided by ultrasound. Surg Gynecol Obstet 142:551, 1976

82. Andersen BN, Hancke S, Nielsen SAD, Schmidt A: The diagnosis of pancreatic cyst by endoscopic retrograde pancreatography and ultrasonic scanning. Ann Surg 185:286, 1977

83. Gronvall J, Gronvall S, Hegedus V: Ultrasound-guided drainage of fluid-containing masses using angiographic catheterization techniques. Am J Roentgenol 129:997, 1977

84. MacErlean DP, Bryan PJ, Murphy JJ: Pancreatic pseudocyst: Management by ultrasonically guided aspiration. Gastrointest Radiol 5:255, 1980

85. Shawker TH, Linzer M, Hubbard VS: Pancreatic size and echo amplitude in chronic pancreatitis. Proceedings from 28th American Institute of Ultrasound in Medicine, J Ultrasound Med 2:2, 1983

86. Isikoff MB, Hill MC: Ultrasonic demonstration of intraductal pancreatic calculi: A report of 2 cases. J Clin Ultrasound 8:449, 1980

87. Weinstein BJ, Weinstein DP, Brodmerkel GJ Jr.: Ultrasonography of pancreatic lithiasis. Radiology 134:185, 1980

88. Matter D, Adloff M, Warter P: Ultrasonically guided percutaneous opacification of a pancreatojejunostomy. Radiology 148:218, 1983

89. Cooperberg PL, Cohen MM, Graham M: Ultrasonographically guided percutaneous pancreatography: Report of two cases. AJR 132:662, 1979

90. Fried AM, Selke AC: Pseudocyst formation in hereditary pancreatitis. J Pediatr 93:950, 1978

91. Kaude JV, McInnis AN: Pancreatic ultrasound following blunt abdominal trauma. Gastrointest Radiol 7:53, 1982

92. Foley LC, Teele RL: Ultrasound of epigastric injuries after blunt trauma. AJR 132:593, 1979

93. Wolfman NT, Ramquist NA, Karstaedt N. Hopkins MB: Cystic neoplasms of the pancreas: CT and sonography. AJR 138:37, 1982

94. Lloyd TV, Antonmattei S, Freimanis AK: Gray-scale sonography of cystadenoma of pancreas: Report of two cases. J Clin Ultrasound 7:149, 1979

95. Carroll B, Sample F: Pancreatic cystadenocarcinoma: CT body scan and gray-scale ultrasound appearance. AJR 131:339, 1978

96. Busilacchi P, Rizzatto G, Bazzocchi M et al: Pancreatic cystadenocarcinoma: Diagnostic problem. Br J Radiol 55:558, 1982

97. Wolson AH, Walls WJ: Ultrasonic characteristics of cystadenoma of the pancreas. Radiology 119:203, 1976

98. Freeny PC, Weinstein CJ, Taft DA, Allen FH: Cystic neoplasms of the pancreas: New angiographic and ultrasonographic findings. AJR 131:795, 1978

99. Herrera L, Glassman CI, Komins JI: Mucinous cystic neoplasm of the pancreas demonstrated by ultrasound and endoscopic retrograde pancreatography. Am J Gastroenterol 73:512, 1980

100. Masterson JB, Bowie JD, Port RB et al: Carcinoma of the pancreas occurring in a child: A case report with description of gray-scale ultrasound findings. J Clin Ultrasound 6:189, 1978

101. Mitty HA, Efremidis SC, Yeh H-C: Impact of fine-needle biopsy on management of patients with carcinoma of the pancreas. AJR 137:1119, 1981

102. Kamin PD, Bernardino ME, Wallace S, Jing B-S: Comparison of ultrasound and computed tomography in the detection of pancreatic malignancy. Cancer 46:2410, 1980

103. Weinstein DP, Wolfman NT, Weinstein BJ: Ultrasonic characteristics of pancreatic tumors. Gastrointest Radiol 4:245, 1979

104. Arger PH, Mulhern CB, Bonavita JA et al: An analysis of pancreatic sonography in suspected pancreatic disease. J Clin Ultrasound 7:91, 1979

105. Gosink BB, Leopold GR: The dilated pancreatic duct: Ultrasonic evaluation. Radiology 126:475, 1978

106. Walls WJ, Templeton AW: The ultrasonic demonstration of inferior vena caval compression: A guide to pancreatic head enlargement with emphasis on neoplasm. Radiology 123:165, 1977

107. Gold J, Rosenfield AT, Sostman D et al: Nonfunctioning islet cell tumors of the pancreas: Radiographic and ultrasonographic appearances of two cases. AJR 131:715, 1978

108. Raghavendra BN, Glickstein ML: Sonography of islet cell tumor of the pancreas: Report of two cases. J Clin Ultrasound 9:331, 1981

109. Shawker TH, Doppman JL, Dunnick NR, McCarthy DM: Ultrasonic investigation of pancreatic islet cell tumors. J Ultrasound Med 1:193, 1982

110. Kuhn F-P, Gunther R, Ruckert K, Beyer J: Ultrasonic demonstration of small pancreatic islet cell tumors. J Clin Ultrasound 10:173, 1982

111. Gunther RW, Klose KJ, Ruckert K et al: Islet-cell tumors: Detection of small lesions with computed tomography and ultrasound. Radiology 148:485, 1983

112. Rice NT, Woodring JH, Mostowycz L, Purcell M: Pancreatic plasmacytoma: Sonographic and computerized tomographic findings. J Clin Ultrasound 9:46, 1981

113. Schnur MJ, Hoffman JC, Koenigsberg M: Gray-scale ultrasonic demonstration of peripancreatic adenopathy. J Ultrasound Med 1:139, 1982

114. Simeone JF, Dembner AG, Mueller PR: Invasion of the pancreas by gastric carcinoma: Ultrasonic appearance. J Clin Ultrasound 8:501, 1980

115. Goldstein HM, Zornoza J, Wallace S et al: Percutaneous fine needle aspiration biopsy of pancreatic and other abdominal masses. Radiology 123:319, 1977

116. Itoh K, Yamanaka T, Kasahara K et al: Definitive diagnosis of pancreatic carcinoma with percutaneous fine needle aspiration biopsy under ultrasound guidance. Am J Gastroenterol 71:469, 1979

117. Cohen MM: Early diagnosis of pancreatic cancer using ultrasound and fine needle aspiration cytology. Am Surgeon 45:715, 1979

118. Tatsuta M, Yamamoto R, Yamamura H et al: Cytologic examination and CEA measurement in aspirated pancreatic material collected by percutaneous fine-needle aspiration biopsy under ultrasonic guidance for the diagnosis of pancreatic carcinoma. Cancer 52:693, 1983

119. Goldman ML, Naib ZM, Galambos JT et al: Preoperative diagnosis of pancreatic carcinoma by percutaneous aspiration biopsy. Digestive Diseases 22:1076, 1977

120. Ho C-S, McLoughlin MJ, McHattie JD, Laing-Che T: Percutaneous fine-needle aspiration biopsy of the pancreas following endoscopic retrograde cholangiopancreatography. Radiology 125:351, 1977

121. Smith EH, Bartrum RJ, Chang YC: Ultrasonically guided percutaneous aspiration biopsy of the pancreas. Radiology 112:737, 1974

122. Phillips G, Schneider M: Ultrasonically guided percutaneous fine-needle aspiration biopsy of solid masses. Cardiovasc Intervent Radiol 4:33, 1981

123. Ohto M, Karasawa E, Tsuchiya Y et al: Ultrasonically guided percutaneous contrast medium injection and aspiration biopsy using a real-time puncture transducer. Radiology 136:171, 1980

124. Taylor KJW, Brand MH: Ultrasonic biopsy guidance in the management of patients with pancreatic cancer. J Clin Gastroenterol 1:267, 1979

125. Lieberman RP, Crummy AB, Matallana RH: Invasive procedures in pancreatic disease. p.192. In Raymond HW, Zwiebel WJ (eds): Seminars in Ultrasound. Vol 1. Grune and Stratton, New York, 1980

126. Silverstein W, Isikoff MB, Hill MC, Barkin J: Diagnostic imaging of acute pancreatitis: Prospective study using CT and sonography. AJR 137:497, 1981

127. Williford ME, Foster WL Jr., Halvorsen RA, Thompson WM: Pancreatic pseudocyst: Comparative evaluation by sonography and computed tomography. AJR 140:53, 1983

128. Kressel HY, Margulis AR, Gooding GW et al: CT scanning and ultrasound in the evaluation of pancreatic pseudocysts: A preliminary comparison. Radiology 126:153, 1978

129. Pollock D, Taylor KJW: Ultrasound scanning in patients with clinical suspicion of pancreatic cancer: A retrospective study. Cancer 47:1662, 1981

130. Hessel SJ, Siegelman SS, McNeil BJ et al: A prospective evaluation of computed tomography and ultrasound of pancreas. Radiology 143:129, 1982

131. Whalen JP: Radiology of the abdomen: Impact of new imaging methods. AJR 133:585, 1979

132. Cotton PB, Lees WR, Vallon AG et al: Gray-scale ultrasonography and endoscopic pancreatography in pancreatic disease. Radiology 134:453, 1980

4

The Urinary Tract

In the past decade ultrasound of the kidney has become a valuable and frequently performed examination. Initially ultrasound was used to evaluate renal masses to determine whether they were cystic or solid. Now, the more common applications of renal ultrasound have been expanded to include (1) evaluation for hydronephrosis, (2) evaluation of the nonvisualized kidney on excretory urography, (3) evaluation of a flank mass in a neonate or child, (4) evaluation for a renal abscess, and (5) others. Although the sonogram is best performed with direct reference to a previous intravenous urogram in the case of a mass, it may be performed without the aid of the urogram when radiation exposure is unwarranted, such as during pregnancy, when the patient is allergic to radiographic contrast material, and also when poor renal function precludes an adequate intravenous urographic study.

In more recent years urinary tract ultrasound has been expanded to include investigation of the bladder and prostate, as well as the renal transplant. The clinical usefulness of this modality depends to a significant degree on how well the urinary tract structure and its surroundings are visualized. This, in turn, is dependent on sonographic technique and the examiner's knowledge. As with other organ systems, the use of the newer real-time systems has vastly improved and facilitated the ultrasound examination of the urinary tract.

TECHNIQUE

Kidney

PREPARATION

There is no specific preparation required prior to a renal ultrasound examination. Occasionally sedation is necessary in very young pediatric patients. The requirement for sedation is much less frequent than in former years because the examination is primarily performed by real-time systems that can allow more movement on the patient's part without compromising the study.

REAL-TIME ULTRASOUND EXAMINATION

The evaluation of the kidneys has by and large become a real-time examination. It is much faster to find the kidney, determine its long axis, and complete a satisfactory study using real-time systems. There is more flexibility as far as the real-time transducer is concerned and the system is portable, enabling the performance of high-quality studies out of the ultrasound laboratory.

The right kidney is best visualized with the patient supine or in the left lateral decubitus position using the liver as an acoustic window (Fig. 4-1). The left kidney is

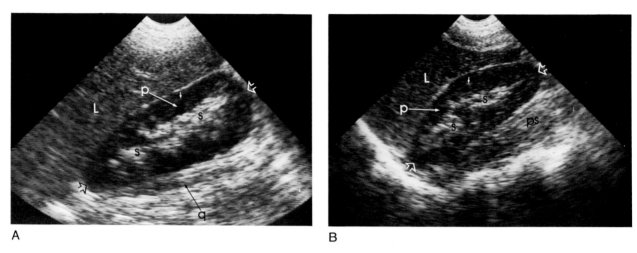

A   B

Fig. 4-1. Normal right kidney. Supine **(A)** and left lateral decubitus **(B)** longitudinal scans with the transducer in the anterior axillary line. The renal pyramids *(p)* are seen as triangular, poorly defined hypoechoic areas in the region of the medulla. The arcuate artery (small arrow) can be seen as an echodense dot at the corticomedullary junction. The renal cortex, between the medulla and renal capsule, is similar in density to the liver *(L)*. The width of the cortex can be determined by measuring the distance from the corticomedullary interface to the renal capsule. The renal sinus *(s)* is the echodense central area. The renal length (open arrows) can be determined by measuring from the superior to the inferior pole. (*ps*, psoas muscle; *q*, quadratus lumborum muscle.)

best scanned in the right lateral decubitus position using the spleen or fluid-filled stomach as an acoustic window[1] (Fig. 4-2). The right kidney may be best visualized by scanning in the anterior axillary line while the left may be best seen by scanning in the posterior axillary line[2] (Figs. 4-1 and 4-2). In the decubitus position, the true frontal plane of the kidney is viewed so that lesions in the

kidney and perirenal and pararenal spaces can be easily located.[3] The coronal view, additionally, has the advantage of allowing easier differentiation between a parapelvic cyst and hydronephrosis.[4] The medial and lateral borders of the kidneys are better visualized in the decubitus position.[5]

Although it is possible to evaluate the kidneys in the

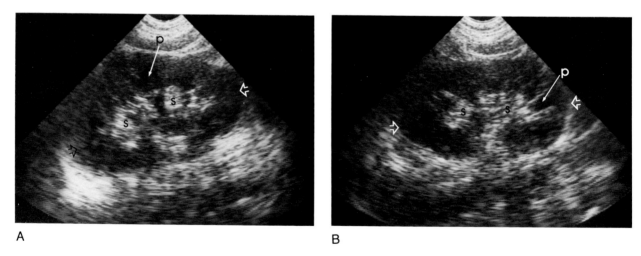

A   B

Fig. 4-2. Normal left kidney. Supine **(A)** and right lateral decubitus **(B)** longitudinal scans with the transducer in the posterior axillary line. The renal pyramids *(p)* are seen as triangular, poorly defined hypoechoic areas in the region of the medulla. The renal cortex, between the medulla and renal capsule, is similar in density to liver and spleen. The width of the cortex can be determined by measuring the distance from the corticomedullary interface to the renal capsule. The renal sinus *(s)* is the echodense central area. The renal length (open arrows) can be determined by measuring from the superior to the inferior pole.

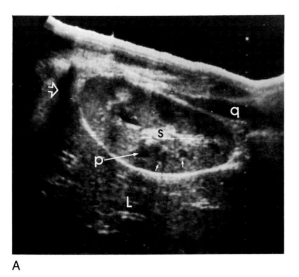

A

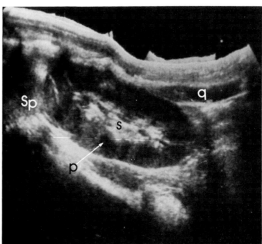

B

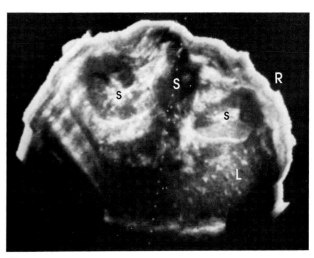

C

Fig. 4-3. Normal kidneys. Prone longitudinal scans **(A,B)** and transverse scan 11 cm **(C)** above the iliac crest. The right kidney is seen on **(A)** posterior to the liver *(L)*. Note the acoustic shadows (open arrow) caused by the ribs. The renal cortex is similar in density to the liver *(L)* and spleen *(Sp)*. The renal pyramids *(p)* are seen as triangular hypoechoic areas in the region of the medulla. The arcuate artery (small arrows) can be seen as an echodense dot at the corticomedullary junction. The width of the cortex can be determined by measuring the distance from the corticomedullary interface to the renal capsule. The renal length can be determined by measuring from the superior to the inferior pole. (*s*, renal sinus; *S*, spine; *q*, quadratus lumborum muscle; *R*, right.)

prone position, there are more problems associated with optimal visualization in this position than in the decubitus positions (Fig. 4-3). In the prone position, the paraspinal muscles may attenuate much of the sound beam and the lower ribs cast acoustic shadows, lending to a suboptimal examination.[1] If the patient can only be scanned in the prone position, a pillow or rolled sheet placed under the anterior abdomen at the level of the kidneys will improve the renal image because the compression reduces the thickness of the soft tissues overlying the kidneys, thus lessening the sound attenuation.[6] Also, the scattering and absorption of the sound beam will be reduced.[6] Similarly, in the decubitus position, there is less interference from adjacent tissue and closer correlation with the functional anatomy of the kidney.[7] In the prone or supine positions, the dorsal and ventral borders of the kidneys are better visualized.[5]

Scans are generally obtained in the position that

allows optimal visualization. The primary positions are described above. If the patient cannot be examined decubitus, then coronal scans through each flank can be obtained in the supine position. Many times it is helpful to examine the kidney in more than one position.

As with all ultrasound studies, the highest frequency transducer should be used that allows adequate visualization of parenchymal detail in each projection. For adults, this is generally a 3 to 5 MHz transducer; in children, a 5 to 7.5 MHz scanhead may be employed.

Optimal demonstration of renal parenchymal anatomy and renal mass lesions requires appropriate gain settings. The gain setting will vary with the kind of machine and transducer used; determination of the gain setting, therefore, is a skill that requires significant experience with the equipment.[8] The ultrasound beam is attenuated exponentially during its passage through tissue. To compensate for the attenuation, selective amplifica-

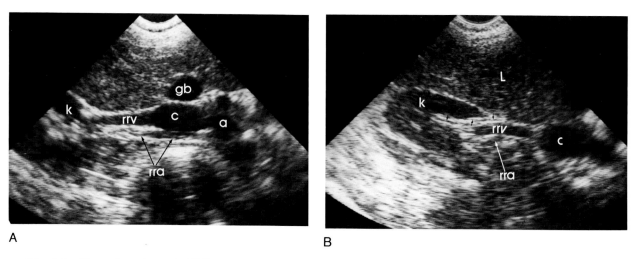

Fig. 4-4. Normal renal vessels. Oblique transverse supine (**A**) and left lateral decubitus (**B**) real-time scans through the right renal hilum. The renal vein *(rrv)* is seen anterior to the artery *(rra)*. (*c*, inferior vena cava; *a*, aorta; *gb*, gallbladder; small arrows, segmental arterial branches; *k*, right kidney; *L*, liver.)

tion of the distant echoes compared to the proximal ones is obtained by the time gain compensation (TGC). The operator must set the proper TGC to achieve even-sized echoes throughout the homogeneous tissue.[9] The gain should be high enough to fill the cortex but low enough so that the medulla is not obliterated[8] (Figs. 4-1 to 4-3).

There are several components to a complete renal ultrasound. Each kidney should be scanned carefully in the longitudinal and transverse planes. The maximum superior–inferior length of the kidney should be obtained during held inspiration. (Figs. 4-1 to 4-3). Several measurements should be taken and averaged. The renal cortical echodensity should be compared to that of liver at a comparable level and evaluated for uniformity (Figs. 4-1 and 4-3). The renal medullary pyramids should be identified in most patients, and in many cases a cortical thickness measurement can be obtained by measuring from the corticomedullary junction (Figs. 4-1 to 4-3). The corticomedullary junction is identified by the arcuate vessel interface. The renal sinus should be identified looking for signs of hydronephrosis. The renal artery and renal vein are often seen during real-time examination, with the artery being the posterior vessel (Fig. 4-4). Whether there is respiratory motion of the kidney should be noted. Generally, the examination is complete if there is no solid mass or hydronephrosis. If hydronephrosis is present, the examiner needs to try to identify the ureter. If the bladder is distended, the kidney can be rescanned for evidence of hydronephrosis after voiding. In the presence of a solid renal mass, the examination is not complete without evaluation of the renal vein and the inferior vena cava, as well as the liver.

STATIC ULTRASOUND

The examination utilitizing static ultrasound does not differ significantly from the real-time examination. It takes longer to localize the long axis of the kidney, as well as to do the examination in general. In the decubitus positions, it is sometimes difficult to sector through the interspaces with the static transducer as there is less flexibility than observed with the real-time system. Scans are generally obtained at 1 cm intervals through the kidneys in transverse and longitudinal projections.

PEDIATRIC

The renal ultrasound examination of the child does not differ greatly from the adult examination. But in the neonate there are some differences. It is critical to maintain body temperature, so heaters and warm gel are used. With the real-time systems, this examination can be performed in the neonatal intensive care unit. Sedation is rarely indicated. At times, it may be advantageous to examine the neonatal kidneys using a coronal approach.[10] With this technique there is little manipulation of the infant, less hindrance from monitoring devices or tubes, and improved visualization of the retroperitoneal structures due to less interference by bowel gas.

When evaluating a neonate with a renal mass, it is important to examine the contralateral kidney because there is a high incidence of abnormalities, as well as implications of bilateral disease.[11] The enlarged kidney may function as a sonic window through which to view the contralateral one. With the patient in an anterior oblique position with the enlarged kidney anteriorly, longitudinal oblique scans via a flank approach can be performed.[11]

Renal Transplant

PREPARATION

When possible, it is best to examine the transplant patient with a distended bladder. This not only gives an anatomical landmark but also increases sound transmission. If hydronephrosis appears to be present, the patient should be rescanned after voiding.

ULTRASOUND TECHNIQUE

Because the transplanted kidney is very superficial, a higher frequency transducer may be employed than with an examination of the native kidneys. As a rule, a 5 MHz scanhead can be used with adequate penetration. As with the routine renal ultrasound, the scan technique must be optimized to obtain parenchymal detail (Fig. 4-5). The sensitivity settings of the receiver unit and output of the transducer should be adjusted for each patient to allow optimal delineation of the renal cortex and medulla.[12]

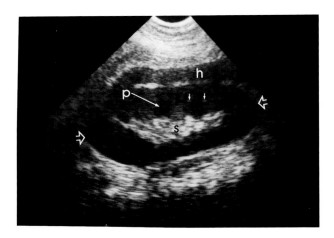

Fig. 4-5. Normal renal transplant. Longitudinal scan along the long axis of a transplanted kidney. The renal pyramids (p) are seen as poorly defined hypoechoic areas. The arcuate artery (small arrows) can be seen as echodense dots at the corticomedullary junction. The width of the cortex is measured between the medulla and the renal capsule. The renal sinus (s) appears echodense. The renal length (open arrows) is measured in its long axis. The gain has been set properly so the cortex is filled in with echoes but the medulla is not obliterated. The hypoechoic mass (h) anterior to the kidney was a postrenal biopsy hematoma.

This examination is especially facilitated by the real-time system because the renal axis is extremely variable. The first step of the examination is to locate the long axis of the kidney and perform the subsequent scans relative to that axis (Fig. 4-5). Besides evaluating the renal parenchyma and sinus, the maximum superior–inferior length of the kidney should be measured. At times, the transverse and anterior-posterior measurements are also necessary. These measurements are all relative to the kidney's axis, not the patient's position, as the long axis may be in the transverse plane while the transverse scans of the kidney may be performed in the longitudinal plane. No study of the renal transplant is complete without evaluating the perirenal and pelvic areas for fluid collections. At times, it may be helpful to have the patient void and rescan the renal sinus if there is a question of hydronephrosis.

A baseline ultrasound should be performed in the early postoperative period before the patient is discharged, or if there is a problem. The baseline scan is used to assess size, texture, and the like; its greatest value being its use as a comparison if the patient returns with problems.

If the scan is performed in the very early postoperative period, the study can be performed by draping the scanhead and cable with a sterile glove and bag and using either sterile gel or sterile antibiotic ointment as an acoustic coupler. A scan performed in the late postoperative period need not be performed with sterile technique.

Bladder and Ureters

PREPARATION

In order for the bladder to be evaluated adequately, it should be distended with fluid. If this cannot be accomplished with oral fluids, a Foley catheter can be used to fill the bladder in a retrograde fashion. A full bladder also facilitates the identification of dilated ureters.

ULTRASOUND TECHNIQUE

Ureters are usually not identified by ultrasound unless dilated. They are certainly easier to follow using real-time systems than static systems. The proximal ureter is best seen from the flank (coronal) or prone position, with the distal ureter seen through the distended bladder. The middle portion of the ureter is the most difficult to see because of overlying bowel gas.

The bladder should be examined with the patient in the supine position, utilizing longitudinal and transverse planes angling caudad and cephalad. The configuration of the bladder on the transverse scans should be symmetrical. The bladder wall should be a thin echogenic interface. A high-frequency transducer should be used.

Prostate

PREPARATION

A distended urinary bladder is necessary for adequate evaluation of the prostate using the transabdominal approach.

ULTRASOUND TECHNIQUE

The prostate may be evaluated using various sonographic techniques. Using the transabdominal suprapubic approach, real-time or static systems may be employed. The transducer may need to be angled caudad under the symphysis in order to visualize the prostate. Scans should be obtained both longitudinally and transversely.

The prostate may also be examined using the endoscopic approach (Fig. 4-6). This may be performed transurethrally or transrectally. The transrectal approach may be done with a radial static or linear array real-time system. The patient is placed in the lithotomy, knee-chest, or lateral decubitus position. After a digital rectal examination—to exclude an obstructing lesion—the anus and probe are coated with gel. The endoscope is inserted into the rectum and nonaerated water is placed into a condom around the probe to maximize acoustic coupling.[13] With the radial static probe, the endoscope is moved superiorly at 0.5 cm sequential intervals until the seminal vesicles are imaged. With the real-time linear transducer, the endoscope is rotated clockwise and counterclockwise (Fig. 4-6).

NORMAL ANATOMY

Kidney

The kidney is covered by a fibrous capsule closely applied but not adherent to the parenchyma. Surrounded by fat, the kidney is bounded anteriorly and posteriorly by the fibrous sheath, Gerota's fascia, and laterally the anterior and posterior leaves fuse to form the lateroconal fascia, which becomes continuous with the peritoneum along the abdominal wall.[2] The perirenal space is closed superiorly and laterally and does not communicate across the midline. It is open or potentially open inferiorly. As such, inflammation could track inferiorly or track back superiorly into the posterior pararenal space.

ADULT

Cortex. The normal adult renal cortex is homogeneously echogenic with low-level echoes similar in density to that of liver parenchyma[8] (Figs. 4-1 to 4-3).

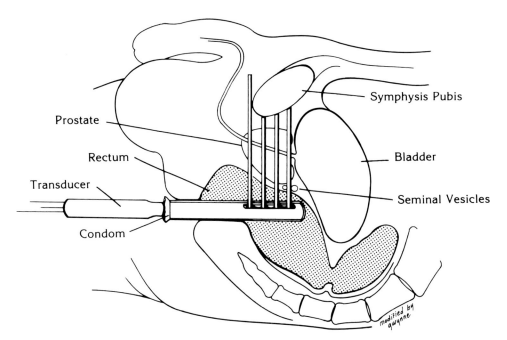

Fig. 4-6. Anatomic drawing—Endoscopic approach. The transducer with a condom over the tip is placed in the rectum. The prostate, seminal vesicles and fluid-filled bladder are visualized by either moving the transducer superior to inferior (radial) or rotating the transducer clockwise or counterclockwise (real-time). (Modified from Rifkin MD, Kurtz AB: Ultrasound of the prostate. p. 95. In Sanders RC, Hill MC (eds): Ultrasound Annual 1983. Raven Press, New York, 1983.)

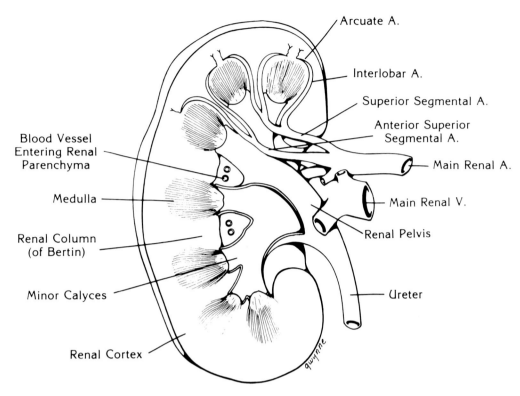

Fig. 4-7. Kidney section. Cut section through the right kidney showing the internal anatomy.

Medulla. The normal medullary pyramids are hypoechoic and are usually 1.2 to 1.5 cm thick[14] (Figs. 4-1 to 4-3, and 4-7). The arcuate vessels at the corticomedullary junction are recognized as discrete high-level echoes; they serve as a marker for evaluation of cortical thickness[8,9,15,16] (Figs. 4-1 to 4-3, and 4-7). These arcuate vessels can be identified in 25 percent of patients.[8] Renal columns of Bertin are cortical tissue extending into the space between adjacent pyramids[14] (Figs. 4-7 and 4-8).

Renal Sinus. The renal sinus contains the collecting system, renal vessels, lymphatics, fat, and fibrous tissue (Fig. 4-7). The renal sinus appears as an ovoid intense echo collection in the kidney on longitudinal axis and a rounded echodense area on transverse plane[17,18] (Figs. 4-1 to 4-4). If the collecting system is bifid, two lobulations of echodensity may be seen[2] (Fig. 4-9).

Length. The ultrasound renal dimensions are smaller than those noted by radiography because there is neither

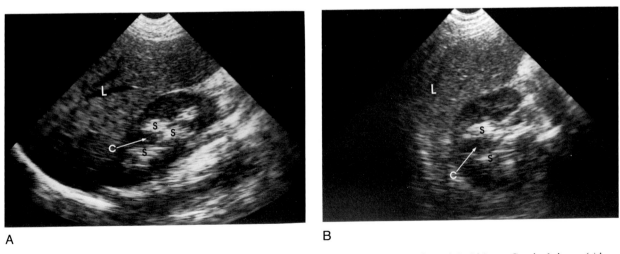

A   B

Fig. 4-8. Renal column of Bertin. Longitudinal **(A)** and transverse **(B)** scans of the right kidney. Cortical tissue *(c)* is seen to extend into the renal sinus *(s)* area. (*L*, liver.)

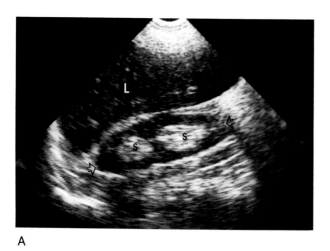

A

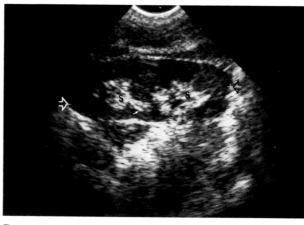

B

Fig. 4-9. Bifid collecting system. Longitudinal scans of the right **(A)** and left **(B)** kidney in two different patients. Two separate echodense areas *(s)* are seen in the area of the renal sinus on **(A)**. In **(B)** the echodense renal sinus *(s)* echoes merge centrally (arrow). This is produced by a bifid collecting system. (*L*, liver; open arrows, renal length.)

geometric magnification nor change in size related to an osmotic diuresis from contrast.[19] At autopsy, the average adult kidney is 11 to 12 cm in length, and 6 cm wide; on radiography, the average length is 12.5 to 13.5 cm with a width of 6 cm.[19] The normal renal ultrasound size has been reported to be 10 cm in length, 5 cm wide, and 2.5 cm thick[20] (Figs. 4-1 to 4-3). The normal size is dependent on a number of variables: individual age, sex, body habitus, and state of hydration.

Various investigators have evaluated the sonographic renal size. In the prone position, one study found the right mean length to be 10.74 cm ($\pm$1.35 standard deviation) with the left 11.10 cm ($\pm$1.15 standard deviation).[19] Another study correlated the renal length (RL) to the distance between the first four lumbar transverse processes (4TP) (Figs. 4-3 and 4-10). To determine the lumbar length, a longitudinal scan in the paraspinal location is performed with the patient prone[21] (Fig. 4-10). The ratio RL/4TP was found to be 1.04 $\pm$ 0.22 on ultrasound.[21] Ninety-five percent of normal patients were found to fall within this range.[21]

There are pitfalls in using ultrasound to obtain renal size. Scanning must be done carefully to obtain the longest axis possible.[19] In addition, the renal inclination (the angle the kidney makes with the horozontal plane) must be taken into account when obtaining the maximum renal length[22] (Fig. 4-11).

Determination of renal volume is a more sensitive means of detecting renal size abnormalities than any single linear measurement of the kidney.[23,24] The formula for calculating the renal volume is based on a three-dimensional ellipsoid formula adjusted by a correction factor for the magnitude of difference as com-

pared to renal volume estimated by water displacement:[25]

$$V = 0.49 \times L \times W \times AP.$$

L represents renal length with W the average measurement from the widths at the hilum and 1 cm above and

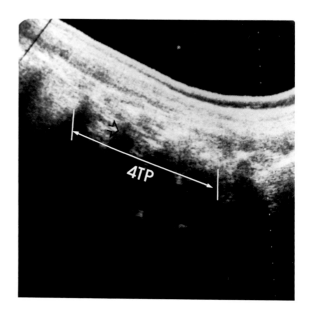

Fig. 4-10. Lumbar length. Longitudinal prone scan to the right of midline next to the spine. The distance between four lumbar vertebral transverse processes *(4TP)* can be measured. This can be correlated with the renal length. The processes cast an acoustic shadow (open arrow).

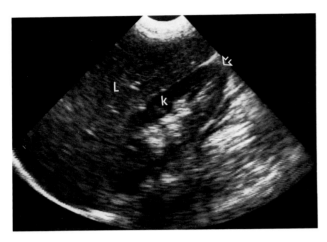

Fig. 4-11. Renal inclination. Longitudinal supine scan, right. Note the severe anteroposterior angulation of this right kidney *(k).* The inferior pole (open arrow) is quite anterior. *(L,* liver.)

1 cm below the hilum. AP is the anteroposterior dimension.

PEDIATRIC

In the normal neonate, there is accentuated corticomedullary differentiation demonstrated up to age 6 months[26] (Fig. 4-12). The enhanced corticomedullary differentiation can be explained by an increase in renal cortical echo production possibly combined with a slight decrease in echo production from the renal pyramids. The variation of size and maturity of individual nephrons and glomeruli may contribute to the increased echogenicity of the renal cortex in the neonatal kidney.

In the neonatal period, the glomeruli occupy 18 percent of the volume of the cortex as compared to 8.6 percent in the adult.[27] Histologically, the glomerular loops are matted together invaginated and surrounded by high, columnar epithelium; as they mature, this epithelial layer is lost and the loops expand.[26] The increased echogenicity of the renal cortex is due to the glomeruli that occupy a proportionately greater volume of the renal cortex during the first 2 months of life.[27]

The pyramids are triangular and arranged with their apices pointing toward the central collecting system (Fig. 4-12).[28] The prominent and hypoechoic renal pyramids can be explained by the larger volume of the medulla in the neonate, which results in a ratio of cortex to medulla of 1.64 : 1 in the neonate as compared to 2.59 : 1 in the adult.[27] The arcuate artery is seen as a bright reflective dot at the base of the pyramid denoting the corticomedullary junction and serves as a marker for assessment of parenchymal thickness. The bright echoes returned from the urothelial surface of the collecting system calyces and infundibula have an echogenicity that is less marked than typically seen in the adult kidney, probably representing the paucity of renal sinus fat in the neonate. Fetal lobulations are prominent features at this age and produce pronounced identations of the renal contour.[28] There is rapid growth of the kidney during the first 2 months of life, which is mainly due to disproportionate growth of the renal tubules as they increase in length.[27] By age two, the pediatric kidney takes on the adult sonographic features.[27]

Length. The ultrasound length versus the patient's age is a useful screening tool if the patient is specifically

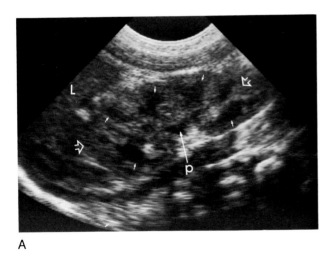

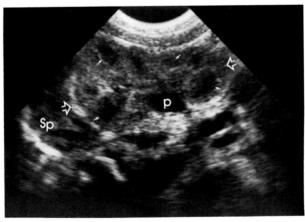

A   B

Fig. 4-12. Normal neonatal kidney. Longitudinal scans of the right **(A)** and left **(B)** kidneys. The renal pyramids (small arrows) are much more prominent in the neonate than the adult. The renal pelvis *(p)* can be seen as a central lucent area. The renal margins (open arrows) are much more difficult to define on freeze-frame images than at real-time. The renal parenchyma blends with the liver *(L)* or the spleen *(Sp).*

TABLE 4-1. Summary of Grouped Observations — Mean Renal Length

Average Age[a]	Interval[a]	Mean Renal Length (cm)	SD	n
0 mo	0–1 wk	4.48	0.31	10
2 mo	1 wk–4 mo	5.28	0.66	54
6 mo	4–8 mo	6.15	0.67	20
10 mo	8 mo–1 yr	6.23	0.63	8
1 ½	1–2	6.65	0.54	28
2 ½	2–3	7.36	0.54	12
3 ½	3–4	7.36	0.64	30
4 ½	4–5	7.87	0.50	26
5 ½	5–6	8.09	0.54	30
6 ½	6–7	7.83	0.72	14
7 ½	7–8	8.33	0.51	18
8 ½	8–9	8.90	0.88	18
9 ½	9–10	9.20	0.90	14
10 ½	10–11	9.17	0.82	28
11 ½	11–12	9.60	0.64	22
12 ½	12–13	10.42	0.87	18
13 ½	13–14	9.79	0.75	14
14 ½	14–15	10.05	0.62	14
15 ½	15–16	10.93	0.76	6
16 ½	16–17	10.04	0.86	10
17 ½	17–18	10.53	0.29	4
18 ½	18–19	10.81	1.13	8

[a] Years unless specified otherwise.

(Rosenbaum DM, Korngold E, Teele RL: Sonographic assessment of renal length in normal children. AJR 142:467, © Am Roent Ray Soc, 1984.)

referred for renal ultrasound. As with the adult, the radiographic technique yields some variability in apparent size of the kidney due to differences in centering of the tube and its distance from the patient, phase of respiration, and osmotic effect of iodinated contrast. The neonatal kidney ranges from 3.3 to 5.0 cm (left being 2 to 5 mm longer) with a width of 2 to 3 cm and a sagittal diameter of 1.5 to 2.5 cm.[28,29] Investigators have found the following formula and table (Table 4-1) useful in calculating normal renal length:[30]

>1 yr − Renal length (cm) = 6.79 + 0.22 × age (yrs)
<1 yr − Renal length (cm) = 4.98 + 0.155 × age (mo)

Ultrasound renal volume correlates better with urologic volume than ultrasound does with urographic renal length. Ultrasound renal volume may therefore be important in following growth patterns in children. The ultrasound length is more accurate than the urographic length. Renal length is defined as the maximum midsagittal length.[31]

Renal Transplant

The sonographic features of the renal cortex, medulla, and sinus of the transplant are very similar to the native kidney (Fig. 4-5). The length tends to be longer, averaging around 11 cm.

RENAL SIZE

Renal size in terms of volume can be calculated from the formula $V = L \times AP \times W \times 0.49$, where L is length, AP is anteroposterior and W is width.[12] From the time of transplant, the kidney begins to hypertrophy. By the end of the second week, there is a 7 to 25 percent increase in volume (mean 10 percent) with 14 to 32 percent (mean 22 percent) by the end of the third week.[12]

PARENCHYMA

To evaluate the renal parenchyma, the following should be assessed: cortical echogenicity, distribution of cortical echoes, characteristic corticomedullary junction, and size and appearance of the pyramids[12] (Fig. 4-5).

PERIRENAL FLUID

Normally, there is no fluid seen around the kidney or within the pelvis of the transplant patient.

Bladder

The various shapes of the normal bladder have been described.[36] At the neck, it is semilunar, while being kidney-bean shaped retropubic and bell shaped suprapubic. The bladder, when distended with fluid, is seen as a symmetrical anechoic structure (Fig. 4-13). It has a sausage shape on longitudinal plane, with a somewhat rounded appearance on transverse scan (Fig. 4-13). The wall of the bladder is seen as a thin, smooth, uniform echogenic line that is usually 3 to 6 mm thick.[33] The seminal vesicles are seen as two small oval, hypoechoic structures posterior to the bladder and superior to the prostate[33] (Fig. 4-13).

During all ultrasound examinations of the bladder, certain entities should be assessed. Wall irregularity will appear as an abnormal density or discontinuity of the wall echoes. Bladder shape should be assessed; with bladder deformity, there is distortion of the normal shape or wall rigidity due to tumor infiltration. Bladder capacity should be noted. The bladder volume can be calculated by using the formula $V = \text{trans} \times AP \times \text{length}$.[34] The normal volume may be up to 500 ml with-

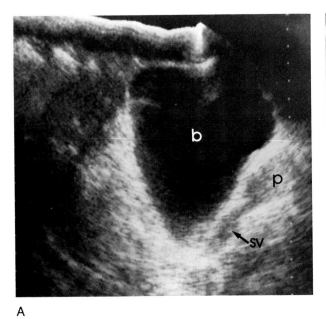

A

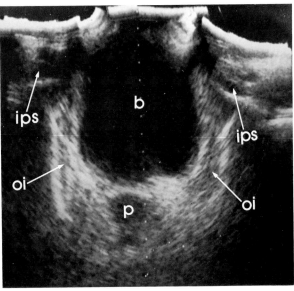

B

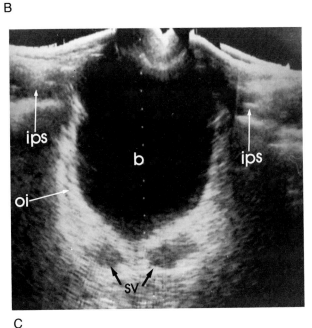

C

Fig. 4-13. Normal bladder. **(A)** Longitudinal scan, male. The distended bladder *(b)* is seen as a triangular anechoic structure with a thin, smooth, echogenic wall. The seminal vesicles *(sv)* are seen as echodense structures that are banana-shaped in this projection. The prostate *(p)* is seen in a retrovesicular location. Transverse scans with **(B)** lower than **(C)** within the pelvis. The normal prostate *(p)* is seen on the lower scan as a rounded, well-defined echodense structure. The paired seminal vesicles *(sv)* are seen as two rounded echodense structures on the higher scan **(C)**. (*oi*, obturator internus muscle; *ips*, iliopsoas muscle.)

out major discomfort.[35] There is reduced capacity caused by bladder contraction secondary to tumor infiltration or large tumor in the lumen.[36]

Ureters

The ureters arise as budlike outgrowths from the mesonephric or Wolffian ducts. The buds lengthen to produce a long, definitive tubular structure found in the adult. The average size is 30 cm long with a diameter of 5 mm. The course of the ureter is retroperitoneal. After entering the pelvis, the ureter passes anterior to either the common iliac or external iliac artery.[37] The normal ureter is not seen sonographically.

Prostate

The normal prostate is a retroperitoneal structure encircling the neck of the bladder and urethra superior to the urogenital diaphragm between the symphysis (anteriorly) and the rectum (posteriorly). The bladder is cephalad and slightly anterior. The inferior and posterolateral margins are the urogenital diaphragm, and levator ani and obturator internus respectively. The prostate averages 20 g in weight and has a thin fibrous capsule.[13] It is 4 cm maximum transversely, 2 cm anteroposteriorly and 3 cm craniocaudad.[13] It contains five lobes: posterior, middle, anterior and two lateral lobes. These lobes are not well defined. The anterior lobe is anterior to the prostatic urethra; the middle lobe is separated by the urethra anteriorly and the ejaculatory ducts posteriorly; the posterior lobe extends from the ejaculatory ducts posteriorly; and the lateral lobes are contiguous with the other divisions dorsal to the urethra. Some authors simply divide the gland in three lobes—median and two lateral.[38]

The normal prostate gland is seen in a retrovesicular location on the longitudinal axis of a distended bladder (Fig. 4-13). It is an oval or trapezoid structure measuring 3×3 cm between the bladder and rectum dorsally.[13] It is diffusely homogeneous in its echogenicity (low level echotexture) and has a well-defined capsule.[13,39] The prostate contour is smooth and well delineated. Centrally, increased echoes are sometimes noted, representing the urethra or periurethral glands[40,41] (Fig. 4-13).

There is a highly significant correlation between the prostatic weight estimated by suprapubic ultrasound and the organ's weight at surgery.[13,42] The volume of the gland can be determined by the formula $\frac{4}{3}\pi r^3$, with r being the average of the anteroposterior and transverse diameters[13,42] (Fig. 4-13). Because the specific gravity of prostatic tissue is 1 to 1.05 g/cm³, it is multiplied by the size to obtain the weight in grams.[13] An accurate estimation of the prostatic weight, as determined by ultrasound, can help the surgeon in deciding the approach for prostatectomy—suprapubic or transurethral.[13,41,42] A gland 50 to 60 g or smaller can be adequately resected transurethrally.[13]

RENAL ABNORMALITIES

Congenital

RENAL CYSTIC DISEASE

Ultrasound provides the initial diagnostic basis for patients with cystic kidney disease, distinguishing solid from cystic lesions and defining the type of cystic disease. Because these cysts are nonfunctional, they are not directly visualized on excretory urography, which is dependent on renal function. Ultrasound is an anatomic study and does not depend on renal function.[43] Real-time ultrasound is particularly suitable for renal imaging since it is noninvasive, lacks ionizing radiation, and can be performed portably.[44]

Multicystic Dysplastic Kidney. There have been several theories proposed for the production of a multicystic

kidney.[45-47] This kidney may represent hydronephrosis secondary to atresia of the ureter, pelvis, or both during the metanephric stage of intrauterine development.[43,46,47] There is a spectrum from unilateral multicystic kidney, through segmental and focal multicystic dysplasia, to bilateral multicystic kidney disease.[46] In the classic multicystic kidney, there is complete ureteral obstruction (atresia) early in fetal life (8 to 10 weeks of gestation).[47] Ureteral branching is interferred with and there is decreased branching of the collecting tubules and inhibition of induction and maturation of the nephron. The collecting tubules enlarge and the terminal portions develop into cysts. The cysts do not communicate and a reniform shape is maintained. If obstruction is incomplete, occurring after nephrogenesis is complete (36th week gestational age), the pelvis and calyces are dilated and the normally developed nephrons and ducts may be dilated but without dysgenesis.[47] The glomeruli and tubules continue to function resulting in hydronephrosis; the altered excretory function inhibits cellular development of the renal parenchyma. In incomplete obstruction (10th to 36th week gestation) there are varying degrees of cyst, pelvis and calyceal dilatation, and dysplastic changes.[47] If the upper ureter alone is atretic the proximal hydronephrotic pelvis may communicate with the multiple cysts. This is indistinguishable from hydronephrosis. If there is atresia of the pelvis too, the usual form of pelvoinfundibular atresia results.[45]

The multicystic dysplastic kidney is the most common cause of an abdominal mass in the newborn.[43] Although this lesion is usually unilateral, a significant number (15 percent) have abnormalities in the other kidney.[48] The

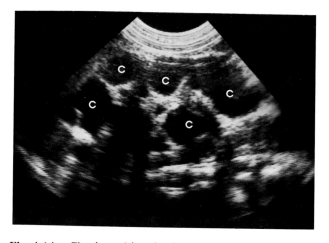

Fig. 4-14. Classic multicystic kidney. Longitudinal scan of a flank mass in a newborn. A large structure containing multiple cysts *(c)* (anechoic areas) is seen. No renal parenchyma or sinus is identified. There is no communication between the cysts. (From Seeds JW, Mittelstaedt CA, Mandell J: Pre- and postnatal ultrasound diagnosis of congenital obstructive uropathies. Urol Clin North Am 13:131, 1986.)

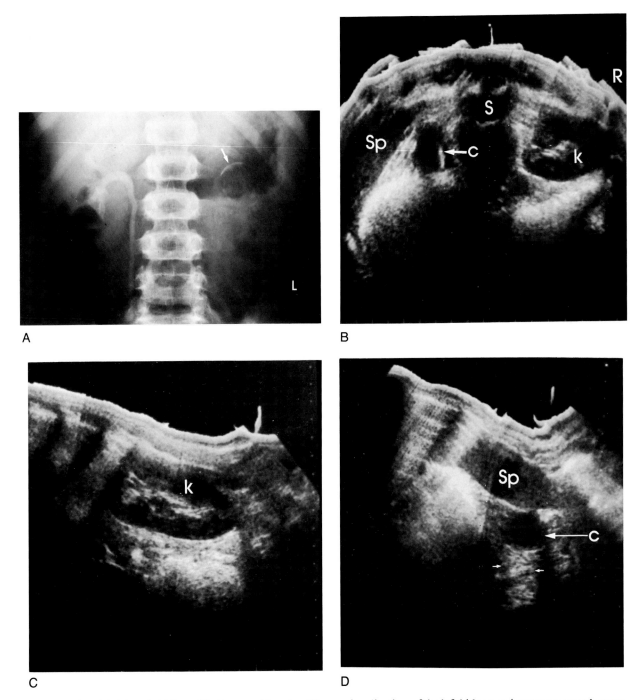

Fig. 4-15. Multicystic kidney. Eight-year-old male with nonvisualization of the left kidney on intravenous pyelogram **(A)**. A mass with a calcified rim (arrow) is seen on the left *(L)*. **(B)** Transverse prone scan. A normal-appearing right *(R)* kidney *(k)* is seen. An anechoic mass *(c)* is seen in the left renal fossa. (*Sp*, spleen; *S*, spine.) **(C)** Longitudinal prone scan of the right kidney *(k)*. The kidney is normal appearing but enlarged. **(D)** Longitudinal prone scan through the left renal fossa. A well-defined anechoic mass *(c)* is seen with acoustic enhancement (arrows). (*Sp*, spleen.) At surgery and pathologically this was felt to represent a multicystic kidney.

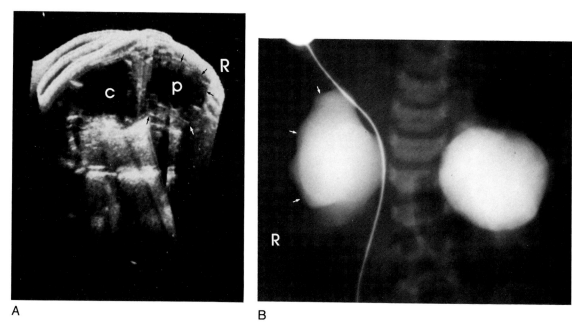

A   B

Fig. 4-16. Multicystic kidney and hydronephrosis. Neonate with renal failure. **(A)** Transverse prone scan. A single cystic (anechoic) structure *(c)* is seen on the left. No parenchyma is seen nor is there a renal sinus. On the right, *(R)* a large cystic (anechoic) structure *(p)* is seen but renal parenchyma (arrows) is seen. Cyst punctures were performed and contrast injected **(B)**. Calyces (arrows) are seen on the right *(R)*. At surgery, the left was a multicystic kidney with ureteropelvic junction obstruction on the right. (From Seeds JW, Mittelstaedt CA, Mandell J: Pre- and postnatal ultrasound diagnosis of congenital obstructive uropathies. Urol Clin North Am 13:131, 1986.)

left kidney is affected twice as often as the right.[48] The ultrasound findings of the classic multicystic kidney include (1) cysts of varying shape and size with the largest peripheral (nonmedial location of largest cyst, 100 per-

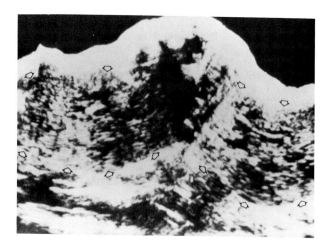

Fig. 4-17. Infantile polycystic kidney disease (IPKD). Newborn with bilateral flank masses. Transverse scan with both kidneys (arrows) enlarged with increased echogenicity throughout the parenchyma. The increased echogenicity is due to the ectatic tubules of IPKD. (From Grossman H, Rosenberg ER, Bowie JE et al: Sonographic diagnosis of renal cystic diseases. AJR 140:81, © Am Roent Ray Soc, 1983.)

cent accurate);[45] (2) absence of connection between adjacent multiple cysts (93 percent accurate);[45] (3) presence of interfaces between cysts (100 percent accurate);[45] (4) absence of identifiable renal sinus (100 percent accurate);[45] (5) absence of renal parenchyma surrounding cysts (74 percent accurate);[45] and (6) presence of eccentric echogenic areas (tiny cysts)[45,47] (Fig. 4-14). The septa separating the cysts and cores of rudimentary tissue (renal) may contain dysplastic glomeruli with tubular atrophy.[43] The lesion may not be identified until childhood or adulthood (Fig. 4-15). Ultrasound followed by nuclear medicine appears to be a logical diagnostic sequence in the evaluation of neonates with a flank mass. The differentiation between hydronephrosis and multicystic kidney is important clinically because the therapeutic approach and indications for surgery differ. As a rule, there is no function seen in a multicystic kidney on a nuclear medicine scan in either early or delayed images.[45]

Unilateral hydronephrosis is a differential diagnosis of the ultrasound findings described with multicystic kidney.[10] Ultrasound is accurate in differentiating classic multicystic kidney from moderate hydronephrosis, but it is often difficult to differentiate severe hydronephrosis from the hydronephrotic form of multicystic kidney.[47] The severity of the dysplastic changes are dependent on the completeness of the obstruction and the gestational

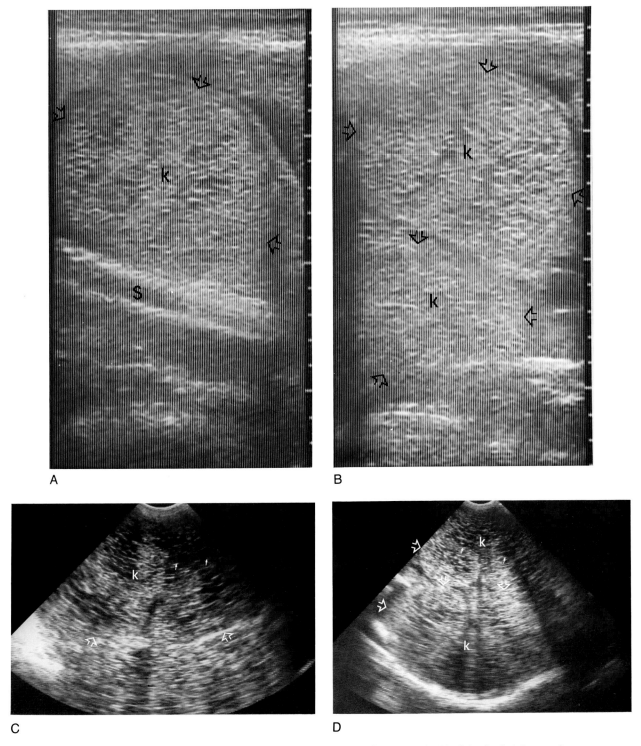

Fig. 4-18. Infantile polycystic kidney disease. Fetal scan: Longitudinal scans (**A,B**) of the fetal abdomen demonstrate massive renal enlargement (*k*, arrows). The kidneys fill the entire abdomen and there are multiple small internal cystic areas. (*S*, fetal spine.) Neonatal scan: Left (**C** more magnified than **D**) and right (**D**) longitudinal scans show tremendous nephromegaly with multiple tiny internal cystic areas (small arrows). Both kidneys (*k*, open arrows) can be seen on (**D**).

age at the time of the obstruction. The ultrasound criteria helpful in the diagnosis of hydronephrosis include (1) visible renal parenchyma surrounding the central cystic component; (2) small peripheral cysts (calyces) budding off a large central cyst; (3) cystic spaces of uniform size that are confluent with each other and the renal pelvis; (4) visualization of a dilated ureter; and (5) single large cyst[43,47] (Fig. 4-16).

Infantile Polycystic Kidney Disease. Blyth and Ockenden have subdivided infantile polycystic disease into four groups: (1) perinatal (Potter I) in which greater than 90 percent of the renal tubules are involved with minimal periportal fibrosis; (2) neonatal; (3) infantile; and (4) juvenile in which 10 percent or less of the renal tubules are involved with hepatic fibrosis and portal hypertension.[49] This form of cystic disease is uncommon and inherited in an autosomal recessive fashion. The infant presents with organomegaly secondary to the large kidneys, which are enlarged due to the ectatic tubules that are 1 to 2 mm in diameter. On microdissection, these collecting tubules have cystic dilatation and hyperplasia. The ectatic tubules are so small that they are not seen with ultrasound, but the interfaces produced by the walls of the tubules cause increased echogenicity throughout the parenchyma.[43,50] The kidneys are seen to be diffusely echogenic such that there is poor definition of the renal sinus, medulla, and cortex[49] (Figs. 4-17 and 4-18). The echogenicity and irregular cortical surface make it difficult to discern the border of the kidney.[49,50] While in the normal newborn, there is increased echogenicity of the cortex, there are sharply delineated hypoechoic medullae (Fig. 4-12). In infantile polycystic disease, the increased echoes from the tubules in the cortex and medulla lead to a loss of the corticomedullary junction.[43]

Juvenile polycystic disease is part of the spectrum of infantile polycystic kidney diseases. The degree of involvement of the kidney relative to the liver, and the rapidity of progression is determined by the age at which the disease presents. In the infant, there is kidney failure; the older child may have systemic hypertension or portal hypertension with varices. The ultrasound pattern depends on the clinical course and pathology. All demonstrate increased echogenicity to the cortex and medulla of the kidney due to the ectatic tubules leading to an indistinct corticomedullary junction. The liver findings are variable. Periportal involvement of the liver seen with this disease may lead to hepatic fibrosis and portal hypertension.[49] The echogenicity of the liver may be increased if there is significant periportal fibrosis and bile duct ectasia is present[43] (Fig. 4-19).

Adult Polycystic Kidney Disease. This form of polycystic disease is inherited as autosomal dominant with a

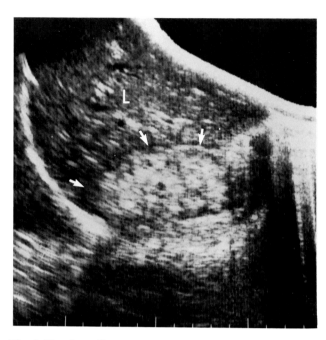

Fig. 4-19. Juvenile polycystic disease. Four year old with hematemesis due to esophageal varices; a biopsy of liver was diagnostic for infantile polycystic kidney disease of the liver and kidney. On a longitudinal scan of the right kidney (arrows), there is increased echogenicity throughout the parenchyma as compared to liver *(L)* and loss of corticomedullary junction (similar findings in left kidney). (From Grossman H, Rosenberg ER, Bowie JD et al: Sonographic diagnosis of renal cystic diseases. AJR 140:81, © Am Roent Ray Soc, 1983.)

high degree of penetrance. The penetrance of the gene is such that there is morphologic evidence of the disease seen in most patients by 80 years of age.[51,52] It occurs in 1 of 500 persons with 5 to 8 percent of patients requiring dialysis or transplantation.[14] The disease usually becomes clinically manifested in the fourth decade although there is sometimes presentation as a child.[43] In this type of cystic disease, there are cystic dilatations of the proximal convoluted tubules and Bowman's capsule as well as the collecting tubules. Classically, the cysts enlarge with age such that the patient presents when renal function begins to decrease.[50]

The most frequent complication of this disease is infection and renal calculi.[53] In addition, there may be cyst rupture, hemorrhage, and ureteric obstruction.[54] There can be calcification associated with the cysts but it is not distinctive. It may appear as a thin rim, ring-like, curvilinear, or small flecks and irregular amorphous concretions.[54] The most common cause of death associated with this disease is uremia (59 percent), with cerebral hemorrhage (13 percent) and cardiac disease being less frequent causes.[53] In 25 to 50 percent of patients there are liver cysts; occasionally, cysts are also seen in the

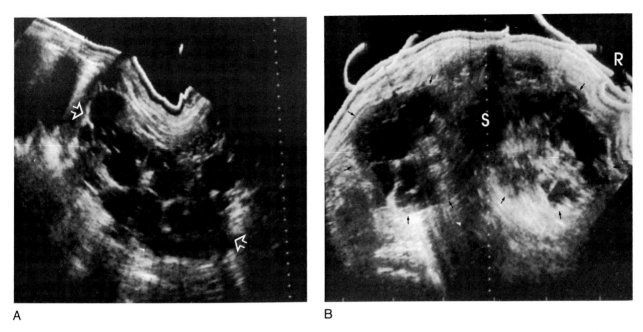

A   B

Fig. 4-20. Adult polycystic kidney disease. **(A)** Longitudinal prone scan demonstrates multiple anechoic areas in a very enlarged kidney (16 cm). The renal margins are indistinct (open arrows). (The other kidney looked similar). **(B)** Transverse prone scan of both kidneys (arrows). Multiple cysts are seen bilaterally. (*S*, spine; *R*, right.)

pancreas (9 percent), lungs, spleen, ovaries, testes, epididymis, thyroid, uterus, and bladder.[53,56]

On ultrasound kidneys affected with polycystic disease are enlarged with discrete cysts in the cortical region[43,55,56] (Fig. 4-20). The renal contour is poorly demarcated from surrounding tissue that may be secondary to multiple peripheral cysts that distort the renal capsule, to perirenal fibrosis, or to an organized hemorrhage in peripheral cysts that cause a decrease in specular reflections from the renal capsule.[14] When involvement of the kidneys is identified with ultrasound, one should carefully scan the liver, pancreas, and spleen for evidence of cystic involvement (See Figs. 3-17, 1-54). In addition, ultrasound can be used to screen family members in order to diagnosis polycystic disease that is not clinically manifested[51,52,55] (Fig. 4-21). This would also help to provide genetic counseling prior to procreation and to learn more about the natural history of the disease.

Although polycystic kidney disease is described as a bilateral process, there have been reports of unilateral disease and of segmental disease.[57–59] Both of these would be difficult to diagnose by ultrasound alone. The differential diagnosis would have to include segmental polycystic disease (very uncommon), localized hydronephrosis, and multilocular cyst.[57]

The adult type of polycystic kidney disease can occur in the neonate.[60] On ultrasound the kidneys are noted to be normal in shape but markedly enlarged and homo-geneously echogenic[60] (Fig. 4-22). Corticomedullary junction differentiation is absent, and no clear cut calyces or papillae are identified. The clue is the absence of impaired renal function.

Medullary Cystic Disease. The pathogenesis of medullary cystic disease or nephronophthisis is obscure as is its mode of inheritance. It is familial with both dominant and recessive modes of transmission. Clinically, these patients present with renal failure, polyuria, thirst, renal salt wasting, hyposthenuria, severe anemia, and a positive family history with a normal urinary sediment but no edema or hypertension.[61,62] The onset of clinical symptoms is usually at age 3 to 5 years to early adulthood with progressive renal insufficiency over the next 5 to 10 years.[62] The pathology is variable with renal biopsies showing interstitial fibrosis and cellular infiltration, tubular atrophy and dilatation, and periglomerular fibrosis. As such, a needle biopsy is not really diagnostic. At postmortem, the kidneys are found to be small with cysts less than 1 mm to greater than 1 cm in the medullary and corticomedullary regions.[61]

The radiographic diagnosis is difficult if the renal function is poor and the cysts are small in size. Most frequently, there is poor opacification of the renal collecting system. On high-dose nephrotomography, sometimes the diagnosis can be made by the identification of well-defined corticomedullary lucencies in association with a thin cortex. The retrograde pyelogram findings

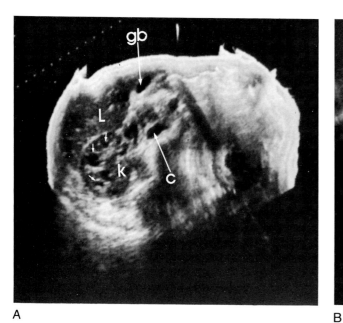

A

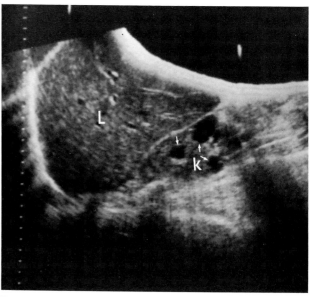

B

Fig. 4-21. Adult polycystic kidney disease (APKD). Twenty-year-old patient without symptoms but with a positive family history for APKD. Transverse **(A)** and longitudinal **(B)** supine scans reveal multiple cysts (arrows) within the right renal cortex. The left kidney appeared similar. (*L*, liver; *k*, right kidney; *c*, inferior vena cava; *gb*, gallbladder.)

are variable in demonstrating communication between the collecting system and cysts.[61]

The ultrasound findings represent a spectrum of irregularly widened central echoes with small cysts and well-

defined cystic structures when larger medullary cysts predominante[63] (Fig. 4-23). The most characteristic ultrasound findings are small cysts confined to the medullary portions of both kidneys.[43,61] There may only be irregular widening of the central echoes with small cysts.[63] The presence of a few small medullary or corti-

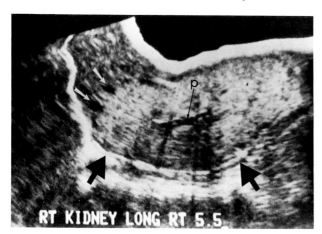

Fig. 4-22. Adult polycystic kidney disease. Neonate. Longitudinal scan with a markedly enlarged right kidney (black arrows) with no identifiable calyces. The slit-like renal pelvis *(p)* is seen as anechoic elongated area in the center of the kidney. The parenchyma has a homogeneously hyperechoic pattern. Small cystic areas in the renal periphery are seen (white arrows). The child's father had adult polycystic kidney disease. (From Hayden CK Jr., Swischuk LE, Davis M, Brouhard BH: Puddling: A distinguishing feature of adult polycystic kidney disease in the neonate. AJR 142:811, © Am Roent Ray Soc, 1984.)

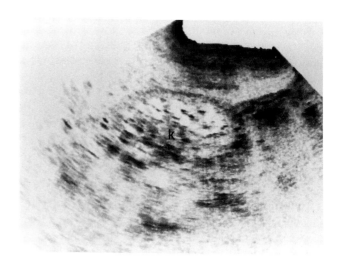

Fig. 4-23. Medullary cystic disease. Multiple 1 to 2 cm cysts confined to the medullary portion of the kidney *(k)* are seen. The kidneys are small, measuring 6 cm, with a regular cortical outline. (From Rego JD Jr., Laing FC, Jeffrey RB: Ultrasonographic diagnosis of medullary cystic disease. J Ultrasound Med 2:433, 1983.)

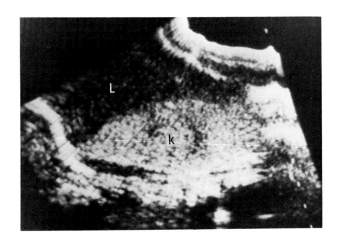

Fig. 4-24. Congenital nephrosis. Longitudinal scan of the right abdomen. An enlarged kidney (7 to 8 cm in length) is seen with a strikingly increased echogenicity and a coarse granular pattern. (*k*, kidney; *L*, liver.) (From Graif M, Lison M, Strauss S et al: Congenital nephrosis: Ultrasonographic features. Pediatr Radiol 12:154, 1982.)

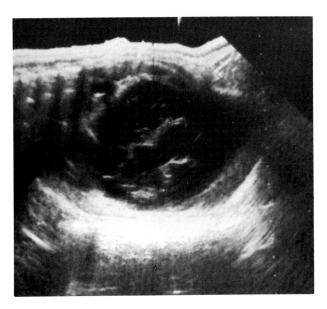

Fig. 4-25. Multilocular renal cyst. Longitudinal scan of the left kidney in a 3-month-old infant. Multiple cystic (anechoic) areas are seen. Unlike multicystic kidney, this kidney functioned at intravenous pyelography. (From Seeds JW, Mittelstaedt CA, Mandell J: Pre- and postnatal ultrasound diagnosis of congenital obstructive uropathies. Urol Clin North Am 13:131, 1986.)

comedullary cysts in a normal sized or moderately small kidney coupled with loss of corticomedullary differentiation and increased parenchymal echogenicity should suggest the diagnosis of juvenile nephronophthisis in a child with severe uremia.[62]

The differential diagnosis for cysts in a medullary location are limited including fluid that may or may not communicate with the pelvocalyceal system. Those that communicate should be visualized on excretory urography and include pyogenic cysts, abscesses, diverticula, papillary necrosis, and medullary sponge kidney. Those without communication would include simple cyst and medullary cystic disease, as well as parapelvic cysts, which are usually not multiple. In polycystic kidney disease, the cysts are variable in size and location and are associated with enlarged kidneys with irregular cortical outlines.[61] The simplicity and reliability of ultrasound make it superior to other modalities in such cases, particularly when a positive family history is lacking or medullary cysts are not seen in biopsy samples.[62]

Congenital Nephrosis. This entity is sometimes termed microcystic disease of the kidney. It is inherited in an autosomal recessive fashion. The infant presents with a low birth weight, is associated with a large placenta, failure to thrive, proteinuria, and edema. The kidneys are diffusely enlarged and microscopy shows dilatation of the proximal tubules and widening of Bowman's spaces. On ultrasound, the kidneys would be enlarged with marked echogenicity and loss of a distinctive cortex, medulla, and renal sinus[64] (Fig. 4-24). The differen-

tial diagnosis would have to include infantile polycystic kidney disease.[64]

Multilocular Renal Cyst. There are several theories for the etiology of a multilocular cyst and it has several names including benign cystic nephroma, cystic Wilms' tumor, cystic hamartoma, cystic lymphangioma, and Perlmann's tumor. Generally, the Wilms' tumor present is relatively benign. This lesion is rare, nonhereditary and limited to one area of the kidney with normal functioning tissue elsewhere in the kidney. The involved part of the kidney is bulky, and well encapsulated, consisting of multiple noncommunicating cysts that are sharply separated from surrounding normal tissue. On ultrasound a large tumor with multiple fluid-filled masses is seen separated by highly echogenic septations with normal renal tissue in the rest of the kidney[43] (Fig. 4-25). On excretory urography, the mass is nonfunctional with the rest of the kidney normal but with distortion or hydronephrosis.[43] (This entity, which goes by many names, is discussed further under Primary Renal Tumor, within the subheadings of Multilocular Cystic Nephroma and Wilms' Tumor.)

Simple Cyst. This lesion arises in the renal cortex, and is more often single than multiple. The etiology is

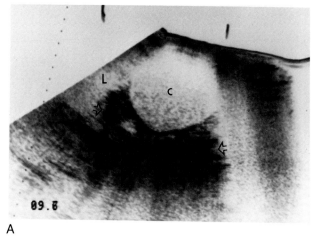

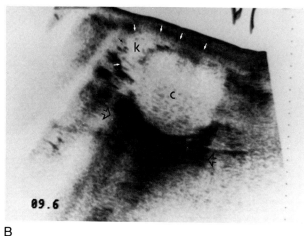

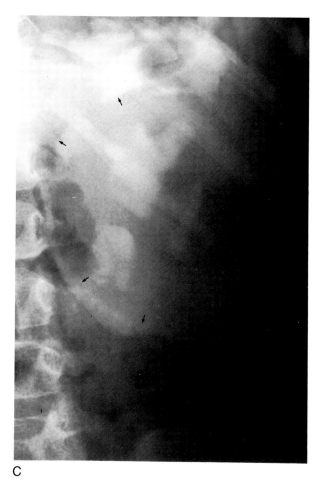

Fig. 4-26. Renal cyst—Child. This child (8 years old) was referred for splenomegaly. On longitudinal supine scan (**A**) a cystic *(c)* (hypoechoic) mass is seen inferior to left lobe of liver *(L)*. The mass has multiple internal echoes but exhibits pronounced acoustic enhancement (open arrows). (**B**) Prone longitudinal scan, left kidney. The mass *(c)* appears to be related to the kidney (*k*, arrows). Acoustic enhancement (open arrows) is noted. (**C**) Intravenous pyelography. A well-defined, smooth mass effect is seen (arrows). At surgery, this was a hemorrhagic renal cyst.

unknown and it is not hereditary. The highest incidence is after age 30 years but it can be seen in children. On ultrasound the characteristic cyst is anechoic, well-defined, and exhibits acoustic enhancement[43] (Fig. 4-26). There is further discussion of simple cysts under the Renal Mass section later in this chapter.

Parapelvic Cyst. These cysts arise in the hilum of the kidney and do not communicate with the collecting system. Their pathogenesis is uncertain. They are usually seen in adults as incidental findings but sometimes can present as a mass on excretory urography. On ultrasound, a medially placed cystic mass is seen with echo-

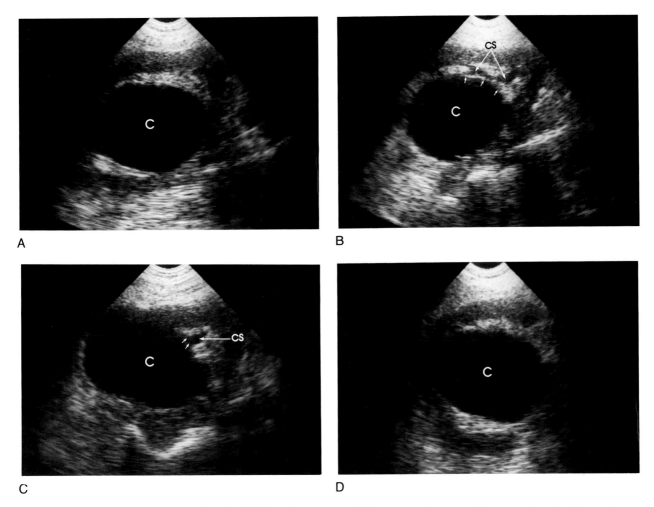

Fig. 4-27. Parapelvic cyst. Longitudinal **(A,B)** and transverse **(C,D)** scans. A large medially placed cystic *(C)* mass is seen. It does not communicate (small arrows) with the collecting system *(cs)* but does compress it.

genic walls (Fig. 4-27). The mass may displace the pelvocaliceal complex and must be differentiated from hydronephrosis by its noncommunication.[43] There is further discussion of parapelvic cysts under the Renal Mass section later in this chapter.

Ureteropelvic Junction Obstruction. At times, a neonate, infant, or child may be referred to ultrasound for evaluation of a palpable mass that represents a ureteropelvic junction (UPJ) obstruction. This lesion is frequently diagnosed on an antenatal ultrasound with a neonate referred to ultrasound on that basis. These infants often do not have a palpable mass.

There are a number of reported causes for congenital UPJ obstruction. These include extrapelvic adhesions, an abnormally situated junction between the renal pelvis and ureter, aberrant vessels to the lower pole of the kidney, folds of mucosa in the upper ureter, and intrinsic

and functional abnormalities of the pelvoureteral junction.[65]

The diagnosis is made on ultrasound by identifying a large dilated anechoic renal pelvis that communicates with the calyces without a dilated ureter[48] (Figs. 4-28 to 4-30). At times, the renal pelvis may be so enormous that the calyces cannot be identified (Figs. 4-28 to 4-30). Still, the diagnosis of UPJ obstruction should be entertained. Functional data concerning the affected kidney may be obtained by excretory urography or nuclear medicine. With nuclear medicine, differential function curves can be performed on each kidney so that the clinician may know the amount of renal function contributed by the affected kidney. If the diagnosis of UPJ obstruction can be made early in life and corrective surgery performed, a great deal of renal function can be saved. Often there is less function the older the child is when the diagnosis is made.

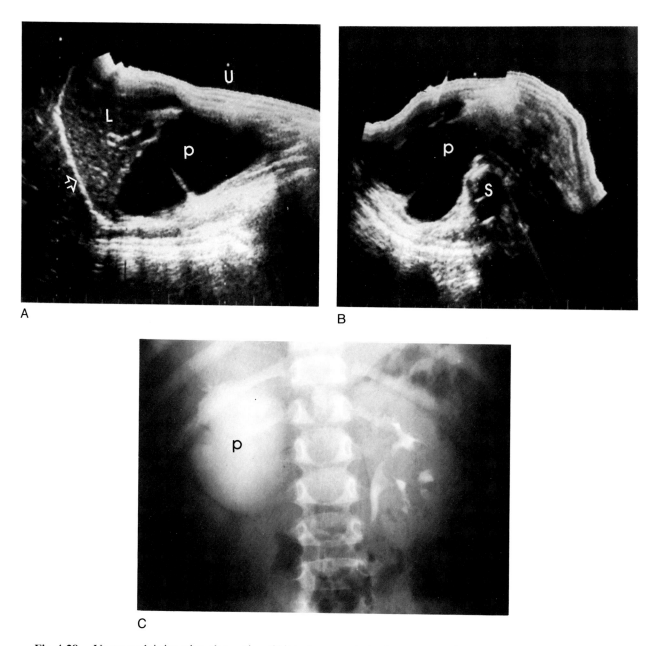

Fig. 4-28.   Ureteropelvic junction obstruction. Child who was noted to have a mass when she presented with a rash. **(A)** Longitudinal supine scan at 4 cm to right of midline. A large anechoic area *(p)* was seen in the region of the kidney. (*L*, liver; open arrow, diaphragm; *U*, level of the umbilicus). **(B)** Transverse scan at 4 cm above the umbilicus. A septated anechoic mass *(p)* is seen. (*S*, spine.) **(C)** Intravenous pyelogram. A dilated right renal pelvis *(p)* is seen. Dilated calyces are not seen. (Figs. **A** and **C** from Mandell VS, Mandell J, Gaisie G: Pediatric urologic radiology—Intervention and endourology. Urol Clin North Am 12:151, 1985.)

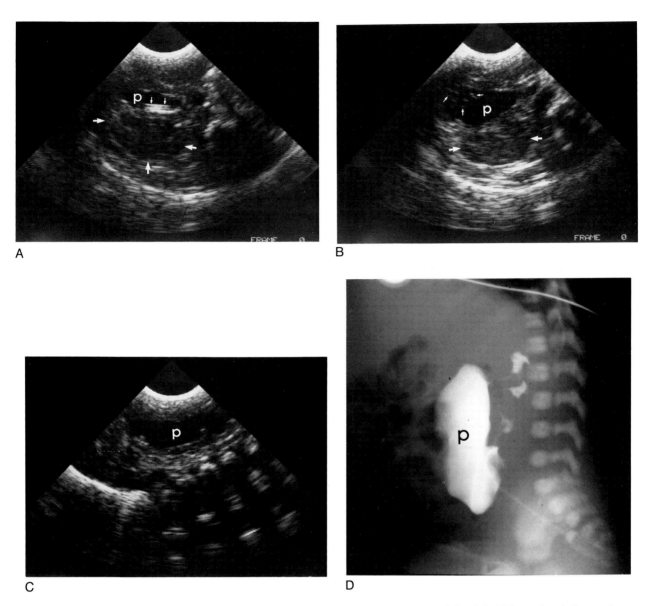

Fig. 4-29. Ureteropelvic junction obstruction with shunt. **(A)** Transverse scan of the right kidney after delivery of a neonate who had a pelvo-amniotic shunt placed in utero. The patient's mother had presented with polyhydramnios and a fetus with a large abdominal cystic mass. The shunt (arrows) is seen as two echogenic lines within the renal pelvis *(p)*, which is anterior to the renal parenchyma (large arrows). Transverse **(B)** and longitudinal **(C)** scans of the kidney during injection of contrast through the shunt tube. The renal pelvis *(p)* is more dilated than in **(A)**. Microbubbles (arrows) can be seen in **(B)** due to the injection. (large arrows, renal parenchyma) **(D)** Lateral portable view of the antegrade pyelogram. The renal pelvis *(p)* is dilated and rotated anteriorly.

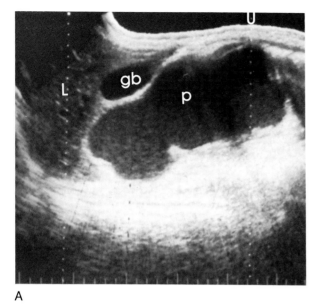

A

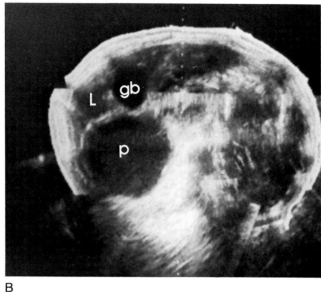

B

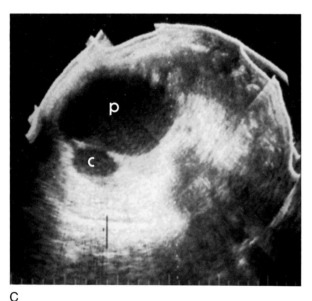

C

Fig. 4-30. Ureteropelvic junction obstruction. Sixteen-year-old pregnant patient, presenting too large for dates for her 8-week pregnancy. **(A)** Longitudinal scan 6 cm to right of midline. A large anechoic *(p)* structure is seen in the renal fossa. (*gb*, gallbladder; *L*, liver; *U*, level of the umbilicus.) Transverse scans at 12 **(B)** and 4 **(C)** cm above the umbilicus. An anechoic area *(p)* is seen in the right renal fossa. Dilated calyces *(c)* are seen posteriorly on **(C)**. Note that while there is acoustic enhancement there are many internal echoes. The patient later developed pyonephrosis. (*L*, liver; *gb*, gallbladder.)

COLLECTING SYSTEM DUPLICATION

The occurrence of collecting system duplication has been reported to be 0.5 to 10 percent of live births with an incidence on urography of 6 percent. The diagnosis is usually made by excretory urography. However, ultrasound may be done in the place of excretory urography to evaluate for presence of kidneys, exclude hydronephrosis, and exclude a duplication anomaly.[66]

The ureters develop from separate ureteric buds that have grown from a single Wolffian duct. The ureter to the lower pole enters the bladder at the trigone. The ureter draining the upper pole enters the bladder below

this point. Occasionally, the upper pole ureter ends ectopically outside the bladder. In males, the ureter end proximal to the external urinary sphincter may enter the vesical neck, prostatic urethra, seminal vesicle, vas deferens, or ejaculatory duct. An ectopic ureter is much more common in females and usually drains into the vesical neck or beyond the sphincter into the urethra, vagina, or uterus. The upper pole ureter frequently ends in the internal sphincter or in association with a ureterocele. This results in hydroureteronephrosis of the upper pole. The renal cortex of the upper pole is usually a functionless shell of dysplastic tissue. The excretory urogram is diagnostic in only 50 percent of cases.[67]

Ultrasound can be helpful in the diagnosis of a duplicated collecting system by identifying two echodensities in the area of the renal sinus (Fig. 4-9). If dilatation is present, the system affected would have the sonographic characteristics of hydronephrosis (Fig. 4-31). The presence of an associated dilated ureter should be determined and its course followed (Fig. 4-32). If dilated ureters are seen within the pelvis, a search for a ureterocele should be made. (Ureteroceles are discussed later in this chapter under the Bladder and Ureter section.)

ABNORMALITIES OF AMOUNT OF RENAL TISSUE

If agenesis is bilateral and total, death will result. If agenesis is unilateral, there may be adequate renal function. Agenesis is presumed to be due to unilateral absence of the nephrogenic primordium, or to failure of the Wolffian duct to make contact with the mesodermal mass. Occasionally, there is a small undifferentiated mass present. The renal artery and vein may be absent or rudimentary. With hypoplasia, there is failure of the kidney to develop to normal size. This entity is most commonly unilateral. There are a reduced number of renal lobules and calyces.[14]

It is extremely difficult for ultrasound to diagnose agenesis. If no identifiable kidney is seen in the renal fossa, an ectopic kidney cannot be excluded. This diagnosis is better made by a renal nuclear medicine study. On the other hand, if a very small kidney is identified in the renal fossa, with hypertrophy of the contralateral kidney, one may suspect hypoplasia on the basis of ultrasound (Fig. 4-33). It is important to note that if only one kidney is visualized, there is a 69.9 percent incidence of genital abnormalities.[68]

ANOMALIES OF POSITION, FORM, AND ORIENTATION

The kidneys may not lie in the normal renal fossa. A kidney may lie either just above the pelvic brim or sometimes within the pelvis (Fig. 4-34). Rarely, a kidney may even be intrathoracic with the left hemithorax being the most common location.[69] The theory for the intrathoracic location is related to the abnormally high ascent of the embryonic kidney, which comes in contact with the diaphragm and affects its development.[69] The kidney may resemble a Bochdalek hernia, neurogenic mass including neuroblastoma, ganglioneuroma, neurofibroma, neurogenic cyst, and mengingocele as well as a pericardial cyst or sequestration. The congenitally high ectopic kidney characteristically has a thin membrane diaphragm layer above the superior pole in contrast to a thoracic kidney in association with either traumatic or Bochdalek hernia[69] (Fig. 4-35). These patients may be referred to ultrasound for evaluation of a pelvic mass. If

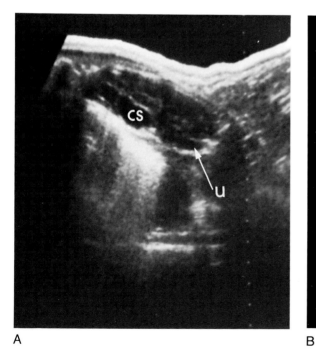
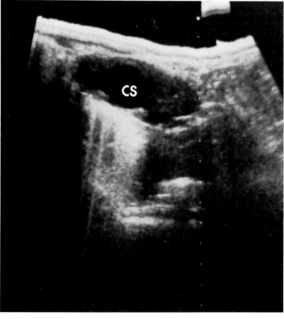

A   B

Fig. 4-31. Dilated duplicated collecting system. Longitudinal prone scans of the left kidney with (**A**) more medial than (**B**). A dilated upper collecting system *(cs)* is seen. (*u*, ureter.) *(Figure continues.)*

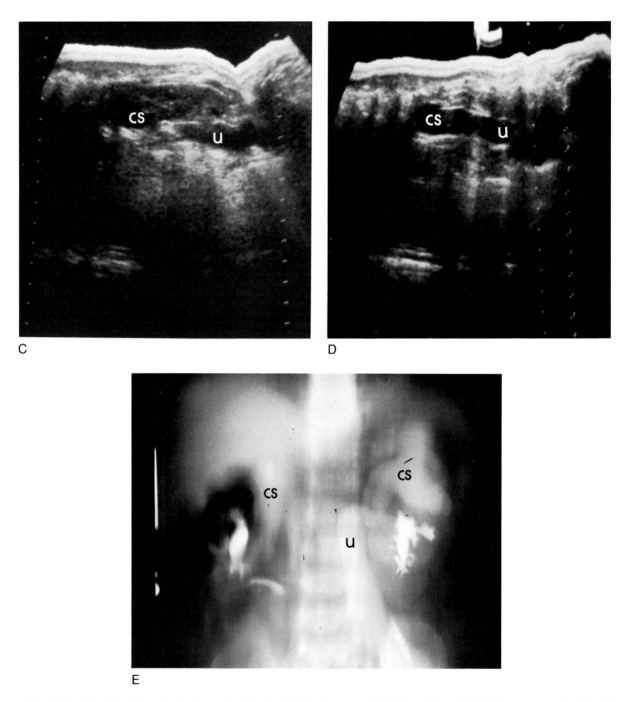

Fig. 4-31 *(Continued).*   Similarly on the right longitudinal scans medial **(C)** and lateral **(D)** is demonstrated a dilated upper pole collecting system *(cs).* The dilated ureter *(u)* is seen on the medial scan **(C). (E)** Intravenous pyelogram. The dilated upper collecting systems *(cs)* are seen as well as the left ureter *(u).*

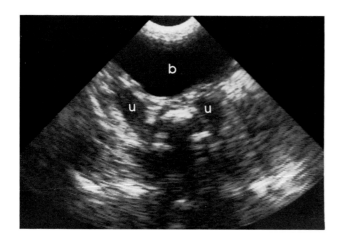

Fig. 4-32. Dilated ureters. Neonate with bilateral hydrone-phrosis and reflux. Transverse scan of fluid-filled bladder *(b)* with bilaterally dilated ureters *(u)* seen as rounded anechoic areas on either side of midline. (From Seeds JW, Mittelstaedt CA, Mandell J: Pre- and postnatal ultrasound diagnosis of congenital obstructive uropathies, Urol Clin North Am 13:131, 1986.)

the mass seen by ultrasound resembles kidney, ectopia should be suspected and both renal fossa should be scanned for confirmation. If the primary question is one of renal ectopia, the patient is better served by a renal nuclear medicine study.

Crossed renal ectopia is relatively uncommon, with fusion of the ectopic kidney being more common than the unfused variety.[70,71] With the unfused type, one kidney is in the normal position and the other is most often located at or below the level of the sacral promentory. With both kidneys on the same side of the abdomen, one of the two ureters crosses the midline to the vesical orifice on the contralateral side.[71] The lesion itself produces no symptoms and typically comes to attention during workup of a patient for other problems, so the examiner should be aware of its appearance. Because ultrasound is used frequently as an initial imaging technique, failure to recognize the abnormality can cause misdiagnosis.

A crossed-fused kidney may mimic a single kidney with a duplicated system or a kidney with a renal mass[71]

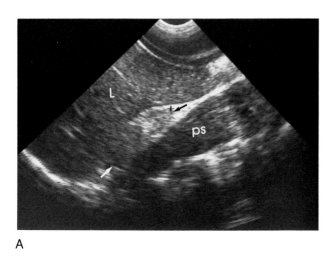

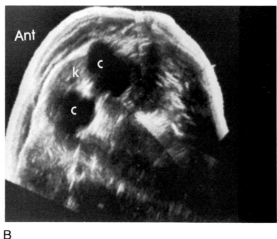

A   B

Fig. 4-33. Hypoplastic kidney. Sixteen-year-old with hyper-tension. **(A)** In the right renal fossa on longitudinal scan, a very small structure *(k)* was seen. (*ps,* psoas muscle; *L,* liver.) **(B)** Right lateral decubitus position, transverse scan of left kidney. Multiple anechoic areas (*c,* cysts) were seen in the area of the left kidney *(k)*. (*Ant,* anterior.) **(C)** Enhanced CT scan. A very small kidney *(k)* is seen on the right with contrast seen in the ureter (arrow). The left kidney demonstrates multiple low-density areas (*c,* cysts).

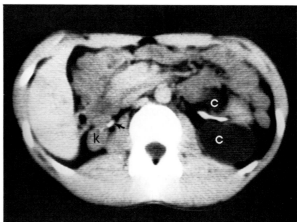

C

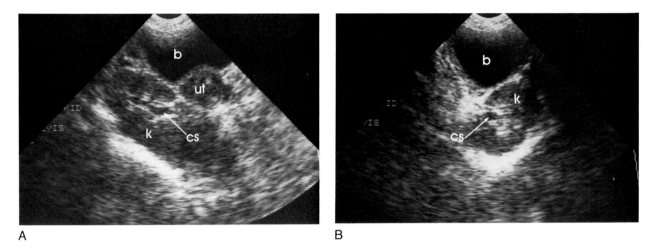

A   B

Fig. 4-34.   Pelvic kidney. **(A)** Longitudinal scan to the left of the midline. The kidney *(k)* is seen superior to bladder *(b)*. It is difficult to define the inferior pole. (*ut*, uterus; *cs*, collecting system.) **(B)** Transverse scan. The kidney *(k)* is seen slightly to left of midline. (*b*, bladder; *cs*, collecting system.)

(Fig. 4-36). The characteristic anterior and/or posterior notch provides the major clue to the correct diagnosis[71] (Fig. 4-37). In addition the kidney will be much too long for a single kidney. In cases of renal agenesis or ectopia, colonic flexure and small bowel may occupy the contralateral renal fossa, mimicking a mass or a hydrone-phrotic kidney.[71,72] The colon filled with stool or fluid may simulate a kidney or a mass.[72]

A horseshoe kidney occurs in 1 of 500 to 1 of 100 autopsies and as such represents a common anomaly.[14,73,74] The majority of these kidneys are fused at the lower pole with 10 percent fused in the upper pole. The

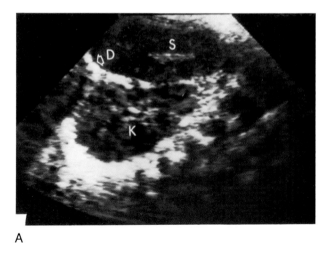

A

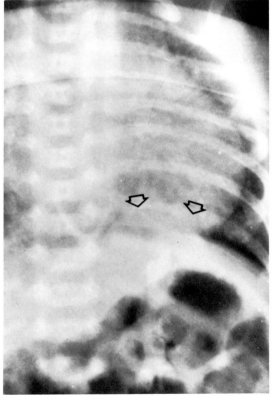

B

Fig. 4-35.   Thoracic kidney. **(A)** Longitudinal real-time scan showing a left chest mass that is an intrathoracic kidney *(K)*. (*D*, diaphragm; *S*, spleen.) **(B)** Postcardiac catheterization anteroposterior film confirms the presence of a high left renal ectopia (arrows, upper pole, left kidney.) (From Sumner TE, Volberg FM, Smolen PM: Intrathoracic kidney—Diagnosis by ultrasound. Pediatr Radiol 12:78, 1982.)

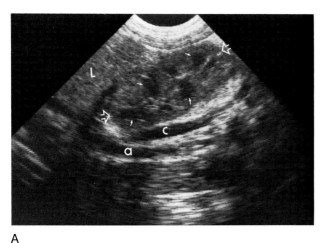

A

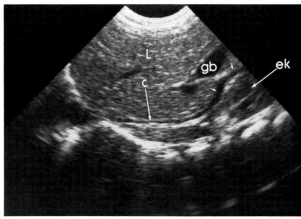

B

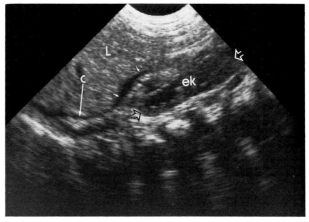

C

Fig. 4-36. Crossed fused ectopia. Neonate **(A)** Longitudinal coronal left lateral decubitus scan of the right kidney. The kidney (open arrows) is identified in the renal fossa anterior to the inferior vena cava *(c)* and aorta *(a)*. (Small arrows, pyramids; *L*, liver.) Longitudinal scans with **(B)** more superior than **(C)**. The inferior vena cava *(c)* is displaced (small arrows) anteriorly and to the left by the crossed-fused kidney *(ek*, open arrows). (*gb*, gallbladder; *L*, liver) *(Figure continues.)*

bridge at the lower poles have the ureters passing anteriorly. This anomalous kidney is not more prone to disease. However, renal calculi are slightly more frequent.[14] These kidneys can also be associated with ectopia; that is they can be located in a pelvic location.[73]

The patient with a horseshoe kidney is often referred to ultrasound for evaluation of a pulsatile mass. On the sonogram, a mass is seen anterior to the abdominal aorta (Fig. 4-38). Instead of immediately considering pancreatic enlargement or lymphadenopathy, the examiner should think about a horseshoe kidney. Using real-time ultrasound, the renal axes should be obtained. The lower poles can be followed into the mass by oblique scanning. The isthmus across the lower poles usually is seen at the fourth to fifth lumbar area[75] (Fig. 4-38). It appears as solid renal tissue.

At times, a patient may have an exaggerated anteroposterior axis to the kidney such that the lower pole is very superficial (Figs. 4-11, 4-39). This patient is often referred to ultrasound for evaluation of a palpable abdominal mass.[76] The kidney is embedded in perirenal fat and lies on the anterior surface of the paravertebral and

psoas muscles. The fat is most abundant behind and inferior to the lower pole of the kidney.[76] The normal axis is parallel to the spine with the lower pole slightly more anterior than the upper pole. Using real-time scanning, one can quickly establish that the mass is indeed the normal lower pole of the kidney (Fig. 4-39). However, careful scanning of the renal fossa should be performed to exclude a mass that is displacing the kidney anteriorly.

Obstructive Uropathy

Hydronephrosis represents dilatation of the renal pelvis and calyces associated with progressive atrophy of the kidney due to obstruction of the outflow of urine. The high pressure in the renal pelvis is transmitted back through the collecting ducts into the cortex causing renal atrophy, also compressing the renal vasculature of the medulla causing a decrease in the inner medullary plasma flow.[14]

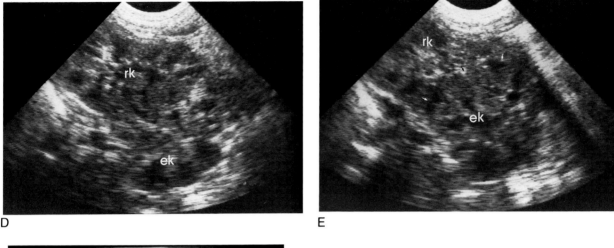

D   E

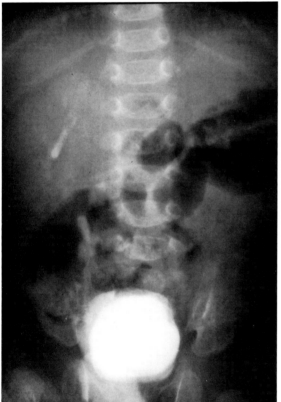

F

Fig. 4-36 *(Continued).* Longitudinal coronal left lateral decubitus scans **(D,E)** lower than the renal fossa, and more medial. A mass (*ek*, arrows) (crossed fused kidney) is seen continuous with the right kidney *(rk).* **(F)** Intravenous pyelogram documenting the finding.

There are numerous causes for hydronephrosis. In addition to identifying the presence of hydronephrosis, the cause should be investigated. The congenital anomalies include posterior urethral valves, urethral strictures, meatal stenosis, bladder neck obstruction, ureteropelvic junction narrowing or obstruction, and severe vesicoureteral reflux. The acquired organic causes for obstruction include calculi, benign prostatic enlargement, tumors (bladder, prostate, contiguous malignant disease, carcinoma of the cervix or uterus), inflammation (prostatitis, ureteritis, urethritis), sloughed papillae or blood clot, normal pregnancy, and functional disorders (neurogenic).[14] Intrinsic causes may include calculus, blood clot, tumor, stricture, ureterocele, pyelonephritis; or congenital etiologies such as UPJ obstruction, posterior urethral valves, or ectopic ureterocele.[53] Extrinsic

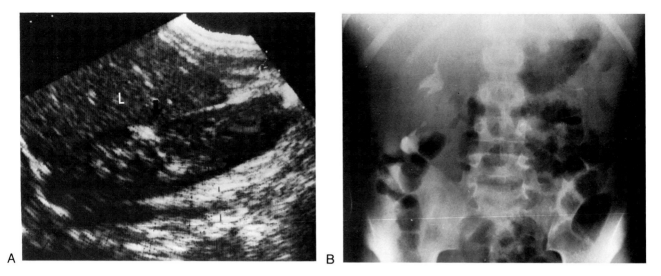

Fig. 4-37. Crossed fused ectopia. Ectopia. **(A)** Longitudinal scan through right renal fossa, demonstrating a reniform structure with a notch (arrow). (*L*, liver.) **(B)** Abdominal radiograph after a contrast CT, showing crossed-fused ectopia. (From McCarthy S, Rosenfield AT: Ultrasonography in crossed renal ectopia. J Ultrasound Med 3:107, 1984.)

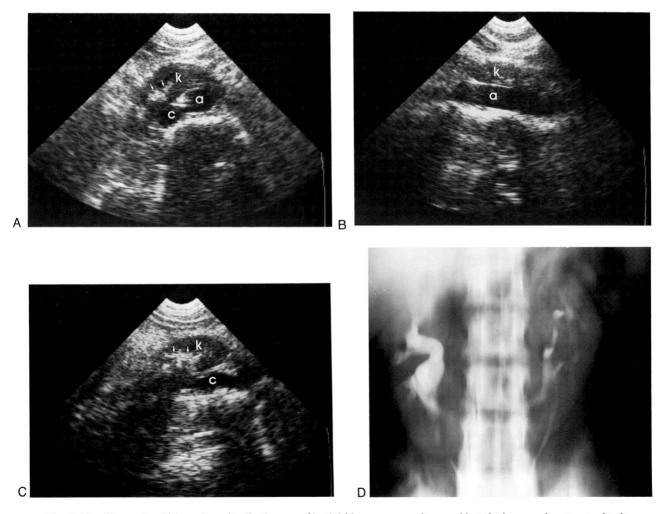

Fig. 4-38. Horseshoe kidney. Longitudinal scans of both kidneys appeared normal but the lower poles appeared to be oriented medially. Transverse scan **(A)** demonstrates a mass *(k)* anterior to aorta *(a)* and inferior vena cava *(c)*. The transducer is angled slightly oblique. Echodense renal sinus echoes (arrows) can be seen. Longitudinal scans reveal a mass *(k)* anterior to the aorta *(a)* **(B)** and inferior vena cava *(c)* **(C)**. Renal sinus echoes (arrows) are seen on **(C)**. **(D)** Intravenous pyelogram confirms the ultrasound findings of a horseshoe kidney.

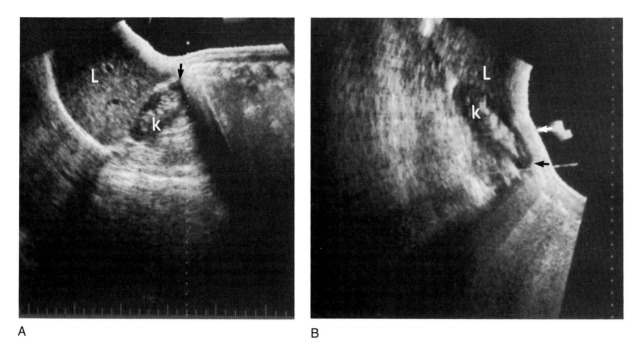

A   B

Fig. 4-39.   Palpable kidney. Thin, young woman with a palpable right abdominal mass. **(A)** Longitudinal supine scan, right kidney *(k)*. Note how anteriorly (arrows) the inferior pole of kidney is. (*L*, liver.) **(B)** Erect, longitudinal scan. The kidney *(k)* is even more superficial. The level (white arrow) of the lower pole in the supine position was marked. In the erect position, the lower pole (black arrow) of the kidney has moved downward. (*L*, liver.)

causes are multiple and include neoplasm, trauma, postoperative, neurogenic bladder, retroperitoneal fibrosis, pregnancy, gynecologic problems (endometrioma, tuboovarian abscess, etc.), and bladder outlet obstruction (caused by neoplasm, prostatic enlargement, and/or urethral problems).[53]

Ultrasound is an accurate modality to screen for hydronephrosis.[77,78] Normally, there is no separation of the dense echo collection in the region of the renal sinus (Figs. 4-1 to 4-3). With mild hydronephrosis, there is slight separation with a lucency noted[67] (Fig. 4-40). With moderate hydronephrosis, there is further separation of the echoes by lucency (Fig. 4-41). In severe hydronephrosis, there is a huge lucent sac seen with marked thinning of the renal parenchyma.[79] (Fig. 4-42). The amount of collecting system dilatation depends on pa-

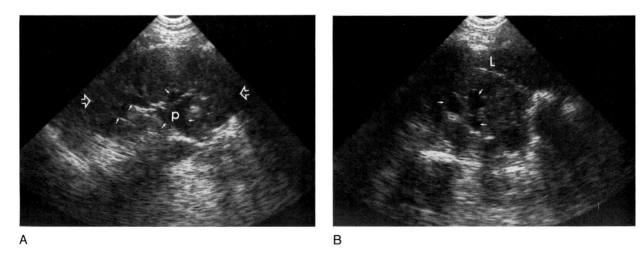

A   B

Fig. 4-40.   Mild hydronephrosis. Longitudinal **(A)** and transverse **(B)** left lateral decubitus scans of the right kidney (open arrows) demonstrate mild dilatation of the collecting system (small arrows). (*p*, pelvis; *L*, liver.)

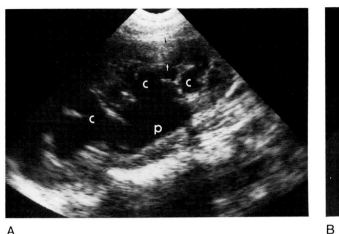

A

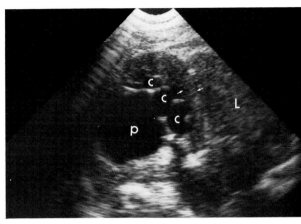

B

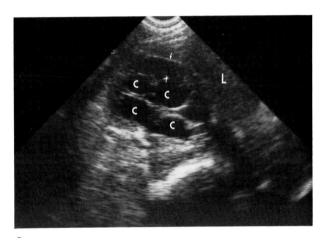

C

Fig. 4-41. Moderate hydronephrosis. Longitudinal **(A)** and transverse **(B,C)** left lateral decubitus scans of the right kidney reveal moderate dilatation of the collecting system (*p*, pelvis; *c*, calyces; *L*, liver). There is a small amount of parenchyma (arrows).

rameters such as duration of obstruction, renal output and presence or absence of spontaneous collecting system decompression.[81] The amount of residual renal cortex identified is of more prognostic significance than the size of the hydronephrotic sac.[53]

There have been reports concerning the influence of hydration and bladder distension on the sonographic diagnosis of hydronephrosis. Findings of moderate bilateral hydronephrosis may be encountered in a dehydrated patient undergoing rehydration. In addition, the filled bladder in a patient undergoing hydration may result in the ultrasound appearance of hydronephrosis (Fig. 4-43). The differentiation between volume depletion and obstructive uropathy is difficult clinically. The ultrasound should be done with an empty bladder and before initiation of rehydration.[80] And, dilatation of the collecting system does not always equate with obstruction.[8] It can be seen with retroperitoneal fibrosis, diabetes insipidus, previous obstruction, ureterovesical reflux, or infection.

The renal sinus is composed of the collecting system structures, vessels, lymphatics, and fibrofatty tissue.

Nonhydronephrotic fragmentation of the central renal complex is usually attributed to nephrolithiasis, renal sinus lipomatosis, and some forms of cystic disease. There are certain entities associated with false negative diagnoses of hydronephrosis. These include staghorn calculus filling the collecting system (acoustic shadow obscures the dilatation) (Figs. 4-44 and 4-45); acute renal obstruction (system not dilated); spontaneous decompression of an obstructive system; numerous cysts with superimposed hydronephrosis; misinterpretation of hydronephrosis or cystic disease; retroperitoneal fibrosis; misinterpretation of calyectasis as large lucent pyramids; fluid-depleted patient with partial obstruction; intermittent obstruction; and technical factors (obesity, adjacent gas, uncooperative patient).[81]

There are false positive causes for the diagnosis of hydronephrosis. These include normal variants (distensible collecting system, extrarenal renal pelvis [Fig. 4-46], full bladder, congenital megacalyces, calyceal diverticulum); increased urine flow (overhydration, medications, osmotic duiresis during or immediately after urography, diabetes insipidus, diuresis in nonoliguric

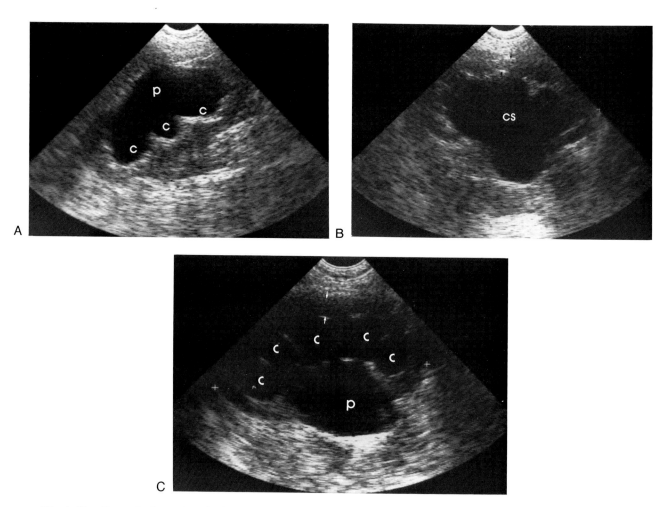

Fig. 4-42. Severe hydronephrosis. Case 1: Longitudinal **(A)** left lateral decubitus scan of the right kidney and longitudinal **(B)** right lateral decubitus scan of the left kidney. The collecting system *(cs)* on the left is more dilated than the right such that there is only a large cystic area. Calyces *(c)* and renal pelvis *(p)* are not distinguished and there is very little parenchyma (arrows). Case 2: **(C)** Similarly to Case 1, this longitudinal scan reveals little renal parenchyma (arrows) with massive dilatation of the collecting system (*p*, pelvis; *c*, calyces).

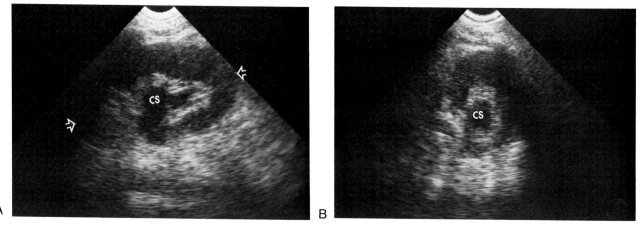

Fig. 4-43. Hydronephrosis and bladder distension. Longitudinal **(A)** and transverse **(B)** scans of the left kidney with dilatation of the collecting system *(cs)*. (Open arrows, renal poles.) The patient was noted to have a distended bladder. *(Figure continues.)*

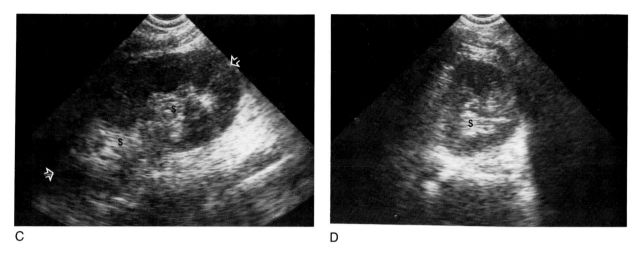

C   D

Fig. 4-43 *(Continued).* After voiding, the kidney was rescanned in longitudinal **(C)** and transverse **(D)** projections and no hydronephrosis was seen. (*s*, renal sinus; open arrows, renal poles.)

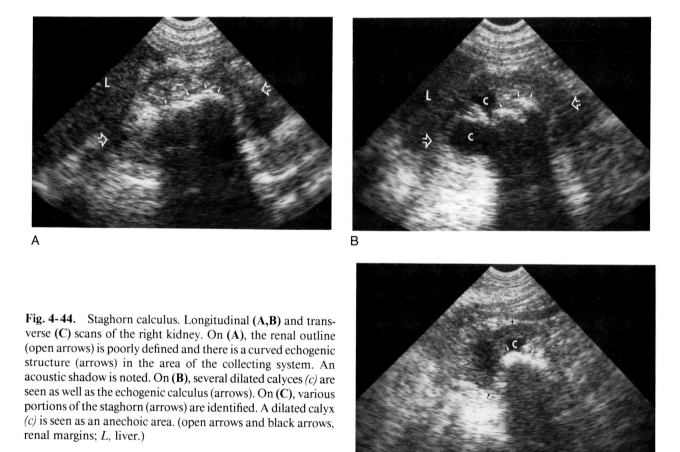

A   B

Fig. 4-44. Staghorn calculus. Longitudinal **(A,B)** and transverse **(C)** scans of the right kidney. On **(A)**, the renal outline (open arrows) is poorly defined and there is a curved echogenic structure (arrows) in the area of the collecting system. An acoustic shadow is noted. On **(B)**, several dilated calyces *(c)* are seen as well as the echogenic calculus (arrows). On **(C)**, various portions of the staghorn (arrows) are identified. A dilated calyx *(c)* is seen as an anechoic area. (open arrows and black arrows, renal margins; *L,* liver.)

C

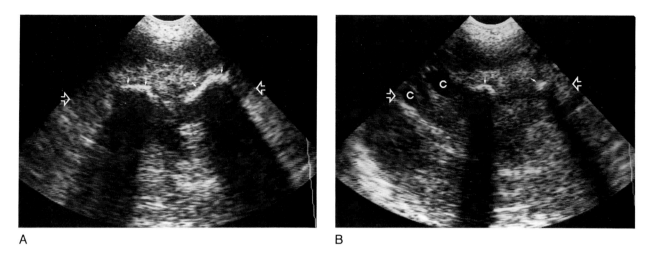

A

B

Fig. 4-45. Staghorn calculus. Longitudinal scans **(A,B)** of the left kidney demonstrate echodensities (small arrows) in the area of the renal sinus. There is marked posterior acoustic shadowing and as such it is difficult to assess for a dilated collecting system. (*c*, calyces.)

azotemia); inflammatory disease (acute pyelonephritis, chronic pyelonephritis, tuberculosis); renal cystic disease (single cyst, parapelvic cyst [Fig. 4-27], adult polycystic kidney disease [Figs. 4-20, 4-21], medullary cystic disease [Fig. 4-23], multicystic-dysplastic kidney); and other causes like postobstructive or postsurgical dilatation, vesicoureteral reflux, papillary necrosis, and renal sinus lipomatosis.[18,53,81]

CONGENITAL CAUSES

Ureteropelvic Junction Obstruction. Ureteropelvic junction (UPJ) obstruction is a common cause of severe pyelocaliectasis in the child.[82,83] The patient may present with a flank mass or urinary tract infection. On ultrasound the dilated renal pelvis without ureteral dilatation would be seen[83] (Figs. 4-28 to 4-30). With severe UPJ obstruction, the calyces and pelvis become one large lucent mass.[82] This entity was more extensively discussed earlier in the chapter under the Congenital section.

Duplex Collecting System. With a duplex system, hydronephrosis involving either or both systems is visible (Figs. 4-31 and 4-47). Dilatation of a duplex collecting system is fairly common with the upper system more often dilated. Occasionally, there can be hydronephrosis of the lower pole system resulting in nonvisualization of

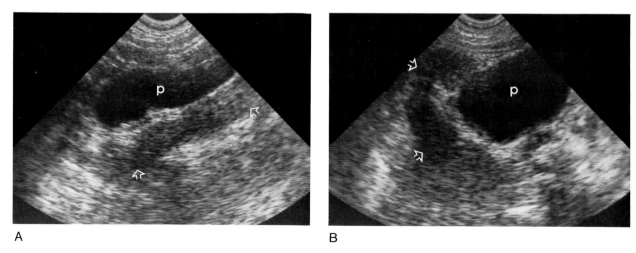

A

B

Fig. 4-46. Extrarenal pelvis. Longitudinal **(A)** and transverse **(B)** scans of the right kidney. A large anechoic area *(p)* is seen representing the dilated extrarenal pelvis. It is seen anterior to the renal parenchyma (open arrows) on the medial longitudinal view **(A)** and medial on the transverse view **(B)**. The calyces were not dilated and the patient was asymptomatic.

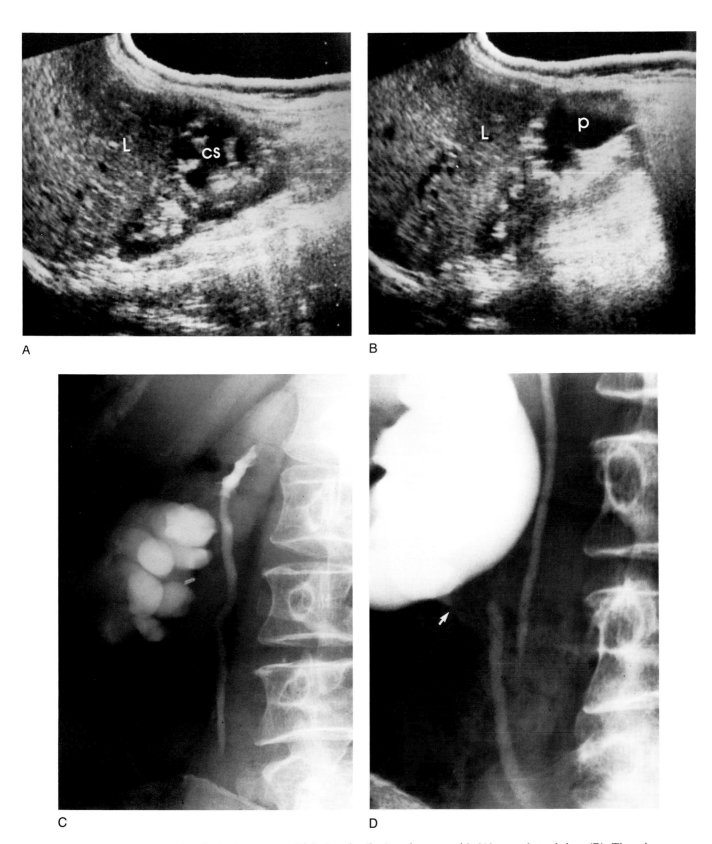

Fig. 4-47. Hydronephrotic duplex system. Right longitudinal static scans with **(A)** more lateral than **(B)**. There is dilatation of the lower pole collecting system *(cs)* with dilatation of the pelvis *(p)* seen on **(B)**. (*L*, liver.) **(C,D)** Intravenous pyelogram demonstrating the bifid system on the right with hydronephrosis of the lower collecting system. On **(D)**, high grade obstruction (arrow) is noted at the lower pole consistent with a ureteropelvic junction obstruction.

the lower pole on intravenous pyelogram simulating a mass.[84] With ultrasound, the typical hydronephrosis pattern is seen (Fig. 4-47). Dilatation of the upper or lower pole system may be caused by reflux. There is significant dilatation of the ureter and upper system in 85 percent of those with ureteroceles.[67] With real-time imaging, churning of urine within the ureter or within the calyces may be visible.[85] There may be ureteropelvic junction obstruction of either system if a dilated ureter is not seen. The examiner should search for a ureterocele when dilatation of an upper duplicated system is seen.

Infundibulopelvic Stenosis.

Infundibulopelvic stenosis is characterized by caliceal dilatation, infundibular stenosis, and hypoplasia or stenosis of the renal pelvis.[86] It is a rare congenital form of hydrocalycosis in which dilated calyces drain through a stenotic infundibulum into a variably hypoplastic or stenosed renal pelvis. It belongs to a spectrum of obstructive dysplasic renal diseases, from generalized pyelocaliectasis secondary to ureteral or ureteropelvic stenosis at one end, to functionless dysplastic kidney at the other.[86] Hydrocalycosis denotes dilatation of one or more calyces secondary to infundibular stenosis, which may be intrinsic or extrinsic. The extrinsic variety is usually congenital and in most cases results from vascular compression of the infundibulum draining the calyces. The acquired type is caused by trauma or a space-occupying lesion. Hydrocalycosis secondary to intrinsic stenosis may be congenital or secondary to an acquired lesion such as infection, tumor, or trauma. On the sonogram a variable degree of caliceal dilatation without associated pelvic dilatation is seen (Fig. 4-48). The differential diagnosis of infundibular stenosis must include the usual type of hydronephrosis as well as megacalycosis and any space-occupying lesion of the renal hilum, such as a parapelvic cyst or tumor.

Renal Cystic Disease.

At times, it may be difficult to differentiate severe hydronephrosis from severe renal cystic disease. The identification of a dilated renal pelvis is the most reliable indicator of hydronephrosis.[87] If no dilated renal pelvis is seen, then the diagnosis is more likely cystic disease. When there is end-stage hydronephrosis, the differentiation may be particularly difficult. With severe hydronephrosis there is often less normal renal parenchyma. To differentiate the two entities one should look for the following: (1) hepatic cysts, bilateral involvement, calculi, uniform size of cysts — suggestive of cystic disease; or (2) central circular lucency with small interconnecting lucencies (collecting system) — suggestive of hydronephrosis.[87]

Miscellaneous Causes of Hydronephrosis.

Hydronephrosis may be secondary to ureteral obstruction. Ureterovesical obstruction is most commonly secondary to extrinsic compression. This may be due to a pelvic lymphoma, pelvic abscess, ovarian mass, or a large abdominal mass. The dilated ureters are seen as tubular lucencies extending from the kidney to the bladder. On a transverse scan, they are seen as circular lucencies posterior to the bladder (Fig. 4-32). If ureteral dilatation is seen proximal to an adynamic narrowed segment of the distal ureter, primary megaureter may be the diagnosis. With a stenotic ureteral orifice, there may be ballooning of the submucosal segment such as a ureterocele, which may prolapse into the bladder outlet causing the obstruction. In most cases of ureteral obstruction, ultrasound is not capable of locating the exact site of the obstruction.[83]

Bladder outlet, urethral obstruction, or nonobstructive dilatation is usually bilateral. The bladder outlet may be obstructed by congenital anomalies such as duplication, septation, or tumor. Urethral obstruction may be due to an anatomic lesion such as posterior urethral valves, or posttraumatic urethral stricture. Functional urethral obstruction may be produced by spasm of the external urinary sphincter (neurogenic bladder).[83]

There may be some degree of hydronephrosis associated with other congenital abnormalities not previously mentioned. With renal dysmorphism and dysplasia, there may be some dilatation with obstruction. In congenital megacalyces, there are congenital, abnormally dilated, blunted supernumerary calyces that may be associated with a nonobstructive, nonreflux dilatation. In Eagle-Barrett syndrome (prune belly or abdominal muscle deficiency), there is dilatation of the calyces, ureters, bladder, posterior urethra, and occasionally the anterior urethra. The degree of dilatation is variable but often is marked. Seventy percent of these patients have vesicoureteral reflux that contributes to the dilatation.[83]

CORRELATIVE IMAGING AND ACCURACY

Real-time is the preferred ultrasound method for scanning due to the greater flexibility and shorter scan time. In one series comparing the accuracy of real-time versus static scanning, real-time demonstrated an overall accuracy of 94 percent, as opposed to 93 percent for static scanning.[79] Other authors have reported a sensitivity of 98 percent for ultrasound when compared to urography.[78,88] Ultrasound is most accurate (100 percent) in moderate to severe hydronephrosis.[78] The inaccuracies are in the area of minimal hydronephrosis. This pattern may be seen normally without hydronephrosis with a

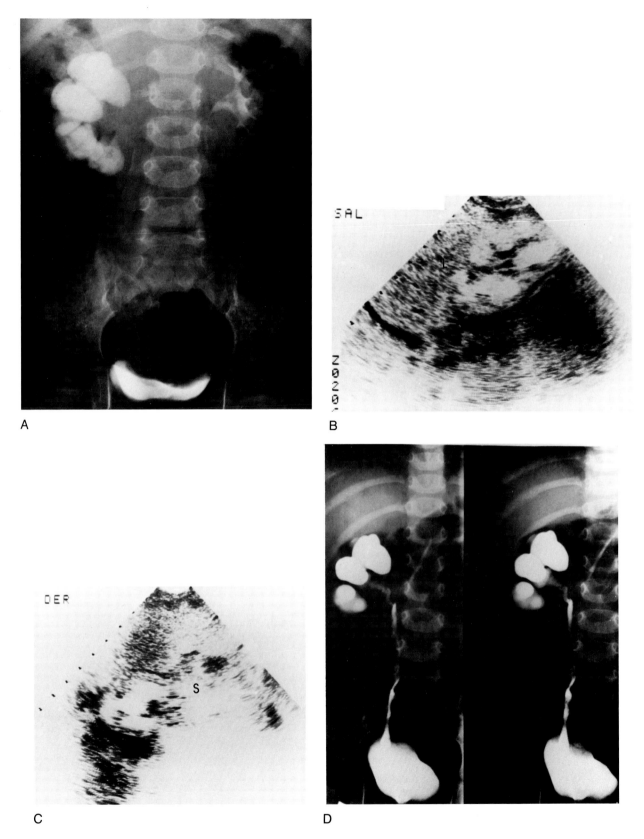

Fig. 4-48. Infundibulopelvis stenosis. **(A)** Excretory urogram 20 minutes after injection. The left kidney is normal. There is severe dilatation of all calyces of the right kidney. Part of the right ureter is seen, but the right pelvis is not seen. Longitudinal **(B)** and transverse **(C)** scans of the right kidney show severe caliceal dilatation. The renal pelvis is not identified. (*L*, liver; *S*, spine.) **(D)** Retrograde ureteropyelogram. A hypoplastic renal pelvis and severe caliceal dilatation are demonstrated. (From Lucaya J, Enriquez G, Delgado R, Castellote A: Infundibulopelvic stenosis in children. AJR 142:471, © American Roentgen Ray Society, 1984.)

full renal pelvis. It may also be seen with multiple para-pelvic cysts.

How accurate is ultrasound in diagnosing hydronephrosis in the patient with chronic renal disease and decreased renal output? Whenever there is obstruction of the urinary outflow, there is elevation of the hydrostatic pressure proximal to the obstruction with eventual transmission of the pressure through the renal tubules to the glomerulus. The ultimate effect on the glomerular filtrate rate is variable, depending on a balance among blood flow, filtration pressure and intratubular pressure, site of obstruction, degree and duration of the obstruction, and rapidity of onset. This is reflected in the extent of the dilatation of the collecting system. Whatever the cause, the precipitous effect of all these variables coupled with dehydration and sepsis apparently results in a markedly decreased urinary output and thus little or no dilatation. As such minimal dilatation in a patient with chronic renal disease may actually represent significant hydronephrosis.[89,90]

Ultrasound appears to be more accurate than nuclear medicine with regard to hydronephrosis. In one study, ultrasound demonstrated a sensitivity of 90 percent with a specificity of 98 percent and an accuracy of 97 percent.[91] Nuclear medicine had a specificity of 89 percent with an accuracy of 88 percent.[91] Nuclear medicine was less sensitive in detecting obstruction, particularly in the presence of chronic renal disease but offered additional information regarding relative blood flow, total effective renal plasma flow, and interval change in renal parenchymal function. While each technique had its advantages, ultrasound was highly sensitive and specific regardless of the degree of renal function impairment.[91]

PREGNANCY

Hydronephrosis is often seen in pregnancy. The incidence of right hydronephrosis is greater (90 percent) than that on the left (67 percent).[92,93] The calyceal diameter of both kidneys is found to increase gradually through pregnancy, with the right increasing more rapidly than the left. There is less likely to be pathologic dilatation when minimal dilatation is seen in an asymptomatic patient.[92] As such, the finding of dilatation should be interpreted with caution because there are sequential variations. Neither parity nor history of urinary tract problems are found to be relevant to the degree of dilatation.

The etiology of hydronephrosis in pregnancy is controversial. Mechanical pressure of the gravid uterus is felt to be the most important pressure on the ureter as it crosses the pelvic brim.[92] This is thought to cause partial obstruction of flow of urine, increasing the pressure in the proximal ureter and subsequent ureteral and pelvic dilatation. Other theories for the production of the hydronephrosis are hormonal. The high progesterone level of pregnancy produces smooth muscle relaxation of the ureteral walls that is analogous to progesterone induced smooth muscle relaxation of the uterus.[93]

RENAL COLIC

One group of investigators have evaluated the role of ultrasound in patients with renal colic.[94,95] To adequately assess these patients, they are hydrated to emphasize mild early caliectasis and ureterectasis plus to fill the bladder. The kidneys are evaluated for calculi, hydronephrosis, and perinephric fluid; the pelvis for the distal ureter, hydroureter, ureterovesical junction calculi, ureterovesical junction edema, and the presence of ureteral jets (discussed under the section on ureters). The criterion for a positive examination is visualization of a urinary tract calculus or unilateral hydronephrosis with or without ureterectasia[95] (Fig. 4-49). This has a sensitivity of 100 percent with a specificity of 95 percent.[95] Eighty-nine percent of those with proven calculi have unilateral hydronephrosis and 17 percent have perirenal fluid.[95] Stones are seen with ultrasound that are not visualized by radiography. The use of ultrasound in the initial evaluation of renal colic is recommended.

URINOMA

The possibility of urinary extravasation or urinoma should be considered if a lucent lesion is seen around a hydronephrotic kidney and a renal nuclear medicine scan confirms the finding. Such urinary leaks are caused by renal injuries, an operation, infection, tumor, calculous erosion, or ureteral obstruction of acute or gradual onset. When the urinary tract is obstructed acutely by a pathologic process or abdominal compression or both, the resultant increase in intraluminal pressure, augmented by a sudden diuretic load of urographic contrast may lead to a rupture at the weakest point. In an otherwise healthy upper urinary tract, the point of rupture is at the caliceal fornices and extravasation of urine dissects into the loose connective tissue of the renal sinus and is absorbed by the lymphatics. This extravasation is transient and relatively innocuous. Extravasation of urine from a tear in the collecting system affected by chronic obstruction, infection, calculous erosion, or tumor usually has grave significance and requires surgery. This urinary extravasation may cause retroperitoneal fibrosis, stricture of the upper ureter or a perinephric abscess. This urine infiltrates the retroperitoneal perirenal area producing a fibroblastic cavity that confines the urine in about 5 to 12 days and produces dense connective tissue encapsulation in 3 to 6 weeks.[96] This cavity is called a urinoma or perirenal pseudocyst.[96] This urinoma or uriniferous perirenal pseudocyst is usually located in the perirenal space between Gerota's fascia and the renal capsule.[97] It is elliptical in shape and orients inferomedially often displacing the adjacent kidney upward.

Ultrasound is a sensitive method for demonstrating

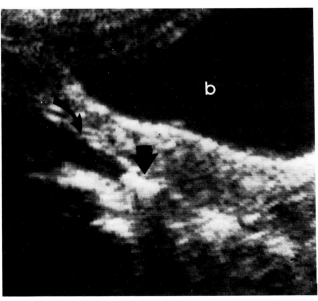

A

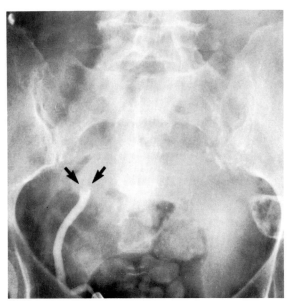

B

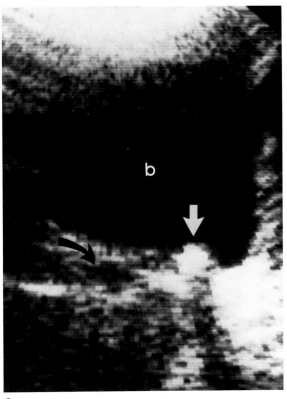

C

Fig. 4-49. Ureterovesical calculus. Case 1: Distal ureteral calculus. **(A)** Longitudinal scan near the bladder *(b)* demonstrates an echogenic calculus (large arrow) with posterior shadowing within the distended ureter (curved arrow). **(B)** Retrograde ureterogram confirms the presence of a nonopaque calculus (arrows) within the distal right ureter. **(C)** One week later, longitudinal scan demonstrates the calculus (straight arrow), which has moved to the ureterovesical junction. Note the dilated ureter (curved arrow). (*b*, bladder.) *(Figure continues.)*

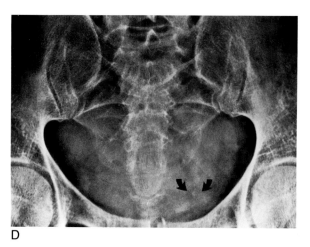

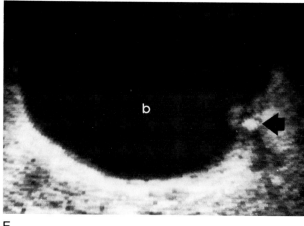

Fig. 4-49 *(Continued).* Case 2: Ureterovesical junction calculus. **(D)** Abdominal radiograph shows a small left-sided pelvic calcification (curved arrows). **(E)** Transverse scan demonstrating an echogenic calculus (arrow) with posterior acoustic shadowing. Note the mound of edematous tissue at the ureterovesical junction. (*b*, bladder.) (From Erwin BC, Carroll BA, Sommer FG: Renal colic: The role of ultrasound in initial evaluation. Radiology 152:147, 1984.)

such collections of urine or urinomas. A hypoechoic or anechoic mass is seen associated with the kidney (Figs. 4-50 to 4-52). However, the ultrasound diagnosis of a urinoma is not specific. The differential diagnosis of such an ultrasound pattern must include lymphocele, hematoma, abscess, cyst, pancreatic pseudocyst, or even ascites. The diagnosis of urinoma may be confirmed by nuclear medicine, excretory urography, or ultrasound guided aspiration of the fluid. A negative nuclear medicine study or excretory urography does not exclude urinoma. The aspirated fluid should be sent for biochemical analysis. At times it is difficult to differentiate the above entities by this method in the poorly functioning kidney when the urea concentration in the urine and serum are similar.[96]

EVALUATION OF THE NONFUNCTIONING KIDNEY

Since ultrasound is independent of renal function, it is the ideal modality for evaluation of the kidney not visualized on excretory urography.[98-101] Ultrasound has the capability to confirm the presence of a kidney and evaluate its size and configuration regardless of renal function.[98] In the child, the differential diagnosis would include ureteropelvic junction obstruction (Figs. 4-28 to 4-30), multicystic kidney (Figs. 4-14 to 4-16), unilateral renal vein thrombosis, and Wilms' tumor. In the adult, 75 percent of cases will be due to hydronephrosis with tumor also included in the differential.[100] Other etiologies to be considered in the differential diagnosis of a

nonvisualized kidney would include chronic infarction, unilateral polycystic kidney disease, agenesis, ectopia, fractured kidney, replacement lipomatosis, and xanthogranulomatous pyelonephritis.[68] (Many of these entities have been discussed or will be discussed later in this chapter).

If the nonvisualized kidney is normal-sized or enlarged, tumor might be a consideration. A renal mass may produce nonvisualization by extensive destruction of the parenchyma or obstruction of either blood flow or urine flow[102] (Fig. 4-53). Renal cell carcinoma is the most common mass that produces nonfunction by parenchymal infiltration, obstruction of the collecting system, vascular thrombosis, or compression, with the most common mechanism—that of renal vein occlusion by tumor extension into the lumen[102] (Fig. 4-53). Other masses producing nonfunction include transitional cell carcinoma, an inflammatory mass, and adult polycystic kidney disease (Fig. 4-20).

There are other causes of nonvisualization of a normal or enlarged kidney. This includes primary cortical disease or medullary involvement or disease processes affecting the pyelocalyceal region.[102] Disease processes such as leukemia and amyloid can affect any portion of the kidney. (These entities are discussed later in this chapter.)

With a small nonvisualized kidney, the offending process may be unilateral or bilateral. The most common mechanical causes of a small nonfunctioning kidney are infarction, ischemia, infection, glomerulonephritis, and nephrosclerosis.[102]

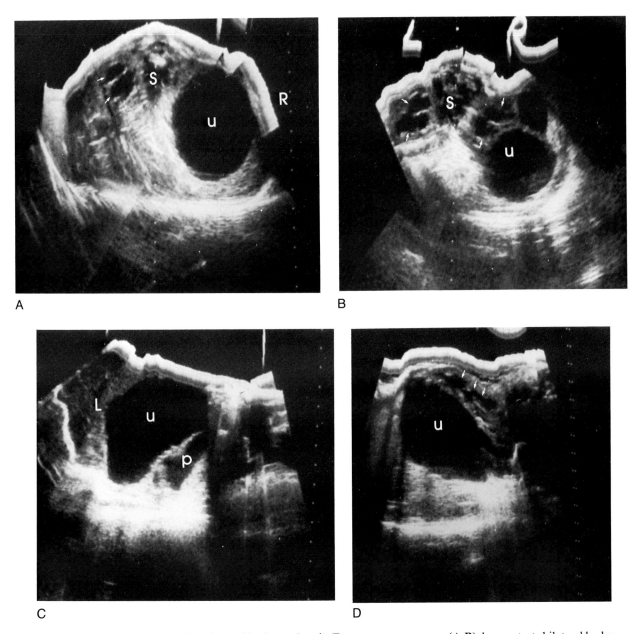

Fig. 4-50. Urinoma. Infant with bilateral hydronephrosis. Transverse prone scans **(A,B)** demonstrate bilateral hydronephrosis (arrows) with a large cystic mass *(u)* on the right *(R)*. (*S*, spine) Longitudinal supine **(C)** and prone **(D)** scans of
the right kidney. A urinoma *(u)* is seen as an anechoic mass superior to the hydronephrotic kidney. (*L*, liver; *p*, pelvis;
arrows, calyces). (Figs. **C** and **D** from Seeds JW, Mittelstaedt CA, Mandell J: Pre- and postnatal ultrasound diagnosis of
congenital obstructive uropathies. Urol Clin North Am 13:131, 1986.)

PYONEPHROSIS

Pyonephrosis is a known and serious complication of
hydronephrosis that develops as a direct consequence of
urinary stasis and secondary infection. It is defined as the
presence of pus in a dilated collecting system.[103] It is seen
with a spectrum of disease processes from infected hydronephrosis to xanthogranulomatous pyelonephritis.

Renal function may have virtually ceased in this entity
with *Escherichia coli* the most common offending organism. As renal function decreases, bacteria and pus fill
the collecting system.[104] Pathologically, there is purulent
exudate composed of sloughed urothelium and a variety
of inflammatory cells. The amount of tissue and cellular
debris varies and is determined by the type and severity
of the inflammatory process.[105]

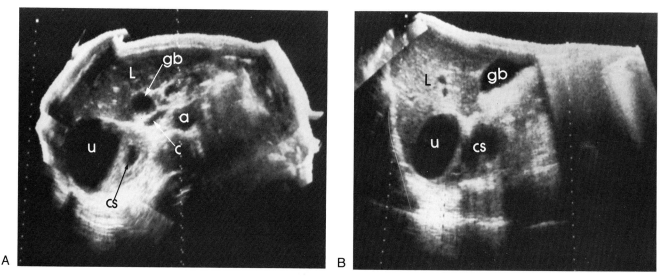

Fig. 4-51. Urinoma. Adult with prostatic carcinoma and hydronephrosis. Supine transverse (**A**) and longitudinal (**B**) scans demonstrate an anechoic mass *(u)* that is superior and lateral to the hydronephrotic right kidney. *(cs,* dilated collecting system; *gb,* gallbladder; *L,* liver; *c,* inferior vena cava; *a,* aorta; *S,* spine.)

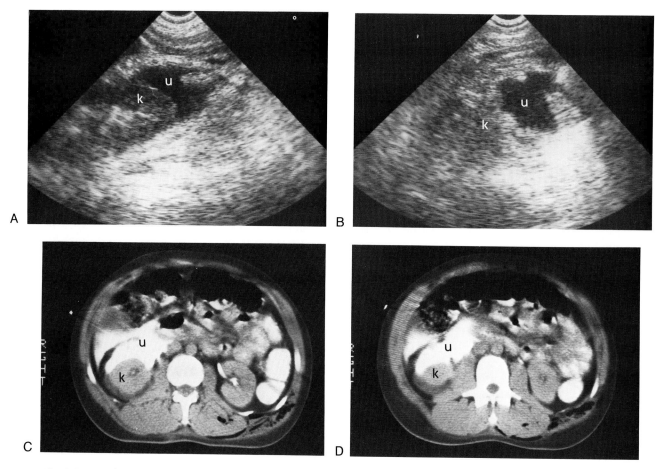

Fig. 4-52. Urinoma. Young adult who was in an automobile accident and suffered renal trauma. Longitudinal (**A**) and transverse (**B**) supine scans demonstrate an anechoic mass *(u)* inferior and medial to the right kidney *(k)*. (**B**) is just below the lower pole of the kidney. No hydronephrosis is noted. (**C,D**) CT scans with (**D**) at the level of the lower pole of the kidney *(k)*. Extravasation *(u)* of contrast can be seen anterior and medial to the right kidney.

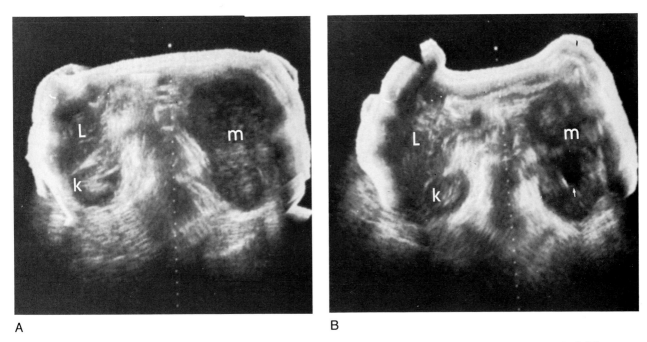

A   B

Fig. 4-53. Nonvisualized kidney—Tumor. Renal cell carcinoma. Transverse supine scans at 8 **(A)** and 12 **(B)** cm above the iliac crest. A large solid mass *(m)* is seen to fill the left abdomen. The left kidney as such is not identified. The mass is mainly echogenic but does have some lucent (arrow) areas. (*L*, liver; *k*, right kidney.) The left kidney did not visualize on intravenous pyelogram.

Prompt and reliable diagnosis of this entity and its differentiation from hydronephrosis is of the utmost importance in clinical practice because the medical implications and therapeutic management differ. The diagnosis of pyonephrosis should be suspected with the appearance of the clinical symptoms of fever and flank pain, combined with radiographic evidence of hydrone-phrosis. The ultrasound diagnosis is based on the presence of internal echoes dispersed or dependent within a dilated pelvocalyceal system with a shifting urine-debris level within the obstructed pyelocalyceal system[103,105,106] (Fig. 4-54). Additional ultrasound findings with pyonephrosis include persistent dependent echoes; shifting urine-debris level; dense peripheral echoes with shadow-

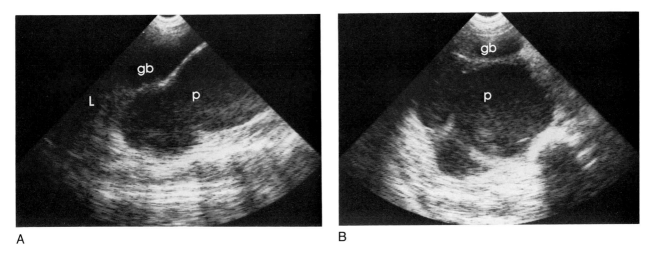

A   B

Fig. 4-54. Pyonephrosis. Same pregnant patient as Figure 4-30. The patient became septic and there are noted to be increased echoes (nonlayering) now seen within the renal pelvis *(p)* on longitudinal **(A)** and transverse **(B)** scans. The dilated system was drained via percutaneous catheter with ultrasound guidance. (*gb*, gallbladder; *L*, liver.)

ing secondary to gas-forming organisms; and poor transonicity with echoes completely filling the pelvis and calyces.[103,104] The ultrasound diagnosis has been found to be 97 percent specific in simple hydronephrosis with the diagnosis of pyonephrosis 90 percent specific.[105] Using ultrasound guidance, aspiration of the collecting system may be performed to make a definitive diagnosis. If pus is obtained, a percutaneous catheter may be inserted for drainage of the infected urine and evaluation of residual kidney function before surgery. The catheter can be used for diagnostic nephrostogram, ureteral perfusion, therapeutic dissolution of stones, and indefinite drainage of the kidney.[103]

PERCUTANEOUS NEPHROSTOMY

Percutaneous nephrostomy has become a well-established technique for permanent or temporary urinary diversion.[107-115] The application of ultrasound and percutaneous puncture techniques in the diagnosis of various fluid-filled renal anomalies permit rapid delineation of anatomic detail, more definitive physiological evaluation, and drainage when necessary in a safe and cost-effective manner.[116] The indications for the procedure are multiple.[116,117] In the azotemic patient with bilateral obstruction or obstruction of a single functioning kidney, this procedure is the initial treatment of choice for severe obstructive renal failure. The treatment of pyonephrosis with percutaneous drainage provides the most gratifying setting for this procedure. The septicemic patient with gram-negative shock, shows prompt clinical improvement and develops clear urine within 24 to 48 hours. Other indications for percutaneous nephrostomy would include uncertain functional capacity of an obstructed kidney; contraindications to immediate surgery; and expected brief duration of the obstruction. A ureteral fistula may close if a percutaneous catheter drains the urine. This catheter can be used for calculus irrigation and possibly even calculus extraction and/or an antegrade pyelogram.[107] Additionally, it can also be used for ureteral stent insertion. A stent is a catheter that extends from the pelvocalyceal system across the ureteral narrowing to provide internal drainage into the bladder or an intestinal conduit.[113] A stent is seen on ultrasound as a tubular structure within the collecting system (Fig. 4-55). Ultrasound can be used to evaluate for hydronephrosis following stent placement.

The indications for percutaneous nephrostomy in neonates, infants, and children include preservation of renal function while awaiting growth of the infant, preservation of renal function in anticipation of relief of transient obstruction, drainage of pyonephrosis, and assessment of reversibility of the impaired renal function.[118]

The procedure itself may be performed with ultrasound alone, with a combination of ultrasound and fluoroscopy, or with fluoroscopy alone.[113] By using the combined approach, there is less radiation and fewer needle sticks.[112,119] The choice of the guidance is influenced heavily by the background and biases of the operator and to a lesser extent by the imaging equipment available. To establish a functioning nephrostomy requires three basic steps: (1) a needle or trocar puncture of the pelvocalyceal system; (2) replacement of the needle or trocar by a catheter with or without the aid of intermediary instruments; and (3) optimal positioning of the catheter within the system.[113] (A more detailed description of the procedure is given in Chapter 10.)

The success rate of the procedure has been reported to be 97 to 100 percent.[113] Its success depends on the placement and the maintenance of adequate drainage. There is a 4 percent incidence of significant complications with a 0.2 percent incidence of mortality (surgical mortality 6 percent). The only relative contraindication is bleeding diathesis.[113]

Inflammatory Disease

ACUTE PYELONEPHRITIS

Infection is the most common disease of the urinary tract and constitutes 75 percent of patients' problems requiring urologic evaluation.[120] Most bacterial pyelonephritis occurs via an ascending route beginning at the level of the bladder and ascending to the kidney. The avenue for such spread is via the subepithelial lymphatic channels of the bladder and ureter and then the renal interstitium. The spread is facilitated by the presence of obstruction, ureteric reflux, or a deformed urinary tract.[120] The most common organism is *E. coli,* which usually responds well to therapy with antibiotics.[106] Patients with such conditions as neurogenic bladder, bladder malignancy, a history of debilitating disease, chemotherapy or intravenous abuse, prolonged catheter drainage and reflux, altered host resistence, trauma, diabetes and urinary tract infection, as well as pregnancy have an increased incidence of this disease process.[106,121]

The combination of parenchymal, caliceal, and pelvic inflammation constitutes pyelonephritis. The kidney is enlarged by inflammatory edema and contains foci of intense inflammation with microabscess formation with infiltration by polymorphonuclear cells throughout the involved interstitial tissue. This results in purulent casts in the collecting tubules, and often inflammatory reaction in the pelvic and caliceal epithelium.[121] The upper urinary tract infection may first involve only the lining membranes of the renal pelvis. Then, infection spreads through the pyramids to the cortex to produce pyelonephritis. Focal areas of inflammation that progress to

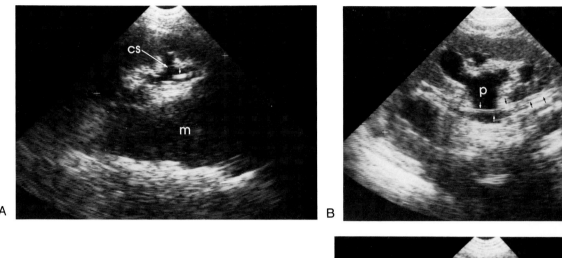

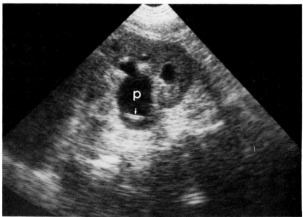

Fig. 4-55. Ureteral stent. Case 1: Non-Hodgkin's lymphoma with paraortic nodes. Longitudinal **(A)** prone scan of the left kidney. The collecting system *(cs)* is dilated with a tubular structure (stent, arrow) seen within it. There is a large solid lymphomatous mass *(m)* anterior to the kidney. Case 2: There is moderate hydronephrosis noted in this patient poststent placement on these longitudinal **(B)** and transverse **(C)** scans of the right kidney. The dilated calyces and pelvis *(p)* are seen as well as the stent (arrows) within the pelvis and ureter.

suppuration forming microabscesses may coalesce to form carbuncles. This may extend to the perinephric space.[120]

On ultrasound the affected kidney is noted to be en-larged with an increased anechoic corticomedullary area with multiple scattered low-level echoes[106,120-124] (Fig. 4-56). This pattern is produced by the multiple small abscesses and necrosis in the outer part of the medulla

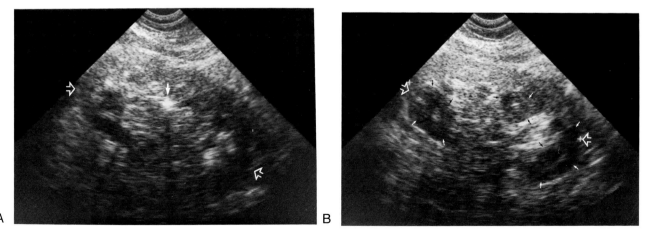

Fig. 4-56. Acute pyelonephritis. Longitudinal **(A,B)** scans of the left kidney. The kidney is enlarged (open arrows) with poor definition between the renal sinus and parenchyma. There appears to be a calculus (arrow) with shadowing within the collecting system on **(A)**. On **(B)**, there are increased anechoic corticomedullary areas (small arrows) with multiple scattered low level echoes.

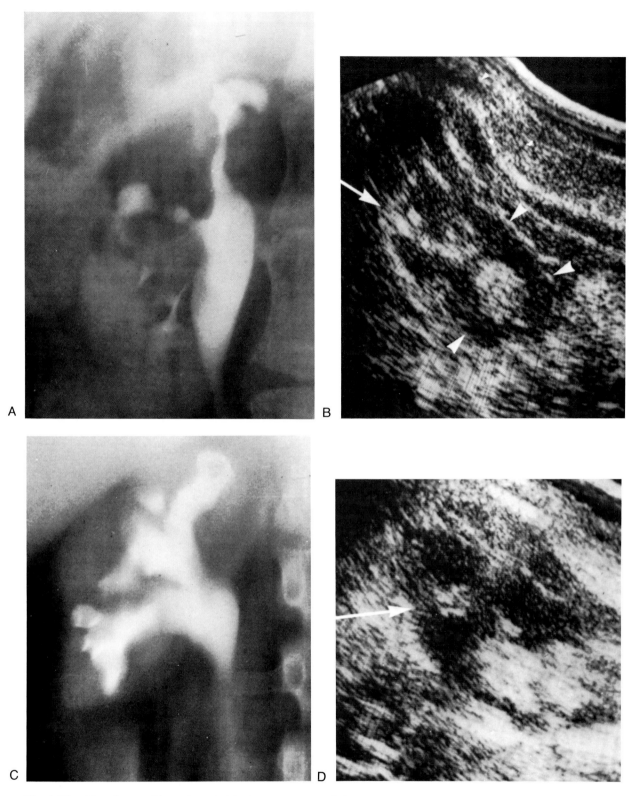

Fig. 4-57. Chronic atrophic pyelonephritis. Case 1: **(A)** There is focal scarring and calyceal retraction in the upper pole of the right kidney, typical of chronic atrophic pyelonephritis. **(B)** Right kidney (arrowheads) with patient prone. There is focal loss of parenchyma, extension of a calyx from renal sinus to renal margin, and associated focal increased echogenicity due to fibrosis (arrow) in the upper pole. Case 2: **(C)** There is focal scarring in both upper and lower poles of the right kidney with associated calyceal blunting. **(D)** Right kidney prone. Focal scarring and extension of the renal sinus to the renal margin in the upper pole of the right kidney (arrow) and increased echogenicity and loss of parenchyma in the lower pole are apparent. (From Kay CJ, Rosenfield AT, Taylor KJW, Rosenberg MA: Ultrasonic characteristics of chronic atrophic pyelonephritis. AJR 132:47, © American Roentgen Ray Society, 1979.)

and cortex.[122] The backwall of the affected kidney is stronger than that of the corresponding normal kidney because the infected kidney has an increased fluid content[122] (Fig. 4-56).

CHRONIC ATROPHIC PYELONEPHRITIS

There are several etiologies for chronic atrophic pyelonephritis. This process may involve the full thickness of the kidney with retraction of the papilla, dilatation of the surrounding calyx, depression of the surface and loss of renal parenchyma, and, most commonly, vesicoureteral reflux. There may be a focal or multifocal process with loss of renal parenchyma, retraction of one or more calyces, decrease in renal size and increased echoes from fibrosis.[125] The focal fibrosis produces increased echoes in the involved area of the medulla and cortex (Fig. 4-57). With retraction of a calyx, if it is not distended, an echogenic zone is seen to extend beyond the normal area of the renal sinus[125] (Fig. 4-57). Focal abnormalities associated with other disease processes such as acute or chronic glomerulonephritis, diabetic glomerulosclerosis, acute tubular necrosis, and Alport's disease usually produce a generalized increase in cortical echoes and preserve the lucent medulla leading to accentuated normal anatomy.

MEGALOCYSTIC INTERSTITIAL NEPHRITIS

Megalocystic interstitial nephritis is a very rare condition similar to renal malacoplakia, which mainly involves the renal cortex and to some extent the medullary

region. The precise etiology is not completely understood but it does appear to be an immunoresponse to certain strains of bacteria, mainly *E. coli* or *Aerobacter aerogenes.* In the absence of obstruction, the excretory urogram shows decreased or normal function depending on the stage of the disease. On ultrasound an enlarged kidney is seen with an overall increased transonic response (Fig. 4-58). The calyceal echoes are splayed and compressed centrally by peripheral, ill-circumscribed masses that contain low-level echoes.[126]

ACUTE FOCAL BACTERIAL NEPHRITIS

Acute focal bacterial nephritis or acute lobar nephronia is an inflammatory mass without drainable pus.[127,128] The offending organism is usually a gram-negative bacteria that probably ascends through ureteral reflux.[127] The patient generally presents with fever, chills, and flank pain.[129] Excretory urography during the acute renal infection often is normal but may show diffuse enlargement, delayed calyceal filling, dilatation, or distortion of the collecting system[127,129] (Fig. 4-59A). Focal renal enlargement is a rare urographic abnormality with acute pyelonephritis.[127]

The ultrasound appearance of acute focal bacterial nephritis is characteristic: a poorly defined mass is seen containing echoes of a lower amplitude than normal renal cortex, which may disrupt the corticomedullary junction[120,121,124,127-129] (Figs. 4-59B and C). When the lesion is followed with ultrasound while under antibiotic therapy, anechoic areas may be seen representing liquefaction. With further follow-up, the mass should resolve

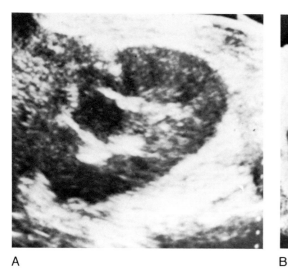 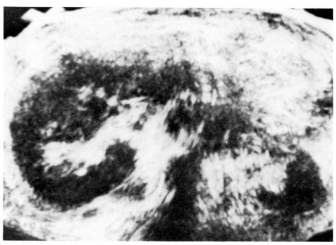

A   B

Fig. 4-58. Megalocystic interstitial nephritis. **(A)** Supine longitudinal scan, right kidney. No focal cystic components are seen. Notice enhanced sonic transmission by the kidney. **(B)** Transverse views of both kidneys reveal massive uniform enlargement of the right kidney and thickening of the capsular area. (From Gonzalez AC, Karciogla Z, Waters BB, Weens HS: Megalocystic interstitial nephritis: Ultrasonic and radiographic changes. Radiology 133:449, 1979.)

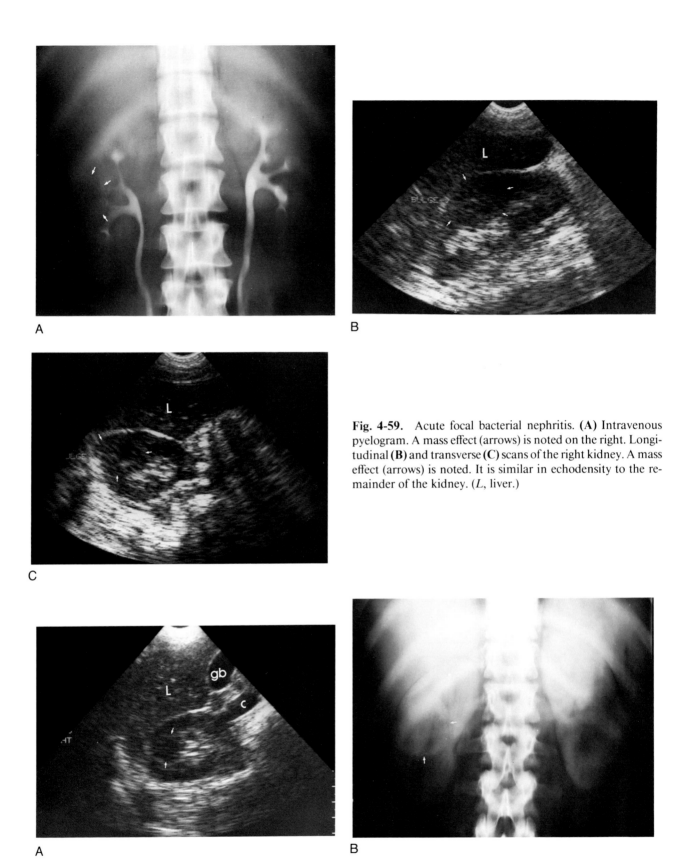

Fig. 4-59. Acute focal bacterial nephritis. **(A)** Intravenous pyelogram. A mass effect (arrows) is noted on the right. Longitudinal **(B)** and transverse **(C)** scans of the right kidney. A mass effect (arrows) is noted. It is similar in echodensity to the remainder of the kidney. (*L*, liver.)

Fig. 4-60. Acute focal bacterial nephritis. Follow-up scan to Figure 4-59. **(A)** Transverse scan. The mass effect (arrow) in the right kidney has decreased in size on antibiotic therapy. (*L*, liver; *gb*, gallbladder; *c*, inferior vena cava.) **(B)** Intravenous pyelogram. Only a slight mass effect (arrows) is seen on the right.

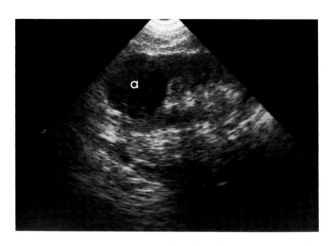

Fig. 4-61. Renal abscess. Longitudinal right lateral decubitus scan of the left kidney. A well-defined hypoechoic rounded mass *(a)* is seen in the upper pole of the kidney. No acoustic enhancement is seen.

(Fig. 4-60). If the mass becomes progressively more lucent, then the diagnosis of an abscess must be entertained and an aspiration may be performed. An abscess is an anechoic mass with irregular margins and good acoustic enhancement; the number of internal echoes depends on the debris[129] (Fig. 4-61). Ultrasound cannot absolutely differentiate acute lobar nephronia from abscess or even tumor. If there is a question of abscess, a needle aspiration may be performed.[129,130]

XANTHOGRANULOMATOUS PYELONEPHRITIS

Xanthogranulomatous pyelonephritis, characterized by destruction and replacement of normal parenchyma by sheets of lipid-laden histiocytes, is a rare form of inflammatory disease in patients with obstructive uropathy secondary to long standing calculi.[131,132] As such, the most common etiologies include chronic infection and obstruction of the ureteropelvic junction generally by a staghorn calculus. As a rule, there is a long history of urinary tract infections with *Proteus mirabilis* and *E. coli* the most often organisms involved.[132,133] There are renal calculi in 50 to 80 percent of cases with resultant hydronephrosis.[131,134] The patients generally have signs and symptoms of malaise, flank pain, mass, weight loss, and urinary tract infection.[132,134] The disease has a higher incidence in diabetics and is rare in black people.[134] There is a slight female predominance.[131] The disease can occur at any age with a peak incidence in the fourth and fifth decades.[132]

Pathologically, this disease is characterized by abscess formation surrounded by inflammatory foam cells, plasma cells, and multinucleated giant cells that give the abscess the characteristic yellow color.[134] The pathologic spectrum is variable dependent on the chronicity of the disease process.[131] Pus filled dilated calyces may predominate with less extensive xanthogranulomatous tissue. Or, there may be replacement of the kidney with xanthogranulomatous tissue that may predominate with less of a purulent component.[131] The process begins within the calyces and pelvis with subsequent mucosal destruction and extension into the adjacent medulla and cortex. The distended calyces compromise the medullary perfusion leading to papillary necrosis.[132]

The ultrasound pattern of xanthogranulomatous pyelonephritis varies with the pattern of involvement — diffuse or segmental.[132] In the typical diffuse pattern, the parenchyma is replaced by multiple circular, apparently fluid-filled masses that surround the central echo complex[131-133,135] (Figs. 4-62 to 4-65). These masses correspond to the debris-filled dilated calyces and/or foci of parenchymal destruction.[132] The kidney is enlarged but the reniform shape is maintained with a smooth contour.[132] The echogenicity of the masses is dependent on the amount of debris and necrosis within them. The central echogenic stone may be difficult to define as may be its associated acoustic shadow.[132] In segmental disease, there are one or more masses surrounding a single calyx that contains a calculus.[132] The masses may be hypoechoic or anechoic with the echogenicity correlating with the amount of necrosis and debris.[132]

FUNGUS BALLS

Renal fungus balls are most commonly due to Candida in patients with altered host resistance, diabetes, malignancy, chronic illness, or those receiving prolonged antibiotic, corticosteroid, or immunosuppressive therapy.[136] The renal involvement is usually secondary to systemic infection. The clinical signs are nonspecific and include flank pain, fever, and chills. On ultrasound one sees an echogenic nonshadowing mass in the collecting system[136] (Fig. 4-66). The differential diagnosis in such an instance would include tumor, blood clot, or pyogenic debris within the collecting system.

ABSCESS

Up to 20 percent of patients with renal abscess have a negative urinalysis and culture.[106] A renal abscess on ultrasound appears as a well-marginated anechoic mass that is round to oval with a wall that is irregular and fine[106,120,137,138] (Figs. 4-61, 4-67 to 4-69). There may be debris within the lesion producing increased echoes. Characteristically, there is acoustic enhancement.[138] The abscess may be highly echogenic due to bright

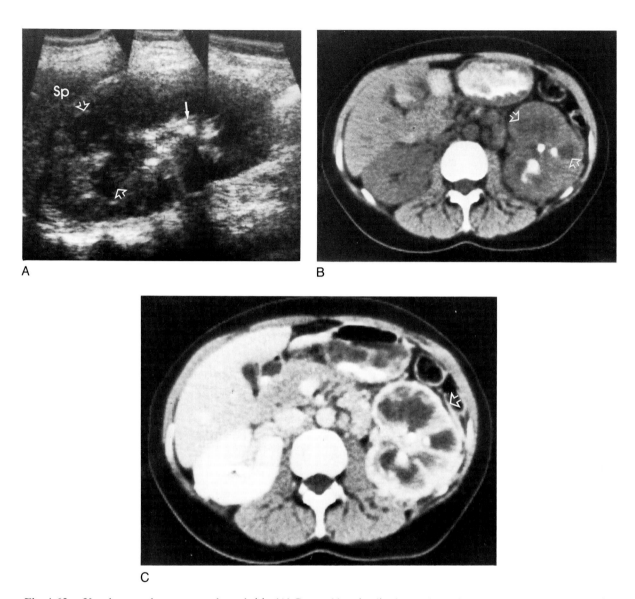

A

B

C

Fig. 4-62.   Xanthogranulomatous pyelonephritis. **(A)** Coronal longitudinal scan through the spleen *(Sp)*. Enlarged left kidney, central echogenic focus with shadowing (arrow) and central mixed echopattern (open arrows) are seen. Note the apparent thickening of the renal parenchyma. **(B)** CT scan through midportion of the kidney (nonenhanced). Multiple calculi are noted in the enlarged left kidney. Areas of diminished attenuation (open arrows) are seen measuring − 5HU to + 5HU in various locations. **(C)** CT scan, enhanced (same level as **B**). Areas of diminished attenuation are now better seen and only minimally enhanced. Surrounding rims of tissue are greatly enhanced, indicative of vascular inflammatory tissue associated with the remaining parenchymal areas. Note thickening of Gerota's fascia surrounding the kidney (open arrow). (From Subramanyam BR, Megibow AJ, Raghavendra BN, Bosniak MA: Diffuse xanthogranulomatous pyelonephritis: Analysis by computed tomography and sonography. Urol Radiol 4:5, 1982.)

echoes caused by microbubbles of gas implying infection by gas-forming organisms[120] (Fig. 4-69). Abscesses smaller than 2 cm may be missed with ultrasound.[139] CT can better define associated fascial thickening or detect subtle alterations in perinephric fat.[139]

To establish a definitive diagnosis, an ultrasound guided aspiration of the lesion may be performed.[130] If pus is obtained, the patient may be referred for percutaneous catheter drainage. When the aspiration is performed, only a small amount of fluid is withdrawn for gram-stain and culture. The remainder of the fluid is left to facilitate catheter placement.[137]

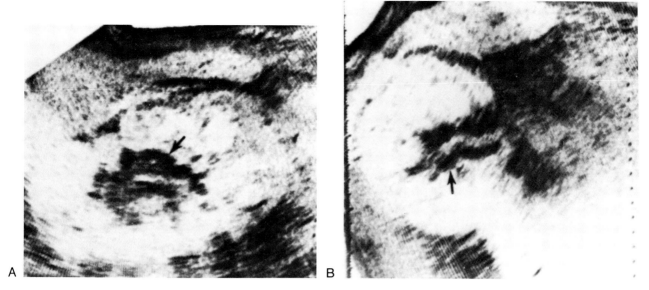

Fig. 4-63. Xanthogranulomatous pyelonephritis. **(A)** Longitudinal supine scan. There is a diffusely enlarged right kidney with central echogenic focus (arrow), acoustic shadowing and scattered parenchymal anechocities. **(B)** Supine transverse scan. Large central echogenic focus (arrow) in right kidney is seen with associated acoustic shadowing. (From Van Kirk OC, Go RT, Wedel VJ: Sonographic features of xanthogranulomatous pyelonephritis. AJR 134: 1035, © Am Roent Ray Soc, 1980.)

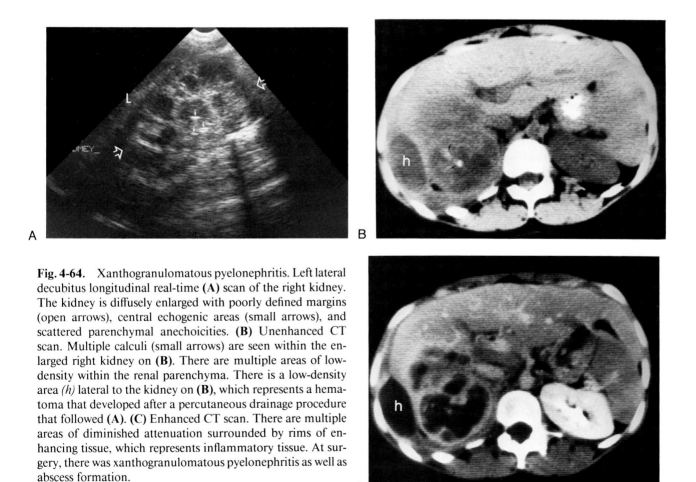

Fig. 4-64. Xanthogranulomatous pyelonephritis. Left lateral decubitus longitudinal real-time **(A)** scan of the right kidney. The kidney is diffusely enlarged with poorly defined margins (open arrows), central echogenic areas (small arrows), and scattered parenchymal anechoicities. **(B)** Unenhanced CT scan. Multiple calculi (small arrows) are seen within the enlarged right kidney on **(B)**. There are multiple areas of low-density within the renal parenchyma. There is a low-density area *(h)* lateral to the kidney on **(B)**, which represents a hematoma that developed after a percutaneous drainage procedure that followed **(A)**. **(C)** Enhanced CT scan. There are multiple areas of diminished attenuation surrounded by rims of enhancing tissue, which represents inflammatory tissue. At surgery, there was xanthogranulomatous pyelonephritis as well as abscess formation.

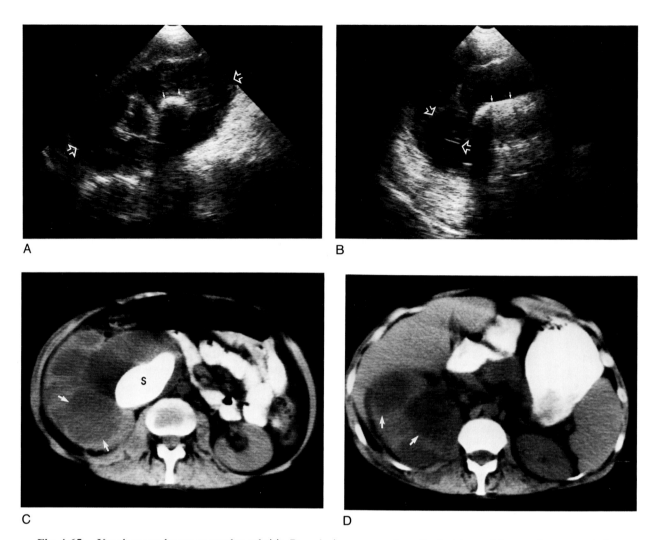

Fig. 4-65. Xanthogranulomatous pyelonephritis. Paraplegic young male patient with past history of recurrent infectious urologic problems. He presented with fever and right flank pain. Supine longitudinal (**A**) and transverse (**B**) scans. The right kidney (open arrows, renal length on (**A**)) is markedly enlarged and hypoechoic but a reniform shape is maintained. There is an echogenic focus (small arrows, calculus) in the region of the renal pelvis. The parenchyma appears to be replaced by multiple hypoechoic areas (open arrows on (**B**)). (**C,D**) Unenhanced CT scans. A large dense calculus *(s)* is seen within the renal pelvis. Multiple poorly defined low density areas (arrows) are seen within the renal parenchyma. This ultrasound pattern is consistent with xanthogranulomatous pyelonephritis.

ABSCESS DRAINAGE

This percutaneous procedure is very similar to that for percutaneous nephrostomy. The indication for the procedure includes the ultrasound diagnosis of a renal abscess with an aspiration yielding pus. This is a rapid, reliable, and safe means of distinguishing abscess from noninflammatory collections.[120,138,140] The basis of effective treatment of intrarenal abscess is early diagnosis and drainage. Percutaneous catheter drainage in combination with antibiotic therapy can be definitive in the treatment of intrarenal abscesses even with perinephric extension.[130] If the patient's condition does not improve or deteriorates, then open surgical drainage can be performed.[130] (There is further discussion of abscess drainage in Chapter 10.)

Renal Medical Disease

Using the current ultrasound equipment permits the identification of three distinct anatomic regions: cortex, medulla, and renal sinus. The corticomedullary junction can be identified by the interface produced by the arcuate vessels. All of the following can be assessed with ultrasound when evaluating a kidney for medical dis-

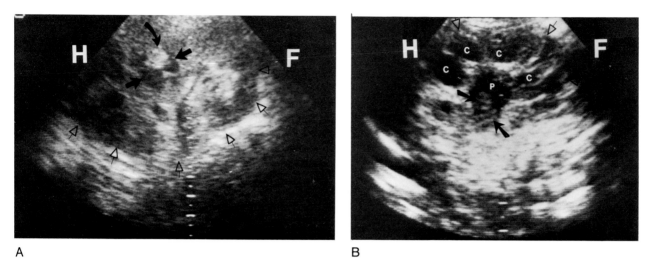

Fig. 4-66. Renal fungus ball. Case 1: **(A)** Unilateral renal fungus ball in an adult diabetic. Real-time coronal scan with the patient in a right lateral decubitus position showing a hyperechoic, nonshadowing mass (curved arrow) within the mildly dilated left upper pole collecting system (straight black arrows) (*H*, patient's head; *F*, patient's feet). Open arrows show renal outline. Case 2: Bilateral renal pelvis fungus balls in a neonate. **(B)** Real-time coronal scan of the right kidney shows an echogenic nonshadowing mass (black arrows) within the renal pelvis *(P)* and mild hydronephrosis (*C*, dilated calyces) (*H*, patient's head; *F*, patient's feet). Open arrows show renal outline. (From Stuck KJ, Silver TM, Jaffe MH, Bowerman RA: Sonographic demonstration of renal fungus balls. Radiology 142:473, 1981.)

ease: renal length; appearance of the renal sinus; detectability and size of the renal pyramids; distinctness of the corticomedullary junction; and cortical echogenicity (by comparing the density to that of liver at a comparable depth and to the renal sinus).[141] The pyramids are considered enlarged if their height exceeds or is thicker than the overlying cortex.[81] The clarity of the corticomedullary junction does not correspond to any histopathologic finding. There is no correlation between the nature and severity of the glomerular lesion on renal biopsy and the

ultrasound findings.[142] However, there is a definite relation between the nature and severity of interstitial changes on biopsy and the echo intensity of the cortex.[142]

RENAL CORTICAL DISEASE

There have been two parenchymal patterns described on ultrasound with renal disease.[8,9,16,142] Type I demonstrates diffuse increase in echogenicity of the cortex with preservation of the corticomedullary junction; the echo

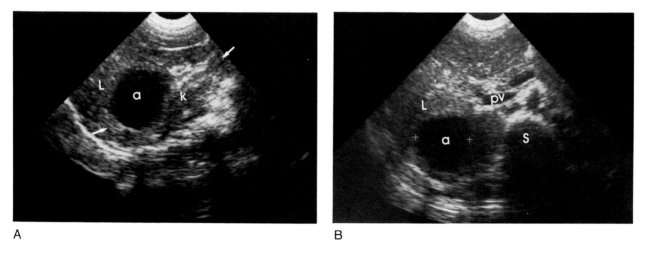

Fig. 4-67. Renal abscess. Child. Longitudinal **(A)** and transverse **(B)** supine scans reveal a well-defined anechoic area *(a)* in the upper pole of the right kidney (*k*, arrows). No acoustic enhancement is seen. It was drained percutaneously. (*L*, liver; *pv*, portal vein; *S*, spine.)

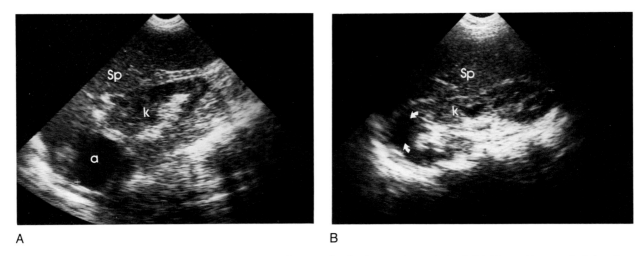

Fig. 4-68.   Renal abscess. **(A)** Right lateral decubitus longitudinal scan through the left kidney (*k*). A well-defined anechoic mass *(a)* is seen in the upper pole. (*Sp*, spleen.) **(B)** Longitudinal scan of the left kidney *(k)* following percutaneous catheter drainage shows that the mass (arrows) is smaller. (*Sp*, spleen.)

intensity in the cortex is equal to or greater than that in the adjacent liver or spleen and equal to that of adjacent renal sinus[8,9] (Fig. 4-70). The increased cortical echoes are seen in disease processes in which there is deposition of collagen or calcium and in some acute processes.[8] Diseases seen to demonstrate a type I pattern include acute and chronic glomerulonephritis, renal transplant rejection, lupus nephritis, hypertensive nephrosclerosis, renal cortical necrosis, methemoglobinuric renal failure, Alport's syndrome, amyloidosis, diabetic nephrosclerosis, and some chronic diseases. With chronic disease, the kidney becomes smaller, the cortex has increased

echogenicity and eventually the medulla will become equally echogenic. Type II represents focal or diffuse loss of the corticomedullary junction definition.[8,9] The type II pattern is seen with such focal lesions as cysts, calyceal diverticuli, renal artery aneurysm, some abscesses, and hematomas.[16]

In the pediatric patient (excluding neonate), echogenic kidneys are associated with medical renal disease in 94 percent of cases[143] (Fig. 4-71). In one series, the cause was glomerular in 30 percent, tubointerstitial in 48 percent, and end-stage in 16 percent.[143] Patients with end-stage disease had small, dense (echogenic) kidneys.

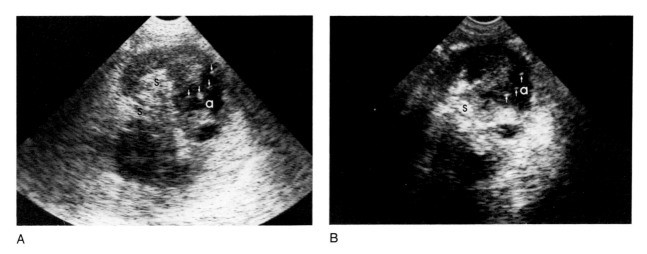

Fig. 4-69.   Renal abscess. Air. A reflective pattern (small arrows) is seen in the area of the poorly defined hypoechoic renal mass *(a)* on right lateral decubitus transverse **(A,B)** scans of the enlarged left lower pole (*s*, renal sinus).

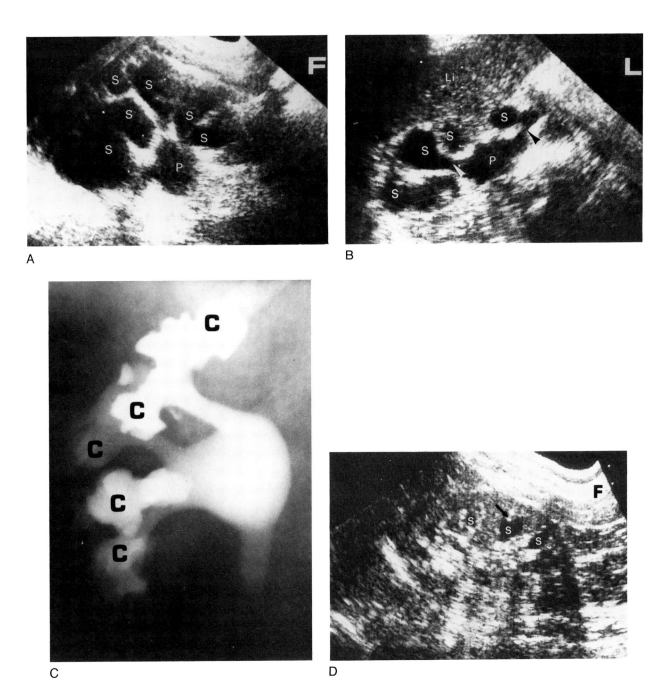

Fig. 4-73. Renal papillary necrosis. Case 1: Analgesic abuser. **(A)** Longitudinal left lateral decubitus scan shows multiple large fluid-filled spaces *(S)* within the kidney arranged in a spokewheel fashion about the renal pelvis *(P)*, which is mildly distended. *(F, patient's foot.)* **(B)** Transverse scan in same position demonstrating the narrow infundibuli (arrowheads) between the fluid-filled clubbed "calyces" *(S)* and the renal pelvis *(P)*. *(Li, liver; L, toward patient's left.)* Case 2: Unilateral disease. **(C)** Right retrograde urogram demonstrating blunted clubbed calyces *(C)*. **(D)** Longitudinal left lateral decubitus scan showing triangular fluid-filled spaces *(S)* about the renal sinus echoes that correlate with the retrograde findings. Note the echo reflection of the arcuate vessels (arrow) at the periphery of the blunted calyx *(F, toward patient's feet).* (From Hoffman JC, Schnur MJ, Koenigsberg M: Demonstration of renal papillary necrosis by sonography. Radiology 145:785, 1982.)

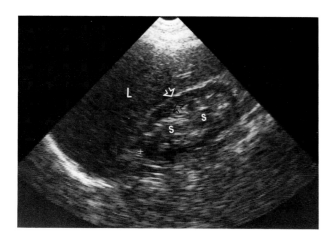

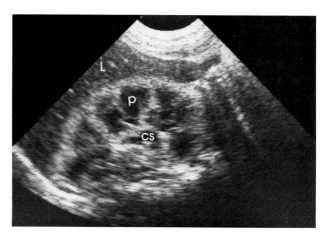

Fig. 4-74. Renal sinus lipomatosis. Longitudinal scan of the right kidney. Note the large renal sinus *(s)* denoted by the echodense area related to the fat in that region. The renal parenchyma (between open arrows) is very thin. (*L*, liver.)

Fig. 4-75. Renal cortical calcification. Left lateral decubitus longitudinal scan of the right kidney in an infant. Note that the density of the renal parenchyma is denser than that of liver *(L)* and the hypoechogenicity of the renal pyramids *(p)* is accentuated. (*cs*, collecting system.)

with nephrocalcinosis including hyperparathyroidism, hypervitaminosis D, milk alkali syndrome, renal tubular acidosis, medullary sponge kidney, hyperoxaluria, and others.[50] To be detected by radiography, the calculi must be quite large.[154,155] Radiography often fails to show early renal calcification.[154,156] Ultrasound can reveal calculi as echogenic structures regardless of chemical composition.[157]

Cortical Calcification. The etiology of nephrocalcinosis is quite variable as has been described. It can be seen with renal tubular disease, enzyme disorders, hypercalcemic states, parenchymal renal disease, vascular phenomena, and may be idiopathic.[158,159] Cushing's syndrome is the least common cause.[158] The most common cause of hypercalcemia in the general population is malignant neoplasm.[159] This may be due to the direct lytic effect on bone by the metastatic tumor. In the absence of bone metastases, tumor-related hypercalcemia may be mediated by the ectopic production of parathyroid hormone, prostaglandins, or osteoid. Hypercalcemia leads to nephrocalcinosis by overloading the renal resorptive mechanism.[159] The high calcium load causes cellular damage followed by calcium salt deposition in the tubular cells, basement membrane, and within the loops of Henle.[159] The classic distribution of nephrocalcinosis is along the corticomedullary junction, but the calcium salts may be deposited elsewhere in the renal parenchyma.

In the cortical type of nephrocalcinosis there are focal or diffuse, punctate or confluent densities in the cortex of the kidney producing, in its most severe form, a dense outline of the kidney[158,159] (Fig. 4-75). The ultrasound pattern may resemble other forms of parenchymal dis-

ease.[155,156] CT would be more sensitive in detecting this pattern of nephrocalcinosis.[155,158]

Primary Hyperoxaluria. Primary hyperoxaluria is a rare hereditary autosomal recessive disorder resulting in an inborn error of glyoxalate metabolism (type I) or hydroxypyruvate metabolism (type II).[153,160] Characteristically, there is hyperoxaluria, calcium oxalate, nephrolithiasis, widespread renal and extrarenal deposits of calcium oxalate crystals (oxalosis), and progressive renal failure leading to death usually before adulthood. Renal parenchymal injury is caused by the calcium oxalate deposits that lead to progressive renal failure.[153] Sixty-five percent of the patient's symptoms, hematuria, are due to renal calculi prior to age of 5.

On ultrasound an increase in the echogenicity of the renal parenchyma in normal sized kidneys is evident[160] (Fig. 4-76). These findings, combined with the urinalysis and ophthaloscopic examination, can be diagnostic and may eliminate the need for biopsy.[160] It is imperative to diagnosis the disease process early so appropriate therapy may be instituted early in order to alter the natural history of the process.

Medullary Nephrocalcinosis. With medullary nephrocalcinosis, the cortical echogenicity is normal but there are focal areas of increased echogenicity corresponding to the renal pyramids[154,156,158,161,163] (Fig. 4-77). The calcification is often not revealed by radiography.[154,164] There is no acoustic shadow associated with these densities, which suggests that macroscopic aggregates of calcium are necessary to produce an acoustic shadow posterior to the echogenic pyramids.[164] The cal-

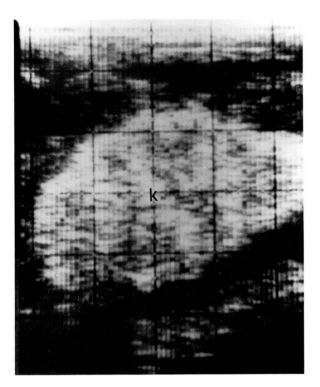

Fig. 4-76. Primary hyperoxaluria. Longitudinal scan of intensely echogenic kidney (k) of normal size demonstrating corticomedullary distinction. Gain has been turned down making the liver appear anechoic. (From Brennan JN, Diwan RV, Makker SP et al: Ultrasonic diagnosis of primary hyperoxaluria in infancy. Radiology 145:147, 1982.)

cifications can be unequivocally localized to the medulla if the arcuate vessels are seen capping the base of the echogenic wedge-shaped area.[164]

Reported cases of medullary nephrocalcinosis have included distal tubular acidosis, furosemide therapy (in infants), prolonged adrenocorticotropic hormone (ACTH) therapy, secondary hyperparathyroidism, Cushing's syndrome, oral pharmocologic doses of vitamin E and calcium, Bartter's syndrome, and hyperparathyroidism.[158,161-166] Furosemide therapy can cause alkalosis and hypercalciuria and as such has been implicated as a cause of nephrocalcinosis.[165] Bartter's syndrome consists of hyperplasia of the juxtaglomerular apparatus, hyperaldosteronism, hypokalemic alkalosis, and a normal blood pressure.[163]

Renal Vascular Calcifications. Calcification in the renal arterial network should be considered when echogenic foci with shadowing are seen in the area of the renal sinus (Fig. 4-78). This diagnosis should be considered in the sonographic differential diagnosis especially in patients with long-standing diabetes, hypertension, or other systemic disease associated with accelerated

atherosclerotic vascular disease.[167] Real-time scanning can help to differentiate these echodensities from calculi as they are seen to pulsate.

Increased echoes in the interlobar and arcuate arteries due to calcification in the lamina elastica of the arteries has been reported in hypertensive children[168] (Fig. 4-79). This calcification was not visible on the radiograph. So, when evaluating a child with renal disease the examiner should look for this.

Collecting System Calcification. Ultrasound has a potential value in the investigation of opaque and nonopaque filling defects within the renal pelvis and in patients with urologic nonvisualization who have a high risk of uric acid lithiasis. The nonopaque stone may be uric acid or urate although there is the rare instance of xanthine and mucoid matrix stones. Uric acid calculi account for 8 percent of all renal stones.[169] Patients at risk for uric acid stones include ileostomy patients, those with myeloproliferative disorders (especially those being treated with cytotoxic agents), gout, and other disorders of uric acid metabolism.[169] By radiography, it is difficult to distinguish nonopaque stones from transitional cell tumor in the renal pelvis and calyces.

On ultrasound all stones, regardless of composition, appear echodense with acoustic shadowing[157] (Figs. 4-44, 4-45, 4-80 to 4-82). The intensity of the shadow does not depend on either the size or composition of the stone.[170] At times, the echodensity of the collecting system stone may be difficult to distinguish from the echoes of the renal sinus. The key is the acoustic shadow. For optimal visualization of this shadow, the following should be undertaken: (1) careful control of the overall gain setting (usually lower) in order to demonstrate the shadow; and (2) use of a transducer with the narrow part of its focal zone in the region of the suspected stone.[18]

Calyceal Diverticuli Calcification. Calyceal diverticuli are uncommon parenchymal cystic lesions believed to be Wolffian duct remnants secondary to failure of regression of the ureteric bud. They are connected to the system by the renal pelvis, infundibulum, or minor calyx. They may develop stones, and are a site for recurrent infection or rupture. Gravity dependent echogenic debris within a cystic structure is seen with milk of calcium or stones in a calyceal diverticulum[171-173] (Fig. 4-83). Or, an echogenic structure with associated shadowing may be seen with stones.[173] This may simulate calcification within the wall of a cystic mass.[173] As such, one should obtain scans in various positions to demonstrate movement.

Milk of calcium has been seen to be associated with primary hyperparathyroidism and possibly milk alkali syndrome.[172] The milk of calcium represents primarily

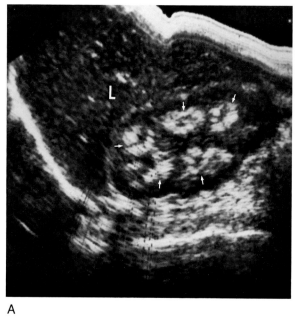

A

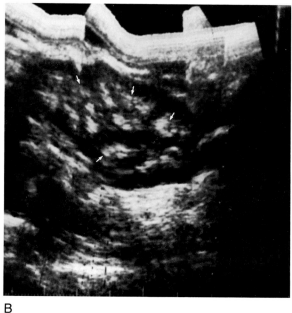

B

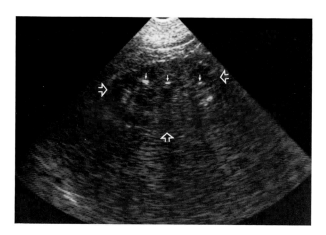

C

Fig. 4-77. Medullary nephrocalcinosis. Longitudinal supine scan of the right kidney **(A)** and longitudinal right lateral decubitus scan of the left **(B)** kidney demonstrate echodense areas (arrows) in the region of the renal pyramids. (*L*, liver.) **(C)** Unenhanced CT scan documents the calcification (arrows). The calcifications were not visible on a radiograph. The patient was found to have hypercalcemia and was treated. On follow-up scans two years later, when the patient's serum calcium was within normal limits, there had been no real change in the sonographic appearance of the kidney.

Fig. 4-78. Renal vascular calcifications. Adult diabetic with hypertension and chronic renal failure. Longitudinal scan of the left kidney (open arrows). Multiple linear echodensities (small arrows) are seen in the area of the renal arterial network. These were seen to pulsate at real-time examination.

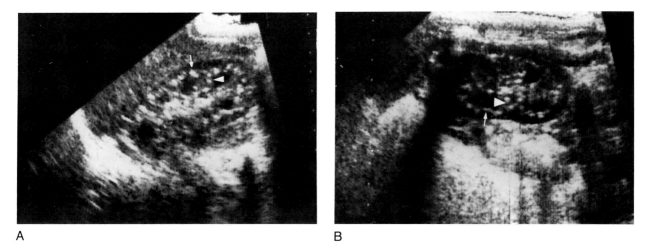

Fig. 4-79. Renal vascular calcification. Hypertensive child. Longitudinal scans of the right (supine) **(A)** and left **(B)** (prone) kidneys. The arcuate arteries (arrows) and interlobar arteries (arrowheads) are abnormally visible. (From Garel LA, Pariente DM, Gubler MC et al: The dotted corticomedullary junction: A sonographic indicator of small-vessel disease in hypertensive children. Radiology 152:419, 1984.)

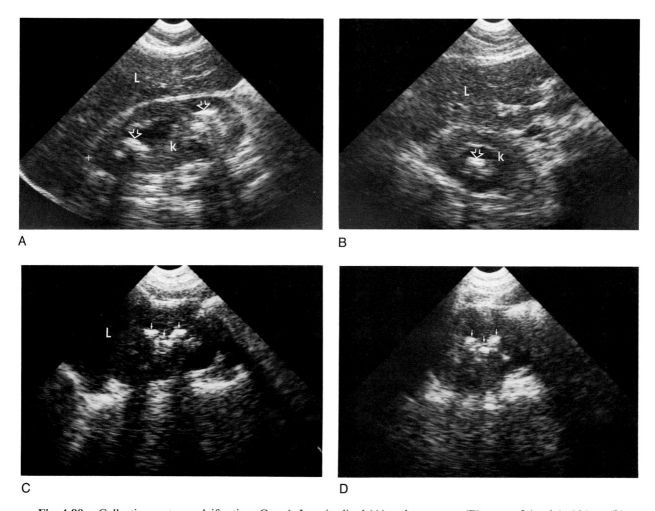

Fig. 4-80. Collecting system calcification. Case 1: Longitudinal **(A)** and transverse **(B)** scans of the right kidney *(k)* demonstrate collecting system calculi (open arrows) both in the upper and lower poles. There is dilatation of the collecting system. (*L*, liver.) Case 2: Longitudinal **(C)** and transverse **(D)** views of the right kidney. Multiple echodense collecting system stones (arrows) are seen. (*L*, liver.)

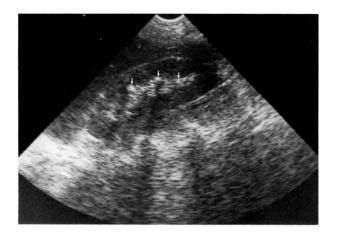

Fig. 4-81. Collecting system calculi. Patient with acute monomyelocytic leukemia and urate nephropathy. Longitudinal scan of the right kidney reveals echodensities (arrows, calculi) in the region of the collecting system with associated shadowing. These were urate stones.

small crystals of calcium carbonate although calcium phosphate, calcium oxalate, ammonia phosphate, and calcium hydroxyapatite are also seen.[172,174] In most cases there is obstruction and low-grade inflammation in a calyceal diverticulum. At least partial obstruction to urine flow with stasis seems to be a requirement for the formation of milk of calcium.[174] It is less commonly associated with ureteropelvic junction obstruction, hydronephrosis and/or a nonfunctioning kidney.[174] Most patients are asymptomatic.

At times, calyceal calculi may be confused with gallstones on the radiograph[175] (Fig. 4-83). If calcifications

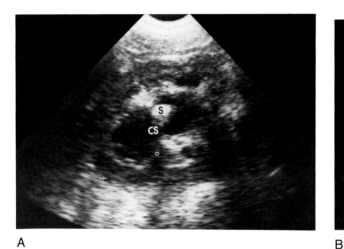

A

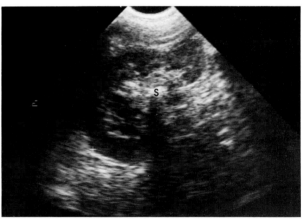

B

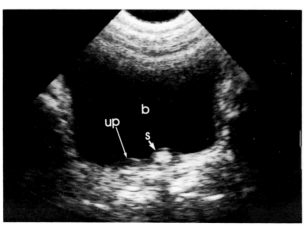

C

Fig. 4-82. Collecting system calculi. Child with hypercalcemia. Longitudinal prone (**A**) scan through the left kidney demonstrates dilatation of the collecting system *(cs)* and calculi *(s)* within. At that time, a dilated distal ureter nor ureteral calculi was seen. (**B**) Longitudinal prone scan, left kidney one week after (**A**). A collecting system calculus *(s)* is seen but the degree of hydronephrosis is decreased. (**C**) Transverse scan of the distended bladder *(b)* at the same time as (**B**) demonstrating a left ureterovesical junction calculus *(s)*. (*up*, right ureteral papilla.)

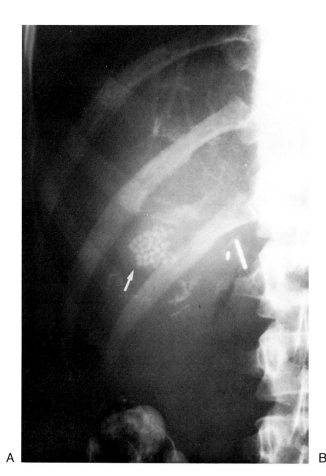

A

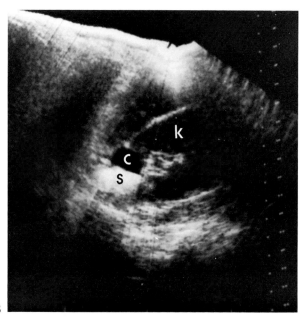

B

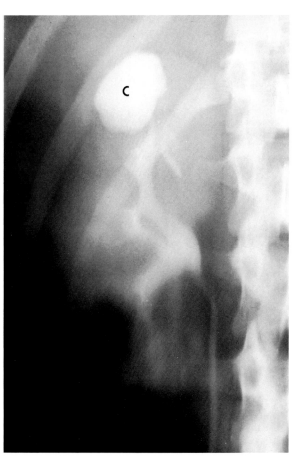

C

Fig. 4-83. Calyceal diverticuli calcifications. Stones. Patient who was postoperative cholecystectomy with appearance of gallstones (arrow) still on a plain film **(A)**. Longitudinal scan **(B)** of the right kidney reveals an anechoic upper pole mass (*c*, calyceal diverticulum) with echodense material (stones, *s*) layering within it. **(C)** Intravenous pyelogram. A calyceal diverticulum *(c)* is visualized in the right upper pole.

are multiple, closely grouped, and faceted, the diagnosis of cholelithiasis is thought to be certain; but these may represent calyceal calculi. Using physiochemical models for stone formation, investigators have shown that if more than one nidus for stone formation is in a saccular structure the surfaces of the adjacent stones form unusual flattened rings of crystals in the plane of contact.[175] It is this flattening at the plane of contact when multiple stones are developing that leads to the formation of faceted stones and can develop in either a hydronephrotic calyx, renal pelvis, or large calyceal diverticulum.[175]

RENAL BIOPSY

The renal biopsy is the singular most important instrument in the diagnosis of renal medical disease. Satisfactory categorization of the biopsy specimen requires light microscopy, electron microscopy, and immunofluorescent studies. The success rate of a percutaneous renal biopsy is dependent on the ability to accurately localize the kidney.[176] Ultrasound has helped immensely with this regard.[177] Initially, the lower pole was localized with static ultrasound, which was time consuming. The lower pole is usually chosen for the biopsy because this area contains the smallest number of large blood vessels and is the least vascular portion of the parenchyma. At the present time, real-time ultrasound has not only increased the speed of the procedure but has also led to a decrease number of passes by the biopsy needle (Fig. 4-84). This procedure is usually done combining the efforts of the nephrologist and sonologist. The sonologist monitors the sterile ultrasound while the nephrologist performs the biopsy using a real-time needle guide. (There is further discussion of this procedure in Chapter 10.)

The complication rate for the renal biopsy procedure has been reported to be 0.7 to 8.1 percent. These complications include oliguria, decreased hematocrit, hematuria, arteriovenous fistula, and abscess. Greater than 50 percent of patients have hematomas revealed by CT, but most are small and not clinically apparent.[141,178]

The procurement of tissue adequate for diagnosis with the minimum of morbidity and mortality is the ultimate goal of the renal biopsy.[117] In one series, surgical and percutaneous biopsies were compared. Adequate tissue was obtained in 100 percent of surgical biopsies and with closed biopsies, adequate tissue was obtained in 82.5 percent.[117] Others report an accuracy of 93 to 96 percent by using ultrasound to guide the renal biopsies.[179,180] A 100 percent accuracy has been described in obtaining renal tissue with a 88.6 percent rate of obtaining glomeruli.[176] After the initial diagnosis is made by biopsy, there is good correlation between cortical echogenicity and severity of histopathologic changes providing a promising noninvasive method for monitoring the progression of renal disease.[141]

Renal Failure

Renal failure is defined as a degree of renal insufficiency causing substantial alteration of plasma biochemistry. Some define it as acute reduction in renal function associated with a rise in serum creatinine of greater than

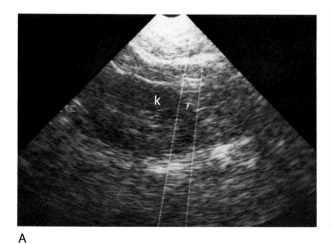
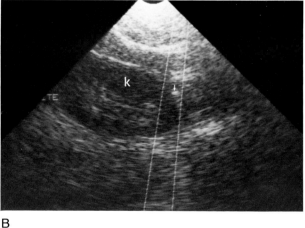

A   B

Fig. 4-84. Renal biopsy. **(A)** With the patient in the prone position, the lower pole of the left kidney *(k)* is localized longitudinally placing it within the biopsy tract (parallel lines) of the biopsy guide. The depth (arrow) from the skin to the renal capsule is measured to be 6 cm. **(B)** With direct real-time visualization, the biopsy needle is inserted until the tip (arrow) is seen at the renal capsule. Then, the needle is released from the needle guide and the biopsy is performed.

2.5 mg/dl.[181] It is termed acute if it develops over days or weeks, and chronic if over months to years. As has been described previously, there is significant correlation between the cortical echopattern and the severity of the histopathologic changes especially with prevalence of global sclerosis, focal tubular atropy, hyaline casts, and leukocyte infiltration. Early in the process, the histologic changes may be isolated within the nephron, vessel, or interstitium. Tubular and interstitial alterations usually follow glomerular changes so the degree of involvement in all three compartments is similar. Increased cortical echoes in advanced stage disease result in combined changes within the glomeruli, tubules, and interstitium.[178]

There have been noted to be characteristic changes in the medulla in response to diurectic states. With increasing diuresis, the pyramids become prominent, anechoic, and easily identified. With increased edema encompassing the peritubular capillaries in the medullary region with medullary congestion, and with increased blood flow through the kidney, the medullary pyramids are easily identified, prominent, and anechoic. While the detection of the medullary pyramids appears to correlate with the histopathologic changes in the cortex, there appears to be a relationship between the number of hyaline casts per glomerulus and nonvisualization of the pyramids. In contrast, the pyramids are echogenic with nephrocalcinosis.[178]

On ultrasound the renal sinus is characteristically echodense primarily due to the hilar adipose tissue, whereas the blood vessels and collecting structures have a secondary contribution. The high amplitude pattern is secondary to the inherent scattering properties of the fat cells and is not due to coexisting fibrous tissue septa. Minor cellular infiltration causes partitioning of the fat cells. With increased septal thickness, the spatial design of the renal sinus is altered. The sinus echoes evolve into an inhomogeneous, patchy, and coarse pattern. As the infiltrative process proceeds, fibrosis follows and atrophy and loss of adipose tissue cells are noted. In the advanced stage, fibrous tissue predominates with a few widely spaced fat cells. So, as the renal sinus is replaced by fibrous tissue, the fat cells are rarely seen and the echogenicity of the renal sinus decreases with loss of a distinct renal sinus[178] (Fig. 4-85).

Renal size is another parameter that can be evaluated in renal failure. The long axis is inclined and the kidney rotated with its hilum facing forward and medial. The upper pole is posterior with the lower pole anterior. The decubitus, coronal scan provides the long dimension of the kidney and the renal hilum is best displayed. Renal lengths obtained on prone or supine views are inaccurate. If the adult kidney is less than 10 cm, it is considered small.[178]

ACUTE RENAL FAILURE

Acute renal failure may be prerenal (renal hypoperfusion secondary to a systemic cause), renal (due to renal medical disease), or postrenal (as a result of outflow obstruction). The prerenal form may be distinguished from the others by laboratory and clinical data. Since the postrenal etiologies (5 percent incidence) are surgically repairable, the diagnosis should be made rapidly with a high degree of accuracy. The renal medical diseases are the most common causes of acute renal failure, with the most common being acute tubular necrosis (ATN). The ultrasound findings in acute renal failure are usually unremarkable. The kidneys may be normal sized or enlarged. The medulla may be readily visible, which probably results from congestion and edema. The main role of ultrasound in acute renal failure is to exclude hydronephrosis.[178]

Some investigators describe several prominent findings with ATN: (1) increased renal size (especially the anteroposterior diameter with the normal anteroposterior dimension 4.26 ± 0.37 cm (mean $\pm$ standard deviation) and (2) sharp delineation of the swollen pyramids[181] (Fig. 4-86). The kidney with ATN is enlarged due to interstitial edema and increased water content; the degree of enlargement depends partly on the severity of functional or histological damage.[181] The kidneys with an increased anteroposterior diameter to length (H/L) ratio may have a longer recovery time (mean 32.4 days) with most requiring hemodialysis while those with a normal H/L ratio may require less recovery time (mean 15.5 days) with few requiring hemodialysis.[181]

The medical causes of acute renal failure are multiple and include all of the following.[178]

1. Acute tubular necrosis
   Ischemia due to major trauma, massive hemorrhage, compartmental syndrome, septic shock, transfusion reaction, myoglobinuria, postpartum hemorrhage, cardiac, aortic and biliary surgery, pancreatitis, and gastroenteritis.
   Nephrotoxicities including hypersensitivity reactions to heavy metals, organic solvents, radiographic contrast, pesticides, fungicides, antibiotics, and other agents.
2. Cortical necrosis
3. Acute interstitial nephritis
4. Diseases of the glomeruli and small blood vessels including acute post strep glomerulonephritis, lupus, polyarteritis nodosa, Schönlein-Henoch purpura, subacute bacterial endocarditis, serum sickness, Goodpasture's syndrome, malignant hypertension, hemolytic uremic syndrome, drug-related vasculitis, abruptio, and rapidly progressive glomerulonephritis.

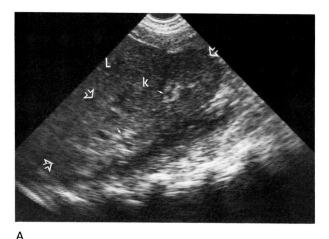

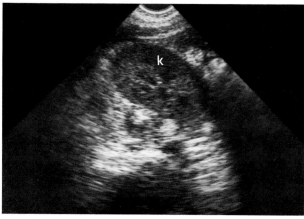

C

Fig. 4-85. Renal failure. Left lateral decubitus longitudinal **(A)** and transverse **(B,C)** scans of the right kidney *(k)*. There is decreased echogenicity of the renal sinus (small arrows) such that it is barely distinguished. It is difficult to distinguish renal parenchyma (open arrows) from the liver *(L)*. On **(C)**, the right renal artery *(rra)* and vein *(rrv)* can be seen but the renal border cannot be distinguished from liver *(L)*.

The causes of acute renal failure in the neonate include bilateral renal agenesis, renal dysplasia, infantile polycystic kidney disease, congenital nephrotic syndrome, congenital nephritis, trauma, hypotension, hemorrhage, hypovolemia, perinatal hypoxia, congestive heart failure, dehydration, septicemia, disseminated intravascular coagulopathy, renovascular accident, drugs, toxins, and obstruction.[182]

Renal Cortical Necrosis. Renal cortical necrosis is a rare form of acute renal failure usually associated with shock, sepsis, myocardial infarction, postpartum hemorrhage, and burns.[183] Ischemia may be due to intravascular thrombosis, toxin production causing capillary endothelium damage, or vasospasm of small vessels. The tubular cells of the cortex undergo necrosis and interstitial fluid and leukocytes infiltrate the periphery of the involved area. The glomeruli may be necrotic and thrombosis of arterioles can be seen. The medulla and the thin rim of subcapsular tissue are preserved. Calcification is often seen at the interface of the necrotic and

viable tissue with its earliest appearance at 6 days after the insult.[183] On ultrasound loss of the normal corticomedullary region with a hypoechoic outer rim of cortex is evident[183] (Fig. 4-87). Both kidneys are of normal size.

Myoglobinuric Renal Failure. Myoglobin causes 5 to 7 percent of all cases of acute renal failure, with renal failure occurring in 33 percent of patients with myoglobinuria. This process results from rhabdomyolysis, which can occur in a variety of conditions. It is seen in drug and in alcohol abusers. Ethanol and heroin have a direct myotoxic effect.[184] It can lead to acute tubular necrosis and renal failure that can be recurrent and can result in permanent renal damage. The theories for the pathogenesis of myoglobinuric renal failure are vascular, nephrotoxic, and tubular destruction.[184] On ultrasound there may be a spectrum of findings. The kidneys may appear normal or they may be enlarged with increased echoes in the cortex with prominent pyramids[184] (Fig. 4-88). Making the correct diagnosis has prognostic significance.

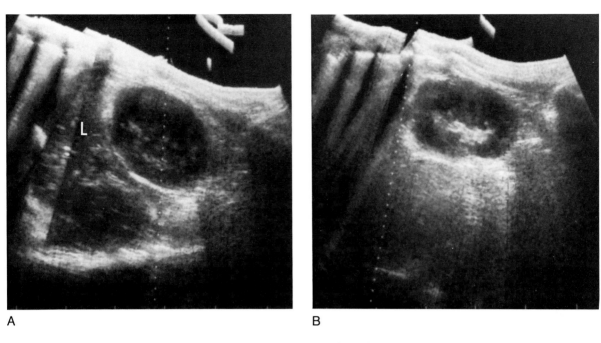

A
B

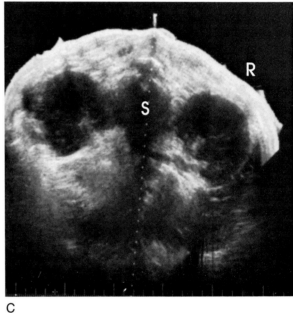

C

Fig. 4-86. Acute tubular necrosis. Longitudinal prone scans of the right (**A**) and left (**B**) kidneys as well as a transverse prone scan (**C**). The kidneys have not increased in length but have markedly increased in their anteroposterior dimension. (*S*, spine; *R*, right; *L*, liver.)

Ethylene Glycol Poisoning. Clinically, with ethylene glycol poisoning, there is a history of antifreeze ingestation with central nervous system, cardiopulmonary, renal, and metabolic manifestations. Ethylene glycol is metabolized in the liver to several intermediary forms producing oxalic acid that is deposited as microscopic calcium oxalate crystals in various organs including the brain, liver, and kidneys. The renal manifestations are potentially reversible renal failure and widespread deposition of calcium oxalate crystals within the tubules and their epithelial lining. On ultrasound the affected kidney is enlarged with increased echogenicity with partial obliteration of the definition of the corticomedullary junction (Fig. 4-89). Once the renal failure resolves, the kidney returns to normal size and echopattern, which may take 66 days.[185]

CHRONIC RENAL FAILURE

There are three main types of chronic renal failure: nephron, vascular, and interstitial abnormalities. After the kidney has been injured for a long period of time in

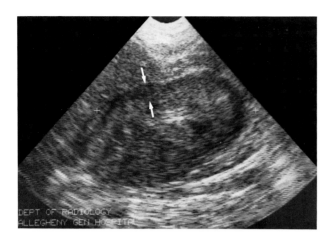

Fig. 4-87. Renal cortical necrosis. Real-time longitudinal scan of the right kidney. A circumferential hypoechoic band (arrows) about 1 cm wide corresponds to the area of cortical necrosis. Similar changes were seen in the left kidney. (From Sefczek RJ, Beckman I, Lupetin AR, Dash N: Sonography of acute renal cortical necrosis. AJR 142:553, © Am Roent Ray Soc, 1984.)

the chronic stage, pathologic changes are seen in all three compartments as they are interrelated. With the exception of cystic disease, the ultrasound findings are not specific for a diagnosis.[178,186] There is no definite correlation between echogenicity of the kidney, kidney size, and degree of decreased renal function.[186] But, if the kidney is more echogenic than normal liver, chronic renal parenchymal disease is likely present[186] (Fig. 4-70). The ultra-

sound appearance of the renal parenchyma corresponds to the degree of the histopathologic changes and the advanced changes in the glomeruli, interstitium and tubules cause and increase in the echoes in the cortex. In the end stage kidney, there is loss of distinction between the cortex and medulla (Fig. 4-90). When correlating length with severity of the pathologic changes, there is noted a relationship between length and prevalence of global sclerosis, focal tubular atrophy, and the number of hyaline casts per glomerulus.[178] In cases of failure, ultrasound is usually performed to exclude obstruction. Fifty-seven percent of kidneys are small or there is a difference of greater than 1.5 cm between the two kidneys[186] (Fig. 4-70). In 43 percent of cases, the kidneys are of normal size.[186]

There are multiple causes of chronic renal failure including:[178]

1. Glomerulonephritis
2. Chronic pyelonephritis
3. Renal vascular disease
4. Metabolic—diabetes, gout, hypercalcemia, hyperoxaluria, cystinosis, Fabry's disease
5. Nephrotoxins
6. Tuberculosis
7. Sarcoid
8. Dysproteinemia—myeloma, amyloid, mixed IgA-IgM cryoglobinemia, Waldenstrom's macroglobinemia
9. Hereditary or congenital—polycystic kidney disease, medullary cystic disease, Alport's syndrome, cys-

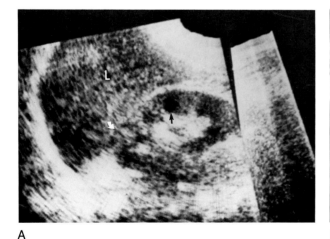

A

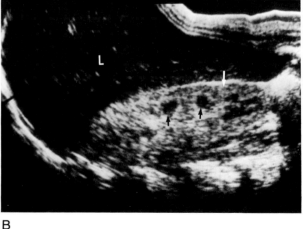

B

Fig. 4-88. Myoglobinuric renal failure. **(A)** Longitudinal scan of the right kidney through the right lobe of the liver *(L)*. The kidney is enlarged (14 cm). The renal pyramids are prominent (black arrow). Renal cortical echogenicity is equal to or greater than that of the liver (white arrow). **(B)** Longitudinal scan of an enlarged right (15 cm) kidney with increased cortical echogenicity (white arrows) and prominent renal pyramids (black arrow). Renal cortical echogenicity is much greater than liver *(L)*. (From Pardes JG, Yong HA, Kazam E: Sonographic findings in myoglobinuric renal failure and their clinical implications. J Ultrasound Med 2:391, 1983.)

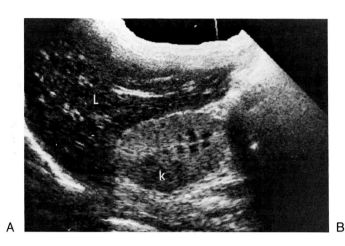

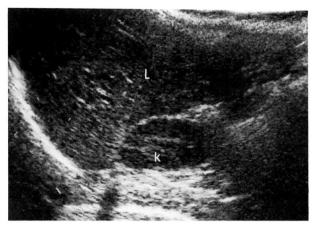

Fig. 4-89. Ethylene glycol poisoning. (A) Longitudinal scan of the right kidney *(k)* revealing intensely echogenic parenchyma with incomplete obliteration of the corticomedullary junction. The kidney is grossly enlarged. *(L,* liver.) (B) Longitudinal scan of right kidney *(k)* obtained after full recovery of renal function demonstrates a normal size and echopattern. *(L,* liver.) (From Walker JT, Keller MS, Katz SM: Computed tomographic and sonographic findings in acute ethylene glycol poisoning. J Ultrasound Med 2:429, 1983.)

tinosis, hyperoxaluria, chronic tubular acidosis, infantile nephrotic syndrome, dysplastic kidney

10. Miscellaneous — radiation
11. Major blood vessel disease — renal artery thrombosis, embolism or stenosis, bilateral renal vein thrombosis.
12. Hepatorenal syndrome
13. Acute pyelonephritis

Trauma

Trauma may be blunt, penetrating, or secondary to operative intervention. Preexisting renal abnormalities such as ectopia, anomalies, or tumor predispose to sig-

nificant renal damage even when the traumatic event is mild.[70] Renal trauma is generally managed conservatively with indications for surgery being on a clinical basis.

Excretory urography is the radiologic modality most commonly used to evaluate trauma to the upper urinary tract. The radiologic classification of renal trauma is as follows: (1) minor — normal urogram or one showing diminished renal concentration of contrast, a decreased nephrogram, minimal distortion of the calyces, or blood clots in pelvis; (2) major — extravasation of contrast; and (3) catastrophic injury — nonvisualization of the kidney or marked deformity of the pelvocalyceal system with extravasation of contrast (the kidney may or may not be damaged in the presence of significant surrounding retroperitoneal injury).[187] Excretory urography is a satisfactory screening procedure but may fail to provide infor-

Fig. 4-90. Chronic renal failure. Longitudinal scan, left kidney. The outline of the kidney can barely be distinguished (open arrows). It was easier to distinguish renal margins on real-time sonography. There is loss of distinction between cortex, medulla, and renal sinus. This hypertensive patient had long standing chronic renal failure.

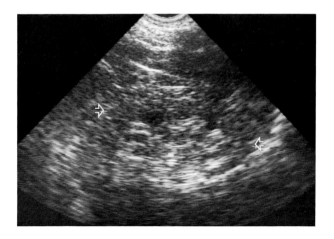

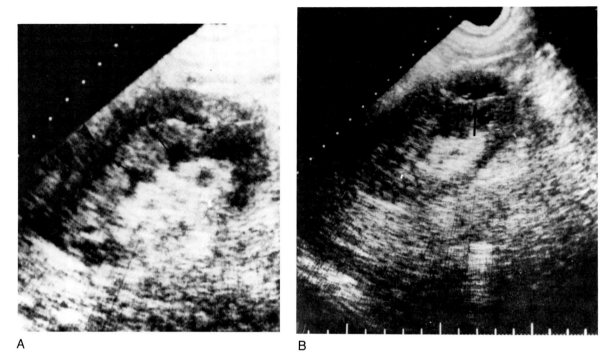

A   B

Fig. 4-91.   Renal trauma. Subcapsular and retroperitoneal hematoma. **(A)** Longitudinal scan demonstrates a perinephric fluid collection around the left kidney (arrows). Increased cortical echoes may be due to acoustic enhancement through the hematoma. **(B)** Transverse scan shows a collection indenting the margin of the left kidney (arrow) consistent with a subcapsular collection. (From Kay CJ, Rosenfield AT, Armm M: Gray-scale ultrasonography in the evaluation of renal trauma. Radiology 134:461, 1980.)

mation on the full extent of the renal injury. Nuclear medicine yields rapid assessment of the extent of parenchymal damage and reveals any significant injury to the renal pedicle.[187]

The information available on ultrasound is anatomic not functional. Bleeding into the retroperitoneal space may be seen as a lucency or a density (primarily depending on how soon after the injury the ultrasound is per-

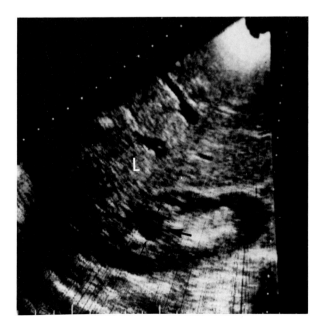

Fig. 4-92.   Renal trauma. Blood clot. Longitudinal scan. A mass containing low-level internal echoes is seen in the upper pole (arrows). This mass was also seen on IVP. (*L*, liver.) (From Kay CJ, Rosenfield AT, Armm M: Gray-scale ultrasonography in the evaluation of renal trauma. Radiology 134:461, 1980.)

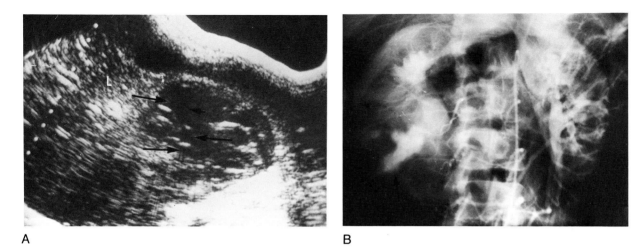

A   B

Fig. 4-93. Renal trauma. Fracture. **(A)** An anechoic line is seen through the upper half of the right kidney (arrows). (L, liver.) **(B)** Aortogram confirms the fracture of the kidney (arrowhead) with associated leakage of contrast material (arrow). (From Kay CJ, Rosenfield AT, Armm M: Gray-scale ultrasonography in the evaluation of renal trauma. Radiology 134:461, 1980.)

formed) (Fig. 4-91). Focal areas of internal hemorrhage and edema may be seen as hypoechoic areas (Fig. 4-91). In a limited number of cases, no findings may be seen on renal ultrasound, with the exception of blood clots in the renal pelvis. Blood clot may be seen in the collecting system as a mass containing low-level echoes, separating the walls of the affected system[187] (Fig. 4-92). A linear reproducible absence of echoes is seen in the area of a traumatized kidney suggesting a renal fracture[187,188] (Fig. 4-93). This must be differentiated from rib artifact where

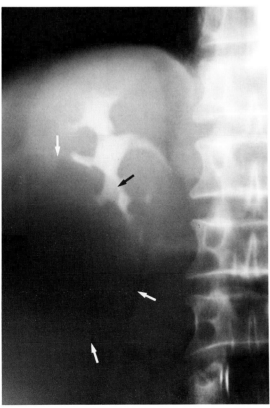

A

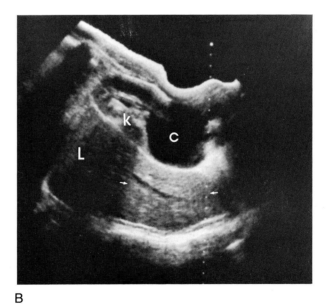

B

Fig. 4-94. Simple cyst. Classic. **(A)** Intravenous pyelogram demonstrating a mass, right lower pole (arrows). **(B)** Prone longitudinal scan, right kidney. A well-defined anechoic mass *(c)* is seen in the lower pole of the right kidney *(k)*. Distal acoustic enhancement (arrows) is seen. (*L*, liver.)

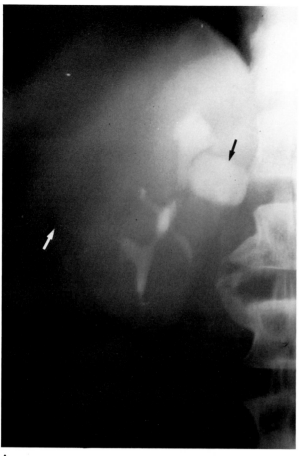

A

Fig. 4-95. Simple cyst. **(A)** Intravenous pyelogram demonstrating a mass effect (white arrow) and a calculus (black arrow). Longitudinal **(B)** and transverse **(C)** scans of the right kidney demonstrate a well-defined anechoic mass *(c)* in the upper pole laterally. Acoustic enhancement (arrows) is seen. A calculus (black arrow) is seen medially on **(C)** but since it is a compound scan its associated shadow is not seen. (*ivc*, inferior vena cava; *L*, liver.)

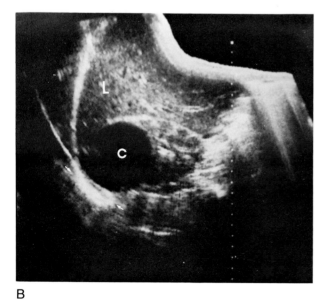

B

C

anechoic areas are seen anterior and posterior to the kidney and from a bifid collecting system.[187] And, urinomas produced by the trauma can be seen as anechoic masses in a perirenal location (Fig. 4-52). Serial ultra-

sound may be used to follow an injury identified on ultrasound.[187] Ultrasound has been reported to be 100 percent accurate if performed with a urogram and disregarding minimal lesions.[189]

Renal Masses

CYST

Simple Cyst. Simple cysts occur in 50 percent of patients over 55 years old.[190-192] They are uncommon in children but are more common with increasing age.[193] They are usually unilocular with an epithelial lining and can be located anywhere in the kidney.

The classic cyst on ultrasound meets the following criteria: (1) clear wall demarcation; (2) spherical or slightly ovoid in shape; (3) absence of internal echoes; and (4) acoustic enhancement beyond the cyst[16,190-195] (Figs. 4-94 and 4-95). An additional finding is a narrow band of acoustic shadowing just beyond the outer margin of the cyst at each border of the acoustic enhancement[192] (Fig. 4-96). This shadowing is secondary to refraction and deflection of the echoes around the curved surface of a cystic mass.[192] Each renal cyst examined with ultrasound should include careful evaluation of irregularity and/or textural changes that might suggest an atypical appearance.[196]

There are several technical factors that can interfere with the recognition of the true anechoic nature of cysts. Reverberation and effects of the beam width can interact with adjacent acoustic reflectors to produce artifactual echoes. Sonic enhancement in the distal tissues varies with time gain compensation, frequency, and position of the focal zone. The operator who is aware of these problems can compensate for them and thereby improve the diagnostic accuracy.[197]

The reverberation from the skin-transducer interface and from the specular reflectors lying anterior to the cyst are recognized as a source of artifact. In a large cyst, such artifacts are usually restricted to the anterior portion of the fluid and rapidly decrease in amplitude after several reflective cycles. They can be suppressed by having the beam strike the reflector at different angles as the cyst can be scanned from an opposite approach through the body (Fig. 4-97). Small cysts are most resistent to artifactual off-axis signals when they lie within the focal zone. These larger changes in transducer output are least likely to result in echo fill-in, especially if there are no specular reflectors in the surrounding media.[197]

The distal sonic enhancement sign is a nonattenuation characteristic of a cystic lesion caused by the time gain compensation and is most visible with greater slopes used with high-frequency transducers. The effect is amplified when the tissue distal to the cyst lies in the intensity peak created by focusing the transducer beam[197] (Fig. 4-98).

The unequivocal diagnosis of a cyst based on ultrasound is 95 to 98 percent accurate with 2 percent due to hematomas, localized hydronephrosis, or septa in cysts.[190-192,194,198] The causes of incorrect diagnoses include lesions less than 2 cm, masses in the left upper pole, diffusely infiltrating urothelial tumors, echogenic fatty lesions or acute abscesses and hematomas.[199] In order to maintain this high degree of accuracy, one must adhere strictly to the criteria listed for a cyst. If a lesion meets only a portion of the criteria, then it is indeterminate for a cyst and further diagnostic tests are warranted. This may be a CT or a cyst puncture. Some authors recommend the use of ultrasound with or without aspiration for all cyst-like renal masses thought to be indeterminate on CT.[200] If, however, the lesion meets all the criteria for a classic cyst on ultrasound, no further investigation is needed.[190] Lesions to be considered if the mass

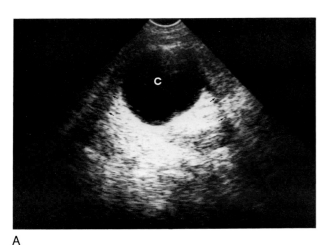

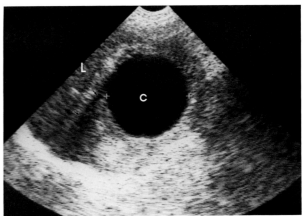

A   B

Fig. 4-96. Simple cyst. Acoustic shadowing. On these transverse **(A)** and longitudinal **(B)** scans of a right renal cyst *(c)*, acoustic shadowing (arrows) is seen paralleling the borders of the mass and on either side of the acoustic enhancement. (*L,* liver.)

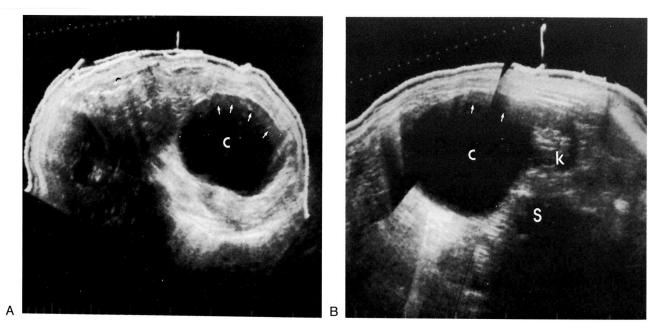

Fig. 4-97. Simple cyst. Reverberation. Transverse supine scan at 10 cm above the umbilicus **(A)** and right lateral decubitus scan **(B)**. Reverberation artifacts (arrows) are seen anteriorly within this left renal cyst *(c)*. (*k*, kidney; *S*, spine.)

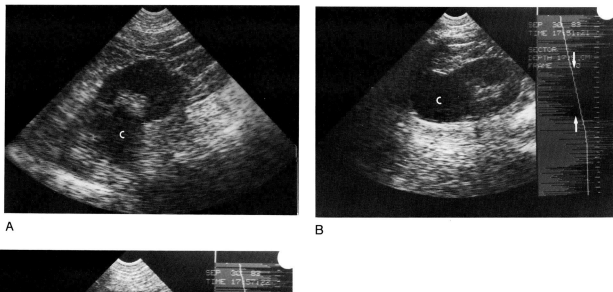

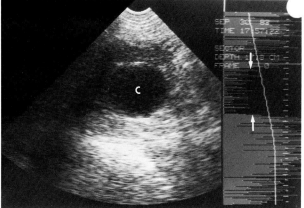

Fig. 4-98. Simple cyst. Change in body position. **(A)** Longitudinal supine scan of the left kidney. A poorly defined hypoechoic mass *(c)* is seen in the midportion of the kidney posteriorly. The patient was placed in the right lateral decubitus position **(B,C)** bringing the mass closer to the focal zone of the transducer. Longitudinal **(B)** and transverse **(C)** scans. The mass *(c)* now appears round, and relatively echofree (see A-mode, arrows) with acoustic enhancement.

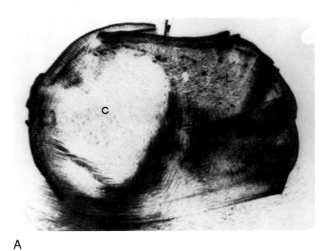
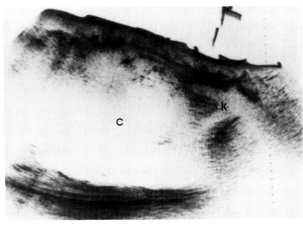

A   B

Fig. 4-99. Hemorrhagic cyst. **(A)** Transverse supine static scan at 12 cm above the umbilicus demonstrating a large cystic *(c)* hypoechoic mass filling the right abdomen. The liver *(L)* is displaced to the left. The mass does contain some internal echoes. **(B)** Prone right longitudinal scan demonstrates the relationship of the mass to the kidney *(k)*. The mass is cystic (noted by the acoustic enhancement) but contains internal echoes.

does not meet all the criteria for a cyst include complicated cyst, abscess, hematoma, renal artery aneurysm, hydronephrosis, and homogeneous or cystic tumor.[195]

Hemorrhagic Cyst. There is a 1 to 11.5 percent incidence of hemorrhage in simple cysts.[192,201] The incidence is even greater in polycystic kidney disease. On ultrasound one may see internal echoes and/or lack of acoustic enhancement (Figs. 4-26 and 4-99). Because these cysts do not meet the classical criteria for a cyst on ultrasound, they would be subject to further investigation:

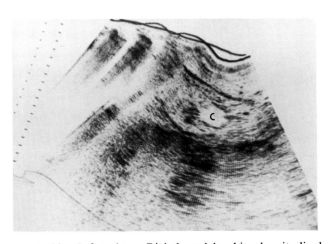

Fig. 4-100. Infected cyst. Right lateral decubitus longitudinal scan of the left kidney. A well-defined anechoic mass *(c)* is seen but no acoustic enhancement is seen. This would be indeterminant for a renal cyst. The fluid was aspirated revealing infection.

aspiration or CT.[202] On a CT scan, these lesions may appear hyperdense.[201-203]

Infected Cyst. As with the hemorrhagic cyst, the infected cyst does not meet the classic ultrasound criteria for a cyst (Fig. 4-100). It often contains internal echoes and the patient is symptomatic. Again, this lesion would be subject to further studies, primarily aspiration under ultrasound guidance. Even if the cyst looks classic for a cyst, infection should be considered in a symptomatic patient.

Atypical Cyst. Septation may be seen within a simple cyst as a linear echodensity (Figs. 4-101 and 4-102). The septae should be evaluated to make sure they are thin. Additionally, there may be multiple septa producing a multilocular mass.

Besides septation, there may be cysts that contain calcification in their wall (Fig. 4-103). The calcification diminishes the sound transmission and may cause the mass to appear solid.[192]

A cyst containing milk of calcium may have a confusing appearance. This cyst usually represents a calyceal diverticulum that has lost its communication with the calyceal system.[192] (This was discussed more extensively under the Renal Medical Disease Section.) On ultrasound, a cystic mass is seen containing a layering linear band of echoes with a shadow[192] (Fig. 4-83).

Parapelvic Cysts. Parapelvic cysts are not true cysts but may be lymphatic in origin or may develop from embryonic rests with no communication with the collecting system. They represent 6 percent of cysts.[148,204]

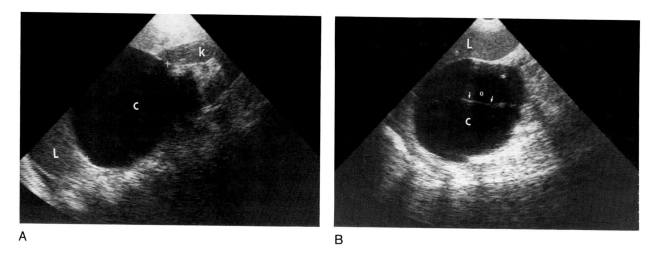

A   B

Fig. 4-101. Atypical cyst. Septation. **(A)** Longitudinal scan of the right kidney. A large well-defined anechoic mass *(c)* is seen in the upper pole of the right kidney *(k)*. *(L, liver)*. On left lateral decubitus longitudinal view **(B)**, a septum (arrows) is seen within the cyst *(c; L, liver)*.

Patients with these cysts are usually asymptomatic but may have hypertension, hematuria, or hydronephrosis or may become secondarily infected. Real-time ultrasound is especially helpful in their evaluation to determine if the cysts communicate with the calyces. At times, these cysts may be difficult to distinguish from hydronephrosis[204,205] (Figs. 4-27 and 4-104).

Tuberous Sclerosis. Tuberous sclerosis is an inherited neurocutaneous disorder in which the characteristic renal lesion is the angiomyolipoma presenting in 40 to 80 percent of patients. Less common manifestations of

this disease are cysts. The cysts in tuberous sclerosis have a hyperplastic eosinophilic epithelial lining that projects into the lumen of the cyst. Their etiology in this disease is unclear. The cysts do not usually cause severe renal impairment but some do. When a child is noted to have the pattern of adult polycystic kidney disease on ultrasound, the examiner should also consider the diagnosis of tuberous sclerosis.[206]

Coexistent Cyst and Tumor. The incidence of tumor and cyst is 2.1 to 7 percent.[196,207,208] Most commonly it is felt that the tumor plays an etiologic role in the cyst

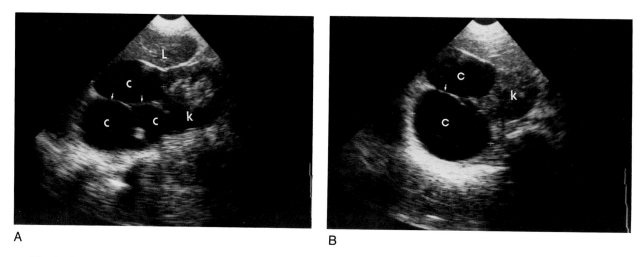

A   B

Fig. 4-102. Atypical cyst. Septation. Right longitudinal **(A)** and transverse **(B)** scans of the right kidney *(k)* demonstrate a multiseptated (arrows) renal cyst *(c)*. *(L, liver; h, hemangioma.)*

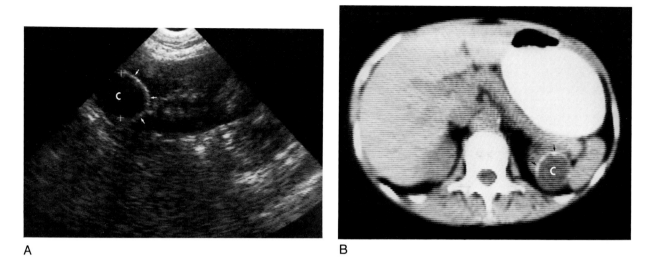

A

B

Fig. 4-103. Atypical cyst. Calcification. **(A)** Longitudinal prone scan of the left kidney demonstrates a well-defined round, anechoic mass *(c)* in the upper pole. The mass has very echodense walls (arrows) without acoustic enhancement. **(B)** Unenhanced CT scan. A low-density mass *(c)* is seen in the upper pole of the left kidney. The walls contain calcification (arrows).

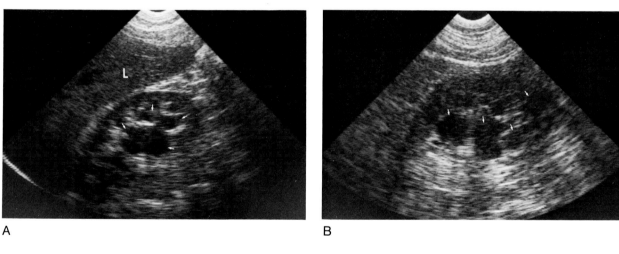

A

B

Fig. 4-104. Parapelvic cysts. Longitudinal scans of the right **(A)** and left **(B)** kidneys. Multiple anechoic areas (arrows) are seen in the region of the renal sinus. They appeared to connect at real-time suggesting hydronephrosis. (*L*, liver.) **(C)** Intravenous pyelogram. No hydronephrosis is seen. Instead, the mass effect of multiple parapelvic cysts is seen.

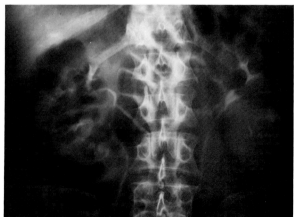

C

formation.[196] In the articles reviewed, none of these cystic lesions could meet all the classical ultrasound criteria for a cyst and as such would be subject to further studies.

Cyst Puncture. The indications for cyst puncture would include the following: (1) a cystic lesion that does not meet the ultrasound critera for a cyst (indeterminate); (2) a cyst that does meet the critera but presents in a patient suspected of infection; and (3) a classic cyst on ultrasound of a patient less than 40-years-old with hematuria or with a high index of suspicion for tumor.

The diagnosis of a cyst with aspiration approaches 100 percent. The incidence of major complications is 1.4 percent.[209] The majority of the complications seen on ultrasound include perirenal hemorrhage. The most common minor complication is hematuria.

To begin the procedure, the patient is usually placed in a prone or semiprone position with a pillow or rolled sheet placed under the stomach. The kidney is scanned in held-respiration and the cyst is localized. A point is picked that is in the center of the lesion. If the lesion is large, then the aspiration procedure may be preformed without direct ultrasound visualization. If the cyst is small or if there is a need to puncture several cysts (such as in the polycystic patient), then the patient is scanned in a sterile fashion while performing the puncture. After the usual sterile preparation of the skin, and local anesthesia, a 22-gauge needle is inserted to the premeasured depth with one swift movement. There is a pop felt when the needle enters the cyst. Fluid is aspirated and sent for cytology. As a rule, clear yellow fluid (looks like urine) is obtained from a simple cyst. If the fluid is hemorrhagic or the fluid is turbid, then the lesion becomes suspicious. If there is any question of infection, the fluid should be Gram-stained and sent for cultures. (There is further discussion of this procedure in Chapter 10.)

ABSCESS (covered under Inflammatory Disease)

INFARCTION

Not all focal parenchymal lesions are tumor. Renal infarction may appear as an area of hyperechoicity (Figs. 4-105 and 4-106). The increase in echoes is probably secondary to an admixture of fibrosis with acoustically dissimilar tissues within the affected region. A focally increased area of parenchymal echoes in association with thinning of the involved cortex has been reported in

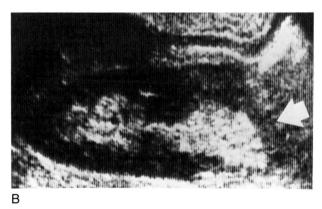

B

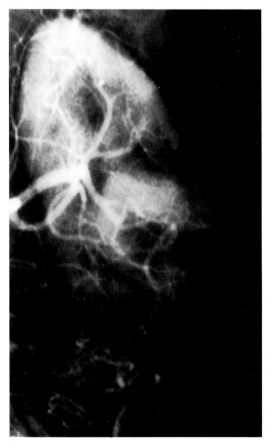

A

Fig. 4-105. Renal infarction. (**A**) Aortogram. An avascular region is seen involving the lower pole of the left kidney. (**B**) Longitudinal scan, left kidney. An echogenic wedge-shaped lower pole renal mass (arrow) is seen. (From Erwin BC, Carroll BA, Walter JR, Sommer FG: Renal infarction appearing as an echogenic mass. AJR 138:759, © Am Roentgen Ray Soc, 1982.)

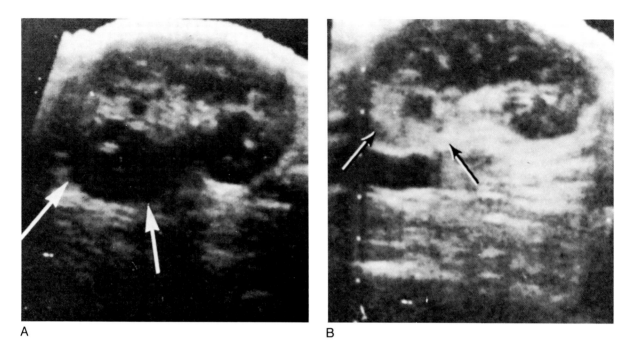

A   B

Fig. 4-106. Renal infarction. Experimental arterial occlusion. Sequence of changes in segmental infarction 27 days after arterial occlusion. **(A)** Scan 8 hours after segmental arterial occlusion. There is bulging along the superoposterior aspect of the kidney (arrows). The infarcted area demonstrates decreased echogenicity. **(B)** Longitudinal scan 27 days later. There is thinning of the renal cortex and increased cortical echogenicity (arrows) in the area of the infarction. (From Spies JB, Hricak H, Slemmer TM et al: Sonographic evaluation of experimental acute renal arterial occlusion in dogs. AJR 142:341, © American Roentgen Ray Society, 1984.)

chronic atrophic pyelonephritis as well as renal infarction.[210] Other lesions in the differential diagnosis of a focal area of increased echogenicity would include solitary and diffuse angiomyolipomata, cavernous renal hemangioma, renal cell carcinoma, angiosarcoma, undifferentiated sarcoma, oncocytoma, and metastatic neoplasm.[210]

Some investigators have evaluated experimentally the sonographic pattern of renal infarction[211] (Fig. 4-106). Within 24 hours after arterial occlusion, a focal hypoechoic mass is seen. Within 7 days, echoes begin to appear within the mass such that it becomes echogenic by 17 days, and total renal arterial occlusion produces no appreciable change in cortical echogenicity. As such, when evaluating specifically for renal infarction, the patient may be best served by a physiologic study.

RENAL COLUMN OF BERTIN

Hypertrophy of a renal column of Bertin may produce a mass effect. It has the following characteristics: (1) it indents the renal sinus laterally; (2) it is clearly defined from the renal sinus; (3) it has a largest dimension of less than 3 cm; (4) it is continuous or contiguous with the renal cortex; and (5) it has an echogenicity close to that of cortex[199,212] (Fig. 4-8). A focal mass that meets all these criteria should be considered a renal column. It may be best seen by scanning the patient in the decubitus position because the column would be in profile.[199] If there is any question, a renal nuclear medicine study may be performed to confirm that the "mass" is composed of functioning tissue.[212]

PRIMARY RENAL TUMORS

Renal Cell Carcinoma. Renal cell carcinoma represents 1 to 3 percent of all visceral cancers and represents 80 to 90 percent of the renal cancers in adults.[14] The lesion is seen in the sixth to seventh decade with a 3:1 male to female ratio.[14] Classically, the patient presents with costovertebral angle pain, mass, and hematuria with hematuria the most reliable presentation. These lesions commonly metastasize widely before they produce local symptoms. Fifty percent go to lungs with 33 percent to bones, followed by nodes, liver, adrenal, and brain.[14] Ten to 15 percent metastasize to the opposite kidney. The average 5 year survival is 45 percent with 70 percent if there are no distant metastases.[14]

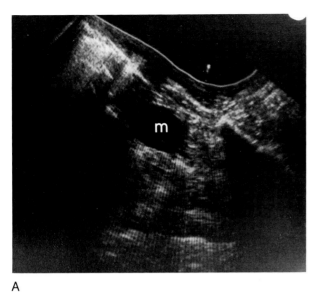

A

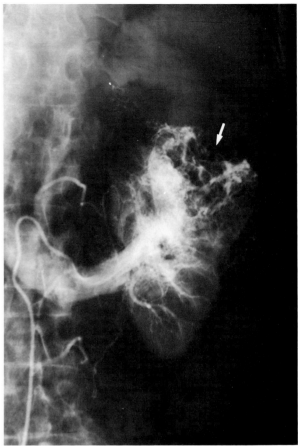

B

Fig. 4-107. Renal cell carcinoma. Anechoic pattern. **(A)** Longitudinal prone scan of a mass *(m)* projecting laterally from the left kidney. The kidney itself is not identified on this scan. The mass is well-defined, round, and anechoic but it does not exhibit acoustic enhancement. As such, it is indeterminate for a cyst; a cyst puncture was performed and no fluid was obtained. The mass was assumed to be solid. **(B)** Angiogram displaying a hypervascular mass (arrows).

The ultrasound appearance of these lesions can be variable. Two basic criteria include a mass that is either more or less echogenic than normal renal parenchyma, and an absence of acoustic enhancement beyond the mass[213] (Figs. 4-53 and 4-107 to 4-111). In one study, 44 percent of these lesions were found to be moderately echogenic with internal echoes similar to normal cortical echoes and commonly noted were irregular margins. Twenty-one percent in the series were more echogenic than the normal renal parenchyma with 35 percent minimally echogenic appearing somewhat similar to a cyst. There was no direct correlation found between echogenicity and vascularity—no linear relationship between the number of echoes and the number of abnormal blood vessels. Also, there was no significant correlation between the pathologic appearance and the ultrasound appearance classified as moderately or markedly echogenic. Seventy-three percent of the minimally echogenic tumors were grossly inhomogeneous, which suggests a sparsity of echoes due to hemorrhage, necrosis, or cystic degeneration.[213]

Other investigators report that the echogenicity of the carcinoma correlates with the degree of neovascular-ity.[214] The degree of vascularity generally paralleled the echogenicity of the lesion with the hypoechoic lesion hypovascular while those with greater echoes or mixed were hypervascular[214] (Figs. 4-107 to 4-111). All angiographic hypervascular tumors and hypovascular tumors with areas of hemorrhage and necrosis are more echoproducing.[215]

Occasionally, a pattern similar to a multilocular cyst may be seen, but the complex cysts are separated by highly echogenic areas also seen infrequently in necrotic and cystic renal cell carcinoma[216] (Fig. 4-112). Cyst aspiration and cytology might make diagnosis.

Five to 10 percent of renal cell carcinomas are papillary, which is a microscopic subclassification that is characterized by slower growth, less extensive involvement at the time of diagnosis, and a better prognosis than the nonpapillary renal parenchymal malignancy.[217,218] There is a high frequency of internal calcifications.[218] On ultrasound 64 percent of papillary tumors have been reported to be hypoechoic with only 23 percent of the nonpapillary tumors being hypoechoic[217] (Fig. 4-113). Data suggests that the papillary carcinomas tend to be hypoechoic due to the large central area of cystic necrosis

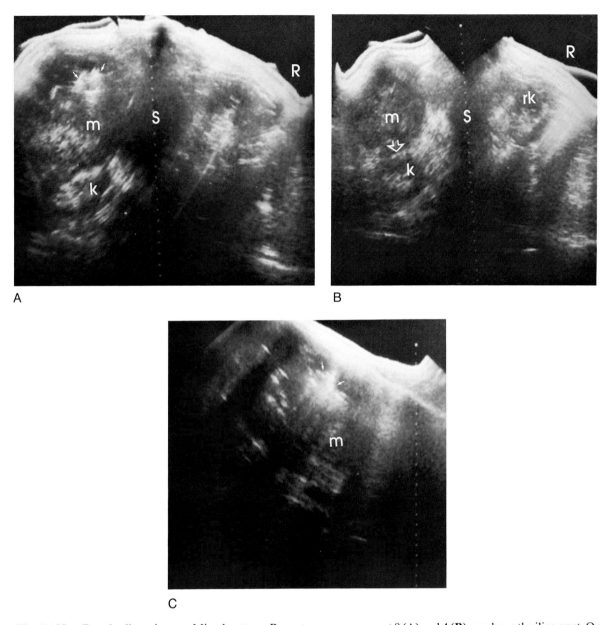

Fig. 4-108. Renal cell carcinoma. Mixed pattern. Prone transverse scans at 8 **(A)** and 4 **(B)** cm above the iliac crest. On **(A)** the mass *(m)* appears to exhibit a mixed echopattern with highly reflective echoes (arrows) close to the transducer much like that seen with bowel gas. On **(B)** a solid mass *(m)* is seen posterior to the left kidney *(k)*. On this view it almost appears separate from the kidney (open arrow). (*rk*, right kidney; *R*, right; *S*, spine.) **(C)** Longitudinal prone scan over the left kidney. A normal reniform shape is not seen. Instead, a highly reflective echopattern (arrows) is seen in the near field. A mass *(m)* is not well outlined in this plane due to the reflection of the sound beam by the air.

in the tumor. Another study reported no consistent ultrasound pattern associated with papillary renal cell carcinoma.[218] In this series, 85 percent of the papillary tumors were confined within the renal capsule (stage I) whereas more than 50 percent of the nonpapillary tumors had extended beyond the limits of the kidney.[217] Most papillary tumors are less vascular and have a better prognosis than the nonpapillary type.[217]

When a solid renal mass is identified on ultrasound, the study is not complete. The contralateral kidney must be examined carefully. In addition, the inferior vena cava, and renal vein should be examined for evidence of tumor extension[219,220] (Fig. 4-114). The prognosis is poorer with tumor extension into the inferior vena cava.[220] The paraortic area should be evaluated for the presence of nodes, and the liver should also be evaluated

A

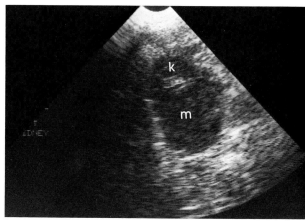

B

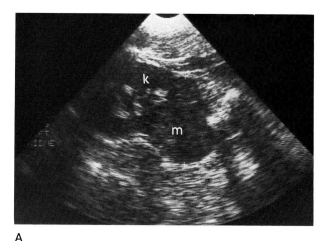

C

Fig. 4-109. Renal cell carcinoma. Echodense pattern. Real-time longitudinal **(A)** and transverse **(B)** scans of the right kidney *(k)* reveal a mass *(m)* with an echopattern similar to renal parenchyma. *(C)* Angiogram. A well-defined mass *(m)* with neovascularity is seen.

for metastases.[220] In staging renal cell carcinoma, ultrasound is correct in 70 percent, with CT correct in 91 percent.[221]

Ultrasound has been shown to have an accuracy of 90 percent in diagnosing solid masses. The causes of incorrect diagnoses have been attributed to lesions less than 2 cm, masses in the left upper pole, diffusely infiltrating urothelial tumors, echogenic fatty lesions, or acute abscess and hematoma. Angiography in the same series was correct in 88 percent of solid lesions.[199]

Oncocytoma. Oncocytomas are uncommon benign tumors that usually occur in middle to old age with males affected more than females (1.7 to 1).[222] They account for 2 to 14 percent of renal tumors that were preoperatively thought to be cancer.[223] These tumors are

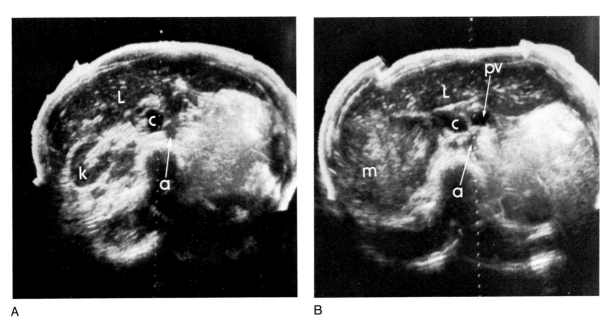

Fig. 4-110. Renal cell carcinoma. Echodense pattern. Transverse scans at 8 (**A**), and 14 cm (**B**) above the umbilicus. In (**A**) the right kidney *(k)* is identified. In (**B**) an echodense mass *(m)* is seen in the renal fossa extending anteriorly and laterally. (*a*, aorta; *c*, inferior vena cava; *pv*, portal vein; *L*, liver.)

usually asymptomatic, although some patients present with pain or hematuria. Although they are usually single, they may be multiple and bilateral.

Oncocytomas have distinct clinical and pathological characteristics. They are not associated with vascular invasion, local recurrence after surgery or distant metastases.[222] Typically, they range from 0.3 to 26 cm in diameter, are well-defined, smooth and homogeneous, often

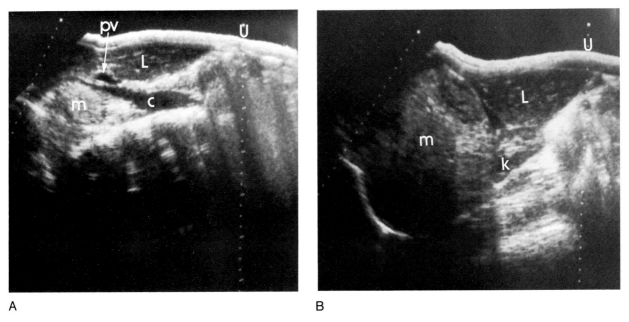

Fig. 4-111. Renal cell carcinoma; same patient as Fig. 4-110. Longitudinal scans in the midline (**A**), and 7 cm (**B**) to the right display the mass *(m)*. The mass is seen to extend posterior to the inferior vena cava *(c)* in (**A**) and superiorly to the right kidney *(k)* in (**B**). The mass is so echo-absorbing that there is decreased penetration of the sound beam seen. (*L*, liver; *pv*, portal vein; *U*, level of the umbilicus.)

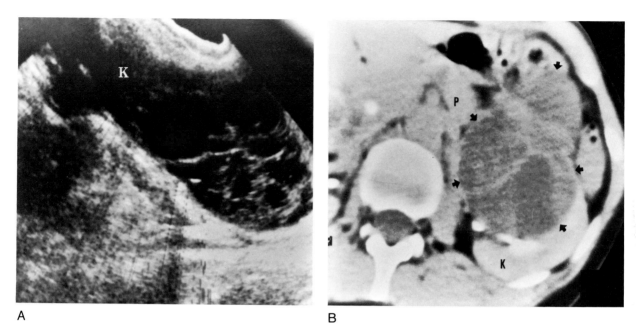

A   B

Fig. 4-112.   Multilocular cystic renal cell carcinoma. **(A)** Prone longitudinal scan, left kidney *(K)*. Multiple fluid-filled cysts are seen separated by thick, echogenic septa. **(B)** CT scan. A large multicystic mass is seen originating from the left kidney *(K)* compressing the kidney dorsally and extending vertically (arrows). *(P,* pancreas.) (From Feldberg MAM, van Waes PFGM: Multilocular cystic renal cell carcinoma. AJR 138:953, © American Roentgen Ray Society, 1982.)

with a central stellate scar.[222,223] So, as the mass enlarges, it may outstrip its blood supply with concomitant infarction, hemorrhage, and necrosis. The central stellate fibrotic scar may form after the central hemorrhage undergoes organization and healing.[223] A comparable renal cell carcinoma will often be well-defined but will not

contain a central scar but instead hemorrhage and necrosis.

On ultrasound an oncocytoma appears as a sold renal mass with low-level echoes similar to a renal cell carcinoma[224] (Fig. 4-115). If a central, echogenic scar is seen in an otherwise homogeneous mass on ultrasound or CT, an oncocytoma should be suspected[222,223] (Fig. 4-116). This criteria appears to apply only if the mass is greater than 3 cm.[222] If the tumor is greater than 6 cm with necrosis or calcification, it cannot be differentiated by ultrasound.[223] The radiologic differentiation of oncocytoma or renal cell carcinoma is important prior to surgery because an oncocytoma is treated by local resection or heminephrectomy without chemotherapy or radiation therapy. If no central scar is seen by ultrasound or CT, an angiogram may be performed. In the case of a typical oncocytoma a spoke-wheel arterial supply or dense tumor blush is extremely suggestive.[222]

Angiomyolipoma. An angiomyolipoma or renal hamartoma is an uncommon benign renal tumor composed of fat cells intermixed with smooth muscle cells and aggregates of thick-walled blood vessels. This lesion is usually unilateral, although it may be multiple. The female to male ratio is 2.3 to 1 to 25 to 2. Eighty percent occur in females with 80 percent on the right side.[225] Twenty-five percent are extrarenal including the renal sinus.[225] The size varies from 1 cm to greater than 20 cm

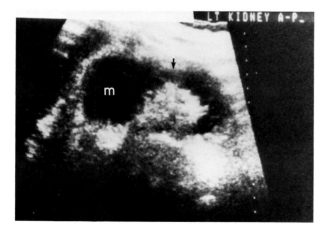

Fig. 4-113.   Papillary renal cell carcinoma. Longitudinal scan, left kidney. A 5 cm mass *(m)* is seen less echogenic than the adjacent renal cortex (arrow). (From Blei CL, Hartman DS, Friedman AC, Davis CJ Jr.: Papillary renal cell carcinoma: Ultrasonic/Pathologic correlation. J Clin Ultrasound 10:429, 1982.)

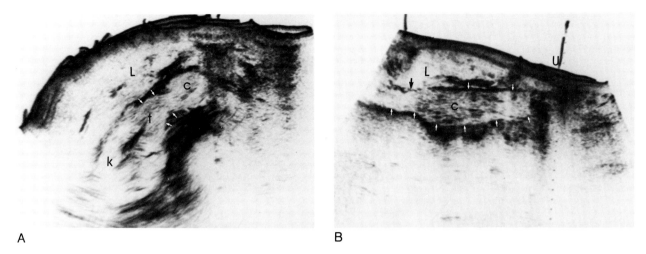

Fig. 4-114. Vascular invasion. Patient with renal cell carcinoma. The inferior vena cava *(c)* is seen distended with echoes on both transverse **(A)** and longitudinal **(B)** scans. On **(A)**, there is distension of the right renal vein (arrows) as well. This represented tumor *(t)* extension. (*L*, liver; *k*, right kidney; *U*, level of the umbilicus.)

with a mean size of 9.4 cm. Sixty to 80 percent of patients with tuberous sclerosis have these lesions, which are usually bilateral and multiple.[225-227] Solitary lesions are not associated with tuberous sclerosis and typically present in the fourth to sixth decade.[225,226]

The clinical presentation of angiomyolipoma is varied.[227] Most are asymptomatic; the symptomatic lesions tend to be much larger and are more likely to contain angiomatous tissue.[228] Hemorrhage within the lesions or within the retroperitoneum is common; it often presents

with acute onset of flank or abdominal pain and/or shock. The small lesions have no known malignant potential and nonoperative management is suggested.[186]

The most characteristic pattern of these lesions seen on ultrasound is that of a hyperechoic lesion (more dense than renal parenchyma)[198,224-230] (Figs. 4-117 and 4-118). Those lesions with a dense pattern appear to have a more myomatous or vascular element. The marked echogenicity is due to the high fat content, multiple nonfat interfaces, hetergeneous cellular architecture, and/or

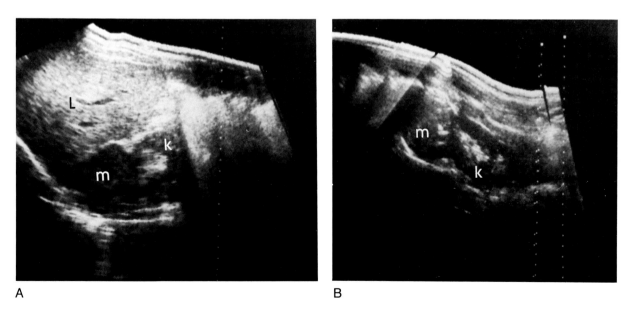

Fig. 4-115. Renal oncocytoma. Longitudinal supine **(A)** and prone **(B)** scans of the right kidney *(k)* reveal a solid mass *(m)* in the upper pole. It is similar in density to renal parenchyma. (*L*, liver.) At angiography, a rounded, well-defined mass was seen with a spoke-wheel pattern of vascularity.

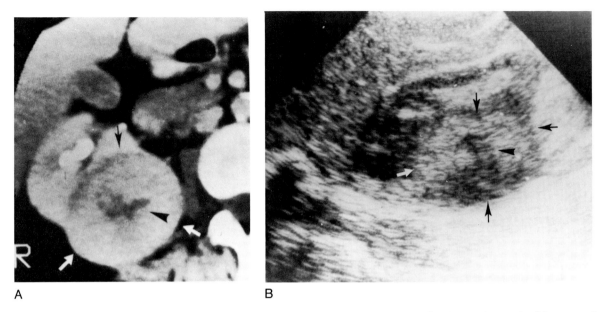

A   B

Fig. 4-116. Renal oncocytoma. Central scar. (A) CT scan demonstrates a well-defined mass (arrows) with a central stellate area of low density (arrowhead) that corresponds to the central scar. (B) Longitudinal scan showing a well-defined solid mass (arrows). The central scar is recognized as a small central hypoechoic zone (arrowhead). (From Quinn MJ, Hartman DS, Friedman AC et al: Renal oncocytoma: New observations. Radiology 153:49, 1984.)

numerous vessels often present within the angiomyolipoma. The less echogenic areas within this tumor may be due to the nonfatty portions of the tumor adjacent to dilated calyces, or areas of hemorrhage, and necrosis. Those with a mixed pattern demonstrate spontaneous hemorrhage and necrosis.[227] Some have a hypoechoic pattern, less dense than the renal sinus. Although the echodense pattern is the most common pattern, it is not pathognomonic for angiolipoma.[227] However, renal cell carcinomas are usually less dense. In a rare case, tumor extension may be seen within the inferior vena cava.[231]

Juxtaglomerular Tumors. The combination of a hypovascular solid renal mass in a patient with elevated renin but no renal arterial lesion should suggest the diagnosis of a juxtaglomerular tumor. These patients present

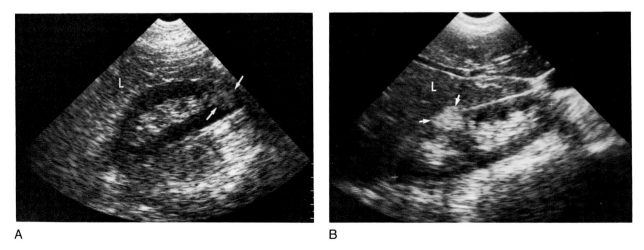

A   B

Fig. 4-117. Renal angiomyolipoma. Case 1: (A) Longitudinal supine scan right kidney. A well-defined echogenic mass (arrows) is seen in the lower pole. (L, liver) Case 2: (B) Longitudinal scan of the right kidney demonstrates an echodense mass (arrows) extending anteriorly from the mid-portion of the kidney. (L, liver.)

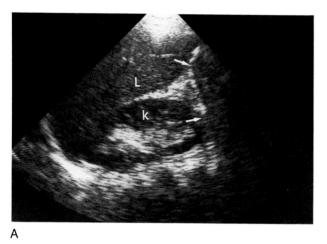

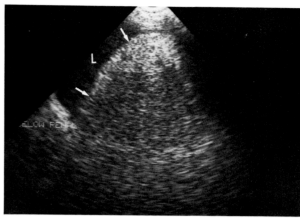

A

B

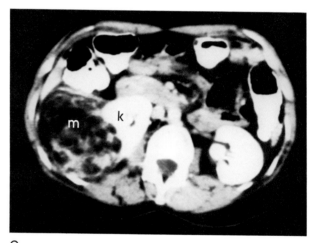

C

Fig. 4-118. Renal angiomyolipoma. Longitudinal scan of the right kidney **(A)** and just below the right kidney *(k)* **(B)**. A large echodense mass (arrows) is seen. It is very echo-absorbing. (*L,* liver.) Enhanced **(C)** CT scan demonstrates a fatty mass *(m)* extending from the right kidney.

with hypertension, more frequent in females with a mean age of 31 years. The renin-producing tumor (reninomas) is a rare but curable cause of hypertension.[232] These patients frequently present with symptoms of moderate to severe headaches, polydypsia, polyuria including enuresis, and intermittent neuromuscular complaints.[232]

These tumors are usually small, solitary, and confined to the kidney with an average size of 2 to 3 cm with most just beneath the renal capsule. Pathologically, there is a pseudocapsule and there are small foci of hemorrhage within the tumor. On ultrasound these lesions are usually echogenic possibly because of the numerous interfaces between the juxtaglomerular cells and the abundant small vascular channels within the tumor[232] (Fig. 4-119). If there is hemorrhage and necrosis, the lesion may be hypoechoic.

Multilocular Cystic Nephroma. This lesion is an uncommon nonfamilial neoplasm that usually affects predominately male children and female adults. Seventy-

three percent of children less than 4 years old are males with 89 percent of patients greater than 4 years old, females.[233] It is usually solitary; rarely is it multiple. It commonly occurs as an asymptomatic mass occasionally with hematuria. The mass is usually seen on a KUB and occasionally there are curvilinear calcifications. The excretory urogram and retrograde pyelogram are helpful when there is pelvic herniation of the tumor or when septae are noted with total body opacification. On an angiogram, the lesion may be avascular, hypovascular, or hypervascular.[233]

The lesion is an uncommon neoplasm characterized by a well-circumscribed encapsulated mass that contains multiple noncommunicating fluid-filled locules with thick internal septations.[224,233,234] This lesion has many names: benign multilocular cystic nephroma, multilocular cyst, cystic nephroma, cystic adenoma, benign cystic differentiated nephroblastoma, cystic partially differentiated nephroblastoma, polycystic nephroblastoma, differentiated nephroblastoma, cystic nephroblastoma, well differentiated polycystic Wilms' tumor, lymphangi-

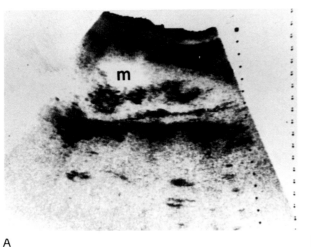

A

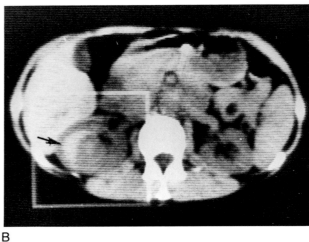

B

Fig. 4-119. Renal juxtaglomular tumor. **(A)** Longitudinal scan. A 5 cm solid hypoechoic mass *(m)* is seen in the upper pole of the right kidney. **(B)** Unenhanced CT scan. The periphery of the mass is isodense with the normal renal parenchyma. A crescent-shaped area of increased attenuation (arrow) is seen representing hemorrhage within the central portion of the mass. (From Dunnick NR, Hartman DS, Ford KK et al: The radiology of juxtaglomerular tumors. Radiology 147:321, 1983.)

oma, and partially polycystic kidney.[233,234] The pathogenesis of this lesion is controversial. The finding of local recurrence, distant metastases, growth of the lesion, and presence of embryonic mesenchyme support the thesis that it is a neoplasm but it is not always benign.[233] Because of the frequency of microscopic foci of nephroblastoma in multilocular nephroma and because of an occasional case of nephroblastoma with focal features of multilocular nephroma it is believed that the development of these two tumors probably progress along separate lines from a common ancestor metanephric blastoma.[233]

The ultrasound findings are related to the amount of stroma and size of the locules. When the cysts are large enough, ultrasound will demonstrate a cluster of echo-free masses separated by intense echoes (connective tissue septa) and this pattern is suggestive of multilocular cystic nephroma[233] (Figs. 4-25 and 4-120). A finely cystic structure with jelly-like contents plus solid components of embryonic tissue give it a solid character at times.[234] If cyst aspiration is performed, clear to yellow fluid is obtained similar to serum. If contrast is injected, only the locule directly punctured by the needle will fill.[233] The treatment is nephrectomy and occasionally removal of the mass.

Wilms' Tumor. Wilms' tumor (nephroblastoma) arises from the metanephric blastoma, the normal fetal precursor of the kidney parenchyma. It is the most common solid renal tumor in patients 1 to 8 years old with a peak at 3 years.[235] Ninety percent of patients are less than

5 years old with 70 percent less than 3 years old.[236] It may be associated with congenital anomalies such as hemihypertrophy, and hamartomas, as well as Beckwith-Wiedemann syndrome. This tumor has also been de-

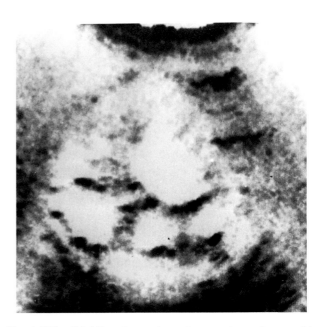

Fig. 4-120. Multilocular cystic nephroma. A renal mass with a multilocular configuration, discrete septae and anechoic spaces with acoustic enhancement is seen. (From Madewell JE, Goldman SM, Davis CJ Jr. et al: Multilocular cystic nephroma: A radiographic-pathologic correlation of 58 patients. Radiology 146:309, 1983.)

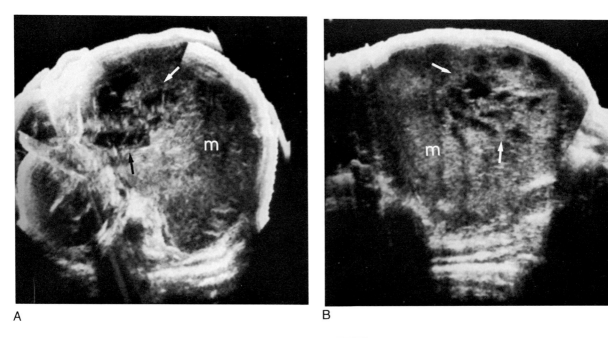

A   B

Fig. 4-121. Wilms' tumor. Transverse (A) and longitudinal
(B) static supine scans reveal a large predominately echodense
mass *(m)* filling the left abdomen. There are some anechoic
internal spaces (arrows). The left kidney is not seen. (C) Enhanced CT scan reveals a large mass *(m)* with mixed density.
There are low-density areas (arrows) seen with enhancement of
the mass. (Fig. A from Mandell VS, Mandell J, Gaisie G: Pediatric urologic radiology — Intervention and endourology. Urol
Clin North Am 12: 151, 1985.)

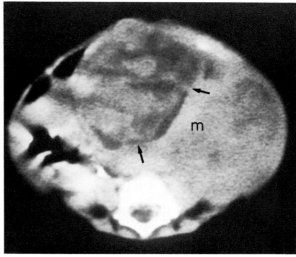

C

scribed in horseshoe kidneys.[74] Affected patients present
with a large asymptomatic flank mass; less frequently
there is abdominal pain, fever, hematuria, or anorexia.
Hypertension is seen in 47 to 90 percent of cases.[83]

Ultrasound can be used to confirm the organ of the
mass, identify large blood vessel involvement, identify
metastases, and define the status of the contralateral kidney. The mass varies from hypoechoic to moderately
echogenic; irregular anechoic areas may be seen corresponding to central necrosis and hemorrhage[83,198,236,237]
(Fig. 4-121). Seventy-one percent of tumors are necrotic
at surgery.[236] Ultrasound can correctly predict the internal consistency of the tumor in 94 percent.[236] The contralateral kidney should be carefully examined because

there is a 5 to 10 percent incidence of bilateral tumors;
bilateral tumors are evident at the time of clinical presentation in two-thirds of cases.[83] Necrotic degeneration
and decreased tumor size are ultrasound features that
correlate with a positive response to therapy.[238] There is
no initial correlation between the ultrasound patterns
and clinical presentation or prognosis.

The multicystic variant of nephroblastoma is infrequently recognized.[239] It presents clinically much as a
typical Wilms' tumor and in the same age group. Pathologically, it is truly a distinct variant of the ordinary
nephroblastoma and has no etiologic relationship to infantile multicystic dysplastic kidney or other benign
multilocular renal cysts. On ultrasound, a multicystic

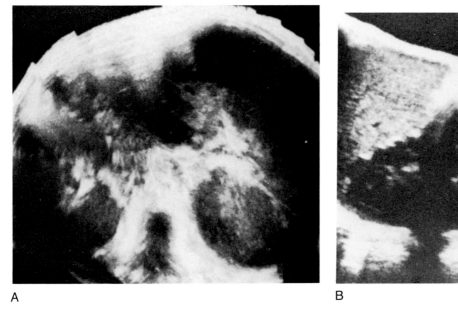

A

B

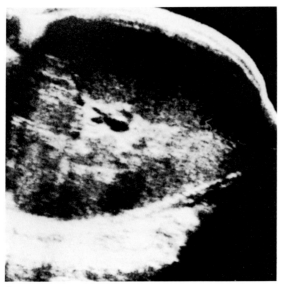

C

Fig. 4-122. Nephroblastomatosis. Transverse (A) and longitudinal scans of the right (B) and left (C) kidneys. Both kidneys are enlarged, particularly the left. There is considerable reduced echogenicity of the cortical region. (From Franken EA Jr., Yiu-Chiu V, Smith WL, Chiu LC: Nephroblastomatosis: Clinicopathologic significance and imaging characteristics. AJR 138:950, © Am Roent Ray Soc, 1982.)

mass is seen[239] (Figs. 4-25 and 4-120). The cysts are of varying sizes. The prognosis of multicystic Wilms' tumor is considered more favorable than its solid counterpart. (This is thought to be the same entity as multilocular cystic nephroma, discussed above, and multilocular renal cyst, discussed in the Congenital section.)

Nephroblastomatosis is a group of pathologic entities characterized by persistent metanephric blastema in the kidney in infants and children.[240] It bears a close relationship to, but not synonymous with bilateral Wilms' tumor. Nephroblastomatosis is thought to occur as a result of arrest in normal nephrogenesis with persistence of residual blastema. This condition is found in 12 to 33 percent of kidneys with Wilms' tumor. It is also found frequently in those conditions associated with a high incidence of Wilms' tumor such as hemihypertrophy, Beckwith-Wiedemann syndrome and major chromosomal anomalies. The relationship of the various types of nephroblastomatosis and Wilms' is unknown but perhaps it is a precursor to Wilms'. The findings described on ultrasound include (1) subcapsular and parenchymal hypoechoic areas, (2) cysts, and (3) nephromegaly with decreased parenchymal echoes (Fig. 4-122). The prognosis of this disease process is undetermined.[240]

At times it may be difficult to differentiate Wilms' tumor from neuroblastoma. Ultrasound shows relative distinctive patterns for the two tumors based on textural differences and will probably be most useful in those equivocal cases in which the site of the tumor origin is uncertain.[241] Wilms' tumor may extend through the renal capsule rather than distort the kidney and mimic neuroblastoma.[242] Ultrasound can correctly differentiate the two tumors based on the echopattern in 88 percent of cases.[241] Typically, Wilms' tumor is sharply marginated with compressed renal tissue forming the pseudocapsule. It is fairly evenly echogenic or evenly echogenic with discrete holes corresponding to areas of cystic necrosis. Neuroblastoma is usually quite heterogeneous with irregular hyperechoic areas intermixed with less echogenic areas[241] (Fig. 4-123).

Mesoblastic Nephroma. Mesoblastic nephroma (fetal renal hamartoma, mesenchymal hamartoma of infancy, congenital Wilms', fibromyxoma, fibrosarcoma, congenital fibrosarcoma) is a rare tumor and is the most common renal neoplasm diagnosed in the early postnatal period.[34,48,243-246] Most patients present with an asymptomatic abdominal mass at less than 3 months old. Occasionally there is hematuria, and/or hypertension. Many infants have been the product of a pregnancy complicated by prematurity and polyhydramnios. Characteristically, a mesoblastic nephroma is a solid tumor with rare cysts or focal areas of hemorrhage and necrosis. The lesion is mixed with smooth muscle or fibroblastic elements, with scattered embryonic tubules and glomeruli. On excretory urography, a mass effect may be seen (Fig. 4-124B). On ultrasound a solid lesion is seen that cannot be differentiated from Wilms' tumor

by ultrasound alone[245] (Fig. 4-124A). It is similar to a noncalcified uterine fibroid—a solid mass with low-level echoes.[246] The prognosis after complete excision is excellent and adjunctive therapy is unnecessary.[246]

Urothelial Tumors: Transitional Cell Carcinoma. Transitional cell carcinoma originates in the renal pelvocalyceal system and represents 7 percent of all renal neoplasms.[247] It constitutes 85 percent of the primary renal pelvic tumors.[248] The lesion is usually first suspected by seeing a defect on an excretory urogram.[247] Several patterns of this lesion on ultrasound have been described: splitting or separation of the central renal echo complex in a fashion similar to hydronephrosis; and a bulky, hypoechoic mass lesion[247-249] (Figs. 4-125 to 4-127). The tumor's echogenicity is similar to renal parenchyma.[224,248]

Ultrasound then is helpful in clarifying the nature of a filling defect seen on urograms. Stones should be dense with an associated acoustic shadow[250] (Figs. 4-44, 4-45, 4-80 to 4-82). Tumors and blood clots appear as echogenic masses without acoustic shadowing.[18] Urothelial tumors are seen as low level echoes that separate the walls of the renal sinus (Figs. 4-125 to 4-127). Blood clots may appear similar to this tumor but should change in its echopattern with time; it should show resolution on follow-up examination[18] (Fig. 4-92).

Urothelial Tumors: Squamous Cell Carcinoma. Squamous cell carcinoma accounts for 15 percent of all

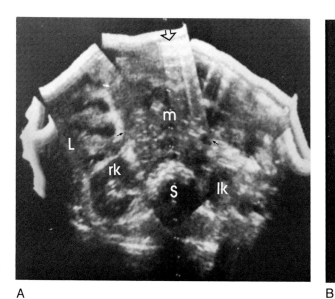
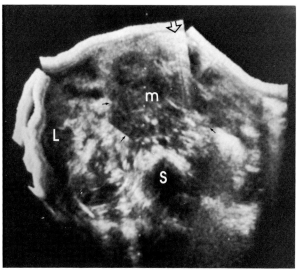

A   B

Fig. 4-123. Neuroblastoma. Transverse static scans at 4 cm **(A)** and 3 cm **(B)** above the umbilicus. A solid mass *(m)* is seen in the midline. It is difficult to define its borders (small arrows) especially on the left but it does extend to the left and right. Bowel gas anterior to the mass causes a reflective pattern (open arrow). (*L*, liver; *rk*, right kidney; *lk*, left kidney; *S*, spine). *(Figure continues.)*

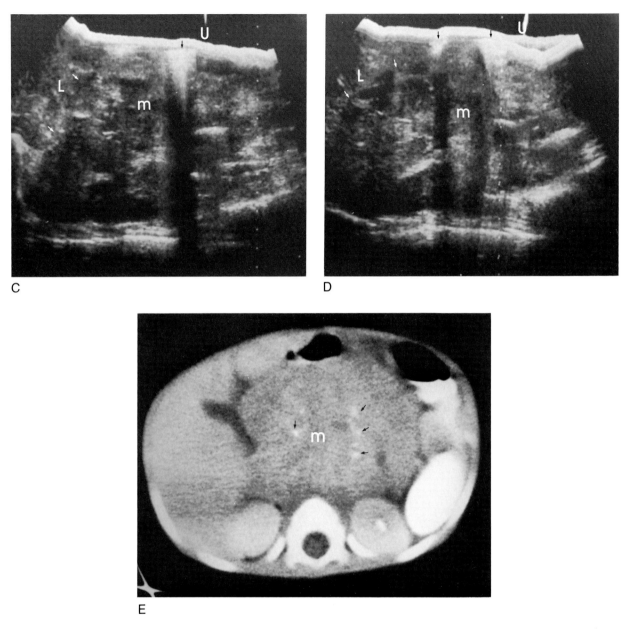

Fig. 4-123 *(Continued).* Longitudinal scans at 1 cm to left of midline **(C)** and midline **(D)** also demonstrate a solid mass *(m)* with poorly defined margins (white arrows). Bowel gas anterior to the mass causes a reflective pattern (black arrows). (*U*, level of the umbilicus; *L*, liver.) **(E)** Enhanced CT scan demonstrates the large mass *(m)* that extends to either side of midline. It does have internal calcification (arrows). The prevertebral vessels cannot be identified.

urothelial tumors with the remainder being 85 percent transitional cell carcinoma.[251] Squamous cell carcinoma is rare and highly malignant with an insidious onset and a tendency to metastasize early with a poor prognosis. Pathologically, a flat, ulcerating mass with extensive indurated infiltration is noted. Twenty-five to 60 percent of cases are associated with previous chronic renal infection and calculi. Ureteropelvic junction obstruction is common. The presence of faceted calculi and marked

hydronephrosis should suggest the diagnosis of squamous cell carcinoma[251] (Fig. 4-128).

SECONDARY RENAL TUMORS

Because a large volume of blood flows through the kidney, it is frequently the site of metastases from carcinomas and sarcomas.[14] The only specific metastasis that selectively metastasizes to kidney is a tumor from the

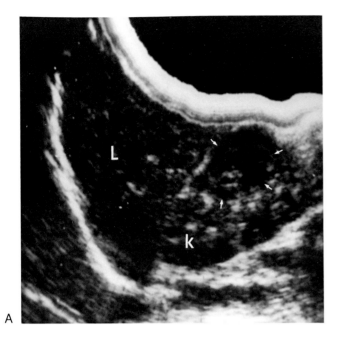

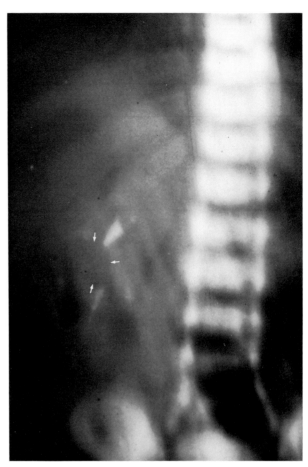

Fig. 4-124. Mesoblastic nephroma. **(A)** Longitudinal scan, right kidney *(k)*. A poorly defined hypoechoic mass (arrows) is seen in the lower pole anteriorly. *(L,* liver.) **(B)** Excretory pyelogram. A mass effect (arrows) is seen on the right.

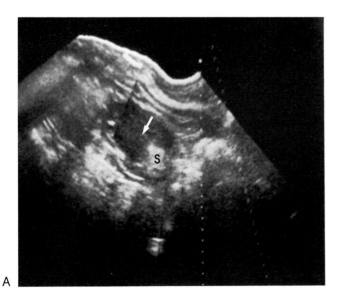

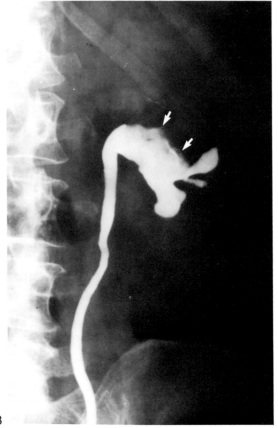

Fig. 4-125. Urothelial tumor: Transitional cell carcinoma. **(A)** Longitudinal scan left kidney. A poorly defined solid appearing mass (arrow) is seen in the upper pole. The echopattern is similar to renal parenchyma. *(s,* renal sinus.) **(B)** Retrograde pyelogram. Irregularity (arrows) of the upper collecting system is seen.

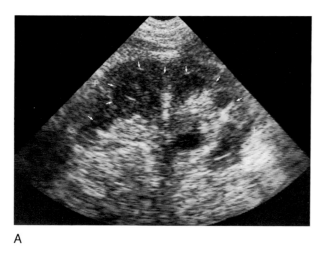

A

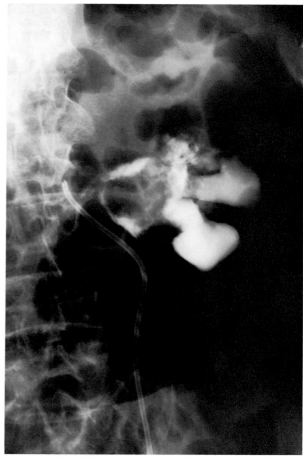

B

Fig. 4-126. Urothelial tumor: Transitional cell carcinoma. Patient with transitional cell carcinoma of the bladder metastatic to the left renal pelvis. **(A)** Longitudinal scan of the left kidney demonstrates a dilated collecting system (arrows) filled with echoes. This represented metastatic tumor. **(B)** Retrograde pyelogram. There is dilatation of the collecting system with filling defects.

contralateral kidney.[14] Metastases are often hypoechoic.[198]

Choriocarcinoma. Choriocarcinoma, a trophoblastic tissue neoplasm, and disease of females in the childbearing years, has a 10 to 50 percent incidence of renal metastases.[252] The most frequent sites of metastases are the lungs and vagina. Once the abdominal viscera are involved—kidneys and brain—the prognosis is fatal. The metastases are characteristically hemorrhagic and necrotic and spread primarily by the hematogeneous route but lymphatic spread and direct extension is seen. On ultrasound a solid hetergeneous mass is seen with sound attenuation[252] (Fig. 4-129). In a young female with hematuria and a renal mass, one should consider choriocarcinoma and screen with HCG titer.[252]

Lymphoma. Excluding the hematopoietic and reticuloendothelial systems, the urinary tract is the most common site of involvement by lymphoma at autopsy. Only lung and breast metastasize to the kidney more often than lymphoma.[253] Rarely are the kidneys the predomi-

nant site of disease at the initial diagnosis. There is renal involvement in 2.7 to 6 percent of cases.[254] The majority evaluated have known lymphoma and are studied for nodal mass size, flank pain, and/or deteriorating renal function.[254] The discrepancy between the incidence of clinical recognition of renal lymphoma and postmortem findings in the past may be due to the fact that the infiltration of the kidneys infrequently causes renal insufficiency or failure. The earliest symptoms are nonspecific with flank pain, or mass, weight loss, and hematuria.[253] Rarely, hypertension and renal failure result from vascular or ureteral compression, extensive parenchymal infiltration by tumor, or superimposed artifact.

The most common form of involvement is that of multiple intraparenchymal nodules with direct invasion from contiguous retroperitoneal lymph node masses observed somewhat less frequently. The gross morphology and consequent radiographic images depend on the mechanism of renal involvement (hematogeneous or direct extension); pattern of intrarenal growth (interstitial or expansile); size, number, and distribution of lesions; and presence of extension beyond the kidney.[253] The

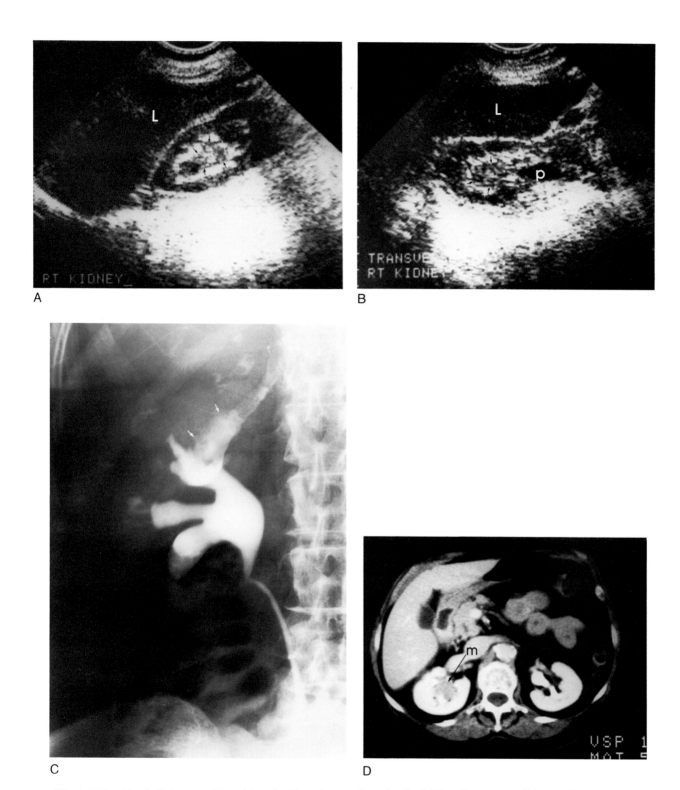

Fig. 4-127. Urothelial tumor: Transitional cell carcinoma. Longitudinal **(A)** and transverse **(B)** scans demonstrate a mass (arrows) within the collecting system of the upper pole of the right kidney. (*L*, liver; *p*, pelvis.) **(C)** Retrograde pyelogram. A filling defect (arrows) is noted in the upper pole. **(D)** Enhanced CT scan. A soft-tissue density mass *(m)* is noted within the right renal collecting system. (Figs. **A**–**C** courtesy of Dr. Aous Al-Khaldi, Department of Radiology, Granville Hospital, Oxford, North Carolina).

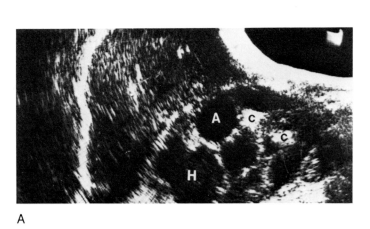

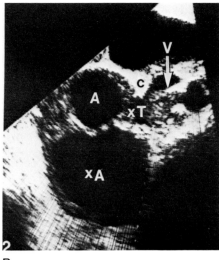

A   B

Fig. 4-128. Urothelial tumor: Squamous cell carcinoma. **(A)** Longitudinal scan, right. (*A*, anechoic dilated renal calyx; *H*, hypoechoic renal calyx containing debris; *C*, calculus.) **(B)** Transverse scan, right. (*A*, dilated calyces; *T*, tumor filling renal pelvis and surrounding a dilated calyx; *C*, calculus; *V*, elevation of the inferior vena cava by tumor areas biopsied.) (From Wimbish KJ, Sanders MM, Samuels BI, Francis IR: Squamous cell carcinoma of the renal pelvis: Case report emphasizing sonographic and CT appearance. Urol Radiol 5:267, 1983.)

kidney normally does not contain lymphoid tissue; it occurs secondary to hematogeneous or contiguous extension. Initially the lymphoma grows between the nephrons that continue to function and because this interstitial proliferation preserves gross morphology, the radiographic detection is difficult. With continued growth, the growth becomes expansile and the lymphomatous mass resembles other neoplasms that enlarge by

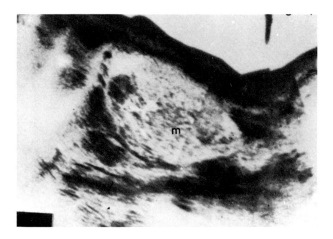

Fig. 4-129. Renal metastasis. Choriocarcinoma. Longitudinal prone scan showing left kidney replaced by a mass *(m)* that has a heterogeneous echopattern and is sound attenuating. (From Kutcher R, Lu T, Gordon DH, Becker JA: Renal choriocarcinoma metastasis: A vascular lesion. Am J Roentgenol 128:1046, © American Roentgen Ray Society, 1977.)

appositional growth. Continued growth and evalesence of small foci result in progressive parenchymal replacement and rarely in the destruction of the entire kidney. Perinephric extension with subsequent vascular and arterial encasement is common.[253] In some, there is diffuse infiltration.

There have been various reports as to the incidence and pattern of renal involvement with lymphoma. In one series, 61 percent of the kidneys were involved with lymphoma with multiple nodules, 11 percent showed invasion from retroperitoneal disease, 7 percent showed solitary nodules and 6 percent demonstrated a bulky single tumor.[255] Another series reported lymphomatous involvement in 48 percent with solitary masses, 29 percent multiple nodules, and 19 percent with almost complete parenchymal replacement by tumor.[253] Renal lymphoma usually occurs late in the disease. In an autopsy series, there was a 13 percent renal involvement in Hodgkin's disease.[254] Renal involvement is more common in non-Hodgkin's disease although the pathologic pattern of renal involvement is similar. Seven and a half to 14 percent of patients with non-Hodgkin's lymphoma have clinically suspected renal involvement with 42 to 65 percent demonstrating involvement at autopsy.[255] Some report renal involvement in 33.5 percent of malignant lymphomas with the kidneys involved rather late in the disease.[256]

The typical ultrasound appearance of lymphoma is that of single or multiple anechoic or hypoechoic masses[198,253,254,256,257] (Fig. 4-130). The anechoic masses may even meet all the criteria for a renal cyst including acoustic enhancement[253,256] (Fig. 4-130). As such, the diagnosis of a cyst should be questioned in a lymphoma patient; further investigation with cyst puncture or gallium scan should be undertaken. In addition to the focal mass pattern, there may be diffuse renal involvement producing renal enlargement and decreased parenchymal echoes[257] (Fig. 4-131). Lymphomatous involvement may be diagnosed more frequently if the ultrasound examination is performed on the lymphoma patient who develops flank pain, a palpable flank mass, decreased renal function, or lymphocyturia.[256]

Leukemia. The incidence of renal infiltration in all forms of leukemia is 63 percent based on an autopsy series.[258] The clinical signs of renal impairment does not necessarily indicate leukemic infiltrates but may be related to other conditions such as hyperuricemia, septicemia, and hemorrhage.[258,259] Leukemic infiltrates should be suspected when there is an elevated blood pressure. The affected kidneys may or may not be palpably en-

larged. The following ultrasound patterns have been described: (1) variable degrees of renal enlargement; (2) loss of definition and distortion of the central sinus echo complex; (3) diffuse coarse echoes throughout the renal cortex with preservation of the renal medullae; and (4) focal renal mass[258] (Figs. 4-132 to 134). Multiple nodular areas of anechocity within enlarged kidneys may be seen; this pattern may revert to normal when the patient is in remission but then recur during a relapse.[259] Ultrasound appears to be more sensitive than urography in delineating the extent of the parenchymal involvement.[258]

The Dialysis Patient

UREMIC RENAL CYSTIC DISEASE

There is a high incidence of bilateral cystic disease in patients who have uremia of chronic renal disease that is being treated by intermittent hemodialysis. Seventy-nine percent of patients have cysts when hemodialysis is

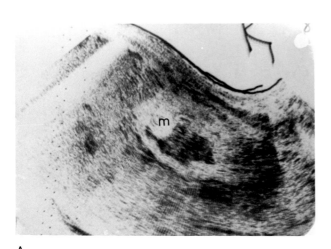

A

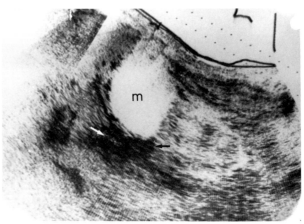

B

C

Fig. 4-130. Renal lymphoma. Poorly differentiated lymphocytic lymphoma, focal masses. Longitudinal scans of the right **(A)** and left **(B,C)** kidneys demonstrate focal anechoic masses *(m)* with two on the left. The mass in **(B)** meets all the criteria for a cyst including acoustic enhancement (arrows). *(Figure continues.)*

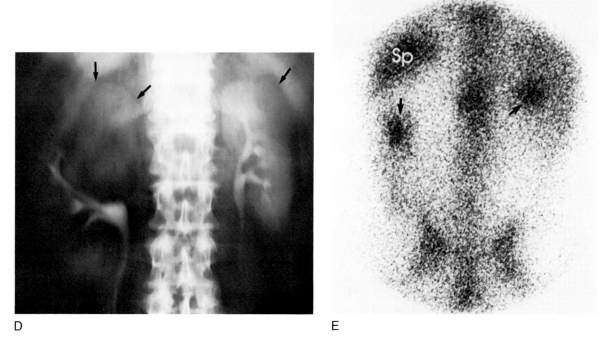

D   E

Fig. 4-130 *(Continued).* **(D)** Intravenous pyelogram. Mass effects (arrows) are seen bilaterally. **(E)** Gallium scan, posterior view. Increased activity (arrows) is seen within both kidneys. *(Sp,* spleen.) (From Shirkhoda A, Staab EV, Mittelstaedt CA: Renal lymphoma imaged by ultrasound and Gallium-67. Radiology 137:175, 1980.)

continued for longer than 3 years.[178,260,261] In less than 3 years treatment with dialysis, 43 percent of patients are affected.[178,260,261] The mean age of such a patient is 40 years.[262]

These cysts are located throughout the kidney and may be multiple, 0.5 to 2 cm, and bilateral.[261] These cysts are lined by flattened cuboidal or papillary epithelium. Proposed etiologies for the production of these cysts includes altered compliance of the tubular basement membrane or an obstructive lesion caused by focal proliferation of the tubular epithelium. Other theories imply that the ducts become obstructed by surrounding

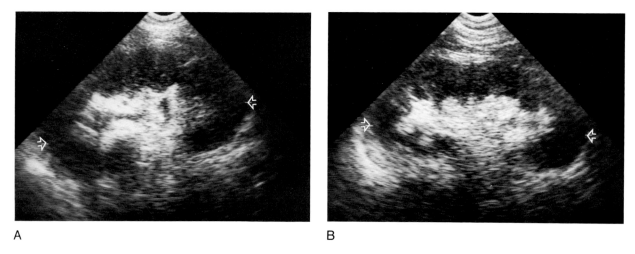

A   B

Fig. 4-131. Renal lymphoma. Non-Hodgkins lymphoma, diffuse. Longitudinal scans of the right (15.7 cm) **(A)** and left (16.7 cm) **(B)** kidneys. The kidneys (open arrows) are markedly increased in length and anteroposterior dimension. No focal masses are seen.

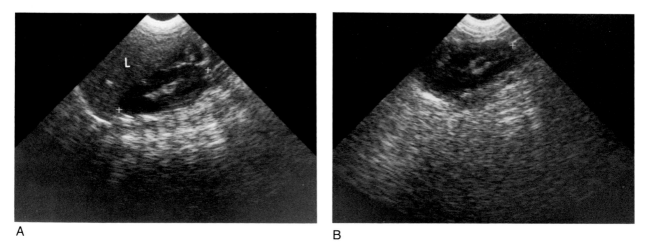

Fig. 4-132. Renal leukemia. Acute lymphocytic leukemia in a child with renal failure. Longitudinal scans of the right **(A)** and left **(B)** kidneys. The kidneys are enlarged with a relatively hypoechoic parenchymal pattern. (*L*, liver.)

interstitial fibrosis or oxalate crystals.[261-263] Still other causative factors include vascular insufficiency and direct toxicity by circulating metabolites.[263]

The kidneys involved are generally low normal for size or atrophic. The renal volume is decreased when there is parenchymal destruction. With cyst development, the kidneys may increase in size[260] (Fig. 4-135). In the absence of complications, the cysts do not significantly increase the renal size.[263] Complications of these cysts

are not uncommon. Hemorrhage into the cysts with macrohematuria and retroperitoneal hemorrhage from cyst rupture are possibilities.[260,263] The dialyzed patient is at risk for hemorrhage as result of frequent anticoagulant therapy for dialysis.[263] Bleeding diatheses of uremic patients also contribute to risk, and unsupported sclerotic blood vessels rupture with minor trauma.[261] Increased awareness of the occurrence of uremic cystic disease and its complications should lead to yearly screening of patients undergoing hemodialysis.[262] If a patient on

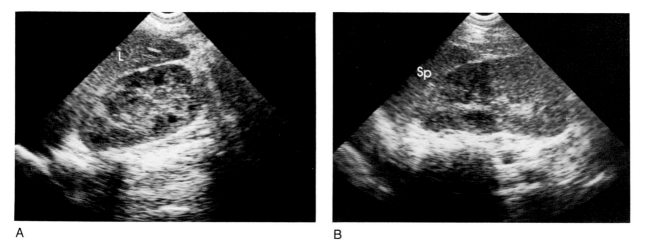

Fig. 4-133. Renal leukemia. Eleven-year-old with acute lymphocytic leukemia and abnormal renal function. Longitudinal scans of the right **(A)** and left **(B)** kidneys reveal nephromegaly with the right being 13.3 cm and the left 12.8 cm. The parenchyma is not lucent but the renal sinus is not well distinguished. After therapy, the patient's renal function improved and on the two week follow-up examination, the right kidney measured 9.5 cm with the left 10 cm. (*L*, liver; *Sp*, spleen.)

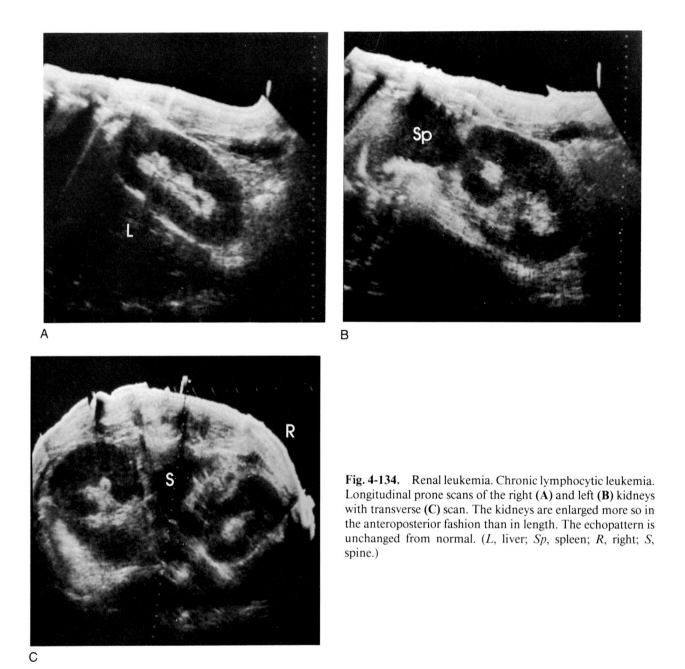

Fig. 4-134. Renal leukemia. Chronic lymphocytic leukemia. Longitudinal prone scans of the right **(A)** and left **(B)** kidneys with transverse **(C)** scan. The kidneys are enlarged more so in the anteroposterior fashion than in length. The echopattern is unchanged from normal. (*L*, liver; *Sp*, spleen; *R*, right; *S*, spine.)

chronic dialysis develops hematuria, flank pain and/or a flank mass, the examiner should evaluate for uremic cystic disease.[260]

RENAL CELL CARCINOMA

Besides the increased incidence of cysts in dialyzed patients, there is also an increased incidence of renal tumors.[260,261,263,264] Forty percent of patients have tumors that are multiple and bilateral.[260,263] Other au-

thors report a 13.3 percent incidence of tumors.[265] These may be papillary adenomas and renal cell carcinoma.[263] Usually there are already cysts present, especially atypical cysts, when the tumors appear. The neoplastic stimulus may be dialysis-related epithelial proliferation of both glomerulus and tubule. Polyamines, which are biologically active hormone-like substances retained in uremia, have been considered responsible for this epithelial proliferation and subsequent tumor formation. So, in addition to evaluating the native kidneys for cysts, solid tumors need to be excluded[261] (Fig. 4-136).

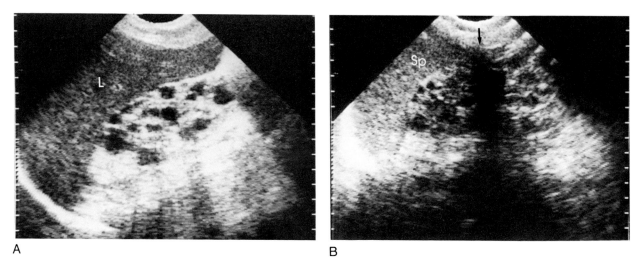

A   B

Fig. 4-135. Uremic renal cystic disease. Longitudinal scans of the right (**A**) (supine) and left (**B**) (decubitus) kidneys. A moderate increase in echogenicity is seen in the right kidney with a slight increase in the left. Multiple small cysts are present bilaterally. The corticomedullary junction and central medullary echo complex is lost. An overlying rib (arrow) causes an attenuation artifact on the left. (*L*, liver; *Sp*, spleen.) (From Kutcher R, Amodio JB, Rosenblatt R: Uremic renal cystic disease: Value of sonographic screening. Radiology 147:833, 1983.)

RENAL TRANSPLANT ABNORMALITIES

Renal transplantation has become the treatment of choice in the management of chronic renal failure. With improved surgical techniques, there is a significantly lower operative mortality and morbidity but the transplant patient still remains at high risk of developing serious and life-threatening postoperative complications.[266]

Because the symptoms of surgical complications such as perinephric and pelvic fluid collections, renal vascular problems, and obstructive uropathy are similar to those associated with transplant rejection and acute tubular necrosis, radiographic (imaging) techniques are important in the evaluation of the transplanted kidney and its site.[266] The correlation of clinical symptomatology, time of presentation of each complication, and diagnostic

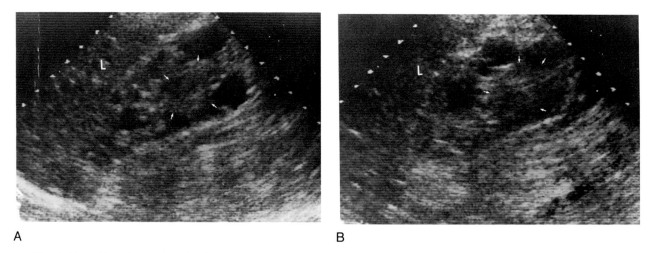

A   B

Fig. 4-136. Uremic renal cystic disease and cell carcinoma. Longitudinal (**A**) and oblique (**B**) scans of the right kidney. Numerous cysts are seen as well as an echogenic mass (arrows) in the mid-to-lower pole. (*L*, liver.) (From Weissberg DL, Miller RB: Renal cell carcinoma and acquired cystic disease of the kidneys in a chronically dialyzed kidney. J Ultrasound Med 2:191, 1983.)

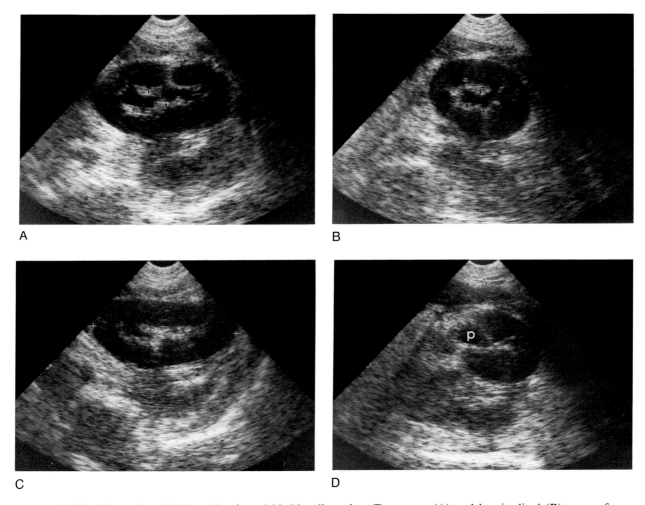

Fig. 4-137. Transplant: Hydronephrosis and bladder distension. Transverse **(A)** and longitudinal **(B)** scans of a transplanted kidney in a transverse lie. There is dilatation of the collecting system (arrows). The patient was found to have a distended bladder. After voiding, repeat transverse **(C)** and longitudinal **(D)** images of the pelvis, demonstrate a kidney without hydronephrosis. (*p*, extrarenal pelvis.)

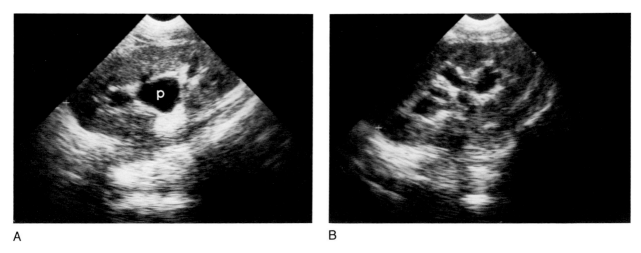

Fig. 4-138. Transplant: Obstruction. Moderate obstruction (without bladder distension). Longitudinal scans **(A,B)** in two different patients demonstrate dilatation of the calyces and renal pelvis *(p)*.

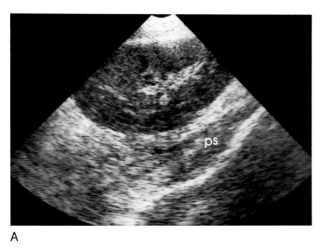

A

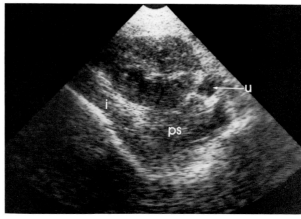

B

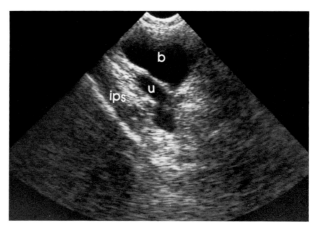

C

Fig. 4-139. Transplant: Hydroureter. No dilatation of the collecting system is seen on longitudinal **(A)** and transverse **(B)** scans of the kidney. The ureter *(u)* is dilated medial to the kidney on **(B)** and posterolateral to the bladder *(b)* on transverse **(C)** scan of the bladder. On a nuclear medicine scan, there was isotope stasis within the ureter. (*ps,* psoas muscle; *i,* iliacus muscle; *ips,* iliopsoas muscle.)

yield of an imaging technique provide the data for an algorithmic radiologic approach to renal transplant complications.[266]

Acute tubular necrosis, rejection, arterial occlusion, arterial stenosis, and renal vein thrombosis all cause acute renal failure in the early posttransplant period. Differentiation of these entities by clinical and laboratory data is not possible. Radiologic procedures with contrast are not recommended because they contribute to further renal damage and seldom produce a specific answer. Multiple nuclear medicine studies provide functional and anatomic information allowing specific diagnosis but are frequently inconclusive. Ultrasound has enhanced the diagnostic armentarium in the renal transplant patient.

Obstructive Uropathy

Compared to normal kidneys, the renal transplant collecting system can be more dilated in the absence of obstruction and the degree of dilatation can be in-

fluenced more by the amount of bladder distension (Fig. 4-137). Patients with the greatest bladder distension may show the greatest degree of hydronephrosis, but hydronephrosis is not always seen with a distended bladder. Ureteral obstruction occurs in 1 to 10 percent of transplants and may be due to a stricture at the ureterovesical junction, torsion, extrinsic compression, ureteral necrosis, or blood clots[267] (Fig. 4-138). The ureter may be large postoperatively due to innervation and possibly relative ischemia. The size of the ureter cannot be used as a criterion for hydroureter (Fig. 4-139). Once hydronephrosis is identified in a transplanted kidney, one needs to search for a possible extrinsic mass[267] (Figs. 4-140 and 4-141).

Acute Tubular Necrosis

Acute tubular necrosis (ATN) is the most common cause of acute posttransplant renal failure, appearing in as many as 50 percent of cadaver kidneys.[178,268,269] Other authors report an occurrence rate of 3 percent of ca-

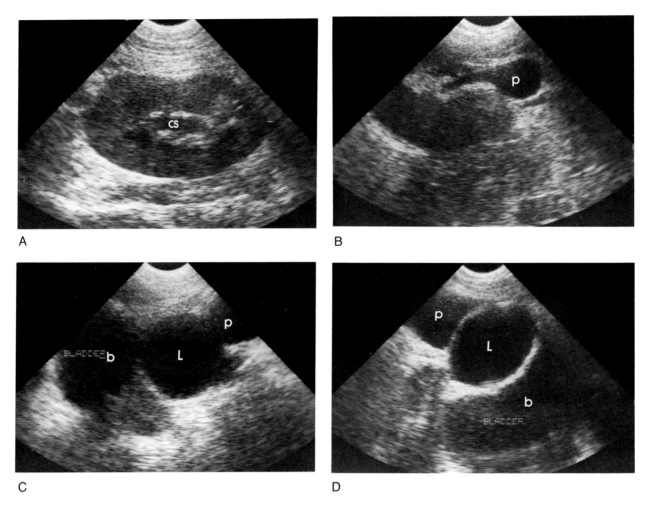

Fig. 4-140. Transplant: Extrarenal pelvis and lymphocele. This kidney was transplanted with its long axis transverse. Long axis (transverse) **(A)** and cross-section (longitudinal) **(B)** scans demonstrate minimal dilatation of the collecting system *(cs)* on **(A)** with a large extrarenal pelvis *(p)* on **(B)**. On transverse **(C)** and longitudinal **(D)** views of the pelvis, the extrarenal pelvis *(p)* and bladder *(b)* are seen with a cystic fluid collection *(L)* between the two. This represented a lymphocele documented by aspiration and percutaneous drainage.

davers and 11 percent live-related-donors.[270] The incidence increases with the length of warm ischemia time.[270] Uncomplicated ATN is reversible and the treatment is maintance of hydration and immunosuppression.

The clinical diagnosis of ATN is most commonly diagnosed by exclusion. Clinically, there is increased creatinine, and the urine output is low. There are no demonstratable changes noted on ultrasound in most patients.[178,271–273] One series[274] reported that 77 percent of patients had decreased echogenicity of the renal sinus. A nuclear medicine renal scan will show an intact vascular supply and in combination with a normal-appearing ultrasound should suggest the diagnosis of ATN.[178]

Infection

Infection is the most common cause of death in the renal transplant patient and the urinary tract is the most common site of the primary infection.[268] But, it is difficult to diagnose. Not only is the immune system suppressed, but the signs and symptoms may be masked for quite a time until sepsis is widespread. The most frequent single cause of failure in the immediate posttransplant period is ATN, which is associated with a high risk of infection.[268]

There has been a report of an emphysematous kidney associated with infection.[268] There was a marked acoustic impedence mismatch of the gas and renal surface,

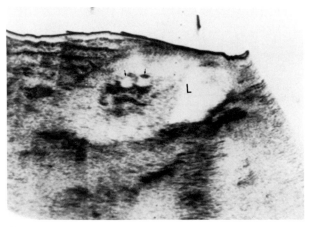

A

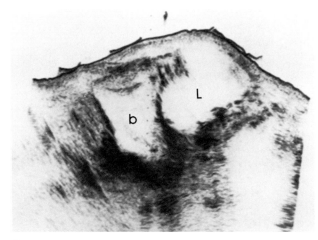

B

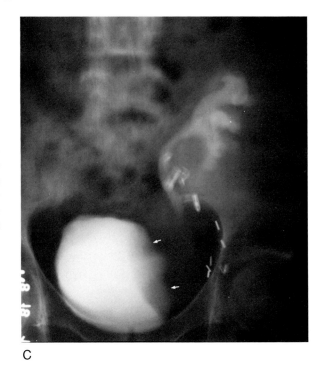

C

Fig. 4-141. Transplant: Obstruction. Lymphocele. **(A)** Longitudinal scan. Dilated calyces (arrows) are seen on this plane of scan as well as an anechoic area *(L)* blending with the lower pole of the kidney. **(B)** Transverse scan below the level of the kidney. The bladder *(b)* is displaced to the right of the cystic mass *(L)*. **(C)** Intravenous pyelogram. There is blunting of the calyces with a mass effect (arrows) on the bladder. The mass represented a lymphocele.

resulting in dense echoes at the acoustic interface with total lack of penetration and the typical reverberation artifacts (Fig. 4-142). In such a case, ultrasound can be used to detect the gas and to monitor therapy if indicated.

Allograft Rejection

Rejection is the most common cause of renal failure after the first posttransplant week. On the basis of clinical and laboratory evidence, the diagnosis is a question.

The triad of fever, graft tenderness, and oliguria are considered the hallmark of rejection.[271] The creatinine, BUN, and creatinine clearance are helpful but lack specificity. Studies with contrast further contribute to renal damage and should be avoided when possible. Nuclear medicine provides functional and anatomic information. Ultrasound demonstrates a spectrum of findings.

Rejection can be divided into acute and chronic based on the nature of the inflammatory lesion on microscopy and not on duration.[272] Rarely is there a hyperacute rejection—in less than 48 hours postoperative. Since rejection is a dynamic process, this spectrum corresponds to the histopathologic changes. While rejection

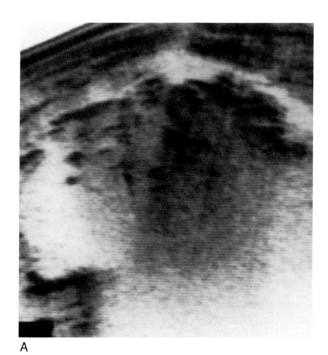 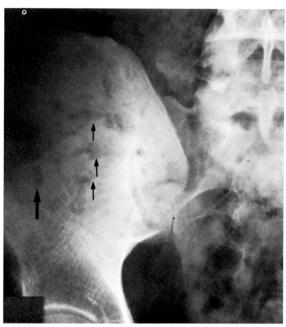

A   B

Fig. 4-142. Transplant: Emphysema. **(A)** Longitudinal scan over kidney. Dense echoes originating from within the renal cortex represent gas. Acoustic shadowing and reverberations are deep to the collections of gas. Some echoes, near the upper pole, may originate in the perinephric region. **(B)** Right lower abdomen. Gas is distributed radially through the transplanted kidney (small arrows) along planes of columns of Bertin. Some gas may be perinephric (large arrow). (From Brenbridge ANAG, Buschi AJ, Cochrane JA, Lees RF: Renal emphysema of transplanted kidney: Sonographic appearance. AJR 132:656, © American Roentgen Ray Society, 1979.)

starts and is most pronounced at the corticomedullary junction, it progresses and involves the entire renal unit.

Early on, there is increased renal size caused by edema, congestion, and mononuclear cell infiltrate.[272,273,275] In 84 percent of cases of acute rejection, there is an abnormal increase in renal volume.[12] An abnormal manifestation of volume includes a sudden increase in volume (greater than 20 percent increase over 5 days) or renal growth during the second week of greater than 25 percent[12] (Fig. 4-143).

Cortical ischemia results in variably sized parenchymal foci of edema, hemorrhage, or infarction.[272,276] The degree of edema, extent of hemorrhage, and presence or absence of infarction is determined by the severity of the impaired cortical perfusion and vascular occlusion. There is uniform or local decrease in the parenchymal echogenicity corresponding to areas of hemorrhage, edema, and hemorrhagic infarct.[12] There are focal zones of lucency in the cortex in 20 percent with patchy lucent areas (cortex and medulla) in 16 percent with coalescence (Figs. 4-144 and 4-145). The cortical echoes may be sparse probably as a result of abundant mononuclear cell infiltrate in the interstitium.[277] There are increased cortical echoes in 58 percent of patients with a decrease in 47 percent.[12]

The pyramids are enlarged in 79 to 88 percent of cases of rejection[12,275] (Fig. 4-146). The pyramids are considered enlarged if their height exceeds the height of the overlying cortex. The enlarged pyramids are due to a combination of edema surrounding the peritubular capillaries and marked congestion of the corticomedullary junction.[178,272,273,276,277] The presence of an indistinct corticomedullary junction is strongly indicative of acute rejection.[278] There is loss of corticomedullary junction definition in 58 percent of cases.[12]

Within the hilar adipose, there is early edema that causes uneven widening of the perilobular tissue. When the changes in the hilar fat are moderate, causing further widening of the intralobular septa, with separation and decrease in size of the fat cells, the ultrasound pattern becomes inhomogeneously dense (Fig. 4-147). With subsequent fibrosis, fat cell atrophy and fat cell loss, there is accentuation of the adipose tissue septation. On the sonogram the renal sinus blends with the adjacent parenchyma[178,273,277] (Fig. 4-148). In 74 percent, there is found to be a decrease in the amplitude of the renal sinus echoes.[12]

Investigators have evaluated this change in the renal sinus with rejection.[279] There appears to be good correlation between histology and the ultrasound changes in

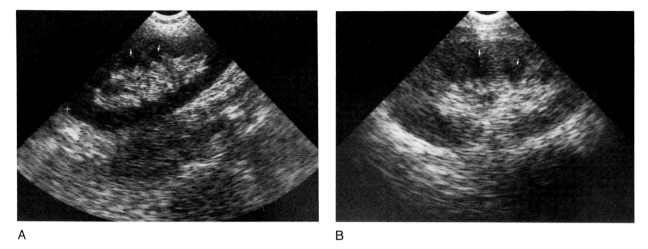

A   B

Fig. 4-143. Transplant rejection: Increased volume. **(A)** Longitudinal baseline scan. The kidney measures 11.3 cm in length and the renal pyramids (small arrows) are not prominent. **(B)** Longitudinal scan during an episode of rejection (at the same degree of magnification as **(A)**). The kidney now measures 13 cm in length and has increased in its anteroposterior dimension as well. The renal pyramids (arrows) are much more prominent on this scan.

Fig. 4-144. Transplant rejection: Zones of lucency. Longitudinal scan with poorly defined hypoechoic area (curved arrows) seen within the cortex. Additionally, the renal sinus echoes *(s)* are poorly defined. (small arrows, pyramids.)

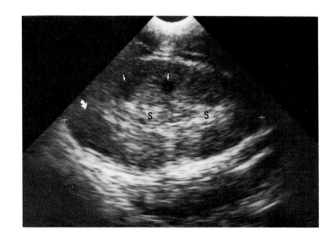

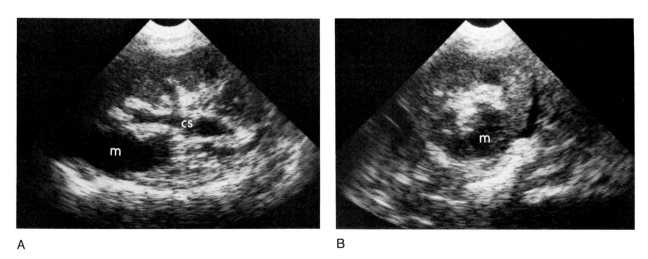

A   B

Fig. 4-145. Transplant rejection: Focal rejection. On longitudinal **(A)** and transverse **(B)** scans, a poorly defined hypoechoic area *(m)* was seen in the superior pole of the kidney. There is slight fullness to the collecting system but this did not represent obstruction. A nuclear medicine study was compatible with rejection. A biopsy performed revealed focal rejection.

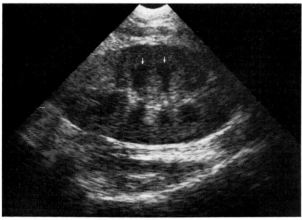

A

B

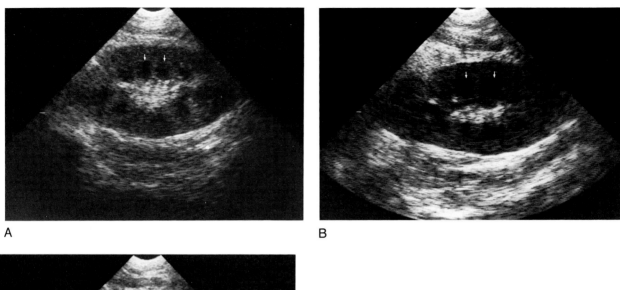

C

Fig. 4-146. Transplant rejection: Enlarged pyramids. Case 1: **(A)** Longitudinal baseline scan. The width of the pyramids (arrows) is equal to the width of the cortex. **(B)** Longitudinal scan with markedly enlarged pyramids (arrows). The height of the pyramids exceeds that of overlying cortex. Case 2: **(C)** Longitudinal scan with pyramidal (arrows) height greater than cortex.

rejection such that it promises to be a reliable predictor of the severity of rejection with a noninvasive, rapid, simple approach. The intense echoes seen in the renal sinus are primarily due to fat. With acute rejection, changes are minimal to none in the renal sinus on ultrasound. With moderate rejection, the echoes in the renal sinus are inhomogeneous, patchy, and coarse (Fig. 4-147). With severe rejection, the renal sinus blends with the parenchyma (Fig. 4-148).

In summary, the spectrum of ultrasound findings with rejection include (1) enlarged pyramids, (2) increased renal volume, (3) increased cortical thickness, (4) de-

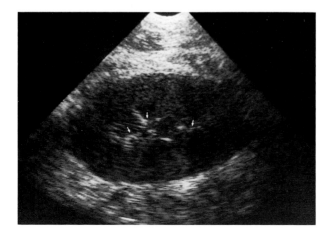

Fig. 4-147. Transplant, moderate rejection: Renal sinus. Longitudinal scan. The renal sinus (arrows) echoes are inhomogeneous, patchy, and coarse. The kidney is increased in its anteroposterior dimension.

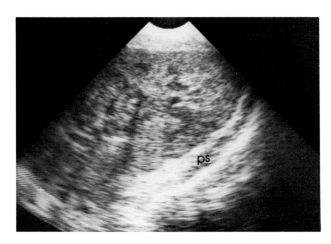

Fig. 4-148. Transplant, severe rejection: Renal sinus. Longitudinal scan. The renal sinus blends with the adjacent parenchyma such that it cannot be distinguished. (*ps*, psoas muscle.)

creased or increased echogenicity of the cortex, (5) areas of decreased parenchymal echogenicity, (6) indistinct corticomedullary junction, (7) decreased amplitude of the renal sinus echoes, and (8) perirenal fluid (58 percent)[12,269,275] (Figs. 4-143 to 4-148). In acute rejection, the following are seen: (1) increased renal size of at least 20 percent, (2) enlarged pyramids, and (3) indistinct corticomedullary junction.[178] In advanced acute rejection, localized hypoechoic areas may be seen in the cortex and medulla. The spectrum in chronic rejection include (1) renal enlargement, (2) cortex and medulla blend, (3) nondifferentiation of the renal sinus, (4) increased echoes throughout the kidney with a course spatial distribution, (5) small kidney, (6) echogenic kidney, and (7) irregular contour to the kidney due to scarring[178,272] (Fig.

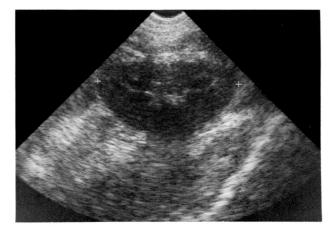

Fig. 4-149. Transplant: Chronic rejection. Longitudinal scan. The kidney is small. There is loss of corticomedullary differentiation as well as renal sinus identification.

4-149). The ultrasound findings are most helpful in conjunction with a nuclear medicine study. Using the ultrasound criteria, the study is 84 percent accurate in diagnosing rejection.[178] There is failure to differentiate acute or chronic rejection in 7 percent.[178]

Investigators have reported problems in evaluating for rejection in the pediatric age group.[280] The ultrasound findings are not helpful if the donor kidney is less than 5 years old. If the donor kidney is greater than 5 years old ultrasound allowed a sensitivity of 97 percent with a specificity of 58 percent by using a combination of three or more of the following ultrasound findings: (1) increased renal volume of 30 percent over baseline, (2) enlarged broadened rectangular medullary pyramids, (3) reduction or absence of the central sinus echoes, and (4) altered echogenicity in the renal parenchyma.[280]

Arterial Occlusion and Stenosis

With arterial occlusion and stenosis, no abnormal echopattern is detected involving the kidney. The only finding is the lack of normal posttransplant hypertrophy.[12] Renal artery stenosis, the most commonly encountered arterial problem, occurs with a 1 to 12 percent incidence.[281] Renal artery thrombosis occurs in 1 to 2 percent.[281] Anastomotic leaks with significant to massive hemorrhage either early or delayed are even less frequent and generally due to technical mishap. A pseudoaneurysm, which is uncommon, appears as a lucent, pulsating mass on real-time scan.[281]

Rupture

Renal rupture occurs secondary to acute rejection as a serious complication in 3.6 to 6 percent of cases.[178,270,282] Most occur during the early posttransplant period with 80 percent within first 2 weeks.[178,282] Clinically, it is associated with tachycardia, hypotension, oliguria, decreased hematocrit, pain, tenderness, and swelling.[282] There is no general agreement concerning its pathogenesis. Ischemic necrosis, hypertension, and previous renal biopsy are among the contributing factors.[282]

Renal rupture most commonly occurs along the convex margin of the kidney with the hematoma developing superiorly and lateral to the kidney, and it is well demarcated. The hematoma infiltrates the retroperitoneal fat and manifests as a fluid collection with numerous high-amplitude echoes in it.[12] On the sonogram there may be gross distortion of the graft contour and a perinephric or parenchymal hematoma[270] (Fig. 4-150).

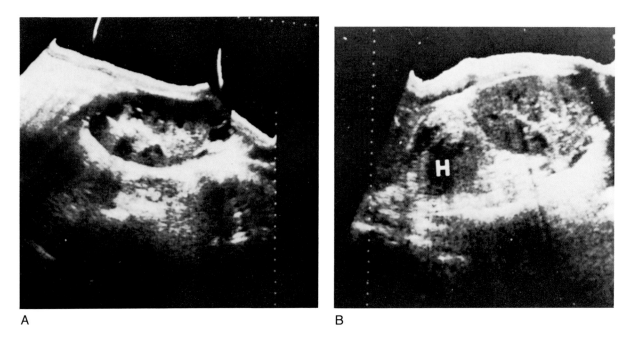

A   B

Fig. 4-150. Transplant rupture: Acute rejection. **(A)** Longitudinal scan during acute renal failure. The kidney is globular. There is uneven enlargement of the pyramids. The renal sinus echoes are patchy in distribution. **(B)** Oblique scan on day of nephrectomy. There is a mixed echopattern mass—hematoma *(H)*—inferior to the upper pole of the transplanted kidney. The kidney shows severe changes of rejection with indistinctness of the corticomedullary boundary and blending of the renal sinus area with remaining parenchyma. (From Hricak H: Renal medial disorders: The role of sonography. p.43. In Sanders RC (ed): Ultrasound Annual 1982. Raven Press, New York, 1982.)

Perirenal Collections

Renal transplant patients are often evaluated with nuclear medicine to assess function. At times, a "halo" or photopenic area is seen around or to the side of the kidney.[283] The differential diagnosis for such an abnormality would include a perirenal hematoma, a lymphocele, urinoma, or inflammatory edema.[283] These patients are often referred to ultrasound for further evaluation.

URINOMA

A urinoma is a serious complication with a 3.23 percent incidence requiring expedient surgery.[270,273] A urine leak is often followed by a wound infection that may lead to loss of the graft, generalized sepsis, and ultimately death. The most common cause of the urinary leak is a defect at the ureteropelvic, ureteroureter, or ureterovesical anatomosis. Ureteropelvic and ureteroureter anatomoses have a high incidence of associated urinomas so are used less frequently. A less common cause is infarction of the kidney with resultant necrosis of the parenchymal and ureteral tip necrosis secondary to vascular compromise.[284]

Patients with urinomas may present with decreased urine output, pain, and swelling over the transplant. These usually occur from 1 day to 3 weeks postoperatively with less than 3 days most common.[266] On ultrasound a hypoechoic mass (often with internal septation) that usually produces hydronephrosis is found[286] (Figs. 4-151 and 4-152). The location of the urinoma is variable.[287] Most are located near the lower pole.[285] Aspiration and biochemical analysis of the lesion may not help if the graft function is poor, since the urea concentration in the urine can be similar to the serum.[284]

LYMPHOCELE

The incidence of lymphoceles is 2 to 18 percent.[270,286] The lymph forming these lesions results from the operation in which the pelvic lymphatics are divided and from the graft kidney.[270,286-290] The lymphatic channels are damaged during the preparation of the pelvic area and the kidney itself has leakage from the injured capsular and hilar lymphatics.[288] The lymph drains into the peritoneal cavity provoking a fibrous reaction, becoming walled off. As the lesion gradually expands, there is pressure on the ureter, bladder, and kidney. The importance of the lesion lies in its effect on surrounding structures

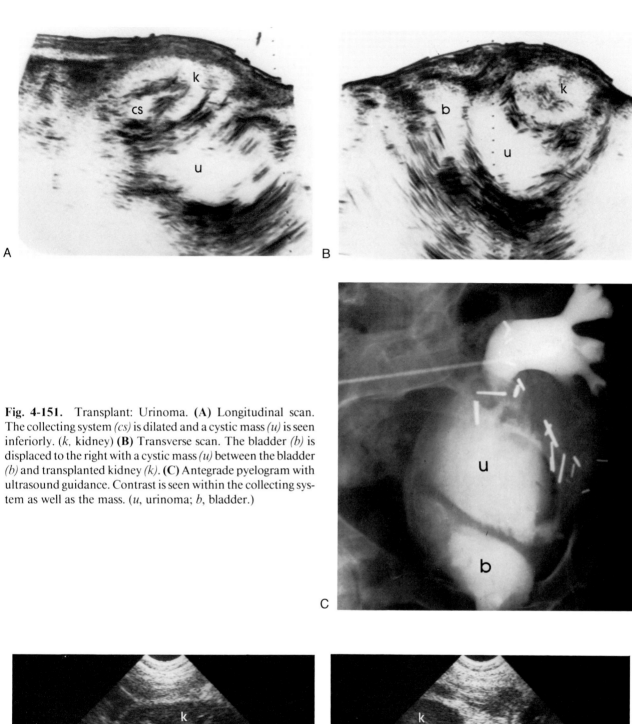

Fig. 4-151. Transplant: Urinoma. **(A)** Longitudinal scan. The collecting system *(cs)* is dilated and a cystic mass *(u)* is seen inferiorly. (*k,* kidney) **(B)** Transverse scan. The bladder *(b)* is displaced to the right with a cystic mass *(u)* between the bladder *(b)* and transplanted kidney *(k)*. **(C)** Antegrade pyelogram with ultrasound guidance. Contrast is seen within the collecting system as well as the mass. (*u,* urinoma; *b,* bladder.)

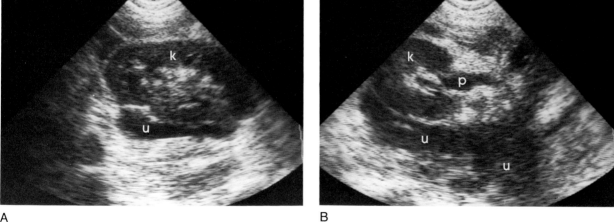

Fig. 4-152. Transplant: Urinoma. Long axis **(A)** and cross-sectional views **(B)** of a transplanted kidney *(k)* in a transverse lie. Fluid *(u)* is seen posterior to the kidney; it extends into the pelvis. (*p,* extrarenal pelvis.)

producing pressure on the iliac veins (producing leg swelling) and pressure on the graft ureter (producing hydronephrosis).[286]

The cardinal features of a lymphocele include progressive decrease in renal function, painless fluctuant swelling over the kidney, soft tissue shadow around the graft, and absence of demonstration of urinary fistula on excretory urogram or nuclear medicine study.[291] Lymphoceles develop 10 days to 2 years postoperatively with the average 5 weeks.[266]

On ultrasound a lymphocele appears as a well-defined cystic area that may be anechoic to hypoechoic[288,289] (Figs. 4-140, 4-141 and 4-153). There may be septation within the lesion. In one series, 67 percent were located inferomedial to the transplant.[266] Sixty-seven percent were cystic with septations, 33 percent were cystic, and 55 percent conformed to the anatomic pelvis.[266] Although ultrasound guided aspiration may help exclude a urinoma and make the diagnosis of a lymphocele, it is usually not definitive in the treatment of the abnormality[270,273] (Fig. 4-153). Lymphoceles are generally treated by marsupialization into the peritoneum or external drainage with breakdown of all loculi.[286,290]

ABSCESS

Patients with an abscess posttransplant present with elevated temperature, increased white blood cell count, proteinuria, and increased creatinine. Steroids may mask the usual signs.[270] These lesions develop from 6 days to 4 months postoperatively, with an average of 2 months.[266] The abscess may be variable in location and echofree to complex in its echopattern[266,273] (Fig. 4-154).

HEMATOMA

The patient with the acute hematoma may present with a minimal decrease in hemoglobin and blood pressure, with decreased urine output and pain and/or a palpable mass. With a chronic hematoma, an increased creatinine and temperature is seen. These develop 4 days

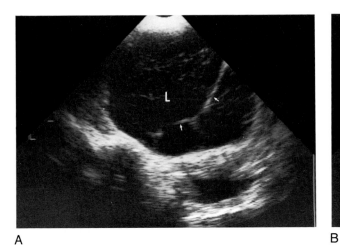

A

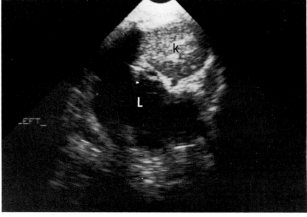

B

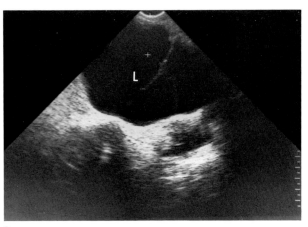

C

Fig. 4-153. Transplant: Lymphocele. Longitudinal **(A)** and transverse **(B)** scans of a cystic pelvic mass *(L)*. While the mass is cystic, it contains many septations (arrows). On **(B)**, the lower pole of the kidney *(k)* is seen along the lateral aspect of the mass. Because there was hydronephrosis, a percutaneous drainage was undertaken. **(C)** Longitudinal scan of the cystic mass *(L)*. A depth was determined (+). *(Figure continues.)*

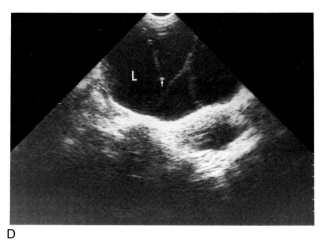

D

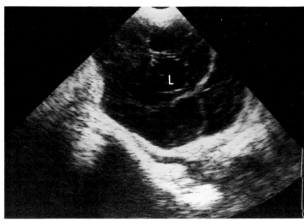

E

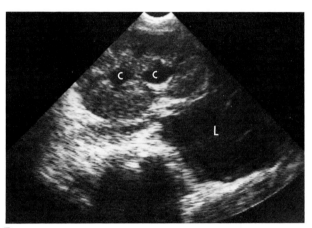

F

Fig. 4-153 *(Continued).* **(D)** After 92 cc of fluid was removed, the lymphocele was rescanned. The mass *(L)* is smaller and the needle tip (arrow) can be seen as a bright echo within the mass. The lymphocele was aspirated as dry as possible. One day later, the mass *(L)* was rescanned longitudinally **(E)**. The mass had reaccumulated and many more septations are present. **(F)** Longitudinal scan of the kidney. Hydronephrosis is present with dilatation of the calyces *(c)* and the mass *(L)* is seen inferior. The patient ultimately underwent surgical drainage.

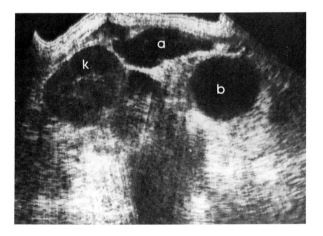

Fig. 4-154. Transplant: Abscess. Oblique scan parallel to inguinal ligament. An irregular complex mass *(a)* is seen between bladder *(b)* and transplanted kidney *(k)* containing echogenic debris. (From Coyne SS, Walsh JW, Tisnado J et al: Surgically correctable renal transplant complications: An integrated clinical and radiologic approach. AJR 136:113, © Am Roent Ray Soc, 1981.)

to 4 months postoperatively with 67 percent less than or equal to 4 days.[266] They may be variably located with a complex echopattern (Figs. 4-155 and 4-156). The ultrasound pattern varies with age, with the acute and chronic ones lucent and the intermediate ones complex[270,273] (Figs. 4-155 and 4-156).

DIFFERENTIATION OF FLUID COLLECTIONS

As noted in the previous discussions, it appears that all the perirenal posttransplant fluid collections look similar on sonograms. How does one differentiate the various collections? One group of investigators have evaluated this.[285] They found that 51 percent of their patients had abnormal fluid collections with 43 percent lymphoceles, 30 percent abscesses, 18 percent urinomas, and 9 percent hematomas.[285] Lymphoceles most commonly caused obstruction and were usually septated. Eighty percent of lymphoceles were septated with 100 percent of hematomas septated.[285] As for size, the lymphoceles

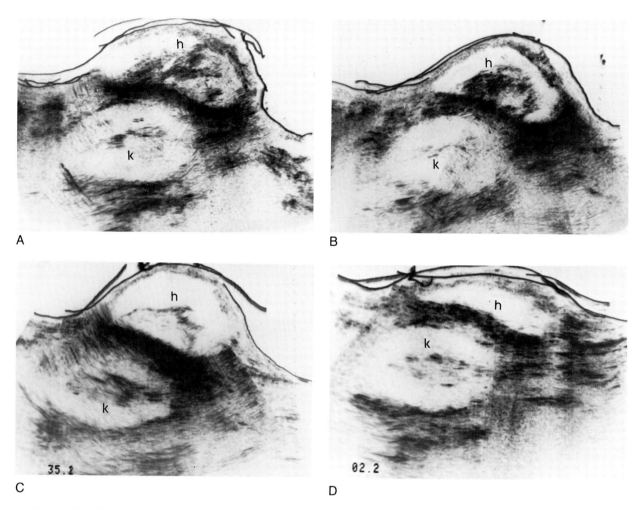

Fig. 4-155. Transplant: Hematoma. Transplant patient who was doing well but developed a mass. **(A)** Longitudinal scan. A relatively superficial echogenic mass *(h)* is seen anterior to the transplanted kidney *(k)*. **(B)** Longitudinal scan 5 days after **(A)**. The mass *(h)* is more lucent. (*k,* kidney.) **(C)** Longitudinal scan 1 month after **(A)**. The mass *(h)* is predominately lucent consistent with evolution of hematoma. **(D)** The hematoma was drained percutaneously. A follow-up scan showed a small remaining hematoma *(h)*. (*k,* kidney.)

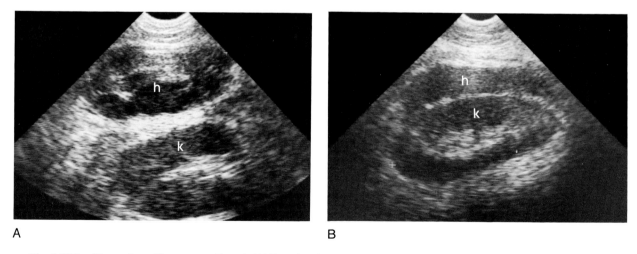

Fig. 4-156. Transplant: Hematoma. Case 1: **(A)** Longitudinal scan post-renal biopsy. A mass *(h)* is seen anterior to the kidney *(k)*. Case 2: **(B)** Long axis view of the transplanted kidney two weeks post-renal biopsy. A hypoechoic mass *(h)* is noted anterior to the kidney *(k)*.

were usually larger than the abscess or urinoma. As for location, most urinomas were located near the lower pole. Ultrasound guided aspiration can provide a diagnosis and facilitate management but one should be careful to avoid bowel. Because of the septation in lymphoceles, they are difficult to aspirate. The patient may be referred to surgery on the basis of deteriorating clinical situation and increasing fluid collection. At times, catheter drainage is possible.

Interventional Procedures

BIOPSY

Renal biopsy may be valuable in determining the cause of posttransplant oliguria and differentiating rejection and ATN.[272,292,293] But, it is invasive and could lead to further deterioration of function. The diagnostic difference is based on a paucity or absence of the characteristic features of rejection—interstitial nephritis, arteritis, or glomerular lesion. It can sometimes be difficult.

The procedure of renal biopsy is generally performed with ultrasound guidance. It is ideal for ultrasound guidance since the kidney lies superficially in the iliac fossa.[283] The superior lateral aspect of the kidney is localized provided the kidney is placed in a cephalad–caudad orientation. If there is a question about orientation, one should localize the most lateral aspect of the kidney away from the renal hilum (as in a transverse lie). The target area may be localized and marked on the skin, or the nephrologist may be guided directly with real-time visualization and a biopsy needle guide. We have found the latter best because it decreases the number of sticks, increases the tissue recovery, and decreases the time of the procedure. Once the needle is seen to enter the kidney, the needle is detached from the needle guide, and the biopsy is performed "free-handed." (For the further discussions see chapter 10.)

OTHER PROCEDURES

Besides renal biopsy, other interventional urologic procedures may be performed on the renal transplant patient. An antegrade pyelogram may be performed if hydronephrosis is increasing in severity by ultrasound and no obvious mass is seen. This can be done with ultrasound guidance using an anterolateral calyx from an angled puncture at the lateral border[294] (Fig. 4-151C). A percutaneous nephrostomy may be performed for temporary drainage, in order to check function, and possibly to remove a calculus.[294] This should be done in a way similar to that described in Chapter 10.

Aspiration and drainage of fluid should be undertaken if the patient's renal function is decreasing, there is fever, mass, or unilateral leg edema.[294] The fluid aspirated is sent for chemical and bacteriologic analysis. An indwelling catheter and repeated puncture increase the risk of the procedure so it is recommended that only fluid aspiration be undertaken. With the second recurrence, surgery is recommended. There is a complication rate of 6 percent.[294] (Fig. 4-153)

Correlative Imaging

Most radiologists would recommend an immediate postoperative nuclear medicine study as the best way to evaluate the renal transplant to assess blood flow, and to evaluate for ATN, rejection, and obstruction. An ultrasound examination should be performed approximately 5 to 7 days postoperatively as a baseline study. The ultrasound examination should assess renal size, hydronephrosis, rejection, and fluid collections. If the patient develops a problem before 3 to 7 days or an abnormality is seen on a nuclear medicine scan (area of decreased or increased activity), then a sonogram should be performed earlier. If need be, the ultrasound may be performed in a sterile fashion using sterile oil on the skin and a sterile glove over the gel-covered scanhead. As for excretory urography, it is used infrequently in the evaluation of the transplant. It is useful in evaluating the course of the ureter, the caliber of the ureter, defining the point of obstruction or localizing the site of extravasated urine seen on the other imaging procedures. Angiography is generally reserved for patients suspected of renal artery stenosis or those with an abnormal perfusion nuclear medicine scan.

With regard to fluid collections, ultrasound is very sensitive in detecting 100 percent of fluid collections in one series.[266] Often a needle aspiration with fluid analysis is needed to differentiate among fluid collections.

During acute renal failure, nuclear medicine may be either suggestive of ATN or equivocal between ATN and rejection. A normal ultrasound supports the diagnosis of ATN.[12] With regard to rejection, to suggest the ultrasound diagnosis, at least two of the described features should be present. Increased renal volume is a more sensitive indicator of increased renal size than a single measurement. If only a single measurement is evaluated, then the anteroposterior diameter and width show the greatest increase as the renal configuration changes from elliptical to globular.[127] The overall accuracy of ultrasound with regard to rejection is 85 percent.[275]

In conclusion, mild episodes of rejection are best recognized by serial nuclear medicine studies interpreted with clinical and laboratory data. An ultrasound examination with decreased echoes in the cortex and increased size are useful when nuclear medicine is inconclusive or suggestive of ATN, or when clinical findings suggest ATN masking rejection.[271] So ultrasound combined with clinical data and nuclear medicine provides a satisfactory answer in the majority of rejection episodes negating biopsy.[275]

ABNORMALITIES OF THE BLADDER AND URETERS

Bladder Abnormalities

CONGENITAL

The bladder develops from a division of the cloaca by a transverse vertical septum. The fetal bladder extends up to the umbilicus where it is in continuity with the allantois stalk. Shortly after birth, the upper half of the bladder narrows as the lower half descends into the pelvis. If a remnant of the allantois remains patent, it presents as a patent urachus that may be an open tube from the bladder to the umbilicus or end as a blind pouch with no connection to bladder.[36]

The urachus connects the apex of the bladder with the allantois through the umbilical cord. Normally, it fibroses at birth and atrophies. Rarely, it remains patent in part or whole. The urachus lies between the transversalis fascia and peritoneum in the space of Retzius'. The urachus proper is 5 to 6 cm long.[36] If the lower part is patent, a bladder diverticulum, or urachal cyst develops.[35]

Urachal Anomalies. Depending on the type of defective obliteration during downward progression of the bladder, various types of congenital urachal anomalies can occur[295] (Fig. 4-157). With a patent urachus, a vesicocutaneous fistula persists throughout from the bladder to umbilicus (Fig. 4-157A). A vesicourachal diverticulum represents the caudal segment of the urachus that is patent, opening into the bladder (Fig. 4-157D). With a urachal sinus, the cephalic portion of the urachus is patent, opening into the umbilicus (Fig. 4-157C). In a urachal cyst, the midportion of the urachus is patent with both cephalic and caudal ends closed, but the cyst can sometimes spontaneously drain its contents into the bladder and/or the umbilicus with increased pressure (Fig. 4-157B).

A urachal cyst typically remains clinically silent until an infection develops in adulthood. The patient often appears with vague abdominal and/or urinary complaints without classic signs of leakage.[295] On ultrasound, a urachal cyst is seen as an echo free tubular structure in the lower mid-abdominal anterior wall[295,296]

(Fig. 4-158). The upper pole is at the level of the umbilicus and the duct extends to the bladder.[295]

Diverticuli. Diverticula of the bladder are a pouch-like eversion or evagination of the bladder wall. The congenital ones are due to focal failure of development of the normal musculature with resultant herniation of the mucosa at this point. The acquired type implies a normal bladder at birth with consequent urethral obstruction causing pouch-like eversions at the point of less resistance to pressure. The clinical significance of this lesion is that it constitutes a site of urinary stasis that tends to become infected.[37]

On ultrasound bladder diverticuli vary greatly in size. They are seen as round, well-defined, thin-walled, distinctly fluid-filled masses with acoustic enhancement[296] (Fig. 4-159). In many, clear demarcation of the communication with the bladder can be seen on the posterior or lateral wall with a straight transverse or longitudinal scan.[296] The diverticulum should disappear when the patient voids.

Exstrophy. Exstrophy of the bladder represents a developmental failure in the anterior wall of the abdomen and bladder so that the bladder either communicates directly through a large defect with the surface of the body in the suprapubic region or as an opened sac. The believed origin is the failure of downgrowth of the mesoderm over the anterior aspect of the bladder; the musculature of the bladder and adjacent abdominal wall never develop and the bladder ruptures anterior to communicate with the skin surface.[37]

Reduplication. Complete reduplication of the bladder is rare. It is difficult to account for replication of the bladder in embryologic terms. The pattern of complete reduplication consists of two separate bladders, each with its own mucosa and muscularis lying side by side, separated by a peritoneal fold. Each bladder receives the ipsilateral ureter and empties into a separate urethra through its own external meatus. There is a common association including reduplication of the genital and distal gastrointestinal system and, less commonly, reduplication or fusion of the lower spine. With reduplication of the bladder, unilateral reflux, obstruction or infection may occur secondary to stenosis, or atresia of the urethra. Ultrasound can be used initially to diagnose and delineate the anatomy[297] (Fig. 4-160).

REFLUX

Vesicoureteral reflux is a common urinary tract abnormality in children. It may occur as a result of a primary maturation abnormality of the trigone and second-

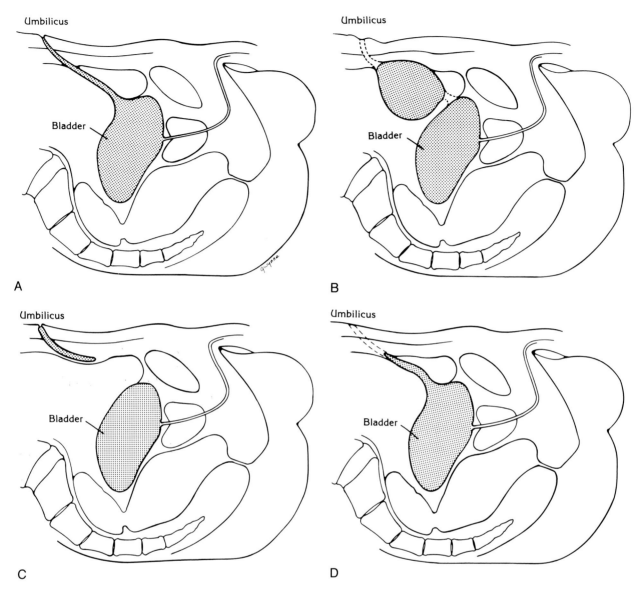

Fig. 4-157. Urachal anomalies. **(A)** Completely patent urachus; **(B)** urachal cyst; **(C)** partially patent urachus. It opens externally but is blind internally (urachal sinus); and **(D)** partially patent urachus. In this instance, it opens internally and is blind externally (vesico-urachal diverticulum).

ary anomalies such as ectopia, posterior urethral valves, paraureteric cyst, prune belly, and neurogenic bladder. Reflux is also often seen into the lower system of a duplex collecting system.[85] High pressure reflux (with or without associated urinary tract infection) may be a major cause of chronic renal failure with marked scarring and atrophic changes in the kidneys. The degree of reflux decreases or disappears in greater than 50 percent of children.[298]

The primary diagnostic procedures to evaluate reflux have included voiding cystourethrography often with excretory urography. Nuclear medicine cystography is a sensitive means to follow reflux. Ultrasound may prove

of value in the management of these children, particularly because this modality provides good visualization of renal size and parenchymal scarring while simultaneously demonstrating reflux.[298]

The ultrasound study for reflux begins with a scan of both kidneys. In the supine position, an 8F straight catheter is placed in the bladder of a male child (8F balloon catheter in the female), residual urine is removed and the patient is returned to the prone position. Cysto-Conray (20 percent) is injected into the bladder after creating turbulence in the contrast by rapidly drawing it in and out of a syringe. Each kidney is scanned while the contrast is injected. The amount of reflux is graded accord-

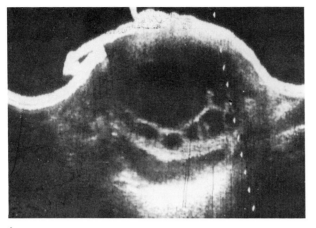

A

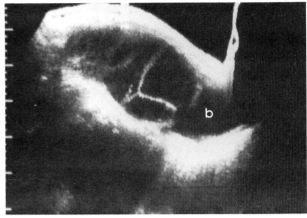

B

Fig. 4-158. Urachal cyst. Infected urachal cyst. Transverse **(A)** and longitudinal **(B)** scans of a predominately cystic mass superior to bladder *(b)* in a 5-year-old girl. The septations are the result of fibrosis and adhesions. (From Friedman AP, Haller JO, Schulze G, Schaffer R: Sonography of vesical and perivesical abnormalities in children. J Ultrasound Med 2: 385, 1983.)

ing to the radiographic classification of Dwoskin and Perlmutter:[298]

Grade I	Lower ureteral filling.
Grade IIA	Ureteral and pelvocalyceal filling without other changes.
Grade IIB	Ureteral and pelvocalyceal filling with mild calyceal blunting without clubbing and without dilatation of the pelvis and tortuousity of the ureter.
Grade III	Ureteral and pelvocalyceal filling, calyceal clubbing and minor to moderate

pelvic dilatation with slight tortuousity of the ureter.

Grade IV	Massive hydronephrosis and hydroureter.

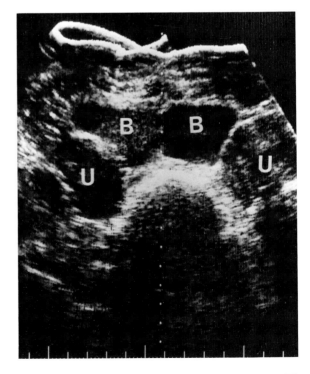

Fig. 4-159. Bladder diverticulum. Transverse scan of the bladder *(b)*. A diverticulum *(d)* is lateral to the left wall of the bladder. (From Morley P: The bladder. p.139. In Rosenfield AT (ed): Clinics in Diagnostic Ultrasound—Genitourinary Ultrasound. Churchill Livingstone, New York, 1979.)

Fig. 4-160. Bladder reduplication. Double bladder *(B)* on transverse scan. Marked reverberation artifact due to obesity. Two widely separated uteri *(U)*. (From Richman TS, Taylor KJW: Sonographic demonstration of bladder duplication. AJR 139:604, © American Roentgen Ray Society, 1982.)

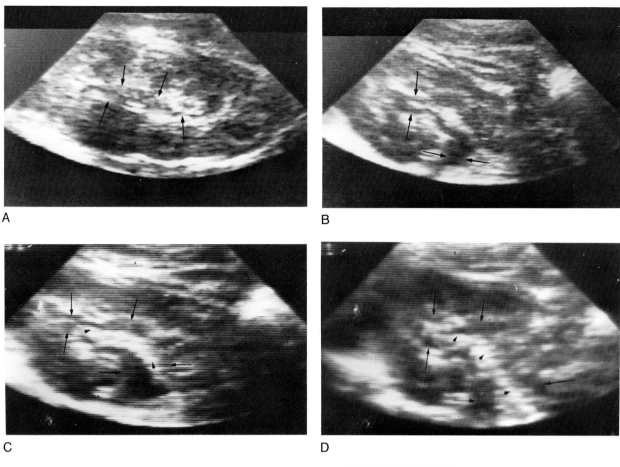

A

B

C

D

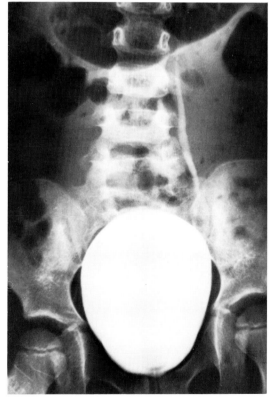

E

Fig. 4-161. Vesicoureteral reflux. Grade IIA reflux. **(A)** Baseline scan, left kidney before bladder filling. Pelvocalyceal system (arrows). **(B – D)** Sequential scans of the left kidney during bladder filling. Progressive dilatation of the pelvocalyceal system (arrows) with echogenic microbubbles (arrowheads) entering the pelvis and the upper pole collecting system. **(E)** Cystogram. Grade IIA reflux bilaterally. (From Kessler RM, Altman DH: Real-time sonographic detection of vesicoureteral reflux in children. AJR 138:1033, © American Roentgen Ray Soc, 1982.)

The sensitivity for Grade IIA reflux or greater on ultrasound imaging is 87 percent while it is 100 percent for Grade IIB or greater in one study.[298] The specificity of this procedure is 100 percent. In each case of reflux, dilatation of the collecting system is preceeded by the appearance of microbubbles even in Grade IIA reflux when cystograms demonstrate no abnormality (Figs. 4-161 to 4-164). There is greater dilatation with increasing grades of reflux.[298]

Ultrasound has potential value in diagnosing as well as following the child with vesicoureteral reflux.[298] This method may prove of value in the management of other children particularly because ultrasound provides good visualization of renal size and parenchymal scarring while simultaneously demonstrating reflux.

DIAGNOSTIC FEATURES

Ultrasound can provide many diagnostic features related to the bladder. The capacity of the bladder, volume of residual urine, changes in bladder outline, changes in wall thickness, and elasticity can be evaluated. The bladder capacity decreases in association with large fixed pelvic masses, in urinary and pelvic inflammatory disease, in patients currently receiving radiation therapy, following radiation therapy, and in advanced stages when the tumor has infiltrated, or after recent surgery. There is increased bladder capacity in bladder neck obstruction and with atonic bladders. Significant residual urine volumes are seen with atonic bladders, bladder neck obstruction, long-standing cystitis, and advanced

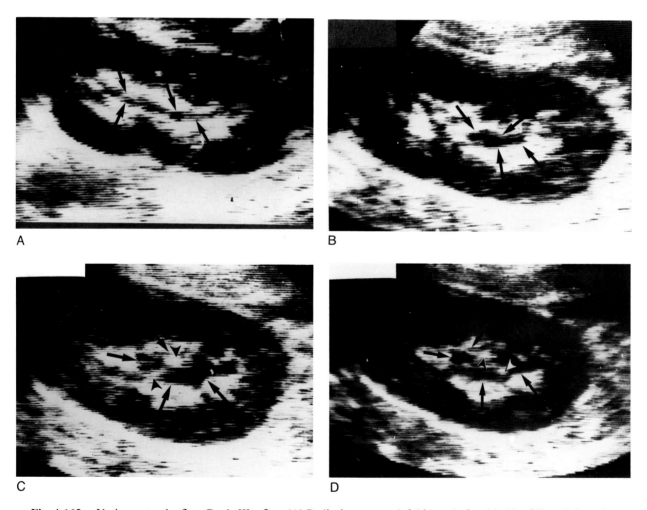

Fig. 4-162. Vesicoureteral reflex. Grade III reflux. **(A)** Preliminary scan, left kidney before bladder filling. Pelvocalyceal system (arrows). **(B–D)** Sequential scans left kidney during bladder filling. Increased pelvocalyceal dilatation (arrows) and echogenic microbubbles (arrowhead) within collecting system. *(Figure continues.)*

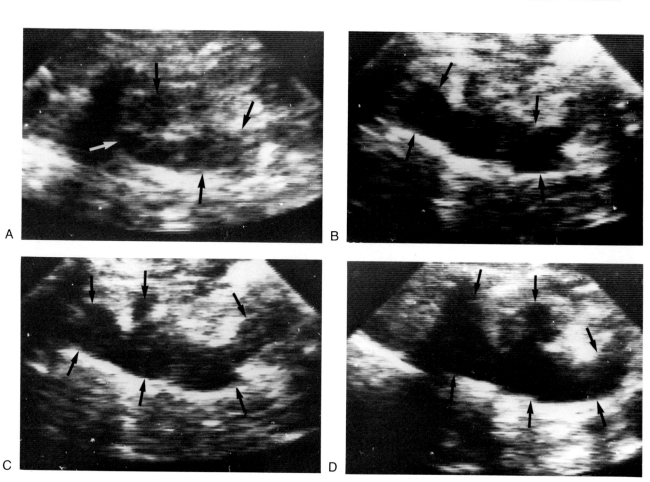

Fig. 4-163. Vesicoureteral reflux. Grade IV reflux. **(A)** Preliminary scan. Small atrophic left kidney (arrows). **(B–D)** Sequential scans of left kidney during bladder filling. Progressive marked pelvocalyceal dilatation (arrows). *(Figure continues.)*

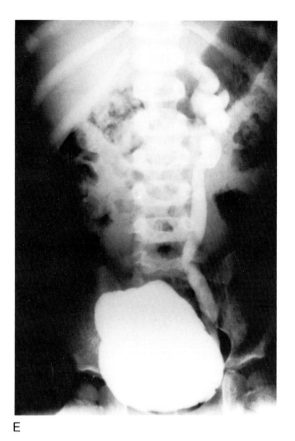

E

Fig. 4-163 *(Continued.* **(E)** Cystogram. Grade IV reflux on left. (From Kessler RM, Altman DH: Real-time sonographic detection of vesicoureteral reflux in children. AJR 138:1033, © American Roentgen Ray Society, 1982.)

invasion by carcinoma. Extrinsic lesions can displace the bladder wall causing changes in bladder shape. Inflammatory changes, tumor infiltration, and recent instrumentation may cause localized loss of elasticity and thickening of the bladder wall with subsequent asymmetry of the bladder outline. Filling defects and irregular bladder wall may be seen with primary bladder tumor, trabeculation, adherent blood blot, granulomatous cystitis, diverticuli, or benign prostatic hypertrophy and extravesical inflammation or neoplastic pathology involving the bladder.[35]

Determination of the amount of residual urine in the

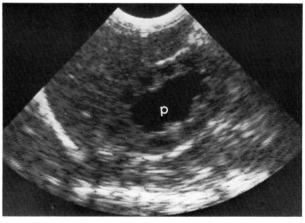

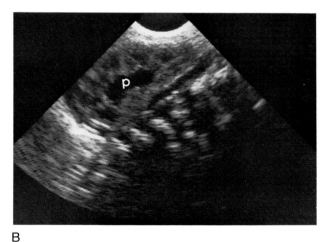

A

B

Fig. 4-164. Vesicoureteral reflux. Grade IV Reflux. This infant presented with palpable abdominal masses. Longitudinal scans of the right **(A)** and left **(B)** kidneys reveal moderate hydronephrosis on the left and severe on the right. (*p,* renal pelvis) *(Figure continues.)*

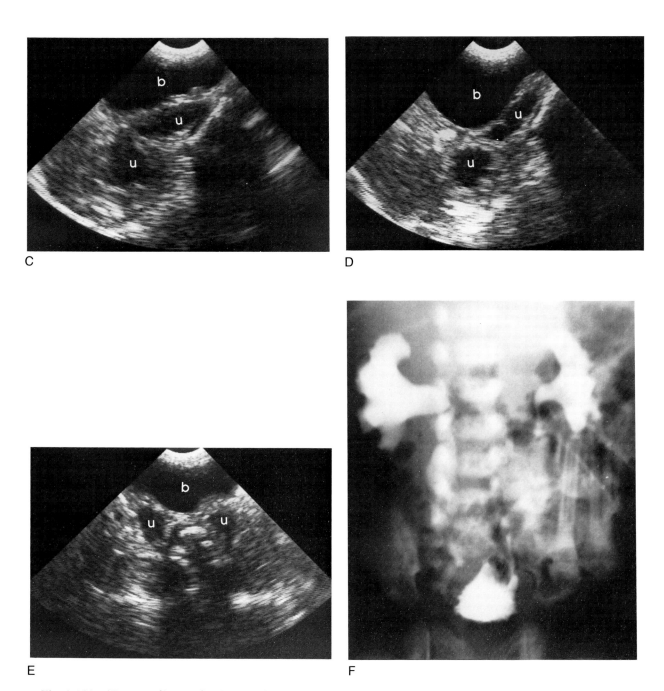

Fig. 4-164 *(Continued). Right* **(C)** and left **(D)** longitudinal scans and transverse scan **(E)** of the pelvis demonstrate dilated ureters *(u)* with a fluid-filled bladder *(b)*. Since the ureters are dilated, it is difficult to follow their long axis. **(F)** Voiding cystourethrogram reveals massive bilateral reflux. (From Seeds JW, Mittelstaedt CA, Mandell J: Pre- and postnatal ultrasound diagnosis of congenital obstructive uropathies. Urol Clin North Am 13:131, 1986.)

bladder has improved the therapy of patients with suspected bladder outlet obstruction. Although prostatic enlargement is usually the etiology of bladder residua, chronic cystitis, and various systemic disorders produce similar symptoms. The most reliable method of measurement is to catheterize the patient and measure the fluid. This runs the risk of both trauma and infection. With ultrasound, one can simply measure the "empty" bladder by taking the maximum width, height and depth (longest anterior–posterior) (Fig. 4-165). This can be applied to the following formula to determine the bladder volume: $V = w \times h \times d$.[299]

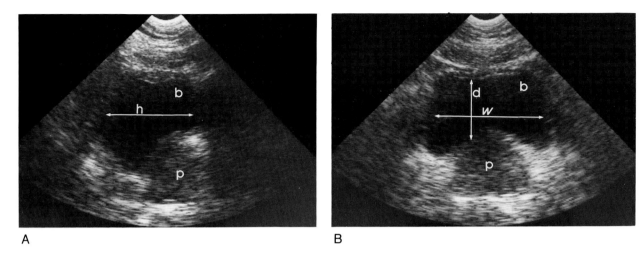

A   B

Fig. 4-165. Bladder volume. Benign prostatic hypertrophy. Longitudinal **(A)** and transverse **(B)** scans of an "empty" bladder *(b)* with measurements for volume. The prostate *(p)* is enlarged with a homogeneous echopattern. (*w*, width; *h*, height; *d*, depth.)

OTHER ABNORMALITIES

Bladder Neck Obstruction. In the male, bladder neck obstruction most commonly is secondary to benign prostatic hypertrophy or carcinoma. With prolonged obstruction, there is progressive hypertrophy of the muscle coat causing thickening and trabeculation of the bladder wall. Ultrasound demonstrates a thickened wall

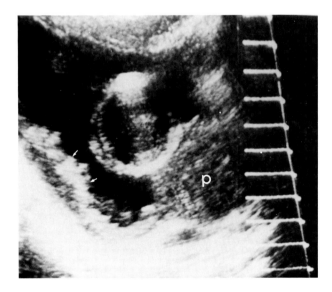

Fig. 4-166. Trabeculated bladder. Longitudinal scan of a bladder with marked trabeculation (arrows) with intravesical enlargement of the prostate *(p)*. A self-retaining catheter is also seen within the bladder. (From Morley P: The bladder. p.139. In Rosenfield AT (ed): Clinics in Diagnostic Ultrasound — Genitourinary Ultrasound. Churchill Livingstone, New York, 1979.)

associated with an irregular inner surface in advanced trabeculation[35] (Fig. 4-166).

Cystitis. Infection of the bladder always implies some predisposing factors that include exstrophy, urethral obstruction, fistulas common to the rectum or vagina, catheterization or instrumentation, cystocele, bladder calculi, bladder neoplasm, trauma, debilitating illness, pyelonephritis, pregnancy, and a derangement of bladder innervation. Up to the middle years, it is more frequent in females presumably due to the shorter urethra, pregnancy, and trauma with coitus.[37]

Bacterial pyelonephritis is frequently preceded by bladder infection with retrograde spread. The common etiology is *E. coli,* followed by *Proteus, Klebsiella,* and *Enterobacter.* With chronicity of the infection, there is fibrous thickening of the tunica propria. The symptoms of this disease include frequency, lower abdominal pain localized over the bladder, and dysuria.[37]

There are several distinct types of cystitis. In encrusted cystitis, there is precipitation of urinary salts, particularly phosphate upon the bladder surface. In bullous cystitis, large vesicles form in the bladder mucosa that collect large amounts of submucosal edema fluid[37] (Figs. 4-167 and 4-168). The changes with catheter-induced cystitis are consistent with bulbous cystitis.[300] The changes include a thickened mucosa that is smooth in the early stages, becoming redundant and polypoid in later stages. The mucosa is usually hypoechoic with the lesion localized to the posterior wall or diffuse and more severe depending on the length of catheterization.[300]

Cystitis is the most commonly encountered pathologic lesion in the bladder but rarely of ultrasound significance. When the process is long-standing, the inflam-

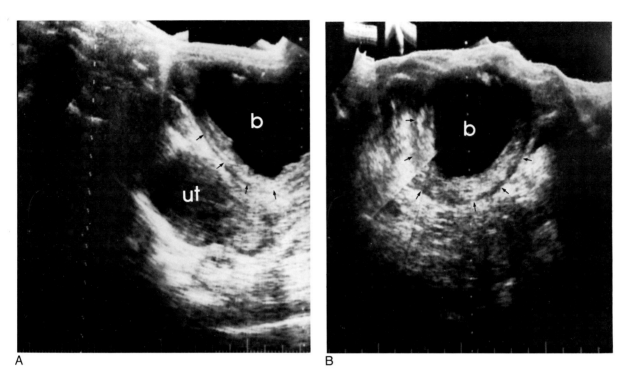

Fig. 4-167. Bullous cystitis. The bladder *(b)* is distended on longitudinal **(A)** and transverse **(B)** scans. The bladder wall is thickened (arrows) with a hypoechoic, irregular wall. (*ut*, uterus.)

matory reaction may cause extreme heaping up of the epithelium and fibrous thickening and loss of elasticity of the bladder wall. This leads to reduced bladder capacity and a rounded, less distensible bladder. Granulation tissue sometimes is seen as an irregular bladder internal surface and the ultrasound findings are indistinguishable from carcinoma[35,301] (Fig. 4-167). With severe purulent cystitis (may develop secondary to neurogenic dysfunction and urine stasis) pus-urine fluid level may be formed with the pus gravitating posteriorly (Figs. 4-169 and 4-170). Mild radiation cystitis is frequently seen producing bladder irritability and is associated with decreased

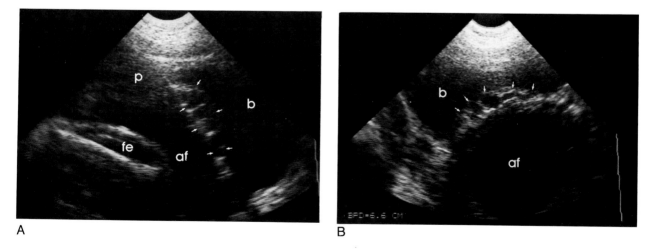

Fig. 4-168. Bullous cystitis. **(A)** Longitudinal and **(B)** transverse scans of the bladder *(b)* in a patient who is 27 weeks pregnant. Multiple cystic areas (arrows) are seen within the posterior bladder wall. (*p*, placenta; *fe*, fetal extremity; *af*, amniotic fluid).

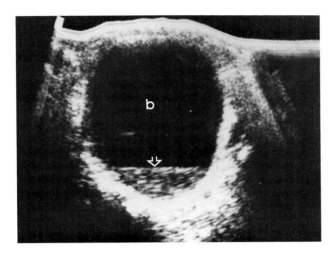

Fig. 4-169. Purulent cystitis. Transverse scan of the bladder *(b)* with a layer of pus (arrow) seen posteriorly. (From Morley P: The bladder. p.139. In Rosenfield AT (ed): Clinics in Diagnostic Ultrasound—Genitourinary Ultrasound. Churchill Livingstone. New York, 1979.)

capacity. In more severe cases, there may be ulceration and sloughing of the bladder wall that may be seen as mucosal irregularity on ultrasound[35] (Fig. 4-171).

Spinal Cord Injury Patients. It is estimated that there are 0.5 to 1 million Americans with spinal cord injuries and there are 20,000 new cases each year.[302] These are mainly due to automobile, diving, and gunshot accidents and are much more common in males than females. The leading cause of death in these patients is

urinary tract complications that arise where the nerve supply to the bladder is disrupted.

Spinal cord injury patients are subject to life long periodic uroradiographic evaluation at intervals of 3 months to 1 year. These patients often undergo excretory urography and voiding cystourethrograms to detect calculi, ureterectasia, hydronephrosis, vesicoureteral reflux, and renal parenchymal disease. Ultrasound is capable of circumventing problems of the radiologic procedures that are common to spinal cord injury patients, such as overlying fecal material or bowel gas. In one series, ultrasound yielded significantly more diagnostic information than radiographic procedures in 36 percent of renal studies and 27 percent of bladder studies.[303]

An ultrasound voiding cystourethrogram can be performed by filling the bladder with a drip infusion of normal saline through an indwelling foley catheter.[303] Using real-time ultrasound, one can watch during infusion for reflux. And one can scan during voiding to look for reflux.

Ultrasound allows a three-dimensional view of the bladder to assess size, shape, and volumetric measurements. These patients are subject to bladder calculi. The earliest sign is an acoustic shadow behind the foley catheter[303] (Figs. 4-172 and 4-173). A calcific crust forms on the foley catheter and then falls off into the bladder, forming a nidus for a stone.[303] Ultrasound is reported to have a 100 percent accuracy for detecting bladder stones.[303]

Ultrasound is unable to see normal ureters consistently. In one series, the ureters were seen in 30 percent of cases with 60 percent of these on real-time.[303] Ultra-

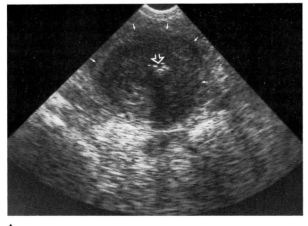
A

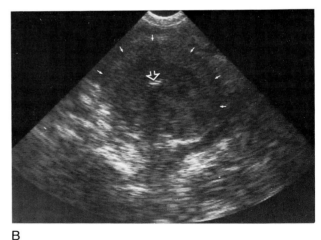
B

Fig. 4-170. Purulent cystitis. Transverse **(A)** and longitudinal **(B)** real-time images reveal a bladder (arrows, bladder outline) completely filled with echoes. Air is seen within the dense fluid collection as linear echodensities (open arrow) that exhibit acoustic shadows.

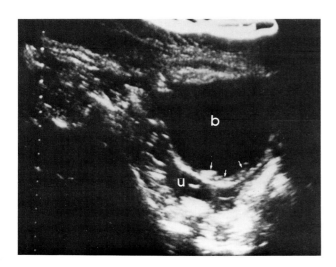

Fig. 4-171. Postradiation cystitis. Mucosal irregularity (arrow) of the posterior bladder *(b)* wall and base is seen. *(u, uterus).* (From Morley P: The bladder. p.139. In Rosenfield AT (ed): Clinics in Diagnostic Ultrasound—Genitourinary Ultrasound. Churchill Livingstone. New York, 1979.)

sound is more successful with ureterectasis (43 percent) than reflux (23 percent).[303] The ureter is best seen with real-time ultrasound, which allows direct observation of peristalsis and/or vesicoureteral reflux. Ureters greater than 8 mm are considered dilated.

Some investigators recommend ultrasound to examine the kidneys and bladder as a replacement for the excretory urogram and voiding cystourethrogram at least at every other periodic examination.[303] Ultrasound has demonstrated 100 percent correlation with excretory urography in parenchymal disease plus over ⅓ of patients give information on ultrasound not available on excretory urogram.[303]

Catheters. Catheters can be easily defined within the bladder on ultrasound. The fluid in the foley balloon is seen as a lucent mass with the catheter walls identified as echodense lines (Fig. 4-172). When possible, it is best to examine the bladder without the catheter in place.[35]

Blood Clots. When blood clots are adherant to the bladder wall they may produce an irregularity along the mucosal surface. This appearance may be similar to that of tumor[35] (Fig. 4-174).

Calculi. Calculi develop primarily in the bladder or pass into the bladder from the upper urinary tract. They are usually single and may be asymptomatic. They may cause inflammatory changes or acute bladder neck obstruction. They are echodense structures producing an acoustic shadow[35,304-306] (Fig. 4-175). The stone need not be calcified to be detected by ultrasound.[306] The

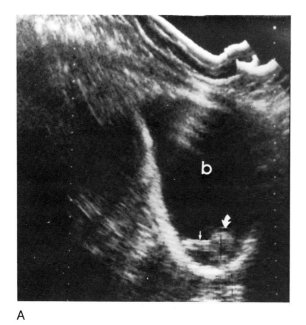

A

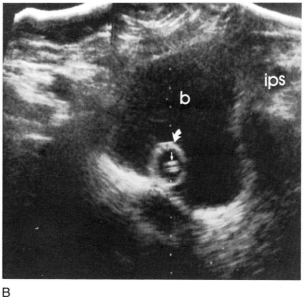

B

Fig. 4-172. Foley catheter. Longitudinal **(A)** and transverse **(B)** scans of the bladder *(b)* with a Foley catheter. The balloon (curved arrow) is seen as an anechoic circle with the catheter seen as two parallel lines (small arrow). Note there is no shadowing associated with the catheter. *(ips,* iliopsous muscle.)

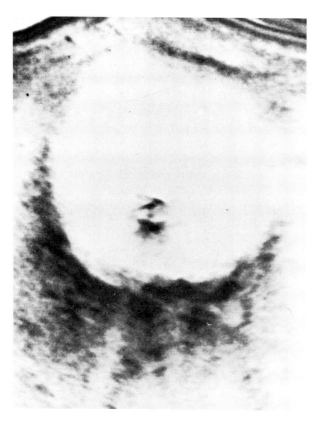

Fig. 4-173. Foley catheter. There are several specular reflectors noted on the foley balloon with acoustic shadowing. (From Brandt TD, Neiman HL, Calenoff L et al: Ultrasound evaluation of the urinary system in spinal-cord-injury patients. Radiology 141:473, 1981.)

calculi shift to the dependent portion of the bladder with change in position.[306]

Endometriosis. Endometriosis occurs in 15 to 30 percent of premenopausal women.[307] It commonly involves the ovaries, fallopian tubes, broad and round ligaments, cervix, vagina, peritoneum, and pouch of Douglas.[308] The urinary tract is involved in 2 to 10 percent with the bladder being the most common urologic site.[307,308] The exact pathogenesis of ectopic endometriosis is unknown. The endometrial element may originate in the uterine wall and reach ectopic positions by direct extension, implantation, or metastasis.[308] Usually the bladder is invaded from without by endometrial tissue penetrating the bladder wall and extending into the bladder lumen. The symptoms of vesical endometriosis are variable. The majority experience a sense of pressure in the suprapubic region usually relieved by voiding with intermittent complaints of urinary urgency, frequency, and burning.[308] Hematuria occurs in 50 percent of cases.[308] The symptoms are cyclic occurring with the menstrual

period. A mass may be palpable in up to 50 percent of patients depending on the size. At least 50 percent of patients have a history of previous pelvic surgery.[308] It is best to time the ultrasound on the day of maximal hormonal stimulation. With vesical endometriosis, a mass along the bladder wall projecting intraluminally may be seen[307,308] (Fig. 4-176). It may be seen as irregular multiple mounds with defined borders. Ultrasound has the advantage of defining the filling defect and its extent.[308]

Neurofibromatosis. Neurofibromatosis is an inherited disorder of the neurilemma cells with characteristic cutaneous, neurologic, and bone lesions. Visceral involvement is uncommon but when it occurs the gastrointestinal tract is frequently affected. Urinary tract involvement is rare. When there is involvement of the bladder, patients often have symptoms of frequency, incontinence, urgency, hematuria, or abdominal pain. The patients are treated conservatively as long as the

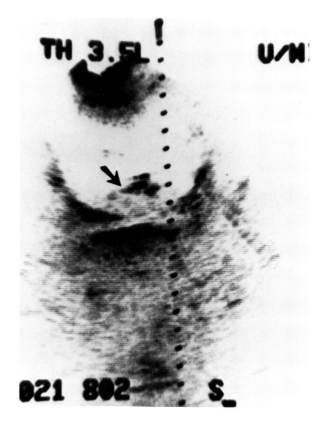

Fig. 4-174. Bladder: Blood clot. Transverse scan. Heterogeneous intraluminal echodensities (arrow) are seen adherent to the bladder wall without acoustic shadowing. (From Bree RL, Silver TM: Sonography of bladder and prevesical abnormalities. AJR 136:1101, © Am Roent Ray Soc, 1981.)

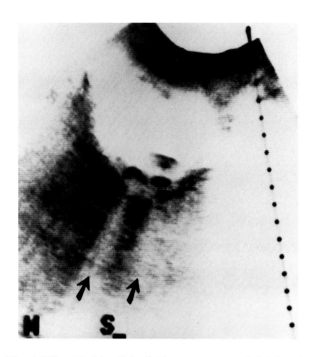

Fig. 4-175. Bladder Calculi. Transverse scan. Brightly echoing intraluminal densities are seen. Acoustic shadowing posteriorly (arrows). (From Bree RL, Silver TM: Sonography of bladder and prevesical abnormalities. AJR 136:1101, © American Roentgen Ray Society, 1981.)

urinary function is maintained. If obstruction develops, an ileal or sigmoid conduit may be necessary.[309]

Although these lesions may be confined to the bladder, there may be diffuse involvement of the pelvis with

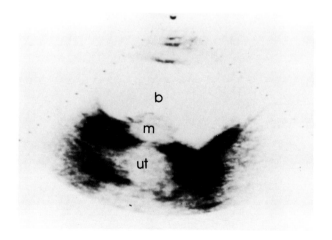

Fig. 4-176. Bladder endometriosis. Transverse scan demonstrating the mass *(m)* situated along the posterior wall of the bladder *(b)*. Note the extent of the mass and its relationship to uterus *(ut)*. (From Kumar R, Haque AK, Cohen MS: Endometriosis of the urinary bladder: Demonstration by sonography. J Clin Ultrasound 12:363, 1984.)

distal urethra, prostate, seminal vesicles, spermatic cords, and testes affected. These tumors are derived from the pelvic autonomic plexuses, which form a complex and interrelated meshwork of nerve fibers innervating the distal ureter, base of the bladder, and other pelvic structures.[309]

Neurofibromatosis may cause massive thickening of the bladder wall on ultrasound (Fig. 4-177). The differential diagnosis would have to include embryonal sarcoma or advanced rhabdomyosarcoma, multiple previous operations, neurogenic bladder, and recurrent cystitis/hemorrhagic cystitis/cytoxan cystitis. Since generalized neurofibromatosis is usually present, the diagnosis is not difficult.[309]

Primary Bladder Tumors. Ninety-five percent of the bladder tumors are epithelial or urothelial. The benign papilloma most commonly occur along the lateral wall with the trigone next in frequency. It is usually small— 0.5 to 2 cm. The malignant tumors of the bladder account for 3 percent of cancer deaths. Ninety percent are transitional cell carcinomas, with 5 percent squamous cell carcinoma, and rarely adenocarcinoma. This malignancy occurs more commonly in males with a 3 to 1 ratio in the 5th to 6th decades.[37] Painless hematuria is the most common presenting symptom in 60 percent of patients.[33,304]

There is a broad spectrum of epithelial bladder tumors from innocuously benign to malignant. Grossly, there may be villous tufts and fronded papillary growths to sessile nodular infiltrating tumors. Local invasion may involve the prostate, seminal vesicles, and retroperitoneum. Forty percent are deeply invasive tumors with metastases to lymph nodes, but hematogeneous spread is late in the disease. The factors affecting curability are depth of infiltration, histologic type, grade of malignancy, and presence of lymphatic or venous permeation of the bladder wall in the region of the tumor.[35,310] The single most important factor is the depth of infiltration, which is defined as the deepest point in the bladder wall to which the tumor has spread.[310] The most important factor in deciding the therapy schedule is the clinically determined stage.[35]

Cystoscopy with biopsy is considered the most accurate method to detect bladder tumors but it is invasive, causes patient discomfort, and often requires anesthesia.[33] Excretory urography, the most commonly used radiologic examination, is relatively insensitive with an accuracy of 70 percent.[33] Ultrasound is helpful as an initial screen of patients with suspected bladder tumors. Nontechnical factors that affect detection include size and location of the tumor, bladder distention, obesity of patient, and operator's skill.[33]

Ultrasound has been shown to reveal certain findings

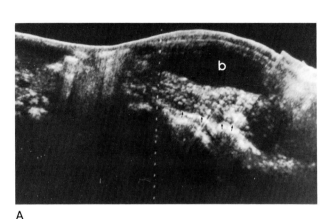
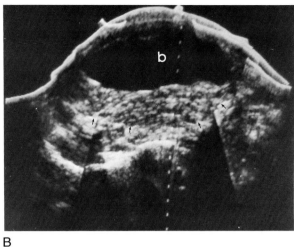

A   B

Fig. 4-177. Bladder neurofibromatosis. Longitudinal (**A**) and transverse (**B**) scans of the bladder *(b)* reveal marked thickening of the posterior and superior walls (arrows). (From Miller WB Jr., Boal DK, Teele R: Neurofibromatosis of the bladder: Sonographic findings. J Clin Ultrasound 11:460, 1983.)

in bladder tumors. Accurate detection depends on the size and location of the neoplasm.[311] Villous tufts appear as small projections of the epithelium that unless numerous, are difficult to define. Small papillomata project from the bladder mucosa and can be pedunculated (Fig. 4-178). If they arise from the bladder base, the pedicle may be obscured. Fronding is seen as a well-defined lesion. A rounded, soft-tissue mass 2 to 4 cm in diameter may be seen with the polypoid type (Fig. 4-179). Massive tumor may be seen obliterating the bladder lumen. The more invasive tumors have a broader-base and spongy

texture or are solid in consistency returning low level echoes (Figs. 4-180 and 4-181). The more sessile ones are irregular on the surface as they frequently are necrotic and ulcerated. The intramural lesions are well defined in

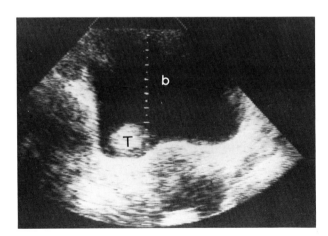

Fig. 4-178. Bladder tumor. Pedunculated. Papillary transitional cell carcinoma. Transverse real-time scan through the bladder *(b)*. A spherical solid mass *(T)* arises from the bladder wall, projecting intraluminally. No acoustic shadowing is seen. (From Bree RL, Silver TM: Sonography of bladder and prevesical abnormalities. AJR 136:1101, © Am Roent Ray Soc, 1981.)

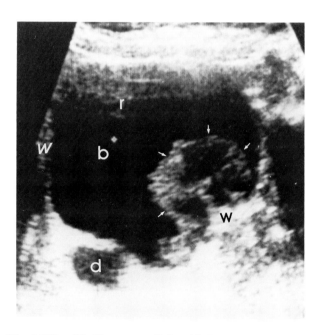

Fig. 4-179. Bladder tumor. Polypoid. Transverse scan of the bladder *(b)* showing a large (3 × 4 cm) polypoid bladder tumor (arrows) with a wide base involving the posterior wall and trigone. The tumor has papillary margins and is of mixed echogenicity. (*d*, diverticulum; *r*, reverberation; *w*, bladder wall.) (From Abu-Yousef MM, Narayana AS, Franken EA Jr, Brown RC: Urinary bladder tumors studied by cystosonography, Part I: Detection. Radiology 153:223, 1984.)

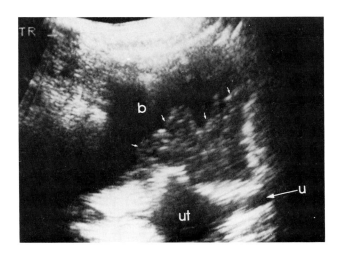

Fig. 4-180. Bladder tumor. Broad-based. Large solid tumor (arrows) obstructing the left ureter *(u)*. The bladder *(b)* wall remains well-defined. The uterus *(ut)* is outlined behind the bladder wall adjacent to the tumor. (From Morley P: The bladder. p.139. In Rosenfield AT (ed): Clinics in Diagnostic Ultrasound—Genitourinary Ultrasound. Churchill Livingstone, New York, 1979.)

outline and demonstrate as being within the bladder wall. An infiltrating wall lesion may produce wall thickening with loss of the concave inner border and little intraluminal mass (Fig. 4-182). Infiltrating tumors occasionally show little intraluminal component and are harder to identify. They vary from high to low level echoes and are usually homogeneous. Exophytic tumors produce focal filling defects of increased or mixed echogenicity arising from the inner surface of the bladder wall. The deeply invasive lesions break through the wall with less definition, as the tumor is seen as a pelvic mass.

Extravesical tumor is usually lower in echodensity than perivesical fat and connective tissue.[35]

Ultrasound is an additional diagnostic tool for detection of bladder tumors and is indicated in cases in which cystoscopy can not be done or is inconclusive. Bladder tumors appear as echogenic structures protruding into the echo free bladder lumen and are easily seen with ultrasound. The detection accuracy is related to the tumor size. Bladder tumors less than 0.5 cm regardless of location and those of any size located in the bladder neck or dome areas are difficult to detect.[311] With tumors > 1 cm the accuracy is 83.3 percent with that of tumors > 2 cm 95 percent.[311] The diagnostic accuracy is 95 percent for tumors greater than 0.5 cm in size and situated on the posterior or lateral wall of the bladder.[311]

It is impossible for ultrasound alone to place bladder tumors in detailed stages. It is usually possible to determine if the tumor is superficial or if it has invaded the bladder muscularis or whether it has spread outside into the pelvic soft tissue. Superficial tumors are usually villous, fronded, or papillary, often with a narrow pedicle (Figs. 4-178 and 4-179). The bladder outline and capacity is normal, as are the pelvic soft tissues. This would correspond to a stage O and A in Jewett's classification.

When the tumor invades the bladder wall, the lesion may vary from a broad-based spongy papillary lesion to a solid, sessile or intramural growth. With involvement of the mucosa and submucosa, a stage T_1 in the TNM system is reached.[310] It is impossible to separate mucosa from submucosa on ultrasound. The underlying echodense bladder wall appears smooth and interrupted by the less echogenic tumor (Fig. 4-183). No bladder deformity or decreased capacity is seen and it is not associated with hydronephrosis.

Superficial muscle involvement (stage B_1 or T_2) causes

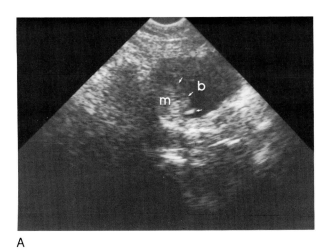

A

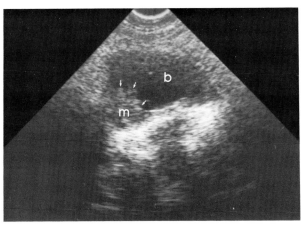

B

Fig. 4-181. Bladder tumor. Recurrent transitional cell carcinoma. Right longitudinal **(A)** and transverse **(B)** scans of the bladder *(b)*. An echodense mass *(m,* arrows) is seen involving the right lateral wall of the bladder.

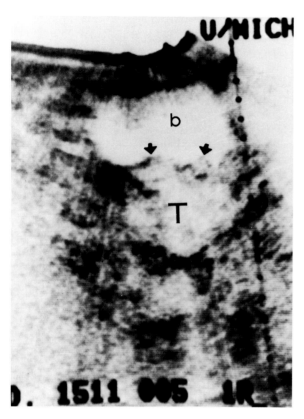

Fig. 4-182. Bladder tumor. Transitional cell carcinoma (stage C). Intraluminal component (arrows) and bulky tumor *(T)* extending posteriorly through bladder *(b)* wall. (From Bree RL, Silver TM: Sonography of bladder and prevesical abnormalities. AJR 136:1101, © Am Roent Ray Soc, 1981.)

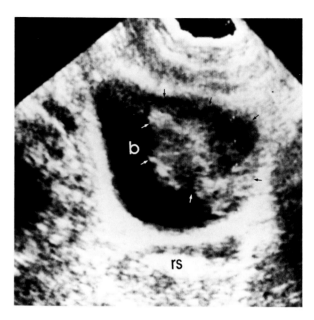

Fig. 4-183. Bladder tumor. Stage T_1, transitional cell carcinoma. Transverse scan of the pelvis shows a large polypoid tumor (white arrows) occupying most of the bladder *(b)* lumen and involving a large area of mucosa. Despite the size of the tumor the muscular wall (black arrows) that underlies the whole extent of the tumor is intact in its entirety, indicating a very superficial tumor. *(rs,* rectosigmoid colon.) (From Abu-Yousef MM, Narayana AS, Brown RC et al: Urinary bladder tumors studies by cystosonography. Part II: Staging. Radiology 153:227, 1984.)

decreased elasticity of the bladder wall adjacent to the tumor. In stage T_2, the superficial invasion of the muscular wall is seen as interruption of the superficial layer of the echogenic wall (Fig. 4-184). There is no associated bladder wall deformity, decreased capacity, or hydronephrosis.

With deeper invasion (stage B_2), the bladder wall is rigid and the bladder capacity is decreased with associated significant residual urine volume. With deep muscular wall involvement, the stage is T_{3A}. In this stage, the whole thickness of the hyperechoic bladder wall is interrupted by the relatively hypoechoic tumor tissue (Fig. 4-185). There is no associated bladder deformity or decreased capacity but hydronephrosis is often associated. Once the tumor extends beyond the bladder wall in the perivesical fat but without involvement of the other perivesical organs, it is stage T_{3B}.[310] The echogenic bladder wall is deformed and there is decreased bladder capacity. The perivesical space is involved by the less echogenic

tumor (Fig. 4-186). Hydronephrosis is usually present. With deep muscle invasion (stage B_2), the ultrasound features are similar to and not always different from tumor that has invaded the perivesical fat (stage C).[35]

Tumors that have invaded the perivesical fat and pelvic soft tissue (stages C and D) are usually sessile though sometimes solid exophytic growths invade deeply. With a stage T_4, there is extension to the perivesical organs — seminal vesicles, prostate, and rectum.[310] The whole thickness of the underlying bladder wall is interrupted by the less echogenic tumor (Fig. 4-187). Hydronephrosis is present. They are identified as in pelvic soft tissues as either or infiltration areas of low-level echoes or as solid tumor masses. The ureter is commonly involved in the lateral wall. The bladder capacity is nearly always decreased and there is significant residual volume.[35] With stage T_N, there are metastases to nodes while stage T_M has distant metastases.[310]

What is the accuracy of ultrasound in staging bladder tumors? With superficial tumors (stages O and A), there is a tendency to overstage the lesion, particularly if the tumor is bulky with a small pedicle. This group can be accurately staged by conventional clinical methods.

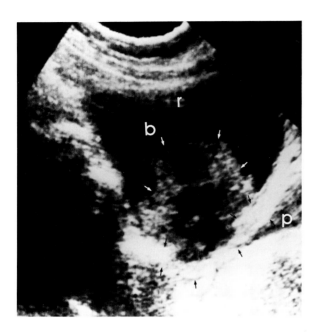

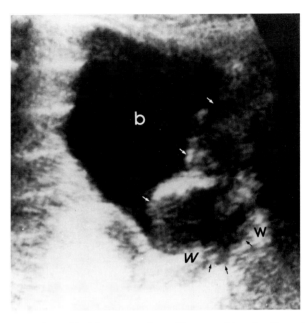

Fig. 4-184. Bladder tumor. Stage T_2, transitional cell carcinoma. Parasagital scan demonstrates a large exophytic mass (white arrows) in the bladder *(b)* trigone. This relatively hypoechoic tumor is seen to infiltrate the superficial layer of the underlying echogenic muscle wall (black arrows). (*p*, prostate; *r*, reverberation.) (From Abu-Yousef MM, Narayana AS, Brown RC et al: Urinary bladder tumors studies by cystosonography. Part II: Staging. Radiology 153:227, 1984.)

Fig. 4-185. Bladder tumor. Stage T_{3A}, transitional cell carcinoma. Longitudinal scan showing an exophytic infiltrating tumor (white arrows) arising from the trigone area. The whole thickness of the underlying muscle wall is infiltrated by the echogenic tumor tissue (black arrows). (*w*, intact muscle wall; *b*, bladder.) (From Abu-Yousef MM, Narayana AS, Brown RC et al: Urinary bladder tumors studies by cystosonography. Part II: Staging. Radiology 153:227, 1984.)

Tumors confined to the bladder wall (stages B_1 and B_2) also are overstaged with ultrasound when compared with conventional methods. With the deeply invasive (stages C and D) tumors, the accuracy of ultrasound in staging rises and the major errors of understaging are rare. The accuracy in staging the superficial tumors is 48 to 55 percent, 78 percent for involvement of the bladder wall and 91 to 100 percent for the deeply invasive group.[35,310] The tumors at the base, posteriorly and lateral walls are more easily staged than those involving the anterior wall and dome.[35]

There are several factors that contribute to ultrasound's efforts to accurately stage these bladder tumors.[310] These include obesity, incomplete bladder distention, anterior location of the tumor, and bullous cystitis. Tumors on the anterior wall are usually poorly imaged because they lie outside of the focal zone of the transducer. Reverberations in the anterior aspect of the bladder may also hide these tumors. Adequate bladder distention is essential but not always possible. Bladder wall edema can obscure the bladder wall.

There are several entities that may mimic the ultrasound appearance of tumor. These include blood clots, benign prostatic hypertrophy (BPH), cystitis, and bladder trabeculae.[33] Blood clots usually move with change

in patient position (Fig. 4-174). BPH is usually in a central location and its relation to the prostate may help differentiate it from a bladder tumor (Fig. 4-188). Bladder trabeculae may also mimic bladder lesions. Trabeculations are usually 1 to 3 mm in size; tumors seldom are this size[33] (Fig. 4-166). In cystitis, there is usually decreased echogenicity, smoother outline and lack of involvement of the muscular wall (Figs. 4-167 to 4-171). As the mucosal involvement is usually more diffuse, the transition from edematous to normal mucosa is usually more gradual. If a focal hyperechoic lesion is seen, it is more likely tumor.

Mesodermal bladder tumors are uncommon benign tumors. They tend to be intramural, encapsulated masses. They are more common in adults though lesions such as angioma are more common in children. The malignant variety of sarcomatous growth is uncommon. They produce a bulky mass that protrudes into the bladder lumen (Fig. 4-189).

Urachal tumors are another bladder related tumor. Eighty percent are in males 50 to 60 years old with vague symptoms.[36] Most are mucinous adenocarcinoma, arising from the intramural (irregularity in dome of bladder) or supravesicular (abdominal mass) portion of the urachus.[36] The supravesicular ones are often cystic and en-

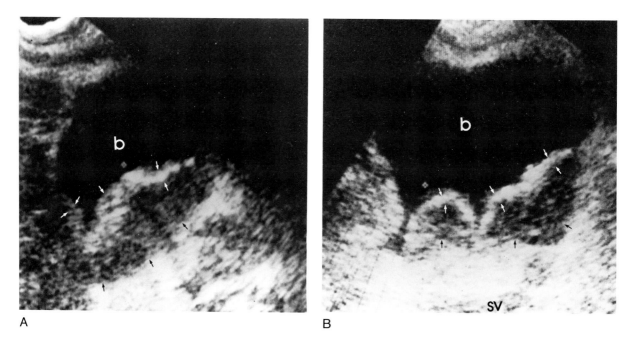

A   B

Fig. 4-186. Bladder tumor. Stage T$_{3B}$, transitional cell carcinoma. Longitudinal (A) and transverse (B) scans showing a large infiltrating mass (black arrows) extending beyond the muscular wall (white arrows) in the perivesical space. The bladder *(b)* itself is markedly deformed. No extension of the tumor to the perivesical organs are seen. *(sv,* seminal vesicles.) (From Abu-Yousef MM, Narayana AS, Brown RC et al: Urinary bladder tumors studies by cystosonography. Part II: Staging. Radiology 153:227, 1984.)

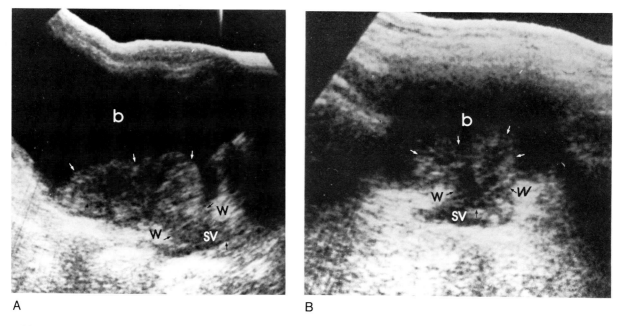

A   B

Fig. 4-187. Bladder tumor. Stage T$_4$ transitional cell carcinoma. Longitudinal (A) and transverse (B) scans at the level of the seminal vesicles *(sv)* show infiltration of the whole thickness of the muscle wall *(w)* by the relatively less echogenic tumor tissue (arrows) with infiltration into the seminal vesicles. There were only two sections that showed deep infiltration of the tumor, which explains how easy it is to understage bladder tumors by cystoscopy and biopsy. (From Abu-Yousef MM, Narayana AS, Brown RC et al: Urinary bladder tumors studies by cystosonography. Part II: Staging. Radiology 153:227, 1984.)

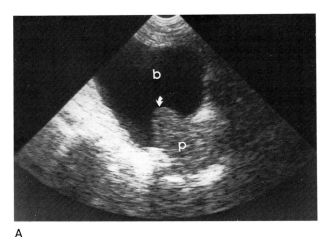 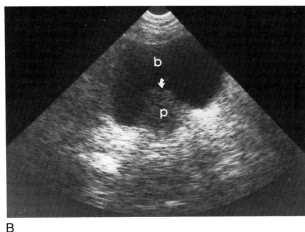

A   B

Fig. 4-188.   Benign prostatic hypertrophy. Longitudinal **(A)** and transverse **(B)** real-time images. An enlarged prostate (arrow, *p*) is seen projecting into the bladder *(b)*. It projects intraluminally on the transverse scan **(B)** and is located retrovesicular on the longitudinal **(A)** scan.

capsulated while the intramural ones are usually small and solid.

Secondary Bladder Tumors. Metastatic bladder tumors usually develop from direct extension, by implantation from a primary lesion of the upper tract or by lymphatic or hematogenous spread. The most common from direct extension are from the cervix, uterus, prostate, and rectum, in that order. Carcinoma of the cervix is particularly prone to spread into the bladder wall particularly in the region of a ureteric orifice (Fig. 4-190). Endometrial carcinoma less commonly involves the bladder. Advanced prostatic carcinoma can extend

into the bladder wall but it more commonly spreads into the seminal vesicles and perivesical connective tissue.[35]

Ureter and Urethral Abnormalities

CONGENITAL

The ureter develops as an outgrowth of the Wolffian (mesonephric) duct during the fourth week of embryonic life.[85,312] Later, the ureter and mesonephric duct

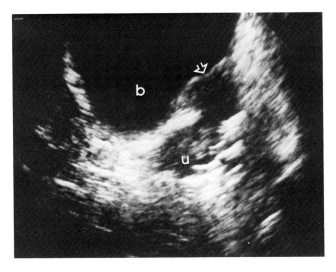

Fig. 4-190.   Metastatic bladder tumor. Stage IV carcinoma of the cervix, invading the bladder (arrow) and surrounding the dilated ureter *(u)*. (*b*, bladder.) (From Morley P: The bladder. p.139. In Rosenfield AT (ed): Clinics in Diagnostic Ultrasound—Genitourinary Ultrasound. Churchill Livingstone, New York, 1979.)

Fig. 4-189.   Bladder Rhabdomyosarcoma. One-year-old boy. Longitudinal scan. A bulky intravesicular tumor *(T)* is seen in the bladder lumen. (From Bree RL, Silver TM: Sonography of bladder and prevesical abnormalities. AJR 136:1101, © American Roentgen Ray Society, 1981.)

separate, entering the bladder at different levels. The caudal end of the ureteric bud is eventually incorporated into the urogenital sinus. There is a 2 to 3 percent incidence of congenital anomalies of the ureter at autopsy.[37] Renal duplication can result from either bifurcation of the bud, incomplete duplication or accessory buds from the Wolffian duct, or complete duplication.[85] In the male, the mesonephric duct empties into the canal of the epididymis, vas deferens, and ejaculatory duct at the lateral aspect of the verumontanum. In the female, the mesonephric duct atrophies, becoming the duct of the epoophora or Gartner's duct, which extends to the anterolateral vaginal wall and ends near the orifice of Bartholin's gland.[312] Developmental anomalies of the lower ureter are frequently associated with renal agenesis or dysplasia and may be associated with anomalies of other mesonephic duct derivation.[313] Ureteral ectopia is more common (70 to 90 percent) in females than males and 10 to 20 percent of cases, regardless of the sex, involve a nonduplicated ureter.[313]

When the ureteric bud originates more cephalad than normal from the mesonephric duct, the ureter may insert into the structures derived from that portion of the mesonephric duct cephalad to the normal origin of the ureteric bud.[313] This includes the posterior urethra, ejaculatory duct, seminal vesicle, and vas deferens. The majority of the extravesicle ectopic ureters in the male are either single, or part of a duplex system, inserting into the posterior urethra (47 to 62 percent) or seminal vesicle (3 to 37 percent). The ejaculatory duct or vas deferens are less frequently involved (40 percent).[313] In the female, the ectopic ureter can implant in the trigone, urethra, perineum, uterus, or vagina.[85]

A more cephalad origin of the ureteric bud from the mesonephric bud also explains renal dysplasia or agenesis often associated with ureteral ectopia. With the more cephalic origin of the ureteric bud, the elongating ureter may fail to meet the nephrogenic blastema in the proper orientation to stimulate normal renal parenchymal development. The incidence and severity of the renal abnormalities increases as the origin of the ureter becomes more cephalad from its normal origin.[313]

Seminal Vesicle Cyst. A seminal vesicle cyst may result from incomplete absorption of the mesonephric duct with the ureter attached to the side of the seminal vesicles or a cyst arising from atresia of the ejaculatory duct. These lesions are diagnosed in the second to third decade of life with symptoms of dysuria, pelvic pain, and ejaculatory disturbances.[35,312] On ultrasound, one sees a cystic structure situated within the seminal vesicle just superior to the prostate and posterior to the bladder[35,296] (Fig. 4-191). These lesions may be quite large and are thin-walled.[296]

Gartner's Duct Cyst. Gartner's duct represents incomplete obliteration of the atrophic mesonephric duct in the female. These cysts may develop in these ducts, lying along the lateral wall of the vagina (Fig. 4-192). They may be asymptomatic or may cause pain, swelling, and dyspareunia.[35,312]

Double or Bifid Ureters. Double and bifid ureters are a relatively common anomaly. It is invariably associated with either totally distinct double renal pelves or anomalous development of a very large kidney, having partially

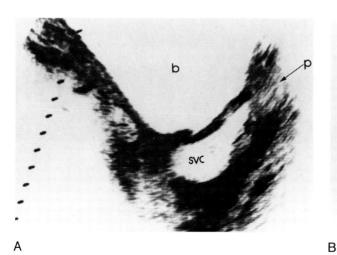
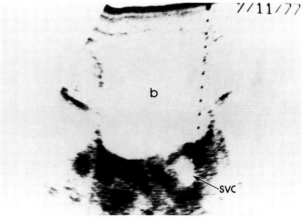

A   B

Fig. 4-191. Seminal vesicle cyst. Longitudinal (**A**) and transverse (**B**) scans demonstrate a cystic 5 × 2.5 × 2.5 cm mass behind the bladder *(b)* and above the prostate *(p)* consistent with a cystic seminal vesicle *(svc)*. (From Weyman PJ, McClennan BL: Computed tomography and ultrasonography in the evaluation of mesonephric duct anomalies. Urol Radiol 1:29, 1979.)

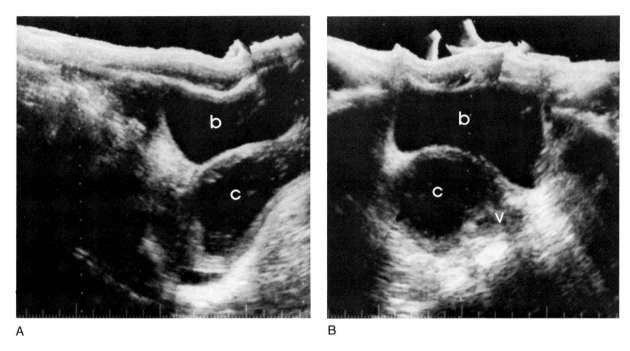

A   B

Fig. 4-192. Gartner's duct cyst. Longitudinal scan 2 cm to the right of midline (**A**) and transverse scan at 2 cm above the symphysis (**B**). A relatively cystic mass *(c)* is seen in the lateral vaginal *(v)* wall. (*b,* bladder.)

bifid pelvis terminating in separate ureters. It is commonly joined within the bladder wall producing a single ureteral orifice. More commonly associated with double ureter, they unite at some point midway to create a "Y".[37]

Miscellaneous Ureteral Anomalies. Other anomalies involving the ureter include anomalous valves, narrowing or strictures, kinks, and torsion.[37] Diverticula are saccular outpouching in the ureteral wall. Hydroureter may be congenital or acquired. The congenital type may be related to an innervation defect of the musculature. The acquired type may be associated with some low ureteral obstruction or pregnancy. Megaloureter, massive enlargement of the ureter, is usually associated with some congenital defect of the kidney, particularly polycystic kidney.[137]

URETEROCELE

An ectopic ureterocele is the third most common cause of hydronephrosis in the neonate.[48] It causes a palpable mass in 50 percent of children.[48] A ureterocele is a cystic dilatation of the submucosal segment of the intravesical ureter with narrowing of the ureteric orifice.[35,67,244,305,314,315] They may cause significant obstruction of the ipsilateral ureter and can obstruct the bladder neck. If associated with an upper pole collecting system, there is often dilatation or hydronephrosis. Most ectopic

ureteroceles insert into the lower urinary bladder or urethra. With simple ureteroceles, the ureter inserts into the bladder in its normal location. This entity has been described in adults.[316]

To make the diagnosis with ultrasound, the examiner must carefully scan the fluid-filled bladder. The demonstration of the ureterocele depends on the sonic reflection of the ureterocele wall interposed between the bladder and the ureterocele fluid contents.[315,317] The intravesical dilatation of the ureterocele is composed of both bladder and ureteric wall and is clearly defined on ultrasound.[35] As such, it is seen as an anechoic thin-walled mass of variable size and shape, projecting into the bladder[296] (Figs. 4-193 and 4-194). When the ectopic ureterocele inserts into the lower bladder or urethra, it is seen quite low in the pelvis and one must angle steeply under the symphysis when scanning (Fig. 4-194). With a simple ureterocele, the anechoic mass is seen in the area of the normal ureteral orifice (Fig. 4-193). This can be confirmed by the presence of ureteral jets.

POSTERIOR URETHRAL VALVES

Posterior urethral valves are the most common cause of urinary obstruction in the male infant and are the second most common cause of hydronephrosis in the neonate. Fifty percent are discovered within the first 3 months of life with 75 percent identified within the first year of life.[243] The obstruction of urinary outflow pro-

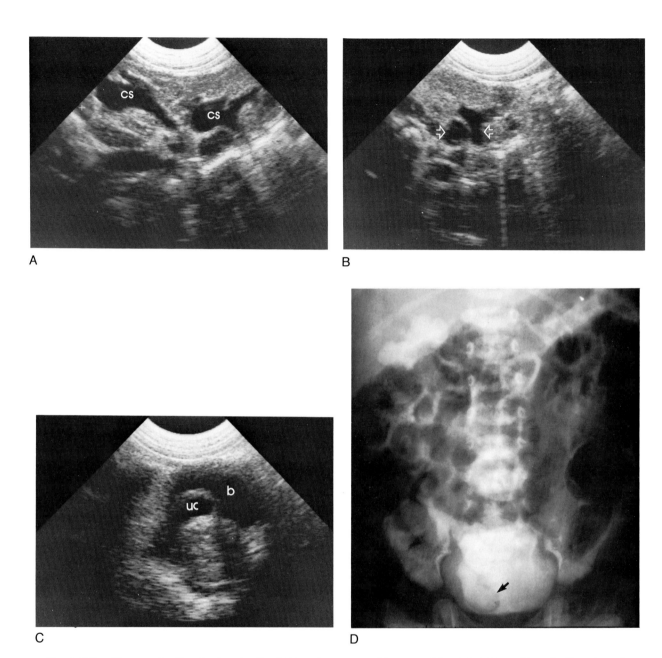

Fig. 4-193. Ureterocele: Simple. Longitudinal (**A**) and transverse (**B**) scans of the right kidney. There is dilatation of a bifid collecting system *(cs)*. On (**B**), the two systems (open arrows) are identified. Transverse (**C**) scan of the bladder *(b)* displays a cystic (anechoic) mass *(uc)* in the area of the right ureteral orifice. This represents a simple ureterocele. (**D**) Intravenous pyelogram confirming the diagnosis. (arrows, ureterocele) (From Seeds JW, Mittelstaedt CA, Mandell J: Pre- and postnatal ultrasound diagnosis of congenital obstructive uropathies. Urol Clin North Am 13:131, 1986.)

duces marked dilatation of the posterior urethra and a thickened trabeculated bladder. The ureters become dilated, elongated, and tortuous with hydronephrosis. The hydronephrosis is usually bilateral but can be asymmetrical depending on the degree of reflux.[48]

Normally there are mucosal folds in the male urethra. These folds are straight extending inferiorly from the verumontanum and dividing into 2 to 4 folds that then diverge from each other. With posterior urethral valves

(type I), a flap of mucosa is seen along the anterior urethral wall, which has a slit-like opening below the verumontanum.[243]

With posterior urethral valves, a spectrum of ultrasound findings are seen. While the normal bladder is seen to have a thin, sharply defined wall, dilatation and thickening of the bladder are almost exclusively seen with an obstructive lesion. The bladder dilates and there is muscular hypertrophy which can be identified on ul-

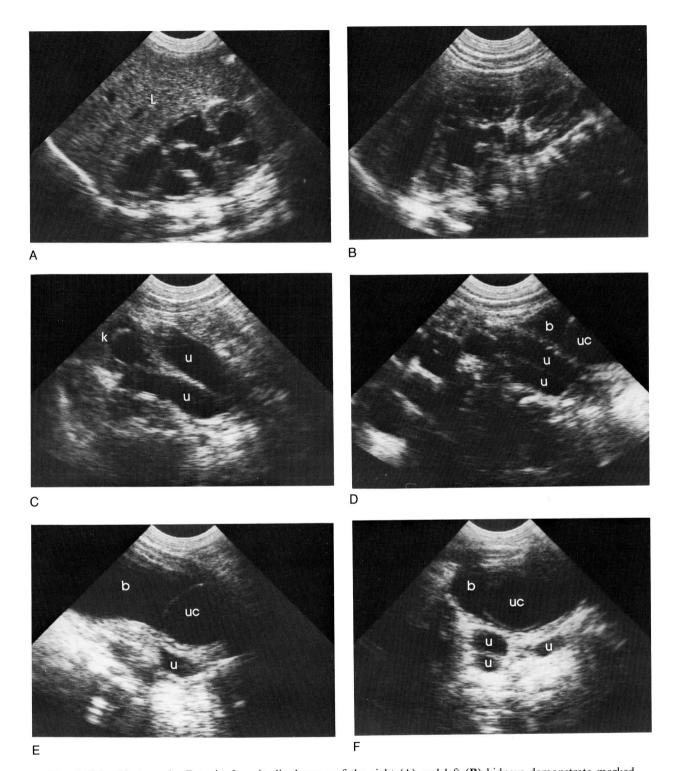

Fig. 4-194. Ureterocele: Ectopic. Longitudinal scans of the right **(A)** and left **(B)** kidneys demonstrate marked dilatation of the collecting system on the right with moderate hydronephrosis on the left. (*L*, liver) On transverse view **(C)** of the right kidney *(k)*, two dilated ureters *(u)* are seen. This was also seen on longitudinal view of the pelvis **(D)**. Two dilated ureters *(u)* are seen. (*b*, bladder; *uc*, ureterocele.) Longitudinal **(E)** and transverse **(F)** views of the bladder *(b)* demonstrate an ectopic ureterocele *(uc)* as a cystic mass in the bladder base. On **(F)**, two dilated ureters *(u)* are seen on the right with one on the left. *(Figure continues.)*

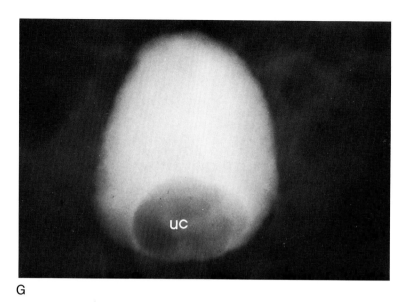

G

Fig. 4-194 *(Continued).* **(G)** Cystogram that confirms the diagnosis. (*uc*, ureterocele.)

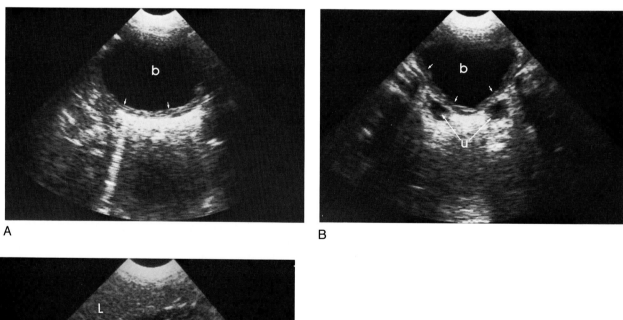

A

B

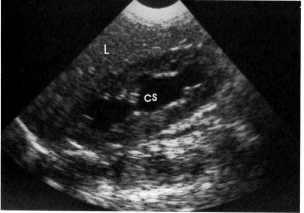

C

Fig. 4-195. Posterior urethral values. Longitudinal **(A)** and transverse **(B)** scans of the bladder *(b)* reveal a thickened bladder wall (arrows). The dilated ureters *(u)* are seen posterior to the bladder in **(B)**. Additionally, there is bilateral hydronephrosis. Longitudinal scan of the right kidney **(C)** demonstrates dilatation of the collecting system *(cs)*. (*L*, liver.)

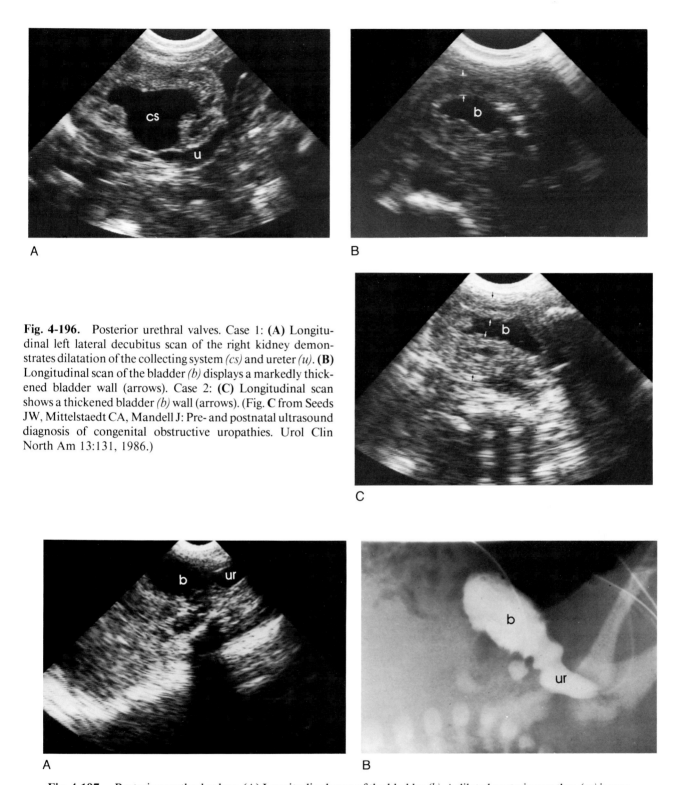

Fig. 4-196. Posterior urethral valves. Case 1: **(A)** Longitudinal left lateral decubitus scan of the right kidney demonstrates dilatation of the collecting system *(cs)* and ureter *(u)*. **(B)** Longitudinal scan of the bladder *(b)* displays a markedly thickened bladder wall (arrows). Case 2: **(C)** Longitudinal scan shows a thickened bladder *(b)* wall (arrows). (Fig. **C** from Seeds JW, Mittelstaedt CA, Mandell J: Pre- and postnatal ultrasound diagnosis of congenital obstructive uropathies. Urol Clin North Am 13:131, 1986.)

Fig. 4-197. Posterior urethral valves. **(A)** Longitudinal scan of the bladder *(b)*. A dilated posterior urethra *(ur)* is seen. **(B)** Voiding cystourethrogram demonstrates the dilated posterior urethra *(ur)*. (*b*, bladder.) (From Seeds JW, Mittelstaedt CA, Mandell J: Pre- and postnatal ultrasound diagnosis of congenital obstructive uropathies. Urol Clin North Am 13:131, 1986.)

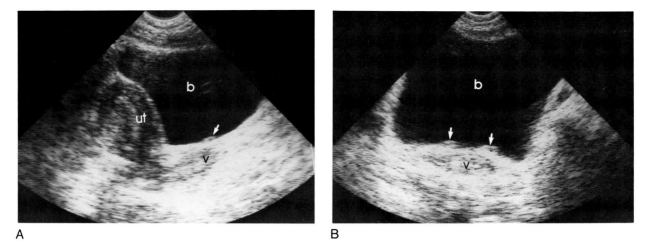

A   B

Fig. 4-198. Ureteral orifice. Longitudinal **(A)** and transverse **(B)** scans of the bladder *(b)*. The papillae of the orifice of the ureters are seen as mucosal elevations (arrows) in the inferior aspect of the bladder on longitudinal scan and on either side of the midline on transverse view. (*ut*, uterus; *v*, vagina.)

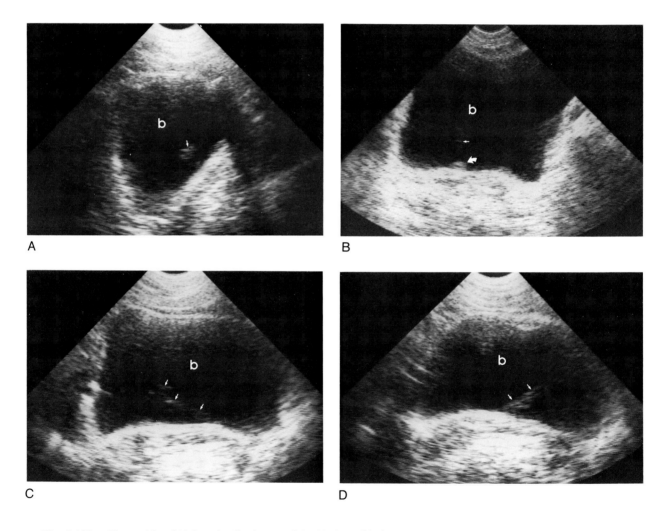

A   B

C   D

Fig. 4-199. Ureteral jet. **(A)** Longitudinal scan of the bladder *(b)* displays a ureteral jet (arrow) as echoes extending from the ureteral orifice. **(B)** Transverse scan of the bladder *(b)* with a jet (small arrow) extending straight anterior from the right ureteral orifice (curved arrow). **(C)** Transverse scan of the bladder *(b)* with a jet (arrows) flowing to the right from the left ureteral orifice. **(D)** Transverse scan of the bladder *(b)* with a jet (arrows) going to the left from the right ureteral orifice. *(Figure continues.)*

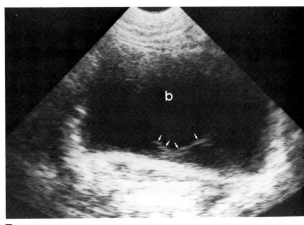

Fig. 4-199 *(Continued).* **(E)** Transverse scan of the bladder *(b)* with bilateral jets (arrows) crossing.

E

trasound (Figs. 4-195 and 4-196). The marked hypertrophy of the bladder muscle may at times simulate a solid echogenic mass.[318] The dilated ureters are seen as lucent tubes medial to the kidney and posterior to the bladder[48] (Fig. 4-195). If a dilated posterior urethra is seen with a distended bladder with a thickened wall, the diagnosis of posterior urethral valves may be made[314,318,319] (Fig. 4-197). Other causes of a dilated posterior urethra include prune-belly syndrome, neurogenic bladder, urethral stricture, and urethral tumor.[319]

DIAGNOSTIC FEATURES: URETERAL JETS

The term "ureteral jets" has been used to describe the appearance of urine entering the bladder. These jets are seen during bladder filling and are not seen when the bladder is full. They are seen at regular intervals (5 to 20 sec), with each jet lasting from a fraction of a second up to 3 seconds.[320 to 322] Each ureter functions independently from the other. At the base of the bladder, there are small elevations of mucosa noted; the jet echoes emanate from these at a 45 degree angle in a caudal direction. On a longitudinal scan, the papilla of the orifice is seen as a mucosal elevation on either side of and at the level of the cervix[322] (Fig. 4-198). The jet starts in the area of the ureteral orifice and flows toward the center of the bladder[320] (Fig. 4-199). The jet extends up to 3 cm and broadens (Fig. 4-199). After a few seconds, the low-intensity echoes become distributed within the bladder and lose their intensity until they are no longer visualized.[320]

There are several theories as to the explanation for the production of the jets and their significance. It has been suggested that the real-time jet and the Doppler shift result from turbulent flow of urine into a static fluid in a closed container (bladder).[322] It is hypothesized that shear forces between the jets and the adjacent static urine create the interface necessary for imaging the jets. The continued changes in these shear forces as a result produce turbulent flow in the urine immediately adjacent to the jet causing a Doppler signal.[322] Other authors have investigated this jet phenomenon and attribute it to acoustic interfaces between fluids of different specific gravities.[320] The clinical importance of the ureteral jet is not yet established. It is impaired in congenital and acquired abnormalities that obstruct the ureter and by abnormal peristalsis.[321]

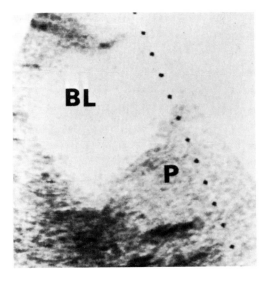

Fig. 4-200. Acute prostatitis. Longitudinal scan in acute prostatitis. The prostate *(P)* is spherical, enlarged, and hypoechoic. *(BL,* bladder.) (From Greenberg M, Neiman HL, Brandt TD et al: Ultrasound of the prostate: Analysis of tissue texture and abnormalities. Radiology 141:757, 1981.)

PROSTATIC ABNORMALITIES

Inflammation

Acute prostatitis is an acute focal or diffuse suppurative inflammation caused by *E. coli* in 80 percent of cases. It is usually due to direct extension from the posterior urethra or urinary bladder. It is one of the most common clinical sequences encountered following surgical manipulation on the urethra or prostate gland such as catheterization, cystoscopy, urethral dilatation, or resection procedures of the prostate.[38] With prostatitis, the local symptoms of low back pain, discomfort, dysuria, frequency, urgency and prostate enlargement and tenderness are seen.[38] On ultrasound the prostate gland is usually enlarged with decreased internal echoes and increased through transmission[41,323] (Fig. 4-200).

Chronic prostatitis is frequently recurrent and is probably the most common cause of relapsing urinary tract infections in males. The mode of development is not well understood. The majority are insidious in onset.[38]

Benign Prostatic Hypertrophy

Benign prostatic hypertrophy (BPH) is common in males over the age of 50 years. Eighty percent of men over 80 years have BPH.[323] It is characterized by the formation of large, fairly discrete nodules in the periurethral region of the prostate. The nodules usually occur

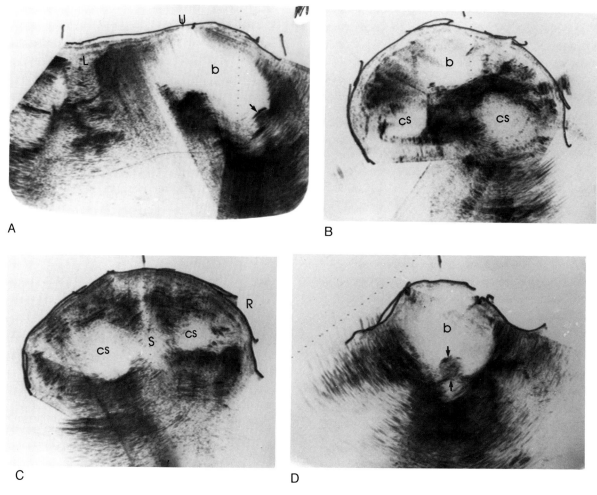

Fig. 4-201. Benign prostatic hypertrophy. Patient referred to ultrasound for evaluation of an abdominal mass. **(A)** Longitudinal static scan reveals a bladder *(b)* distended up to the level of the umbilicus *(U)*. The enlarged prostate (arrow) is seen. (*L*, liver) Transverse scans of the upper abdomen in the supine **(B)** and prone **(C)** positions. The dilated right *(R)* and left collecting systems *(cs)* are seen as well as a distended bladder *(b)*. (*S*, spine.) **(D)** Transverse scan of the bladder *(b)* reveals a mass (arrow) in the area of the prostate. *(Figure continues.)*

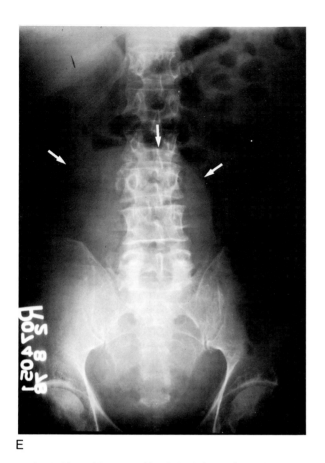

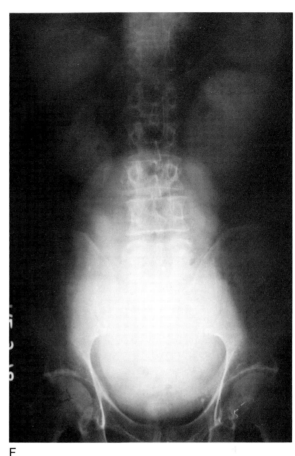

E   F

Fig. 4-201 *(Continued).* **(E)** Plain radiograph demonstrates a large soft tissue density mass (arrows) representing bladder. **(F)** Urogram. The bilateral hydronephrosis and distended bladder are seen.

in the lateral and middle or median lobes and do not involve the posterior portion of the median lobe. The symptoms include frequency, nocturia, difficulty in starting and stopping the stream of urine, overflow, dribble, and dysuria. Secondary bladder changes of hypertrophy, trabeculation, and pseudodiverticuli develop.[38] Five to 10 percent of patients require surgical treatment for relief of urinary tract obstruction.

With BPH, the gland changes in its configuration. The median enlargement increases the anteroposterior diameter of the prostate. If the lateral lobes enlarge, the prostate assumes a more spherical shape. So in BPH, the contour of the enlarged prostate changes from an expanded semilumar shape to round.[324] Proliferative glandular and stromal elements of the periurethral tissues in the lateral and medial lobes create macroscopic nodules that grow in a symmetrical fashion and eventually compress the gland into a pseudocapsule that is seen on ultrasound as a rind of slightly increased echogenicity adjacent to the adenoma. There are usually clearly demarcated capsular margins. If the glandular prolifera-

tion predominates, then the gland appears hypoechoic. With significant stromal proliferative, the glandular tissue is separated by a large amount of collagen, producing increased echogenicity. The gland is usually symmetrically enlarged with sharp margins and a homogeneous texture on ultrasound (Figs. 4-165, 4-188, and 4-201 to 4-203). With diffuse disease, the gland is enlarged with its echogenicity normally homogeneous or diffusely inhomogeneous. Focal disease may be hypoechoic, mixed, or hyperechoic. The majority of focal lesions in BPH are hyperechoic.[13] Intense punctate echoes may represent calcification that is usually secondary to inflammation and ductal obstruction[323] (Figs. 4-202 and 4-203).

Carcinoma

The prostate is the most common reproductive structure to develop neoplastic growth in the older male population. Carcinoma of the prostate is the second most common cancer in men and the third leading cause of

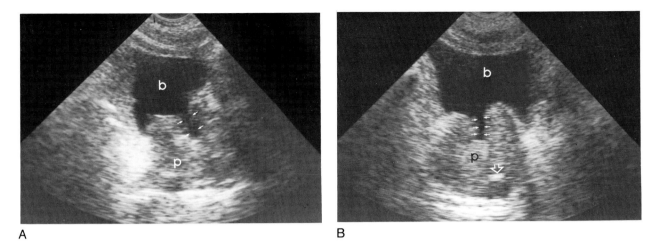

Fig. 4-202. Benign prostatic hypertrophy. Postoperative for transurethral resection of the prostate. Longitudinal (**A**) and transverse (**B**) scans of the bladder *(b)* demonstrate an enlarged prostate *(p)* with a dilated posterior urethra (small arrows). There is a focus of calcification on (**B**) as an echodense area (open arrow).

cancer death.[13,323] It occurs in 10 percent of men age 50 to 59 years and 40 to 50 percent are greater than 70 years old. It is seen in 14 to 40 percent of men over the age of 50 at autopsy.[323] It is more frequent in blacks than whites.[38] The disease has limited clinical symptoms including urinary frequency, dysuria, difficulty in attaining a urine stream, and physical findings of diffuse enlargement or focal mass. Evidence of prostatic malignancy with spread include elevated serum acid phosphatase, retroperitoneal and pelvic lymphadenopathy, and sclerotic bone lesions. Direct prostatic visualization may be achieved with excretory urography, CT, and ultrasound. On CT, the prostate size and, if malignancy is present,

evaluation of local extension and distant metastases particularly to the retroperitoneum and liver can be accomplished. Ultrasound also allows direct visualization of the internal glandular structure and surrounding tissue.

The prevalence of this disease and the lack of reliable diagnostic laboratory tests have led to the development of various imaging modalities. Rectal palpation is the easiest method for local tumor staging but this underestimates the real tumor stage up to 42 percent of cases.[40] On excretory urography, calcification and intravesicular extension can be seen but one cannot distinguish malignancy. CT suggests carcinoma when there is extension beyond the capsule or into the seminal vesicles. Addi-

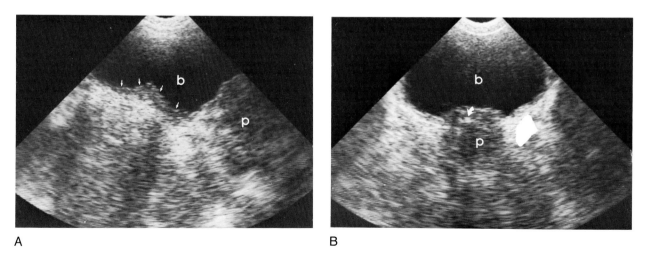

Fig. 4-203. Benign prostatic hypertrophy. Longitudinal (**A**) and transverse (**B**) scans. A markedly enlarged prostate *(p)* is seen. It contains several echogenic foci (curved arrow) with shadowing representing calcification. There is thickening of the bladder wall (small arrows) due to trabeculation. (*b*, bladder.)

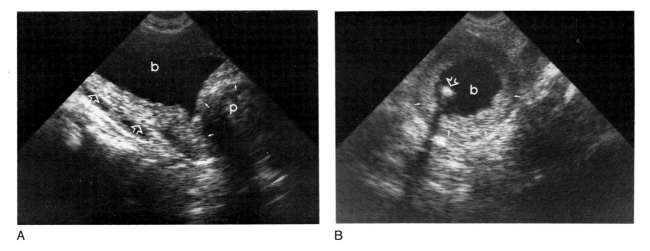

A   B

Fig. 4-204. Benign prostatic hypertrophy and carcinoma. **(A)** Longitudinal scan of the bladder *(b)*. There is a diffusely thickened bladder wall (open arrows). The prostate *(p)* is poorly defined (small arrows). **(B)** Transverse view of the bladder *(b)* with the tip of the Foley catheter (open arrow) seen as an echodense area. The bladder wall is diffusedly thickened (small arrows). Scans of the kidneys revealed bilateral hydronephrosis.

tionally, ultrasound has demonstrated the ability to differentiate changes shown by carcinoma.[325]

On ultrasound, carcinoma is seen as focal areas of increased or decreased echoes with irregular margins[323] (Figs. 4-204 to 4-207). Pathologically, the hypoechoic area is produced by foci of abnormal glands with surrounding desmoplastic reaction characterized by marked deposition of collagen.[323] Seventy-five percent occur in the posterior lobe, which explains the absence of the spherical or oval shape noted in BPH. Carcinoma is

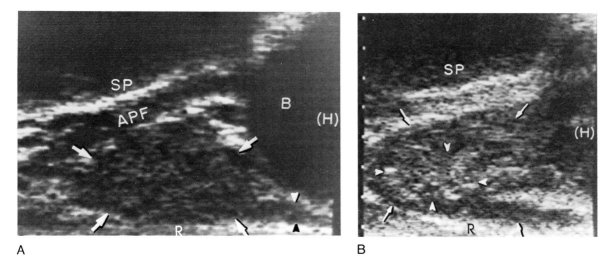

A   B

Fig. 4-205. Prostatic carcinoma. Transrectal linear array scans. **(A)** Normal prostate. The probe is placed in the rectum *(R)* and the sound beam travels toward the anterior structures, i.e. the symphysis pubis *(SP)*. The bladder *(B)* is distended. The image is oriented with the patient in the supine position. The normal sized gland is homogeneously echogenic with defined margins (arrows). The seminal vesicles (arrowheads) are noted as slightly echogenic structures seen in cross-section just superior to the prostate. (*APF,* anterior prostatic fascia; *H,* patient's head.) (Fig. **A** from Rifkin MD: Diagnostic imaging of the lower genitourinary tract. Raven Press, New York, 1985.) **(B)** Prostatic carcinoma. The prostate is minimally enlarged (arrows) with poorly defined nonpalpable echogenic areas scattered throughout the apex of the gland (arrowheads). Echogenic thickness and brightness are grade I in this patient with locally invasive carcinoma. (*H,* toward head; *R,* rectum; *SP,* symphysis pubis). (Fig. **B** from Rifkin MD, Kurtz AB: Ultrasound of the prostate. p.95. In Sanders RC, Hill MC (eds): Ultrasound Annual 1983. Raven Press, New York, 1983.)

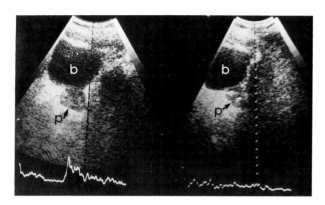

Fig. 4-206. Prostatic carcinoma. Organ-limited. Stage B. Regular prostatic *(p)* contour; echo inhomogenicity. (Left side: transverse scan; Right side: longitudinal scan.) *(b,* bladder.) (From Denkhaus H, Dierkopf W, Grabbe E, Donn F: Comparative study of suprapubic sonography and computed tomography for staging of prostatic carcinoma. Urol Radiol 5:1, 1983.)

suggested when there is distortion, deformity of the prostatic capsule, and the presence of focally dense areas that do not fade with increased altenuation.[326] In advanced disease, there is deformity or destruction of the prostatic capsule and irregular rough dots.[326] And, with advanced carcinoma, there is an asymmetric contour to the gland with an unbalanced elongation of the anteroposterior diameter.[324]

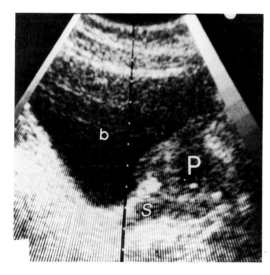

Fig. 4-207. Prostatic carcinoma. Stage C. Seminal vesicle and bladder wall infiltration. Longitudinal scan through the seminal vesicle *(S)* on the left side. The bladder base is infiltrated by tumor tissue. The seminal vesicle is broad and shortened. *(P,* prostate; *b,* bladder.) (From Denkhaus H, Dierkopf W, Grabbe E, Donn F: Comparative study of suprapubic sonography and computed tomography for staging of prostatic carcinoma. Urol Radiol 5:1, 1983.)

Some investigators have evaluated the prostate using a transabdominal approach by assessing echogenicity, location, shape and margin, and integrity of the capsule.[327] Two-thirds of the lesions were found to be echogenic with ⅓ hypoechoic. Seventy-five percent were in the posterior lobe.[327] The lesions had ill-defined borders. They found the transabdominal evaluation of the prostate 80 percent sensitive.[327]

Abdominal and transurethral ultrasound techniques have their limitations. Using the transabdominal approach, the entire prostate gland cannot be fully imaged when it is small or minimally enlarged. The transurethral technique is not routinely used because of its invasive nature.[13,325]

The transrectal ultrasound approach allows the best visualization of the prostate. The first studies employing this technique used radial scanning, producing transverse images of the prostate, allowing evaluation of the prostatic size, texture, and its surrounding tissue.[328] More recently, investigators have been evaluating a linear array, real-time transducer for transrectal evaluation of the prostate. This transducer produces longitudinal scans and the plane of the scan is altered by rotating the scanhead. There are numerous benefits to both radial and real-time transrectal scanning, including: (1) entire gland imaged regardless of size and position, (2) capsule clearly defined and disruption caused by invasion defined, (3) seminal vesicles adequately demonstrated (better with radial than longitudinal real-time), (4) lateral musculature clearly defined, (5) accurately guide percutaneous biopsy (real-time), and (6) prostatic calculi defined (real-time).[13]

No acoustic properties allow consistent separation between benign and malignant disease on ultrasound. Endoscopic prostatic ultrasound appears to yield a significantly higher degree of accuracy than other imaging modalities for evaluation of focal prostatic disease. There are certain characteristics that suggest malignancy. In 92 percent, the margins of the malignancies are poorly defined. Seventy-seven percent of the lesions are hyperechoic (Fig. 4-205). There are no purely hypoechoic tumors seen in one series. There are also certain findings associated with benignancy. Hyperechoic lesions that are bright and thick are seen in 56 percent of benign cases. Foci with shadowing representing calculi are seen in 31 percent of benign cases.[325] Transrectal ultrasound can detect foci representing carcinoma in 95 percent of cases.[13] While this technique cannot be used to screen for carcinoma, in symptomatic patients and others at risk, it may yield substantial clinically significant information.[325]

Ultrasound may be used for staging of prostatic carcinoma. In stage A/B, the tumor is organ-limited and on rectal examination, the prostate can be separated from surrounding tissue. On ultrasound, the contour of the organ is smooth or bulky but preserved (Fig. 4-206). With carcinoma, the echo-pattern is inhomogeneous with local or diffuse increase echo reflection. In stage C/D, the prostate cannot be separated from the surrounding tissue on digital examination. With ultrasound imaging, the prostate outline appears asymmetrical and irregular (Fig. 4-207). The contour cannot be completely separated because there is invasion of surrounding tissue.[40]

Some investigators have compared various modalities with regard to the accuracy of staging prostatic carcinoma. With stage C/D, ultrasound is most accurate with a rate of 81 percent; CT had an accuracy of 30 percent with digital examination 73 percent.[40] Ultrasound did not fare as well with stage A/B; CT was most accurate with a rate of 37 percent, digital examination 22 percent and ultrasound 7 percent.[40] However, CT underestimated the actual tumor stage in 33 percent of cases. It was concluded that ultrasound and rectal examination were the most reliable and practical methods. However, other investigators have recommended CT as it is better suited for staging.[327]

Biopsy

Using transrectal ultrasound guidance for prostatic biopsy allows for accurate placement of the biopsy needle tip into a suspicious area.[13,329] Ultrasound prior to biopsy is recommended to provide confirmation of a palpable mass and to reveal other suspicious areas not clinically suspected.

To perform the procedure with transrectal ultrasound guidance, the patient is placed in the lithotomy or left lateral decubitus position and a condom (placed over tip of probe) covered with gel is inserted into the rectum. Water is instilled to distend the condom. The probe is moved caudad and cephalad and rotated clockwise and counterclockwise to ensure that the entire prostate is examined. A needle is inserted through the perineum in a sterile fashion with direct ultrasound visualization.[13,329] This approach allows more accurate biopsy of nodules.[13,39] The definitive diagnosis depends on the biopsy.

There are numerous benefits to the ultrasound guided prostatic biopsy.[39] The needle can be followed with real-time. The path of the needle can be altered as needed. And, the actual site of the tissue extracted is visualized.

Conclusions

It is suggested that men with palpable or suspected prostatic neoplasm have a transrectal ultrasound examination prior to biopsy.[329] Whenever nonspecific lower urinary tract symptoms are present, ultrasound should be used to evaluate for possible prostatic disease. Ultrasound is not recommended as a screening procedure since differentiation between benign and malignant disease is not possible.[39,329]

REFERENCES

1. Rosenberg ER, Clair MR, Bowie JD: The fluid-filled stomach as an acoustic window to left kidney. AJR 138:175, 1982
2. Finberg H: Renal Ultrasound: Anatomy and Technique. p.7. In Raymond HW, Zwiebel WJ (eds): Seminars in Ultrasound. Vol 2. Grune and Stratton, New York, 1981
3. Bazzocchi M, Rizzato G: The value of the posterior oblique longitudinal scan in renal ultrasonography. Urol Radiol 1:221, 1980
4. Thompson IM, Kovac A, Geshner J: Coronal renal ultrasound: II. Urology 17:210, 1981
5. Albarelli JN, Lawson TL: Renal ultrasonography: Advantages of the decubitus position. J Clin Ultrasound 6:115, 1978
6. Skolnick ML: Enhanced ultrasonic visualization of kidneys via an abdominal compression pillow. J Clin Ultrasound 6:440, 1978
7. Thompson IM, Kovac A, Geshner J, Sarma D: Coronal renal ultrasound: I. Urology 17:92, 1981
8. Rosenfield AT, Taylor KJW, Crade M, DeGraaf CS: Anatomy and pathology of the kidney by gray scale ultrasound. Radiology 128:737, 1978
9. Rosenfield AT, Taylor KJW, Crade M: Renal ultrasound 1979: Gray scale, real-time, Doppler. p.1. In Rosenfield AT (ed): Clinics in Diagnostic—Genitourinary Ultrasound. Churchill Livingstone, New York, 1979
10. Magill HL, Tonkin ILD, Badi H, Riggs W, Jr.: Advantages of coronal ultrasonography in evaluating the neonatal retroperitoneum. J Ultrasound Med 2:289, 1983
11. Jacobs NM, Grant EG, Richardson JD: Neonatal renal enlargement as a sonic window. J Clin Ultrasound 11:521, 1983
12. Hricak H, Cruz C, Eyler WR et al: Acute post-transplant renal failure: Differential diagnosis by ultrasound. Radiology 139:441, 1981
13. Rifkin MD, Kurtz AB: Ultrasound of the prostate. p.95. In Sanders RC, Hill MC (eds): Ultrasound Annual 1983. Raven Press, New York, 1983
14. Robbins SL, Cotran RS: The Kidney. p.1115. In Pathologic Basis of Disease. WB Saunders, Philadelphia, 1979
15. Cook JH III, Rosenfield AT, Taylor KJW: Ultrasonic demonstration of intrarenal anatomy. Am J Roentgenol 129:831, 1977
16. Rosenfield AT: Ultrasound evaluation of renal parenchymal disease and hydronephrosis. Urol Radiol 4:125, 1982
17. Sanders RC, Conrad MR: The ultrasonic characteristics of the renal pelvicalyceal echo complex. J Clin Ultrasound 5:372, 1977

18. Rosenfield AT, Taylor KJW, Dembner AG, Jacobson P: Ultrasound of renal sinus: New observations. AJR 133:441, 1979

19. Brandt TD, Neiman HL, Dragowski MJ et al: Ultrasound assessment of normal renal dimensions. J Ultrasound Med 1:49, 1982

20. Bo WJ, Krueger WA: Anatomic concepts of the urogenital system: Gross and cross-sectional anatomy. p.37. In Resnik MI, Sanders RC (eds): Ultrasound in Urology. Williams & Wilkins, Baltimore, 1979

21. Lewis E, Ritchie WGM: A simple ultrasonic method for assessing renal size. J Clin Ultrasound 8:417, 1980

22. Farrant P, Meire HB: Ultrasonic measurement of renal inclinations: Its importance in measurement of renal length. Br J Radiol 51:628, 1978

23. Rasmussen SN, Haase L, Kjeldsen H, Hancke S: Determination of renal volume by ultrasound scanning. J Clin Ultrasound 6:160, 1978

24. Jones TB, Ruddick LR, Harpen MD et al: Ultrasonographic determination of renal mass and renal volume. J Ultrasound Med 2:151, 1983

25. Hricak H, Lieto RP: Sonographic determination of renal volume. Radiology 48:311, 1983

26. Haller JO, Berdon WE, Friedman AP: Increased renal cortical echogenicity: A normal finding in neonates and infants. Radiology 142:173, 1982

27. Hricak H, Slovis TL, Callen CW et al: Neonatal kidneys: Sonographic anatomic correlation. Radiology 147:699, 1983

28. Scheible W, Leopold GR: High-resolution real-time ultrasonography of neonatal kidneys. J Ultrasound Med 1:133, 1982

29. McInnis AN, Felman AH, Kaude JV, Walker RD: Renal ultrasound in the neonatal period. Pediatr Radiol 12:15, 1982

30. Rosenbaum DM, Korngold E, Teele RL: Sonographic assessment of renal length in normal children. AJR 142:467, 1984

31. Moskowitz PS, Carroll BA, McCoy JM: Ultrasonic renal volumetry in children: Accuracy and simplicity of the method. Radiology 134:61, 1980

32. Harada K, Igari D, Tanahashi Y et al: Staging of bladder tumor by means of transrectal ultrasonography. J Clin Ultrasound 5:388, 1977

33. Abu-Yousef MM, Narayana AS, Franken EA Jr, Brown RC: Urinary bladder tumors studied by cystosonography, Part I: Detection. Radiology 153:223, 1984

34. Slovis TL, Perlmutter AD: Recent advances in pediatric urological ultrasound. J Urol 123:613, 1980

35. Morley P: The bladder. p.139. In Rosenfield AT (ed): Clinics in Diagnostic Ultrasound — Genitourinary Ultrasound. Churchill Livingstone, New York, 1979

36. Han SY, Witten DM: Carcinoma of the urachus. Am J Roentgenol 127:351, 1976

37. Robbins SL, Cotran RJ: The lower urinary tract. p.1186. In Pathological Basis of Disease. WB Saunders, Philadelphia, 1979

38. Robbins SL, Cotran RJ: Male genital system. p.1230. In Pathologic Basis of Disease. WB Saunders, Philadelphia, 1979

39. Rifkin MD, Kurtz AB, Goldberg BB: Sonographically guided transperineal prostatic biopsy: Preliminary experience with a longitudinal linear-array transducer. AJR 140:745, 1983

40. Denkhaus H, Dierkopf W, Grabbe E, Donn F: Comparative study of suprapubic sonography and computed tomography for staging of prostatic carcinoma. Urol Radiol 5:1, 1983

41. Sukov RJ, Scardino PT, Sample WF et al: Computed tomography and transabdominal ultrasound in the evaluation of the prostate. J Comput Assist Tomogr 1:281, 1977

42. Henneberry M, Carter MF, Neiman HL: Estimation of prostatic size by suprapubic ultrasonography. J Urol 121:615, 1979

43. Grossman H, Rosenberg ER, Bowie JD et al: Sonographic diagnosis of renal cystic diseases. AJR 140:81, 1983

44. Sumner TE, Volberg FM, Martin JF et al: Real-time sonography of congenital cystic kidney disease. Urology 20:97, 1982

45. Stick KJ, Koff SA, Silver TM: Ultrasonic features of multicystic dysplastic kidney: Expanded diagnostic criteria. Radiology 143:217, 1982

46. Walker D, Fennell R, Garin E, Richard G: Spectrum of multicystic renal dysplasia: Diagnosis and management. Urology 11:433, 1978

47. Sanders RC, Hartman DS: The sonographic distinction between neonatal multicystic kidney and hydronephrosis. Radiology 151:621, 1984

48. Barth RA, Mindell HJ: Renal masses in the fetus and neonate: Ultrasonographic diagnosis. p.3. In Teele RL (ed): Seminars in Ultrasound, CT and MR — Pediatrics. Vol. 5. Grune and Stratton, Orlando, 1984

49. Boal DK, Teele RL: Sonography of infantile polycystic kidney disease. AJR 135:575, 1980

50. Babcock DS: Medical diseases of the urinary tract and adrenal gland. p.113. In Haller JO, Shkolnik A (eds): Clinics in Diagnostic Ultrasound — Ultrasound in Pediatrics. Churchill Livingstone, New York, 1981

51. Rosenfield AT, Lipson MH, Wolf B et al: Ultrasonography and nephrotomography in the presymptomatic diagnosis of dominantly inherited (adult-onset) polycystic kidney disease. Radiology 135:423, 1980

52. Walker FC Jr, Loney LC, Root ER et al: Diagnostic evaluation of adult polycystic kidney disease in childhood. AJR 142:1273, 1984

53. Ralls PW, Halls J: Hydronephrosis, renal cystic disease, and renal parenchymal disease. p.49. In Raymond HW, Zwiebel WJ (eds): Seminars in Ultrasound. Vol. 2. Grune and Stratton, New York, 1981

54. Kutcher R, Schneider M, Gordon DH: Calcification in polycystic disease. Radiology 122:77, 1977

55. Kelsey JA, Bowie JD: Gray-scale ultrasonography in the diagnosis of polycystic kidney disease. Radiology 122:791, 1977

56. Lawson TL, McClennan BL, Shirkhoda A: Adult poly-

cystic kidney disease: Ultrasonographic and computed tomographic appearance. J Clin Ultrasound 6:297, 1978

57. Kutcher R, Sprayregen S, Rosenblatt R, Goldman M: The sonographic appearance of segmental polycystic kidney. J Ultrasound Med 2:425, 1983

58. Lee JKT, McClennan BL, Kissane JM: Unilateral polycystic kidney disease. AJR 130: 1165, 1978

59. Hantman SS: Unilateral adult polycystic kidney. J Ultrasound Med 1:371, 1982

60. Hayden CK Jr, Swischuk LE, Davis M, Brouhard BH: Puddling: A distinguishing feature of adult polycystic kidney disease in the neonate. AJR 142:811, 1984

61. Rego JD Jr., Laing FC, Jeffrey RB: Ultrasonographic diagnosis of medullary cystic disease. J Ultrasound Med 2:433, 1983

62. Garel LA, Habib R, Pariente D et al: Juvenile nephronophthisis: Sonographic appearance in children with severe uremia. Radiology 151:93, 1984

63. Rosenfield AT, Siegel NJ, Kappelman NB, Taylor KJW: Gray scale ultrasonography in medullary cystic disease of the kidney and congenital hepatic fibrosis with tubular ectasia: New observations. Am J Roentgenol 129:297, 1977

64. Graif M, Lison M, Strauss S et al: Congenital nephrosis: Ultrasonographic features. Pediatr Radiol 12:154, 1982

65. Pope TL Jr., Alford BA, Buschi AJ et al: Nuclear scintigraphy and ultrasound in the diagnosis of congenital ureteropelvic junction obstruction. J Urol 124:917, 1980

66. Schaffer RM, Shih YH, Becker JA: Sonographic identification of collecting system duplications. J Clin Ultrasound 11:309, 1983

67. Mascatello VJ, Smith EH, Carrera GF et al: Ultrasonic evaluation of the obstructed duplex kidney. Am J Roentgenol 129:113, 1977

68. Brown JM: The ultrasound approach to the urographically nonvisualizing kidney. In Raymond HW, Zwiebel WJ (eds): Seminars in Ultrasound. Vol. 2. Grune and Stratton, New York, 1981

69. Sumner TE, Volberg FM, Smolen PM: Intrathoracic kidney—Diagnosis by ultrasound. Pediatr Radiol 12:78, 1982

70. Rosenberg HK: Traumatic avulsion of the vascular supply of a crossed unfused ectopic kidney: Complementary roles of ultrasonography and intravenous pyelography. J Ultrasound Med 3:89, 1984

71. McCarthy S, Rosenfield AT: Ultrasonography in crossed renal ectopia. J Ultrasound Med 3:107, 1984

72. Teele RL, Rosenfield AT, Freedman GS: The anatomic splenic flexure: An ultrasonic renal imposter. Am J Roentgenol 128:115, 1977

73. Trackler RT, Resnick ML, Leopold GR: Pelvic horseshoe kidney: Ultrasound findings and case report. J Clin Ultrasound 6:51, 1978

74. Gray BB Jr., Dawes RK, Atkinson GO Jr., Ball TI Jr.: Wilms' tumor in horseshoe kidneys: Radiologic diagnosis. Radiology 146:693, 1983

75. Mindell HJ, Kupic EA: Horseshoe kidney: Ultrasonic demonstration. Am J Roentgenol 129:526, 1977

76. Bree RL: Anterior position of the lower pole of the right kidney: Potential confusion with right upper quadrant mass. J Clin Ultrasound 4:283, 1976

77. Hasch E: Ultrasound in the diagnosis of hydronephrosis in infants and children. J Clin Ultrasound 2:21, 1974

78. Ellenbogen PH, Scheible FW, Talner LB, Leopold GR: Sensitivity of gray-scale ultrasound in detecting urinary tract obstruction. AJR 130:731, 1978

79. Lee JKT, Baron RL, Melson GL et al: Can real-time ultrasonography replace static B-scan in the diagnosis of renal obstruction? Radiology 139:161, 1981

80. Morin ME, Baker DA: The influence of hydration and bladder distension in the sonographic diagnosis of hydronephrosis. J Clin Ultrasound 7:192, 1979

81. Amis ES Jr., Cronan JJ, Pfister RC, Yoder IC: Ultrasonic inaccuracies in diagnosing renal obstruction. Urology 19:101, 1982

82. Chopra A, Teele RL: Hydronephrosis in children: Narrowing the differential diagnosis with ultrasound. J Clin Ultrasound 8:473, 1980

83. Markle BM, Potter BM: Surgical diseases of the urinary tract. p.135. In Haller JO, Shkolnik A (eds): Clinics in Diagnostic Ultrasound—Ultrasound in Pediatrics. Churchill Livingstone, New York, 1981

84. Nusbacher N, Bryk D: Hydronephrosis of the lower pole of the duplex kidney: Another renal pseudotumor. AJR 130:967, 1978

85. Wyly JB, Resende CMC, Teele RL: Ultrasonography of the complicated duplex kidney: Further observations. In Teele RL (ed): Seminars in Ultrasound, CT, and MR—Pediatrics. Vol. 1. Grune and Stratton, Orlando, 1984

86. Lucaya J, Enriquez G, Delgado R, Castellote A: Infundibulopelvic stenosis in children. AJR 142:471, 1984

87. Ralls PW, Esensten ML, Boger D, Halls JM: Severe hydronephrosis and severe renal cystic disease: Ultrasonic differentiation. AJR 134:473, 1980

88. Jeffrey RB, Federle MP: CT and ultrasonography of acute renal abnormalities. Radiol Clin North Am 21:515, 1983

89. Curry NS, Gobien RP, Schabel SI: Minimal-dilatation obstructive nephropathy. Radiology 143:531, 1982

90. Talner LB, Scheible W, Ellenbogen PH et al: How accurate is ultrasonography in detecting hydronephrosis in azotemic patients. Urol Radiol 3:1, 1981

91. Malave SP, Neiman HL, Spies SM et al: Diagnosis of hydronephrosis: Comparison of radionuclide scanning and sonography. AJR 135:1179, 1980

92. Fried AM, Woodring JH, Thompson DJ: Hydronephrosis of pregnancy: A prospective sequential study of the course of dilatation. J Ultrasound Med 2:255, 1983

93. Peake SL, Roxburgh HB, Langlois SLP: Ultrasonic assessment of hydronephrosis of pregnancy. Radiology 146:167, 1983

94. Erwin BC, Carroll BA, Sommer FG: Ultrasound in renal colic. Proceedings from the 28th Annual American Institute of Ultrasound in Medicine. J Ultrasound Med 2:14, 1983

95. Erwin BC, Carroll BA, Sommer FG: Renal colic: The

role of ultrasound in initial evaluation. Radiology 152:147, 1984

96. Yeh E-L, Chiang L-C, Meade RC: Ultrasound and radionuclide studies of urinary extravasation with hydronephrosis. J Urol 125:728, 1981

97. Itoh S, Yoshioka H, Kaeriyama M et al: Ultrasonographic diagnosis of uriniferous perirenal pseudocyst. Pediatr Radiol 12:156, 1982

98. Shkolnik A: B-mode ultrasound and the nonvisualizing kidney in pediatrics. Am J Roentgenol 128:121, 1977

99. Sanders RC: The place of diagnostic ultrasound in the examination of kidneys not seen on excretory urography. J Urol 114:813, 1975

100. Marangola JP, Bryan PJ, Azimi F: Ultrasonic evaluation of the unilateral nonvisualized kidney. Am J Roentgenol 126:853, 1976

101. Behan M, Wixson D, Kazam E: Sonographic evaluation of the nonfunctioning kidney. J Clin Ultrasound 7:449, 1979

102. Finberg HJ, Billman B, Smith EH: Ultrasound in the evaluation of the nonfunctioning kidney. p.105. In Rosenfield AT (ed): Clinics in Diagnostic Ultrasound—Genitourinary Ultrasound. Churchill Livingstone, New York, 1979

103. Yoder IC, Pfister RC, Lindfors KK, Newhouse JH: Pyonephrosis: Imaging and intervention. AJR 141:735, 1983

104. Coleman BG, Arger PH, Mulhern CB Jr. et al: Pyonephrosis: Sonography in the diagnosis and management. AJR 137:939, 1981

105. Subramanyam BR, Raghavendra BN, Bosniak MA et al: Sonography of pyonephrosis: A prospective study. AJR 140:491, 1983

106. Morehouse HT, Weiner SN, Hoffman JC: Imaging in inflammatory disease of the kidney. AJR 143:135, 1984

107. Sumner TE, Crowe JE, Resnick MI: Ultrasonically guided antegrade pyelography of an obstructed solitary pelvic kidney. J Clin Ultrasound 6:262, 1978

108. Pedersen JF, Cowan DF, Kristensen JK et al: Ultrasonically-guided percutaneous nephrostomy: Report of 24 cases. Radiology 119:429, 1976

109. Barbaric ZL, Wood BP: Emergency percutaneous nephropyelostomy: Experience with 34 patients and review of the literature. Am J Roentgenol 128:453, 1977

110. Sadlowski RW, Finney RP, Branch WT et al: New technique for percutaneous nephrostomy under ultrasound guidance. J Urol 121:559, 1979

111. Baron RL, Lee JKT, McClennan BL, Melson GL: Percutaneous nephrostomy using real-time sonographic guidance. AJR 136:1018, 1981

112. Zegal HG, Pollack HM, Banner MP et al: Percutaneous nephrostomy: Comparison of sonographic and fluoroscopic guidance. AJR 137:925, 1981

113. Stables DP, Johnson ML: Percutaneous nephrostomy: The role of ultrasound. p.73. In Rosenfield AT (ed): Clinics in Diagnostic Ultrasound—Genitourinary Ultrasound. Churchill Livingstone, New York, 1979

114. Burnett KR, Handler SJ, Conroy RM et al: Percutaneous nephrostomy utilizing B-mode and real-time ultrasound guidance: The lateral approach and puncture facilitation with furosemide. J Clin Ultrasound 10:252, 1982

115. Stanley P, Bear JW, Reid BS: Percutaneous nephrostomy in infants and children. AJR 141:473, 1983

116. Bartone FF, Mazer MJ, Anderson JC et al: Diagnosis and treatment of fluid-filled renal structures in children with ultrasonography and percutaneous puncture. Urology 16:432, 1980

117. Bolton WK, Vaughan ED Jr.: A comparative study of open surgical and percutaneous renal biopsies. J Urol 117:696, 1977

118. Winfield AC, Kirchner SG, Brun ME et al: Percutaneous nephrostomy in neonates, infants, and children. Radiology 151:617, 1984

119. Dubuisson RL, Eichelberger RP, Jones TB: A simple modification of real-time sector sonography to monitor percutaneous nephrostomy. Radiology 146:232, 1983

120. Kuligowska E, Newman B, White SJ, Caldarone A: Interventional ultrasound in detection and treatment of renal inflammatory disease. Radiology 147:521, 1983

121. Gold RP, McClennan BL, Rottenberg RR: CT appearance of acute inflammatory disease of the renal interstitium. AJR 141:343, 1983

122. Edell SL, Bonavita JA: The sonographic appearance of acute pyelonephritis. Radiology 132:683, 1979

123. Fiegler W: Ultrasound in acute inflammatory lesions. European J Radiol 3:354, 1983

124. Ben-Ami T: The sonographic evaluation of urinary tract infection in children. In Teele RL (ed): Seminars in Ultrasound, CT, and MR—Pediatrics. Vol. 5. Grune and Stratton, Orlando, 1984

125. Kay CJ, Rosenfield AT, Taylor KJW, Rosenberg MA: Ultrasonic characteristics of chronic atrophic pyelonephritis. AJR 132:47, 1979

126. Gonzalez AC, Karciogla Z, Waters BB, Weens HS: Megalocystic interstitial nephritis: Ultrasound and radiographic changes. Radiology 133:449, 1979

127. Siegel MJ, Glasier CM: Acute focal bacterial nephritis in children: Significance of ureteral reflux. AJR 137:257, 1981

128. Rosenfield AT, Glickman MG, Taylor KJW et al: Acute focal bacterial nephritis (acute lobar nephronia). Radiology 132:553, 1979

129. Lee JKT, McClennan BL, Melson GL, Stanley RJ: Acute focal bacterial nephritis: Emphasis on gray scale sonography and computed tomography. AJR 135:87, 1980

130. Finn DJ, Palestrant AM, DeWolf WC: Successful percutaneous management of renal abscess. J Urol 127:425, 1982

131. Subramanyam BR, Megibow AJ, Raghavendra BN, Bosniak MA: Diffuse xanthogranulomatous pyelonephritis: Analysis by computed tomography and sonography. Urol Radiol 4:5, 1982

132. Hartman DS, Davis CJ Jr., Goldman SM et al: Xanthogranulomatous pyelonephritis: Sonographic-pathologic correlation of 16 cases. J Ultrasound Med 3:481, 1984

133. Van Kirk OC, Go RT, Wedel VJ: Sonographic features of xanthogranulomatous pyelonephritis. AJR 134:1035, 1980

134. Boutros GA, Athey PA: Ultrasonic demonstration of xanthogranulomatous pyelonephritis. J Clin Ultrasound 6:427, 1978

135. Morgan CL, Dempsey PJ, Johnsrude I, Johnson ML: Ultrasound in the diagnosis of xanthogranulomatous pyelonephritis: A case report. J Clin Ultrasound 3:301, 1975

136. Stuck KJ, Silver TM, Jaffe MH, Bowerman RA: Sonographic demonstration of renal fungus balls. Radiology 142:473, 1981

137. Gerzof SG, Gale ME: Computed tomography and ultrasonography for diagnosis and treatment of renal and retroperitoneal abscess. Urol Clin North Am 9:185, 1982

138. Gerzof SG: Percutaneous drainage of renal and perinephric abscess. Urol Radiol 2:171, 1981

139. Hoddick W, Jeffrey RB, Goldberg HI et al: CT and sonography of severe renal and perirenal infections. AJR 140:517, 1983

140. Conrad MR, Sanders RC, Mascardo AD: Perinephric abscess aspiration using ultrasound guidance. Am J Roentgenol 128:459, 1977

141. Hricak H, Cruz C, Romanski R et al: Renal parenchymal disease: Sonographic-histologic correlation. Radiology 144:141, 1982

142. Rosenfield AT, Siegel NJ: Renal parenchymal disease: Histopathologic-sonographic correlation. AJR 137:793, 1981

143. Krensky AM, Reddish JM, Teele RL: Causes of increased renal echogenicity in pediatric patients. Pediatrics 72:840, 1983

144. Hayden CK Jr., Santa-Cruz FR, Amparo EG et al: Ultrasonographic evaluation of the renal parenchyma in infancy and childhood. Radiology 152:413, 1984

145. McCarten KM, Cleveland RH, Simeone JF, Aretz T: Renal ultrasonography in Beckwith-Wiedemann syndrome. Pediatr Radiol 11:46, 1981

146. Subramanyam BR: Renal amyloidosis in juvenile rheumatoid arthritis: Sonographic features. AJR 136:411, 1981

147. Hoffman JC, Schnur MJ, Koenigsberg M: Demonstration of renal papillary necrosis on sonography. Radiology 145:785, 1982

148. Cronan JJ, Yoder IC, Amis ES Jr., Pfister RC: The myth of anechoic renal sinus fat. Radiology 144:149, 1982

149. Ambos MA, Bosniak MA, Gordon R, Madayag MA: Replacement lipomatosis of the kidney. AJR 130:1087, 1981

150. Subramanyam BR, Bosniak MA, Horii SC et al: Replacement lipomatosis of the kidney: Diagnosis by computed tomographic and sonography. Radiology 148:791, 1983

151. Behan M, Kazam E: The echographic characteristics of fatty tissues and tumors. Radiology 129:143, 1978

152. Yeh H-C, Mitty HA, Wolf BS: Ultrasonography of renal sinus lipomatosis. Radiology 124:791, 1977

153. Wilson DA, Wenzl JE, Altshuler GP: Ultrasound demonstration of diffuse hyperoxaluria. AJR 132:659, 1979

154. Alon U, Brewer WH, Chan JCM: Nephrocalcinosis: Detection by ultrasonography. Pediatrics 71:970, 1983

155. Manz F, Jaschke W, Van Kaick G et al: Nephocalcinosis in radiography, computed tomography, sonography and histology. Pediatr Radiol 9:19, 1980

156. Afschrift M, Nachtegaele P, Van Rattinghe R et al: Nephrocalcinosis demonstrated by ultrasound and CT. Pediatr Radiol 13:42, 1983

157. Stafford SJ, Jenkins JM, Staab EV et al: Ultrasonic detection of renal calculi: Accuracy tested in an in vitro porcine kidney model. J Clin Ultrasound 9:359, 1981

158. Foley LC, Luisiri A, Graviss ER, Campbell JB: Nephrocalcinosis: Sonographic detection in Cushing syndrome. AJR 139:610, 1982

159. Shuman WP, Mack LA, Rogers JV: Diffuse nephrocalcinosis: Hyperechoic sonographic appearance. AJR 136:830, 1981

160. Brennan JN, Diwan RV, Makker SP et al: Ultrasonic diagnosis of primary hyperoxaluria in infancy. Radiology 145:147, 1982

161. Cacciarelli AA, Young N, Levine AJ: Gray-scale ultrasonic demonstration of nephrocalcinosis. Radiology 128:459, 1978

162. Sty JR, Starshak RJ, Hubbard AM: Medullary nephrocalcinosis in a newborn: Real-time ultrasound evaluation. J Clin Ultrasound 11:326, 1983

163. Cumming WA, Ohlsson A: Nephrocalcinosis in Bartter's syndrome: Demonstration by ultrasonography. Pediatr Radiol 14:125, 1984

164. Glazer GM, Callen PW, Filly RA: Medullary nephrocalcinosis: Sonographic evaluation. AJR 138:55, 1982

165. Glasier CM, Stoddard RA, Ackerman NB et al: Nephrolithiasis in infants: Association with chronic furosemide therapy. AJR 140:107, 1983

166. Rausch HP, Hanefeld F, Kaufmann JH: Medullary nephrocalcinosis and pancreatic calcifications demonstrated by ultrasound and CT in infants after treatment with ACTH. Radiology 153:105, 1984

167. Kane RA, Manco LG: Renal arterial calcification simulating nephrolithiasis on sonography. AJR 140:101, 1983

168. Garel LA, Pariente DM, Gubler MC et al: The dotted corticomedullary junction: A sonographic indicator of small-vessel disease in hypertensive children. Radiology 152:1419, 1984

169. Pollack HM, Arger PH, Goldberg BB, Mulholland SG: Ultrasonic detection of nonopaque renal calculi. Radiology 127:233, 1978

170. Edell S, Zegel H: Ultrasonic evaluation of renal calculi. AJR 130:261, 1978

171. Schabel SI, Rittenberg GM, Moore TE, Lowrance W: Ultrasound demonstration of milk of calcium in a calyceal diverticulum. J Clin Ultrasound 8:154, 1980

172. Widder DJ, Newhouse JH: The sonographic appearance of milk of calcium in renal calyceal diverticuli. J Clin Ultrasound 10:448, 1982

173. Jacobs RP, Kane RA: Sonographic appearance of calculi in renal calyceal diverticula. J Clin Ultrasound 12:289, 1984

174. Herman RD, Leoni JV, Matthews GR: Renal milk of calcium associated with hydronephrosis. AJR 130:572, 1978

175. Hewitt MJ, Older RA: Calyceal calculi simulating gallstones. AJR 134:507, 1980
176. Mets T, Lameire N, Matthys E, Afschrift M: Sonically guided renal biopsy. J Clin Ultrasound 7:190, 1979
177. Chan JCM, Brewer WH, Still WJ: Renal biopsies under ultrasound guidance: 100 consecutive biopsies in children. J Urol 129:103, 1983
178. Hricak H: Renal medial disorders: The role of sonography. p.43. In Sanders RC (ed): Ultrasound Annual 1982. Raven Press, New York, 1982
179. Goldberg BB, Pollack HM, Kellerman E: Ultrasonic localization for renal biopsy. Radiology 115:167, 1975
180. Saitoh M: Selective renal biopsy under ultrasonic real-time guidance. Urol Radiol 6:30, 1984
181. Nomura G, Kinoshita E, Yamagata Y, Koga N: Usefulness of renal ultrasonography for assessment of severity and cause of acute tubular necrosis. J Clin Ultrasound 12:135, 1984
182. Jain R: Acute renal failure in the neonate. Pediatr Clin North Am 24:605, 1977
183. Sefczek RJ, Beckman I, Lupetin AR, Dash N: Sonography of acute renal cortical necrosis. AJR 142:553, 1984
184. Pardes JG, Yong HA, Kazam E: Sonographic findings in myoglobinuric renal failure and their clinical implications. J Ultrasound Med 2:391, 1983
185. Walker JT, Keller MS, Katz SM: Computed tomographic and sonographic findings in acute ethylene glycol poisoning. J Ultrasound Med 2:429, 1983
186. Moccia WA, Kaude JV, Wright PG, Gaffney EF: Evaluation of chronic renal failure by digital gray-scale ultrasound. Urol Radiol 2:1, 1980
187. Kay CJ, Rosenfield AT, Armm M: Gray-scale ultrasonography in the evaluation of renal trauma. Radiology 134:461, 1980
188. Afschriff M, de Sy W, Voet D et al: Fractured kidney and retroperitoneal hematoma diagnosed by ultrasound. J Clin Ultrasound 10:335, 1982
189. Schmoller H, Kunit G, Frick J: Sonography in blunt renal trauma. Eur Urol 7:11, 1981
190. Pollack HM, Banner MP, Arger PH et al: The accuracy of gray-scale renal ultrasonography in differentiating cystic neoplasms from benign cysts. Radiology 143:741, 1982
191. Pollack HM, Banner MP, Arger PH et al: Comparison of computed tomography and ultrasound in the diagnosis of renal masses. p.25. In Rosenfield AT (ed): Clinics in Diagnostic Ultrasound—Genitourinary Ultrasound. Churchill Livingstone, New York, 1979
192. Elyaderani MK, Gabriele OF: Ultrasound of renal masses. p.21. In Raymond HW, Zwiebel WJ (eds): Seminars in Ultrasound. Vol.2. Grune and Stratton, New York, 1981
193. Bartholomew TH, Slovis TL, Kroovand RL, Corbett DP: The sonographic evaluation and management of simple renal cysts in children. J Urol 123:732, 1980
194. Leopold GR, Talner LB, Asher WM et al: An updated approach to the diagnosis of renal cyst. Radiology 109:671, 1973
195. Green WM, King DL, Casarella WJ: A reappraisal of sonolucent renal masses. Radiology 121:163, 1976
196. Foster WL Jr., Vollmer RT, Halvorsen RA Jr., Williford ME: Ultrasonic findings of small hypernephroma associated with renal cyst. J Clin Ultrasound 11:463, 1983
197. Jaffe CC, Rosenfield AT, Sommer G, Taylor KJW: Technical factors influencing the imaging of small anechoic cysts by B-scan ultrasound. Radiology 135:429, 1980
198. Sanders RC: Kidneys. p.68. In Goldberg BB (ed): Clinics in Diagnostic Ultrasound—Ultrasound in Cancer. Churchill Livingstone, New York, 1981
199. Behan M, Wixson D, Pitts R Jr., Kazam E: Sonographic evaluation of renal masses: Correlations with angiography. Urol Radiol 1:137, 1980
200. Balfe DM, McClennan BL, Stanley RJ et al: Evaluation of renal masses considered indeterminant on computed tomography. Radiology 142:421, 1982
201. Sussman S, Cochran ST, Pagani JJ et al: Hyperdense renal masses: A CT manifestation of hemorrhagic renal cysts. Radiology 150:207, 1984
202. Curry NS, Brock G, Metcalf JS, Sens MA: Hyperdense renal mass: Unusual CT appearance of a benign renal cyst. Urol Radiol 4:33, 1982
203. Zirinsky K, Auh YH, Rubenstein WA et al: CT of the hyperdense renal cyst: Sonographic correlation. AJR 143:151, 1984
204. Cronan J, Amis ES Jr., Yoder IC et al: Peripelvic cysts: An imposter of sonographic hydronephrosis. J Ultrasound Med 1:229, 1982
205. Hidalgo H, Dunnick NR, Rosenberg ER et al: Parapelvic cysts: Appearance on CT and sonography. AJR 138:667, 1982
206. Mitnick JS, Bosniak MA, Hilton S et al: Cystic renal disease in tuberous sclerosis. Radiology 147:85, 1983
207. Murphy JB, Marshall FF: Renal cyst versus tumor: A continuing dilemma. J Urol 123:566, 1980
208. Ambrose SS, Lewis EL, O'Brien DP III et al: Unsuspected renal tumors associated with renal cysts. J Urol 117:704, 1977
209. Thompson IM Jr., Kovac A, Geshner J: Ultrasound followup of renal cyst puncture. J Urol 124:175, 1980
210. Erwin BC, Carroll BA, Walter JF, Sommer FG: Renal infarction appearing as an echogenic mass. AJR 138:759, 1982
211. Spies JB, Hricak H, Slemmer TM et al: Sonographic evaluation of experimental acute renal arterial occlusion in dogs. AJR 142:341, 1984
212. Leekam RN, Matzinger MA, Brunelle M et al: The sonography of renal columnar hypertrophy. J Clin Ultrasound 11:491, 1983
213. Coleman BG, Arger PH, Mulhern CT Jr. et al: Gray-scale sonographic spectrum of hypernephromas. Radiology 137:757, 1980
214. Ladwig SH, Jackson D, Older RA, Morgan CL: Ultrasonic, angiographic, and pathologic correlation of non-cystic-appearing renal masses. Urol 17:204, 1981
215. Maklad NF, Chuang YP, Doust BD et al: Ultrasonic characterization of solid renal lesions: Echographic, angiographic and pathologic correlation. Radiology 123:733, 1977

216. Feldberg MAM, van Waes PFGM: Multilocular cystic renal cell carcinoma. AJR 138:953, 1982

217. Blei CL, Hartman DS, Friedman AC, Davis CJ Jr.: Papillary renal cell carcinoma: Ultrasonic/Pathologic correlation. J Clin Ultrasound 10:429, 1982

218. Press GA, McClennan BL, Melson GL et al: Papillary renal cell carcinoma: CT and sonographic evaluation. AJR 143:1005, 1984

219. McDonald DG: The complete echographic evaluation of solid renal masses. J Clin Ultrasound 6:402, 1978

220. Green B, Goldstein HM, Weaver RM Jr.: Abdominal pansonography in the evaluation of renal cancer. Radiology 132:421, 1979

221. Cronan JJ, Zeman RK, Rosenfield AT: Comparison of computerized tomography, ultrasound, and angiography in staging renal cell carcinoma. J Urol 127:712, 1982

222. Quinn MJ, Hartman DS, Friedman AC et al: Renal oncocytoma: New observations. Radiology 153:49, 1984

223. Goiney RC, Goldenberg L, Cooperberg PL et al: Renal oncocytomas: Sonographic analysis of 14 cases. AJR 143:1001, 1984

224. Charboneau JW, Hattery RR, Ernest EC III et al: Spectrum of sonographic findings in 125 renal masses other than benign simple cyst. AJR 140:87, 1983

225. Scheible W, Ellenbogen PH, Leopold GR, Siao NT: Lipomatous tumors of the kidney and adrenal: Apparent echographic specificity. Radiology 129:153, 1978

226. Totty WG, McClennan BL, Melson GL, Patel R: Relative value of computed tomography and ultrasonography in the assessment of renal angiomyolipoma. J Comput Assist Tomogr 5:173, 1981

227. Hartman DS, Goldman SM, Friedman AC et al: Angiomyolipoma: Ultrasonic-pathologic correlation. Radiology 139:451, 1981

228. Raghavendra BN, Bosniak MA, Megibow AJ: Small angiomyolipoma of the kidney: Sonographic-CT evaluation. AJR 141:575, 1983

229. Lee TG, Henderson SC, Freeny PC et al: Ultrasound findings of renal angiomyolipoma. J Clin Ultrasound 6:150, 1978

230. Duffy P, Ryan J, Aldons W: Ultrasound demonstration of a 1.5 cm intrarenal angiomyolipoma. J Clin Ultrasound 5:111, 1977

231. Kutcher R, Rosenblatt R, Mitsudo SM et al: Renal angiomyolipoma with sonographic demonstration of extension into inferior vena cava. Radiology 143:755, 1982

232. Dunnick NR, Hartman DS, Ford KK et al: The radiology of juxtaglomerular tumors. Radiology 147:321, 1983

233. Madewell JE, Goldman SM, Davis CJ Jr. et al: Multilocular cystic nephroma: A radiographic-pathologic correlation of 58 patients. Radiology 146:309, 1983

234. Carlson DH, Carlson D, Simon H: Benign multilocular cystic nephroma. AJR 131:621, 1978

235. Teele RL: Ultrasonography of the genitourinary tract in children. Radiol Clin North Am 15:109, 1977

236. Gates GF, Miller JH, Stanley P: Necrosis of Wilms' tumor. J Urol 123:916, 1980

237. Jaffee MH, White SJ, Silver TM, Heidelberger KP: Wilms' tumor: Ultrasonic features, pathologic correlation and diagnostic pitfalls. Radiology 140:147, 1981

238. Mulhern CB Jr., Arger PH, Coleman BG et al: Wilms' tumor: Diagnostic therapeutic implication. Urol Radiol 4:193, 1982

239. Wood BP, Muurahaihen N, Anderson VM, Ettinger LJ: Multicystic nephroblastoma: Ultrasound diagnosis (with a pathologic-anatomic commentary). Pediatr Radiol 12:43, 1982

240. Franken EA Jr., Yiu-Chiu V, Smith WL, Chiu LC: Nephroblastomatosis: Clinicopathologic significance and imaging characteristics. AJR 138:950, 1982

241. Hartman DS, Sanders RC: Wilms' tumor versus neuroblastoma: Usefullness of ultrasound in differentiation. J Ultrasound Med 1:117, 1982

242. Fried AM, Hatfield DR, Ellis GT, Fitzgerald KW: Extrarenal Wilms' tumor: Sonographic appearance. J Clin Ultrasound 8:360, 1980

243. Sty JR, Starshak RJ: Sonography of pediatric urinary tract abnormalities. p.71. In Raymond HW, Zwiebel WJ (eds): Seminars in Ultrasound. Vol. 2. Grune and Stratton, New York, 1981

244. Frank JL, Potter BM, Shkolnik A: Neonatal urosonography. p.159. In Rosenfield AT (ed): Clinics in Diagnostic Ultrasound—Genitourinary Ultrasound. Churchill Livingstone, New York, 1979

245. Grider RD, Wolverson MK, Jagannadharao B et al: Congenital mesoblastic nephroma with cystic component. J Clin Ultrasound 9:43, 1981

246. Hartman DS, Lesar MSL, Madewell JE et al: Mesoblastic nephroma: Radiologic-pathologic correlation of 20 cases. AJR 136:69, 1981

247. Arger PH, Mulhern CB, Pollack HM et al: Ultrasonic assessment of renal transitional cell carcinoma: Preliminary report. AJR 132:407, 1979

248. Subramanyam BR, Raghavendra BN, Mudambra MR: Renal transitional cell carcinoma: Sonographic and pathologic correlations. J Clin Ultrasound 10:203, 1982

249. Cunningham JJ: Ultrasonic demonstration of renal collecting system invasion by transitional cell cancer. J Clin Ultrasound 10:339, 1982

250. Mulholland SG, Arger PH, Goldberg BB, Pollack H: Ultrasonic differentiation of renal pelvic filling defects. J Urol 122:14, 1979

251. Wimbish KJ, Sanders MM, Samuels BI, Francis IR: Squamous cell carcinoma of the renal pelvis: Case report emphasizing sonographic and CT appearance. Urol Radiol 5:267, 1983

252. Kutcher R, Lu T, Gordon DH, Becker JA: Renal choriocarcinoma metastasis: A vascular lesion. Am J Roentgenol 128:1046, 1977

253. Hartman DS, Davis CJ Jr., Goldman SM et al: Renal lymphoma: Radiologic-pathologic correlation of 21 cases. Radiology 144:759, 1982

254. Shirkhoda A, Staab EV, Mittelstaedt CA: Renal lymphoma imaged by ultrasound and Gallium 67. Radiology 137:175, 1980

255. Heiken JP, Gold RP, Schnur MJ et al: Computed tomog-

raphy of renal lymphoma with ultrasound correlation. J Comput Assist Tomogr 7:245, 1983

256. Kaude JV, Lacy GD: Ultrasonography in renal lymphoma. J Clin Ultrasound 6:321, 1978

257. Gregory A, Behan M: Lymphoma of the kidneys: Unusual ultrasound appearance due to infiltration of the renal sinus. J Clin Ultrasound 9:343, 1981

258. Kumari-Subaiya S, Lee WJ, Festa R et al: Sonographic findings in leukemic renal disease. J Clin Ultrasound 12:465, 1984

259. Goh TS, LeQuesne GW, Wong KY: Severe infiltration of the kidneys with ultrasonic abnormalities in acute lymphoblastic leukemia. Am J Dis Child 132:1204, 1978

260. Weissberg DL, Miller RB: Renal cell carcinoma and acquired cystic disease of the kidneys in a chronically dialyzed kidney. J Ultrasound Med 2:191, 1983

261. Scanlon MH, Karasick SR: Acquired renal cystic disease and neoplasm: Complications of chronic hemodialysis. Radiology 147:837, 1983

262. Kutcher R, Amodia JB, Rosenblatt R: Uremic renal cystic disease: Value of sonographic screening. Radiology 147:833, 1983

263. McArdle CR, Grumback K: Sonographic and computed tomographic appearances of acquired renal cystic disease. J Ultrasound Med 2:519, 1983

264. Andersen BL, Curry NS, Gobien RP: Sonography of evolving renal cystic transformation associated with hemodialysis. AJR 141:1003, 1983

265. Levine E: Grantham JJ, Slusher SL et al: CT of acquired cystic kidney disease and renal tumors in long-term dialysis patients. AJR 142:125, 1984

266. Coyne SS, Walsh JW, Tisnado J et al: Surgically correctable renal transplant complications: An integrated clinical and radiologic approach. AJR 136:113, 1981

267. Balchunas WR, Hill MC, Isikoff MB, Morillo G: The clinical significance of dilatation of the collecting system in the transplanted kidney. J Clin Ultrasound 10:221, 1982

268. Brenbridge ANAG, Buschi AJ, Cochrane JA, Lees RF: Renal emphysema of transplanted kidney: Sonographic appearance. AJR 132:656, 1979

269. Hricak H, Toledo-Pereyra LH, Eyler WR et al: Evaluation of acute post-transplant renal failure by ultrasound. Radiology 133:443, 1979

270. Johnson ML, Dunne MG, Watts B, Stables D: Ultrasonography in renal transplantation. p.89. In Rosenfield AT (ed): Clinics in Diagnostic Ultrasound—Genitourinary Ultrasound. Churchill Livingstone, New York, 1979

271. Singh A, Cohen WN: Renal allograft rejection: Sonography and scintigraphy. AJR 135:73, 1980

272. Maklad NF, Wright CH, Rosenthal SJ: Gray scale ultrasonic appearances of renal transplant rejection. Radiology 131:711, 1979

273. Maklad NF: Ultrasonic evaluation of renal transplantation. p.88. In Raymond HW, Zwiebel WJ (eds): Seminars in Ultrasound. Vol. 2. Grune and Stratton, New York, 1981

274. Barrientos A, Leiva O, Diaz-Gonzalez R et al: The value of ultrasonic scanning in the differentiation of acute posttransplant renal failure. J Urol 126:308, 1981

275. Frick MP, Feinberg SB, Sibley K, Idstrom ME: Ultrasound in acute renal transplant rejection. Radiology 138:657, 1981

276. Conrad MR, Dickerman R, Love IL et al: New observations in renal transplants using ultrasound. AJR 131:851, 1978

277. Hricak H, Toledo-Pereyra LH, Eyler WR et al: The role of ultrasound in the diagnosis of kidney allograft rejection. Radiology 132:667, 1979

278. Hillman BJ, Birnholz JC, Busch GJ: Correlation of echographic and histologic findings in suspected renal allograft rejection. Radiology 132:673, 1979

279. Hricak H, Romanski RN, Eyler WR: The renal sinus during allograft rejection: Sonographic and histopathologic findings. Radiology 142:693, 1982

280. Slovis TL, Babcock DS, Hricak H et al: Renal transplant rejection: Sonographic evaluation in children. Radiology 153:659, 1984

281. Renigers SA, Spigos DG: Pseudoaneurysm of the arterial anastomosis in a renal transplant. AJR 131:525, 1978

282. Rahatzad M, Henderson SC, Boren GS: Ultrasound appearance of spontaneous rupture of renal transplant. J Urol 126:535, 1981

283. Blumhardt R, Growcock G, Lasher JC: Cortical necrosis in a renal transplant. AJR 141:95, 1983

284. Spigos DG, Tan W, Pavel DG et al: Diagnosis of urine extravasation after renal transplantation. Am J Roentgenol 129:409, 1977

285. Silver TM, Campbell D, Wicks JD et al: Peritransplant fluid collections: Ultrasound evaluation and clinical significance. Radiology 138:145, 1981

286. Brockis JG, Hulbert JC, Patel AS et al: The diagnosis and treatment of lymphoceles associated with renal transplantation. Br J Urol 50:307, 1978

287. Koehler PR, Kanemoto HH, Maxwell JC: Ultrasonic "B" scanning in the diagnosis of complications in renal transplant patients. Radiology 119:661, 1976

288. Kurtz AB, Rubin CS, Cole-Beuglet C et al: Ultrasound evaluation of the renal transplant. JAMA 243:2429, 1980

289. Phillips JF, Neiman HL, Brown TL: Ultrasound diagnosis of post-transplant renal lymphocele. Am J Roentgenol 126:1194, 1976

290. Spigos D, Capek V: Ultrasonically guided percutaneous aspiration of lymphoceles following renal transplantation: A diagnostic and therapeutic method. J Clin Ultrasound 4:45, 1976

291. Rashid A, Posen G, Couture R et al: Accumulation of lymph around the transplanted kidney (lymphocele) mimicking renal allograft rejection. J Urol 111:145, 1974

292. Parker RA, Elliott WC, Muthers RS et al: Percutaneous aspiration biopsy of renal allograft using ultrasound localization. Urol 15:534, 1980

293. Spigos D, Capek V, Jonasson D: Percutaneous biopsy of renal transplants using ultrasonographic guidance. J Urol 117:699, 1977

294. Curry NS, Cochran S, Barbaric ZL et al: Interventional radiologic procedures in the renal transplant. Radiology 152:647, 1984

295. Bouvier JF, Pascaud E, Maihes F et al: Urachal cyst in the adult: Ultrasound diagnosis. J Clin Ultrasound 12:48, 1984

296. Rifkin MD, Needleman L, Kurtz AB et al: Sonography of nongynecologic cystic masses of the pelvis. AJR 142:1169, 1984

297. Richman TS, Taylor KJW: Sonographic demonstration of bladder duplication. AJR 139:604, 1982

298. Kessler RM, Altman DH: Real-time sonographic detection of vesicoureteral reflux in children. AJR 138:1033, 1982

299. Mchean GK, Edell SL: Determination of bladder volumes by gray scale ultrasonography. Radiology 128:181, 1978

300. Abu-Yousef MM, Narayana AS, Brown RC: Catheter-induced cystitis: Evaluation by cystosonography. Radiology 151:471, 1984

301. Rifkin MD, Kurtz AB, Pasto ME, Goldberg BB: Unusual presentations of cystitis. J Ultrasound Med 2:25, 1983

302. Shapeero LG, Friedland GW, Perkash I: Transrectal sonographic voiding cystourethrography: Studies in neuromuscular bladder dysfunction. AJR 141:83, 1983

303. Brandt TD, Neiman HL, Calenoff L et al: Ultrasound evaluation of the urinary system in spinal-cord-injury patients. Radiology 141:473, 1981

304. Cronan JJ, Simeone JF, Pfister RC et al: Cystosonography in the detection of bladder tumors: A prospective and retrospective study. J Ultrasound Med 1:237, 1982

305. Bree RL, Silver TM: Sonography of bladder and prevesical abnormalities. AJR 136:1101, 1981

306. Rosenfield AT, Taylor KJW, Weiss RM: Ultrasound evaluation of bladder calculi. J Urol 121:119, 1979

307. Goodman JD, Macchia RJ, Macasaet MA, Schneider M: Endometriosis of the urinary bladder: Sonographic findings. AJR 135:625, 1980

308. Kumar R, Haque AK, Cohen MS: Endometriosis of the urinary bladder: Demonstration by sonography. J Clin Ultrasound 12:363, 1984

309. Miller WB Jr., Boal DK, Teele R: Neurofibromatosis of the bladder: Sonographic findings. J Clin Ultrasound 11:460, 1983

310. Abu-Yousef MM, Narayana AS, Brown RC et al: Urinary bladder tumors studies by cystosonography. Part II: Staging. Radiology 153:227, 1984

311. Itzchak Y, Singer D, Fischelovitch Y: Ultrasonographic assessment of bladder tumors I: Tumor detection. J Urol 126:31, 1981

312. Arger PH, Zarembok I: Ultrasound efficacy in evaluation of lower genitourinary tract anomalies. J Clin Ultrasound 3:61, 1977

313. Weyman PJ, McClennan BL: Computed tomography and ultrasonography in the evaluation of mesonephric duct anomalies. Urol Radiol 1:29, 1979

314. Friedman AP, Haller JO, Schulze G, Schaffer R: Sonography of vesical and perivesical abnormalities in children. J Ultrasound Med 2:385, 1983

315. Summer TE, Crowe JE, Resnick MI: Diagnosis of ectopic ureterocele using ultrasound. Urol 15:82, 1980

316. Brenner RJ, DeMartini WJ, Gooding GAW, Hedgcock MW: Ultrasonographic demonstration of a simple ureterocele and dilated ureter in an adult. J Clin Ultrasound 6:431, 1978

317. Rose JS, McCarthy J, Yeh H-C: Ultrasound diagnosis of ectopic ureterocele. Pediatr Radiol 8:17, 1979

318. Gilsanz V, Miller JH, Reid BS: Ultrasonic characteristics of posterior urethral valves. Radiology 145:143, 1982

319. McAlister WH: Demonstration of the dilated prostatic urethra in posterior urethral valve patients. J Ultrasound Med 3:189, 1984

320. Kremer H, Dobrinski W, Mikyska M et al: Ultrasonic in vivo and in vitro studies on the nature of the ureteral jet phenomenon. Radiology 142:175, 1982

321. Elejalde BR, de Elejalde MM: Ureteral ejaculation of urine visualized by ultrasound. J Clin Ultrasound 11:474, 1983

322. Dubbins PA, Kurtz AB, Darby J, Goldberg BB: Ureteric jet effect: The echographic appearance of urine entering the bladder. A means of identifying the bladder trigone and assessing ureteral function. Radiology 140:513, 1981

323. Greenberg M, Neiman HL, Brandt TD et al: Ultrasound of the prostate: Analysis of tissue texture and abnormalities. Radiology 141:757, 1981

324. Haradu K, Igari D, Tanahashi Y: Gray scale transrectal ultrasonography of the prostate. J Clin Ultrasound 7:45, 1979

325. Rifkin MD, Kurtz AB, Choi HY, Goldberg BB: Endoscopic ultrasonic evaluation of the prostate using a transrectal probe: Prospective evaluation and accoustic characterization. Radiology 149:265, 1983

326. Kohri K, Kaneko S, Akiyama T et al: Ultrasonic evaluation of prostatic carcinoma. Urol 17:214, 1981

327. Greenberg M, Neimen HL, Vogelzang R, Falkowski W: Ultrasonographic features of prostatic carcinoma. J Clin Ultrasound 10:307, 1982

328. Watanabe H: Prostatic Ultrasound. p.125. In Rosenfield AT (ed): Clinics in Diagnostic Ultrasound—Genitourinary Ultrasound. Churchill Livingstone, New York, 1979

329. Rifkin MD, Kurtz AB, Goldberg BB: Prostate biopsy utilizing transrectal ultrasound guidance: Diagnosis of nonpalpable carcinoma. J Ultrasound Med 2:165, 1983

5

The Retroperitoneum

For years, the retroperitoneum has been a difficult region to image radiographically. Additionally, signs and symptoms of retroperitoneal diseases are frequently vague and poorly localized. With the advent of ultrasound and computed tomography (CT), the identification of retroperitoneal disorders and their spread through the various retroperitoneal compartments are readily assessed.[1]

TECHNIQUE

Preparation

There is no specific prior preparation for an ultrasound examination of the retroperitoneal structures. As the study is sometimes limited by bowel gas, an overnight fast is desirable in order to diminish this problem.

Ultrasound Technique

As with all examinations, the highest frequency transducer should be used to evaluate the structure being scanned.

ADRENAL

Due to the flexibility and maneuverability of the real-time system, ultrasound studies of the adrenal are greatly facilitated by its use, as is the case with many other organ-specific examinations. In addition, bowel gas is less of a problem than with the static system. Although the study may be performed with static systems, it is more technically difficult and involves a longer period of time. The overall success of visualization of the normal adrenal depends on the size of the patient, the amount of perirenal fat, and the bowel gas.[2] It also depends in part on the persistence of the examiner—various projections must be tried before abandoning the examination.

One approach to examination of the adrenal is a specific alignment between the kidney and the ipsilateral paravertebral vessel (inferior vena cava or aorta) and this is best accomplished in the decubitus position [3,4] (Figs. 5-1 to 5-5). The scan is performed in a line connecting the center of the kidney and the paravertebral vessel (Figs. 5-1 and 5-2). This approach visualizes the adrenal in its coronal section, which is in line with the central axis of the kidney.[5] In order to visualize the adrenal, as well as to separate it from the crus of the diaphragm, one needs to sector through the appropriate intercostal space during suspended respiration. Small changes in the receiver sensitivity and/or transducer output are often required to distinguish the adrenal from surrounding retroperitoneal fibro-fatty tissue.[4]

One of the most successful techniques for visualization of the adrenal is the coronal approach (Figs. 5-1, 5-2, 5-4, and 5-5). The scan may be performed in the supine, decubitus, or erect position with the transducer in the middle to posterior axillary line. One should slowly sector from lateral to posterolateral toward the inferior vena cava or aorta, which are used as references in the longitudinal and transverse planes.[6] The right adrenal is best seen by sectoring between the junction of the anterior and midaxillary line in the 9th-10th intercostal space.[7] The left is best visualized by scanning in the

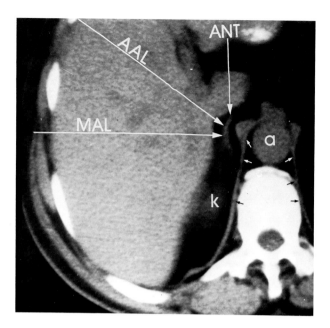

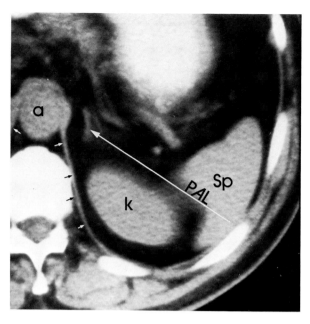

Fig. 5-1. Adrenal scanning approach, right: CT scan. The scan approach for the right adrenal may be a lateral one using the middle axillary line *(MAL)* or anterior axillary line *(AAL)*, or a direct anterior *(ANT)* one in the supine or left lateral decubitus position. In the left lateral decubitus scan, the scan is performed connecting a line from the center of the kidney *(k)* and the inferior vena cava. The adrenal is seen posterior to the inferior vena cava and lateral to the crus. (*a*, aorta; arrows, diaphragmatic crura.)

Fig. 5-2. Adrenal scanning approach, left: CT scan. The scan approach for the left adrenal may be a lateral one using the posterior axillary line *(PAL)* in the right lateral decubitus position. The scan is performed by sectoring through the spleen *(Sp)* and left kidney *(k)* looking for the pulsating aorta *(a)*. The adrenal is seen slightly posterolateral to the aorta and lateral to the crus (arrows).

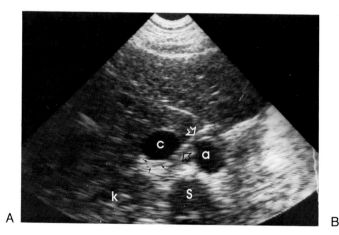

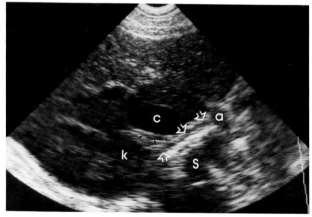

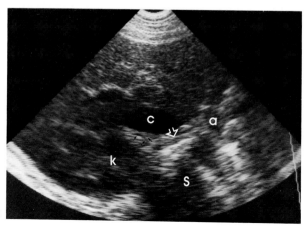

Fig. 5-3. Normal adrenal, right. Anterior approach. Transverse **(A)** and slightly oblique transverse **(B,C)** ultrasound scans. The right adrenal (black arrows) is seen as a lucent structure surrounded by echogenic fat posterior to the inferior vena cava *(c)* and lateral to the diaphragmatic crus (open arrows). (*a*, aorta; *S*, spine; *k*, right kidney.) *(Figure continues.)*

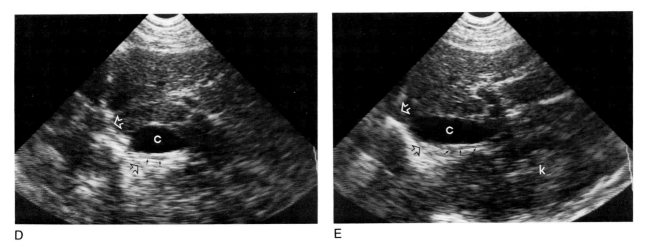

D   E

Fig. 5-3 *(Continued).* On longitudinal scans **(D,E),** the adrenal (black arrows) is seen posterior to the superior margin of the inferior vena cava (c). (open arrows, diaphragm; *k,* right kidney.)

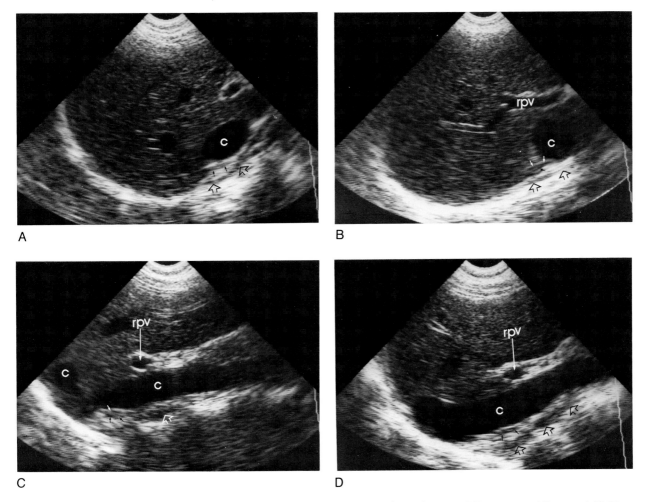

A   B

C   D

Fig. 5-4. Normal adrenal, right. **(A – D)** Lateral approach: Anterior axillary line. **(A,B)** Transverse oblique and **(C,D)** longitudinal slightly oblique scans demonstrate the adrenal (small arrows) as a lucent structure surrounded by echogenic fat posterior to the inferior vena cava *(c)* and lateral to the diaphragm (open arrows). *(rpv,* right portal vein.) *(Figure continues.)*

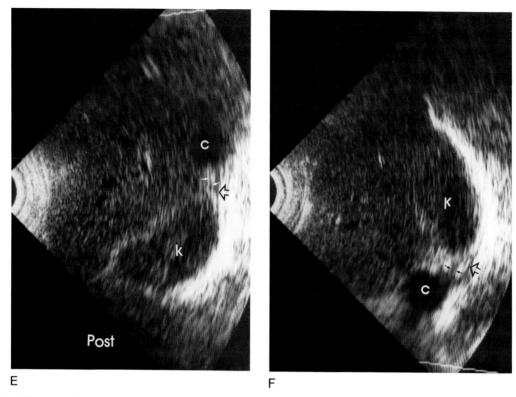

Fig. 5-4 *(Continued).* **(E,F)**Lateral approach: Middle axillary line. Transverse oblique scans demonstrate the adrenal (small arrows) posterior to the inferior vena cava *(c)* and lateral to the diaphragmatic crus (open arrows). (*k,* right kidney; *Post,* posterior.)

posterior axillary line.[7] A deep inspiration is essential in order to scan subcostally either in the midclavicular line or through the flank.[7] The time-gain compensation (TGC) and gain are adjusted using the renal parenchyma as a reference; normally there are fine echoes within the parenchyma.

The normal adrenal glands are not visualized as often in the prone position as in other positions. Masses as large as 3 cm can be detected with this approach.

PARAORTIC NODES

The paraortic nodes are not visualized on ultrasound unless they are enlarged. They may be enlarged secondary to metastatic disease, lymphoma, or inflammation. As such, one needs to be able to identify their presence. They are located anterior to the inferior vena cava and aorta, as well as along the origin of the major vessels (Fig. 5-6). Sometimes enlarged nodes are even seen posterior to the aorta. To search for lymphadenopathy, it is necessary to first identify the aorta and inferior cava and follow their course, looking for masses.[8] In addition, the

courses of these vessels' major branches must be followed. Enlarged nodes may also be found in the porta hepatis, renal hila, and splenic hilum. Sometimes these areas as well as the paraortic area are difficult to visualize due to bowel gas. The study may be facilitated somewhat by the oral administration of water to help transmit the sound beam and displace the gas. In addition, the patient may be scanned in various positions such as supine, lateral decubitus, and erect. Generally, the prone position is not useful in evaluation for paraortic or other abdominal nodes. There is improved visibility of the paraortic and paracaval nodes in the oblique view.[9]

RETROPERITONEUM

In some instances, the entire retroperitoneum needs to be scanned, for example, when looking for a hematoma, an abscess, retroperitoneal fibrosis, lymphoceles, or a tumor. Using a static system, longitudinal and transverse scans are performed from the diaphragm to the iliac crest in the prone position and from the crest to the symphysis in the supine position, with a full bladder. With a real-

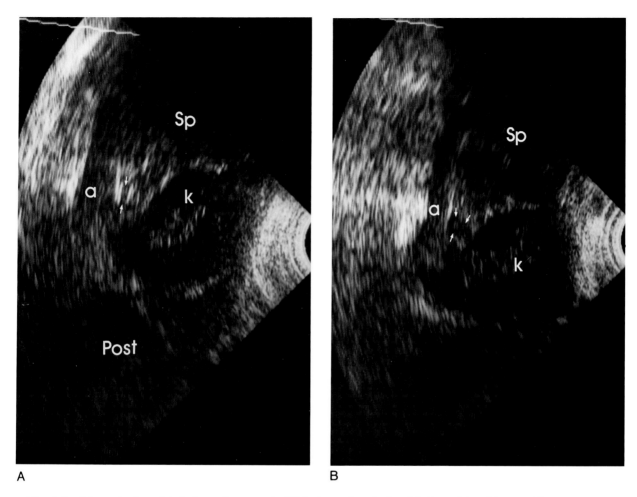

A   B

Fig. 5-5. Normal adrenal, left. Lateral approach. With the patient in the right lateral decubitus position, transverse slightly oblique **(A,B)** scans are taken through the spleen *(Sp)* and left kidney *(k)*, looking for the aorta *(a)*. The adrenal (small arrows) is seen between the kidney, spleen, and aorta. (*Post,* posterior.)

time system, the entire area can be scanned supine and then the upper abdomen can be scanned in the lateral decubitus positions. To be complete, all scans of the retroperitoneum must include the kidneys, as many processes originate from the kidney; the kidneys can be used as landmarks. One should note if the kidneys move with respiration because in a perinephric inflammatory process they will not move. The retroperitoneal muscles should be identified.

DIAPHRAGMATIC CRURA

With the recent improvements in resolution of the ultrasound equipment, extremely small anatomic structures are now being recognized with increasing frequency. The proper identification of these normal structures is important because they often serve as useful anatomic landmarks or may be misinterpreted as abnormalities.

The longitudinal coronal approach improves the visualization of the crura. The right crus is seen in a plane that passes through the right lobe of the liver, the kidney, and the adrenal gland (Figs. 5-7 and 5-8). The left is seen using the spleen and left kidney as windows; the sound is perpendicular to the left crus, so it is to the left of the aorta[10] (Figs. 5-7 and 5-9).

NORMAL ANATOMY

The retroperitoneum is delineated anteriorly by the posterior peritoneum, posteriorly by the transversalis fascia, and laterally by the lateral borders of the quadratus lumborum muscle and peritoneal leaves of the

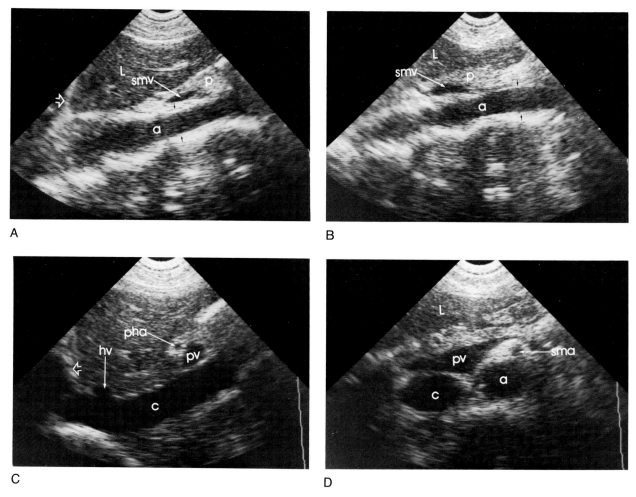

Fig. 5-6. Normal inferior vena cava and aorta. **(A,B)** Longitudinal (long axis) views of the normal aorta *(a, arrows).* **(A)** is at a higher level in the abdomen than **(B)**. (open arrow, diaphragm; *L,* liver; *smv,* superior mesenteric vein; *p,* pancreas.) **(C)** On longitudinal supine view, the inferior vena cava *(c)* is seen as a tubular anechoic structure projecting anterior as it runs cephalad. (open arrow, diaphragm; *hv,* hepatic vein; *pv,* portal vein; *pha,* proper hepatic artery.) **(D)** Transverse supine view of the inferior vena cava *(c)* and aorta *(a).* (*pv,* portal vein; *sma,* superior mesenteric artery; *L,* liver.) There are no nodes normally seen anterior to the inferior vena cava or aorta.

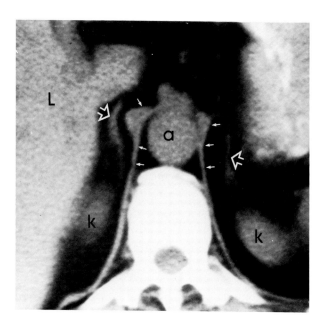

Fig. 5-7. Crura scanning approach. CT scan. The right crus (small arrows) can be seen as a linear soft-tissue density between the adrenal (open arrow) and the aorta *(a)*. It is seen in a plane that passes through the right lobe of the liver *(L)*, kidney *(k)*, and adrenal (open arrow). The left crus (small arrows) is seen, like the right, between the aorta and the adrenal.

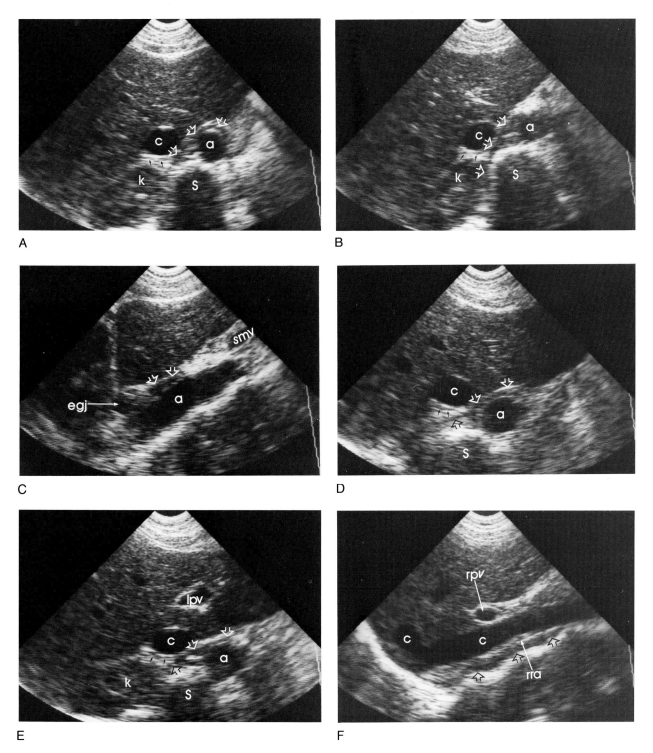

Fig. 5-8. Right crus. **(A,B)** Transverse scans from a directly anterior approach demonstrate the right crus (open arrows) as a hypoechoic linear structure posterior to the inferior vena cava *(c);* it runs between the inferior vena cava and aorta *(a),* as well as anterior to the aorta. The adrenal (small arrows) and right kidney *(k),* can be seen medially. (*S,* spine.) On longitudinal, directly anterior scan **(C),** the crus (open arrows) is seen as a hypoechoic structure anterior to the aorta *(a).* This represents the anterior decussation of the crus. It ends cephalically near the esophagogastric junction *(egj).* (*smv,* superior mesenteric vein.) **(D,E)** Transverse slightly oblique scans from a lateral approach (anterior axillary line) demonstrate the right crus (open arrows) as a hypoechoic structure posterior to the inferior vena cava *(c),* running between the inferior vena cava and aorta *(a)* and anterior to the aorta *(a).* (small arrows, adrenal; *S,* spine; *k,* right kidney; *lpv,* left portal vein.) **(F)** A longitudinal scan from the anterior axillary line demonstrates the right crus (open arrows) as a hypoechoic structure posterior and parallel to the inferior vena cava *(c).* (*rpv,* right portal vein; *rra,* right renal artery.)

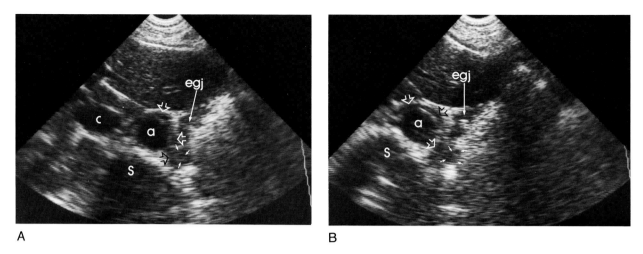

A   B

Fig. 5-9.   Left crus. Multiple transverse **(A,B)** scans from a directly anterior approach demonstrate the left crus (open arrows) as a hypoechoic structure running anterior and lateral to the aorta *(a)*. The esophagogastric junction *(egj)* can be seen anteriorly. (small arrows, adrenal; *S,* spine.)

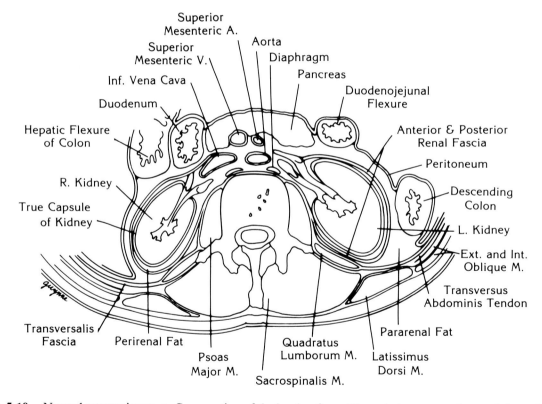

Fig. 5-10.   Normal retroperitoneum. Cross-section of the lumbar fossa. The anterior pararenal space is bounded by the posterior peritoneum and anterior renal fascia and is continuous across the midline. The pancreas, common bile duct, duodenum, superior mesenteric vessels, ascending and descending colon are included in this compartment. The perirenal spaces are separated by connective tissue sheaths surrounding the inferior vena cava and aorta. The lateral fusion of the anterior and posterior renal fascia form the lateroconal fascia. Behind the posterior pararenal space is the transversalis fascia, which forms the anterior border of the retrofascial spaces (including the quadratus lumborum and psoas muscles).

mesentery (Fig. 5-10). In its superior to inferior axes, the retroperitoneum extends from the diaphragm to the pelvic brim[1] (Fig. 5-11). Superior to the pelvic brim, the retroperitoneum can be partitioned into the lumbar and iliac fossae. The pararenal and perirenal spaces are included in the lumbar fossa.

In order to understand the patterns of spread and containment of retroperitoneal pathologic processes, a knowledge of the fascial layers of the retroperitoneum are essential. Though these layers are rarely directly visualized by ultrasound, their presence is suggested by the demonstration of pathologic processes or collections corresponding to known fascial compartments. Portions of the retroperitoneal connective tissue continue below the transversalis fascia of the abdominal wall. As such, pathologic processes can stretch from the anterior abdominal wall to the subdiaphragmatic space, mediastinum, and subcutaneous tissues of the back and flank. The retrofascial space, which includes the psoas, quadratus lumborum, and iliacus muscles (muscles posterior to the transversalis fascia), is often the site of extension of retroperitoneal pathologic processes.[1]

Anterior Pararenal Space

Bounded anteriorly by the posterior parietal peritoneum, and posteriorly by the anterior renal fascia, the anterior pararenal space is delineated laterally by the lateroconal fascia formed by the fusion of the anterior and posterior leaves of the renal fascia (Figs. 5-10 and 5-11). This space merges with the bare area of the liver by the coronary ligament. The pancreas, duodenal sweep, and the ascending and transverse colon are the organs included in the anterior pararenal space (Fig. 5-10).

The ultrasound delineation of the normal anterior pararenal space is limited to identification of the pancreas and adjacent vasculature (Fig. 5-12). The pancreas extends in nearly a transverse plane from the region of the splenic hilum, posterior, inferior, and to the right. The splenic vein is posterior to the superior border of the pancreas. For further discussion of the pancreas and its vasculature, refer to Chapter 3.

The retroperitoneal portions of the intestinal tract lie within this space. The fluid-filled ascending and descending portions of the colon can sometimes be identified as tubular lucent structures. When there are pathologic processes involving the wall of this bowel, there is the production of the "bull's-eye" pattern caused by eccentric thickening. The duodenum can often be seen as a tubular or triangular fluid-filled space along the right lateral margin of the pancreatic head[1] (Fig. 5-12). For further discussion of the gastrointestinal tract, refer to Chapter 9.

Perirenal Space

The perirenal space is surrounded by the anterior and posterior layers of the renal fascia (Gerota's fascia) (Figs. 5-10, 5-11, and 5-13). These layers join and attach to the diaphragm superiorly, but they are united only loosely

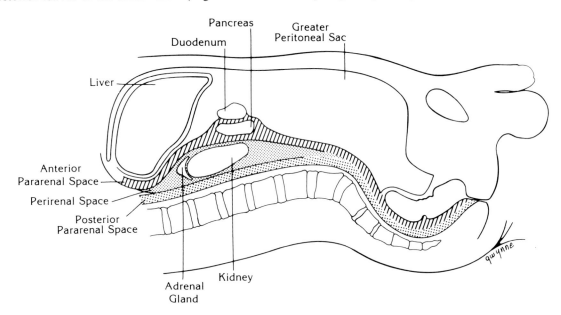

Fig. 5-11. Normal retroperitoneum. Right longitudinal section through the abdomen and pelvis. The anterior pararenal space is bounded anteriorly by the posterior peritoneum and posteriorly by the anterior renal fascia. The perirenal space is located between the anterior and posterior renal fascia. The posterior pararenal space is between the posterior renal fascia and the transversalis fascia. The lumbar fossa extends from the diaphragm to the ilium. It is open inferiorly and merges as it enters the iliac fossa.

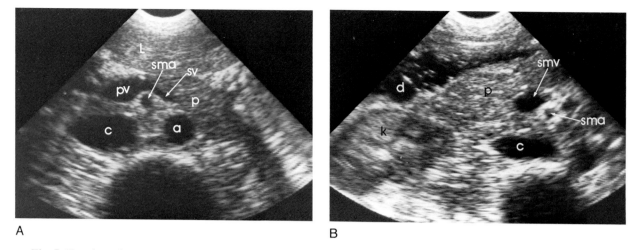

Fig. 5-12. Anterior pararenal space. Transverse erect (**A**) and right lateral decubitus (**B**) scans of the upper abdomen. The ultrasound delineation of the normal anterior pararenal space is usually limited to the identification of the pancreas *(p)* and adjacent vasculature. (*d,* duodenum; *sma,* superior mesenteric artery; *smv,* superior mesenteric vein; *a,* aorta; *c,* inferior vena cava; *k,* right kidney; *sv,* splenic vein; *pv,* portal vein; *L,* liver.)

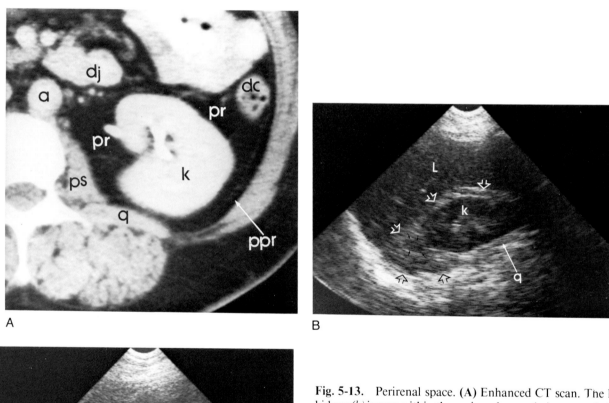

Fig. 5-13. Perirenal space. (**A**) Enhanced CT scan. The left kidney *(k)* is seen within the perirenal space *(pr)* surrounded by perirenal fat. The anterior pararenal space is located anteriorly containing the descending colon *(dc)* and duodenojejunal flexure *(dj).* The posterior pararenal space *(ppr)* is seen posterior to the perirenal space. (*a,* aorta; *ps,* psoas muscle; *q,* quadratus lumborum muscle.) Longitudinal (**B**) and transverse (**C**) ultrasound scans of the right kidney *(k).* In this patient, the perirenal space (open arrows) can be identified by the abundant echodense perirenal fat. (*L,* liver; small arrows, adrenal; *q,* quadratus lumborum muscle.)

inferiorly at the level of the iliac crest, or superior border of the "false"pelvis. Collections in the perinephric space can communicate within the iliac fossa of the retroperitoneum. The lateroconal fascia, the lateral fusion of the renal fascia, proceeds anterior as the posterior peritoneum. The posterior renal fascia fuse medially with the psoas or quadratus lumborum fascia; the anterior renal fascia fuses medially with connective tissue surrounding the great vessels. This space contains the adrenal, kidney, and ureter; the great vessels, which also lie within this space, are largely isolated within their connective tissue sheaths[1] (Fig. 5-13).

The perirenal space contains the adrenal and kidney, which are enclosed in a variable amount of echogenic perinephric fat, the thickest portion being posterior and lateral to the lower pole of the kidney (Fig. 5-13). The kidney is located anterolateral to the psoas muscle, anterior to the quadratus lumborum muscle, and posteromedial to the ascending and descending colon. The second portion of the duodenum is anterior to the kidney hilum on the right. On the left, the kidney is bounded by the stomach anterosuperiorly, the pancreas anteriorly, and the spleen anterolaterally.[1] For further discussion of the kidney and its associated disease processes, refer to Chapter 4, The Urinary Tract.

ADRENAL

Adult Adrenal. The adrenal glands are generally anterior, medial, and superior to the kidneys (Fig. 5-1 and 5-2). On the right, the adrenal is more superior to the kidney while the left is more medial. The medial portion of the right gland is located immediately posterior to the inferior vena cava, at or slightly above the level of the portal vein and lateral to the crus (Figs. 5-1, 5-3, and 5-4). The lateral portion of the gland is posterior and medial to the right lobe of the liver and posterior to the duodenum. The left is lateral or slightly posterolateral to the aorta and lateral to the crus (Figs. 5-2 and 5-5). The superior portion is posterior to the lesser omental space, which is posterior to the stomach; the inferior portion of the left gland is posterior to the pancreas. The splenic vein and artery pass between the pancreas and the left adrenal gland.[2] The right is posterior to the inferior vena cava and the left is to the left of the aorta.[11]

The adrenal glands vary in size, shape, and configuration. The normal adrenal has been reported to be triangular, trapezoid-like, finger-like, or like an inverted "V" or "Y" in shape on a transverse scan.[5,7,12] Others describe the right gland as triangular in shape and the left as semilunar.[5,11] A triangular shape is most frequently described, with the tail extending from the anteromedial aspect of the kidney. The internal texture is medium in

consistency and the cortex and medulla are not distinguished. Normally the adrenal appears as a distinct hypoechoic structure; other times, only the highly echogenic fat is seen.[7] (Figs. 5-3 to 5-5). The size is infrequently greater than 3 cm, with the normal adrenal being 3 to 6 cm long, 3 to 6 mm thick, and 2 to 4 cm wide.[2,4,5,11-13] The distance from the skin to the adrenal is generallly 4 to 8 cm when scanning in the decubitus position. The best ultrasound criterion for adrenal abnormality is a triangular shape ranging from a single convex margin to a perfectly round gland.[3,14]

How often is the adrenal gland visualized on ultrasound? The normal adrenal has been reported to be visualized in 85 percent of cases and the normal adrenal area is seen in 12 percent.[3] The normal gland on the right has been reported to be visualized in 78 to 90 percent with the left visualized 44 to 80 percent.[2,14] Using real-time sonography, the right adrenal can be identified 82 percent of the time longitudinally and 78.5 percent of the time transversely at the midaxillary line in the 9th-10th intercostal space.[7] The left can be seen in 41 percent of longitudinal scans and 21.4 percent of transverse scans when scanning intercostally.[7] When scanning in the anterior axillary line through the flank, the right adrenal gland can be visualized in 53.5 percent of scans; when scanning subcostally oblique in the midclavicular line parallel to the rib cage, it can be visualized in 39.2 percent of scans.[7] On the left side, the adrenal is seen in 12.5 percent of longitudinal scans when scanning in the flank in the posterior axillary line.[7] The least favorable approach for adrenal scanning is the posterior approach, in which the adrenal is seen 1.7 to 3.5 percent of the time.[7] The reasons for poor adrenal visibility are the gland's small size, poor lateral resolution of ultrasound, and small differences in impedance between adrenals and surrounding fatty tissue.[7] Lesions as small as 12 to 20 mm have been identified with real-time ultrasound.[7] When the adrenal area is scanned, a tumor may be ruled out if no round or oval-shaped lesion is seen. This is true even if the normal gland is not visualized. The sensitivity of this sort of scan is 97 percent with a 96.5 percent specificity.[2]

Neonatal Adrenal. In the neonate, the adrenal is characterized by a thin echogenic core surrounded by a thick transonic zone (Figs. 5-14 and 5-15). The thick rim of transonicity represents the hypertrophied adrenal cortex, while the echogenic core is the adrenal medulla. The decreased cortical echogenicity is probably a result of several factors. There are dilated blood-filled cortical sinusoids in the cortex due to vascular congestion. In addition, there is orderly parallel orientation of the cuboidal cells lining the cortical columns. The relative echogenicity of the adrenal medulla is probably secondary to the random orientation of its cell population. This structural disorder produces multiple reflective interfaces resulting in an area of increased echogenicity. Increased amounts of collagen surrounding the central vessels may also add to the medullary echogenicity.[15] The characteristic appearance of the neonatal adrenal is especially important to recognize in renal agenesis, as the adrenal glands may simulate the appearance of the normal kidneys.[15,16]

At birth, the neonatal adrenal cortex is relatively thick (Fig. 5-14). The cortex is composed of two layers: a thick fetal zone occupying 80 percent of the gland and a thin peripheral region that becomes the adult cortex.[15] The fetal cortex synthesizes a considerable amount of the precursors for maternal estrogens and is one of the main consumers of placental progesterone.[15] After birth, the fetal zone of the adrenal cortex undergoes inevitable involution (Fig. 5-15).

There is increased visualization of the neonatal adrenal due to several factors. The infant adrenal is proportionally larger than the adult adrenal. At birth, the adrenal is one third the size of the kidney, whereas in the

adult, it is one thirteenth the size of the kidney. In the neonate, there is a paucity of perirenal fat, which allows for easier resolution of the adrenal. In addition, the neonatal adrenal is closer to the skin surface, which allows for the use of higher frequency transducers, which in turn increases the resolution of small structures.[15] The right adrenal can be seen in 97 percent of cases with the left seen in 83 percent.[15] The length of the neonatal adrenal varies from 0.9 to 3.6 cm (a mean of 1.5 cm) with a width of 0.2 to 0.5 cm (a mean of 0.3 cm).[15]

AORTA

The aorta as a unit is in the perirenal space, although its dense perivascular connective tissue serves as a barrier to extension of perinephric processes. The aorta enters the abdomen posterior to the diaphragm at L-1 and passes posterior to the left lobe of the liver (Fig. 5-6). It has a relatively straight course to L-4 where it bifurcates. It has a slight anterior curve due to the lumbar lordosis. In a thin patient with exaggerated lumbar lordosis, the aorta may lie within 3 to 4 cm to the anterior abdominal

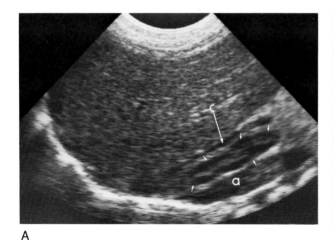

A

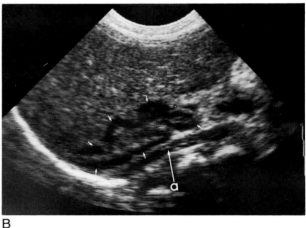

B

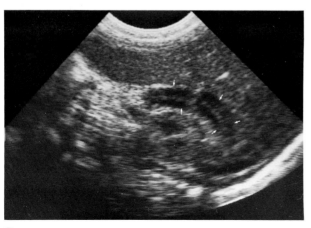

C

Fig. 5-14. Normal neonatal adrenal. Right adrenal. Magnified longitudinal coronal scans (lateral to medial) **(A–C).** The normal adrenal (small arrows) is seen as a structure with an echogenic core and a hypoechoic rim (*c*, inferior vena cava; *a*, aorta.) *(Figure continues.)*

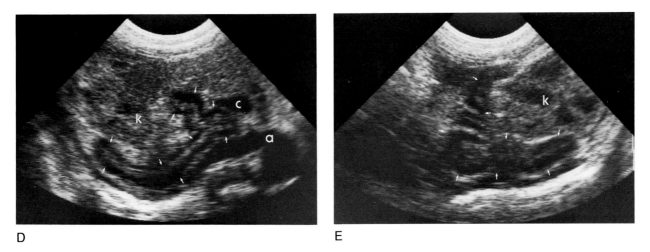

D   E

Fig. 5-14 *(Continued).* Transverse oblique **(D)** scan of the normal adrenal (small arrows) seen as a structure with an echogenic core and a hypoechoic rim. (*c,* inferior vena cava; *a,* aorta; *k,* kidney.) **(E)** Left adrenal. The left adrenal (small arrows) appears similar to the right on transverse oblique **(E)** scan. (*k,* left kidney.)

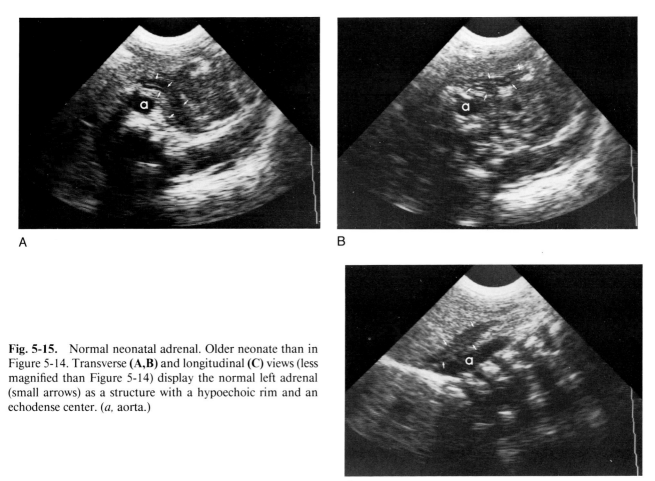

A   B

C

Fig. 5-15. Normal neonatal adrenal. Older neonate than in Figure 5-14. Transverse **(A,B)** and longitudinal **(C)** views (less magnified than Figure 5-14) display the normal left adrenal (small arrows) as a structure with a hypoechoic rim and an echodense center. (*a,* aorta.)

wall and may be mistaken for an aneurysm on physical exam. It generally lies close to the anterior spine, which can be identified as an intense linear echo with distal shadow on longitudinal view and an anterior concave echo on transverse scan (Fig. 5-6). If there is separation between the aorta and the spine, adenopathy, as well as fibrosis or hematoma, should be questioned.[1] For further discussion of the aorta, refer to Chapter 6, Vascular Ultrasound.

INFERIOR VENA CAVA

The inferior vena cava has a more lengthy intraabdominal course than the aorta. It extends from the junction of the two common iliac veins to the right of L-5 and travels cephalad (Fig. 5-6); it then curves anterior toward its termination in the right atrium.[1] For further discussion of this vessel, refer to Chapter 6 on the vascular system.

DIAPHRAGMATIC CRURA

The diaphragmatic crura begin as tendinous fibers from the lumbar vertebral bodies, disks, and transverse processes of L-3 on the right and L-1 on the left (Fig. 5-16). As it proceeds cephalad from its origin, the right crus, which is longer, larger, and frequently more lobular than the left, is closely associated with the anterior aspect of the lumbar vertebral bodies as it blends with the anterior longitudinal vertebral ligament (Figs. 5-7, 5-8, and 5-16). The right renal artery crosses anterior to the crus and posterior to the inferior vena cava at the level of the

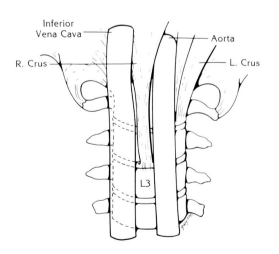

Fig. 5-16. Diaphragmatic crura. The relationship of the diaphragmatic crura, aorta, and inferior vena cava are illustrated. (Modified from Callen PW, Filly RA, Sarti DA, Sample WF: Ultrasonography of the diaphragmatic crura. Radiology 130:721, 1979.)

right kidney. The right crus is bounded by the inferior vena cava anterolaterally and the right adrenal and right lobe of the liver posterolaterally in the upper abdomen (Figs. 5-7 and 5-8). The fibers of the right crus diverge as it ascends superiorly. Laterally, most fibers insert in the central tendon of the diaphragm while the medial fibers ascend on the left side of the esophageal hiatus (Fig. 5-8). The right crus's medial tendinous margin extends anterior and decussates with the left anterior to the aorta.[10]

On a longitudinal scan, the entire right crus can be seen as a solid, longitudinally oriented structure immediately posterior to the inferior vena cava (Fig. 5-8). It should not be confused with the right renal artery.[17] To the left of midline, the right crus is also visualized as a solid, longitudinally oriented form anterior to the aorta.[10]

The left crus courses along the anterior lumbar vertebral bodies in a superior direction and inserts into the central tendon of the diaphragm (Figs. 5-7, 5-9, and 5-16). During its ascent, it is closely associated with the celiac ganglion, left adrenal gland, splenic vasculature, and esophagogastric junction. Occasionally the medial fibers pass over the aorta and stretch obliquely to the fibers of the right, toward the inferior vena cava.[10]

The right crus can be visualized in 50 percent of patients on longitudinal scans and in 90 percent on transverse scans. The left is never seen longitudinally, but can be seen on 50 percent of transverse scans[10] (Fig. 5-9).

NODES

Retroperitoneal nodes are known to surround the aorta and inferior vena cava, and are sometimes located anterior to the spine. When normal, up to 1 cm, they are not seen on ultrasound scans. The common sites include paraortic, paracaval, peripancreatic, renal hilar, and mesenteric. Descriptions of ultrasound patterns associated with nodes include (1) rounded, focal echopoor lesions 1 to 3 cm in size; (2) larger, confluent echopoor masses often displacing the kidney laterally; (3) "mantle" of nodes in a paraspinal location; (4) "floating" or anterior displaced aorta; and (5) mesenteric "sandwich" sign representing anterior and posterior node masses surrounding mesenteric vessels.[1]

Posterior Pararenal Space and Iliac Fossa

The posterior pararenal space is located between the posterior renal fascia and the transversalis fascia (Figs. 5-10, 5-11, and 5-17). It communicates with the properitoneal fat visualized on a radiograph as the "flank stripe," lateral to the lateroconal fascia. Continuing from

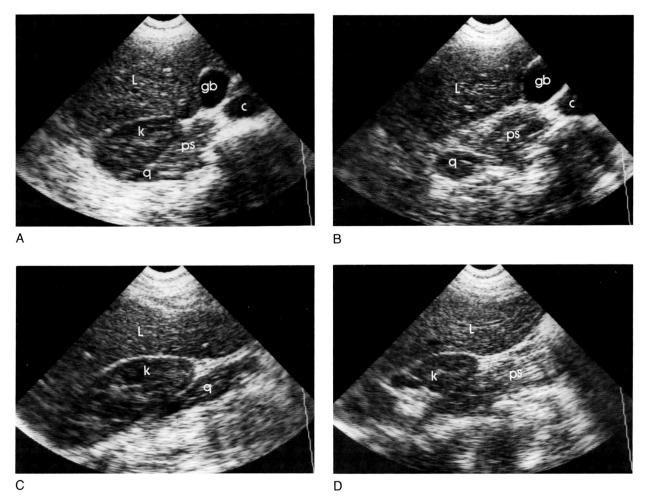

Fig. 5-17. Posterior pararenal space. The structures on the anterior and posterior boundaries of this space can be seen with ultrasound. Anteriorly in the perirenal space, the right kidney *(k)* can be seen with its perirenal fat. Posteriorly are components of the retrofascial space — the psoas and quadratus lumborum muscles at this level. Transverse **(A,B)** and longitudinal coronal **(C,D)** scans display the quadratus lumborum *(q)* muscle, which is a cephalically tapering elliptical hypoechoic structure. The psoas *(ps)* muscle is seen medial to the quadratus. (*c,* inferior vena cava; *gb,* gallbladder; *L,* liver.)

the diaphragm to the iliac crest, this posterior space merges inferiorly with the anterior pararenal space and the retroperitoneal tissues of the iliac fossa. The psoas muscle, the fascia of which merges with the posterior transversalis fascia, makes up the medial border of this posterior space. This space is open laterally and inferiorly.[1] Blood vessels and lymph nodes embedded in fat are found in the posterior pararenal space.

The iliac fossa is that region extending between the internal surface of the iliac wings from the crest to the iliopectineal line (Figs. 5-18 and 5-19). This space is also known as the "false" pelvis and contains the ureter and major branches of the distal great vessels and their accompanying lymphatics.[1] The transversalis fascia extends into the iliac fossa as the iliac fascia. The renal

fascia terminates at the level of the superior margin of the iliac fossa and mixes loosely with the iliac fascia.

Retrofascial Space

The posterior abdominal wall components, muscles, nerves, lymphatics, and areolar tissue behind the transversalis fascia make up the retrofascial space (Fig. 5-20). It can be divided into three compartments—psoas, lumbar (quadratus lumborum), and iliac by the leaves of the transversalis fascia, which invests each muscle and provides a barrier to the spread of infection.[1]

The quadratus lumborum originates from the iliolumbar ligament, the adjacent iliac crest, and the supe-

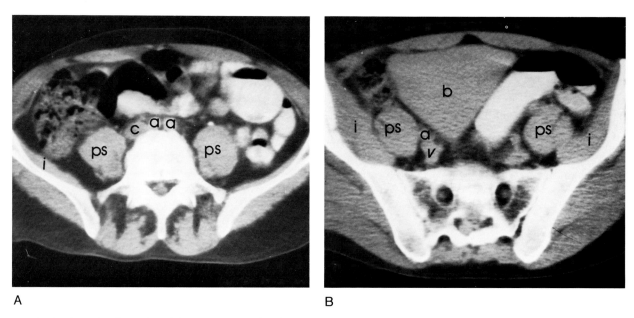

Fig. 5-18. Iliac fossa. **(A,B)** CT scans. The iliac fossa is the space between the peritoneum and transversalis fascia, which invests the iliacus *(i)*, and psoas *(ps)* muscles. (*c,* inferior vena cava; *a,* iliac artery; *v,* iliac vein; *b,* bladder.)

rior borders of the transverse process of the last three or four lumbar vertebra and inserts into the inferior margin of the 12th rib (Fig. 5-20). It is adjoining and posterior to the colon, kidney, and psoas, depending on the level. On ultrasound, this muscle appears on transverse scan as a solid ovoid structure with low-amplitude internal echoes (Figs. 5-17 and 5-21). Longitudinally, it is seen as a cephalically tapering elliptical structure (Figs. 5-17 and

5-21). Occasionally a linear echo can be seen within the muscle substance probably representing a cleft between muscle bundles[18] (Fig. 5-21B).

The psoas muscle spans from the mediastinum to the thigh (Figs. 5-17 to 5-19, and 5-21). With its fascia attaching to the pelvic brim, it extends to the thigh, joining with the inguinal ligament, iliacus fascia, and femoral sheath. It is seen as a tubular hypoechoic structure me-

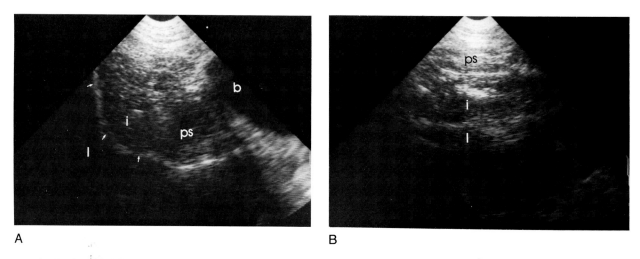

Fig. 5-19. Iliac fossa. Iliacus and psoas muscles. The iliac fossa, that portion of the retroperitoneum between the posterior peritoneum and the transversalis fascia, is located between the internal surface of the iliac wings (*I,* arrows) from the crest to iliopectal line. Right transverse **(A)** and longitudinal **(B)** scans display the structures visualized on ultrasound within this fossa, which include the psoas *(ps),* and iliacus *(i)* muscles. The iliacus appears as a hypoechoic structure medial to the iliac wing. The psoas is seen posterior and medial to the iliacus. The anterior margins of the muscles are not sharply defined at this level. (*b,* bladder.)

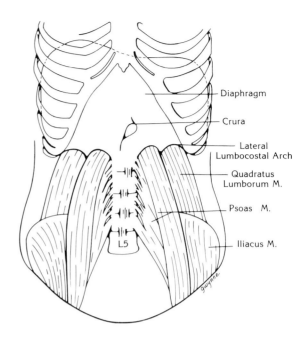

Fig. 5-20. Retrofascial space. The posterior abdominal wall components, muscles, nerves, lymphatics and areolar tissue behind the transversalis fascia constitute this space. (Modified from Koenigsberg M, Hoffman M, Schnur MJ: Sonographic evaluation of the retroperitoneum. p. 79. In Raymond HW, Zweibel WJ (eds): Seminars in Ultrasound. Vol. 3. Grune & Stratton, New York, 1982, by permission.)

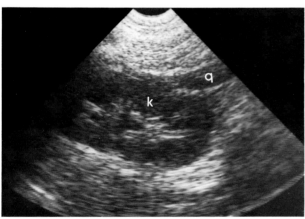

A

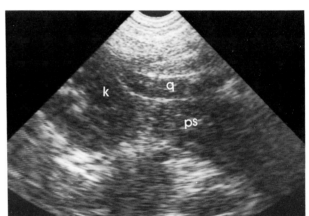

B

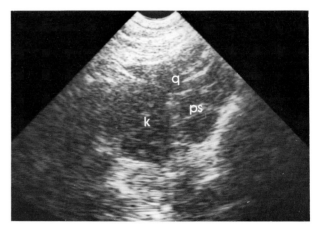

C

Fig. 5-21. Quadratus lumborum and psoas muscles. Prone left longitudinal **(A,B)** and transverse **(C)** scans. The quadratus lumborum muscle *(q)* is seen in its long axis as a cephalically tapering elliptical hypoechoic structure. The psoas muscle *(ps)* is seen more medially. (*k,* left kidney.)

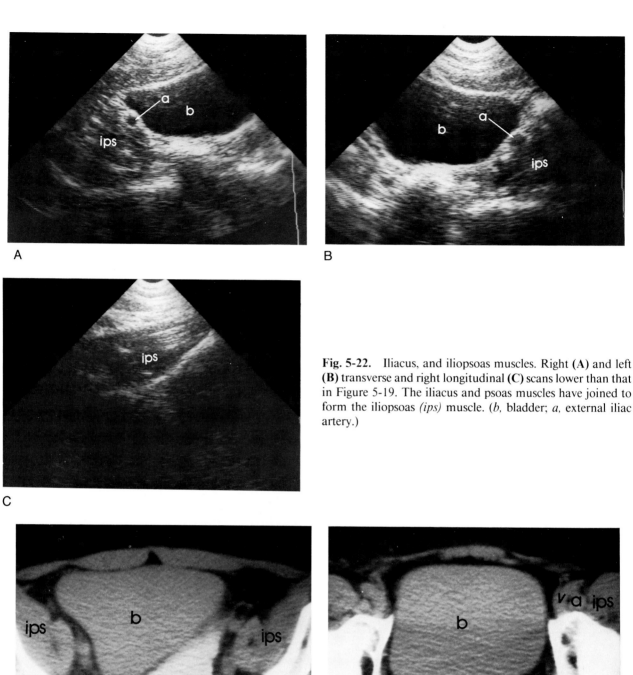

Fig. 5-22. Iliacus, and iliopsoas muscles. Right (**A**) and left (**B**) transverse and right longitudinal (**C**) scans lower than that in Figure 5-19. The iliacus and psoas muscles have joined to form the iliopsoas *(ips)* muscle. (*b,* bladder; *a,* external iliac artery.)

Fig. 5-23. Pelvic retroperitoneum. (**A,B**) CT scans. The pelvic portion of the retroperitoneum lies between the sacrum and pubis, the pelvic peritoneal reflection and pelvic diaphragm, and the fascial investment of the lateral pelvic wall musculature. (*ips,* iliopsoas muscle; *p,* piriformis muscle; *rs,* rectosigmoid colon; *r,* rectum; *sv,* seminal vesicles; *o,* obturator internus muscle; *v,* external iliac vein; *a,* external iliac artery.)

dial and posterior to the kidney on longitudinal scan (Figs. 5-17 and 5-21). On transverse scan, it is a rounded or oval hypoechoic structure lateral to the spine[1](Figs. 5-17 and 5-21).

The iliacus muscle, which makes up the iliac space, extends the length of the iliac fossa (Figs. 5-18 to 5-20). The psoas passes through the iliac fossa medial to the iliacus muscle and posterior to the iliac fascia. The two muscles merge as they extend into the true pelvis (Fig. 5-22). Proximal to their merger, the iliacus appears as a hypoechoic soft tissue layer medial to the iliac wings (Fig. 5-19). The iliopsoas muscle takes on a progressively more anterior location caudally to lie along the lateral pelvic sidewall(Fig. 5-22).

Pelvic Retroperitoneum

The pelvic portion of the retroperitoneum lies between the sacrum and pubis from back to front, pelvic peritoneal reflection above and pelvic diaphragm (coccygeus and levator ani muscles) below, and between the fascial investment of the lateral pelvic wall musculature (obturator internus and piriformis)[1] (Fig. 5-23). There are four subdivisions of this pelvic space: prevesical, rectovesical, presacral, and bilateral pararectal (and paravesical) spaces.[1]

The prevesical space (retropubic space of Retzius') spans from the pubis to the anterior margin of the bladder and is bordered laterally by the obturator fascia (Fig.

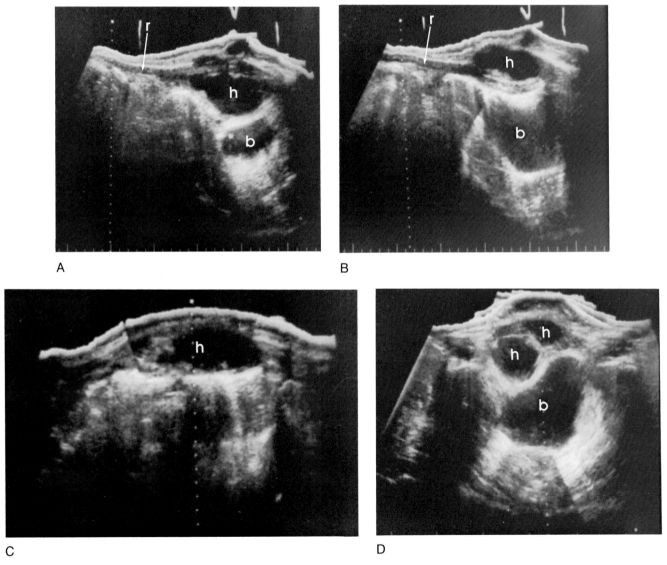

Fig. 5-24. Prevesical space. Postoperative hematoma. On longitudinal scans 2 cm to the right **(A)** and 2 cm to the left **(B)** of midline and transverse scans 6 cm **(C)** and 13 cm **(D)** below the umbilicus, a hypoechoic septated mass *(h)* is seen anterior to the bladder *(b)*. It appears to be continuous with the rectus abdominus *(r)* muscle making it extraperitoneal.

5-24). Connective tissue covering the bladder, seminal vesicles, and prostate is continuous with the fascial lamina within this space. The space is an extension of the retroperitoneal space of the anterior abdominal wall deep to the rectus sheath, which is continuous with the transversalis fascia. The space between the bladder and rectum is the rectovesical space (Fig. 5-25). The presacral space is between the rectum and fascia covering the sacrum and posterior pelvic floor musculature.[1] The bilateral pararectal space is bounded laterally by the piriformis and levator ani fascia and medially by the rectum. The paravesical space extends anteriorly from the bladder, medially to the obturator internus and laterally to the external iliac vessels. The paravesical and pararectal spaces are traversed by the ureters.[1]

The pelvic wall muscles, iliac vessels, ureter, bladder, prostate, seminal vesicles, and cervix are the retroperitoneal structures within the true pelvis (Figs. 5-23 and

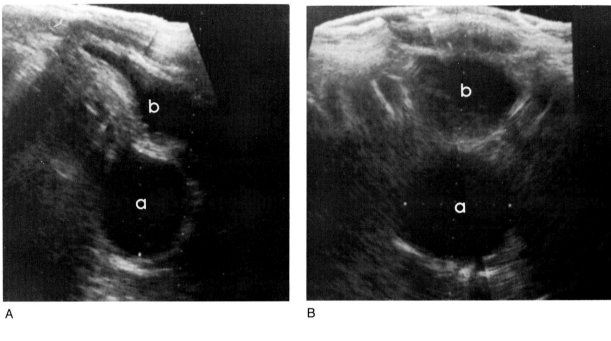

A   B

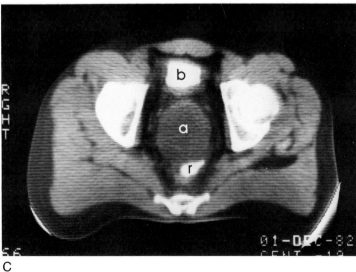

C

Fig. 5-25. Retrovesical space. Postoperative appendectomy abscess. Longitudinal **(A)** and transverse **(B)** scans in a febrile male patient demonstrates a hypoechoic mass *(a)* posterior to the bladder *(b)*. **(C)** Similar to **(B)**, a low-density mass *(a)* is seen posterior to the bladder *(b)* and anterior to the rectum *(r)* on CT scan. This abscess was drained via a transrectal catheter.

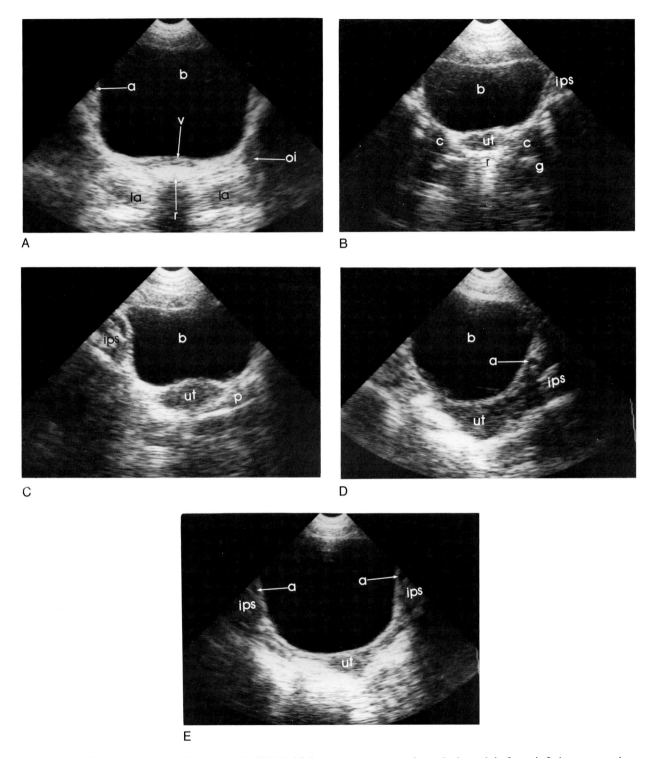

Fig. 5-26. Pelvic retroperitoneum. **(A–E)** Multiple transverse scans through the pelvis from inferior to superior demonstrate the normal pelvic musculature. The distended bladder *(b)* is seen in the midline. (*ips,* iliopsoas muscle; *oi,* obturator internus muscle; *p,* piriformis muscle; *g,* gluteus maximus muscle; *c,* coccygeus muscle; *la,* levator ani muscle; *v,* vagina; *ut,* uterus; *r,* rectum; *a,* external iliac artery.)

5-26). The obturator internus muscle lines the lateral aspect of the pelvis and is seen as a hypoechoic soft tissue structure with a concave medial border along the lateral aspect of the bladder (Fig. 5-26). Posteriorly, the piriformis muscle, a similar appearing structure, is seen extending anterolaterally from the region of the sacrum. Located medial to the obturator internus muscle is the internal iliac vein.[1]

Retroperitoneal Fat

At times it may be difficult to determine the anatomic origin of a right upper quadrant mass. The reflection produced by right upper quadrant retroperitoneal fat (Fig. 5-13B and C) is displaced in a characteristic manner by masses originating from this area. This pattern of displacement helps to localize the origin of the mass. Retroperitoneal lesions cause ventral and often cranial displacement of the echo (see Fig. 1-52). In addition, the lesion can be still further differentiated. Fibro-fatty echoes wedged in a triangular shape by masses in the upper pole of the kidney prove to be adrenal in origin (see Fig. 1-52). Lesions in the liver or in Morison's pouch displace the echoes posterior and inferior (see Fig. 1-53). Therefore, hepatic and subhepatic masses cause posterior displacement of this echo while renal and adrenal lesions cause anterior displacement of it[19,20] (see Figs. 1-52 and 1-53). Extrahepatic masses also shift the inferior vena cava anteromedially, resulting in anterior displacement of the right kidney.[20] This sign is absent or unreliable in a child or cachectic patient with a paucity of retroperitoneal fat. The displacement and identification of the retroperitoneal fat is best seen on longitudinal scans and is inconsistent and poorly seen on transverse scans.[19,20] By knowing the vector of displacement of retroperitoneal fat, one can reliably diagnose the anatomic origin of the mass in the right upper quadrant.

ADRENAL ABNORMALITIES

Ultrasound has been reported to have an overall accuracy of 95 percent in the evaluation of adrenal abnormalities.[3] The best criterion for diagnosing adrenal abnormalities is a change in the triangular shape ranging from a single convex margin to a perfectly round gland[3] (Fig. 5-27). To differentiate an adrenal mass from a renal mass one must define an echo interface separating the mass from the upper pole of the kidney[13] (Fig. 5-28). The kidney may be displaced inferiorly with its upper pole compressed and flattened by the mass.[13] There should be no distortion or splaying of the collecting system.

When the tumor grows inferiorly along the anterior surface of the kidney, there may be little downward displacement of the kidney.[5,21] Instead, there is a pressure deformity of the upper pole and the anterior surface of the kidney is compressed (Fig. 5-29). This may simulate tumor invasion on ultrasound.[5,21] If downward extension anterior to the kidney occurs on the right, the mass may become posterior to the head of the pancreas, com-

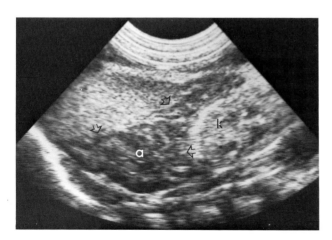

Fig. 5-27. Adrenal hyperplasia. Longitudinal scan of the right adrenal in an infant demonstrates marked enlargement. (a, arrows). The triangular shape of the adrenal is maintained. (k, kidney.) This patient with bilateral adrenal enlargement had a sibling with adrenal hyperplasia and had biochemical changes consistent with this disease process.

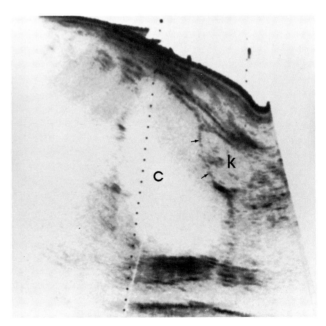

Fig. 5-28. Adrenal cyst. Prone longitudinal scan depicts an anechoic (c) structure that appears to be separate (arrows) from the left kidney (k). The kidney is displaced inferiorly.

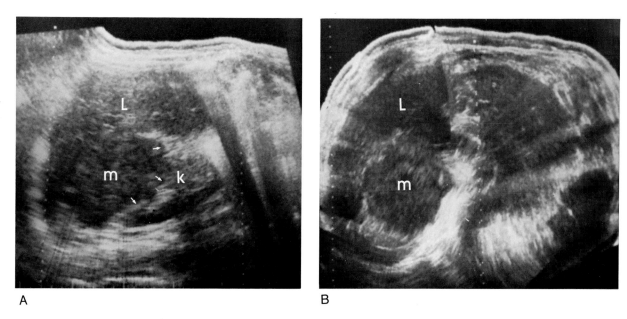

A   B

Fig. 5-29. Adrenal metastasis. Carcinoma of the lung. **(A)** Longitudinal static scan 8 cm to the right of midline. **(B)** Transverse scan 12 cm above the crest. A solid adrenal mass *(m)* is seen compressing (arrows) the upper pole of the right kidney *(k)* and displacing it posteriorly and inferiorly. (*L,* liver.)

press and displace the pancreas forward, and simulate a pancreatic mass on ultrasound.[21]However, with a pancreatic tumor the splenic vein will be displaced anteriorly instead of posteriorly.[21] A large right mass may displace the inferior vena cava forward. Compression of the posterior wall and/or anterior displacement of the inferior vena cava is seen in two thirds of right adrenal tumors.[11] A larger left mass may extend forward and medial to partially surround the aorta.[21]

The usual solid adrenal mass is relatively hypoechoic, due to the rather homogeneous cellular structure, with uniformly distributed echoes.[2,5,12,21] As the mass grows, focal necrosis may develop, proceeding to liquefaction and becoming anechoic. A cavity surrounded by necrotic tissue may show an irregular and shaggy wall.

Adrenal Cyst

Adrenal cysts are relatively infrequent lesions that seldom are manifested clinically. Forty-four percent are endothelial in origin and these can be further subdivided into lymphangiomatous (41 percent) and angiomatous (3 percent) cysts.[22] Pseudocyst (40 percent) is the next most frequent category and is the most likely to present clinically, as these cysts may be of considerable size. Pseudocysts may be secondary to hemorrhage either into the normal adrenal or within an adrenal tumor such as an adenoma — this is the usual cause. Finally, the epithelial cyst represents cystic degeneration of adenomas and

parasitic cysts and constitutes 6 percent of adrenal cysts.[22]

Adrenal cysts may range in size from small to very large. They may be unilocular or multilocular. In 15 percent there may be calcification that is typically peripheral and curvilinear.[5,22] However, the calcification in the wall may be thick and strongly echogenic.[5] The wall of the cyst is thin and smooth. These patients present in the third to fifth decade of life. Because cysts are rarely

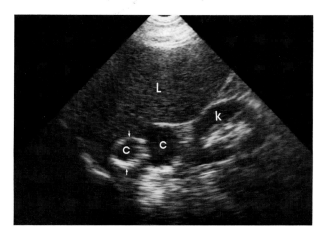

Fig. 5-30. Adrenal cyst. Longitudinal scan shows multiple hypoechoic masses *(c)* in the adrenal area. One (arrows) has a very dense wall felt to represent calcification. Fluid obtained from an aspiration (patient had a known primary tumor) was consistent with adrenal cyst fluid. (*k,* right kidney; *L,* liver.)

symptomatic and thus are frequently encountered incidently, a conservative approach with regard to therapy is
recommended. On ultrasound, the cyst is smooth,
round, and echofree with thin walls and acoustic enhancement[2,5] (Figs. 5-28, 5-30, and 5-31). If the lesion is
purely cystic, an ultrasound-guided aspiration may be
performed to alleviate symptoms of pressure.[22]

Adrenal Hemorrhage

Immediately after birth, the bulk of the primitive adrenal cortex undergoes atrophy. Already dilated vascular
channels in the primitive cortex become more engorged
and more vulnerable to hemorrhage.[5] The neonatal adrenals are susceptible to trauma and hemorrhage be-

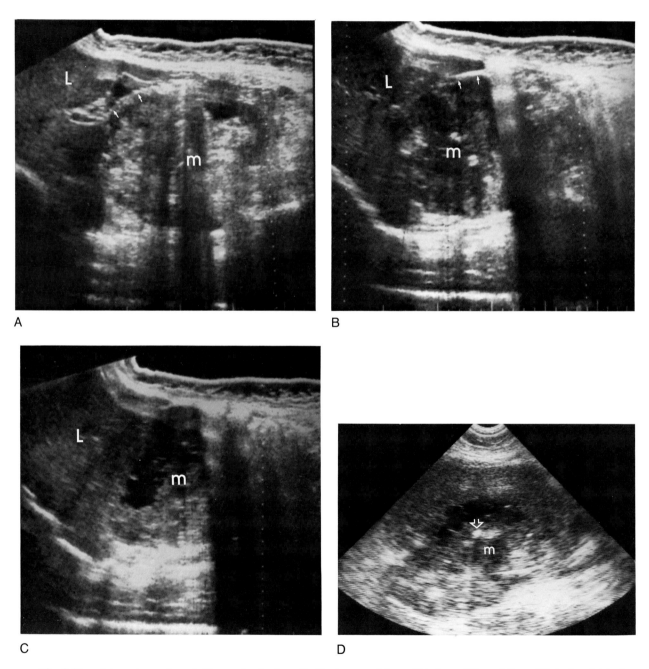

Fig. 5-31. Adrenal pseudocyst. Hemorrhagic. Longitudinal scans at 3 cm (**A**), 5 cm (**B**), and 6 cm (**C**) to the right of
midline. (**D**) Longitudinal real-time scan. A complex mass *(m)* is seen in the right adrenal area. It contains lucent as well
as dense areas; some of the dense areas (open arrow) are thought to be calcification. The retroperitoneal fat (arrows) is
displaced anteriorly and superiorly indicating the retroperitoneal origin of the mass. (*L*, liver.)

cause of their relatively large size and vascularity with the bleeding usually confined to the subcapsular space.[23] The exact cause of adrenal hemorrhage is unknown but there are many factors implicated, including (1) stress and trauma at birth; (2) anoxia; and (3) systemic disease —thrombocytopenia purpura, hemorrhagic disease of the newborn, septicemia, and congenital syphilis.[23,24] Most frequently, these patients present within 2 to 7 days of life with an abdominal mass that is usually located on the right side and hyperbilirubinemia. Seventy percent are on the right side with 5 to 10 percent bilateral.[24]

Adrenal hemorrhage can be diagnosed with a combination of ultrasound and excretory urography without resorting to surgical exploration or invasive diagnostic procedures. On urography, there is downward displacement of the kidney on the affected side and a radiolucent suprarenal mass on body nephrogram phase. There

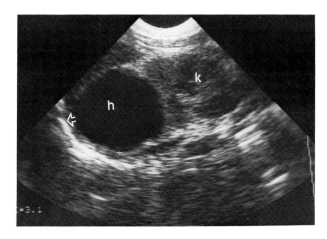

Fig. 5-32. Adrenal hemorrhage. Longitudinal coronal scan on the right. A round, anechoic, suprarenal mass *(h)* is seen. (*k,* right kidney; open arrow, diaphragm.)

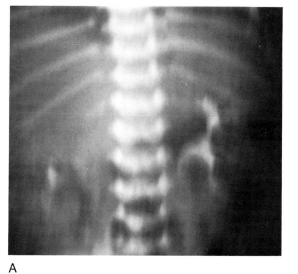

A

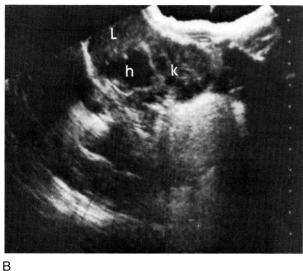

B

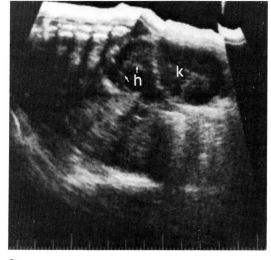

C

Fig. 5-33. Adrenal hemorrhage. (A) Intravenous pyelogram. There is compression of the upper pole of the right kidney. (B) Longitudinal left lateral decubitus scan. A well-defined anechoic mass *(h)* is seen superior to the right kidney *(k).* (*L,* liver.) There is downward displacement of the right kidney. (C) Prone longitudinal scan. The previously noted anechoic mass *(h)* appears to have an echogenic component (arrows) on this view. (*k,* right kidney.)

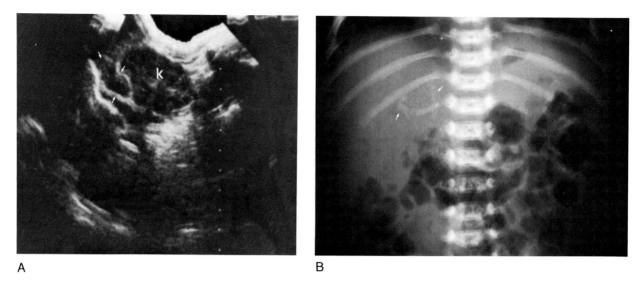

A   B

Fig. 5-34. Adrenal hemorrhage, follow-up. Follow-up scan, 1 month after Figure 5-33. **(A)** Only a small mass (arrows) is seen in the area of the previous hemorrhage. (*k,* right kidney.) **(B)** Radiograph. The typical calcifications (arrows) associated with adrenal hemorrhage are seen.

is an anechoic suprarenal mass seen on ultrasound scans[2,23-25] (Figs. 5-32 and 5-33). There can be an echogenic component to the mass depending on the age of the hemorrhage; the echopattern is related to the state of liquefaction[2,5,23-25] (Fig. 5-33C). On follow-up examination, 2 to 4 weeks after the hemorrhage, typical suprarenal curvilinear calcifications can be seen radiographically, with a decrease in size of the mass seen on ultrasound scans[24] (Fig. 5-34).

elements.[2,5,27,26] Hemorrhage and/or calcification may be present.[28] There is no malignant potential and the lesions are nonfunctioning.[28] The etiology of this lesion is unknown; the cause is suggested to be metaplasia of the mesenchymal stem cells, which are precursors both to adrenal and myeloid tissue. Chronic infection and trauma have been proposed as additional causative factors.[27] The lesion may vary from microscopic to 30 cm in diameter.[28] Most cases occur in the fourth to sixth

Primary Adrenal Tumors

CORTICAL TUMORS

Adenoma. In 2 percent of adult autopsies, adrenal adenomas are noted; most are nonsteroid producing, but they may be part of an endocrine neoplastic syndrome. They are usually 1 to 5 cm and poorly encapsulated.[26]

Carcinoma. Adrenal carcinomas usually produce steroids (90 percent) and are associated with one of the hyperadrenal syndromes. These lesions are rare, with many larger than 20 cm (Fig. 5-35). There is a strong tendency for these lesions to invade the adrenal vein, inferior vena cava, and lymph glands. Metastases to regional and periaortic nodes are common with distant hematogeneous spread to the lungs and viscera.[26]

Myelolipoma. Adrenal myelolipoma is a rare cortical tumor (0.08 to 0.2 percent incidence at autopsy) composed of varying proportions of fat and bone marrow

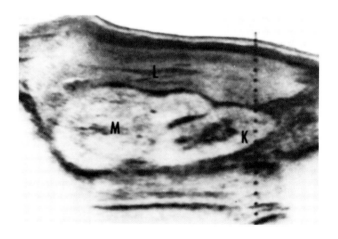

Fig. 5-35. Adrenal carcinoma. Supine longitudinal scan through a primary right adrenal carcinoma *(M)*. Note the cleavage plane between the undersurface of the liver *(L)* and the upper pole of the kidney *(K)*. (From Bernardino ME, Goldstein HM, Green B: Gray scale ultrasonography of adrenal neoplasm. AJR 130:741, © Am Roent Ray Soc, 1978.)

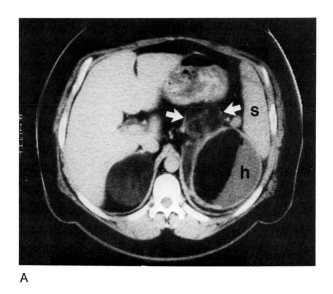

A

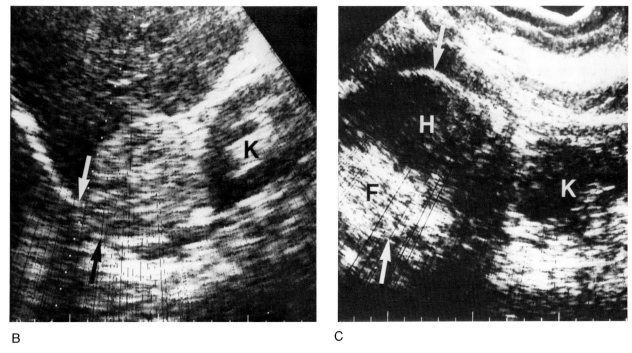

B   C

Fig. 5-36. Adrenal myelolipoma. Bilateral myelolipomas. **(A)** CT scan shows that the areas of lowest density within the right-sided myelolipoma are slightly higher than normal fat, and subtle areas of inhomogenicity are also evident. The left-sided myelolipoma contains areas of density equivalent to normal fat, and hemorrhage *(h)* has produced a blood-fat interface. Also on the left, there is extension of the tumor (arrows) beyond an apparent pseudocapsule and anterior displacement of the spleen *(S)*. **(B)** Right longitudinal ultrasound scan shows that the homogeneously fat myelolipoma has a relatively even pattern of high-amplitude echoes. A propagation speed artifact results in apparent discontinuity and posterior displacement of the diaphragm (arrows) deep to the mass. These ultrasound appearances are highly suggestive of a fatty mass. *(K,* right kidney.) **(C)** Coronal scan of the left myelolipoma (arrows) shows two distinct components: low-level echoes laterally corresponding to hemorrhage *(H)* and high-amplitude echoes medially caused by fat *(F)*. The fatty component was recognized only in retrospect after review of the CT scan **(A)**. *(K,* left kidney.) (From Vick CW, Zeman RK, Mannes E, et al: Adrenal myelolipoma: CT and ultrasound findings. Urol Radiol 6:7, 1984.)

decades with equal frequency among men and women.[28] The patient may be asymptomatic or may complain of pain due to hemorrhage, necrosis, or pressure on surrounding structures.[28]

The ultrasound appearance of an adrenal myelolipoma depends on its variable tissue components.[28] It is usually a well-defined discrete mass that may have a pseudocapsule and occasional involvement of extracapsular cortical tissue. It has been described as markedly echogenic on ultrasound [27,28] (Fig. 5-36). An additional finding that suggests a fat content is the apparent discontinuity and posterior displacement of an acoustic interface (e.g., diaphragm) distal to the fatty lesion[28] (Fig. 5-36). CT is recommended to confirm the fatty nature of the lesion (Fig. 5-36). The differential diagnosis includes lipoma, lymphangioma, myelolipoma, angiomyolipoma, increased abdominal fat deposition, retroperitoneal teratoma, and liposarcoma.[28]

MEDULLARY TUMORS

Pheochromocytoma. Pheochromocytomas are uncommon tumors occurring in 0.5 to 1.0 percent of those patients with hypertension. Ninety percent occur between the diaphragm and pelvic floor. These lesions arise from chromaffian cells with most in the adrenal; the remainder (7 to 10 percent) originate in the autonomic tissue, particularly the organs of Zuckerkandl and in the parasympathetic ganglia.[29,30] Pheochromocytomas are malignant 5 to 10 percent of the time and are multiple 3 to 5 percent of the time. The multiple lesions are frequently associated with heredofamilial syndromes. Clinically, the affected patients present with hypertension (50 percent paroxysmal) in the fourth to fifth decades. The diagnosis can be confirmed by biochemical assay for catecholamines and metabolites in the urine.[30]

On ultrasound, pheochromocytomas may appear as purely solid masses of homogeneous or heterogeneous echoes (Fig. 5-37). Hypoechoic areas indicate necrosis and hyperechoic regions indicate hemorrhage (Fig. 5-37). These lesions are usually quite large and sharply marginated and have a significant solid component with or without central necrosis or hemorrhage.[29]

Neuroblastoma. Neuroblastoma is one of the most common tumors of childhood with 80 percent occurring in patients less than 5 years of age and 35 percent in those less than 2 years. There is a striking correlation between age and prognosis. After one year, the tumor acts malignant; before one year there is a remarkable tendency to spontaneous regression. The lesion may regress in the following manner: (1) disappear by cytolysis; (2) undergo hemorrhage and then necrosis, leading to fibrocalcific residuals; and/or (3) cytodifferentiation into ganglioneuroma and ganglioneuroblastoma.[30] Most of these lesions (50 to 80 percent) occur in the adrenal glands, with the posterior mediastinum being the second most common site. The tumor metastasizes rapidly and widely through local infiltration and node metastases and is spread by blood to the liver, lungs, and the bones.

There are varying levels of differentiation found. A ganglioneuroma is composed of a fibrous background and is completely differentiated. A ganglioneuroblastoma is intermediate in differentiation. Ganglioneuromas are uncommon neurogenic neoplasms, 60 percent of which occur in patients less than 20 years of age with a slight female predominance.[31] They are most frequently in the thorax, with 43 percent in the mediastinum, 32 percent in the abdomen, and 8 percent in the neck.[31] The intra-abdominal lesions are usually extraadrenal. The clinical presentation of neuroblastoma is related to the rapid growth and its secretory products. There is a loss of energy and weight, pallor, abdominal protrusion, irregular fever, and generalized malaise. Greater than 90 percent of lesions produce catecholamines. In three fourths of cases, the patients present with the metastases before the diagnosis of the primary lesion is made.[30]

Ultrasound is helpful in the detection of these tumors, as 70 percent arise in the abdomen. However, ultrasound is limited when the lesion arises or extends into the chest and/or paraspinal area with extradural extension.[32] These lesions generally are heterogeneously echogenic with poorly defined margins[2,32] (Fig. 5-38; see Fig. 4-123). Some exhibit internal calcifications.[32] Twenty percent of neuroblastomas demonstrate internal calcification on CT[31] (see Fig. 4-123). Many contain discrete anechoic areas. Neuroblastomas and ganglioneuroblastomas frequently contain focal areas of necrosis, hemorrhage, and calcification.[31] As a result of this heterogeneous makeup, these masses contain more echoproducing interfaces than the ganglioneuroma (Fig. 5-38). Other distinguishing factors between neuroblastomas and ganglioneuroma include the tendency of neuroblastoma to cross the midline and to have ill-defined edges.[31] A careful examination should be performed to delineate the relationship of the mass to important vascular structures such as the inferior vena cava and aorta[33] (Fig. 5-38; see Fig. 4-123). Although the mass may have well-defined margins, it also may adhere to adjacent structures, thus leading to involvement of those adjacent structures.[31] The differential diagnosis of such a retroperitoneal mass in a child includes benign and malignant mesenchymal tumors, tumors of neurogenic origin such as schwannoma, neuroblastoma, pheochromocytoma, Wilms' tumor, lymphoma, and metastases from testicular neoplasm.[31]

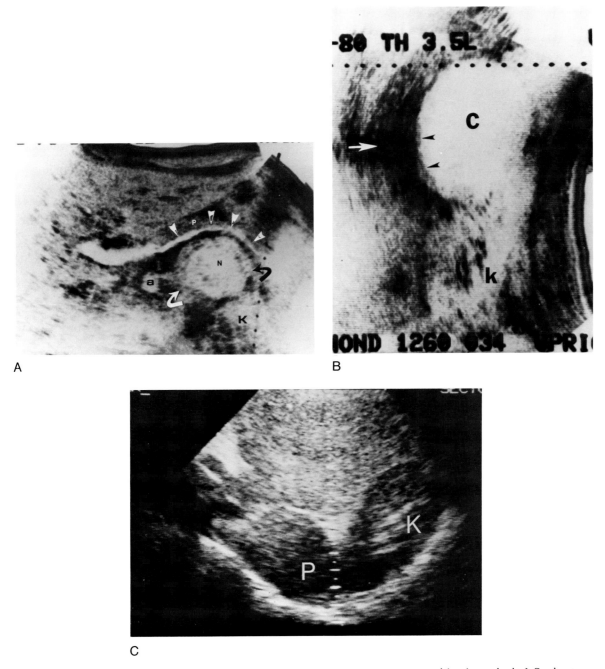

Fig. 5-37. Adrenal pheochromocytoma. **(A)** Case 1. Necrotic pheochromocytoma with echogenic rind. Supine transverse scan. A hetergeneous solid mass (curved arrows) displaces the splenic vein (arrowheads) anteriorly. An echogenic rind surrounds a necrotic hypoechoic center *(N)*. (*P,* pancreas; *a,* aorta; *K,* kidney.) **(B)** Case 2. Cystic pheochromocytoma. Upright posterior longitudinal scan. A thin-walled cystic mass *(C)* with irregular margins (arrowheads) is seen. There is marked distal sound enhancement (arrow) and displacement of the left kidney *(k)* posterocaudally. **(C)** Case 3. Solid pheochromocytoma. Longitudinal oblique real-time scan through the right upper quadrant in the left lateral decubitus position. A homogeneously solid entirely suprarenal right pheochromocytoma *(P)* is seen. (*K,* kidney.) (From Bowerman RA, Silver TM, Jaffe MH, et al: Sonography of adrenal pheochromocytomas. AJR 137:1227, © Am Roent Ray Soc, 1981.)

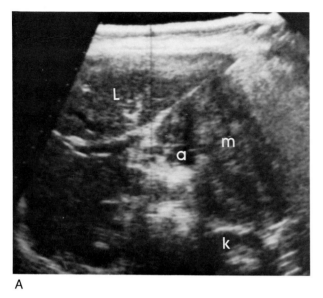

A

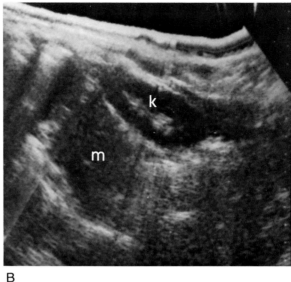

B

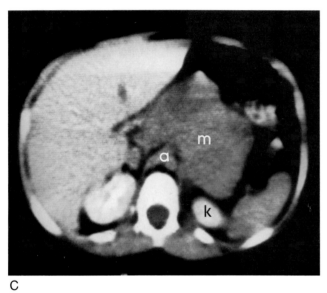

C

Fig. 5-38. Adrenal ganglioneuroma. **(A)** Transverse supine scan 13 cm above the umbilicus. A solid mass *(m)* is seen anterior, lateral, and posterior to the aorta *(a)*. It is separate from the posteriorly displaced left kidney *(k)*. (*L,* liver.) **(B)** Prone longitudinal scan that clearly demonstrates the solid mass *(m)* anterior and separate from the left kidney *(k)*. **(C)** CT scan, enhanced. A soft-tissue density mass *(m)* is seen anterior to the left kidney *(k)* with a very similar appearance to **(A)**. (*a,* aorta.)

Metastatic Adrenal Tumors

Delineation of small adrenal masses in the normal adrenal gland presents a great challenge to the sonologist. Small and moderately sized (4 to 5 cm) masses characteristically are anteromedial to the upper pole of the kidney (Figs. 5-29 and 5-39). They may indent the posterior wall of the inferior vena cava.[2,34] The kidneys are displaced inferiorly by larger adrenal masses. Adrenal tumors are usually round or oval in shape; the large ones are usually irregular. The tumors are usually somewhat hypoechoic[35-37] (Figs. 5-29 and 5-39). There may be strong areas of echoes with necrosis and hemorrhage.[2]

The adrenal glands are the fourth most common site in the body for metastases after the lungs, the liver, and the bones.[36] Most commonly metastases to the adrenal are from squamous cell carcinoma of the lung (33 per-

cent), with 30 percent from breast carcinoma and the remainder from melanoma, gastric carcinoma, and tumors of the colon, pancreas, kidney, and thyroid.[38] Up to 33 percent of patients with bronchogenic carcinoma of the lung have adrenal metastases.[37] In an autopsy series, there was a 25-percent incidence of adrenal involvement in non-Hodgkin's lymphoma.[36] As such, lymphoma should be a major consideration when a hypoechoic solid mass is identified in the adrenal gland[35] (Fig. 5-40).

Correlative Imaging

How do CT and ultrasound compare in imaging of the adrenal gland? Most institutions use CT when the primary question is whether or not there is an adrenal mass.

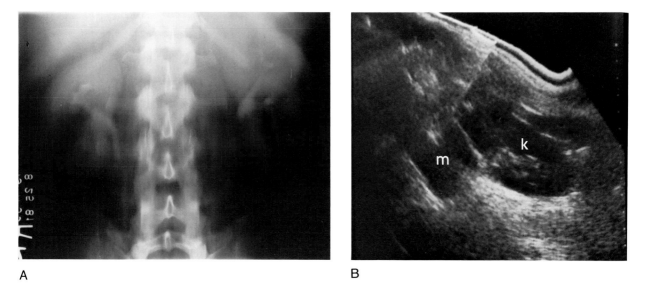

A

B

Fig. 5-39. Adrenal metastases. Carcinoma of the lung. **(A)** The intravenous pyelogram does not show evidence of a right adrenal mass. **(B)** Prone longitudinal static scan on the right with a solid mass *(m)* anterior to the kidney *(k)* in the area of the adrenal.

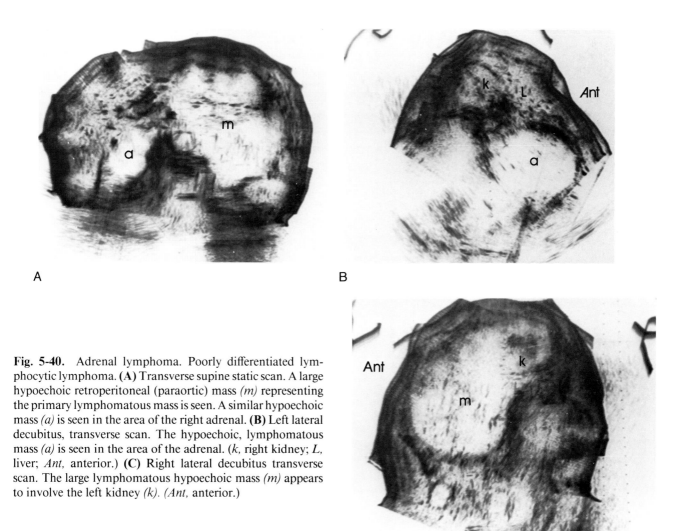

A

B

Fig. 5-40. Adrenal lymphoma. Poorly differentiated lymphocytic lymphoma. **(A)** Transverse supine static scan. A large hypoechoic retroperitoneal (paraortic) mass *(m)* representing the primary lymphomatous mass is seen. A similar hypoechoic mass *(a)* is seen in the area of the right adrenal. **(B)** Left lateral decubitus, transverse scan. The hypoechoic, lymphomatous mass *(a)* is seen in the area of the adrenal. (*k,* right kidney; *L,* liver; *Ant,* anterior.) **(C)** Right lateral decubitus transverse scan. The large lymphomatous hypoechoic mass *(m)* appears to involve the left kidney *(k). (Ant,* anterior.)

C

CT can detect normal adrenal glands in the majority of patients. In contrast, with ultrasound it is much more difficult to identify the normal gland on a consistent basis. In addition, CT is able to detect slight or subtle enlargement. CT is reported to have a sensitivity of 82 to 84 percent, a specificity of 95 to 98 percent, and an accuracy of 90 to 91 percent in the evaluation of the adrenal.[14,39,40] In the same studies, ultrasound had a sensitivity of 79 to 90 percent, a specificity of 61 to 97 percent, and an accuracy of 70 to 95 percent.[39]

Ultrasound does have a use in adrenal imaging. It is the modality of choice for evaluation of the neonatal adrenal as well as that of the cachectic patient. At times it may be difficult to define the adrenal as the origin of a mass on CT. By using longitudinal scans, various body positions, and the "retroperitoneal fat sign," ultrasound can often definitely identify the adrenal as the source of the mass.

RETROPERITONEAL ABSCESSES

Abscesses remain a problem in clinical practice despite advances in antibiotics and surgical technique. They present with increasing frequency in our enlarging population of patients who are immunocompromised due to steroids or chemotherapy, or in renal transplants, leukemia patients, and alcoholics.[41] Conventional radiography has inherent limitations in the delineation of retroperitoneal abscesses, which can explain the increased morbidity from and mortality (100 percent if untreated) for these lesions as compared to the morbidity from and mortality for intraperitoneal abscesses.[42] Early diagnosis is crucial because surgical treatment prior to development of septicemia offers the greatest patient benefit.[42]

Retroperitoneal abscesses are usually secondary to infection (appendicitis, pyelonephritis, perinephric abscesses, bacterial spondylitis), trauma, bowel perforation, surgery, or malignancy in adjacent retroperitoneal or intraperitoneal structures.[42-44] The most common presenting symptom is pain in the lower abdomen or flank. Less commonly, there is pain referred to the hip or thigh.[42] All patients present with fever and 50 percent have a palpable flank mass or swelling.[42]

Retroperitoneal inflammatory disease is often elusive to detection by clinical and radiographic methods.[44] In one study, 90 percent of patients had radiographic signs of abnormality but the diagnosis was not made until postmortem in 25 to 30 percent of cases.[42] Almost half (40-50 percent) of patients with a retroperitoneal abscess die from the disease.[44] Ultrasound provides direct visualization of the abnormal retroperitoneal fluid collection. While this modality cannot differentiate the different retroperitoneal fluid collections by echopattern alone, it

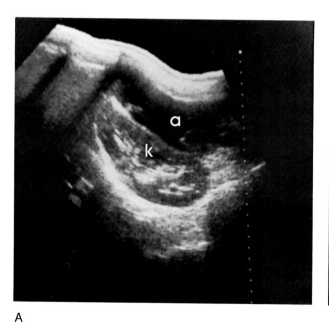
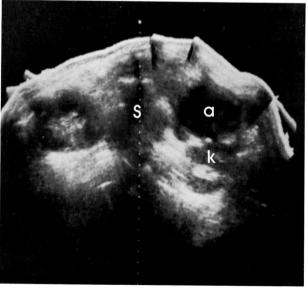

A   B

Fig. 5-41. Retroperitoneal abscess. **(A)** Prone longitudinal static scan. A poorly defined hypoechoic mass *(a)* is seen posterior to the right kidney *(k)*. **(B)** Prone transverse static scan. The hypoechoic mass (*a,* abscess) is seen posterior to the right kidney *(k)*, displacing it anteriorly. (*S,* spine.) The patient had a history of urinary tract infection and the abscess was in the posterior pararenal space.

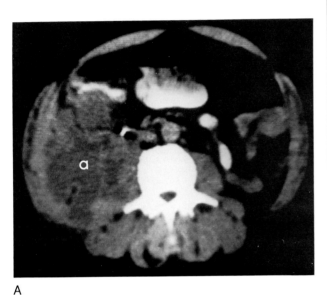

A

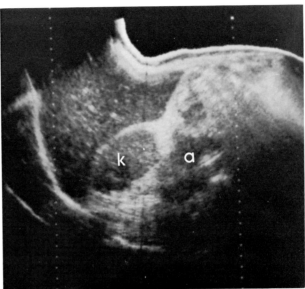

B

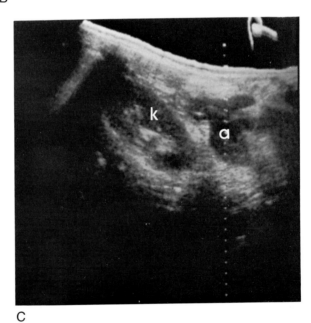

C

Fig. 5-42. Retroperitoneal abscess. **(A)** CT scan. A large mass *(a)* with a mixed density in the region of the psoas muscle is seen below the level of the kidney. **(B)** Longitudinal supine static scan. A poorly defined mass *(a)* is seen inferior to the right kidney *(k)*. **(C)** Prone longitudinal static scan. The abscess *(a)* is more easily seen inferior to the kidney *(k)*. It was aspirated for diagnosis.

can localize the lesion for percutaneous aspiration, which will lead to a definitive diagnosis.[42] Ultrasound can define the limits of the mass, identify displacement of adjacent organs, and demonstrate acoustic enhancement confirming that the mass is indeed fluid-filled.[44] The fluid content of the space-occupying abscess allows it to assume a volumetrically economical shape, usually spherical or ellipsoid.[41] Its shape depends on its location. The fluid collection varies from uniformly echofree to mildly echogenic to highly echogenic[41] (Figs. 5-41 to 5-44). The mass may even have septation. The walls are usually convex and well defined, but irregular.

The most common abscesses in the anterior pararenal space are enteric in origin and result from pancreatitis, diverticulitis, or ulcer perforation. The abscesses in the perirenal space often occur postoperatively.[45] Perirenal abscesses have more irregular walls, are lobular in contour, and contain internal echoes. They often extend along the fascial plane to assume an elongated shape. They are commonly found in the psoas, as the abscess extends along the belly of the muscle.[45]

The indications for percutaneous drainage of a retroperitoneal abscess would include the identification of an abscess on ultrasound or CT and confirmation of the diagnosis by percutaneous aspiration. The contraindications are few and include anticoagulant therapy and he-

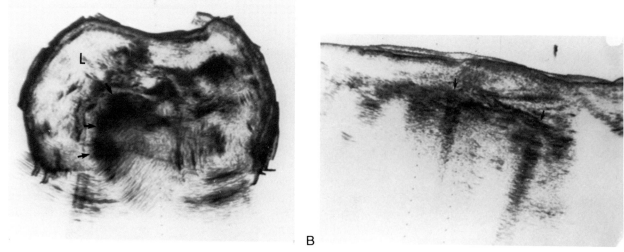

Fig. 5-43. Retroperitoneal abscess. **(A)** Transverse supine static scan at 11 cm above the umbilicus. No mass is identified, but a very reflective pattern (arrows) is seen in the right renal fossa. The kidney cannot be identified. (*L,* liver.) **(B)** Prone longitudinal static scan. In the area of the right kidney there is only a reflective pattern (reverberation artifacts, arrows) much like that seen with bowel gas. The kidney cannot be seen or an abscess mass as such. This represented a large retroperitoneal abscess containing air.

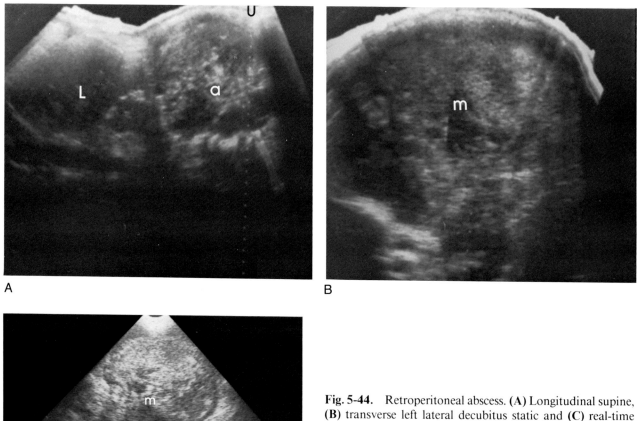

Fig. 5-44. Retroperitoneal abscess. **(A)** Longitudinal supine, **(B)** transverse left lateral decubitus static and **(C)** real-time scans demonstrate a large solid appearing echodense mass (*a, m* in **B** and **C**) which represents a retroperitoneal abscess. (*L,* liver; *U,* level of the umbilicus.)

matologic disorders that cause bleeding diatheses.[45] The catheter drainage may be accomplished by the modified Seldinger technique, which is similar to angiography. The patient's fever usually subsides within 24 to 48 hours following drainage, with the white blood cell count returning to normal within a week. If the patient does not improve within 48 to 72 hours after drainage is begun and with appropriate antibiotics, a scan is obtained to ascertain the location of the catheter and to evaluate the presence of undrained fluid. The catheter is usually removed 1 to 2 days after drainage stops (usually 10 to 14 days following the drainage procedure). Before the catheter is withdrawn, the area is scanned to ensure that resolution is complete.[45]

RETROPERITONEAL HEMORRHAGE

In the child, a retroperitoneal hematoma is usually secondary to trauma or hemophilia. The patient presents with flank pain and/or stiffness referred to the leg, hip, or groin. There may be a flexure contracture of the hip secondary to muscle spasm. Although such bleeding may be clinically apparent, exact location sometimes is difficult to establish particularly when there is involvement of the retroperitoneal space, pelvic structures, muscle bundles, bowel loops, or mesentery.[46]

Early diagnosis of a psoas hematoma is extremely important in hemophilia because prompt therapy with plasma concentrate and appropriate plasma factor is highly effective in preventing femoral nerve entrapment and resulting nerve deficit.[43,47] A small hematoma in a large muscle generally is resorbed without complication. A similar hematoma in a tight fascial compartment may cause significant ischemic myopathy and neuropathy.[46] Bleeding into the psoas causes it to enlarge and become more rounded.[43,47] The hematoma within the muscle is inseparable from the muscle (Figs. 5-45 and 5-46). Acutely after development, the hemorrhage may appear anechoic.[43,47] A hematoma cannot be distinguished from an abscess by ultrasound alone.

In the adult, a retroperitoneal hematoma may be secondary to trauma, bleeding diastheses, or a leaking aortic

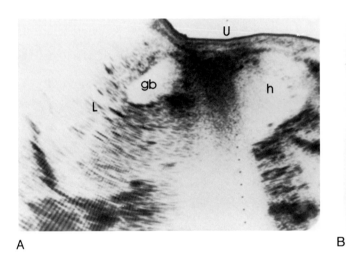

A

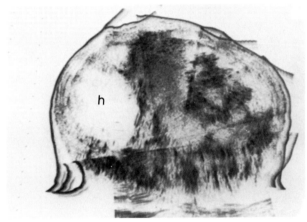

B

Fig. 5-45. Retroperitoneal hematoma. Hemophiliac. **(A)** Longitudinal static scan to the right of midline. A large hypoechoic mass *(h)* is seen in the region of the psoas/iliopsoas muscles. *(gb,* gallbladder; *L,* liver; *U,* level of the umbilicus.) **(B)** Transverse static scan through the retroperitoneal hematoma *(h),* which projects quite anteriorly and is hypoechoic. **(C)** Prone static longitudinal scan. The retroperitoneal hematoma *(h)* is seen as a hypoechoic mass inferior to the right kidney *(k). (C,* iliac crest level.) (Fig. C from Shirkhoda A, Mauro MA, Staab EV, Blatt PM: Soft-tissue hemorrhage in hemophiliac patients: computed tomography and ultrasound study. Radiology 147:811, 1983.)

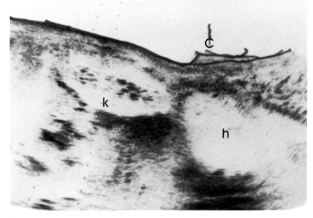

C

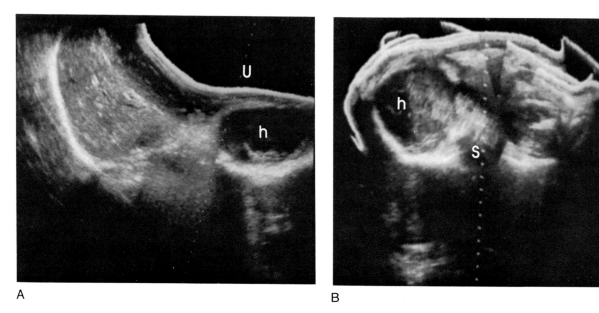

A   B

Fig. 5-46. Retroperitoneal hematoma. Hemophiliac. Right longitudinal static scan **(A)**. A hypoechoic mass *(h)* is seen in the area of the psoas/iliopsoas muscles. (*U,* level of the umbilicus.) **(B)** Transverse supine scan at 4 cm below the umbilicus. A hypoechoic mass *(h)* is seen in the area of the iliopsoas muscle. (*S,* spine.)

aneurysm (Fig. 5-47). A neoplasm may also rupture and bleed. The hematoma may be well localized or poorly defined as an infiltrative process. If the hemorrhage is recent in onset, it is typically anechoic. As clotting occurs, the pattern may change to complex with cystic and solid components; the degree of complexity varies with the ratio of clot to liquid blood within the hematoma.[6]

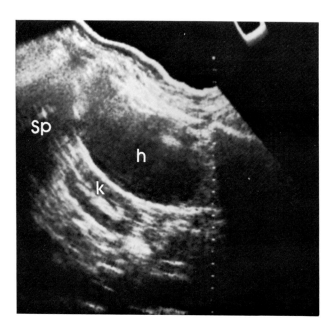

Fig. 5-47. Retroperitoneal hematoma. This patient was anticoagulated and experienced a drop in her hematocrit. A prone longitudinal static scan demonstrates a hypoechoic mass *(h)* posterior to the left kidney *(k)*. (*Sp,* spleen.)

RETROPERITONEAL FIBROSIS

Retroperitoneal fibrosis represents dense fibrous tissue proliferation in the form of a plaque-like or bulky mass 2 to 6 cm thick and generally confined to the central and paravertebral regions.[48] It is usually found to extend from the perirenal space between the hila of the kidneys to the dome of the bladder. It has a potential to envelop rather than displace hollow structures such as ureters and blood and lymphatic vessels. It is an uncommon but progressive and serious illness that is usually clinically silent until it causes ureteral or vascular obstruction.[48] Its progressive course often results in significant obstructive uropathy.

The etiology of this disease process is obscure. In 70 percent of cases, it is idiopathic. There is evidence that there may be a hypersensitivity reaction to methysergide, which may be a cause; regression of the disease is variable after removal of the drug from the patient's therapy. Patients with primary or metastatic retroperitoneal neoplasm are seen to exhibit retroperitoneal fibrosis. The malignancy, irrespective of its type and/or source, apparently stimulates a fibrotic type of reaction indistinguishable from that of idiopathic fibrosis.[49]

Clinically, these patients present with back, flank, or abdominal pain often accompanied by nonspecific complaints of weight loss, nausea and vomiting, and malaise.[48,49] There is a palpable abdominal or rectal mass in 30 percent of patients.[49] Hypertension and anuria are relatively common.[49] It has a peak incidence in the fifth to sixth decades with a male-to-female ratio of 2 : 1.[48,49] Clinical and radiographic features of retroperitoneal fibrosis are often varied and nonspecific.[49]

Excretory urography and retrograde studies are commonly used for the diagnosis. Bilateral or unilateral hydroureter associated with abdominal narrowing of ureteral caliber or an encased appearance represent the diagnostic findings.[49] The combination of proximal hydroureter and medial deviation of the middle third of the ureter is thought to be almost pathognomonic.[49]

On ultrasound, this lesion is seen either as a large bulky mass with ill-defined irregular margins or a flat large mass with smooth margins located centrally and in the paravertebral region extending to the level of the sacral promontory and to the renal vessels.[48-51] It may be anechoic to hypoechoic[48-53] (Figs. 5-48 and 5-49). The anterior margin appears to respect the peritoneal boundary and is clearly delineated, whereas the posterior margin is poorly defined and not easily separated.[49,53] In one series, 87 percent of patients had associated hydronephrosis; this is often found to be the case.[48,51] It has a tendency to envelop but not displace structures such as the aorta, the inferior vena cava, and the ureters.[49,51,53] Its appearance is similar to retroperitoneal sarcoma, nodal metastases, lymphoma, and retroperitoneal hematoma.[49,51,53]

RETROPERITONEAL LYMPHOCELE

Lymphoceles, which are lymph-filled spaces without a distinct epithelial lining, usually occur secondary to surgery. The most common source is the pelvic lymphatics although they may come from the paraortic or renal hilar lymphatics.[54] There has been a report of a 3-percent incidence following pelvic lymphadenectomy for staging prostatic carcinoma.[55] They also occur following radical gynecologic procedures, extensive urologic operations, and renal transplants. A pelvic lymphocele represents an imbalance between inflow of lymph from the channels of the lower extremities, pelvic organs, and abdominal wall and outflow from the surgical bed into the central lymphatic structure.[55]

The characteristic pelvic location for this lesion is lateral to the bladder [55] (Figs. 5-50 and 5-51). Although commonly located extraperitoneally in the pelvis, upper abdominal lymphoceles have been reported secondary to aortofemoral bypass, simple nephrolithotomies, and paraortic/renal hilar node dissections. The anterior surface of the lymphocele may be within 3 cm of the anterior abdominal wall. The most common clinical presentation is a constellation of fullness and flank pain with or without pain extending into the pelvis and leg.[54]

Small (cross-sectional area less than 30 cm^2) anechoic lymphoceles most likely result in long-term spontaneous resolution. Those that are larger or complex result in complications requiring surgical intervention. These lesions usually have an ellipsoid shape with well-defined walls and never contain debris; they may be multilocular but are most often unilocular.[56] They are characterized

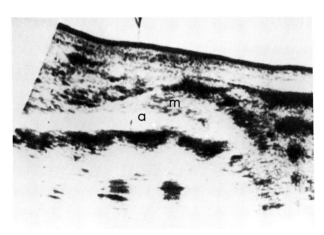

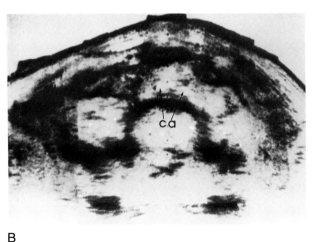

A

B

Fig. 5-48. Retroperitoneal fibrosis. **(A)** Longitudinal static scan demonstrating a smooth-bordered, slightly echofilled mass *(m)* anterior to the sacral promontory adjacent to the aorta *(a)*. **(B)** Transverse static scan. A lobulated mass surrounds the psoas muscle, inferior vena cava *(c)*, and aorta *(a)* caused by retroperitoneal fibrosis. (From Sanders RC, Duffy T, McLoughlin MG, Walsh PC: Sonography in the diagnosis of retroperitoneal fibrosis. J Urol 118:944, ©1977 The Williams & Wilkins Co., Baltimore.)

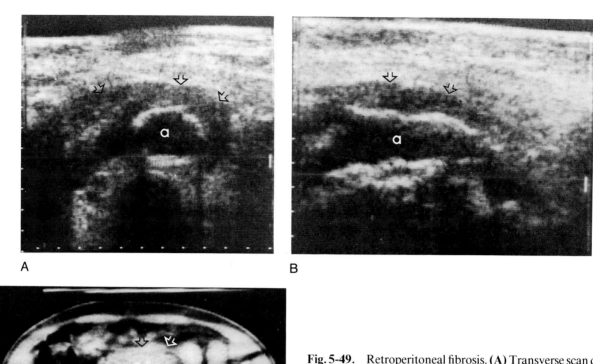

A   B

C

Fig. 5-49. Retroperitoneal fibrosis. (A) Transverse scan demonstrating a hypoechoic mass (arrows) encompassing the aorta *(a)* and the inferior vena cava. (B) Midline longitudinal scan. A hypoechoic mass (arrows) is seen anterior to the aorta *(a)*. (C) CT scan. The same mass (arrows) is seen surrounding the aorta *(a)*. (From Center S, Schwab R, Goldberg BB: The value of ultrasonography as an aid in the treatment of idiopathic retroperitoneal fibrosis. J Ultrasound Med 1:87, 1982.)

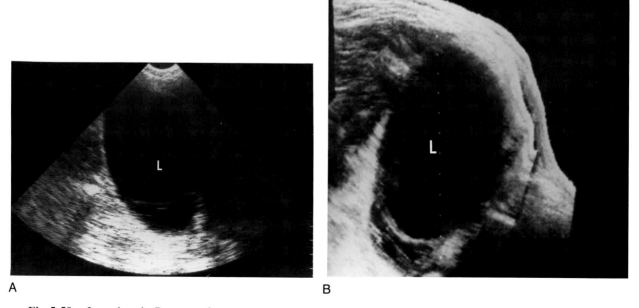

A   B

Fig. 5-50. Lymphocele. Postoperative prostatectomy patient with pelvic node dissection. An anechoic mass *(L)* is seen in the right pelvis on these transverse (A) and transverse oblique (B) scans.

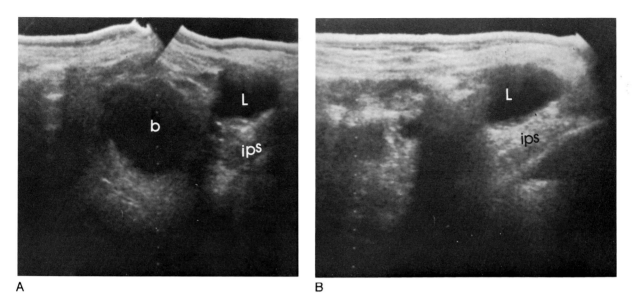

A   B

Fig. 5-51. Lymphocele. Postoperative ovarian carcinoma patient with node dissection. **(A)** Transverse supine scan at 8 cm above the symphysis. An anechoic mass *(L)* is seen to the left of bladder *(b)* and anterior to the iliopsoas *(ips)* muscle. **(B)** Longitudinal static scan 6 cm to the left of midline. The anechoic lymphocele *(L)* is seen anterior to the iliopsoas *(ips)* muscle.

by increased through transmission and no internal echoes, although thin septation has been seen (see Fig. 4-153). While ultrasound alone cannot differentiate lymphocele from hematoma, seroma, or abscess, a percutaneous aspiration may give a definitive diagnosis.[55] The fluid in lymphoceles is clear.

LYMPHADENOPATHY

Lymph nodes are an important component of the widely dispersed lymphoreticuloendothelial system and are distributed throughout the body. These discrete structures are ovoid in shape and measure 1 mm to between 1 and 2 cm in length. They are surrounded by a connective tissue capsule. Lymph nodes are rarely the site of primary disease but are secondarily involved in virtually all systemic infections and in many neoplastic disorders.[57]

Lymphoma

Malignant lymphomas are classified as Hodgkin's or non-Hodgkin's. Forty percent of newly diagnosed lymphomas are Hodgkin's disease with the remainder being non-Hodgkin's (nodular or diffuse). Effective therapeutic management using both radiation and chemotherapy in these patients requires not only accurate histologic

classification but also reliable definition of the anatomic regions involved.[58-60]

Classically, the modality of lymphangiography has been proven to be accurate in the diagnosis of paraortic and paracaval adenopathy, but fails to detect disease in other sites such as mesenteric, perisplenic, and perihepatic sites, as well as those in extranodal sites such as the liver and spleen. Ultrasound can detect retroperitoneal disease and provide additional information about the extent of abdominal involvement.[59,60] It is reported to be 80- to 90-percent accurate in detecting retroperitoneal nodal lymphoma.[58]

To evaluate for abdominal lymphoma or to determine the presence or absence of lymphadenopathy, the abdomen and pelvis must be scanned carefully[61] (Figs. 5-40, 5-52 to 5-57; see Fig. 2-83). Both the hepatic and splenic hila should be checked, and the liver, spleen, and kidneys should be scrutinized for changes in echopattern (see Figs. 1-96, 1-97, 1-99, 2-83, 4-130, 4-131, 8-11, and 8-12). There should be a search for nodes in the abdomen, at the origin of the celiac and the superior mesenteric arteries, and in the paraortic and renal hilar areas (Figs. 5-53 to 5-56). The pelvis should be scanned with careful attention to the iliac areas (Fig. 5-57).

PARAORTIC NODES

There is involvement of the paraortic nodes in 25 percent of Hodgkin's patients and 40 percent of non-Hodgkin's patients. Greater than 12 percent of patients with

Hodgkin's will demonstrate normal lymphangiograms with celiac, perisplenic, or mesenteric nodes. In patients with non-Hodgkin's disease, greater than 40 percent with normal lymphangiograms have mesenteric disease. The accuracy of ultrasound in the detection of retroperitoneal nodes has been reported to be 80 to 90 percent.[59,60,62] The detected nodal size is correct in 98.2 percent of cases, with nodes larger than 2 cm detected.[62] Bowel gas can obscure retroperitoneal structures and mesenteric and retroperitoneal fat can degrade the ultrasound resolution, but there is a relatively high degree of accuracy in detection of nodes and extranodal disease,

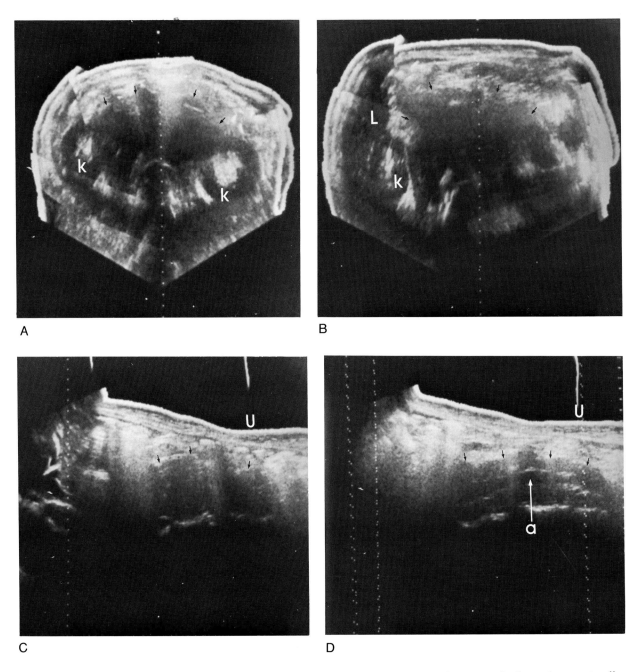

A

B

C

D

Fig. 5-52. Hodgkin's lymphoma. **(A,B)** Transverse and **(C,D)** longitudinal scans. The prevertebral vessels are not well seen and a mass effect (arrows) is seen. (*L,* liver; *k,* kidney; *U,* level of the umbilicus.) The aorta *(a)* lumen is seen to be encompassed by a mass (arrows) on **(D)**. *(Figure continues.)*

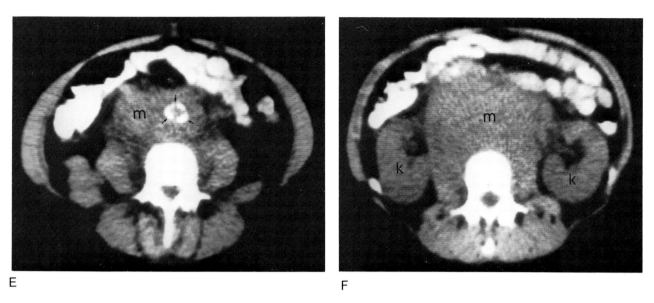

E

F

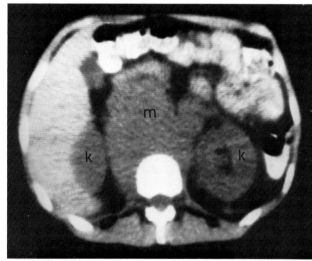

G

Fig. 5-52 *(Continued).* **(E–G)** CT scans. The aorta and inferior vena cava are not seen on **(F,G).** On **(E),** the aorta can be identified by the calcification (arrows) within the mass *(m)* surrounding it. (*k*, kidney.)

which suggests that ultrasound has a useful role in the initial staging process.[59,60]

The ultrasound appearance of lymphomatous nodes varies from hypoechoic to anechoic with very good sound transmission.[59,60,63–65] (Figs. 5-40, 5-52, 5-54, and 5-57; see Fig. 2-83). Lymphomatous masses may be relatively echofree because of their homogeneous structure, which does not have sufficient interfaces to produce echoes.[63] At times the crus may be confused with nodes. Adenopathy secondary to nonlymphomatous disease or inflammatory process such as retroperitoneal fibrosis is indistinguishable. There is no correlation between the ultrasound apearance of the nodes and the histology of the lymphoma. However, the largest paraortic nodes

usually result from non-Hodgkin's lymphoma[59,60] (Figs. 5-40 and 5-53).

Various ultrasound patterns of malignant lymphoma have been described, including (1) a mantle-like plaque of tumor seated on the vertebral body especially in the paraortic and paravertebral region (Figs. 5-52 and 5-53); (2) a conglomerated mass of tumor from mesenteric nodes surrounded by gastrointestinal gas; (3) organ compression or displacement by a mass of abdominal nodes; (4) compression or obscuration of the outlines of the aorta or inferior vena cava (Figs. 5-52 to 5-54); and (5) hypoechoic to anechoic images on ultrasound scans[63–67] (Figs. 5-52 to 5-57). Care should be taken to differentiate lymphadenopathy from collateral channels

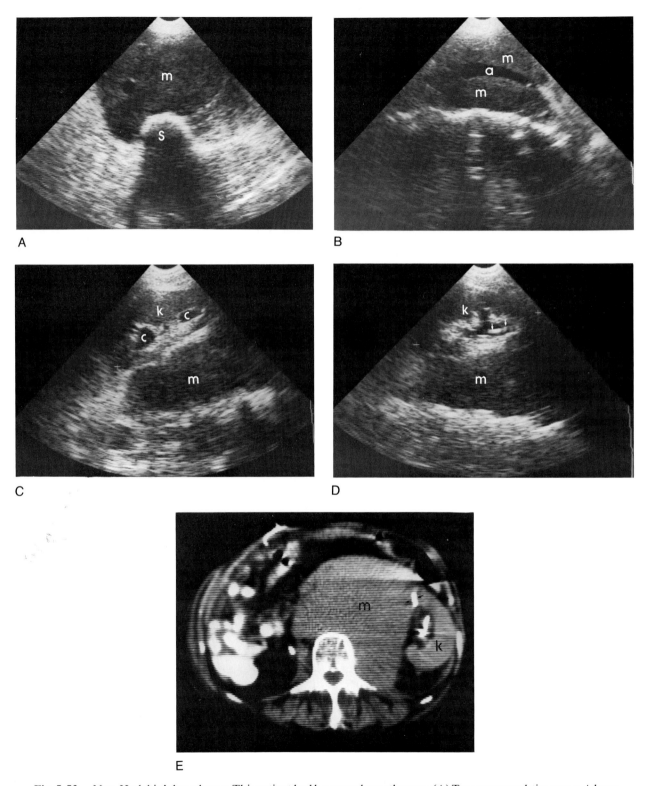

Fig. 5-53. Non-Hodgkin's lymphoma. This patient had been on chemotherapy. **(A)** Transverse real-time scan. A large hypoechoic mass *(m)* is seen, without identification of the aorta or inferior vena cava. *(S,* spine.) **(B)** Longitudinal real-time scan. The mass *(m)* surrounds the aorta *(a)*. **(C,D)** Prone longitudinal scans. The hydronephrotic left kidney *(k)* is seen with a stent (arrows) in the collecting system on **(D)**. The lymphomatous mass *(m)* is seen anteriorly. *(c,* calyces.) **(E)** CT scan. A large soft-tissue density mass *(m)* is seen in the prevertebral area displacing the left kidney *(k)* to the left. The stent (arrows) is also demonstrated.

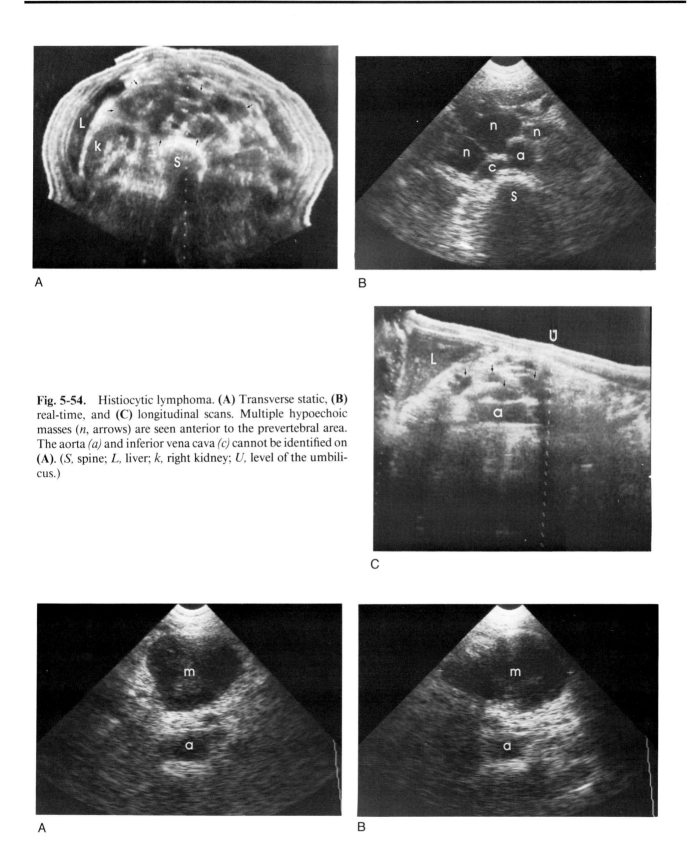

Fig. 5-54. Histiocytic lymphoma. **(A)** Transverse static, **(B)** real-time, and **(C)** longitudinal scans. Multiple hypoechoic masses (*n*, arrows) are seen anterior to the prevertebral area. The aorta *(a)* and inferior vena cava *(c)* cannot be identified on **(A)**. (*S,* spine; *L,* liver; *k,* right kidney; *U,* level of the umbilicus.)

Fig. 5-55. Lymphocytic lymphoma. **(A,B)** Transverse scans of the paraortic area in the midabdomen show a globular hypoechoic mass *(m)* anterior to the aorta *(a).*

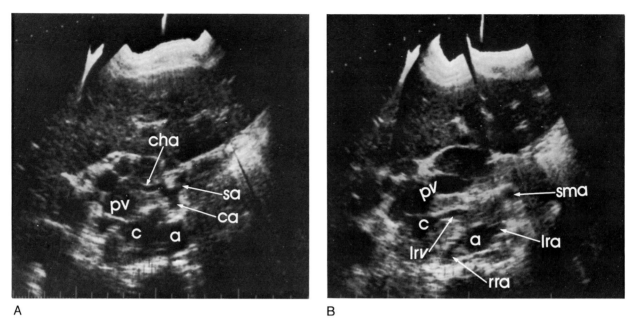

A   B

Fig. 5-56. Peripancreatic lymphadenopathy. Lymphocytic leukemia. **(A,B)** Transverse scans. Multiple masses compressing and displacing the prevertebral vessels and their branches are seen in the pancreatic area. (*a,* aorta; *c,* inferior vena cava; *pv,* portal vein; *lrv,* left renal vein; *rra,* right renal artery; *cha,* common hepatic artery; *ca,* celiac artery; *sma,* superior mesenteric artery; *sa,* splenic artery.)

produced by portal and systemic venous systems, as both may have a lucent appearance.[68] Real-time or Doppler systems might help if pulsation is present. When portal hypertension and retroperitoneal masses are present, the possibility of varices should be considered.

PERIPANCREATIC LYMPHADENOPATHY

Enlarged nodes may appear as well-defined hypoechoic ovoid or rounded masses in the retropancreatic location or may surround and silhouette the region of

the pancreatic head and body[69] (Fig. 5-56). Peripancreatic nodes represent paraduodenal, anterior paracaval, and superior mesenteric vessel nodes. These nodes are infrequently opacified on contrast lymphangiogram scans.

Two major ultrasound patterns of peripancreatic lymphadenopathy have been described: (1) well-defined rounded or ovoid masses lateral and posterior to the pancreas but anterior to the level of the inferior vena cava, left renal vein, and aorta and easily distinguished from the pancreas; and (2) large confluent masses insep-

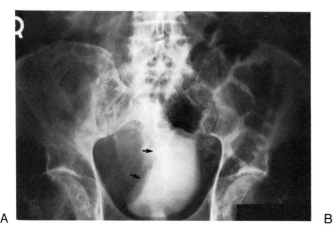

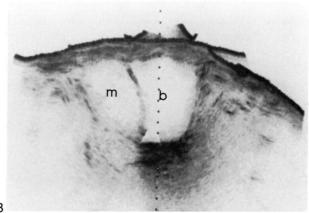

A   B

Fig. 5-57. Pelvic lymphoma. Diffuse histiocytic lymphoma. **(A)** Intravenous pyelogram. An extrinsic mass effect (arrows) is seen on the bladder. **(B)** Transverse static scan. A hypoechoic mass *(m)* is seen to the right of the bladder *(b).* An ultrasound guided percutaneous biopsy was consistent with lymphoma.

arable from and engulfing the pancreatic head.[69] These lesions lie posterior to the splenic vein and the confluence of the splenic and portal veins.

MESENTERIC LYMPHADENOPATHY

The demonstration of mesenteric nodal involvement merits considerable attention because of the revision in therapy and prognosis that follows. For an indepth discussion, refer to Chapter 7. There is mesenteric adenopathy in greater than 50 percent of non-Hodgkin's and less than 4 percent of Hodgkin's lymphoma. The pattern of the adenopathy resembles retroperitoneal nodes, however there is usually no "silhouette" sign involving the aorta and inferior vena cava.[59] Instead, the characteristic appearance is the presence of a lobulated confluent mass infiltrating the mesenteric leaves and encasing the superior mesenteric artery and vein, producing a "sandwich" appearance.[70]

Burkitt's Lymphoma

Burkitt's lymphoma is a clinically and histologically distinct tumor first described in African children.[71] It arises from the B-lymphocytes and has a rapid doubling time but responds dramatically to a combination chemotherapy.[71] Though it is potentially curable, the chemotherapy can produce rapid tumor lysis with subsequent life-threatening metabolic abnormalities, especially in a patient with a large tumor or compromised renal function.

There is a 69 percent incidence of abdominal involvement in Burkitt's lymphoma. The abdominal masses tend to be large, solitary, and acoustically homogeneous. Most are found in the pelvis and upper abdomen as well as in the retroperitoneum.[72] There is a high incidence of ileocecal, mesenteric, or ovarian involvement.[72] The terminal ileum is the most common site of gastrointestinal involvement.[71] These patients usually do not have the typical mantle of enlarged nodes seen in other types of lymphoma. The absence of lymph node disease and the presence of a bulky homogeneous extranodal tumor are characteristic ultrasound findings.[72]

The tumor bulk is the major prognostic factor in identifying those patients likely to have metabolic complications resulting from chemotherapy. Because of the poor prognosis associated with large abdominal masses, there is usually surgical debulking prior to chemotherapy. Ultrasound can be used to demonstrate tumor size, location, and relationship between the tumor and normal

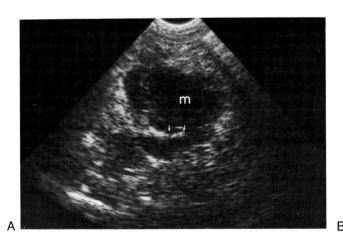

A

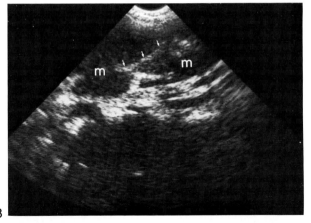

B

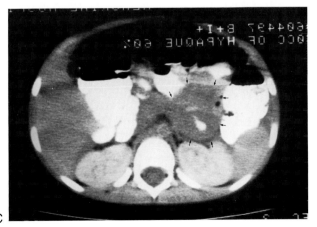

C

Fig. 5-58. Burkitt's lymphoma. (A) Transverse real-time scan. A large hypoechoic mass *(m)* is seen with a target pattern on the left. The echodense area (arrows) represents involved bowel lumen. (B) Longitudinal scan through the hypoechoic mass *(m)*. The bowel lumen (arrows) is within the mass. (C) CT scan demonstrating a soft-tissue mass (arrows) on the left involving bowel.

organs. The tumor pattern varies from lucent to hyperechoic[63,71] (Fig. 5-58). In 76 percent of cases, the tumor is well defined, sharply marginated, and homogeneous. In 13 percent, there is ascites.[72]

Once Burkitt's lymphoma is suspected on the basis of the ultrasound scan, the kidneys should be assessed, as there is a 5-percent incidence of direct renal involvement with this disease.[71,72] If there is abnormal renal function, an increased risk of metabolic complications with chemotherapy exists. Hydronephrosis is a recognized complication of nodal masses. There also may be tumor infiltration, poorly defined anechoic masses, or enlarged kidneys as a result of diffuse infiltration. If there is decreased renal function and a normal ultrasound appearance, uric acid nephropathy may be considered.[72]

Metastatic Lymphopathy

Metastatic disease can occur by lymphatic or hematogeneous spread. It may be secondary to carcinoma of the breast, lung, or testis. Many times there is primary recurrence from previously resected urologic or gynecologic tumors.[6] Although the echopattern of these nodes which are enlarged secondary to metastatic disease, may be varied, they are less commonly hypoechoic with metastatic disease than with lymphoma (Figs. 5-59 to 5-62). In one study it was found that 83 percent of lymphomatous nodes and only 53 percent of those secondary to soft tissue tumors were anechoic.[73] If ascites is found invasion of the peritoneal surface is indicated.

Biopsy

Nodal biopsy is performed for confirmation of the lymphangiographic findings and for histologic diagnosis in lieu of surgery.[74] In patients with lymphoma, 54 to 85 percent of biopsy specimens provide adequate cytology for a correct diagnosis.[74,75] As far as carcinoma to nodes is concerned, a fine-needle biopsy is diagnostically correct 72 percent of the time.[75]

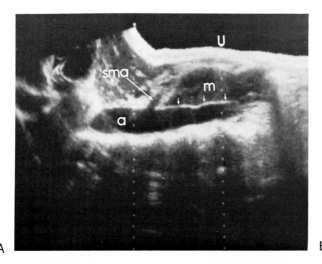

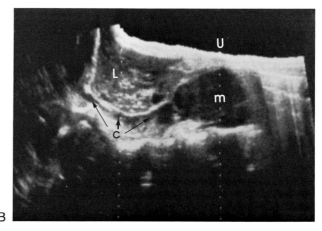

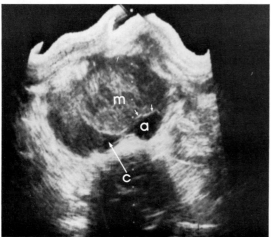

Fig. 5-59. Metastatic disease. Patient with known prostatic carcinoma and a pulsatile mass. Longitudinal scans in the midline (**A**) and 1 cm to the right of midline (**B**) as well as transverse scan 8 cm below the xyphoid (**C**) demonstrate an extra-aortic mass *(m)*. The outer wall (arrows) of the aorta is the densest outline and the mass is external to this wall making it extra- or paraortic. In addition, there is compression of the inferior vena cava *(c)* seen in **B** and **C**. Percutaneous biopsy proved this to be prostatic carcinoma. (*L,* left lobe of the liver; *U,* level of the umbilicus; *sma,* superior mesenteric artery.)

Correlative Imaging

At most institutions, CT is the preferred modality for identification, staging, and follow-up of lymphoma. CT can detect smaller nodal enlargments than ultrasound can and is less likely to be nondiagnostic. In one study, 50 percent of the ultrasound scans ordered for staging the abdomen and pelvis were not sufficiently visualized for diagnostic conclusion.[76] On ultrasound scans, the presence or extent of the disease in nodal sites caudal to the pancreas was underestimated more commonly than in other areas.[76] Others report ultrasound to have an accu-racy of 80 to 90 percent, a specificity of greater than 90 percent, and a sensitivity of 60 to 70 percent in the staging of lymphoma.[61]

PRIMARY RETROPERITONEAL TUMORS

Most of the primary retroperitoneal tumors arise from the kidney and adrenal gland with primary tumors other than lymphoma derived from mesenchymal and neurogenic tissue. Most are malignant.[6,77] Components may

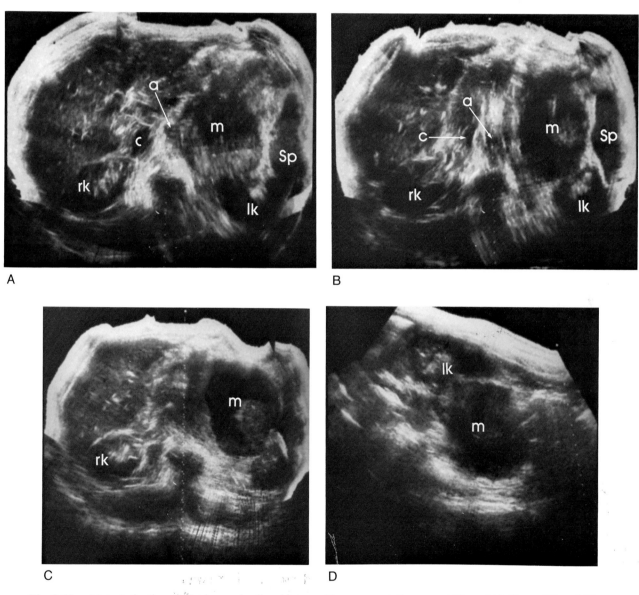

Fig. 5-60. Metastatic disease. Embryonal cell carcinoma. Transverse static scans at 13 cm **(A)**, 11 cm **(B)** and 10 cm **(C)** above the umbilicus. A large mass *(m)* of mixed echodensity is seen. The left kidney *(lk)* appears displaced posteriorly and to the right. (*a*, aorta; *rk*, right kidney; *Sp*, spleen; *c*, inferior vena cava.) **(D)** Prone longitudinal scan. A hypoechoic mass *(m)* is seen anterior to the left kidney *(lk). (Figure continues.)*

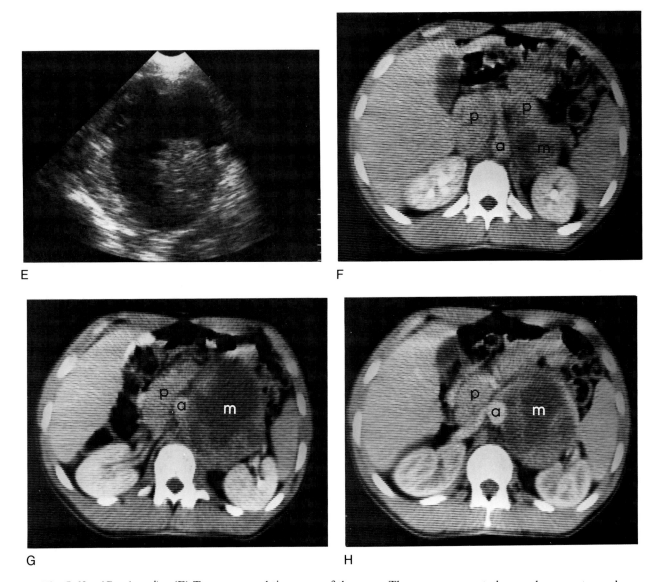

E

F

G

H

Fig. 5-60 *(Continued).* **(E)** Transverse real-time scan of the mass. The mass appears to have a dense center and a hypoechoic periphery. **(F–H)** Enhanced CT scans. The mass *(m)* with a mixed density is seen lateral to the aorta *(a)*. It appears separate from the pancreas *(p)*.

include fibrous tissue, muscle, fat, nerves, blood, and lymph vessels, as well as embryonic rests from the genitourinary or gastrointestinal systems.[6]

The most frequently described primary retroperitoneal tumor is the liposarcoma, which is often quite echoreflective depending on its fat content[1,6] (Fig. 5-63). It is an uncommon tumor, but the third most common malignant tumor of soft tissue and the second most frequent retroperitoneal malignant tumor. Thirteen percent of liposarcomas occur in the retroperitoneum with greater than one third of these originating from the perirenal fat.[77] The diagnosis is rarely made preoperatively. On ultrasound, a mass with a complex echopattern and

an irregularly thickened wall is seen[77] (Fig. 5-63). On the basis of ultrasound, liposarcoma cannot be differentiated from leiomyosarcoma and other retroperitoneal sarcomas.

Sarcomas other than liposarcoma present as complex or centrally necrotic soft tissue masses or as homogeneous soft tissue masses; on ultrasound, there are increased or decreased internal echoes or there is an echodense central area with a hypoechoic periphery[1,78] (Fig. 5-64). Leiomyosarcomas tend to undergo necrosis and cystic generation. Fibrosarcomas (Fig. 5-65) and rhabdomyosarcomas (Fig. 5-66) are quite invasive and infiltrate widely into muscle and adjoining soft tissue.[6]

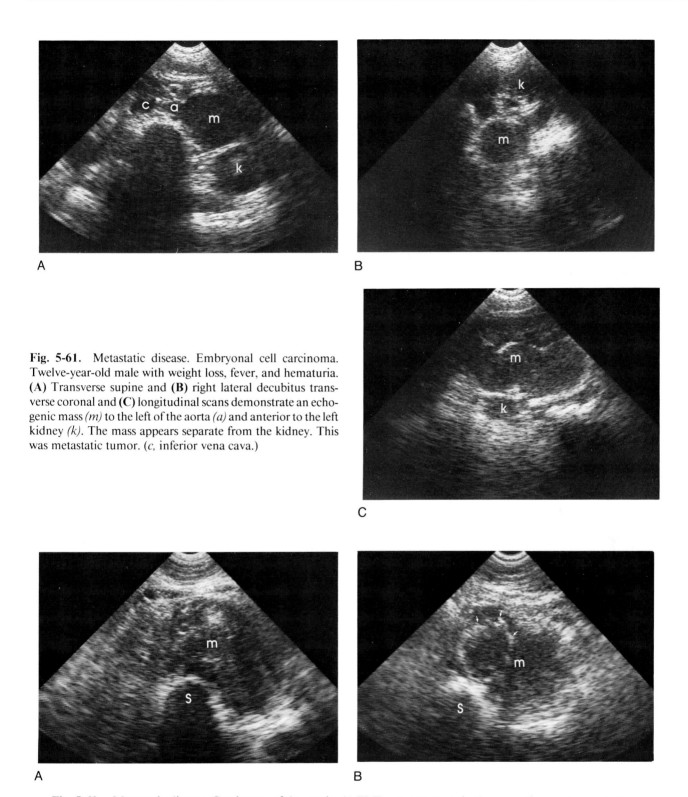

Fig. 5-61. Metastatic disease. Embryonal cell carcinoma. Twelve-year-old male with weight loss, fever, and hematuria. **(A)** Transverse supine and **(B)** right lateral decubitus transverse coronal and **(C)** longitudinal scans demonstrate an echogenic mass *(m)* to the left of the aorta *(a)* and anterior to the left kidney *(k)*. The mass appears separate from the kidney. This was metastatic tumor. (*c*, inferior vena cava.)

Fig. 5-62. Metastatic disease. Carcinoma of the cervix. **(A,B)** Transverse scans in the paraortic area demonstrate a large solid mass *(m)*. The echodensities (arrows) in **(B)** represent calcifications. The aorta and inferior vena cava cannot be identified. (*S,* spine.) *(Figure continues.)*

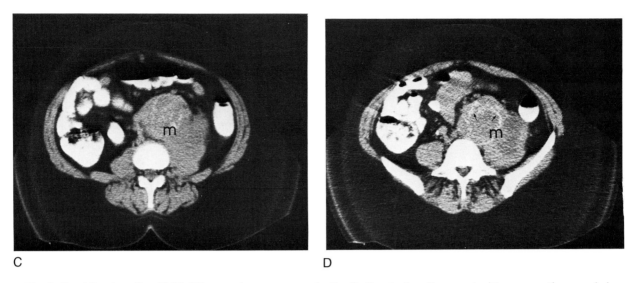

C   D

Fig. 5-62 *(Continued).* **(C,D)** CT scans demonstrate a similar finding to the ultrasound with a paraortic mass *(m)* which contains some calcification (arrows).

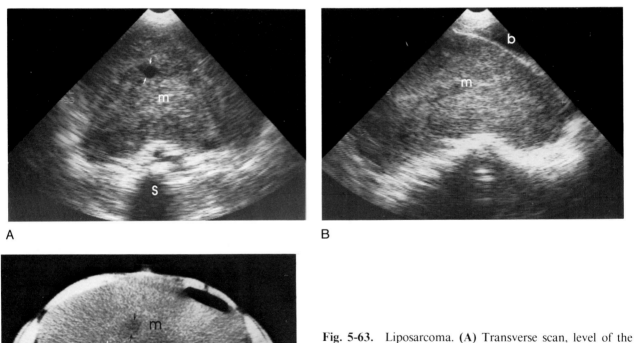

A   B

C

Fig. 5-63. Liposarcoma. **(A)** Transverse scan, level of the umbilicus. An echodense mass *(m)* is seen anterior to the spine *(S)*. The aorta is not seen. There is a small anechoic area (arrows) within the mass. **(B)** Longitudinal scan. The echodense mass *(m)* extends from the pelvis upward. The bladder *(b)* is seen anteriorly. **(C)** CT scan similar to **(A)**. The mass *(m)* is lower in density than soft-tissue and contains a low-density area (arrows).

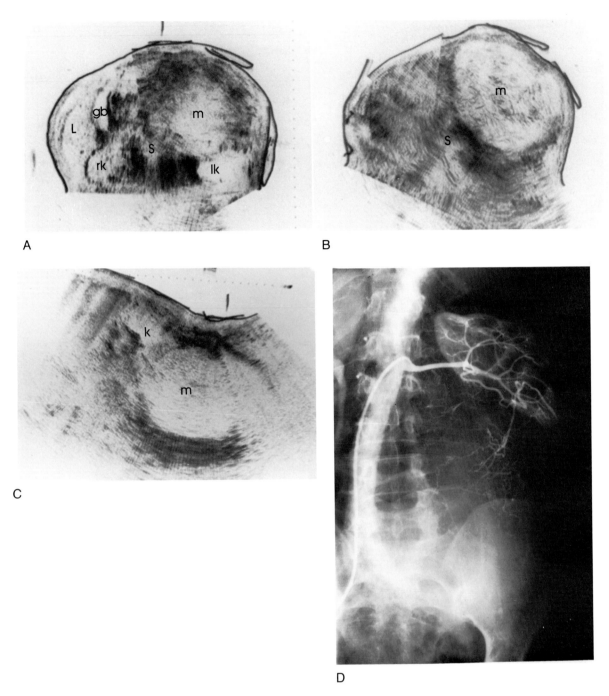

Fig. 5-64. Leiomyosarcoma. Transverse scans at 8 cm **(A)** and 2 cm **(B)** above the umbilicus. An echodense mass *(m)* is seen on the left. (*gb,* gallbladder; *S,* spine; *L,* liver; *gb,* gallbladder; *rk,* right kidney; *lk* left kidney.) **(C)** Prone longitudinal scan. The mass *(m)* appears to be involving the lower pole of the left kidney *(k).* **(D)** Angiogram. The abnormal vessels feeding the mass appear to be originating from the renal vasculature. The tumor represented a leiomyosarcoma of the renal capsule.

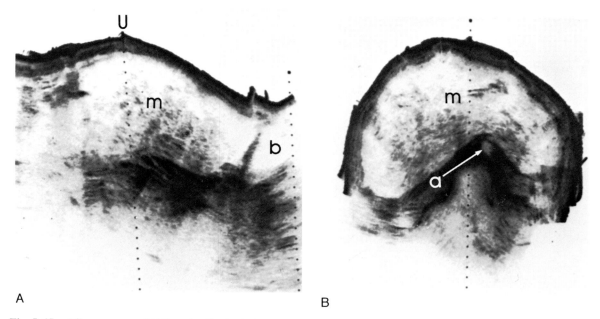

A   B

Fig. 5-65. Fibrosarcoma. **(A)** Longitudinal midline scan and **(B)** transverse scan 12 cm above the umbilicus demonstrate a large mass *(m)* of mixed density. It is more lucent than dense. (*b,* bladder; *U,* level of the umbilicus; *a,* aorta.)

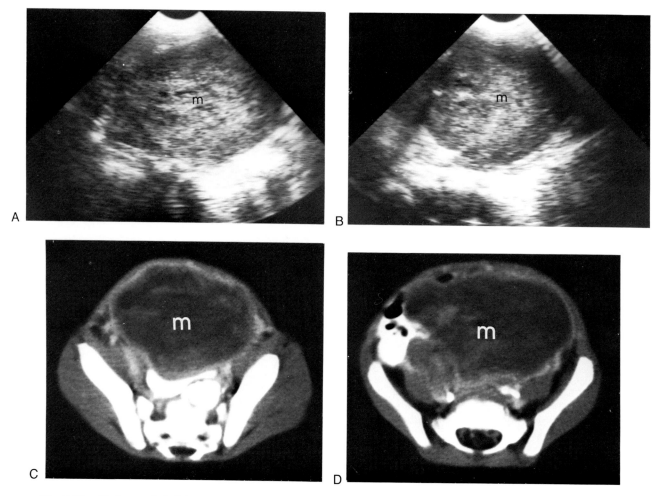

Fig. 5-66. Embryonal rhabdomyosarcoma. Large abdominal mass in 14-month-old male. **(A)** Longitudinal and **(B)** transverse scans of the abdomen reveal a solid, echodense mass *(m)* filling the entire lower abdomen. No anatomic structures are identified. **(C,D)** CT scans. The mass *(m)* appears to be low in density on CT and fills the entire lower abdomen.

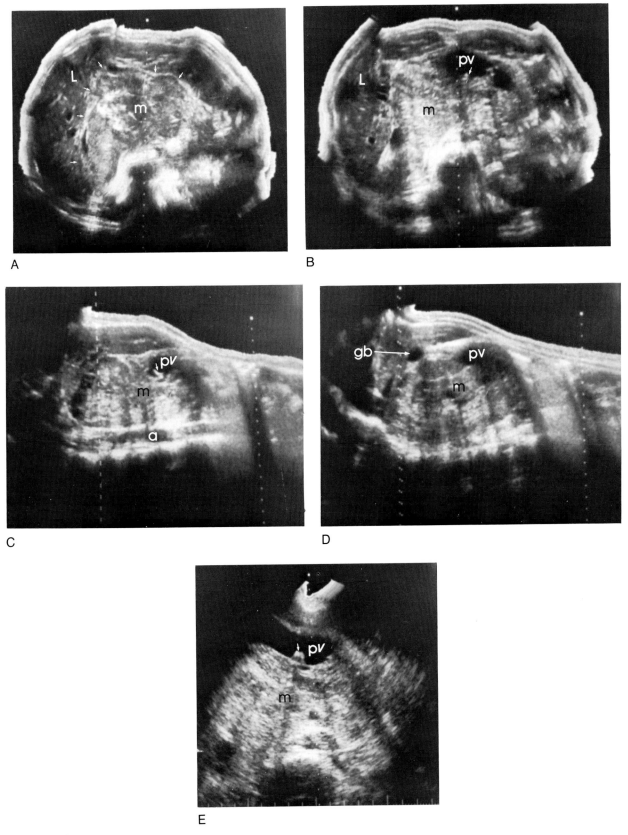

Fig. 5-67. Retroperitoneal paraganglioma. Transverse scans at 16 cm **(A)** and 10 cm **(B)** above the umbilicus and longitudinal scans in the midline **(C)** and 2 cm to the right of midline **(D)** demonstrate a large echodense prevertebral mass *(m)*. The portal vein *(pv)* appears dilated and located anterior to the mass on **(E)**, a cone-down transverse view. It contains an echodense tumor nodule (arrows) **(B,C,E)** that moved on real-time scan but was attached to the wall of the portal vein. This patient had metastases to the liver, lung, and portal vein. (*gb*, gallbladder; *a*, aorta; *L*, liver.)

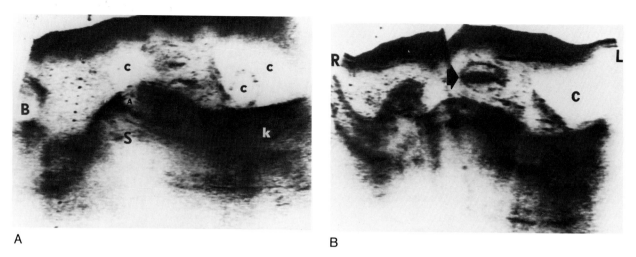

Fig. 5-68. Teratoma. **(A)** Oblique scan from the pelvis at the level of the bladder *(B)* to the left upper quadrant over the left kidney *(k)*. Excellent acoustic enhancement is noted behind the entire amorphous mass. The full length of the mass is well appreciated on the scan. *(S, spine; A, aorta; C, cyst.)* **(B)** 45° oblique scan from the right side of the pelvis *(R)* to the left upper quadrant *(L)*. The mass (arrow) is seen with a ringlike reflective perimeter and an ovoid hyperechoic center which represents a fatty mass within the cyst *(C)*. (From Weinstein BJ, Lenkey JL, Williams S: Ultrasound and CT demonstration of a benign cystic teratoma arising from the retroperitoneum. AJR 133:936, © Am Roent Ray Soc, 1979.)

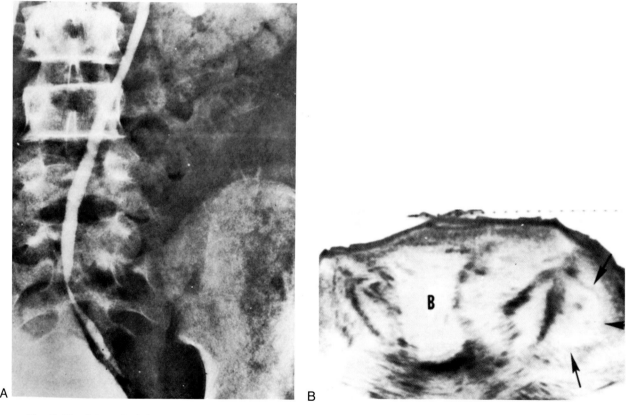

Fig. 5-69. Musculoskeletal tumor. Ewing's sarcoma of the iliac crest. **(A)** Intravenous pyelogram demonstrating a permeative destructive process of the left iliac bone with considerable mass effect on the left ureter and urinary bladder. **(B)** Transverse scan showing a huge intrapelvic mass displacing the bladder *(B)*. Note smaller extrapelvic component (arrows). (From deSantos LA, Goldstein HM: Ultrasonography in tumors arising from the spine and bony pelvis. Am J Roentgenol 129:1061, © American Roentgen Ray Society, 1977.)

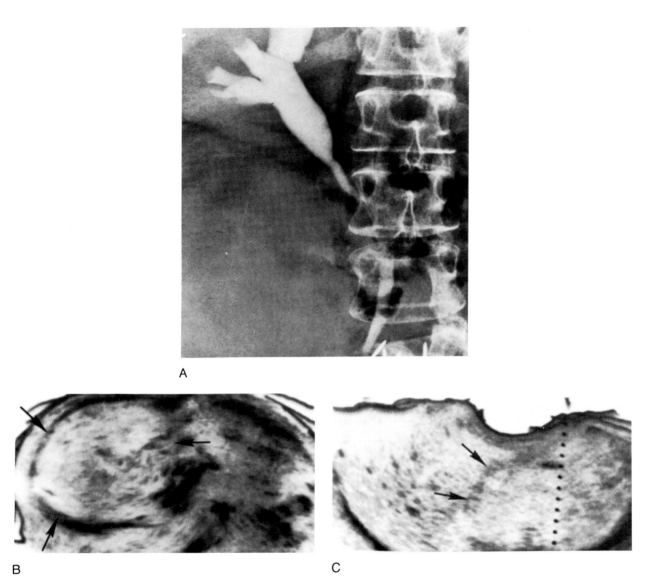

A

B   C

Fig. 5-70. Musculoskeletal tumor. Giant cell tumor of the fifth lumbar vertebra. **(A)** Intravenous urogram demonstrating destructive bony changes and a large soft tissue mass. Note upward rotation of the kidney and marked medial displacement of the right ureter. **(B)** Transverse scan 1 cm below the umbilicus defining a large intraabdominal mass on the right (arrows). **(C)** Longitudinal scan 8 cm to the right of midline. A large mass is seen extending to the right hepatic margin. The interface at the mass-liver junction (arrows) indicates an extrahepatic location of the mass. (From deSantos LA, Goldstein HM: Ultrasonography in tumors arising from the spine and bony pelvis. Am J Roentgenol 129:1061, © American Roentgen Ray Society, 1977.)

Neurogenic tumors are common in the paravertebral region where they arise from nerve roots or sympathetic chain ganglia (Fig. 5-67). Generally, retroperitoneal tumors are rapidly growing; the larger tumors are more likely to show evidence of necrosis and hemorrhage. The concurrence of the mass and ascites indicates invasion of the peritoneal surface.[1]

Teratomas are usually differentiated tumors containing tissues from the three germ layers. Most occur in the vicinity of the upper pole of the left kidney. The retro-peritoneal space is the fourth most frequent site of origin; they most commonly occur in the ovaries, testes, anterior mediastinum, retroperitoneum, and sacrococcygeal region.[79,80] The incidence of malignancy is 6 to 10 percent (90% benign) with 50 percent occurring in the pediatric age group.[79,80] Teratomas are characteristically heterogeneously mixed with solid areas, calcification, and cystic spaces[1,79] (Fig. 5-68). They can appear cystic.[80]

Some musculoskeletal tumors frequently have a soft tissue component in association with the bony abnor-

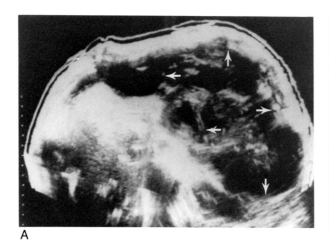
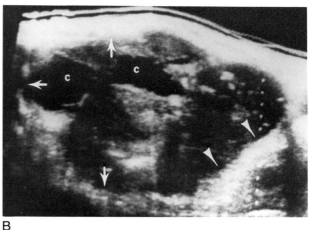

A   B

Fig. 5-71. Hemangiopericytoma. **(A)** Transverse scan at 3 cm inferior to the xyphoid. A large mixed solid and cystic mass is seen occupying the entire left abdomen (arrows). **(B)** Longitudinal scan at 4 cm to left of midline. A mixed solid and cystic mass (arrows) is seen extending into the left iliac fossa (arrowheads). Note internal cystic region with ragged border *(C)*. (From Grant EG, Gromvall S, Sarosi TE, et al: Sonographic findings in four cases of hemangiopericytoma: correlation with computed tomographic, angiographic, and pathologic findings. Radiology 142:447, 1982.)

mality. These include sacrococcygeal teratoma, giant cell tumor, and Ewing's sarcoma.[81] In Ewing's sarcoma, there is an extraosseous component in 90 percent of cases.[81] Ultrasound can be useful in evaluation of such pelvic and abdominal soft tissue masses (Figs. 5-69 and 5-70). This helps in assessment of the extent of disease, radiation planning, and the follow-up.[81]

Hemangiopericytomas are unusual vascular neoplasms that arise from the pericytes of Zimmermann.

These cells are found in close apposition to capillaries and are thought to have some contractile capabilities. These lesions can occur anywhere in the body but are most common in the lower extremity and pelvic retroperitoneum. The peak incidence is in the fifth to sixth decades with equal sex distribution.[82] The majority are said to be benign with a high 5-year-survival rate.[82] The signs and symptoms are insidious so that the mass is quite large before symptoms present.

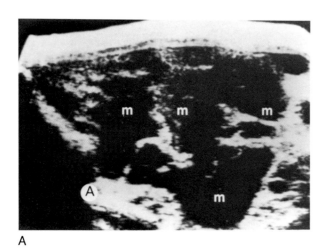
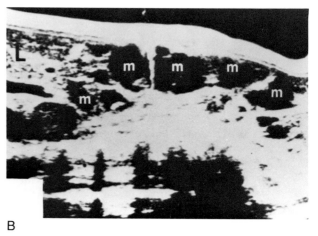

A   B

Fig. 5-72. Lymphangiomyomatosis. **(A)** Transverse sonogram of the true pelvis showing multiple cystic masses *(m)*. **(B)** Longitudinal parasagittal section through the liver *(L)* at the level of the inferior vena cava showing multiple masses *(m)* extending from the interior portion of the liver to the true pelvis. Note the thick septae between the masses. Some masses are anechoic while others have low level echoes within them. (From Walsh J; Taylor KJW, Rosenfield AT: Gray-scale ultrasonography in retroperitoneal lymphangiomyomatosis. Am J Roentgenol 129:1101, © Am Roent Ray Soc, 1977.)

The ultrasound pattern of hemangiopericytomas may be varied. One may see a well-defined predominatedly cystic mass, a mixed solid and cystic mass, or a solid mass with acoustic shadowing[82] (Fig. 5-71). Ultrasound can be used to define the limits of the mass and to offer a way to follow the mass while the patient is undergoing therapy.[82]

Lymphangiomyomatosis is a rare tumor-like condition characterized by smooth muscle proliferation involving the major lymphatic trunks in the mediastinum and retroperitoneum, lymph nodes in these areas, and lymphatics. It is an uncommon myoproliferative disorder confined to females of reproductive age. The lesion consists of one or more nodules of tumor-like proliferation of smooth muscle fascicles divided from each other by lymph channels. The smooth muscle meshwork involves the walls of preexisting lymphatic channels and replaces sinusoids of lymph nodes. Lymphatic obstruc-

tion leads to distended collateral vessels and small and large lymph cysts. Ultrasound demonstrates cystic structures of varying size lying along the course of the aorta and inferior vena cava (Fig. 5-72). The cyst walls are thick and often continuous with the walls of the nearby cyst, giving a septated appearance. There are low-level internal echoes.[83]

Abdominal lipoblastomatosis is a rare benign tumor of embryonal adipose tissue.[84] The majority of these tumors are found superficially in the upper and lower extremities and are occasionally found in the neck, trunk, mediastinum, and retroperitoneum. Ninety percent occur in infants less than 3 years of age. The tumor consists of lobules of immature adipose tissue with myxoid stroma separated by richly vascularized connective tissue septa. Ultrasound has delineated a myxoid mass embedded within highly echogenic fat[84] (Fig. 5-73).

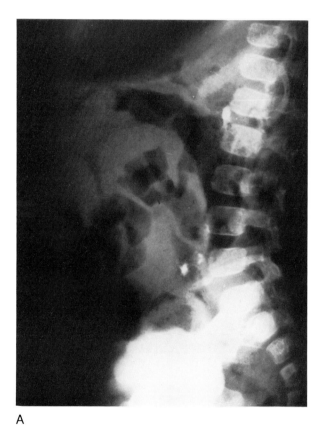

A

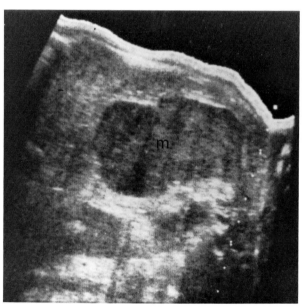

B

Fig. 5-73. Lipoblastomatosis. Case 1. **(A)** Lateral view of the abdomen during excretory urography. An apparently bilobed mass is seen inferior to the right kidney surrounded by a lucent rim of fat. The difference between the fatty and solid tumor tissue is accentuated by total body opacification. There is a small amount of residual barium anterior to L-5. **(B)** Longitudinal scan. There is clear differentiation in echogenicity between the central myxoid masses *(m)* and the adjacent fat. *(Figure continues.)*

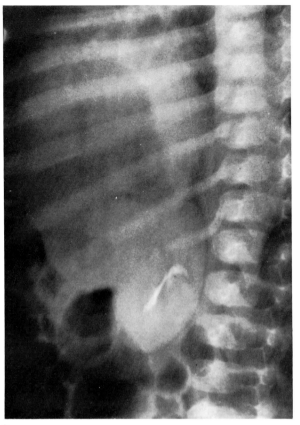

C

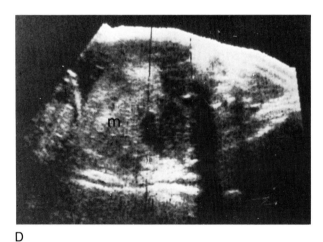

D

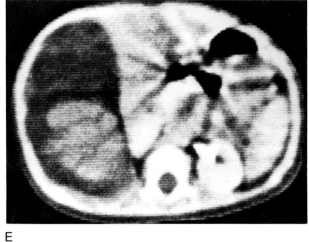

E

Fig. 5-73 *(Continued).* Case 2. **(C)** Right posterior oblique 10-minute radiograph from an excretory urogram. The intact right kidney is displaced caudally by an avascular radiolucent mass in the right upper quadrant. **(D)** Longitudinal scan demonstrating a large highly echogenic mass of fatty tissue *(m)* with a smaller hypoechoic mass of myxoid tissue inferiorly. **(E)** CT scan 5.3 cm below the xyphoid. A large fat-containing mass is seen in the right abdomen, within which is a smaller, denser area subsequently shown to be myxoid tissue. The lateral border of the right lobe of the liver is markedly displaced but was separate from the tumor. (From Fisher MF, Fletcher BD, Dahms BB, et al: Abdominal lipoblastomatosis: radiographic, echographic and computed tomographic findings. Radiology 138:593, 1981.)

REFERENCES

1. Koenigsberg M, Hoffman JC, Schnur MJ: Sonographic evaluation of the retroperitoneum. p. 79. In Raymond HW, Zwiebel WJ (eds): Seminars in Ultrasound. Vol. 3. Grune and Stratton, New York, 1982
2. Yeh H-C: Ultrasound and CT of the adrenals. p. 97. In Raymond HW, Zwiebel WJ (eds): Seminars in Ultrasound. Vol. 3. Grune and Stratton, New York, 1982
3. Sample WF: Adrenal ultrasonography. Radiology 127:461, 1978
4. Sample WF: A new technique for evaluation of the adrenal gland with gray scale ultrasonography. Radiology 124:463, 1977

5. Yeh H-C: Adrenal sonography. p. 101. In Leopold GR (ed): Clinics in Diagnostic Ultrasound: Ultrasound in Breast and Endocrine Disease. Churchill Livingstone, New York, 1984
6. Goldberg BB, Pollack HM, Bancks NH: Retroperitoneum. p. 188. In Resnick MI, Sanders RC (eds): Ultrasound in Urology. Williams and Wilkins, Baltimore, 1979
7. Gunther RW, Kelbel C, Lenner V: Real-time ultrasound of normal adrenal glands and small tumors. J Clin Ultrasound 12:211, 1984
8. Ritchie WGM: Sonographic demonstration of abdominal visceral lymph node enlargement. AJR 138:517, 1982
9. Pardes JG, Kazam E, Kneelard JB et al: Sonography of the retroperitoneum: value of the oblique coronal view. Proceedings of the American Institute of Ultrasound in Medicine. J Ultrasound Med 2:3, 1983
10. Callen PW, Filly RA, Sarti DA, et al: Ultrasonography of the diaphragmatic crura. Radiology 130:721, 1979
11. Bernardino ME, Goldstein HM, Green B: Gray scale ultrasonography of adrenal neoplasm. AJR 130:741, 1978
12. Yeh H-C, Mitty HA, Rose J et al: Ultrasonography of adrenal masses: usual features. Radiology 127:467, 1978
13. Ghorashi B, Holmes JH: Gray scale sonography appearance of an adrenal mass: a case report. J Clin Ultrasound 4:121, 1976
14. Sample WF: Ultrasonography of the adrenal gland. p. 73. In Resnick MI, Sanders RC (eds): Ultrasound in Urology. Williams and Wilkins, Baltimore, 1979
15. Oppenheimer DA, Carroll BA, Yousem S: Sonography of the normal neonatal adrenal gland. Radiology 146:157, 1983
16. Silverman PM, Carroll BA, Moskowitz PS: Adrenal sonography in renal agenesis and dysplasia. AJR 134:600, 1980
17. Sample WF, Sarti DA: Computed body tomography and gray scale ultrasonography: anatomic correlation and pitfalls in the upper abdomen. Gastrointest Radiol 3:243, 1978
18. Callen PW, Filly RA, Marks WM: The quadratus lumborum muscle: a possible source of confusion in sonographic evaluation of the retroperitoneum. J Clin Ultrasound 7:349, 1979
19. Gore RM, Callen PW, Filly RA: Displaced retroperitoneal fat: sonographic guide to right upper quadrant mass localization. Radiology 142:701, 1982
20. Graif M, Manor A, Itzchak Y: Sonographic differentiation of extra- and intrahepatic masses. AJR 141:553, 1983
21. Yeh H-C, Mitty HA, Rose J et al: Ultrasonography of adrenal masses: Unusual manifestation. Radiology 127:475, 1978
22. Scheible W, Coel M, Siemers PT, Siegel H: Percutaneous aspiration of adrenal cysts. Am J Roentgenol 128: 1013, 1977
23. Pery M, Kaftori JK, Bar-Maor JA: Sonography for diagnosis and follow-up of neonatal adrenal hemorrhage. J Clin Ultrasound 9:397, 1981
24. Mittelstaedt CA, Volberg FM, Merten DF, Brill PW: The sonographic diagnosis of neonatal adrenal hemorrhage. Radiology 131:453, 1979
25. Mineau DE, Koehler PR: Ultrasound diagnosis of neonatal adrenal hemorrhage. AJR 132:443, 1979
26. Robbins SL, Cotran RS: The endocrine system—adrenal cortex p. 1387. In Pathologic Basis of Disease. W.B. Saunders, Philadelphia, 1979
27. Behan M, Martin EC, Muecke EC, Kazam E: Myelolipoma of the adrenal: two cases with ultrasound and CT findings. Am J Roentgenol 129:993, 1977
28. Vick CW, Zeman RK, Mannes E, et al: Adrenal myelolipoma: CT and ultrasound findings. Urol Radiol 6:7 1984
29. Bowerman RA, Silver TM, Jaffee MH, et al: Sonography of adrenal pheochromocytomas. AJR 137:1227, 1981
30. Robbins SL, Cotran RS: The endocrine system: Adrenal medulla p. 1402. In Pathologic Basis of Disease. W.B. Saunders, Philadelphia, 1979
31. Jasinski RW, Samuels BI, Silver TM: Sonographic features of retroperitoneal ganglioneuroma. J Ultrasound Med 3:413, 1984
32. White SJ, Stuck KJ, Blane CE, Silver TM: Sonography of neuroblastoma. AJR 141:465, 1983
33. Berger PE, Kuhn JP, Munschauer RW: Computed tomography and ultrasound in the diagnosis and management of neuroblastoma. Radiology 128:663, 1978
34. Crade M, Taylor KJW, Rosenfield AT: Discovery of an adrenal tumor by ultrasound: case report. J Clin Ultrasound 6:191, 1978
35. Cunninghan JJ: Ultrasonic findings in "primary" lymphoma of the adrenal area. J Ultrasound Med 2:467, 1983
36. Antoniou A, Spetseropoulos J, Vlahos L, Pontifex G: The sonographic appearance of adrenal involvement in non-Hodgkin's lymphoma. J Ultrasound Med 2:235, 1983
37. Forsythe JR, Gosink BB, Leopold GR: Ultrasound in the evaluation of adrenal metastases. J Clin Ultrasound 5:31, 1977
38. Gooding GAW: Ultrasonic spectrum of adrenal masses. Urology 13:211, 1979
39. Abrams HL, Siegelman SS, Adams DF, et al: Computed tomography versus ultrasound of the adrenal gland: a prospective study. Radiology 143:121, 1982
40. Sample WF, Sarti DA: Computed tomography and gray scale ultrasonography of the adrenal gland: a comparative study. Radiology 128:377, 1978
41. Gerzof SG: The role of ultrasound in the search for intraabdominal and retroperitoneal abscesses. p. 101. In Taylor KJW, Viscomi GN (eds): Clinics in Diagnostic Ultrasound: Ultrasound in Emergency Medicine. Churchill Livingstone, New York, 1981
42. Wicks JD, Silver TM, Thornbury JR: Complementary use of radiography, ultrasonography and gallium-67 scintigraphy in the diagnosis of a retroperitoneal abscess. Urol Radiol 1:25, 1979
43. Kumari S, Pillari G, Phillips G, Pochaczevsky R: Fluid collections of the psoas in children. p. 139. In Raymond HW, Zwiebel WJ (eds): Seminars in Ultrasound Vol. 3. Grune and Stratton, New York, 1982
44. Laing FC, Jacobs RP: Value of ultrasonography in the detection of retroperitoneal inflammatory masses. Radiology 123:169, 1977
45. Gerzof SG, Gale ME: Computed tomography and ultraso-

nography for diagnosis and treatment of renal and retroperitoneal abscess. Urol Clinic No Am 9:185, 1982

46. Shirkhoda A, Mauro MA, Staab EV, Blatt PM: Soft-tissue hemorrhage in hemophiliac patients: computed tomography and ultrasound study. Radiology 147:811, 1983

47. Kumari S, Fulco JD, Karayalcin G, Lipton R: Gray scale ultrasound: Evaluation of iliopsoas hematoma in hemophiliacs. AJR 133:103, 1979

48. Fagan CJ, Amparo EG, Davis M: Retroperitoneal fibrosis. p. 123. In Raymond HW, Zwiebel WJ (eds): Seminars In Ultrasound. Vol. 3. Grune and Stratton, New York, 1982

49. Fagan CJ, Larrieu AJ, Amparao EG: Retroperitoneal fibrosis: ultrasound and CT features. AJR 133:239, 1979

50. Sanders RC, Duffy T, McLoughlin MG, Walsh PC: Sonography in the diagnosis of retroperitoneal fibrosis. J Urol 118:944, 1977

51. Center S, Schwab R, Goldberg BB: The value of ultrasonography as an aid in the treatment of idiopathic retroperitoneal fibrosis. J Ultrasound Med 1:87, 1982

52. Jacobson JB, Redman HC: Ultrasound findings in a case of retroperitoneal fibrosis. Radiology 113:423, 1974

53. Bowie JD, Bernstein JR: Retroperitoneal fibrosis: Ultrasound findings and case report. J Clin Ultrasound 4:435, 1976

54. Fried AM, Williams CB, Litvak AS: High retroperitoneal lymphocele: unusual clinical presentation and diagnosis by ultrasonography. J Urol 123:583, 1980

55. Spring DB, Schroeder D, Babu S, et al: Ultrasonic evaluation of lymphocele formation after staging lymphadenectomy for prostatic carcinoma. Radiology 141:479, 1981

56. Doust BD, Thompson R: Ultrasonography of abdominal fluid collections. Gastrointest Radiol 3:273, 1978

57. Robbins SL, Cotran RS: Lymph nodes and spleen. p. 757. In Pathologic Basis of Disease. W.B. Saunders, Philadelphia, 1979

58. Carroll BA, Ta HN: The ultrasound appearance of extranodal abdominal lymphoma. Radiology 136:419, 1980

59. Carroll BA: Ultrasound of lymphoma. p. 114. In Raymond HW, Zwiebel WJ (eds): Seminars in Ultrasound. Vol. 3. Grune and Stratton, New York, 1982

60. Carroll BA: Lymphoma. p. 52. In Goldberg BB, (ed): Clinics in Diagnostic Ultrasound: Ultrasound in Cancer. Churchill Livingstone, New York, 1981

61. Rochester D, Bowie JD, Kunzmann A, Lester E: Ultrasound in the staging of lymphoma. Radiology 124:483, 1977

62. Brascho DJ, Durant JR, Green LE: The accuracy of retroperitoneal ultrasonography in Hodgkin's disease and non-Hodgkin's lymphoma. Radiology 125:485, 1977

63. Kaude JV, Joyce PH: Evaluation of abdominal lymphoma by ultrasound. Gastrointest Radiol 5:249, 1980

64. Asher WM, Friemanis AK: Echographic diagnosis of retroperitoneal lymph node enlargement. Am J Roentgenol 105:438, 1969

65. Neiman HL: Retroperitoneum. p. 90. In Goldberg BB (ed): Clinics in Diagnostic Ultrasound: Ultrasound in Cancer. Churchill Livingstone, New York, 1981

66. Kobayashi T, Takatani O, Kimura K: Echographic pat-

terns of malignant lymphoma. J Clin Ultrasound 4:181, 1976

67. Leopold GR: A review of retroperitoneal ultrasonography. J Clin Ultrasound 1:82, 1973

68. Creed H, Reger K, Pond GD, Aapro M: Potential pitfall in CT and sonographic evaluation of suspected lymphoma. AJR 139:606, 1982

69. Schnur MJ, Hoffman JC, Koenigsberg M: Gray scale ultrasonic demonstration of peripancreatic adenopathy. J Ultrasound Med 1:139, 1982

70. Mueller PR, Ferrucci JT Jr, Harbin WP, et al: Appearance of lymphomatous involvement of the mesentery by ultrasonography and body computed tomography: the "sandwich sign". Radiology 134:467, 1980

71. Dunnick NR, Reaman GH, Head GL, et al: Radiologic manifestation of Burkitt's lymphoma in American patient. AJR 132:1, 1979

72. Shawker TH, Dannick NR, Head GL, Magrath IT: Ultrasound evaluation of American Burkitt's lymphoma. J Clin Ultrasound 7:279, 1979

73. Hillman BJ, Haber K: Echographic characteristics of malignant lymph nodes. J Clin Ultrasound 8:213, 1980

74. Zornoza J, Jonsson K, Wallace S, Lukeman JM: Fine needle aspiration biopsy of retroperitoneal lymph node and abdominal masses: an updated report. Radiology 125:87, 1977

75. Zornoza J, Cabranillas FF, Altoff TM, et al: Percutaneous needle biopsy in abdominal lymphoma. AJR 136:97, 1981

76. Neumann CH, Robert NJ, Rosenthal D, Canellos G: Clinical value of ultrasonography for the management of non-Hodgkin's lymphoma patients as compared with abdominal computed tomography. J Comput Assist Tomogr 7:666, 1983

77. Chung W-M, Ting YM, Gagliardi RA: Ultrasonic diagnosis of retroperitoneal liposarcoma. J Clin Ultrasound 6:266, 1978

78. Karp W, Hufstrom LO, Jonsson PE: Retroperitoneal sarcoma: ultrasonographic and angiographic evaluation. Brit J. Radiol 53:525, 1980

79. Aston JK: Ultrasound demonstration of retroperitoneal teratoma. J Clin Ultrasound 7:377, 1979

80. Weinstein BJ, Lenkey JL, Williams S: Ultrasound and CT demonstration of a benign cystic teratoma arising from the retroperitoneum. AJR 133:936, 1979

81. deSantos LA, Goldstein HM: Ultrasonography in tumors arising from the spine and bony pelvis. Am J Roentgenol 129:1061, 1977

82. Grant EG, Gromvall S, Sarosi TE, et al: Sonographic findings in four cases of hemangiopericytoma: correlation with computed tomographic, angiographic, and pathologic findings. Radiology 142:477, 1982

83. Walsh J, Taylor KJW, Rosenfield AT: Gray scale ultrasonography in retroperitoneal lymphangiomyomatosis. Am J Roentgenol 129:1101, 1977

84. Fisher MF, Fletcher BD, Dahms BB, et al: Abdominal lipoblastomatosis: radiographic, echographic and computed tomographic findings. Radiology 138:593, 1981

6

Vascular Ultrasound

The vascular system is ideally suited for ultrasound evaluation, especially with the high resolution real-time systems. The structures that make up the vascular system contain fluid. Thus, they are anechoic, making them easy to see with ultrasound. Many are pulsatile or change with respiration, another feature that can be studied with real-time ultrasound. This aspect of sonographic evaluation was not possible until recent years. By adding the study of motion to an evaluation of the vascular system, real-time scanning has broadened ultrasound's capability.

TECHNIQUE

Preparation

As with other ultrasound studies of the abdomen, it is beneficial to have the patient fast at least 8 hours prior to the study, because there is less bowel gas after fasting. However, a satisfactory study may be obtained without fasting, depending on the patient's body habitus.

Scan Technique

Although vascular studies may be performed on static systems, there is less information available than with real-time systems. The examiner can evaluate the pulsatile motion of the aorta and its branches with real-time ultrasound and look for moving intimal flaps if a dissection is questioned. In addition, the long axis of the aorta can be quickly identified, and true transverse scans of the aorta at 90° to the long axis can be easily obtained. It is difficult to quickly assess the long axis of the aorta and obtain true transverse scans of the aorta on static systems. On the other hand, static systems do have the advantage of showing a larger field of view than real-time systems. Many investigators use a combination of the two systems. Real-time ultrasound is used to evaluate motion of the aorta and obtain the long axis and true transverse axis. Then the scans are taken and photographed on the static system. Over the years, we have gone almost exclusively to real-time ultrasound for evaluation of the vascular system.

AORTA

To evaluate the aorta with ultrasound, several techniques have been employed. First, there is the supine technique. Using the real-time transducer, the long axis of the aorta is identified. This is usually just to the left of the midline. The axis of the aorta may parallel the left of the spine or it may be tortuous. Beginning at the level of the diaphragm, the aorta is studied and photographed. The transducer is slowly moved inferiorly on the aorta while maintaining the long axis. This may require rotating the scanhead slightly. In most cases in which the aorta is tortuous, it curves to the left; but, at times, it is tortuous to the right. Scans of the long axis of the aorta are obtained by overlapping consecutive scans (Fig. 6-1). The lumen and walls are evaluated. Once the aortic bifurcation is reached the axis of the transducer is altered so its long axis is between the umbilicus and inguinal region. This is for the purpose of obtaining views of

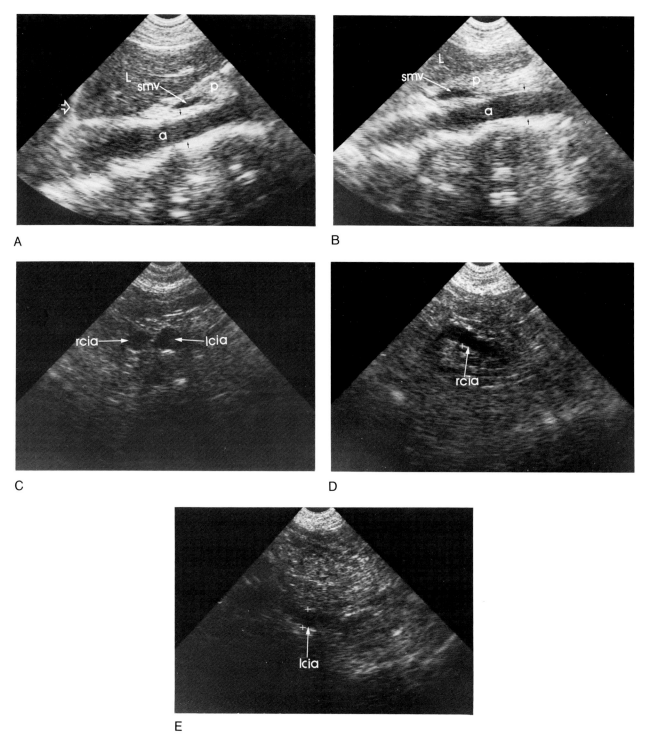

Fig. 6-1. Normal aorta and common iliac arteries. **(A,B)** Longitudinal (long axis) views of the normal aorta *(a)* are obtained. **(A)** is from a higher level in the abdomen than **(B)**. To obtain an anteroposterior measurement, the aorta is measured from outside to outside wall (arrows). (open arrows, diaphragm; *L*, liver; *smv*, superior mesenteric vein; *p*, pancreas.) Once the aortic bifurcation is reached transversely **(C)**, the axis of the transducer is angled such that the long axis **(D,E)** of each common iliac artery is obtained. Often, only a short segment is seen normally. To obtain an anteroposterior measurement, the iliac arteries are measured from outside wall to outside wall. (*rcia*, right common iliac artery; *lcia*, left common iliac artery.)

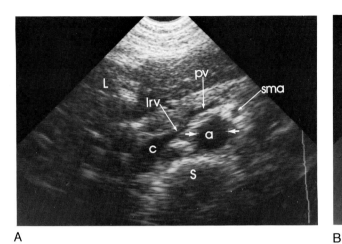 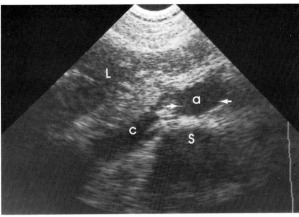

A B

Fig. 6-2. Normal aorta. (A) This is a transverse scan taken 90° to the long axis of the aorta *(a)*. Note that the transverse measurement (arrows) is smaller (1.6 cm) than in (B). (*c*, inferior vena cava; *pv*, portal vein; *lrv*, left renal vein; *sma*, superior mesenteric artery; *S*, spine; *L*, liver.) (B) This is an oblique transverse scan of the aorta *(a)* in (A) giving the aorta an apparently large transverse dimension (arrows) (2.2 cm). This would be the same effect as taking a straight transverse scan of a tortuous aorta. (*c*, inferior vena cava; *L*, liver; *S*, spine.)

both common iliac arteries (Fig. 6-1). Because a significant number of aortic aneurysms involve the iliacs, this should be part of the aortic evaluation. As with the aorta, long axis views of both iliacs are obtained and marked appropriately as to right or left.

To obtain true transverse views, the transducer must be rotated 90° to the long axis. If this is not done, and a straight transverse of the abdomen is obtained, the transverse section through the aorta will be artificially enlarged if the aorta is tortuous (Fig. 6-2). Instead of being a transverse section, it is an oblique view. True transverse sections are taken through the entire aorta, beginning at the diaphragm. These should be taken every 1 cm. Once the aortic bifurcation is reached, a true transverse section through each iliac should be obtained. Throughout the entire examination, the examiner should be assessing the motion of the aorta, identifying thrombus within the aorta, and looking for intimal flaps. In addition, the examiner should note if there are any paraortic masses.

Measurements of the aorta should be obtained in the anteroposterior plane as well as the transverse axis (Figs. 6-1 and 6-2). These are outside-to-outside wall measurements, which correlate best with surgery. The examiner should try to assess the longitudinal length of the aortic aneurysm. This may be difficult at times because the beginning of the aneurysm may not be identified. If at all possible, an attempt should be made to identify the level of the renal arteries. Although the majority (95 percent) of abdominal aneurysms are below the renal arteries, it is still beneficial to correctly identify the level.[1] The renal arteries may be best seen on a transverse view of the aorta

(Figs. 6-3 and 6-4). The examiner should identify the superior mesenteric artery, then the renal veins. At approximately that same level, the renal arteries should be seen as lateral branches of the aorta. The right renal artery passes posterior to the inferior vena cava while the left renal artery passes directly towards the kidney from the aorta (Figs. 6-3 and 6-4).

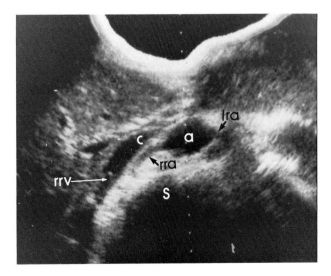

Fig. 6-3. Renal arteries. Transverse scan demonstrates the renal arteries, which are seen as lateral branches of the aorta *(a)*. (*rra*, right renal artery; *lra*, left renal artery; *c*, inferior vena cava; *rrv*, right renal vein; *S*, spine.)

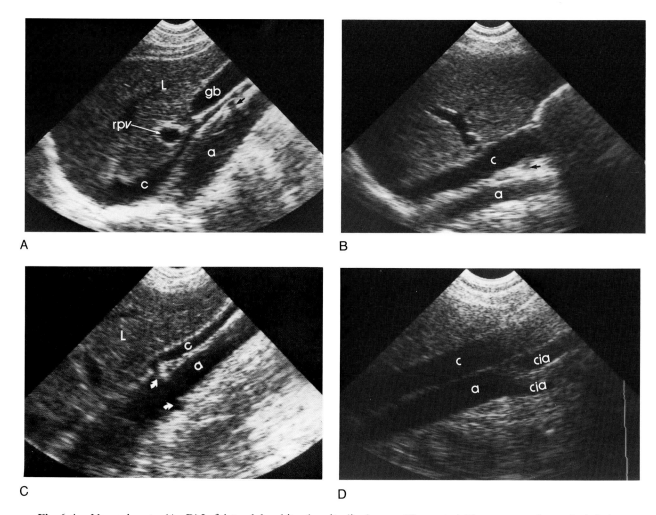

A

B

C

D

Fig. 6-4. Normal aorta. (A–D) Left lateral decubitus longitudinal scans. The aorta *(a)* is seen posterior to the inferior vena cava *(c)* in these projections. The right renal artery (arrow) is seen as a circular lucency posterior to the inferior vena cava on (A,B). On (C), the two renal arteries (arrows) can be seen. Unlike (B) where the bifurcation is "gassed out," the aortic bifurcation or common iliac arteries *(cia)* are seen on (D). (*L*, liver; *rpv*, right portal vein; *gb*, gallbladder.)

In some cases it may be beneficial to examine the patient in the left-lateral decubitus position or to scan coronally.[2] There may be bowel gas obscuring visualization of the aorta or the examiner may be handicapped by the patient's body habitus. With the patient in this decubitus position, the liver is used as an acoustic window and the exam is less limited by overlying bowel gas. This is also true for the coronal scan when one scans in the mid-axillary line with the patient in the supine position. The long axis of the aorta may be obtained by placing the transducer longitudinally on the patient's right flank. The aorta will be seen posterior to the inferior vena cava (Fig. 6-4). In 80 percent of patients, the renal arteries may be identified employing this technique.[1] This position is also often better for identification of the bifurcation of the aorta.[3] The patient can even be scanned in the right-lateral decubitus position, if the spleen is enlarged and can be used as an acoustic window.[3]

AORTIC BRANCHES

If specific branches of the aorta are being evaluated, the examiner should start the study with the origin at the aorta. With the celiac artery, one would begin with a transverse scan high in the abdomen (Fig. 6-5). The celiac artery immediately branches into the common hepatic, left gastric and splenic arteries. These too can be adequately identified in most cases. Measurements of size can be obtained both in the longitudinal and transverse plane. This is true for the superior mesenteric artery, and renal arteries (Figs. 6-3, 6-4C, and 6-5).

All examinations of the aorta should include as their endpoint the iliac bifurcation unless: (1) iliac enlargement is suspected by the clinician or detected by ultrasound and (2) the patient had an aortofemoral or aorto-iliac graft.[4] The iliac arteries descend posteriorly into the pelvis and often there is overlying bowel gas obscuring

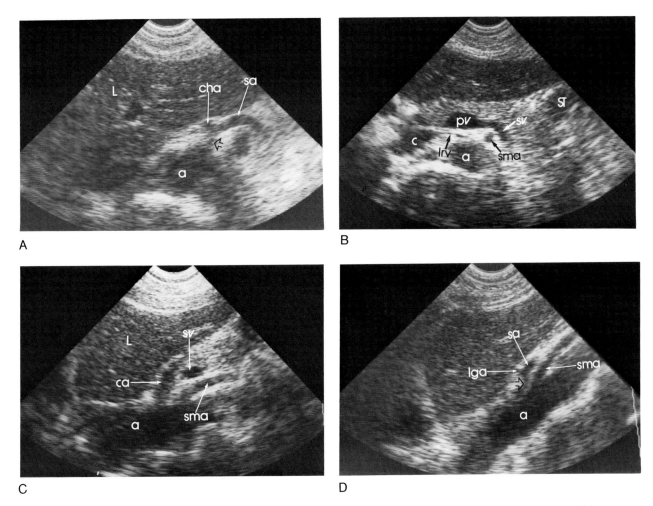

Fig. 6-5. Normal celiac and superior mesenteric arteries. **(A)** Transverse scan. The celiac artery (open arrow) is seen branching from the aorta *(a)* anteriorly. The common hepatic *(cha)* and splenic *(sa)* arteries are seen branching from the celiac artery. *(L,* liver) **(B)** Transverse scan at a lower level than **(A)**. The superior mesenteric artery *(sma)* is seen anterior to the aorta *(a)*. *(c,* inferior vena cava; *sv,* splenic vein; *pv,* portal vein; *lrv,* left renal vein; *ST,* stomach.) **(C,D)** Longitudinal scans. The celiac artery *(ca,* open arrow) is the first anterior branch of the abdominal aorta *(a)* with the superior mesenteric artery *(sma)* the second. *(lga,* left gastric artery; *sv,* splenic vein; *sa,* splenic artery; *L,* liver.)

their discrete margins (Figs. 6-1 and 6-4D). Graft limbs produce distinct echoes that facilitate delineation of vessel boundaries. Moderate to large aneurysms tend to displace bowel.

INFERIOR VENA CAVA

Like the aorta, the inferior vena cava can be evaluated in the supine or left-lateral decubitus positions. The scan of this structure should start at the diaphragm and slowly work down along the inferior vena cava until its origin in the iliacs is identified. The inferior vena cava should increase in caliber with a held breath or expiration, but should decrease in size with inspiration or the Valsalva maneuver. The wall should be thin and there should be no masses within the lumen (Figs. 6-4A and 6-4B; see

Fig. 6-6). The retrohepatic portion of the inferior vena cava is the easiest portion to see because the liver (as an acoustic window) is anterior (see Fig. 6-6A). The origin of the inferior vena cava is difficult to see because of bowel gas. It can be better visualized in the left lateral decubitus position[2] (Figs. 6-4A and 6-4B). In that position, it is sometimes easier to also evaluate for intraluminal thrombus or extrinsic compression.[2] Once the longitudinal views of the inferior vena cava are obtained, then the transverse scans can be produced.

INFERIOR VENA CAVA BRANCHES

Various branches of the inferior vena cava can be identified. The renal veins should be routinely identified (Figs. 6-3, 6-6C, and 6-6D). The left renal vein can be

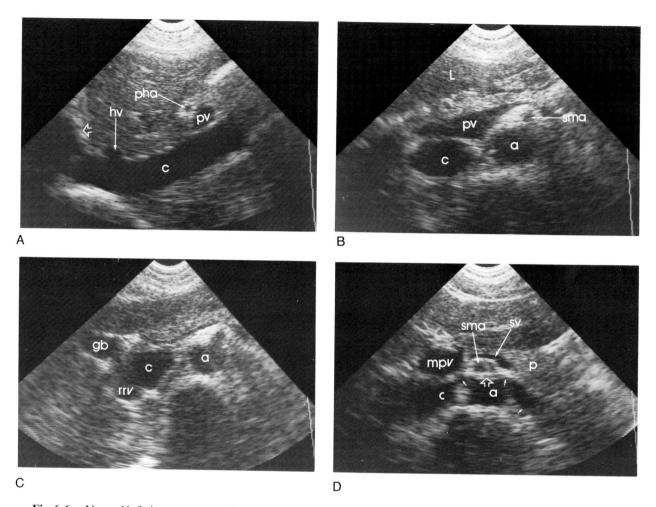

A

B

C

D

Fig. 6-6. Normal inferior vena cava and renal veins. **(A)** Longitudinal supine view of normal inferior vena cava *(c)*. It is seen as a tubular anechoic structure projecting anteriorly as it runs cephalad. (open arrow, diaphragm; *hv,* hepatic vein; *pv,* portal vein; *pha,* proper hepatic artery.) **(B)** Transverse supine view of the inferior vena cava *(c)*. (*a,* aorta; *pv,* portal vein; *sma,* superior mesenteric artery; *L,* liver.) **(C)** Transverse scan of right renal vein. The vein *(rrv)* is seen extending from the inferior vena cava *(c)* toward the renal hilum. (*a,* aorta; *gb,* gallbladder.) **(D)** Transverse scan of the left renal vein (arrows) shows it extending from the inferior vena cava *(c)* to the left renal hilum, between the superior mesenteric artery *(sma)* and the aorta *(a)*. It appears compressed (open arrow) between these two. (*mpv,* main portal vein; *sv,* splenic vein; *p,* pancreas.)

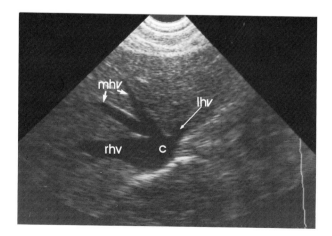

Fig. 6-7. Normal hepatic veins. High transverse scan. The right *(rhv)*, middle *(mhv)*, and left *(lhv)* are seen draining into the inferior vena cava *(c)*. There are two middle hepatic veins in this person.

seen posterior to the superior mesenteric artery and anterior to the aorta on a transverse view (Figs. 6-5B and 6-6D). The right renal vein can be seen just to the right of the inferior vena cava at the level of the renal hilum (Figs. 6-3 and 6-6C). The hepatic veins can also be identified as they drain the liver into the inferior vena cava. They are best identified on a high transverse view through the inferior vena cava and liver. The right, middle, and left hepatic branches should be seen (Fig. 6-7). (For more in-depth discussion of the hepatic veins, see Chapter 1.)

NORMAL ANATOMY

Aorta

The aorta is normally seen as an anechoic, pulsatile, tubular structure anterior to the left portion of the spine. Its long axis is usually posterior (superiorly) and anterior (inferiorly) (Fig. 6-1). Both walls appear to pulsate on real-time ultrasound. Its anteroposterior dimension is on the average 2 cm at the level of the diaphragm and decreases to 1.5 cm at the bifurcation (Fig. 6-1). It is considered abnormal in size if its dimension exceeds 3 cm and/or there is a localized dilatation of the lumen. On transverse sections, the aortic lumen is usually round with its width greater than its anteroposterior dimension (Fig. 6-2).

Aortic Branches

The aortic branches can be readily identified with real-time ultrasound (Fig. 6-8). The celiac artery, the first abdominal anterior branch, is seen exiting from the aorta and immediately branching into the common hepatic, left gastric, and splenic arteries (Fig. 6-5). These should be routinely identified on a transverse scan. The superior mesenteric artery, the second anterior branch, is best seen on a transverse scan below the level of the celiac artery (Fig. 6-5). It is seen anterior to the aorta and posterior to the body of the pancreas. On a longitudinal view it can be seen leaving the aorta as the second branch. The mean luminal measurement of the superior mesenteric artery is 7 mm.[5] The distance between the anterior wall of the aorta and the posterior wall of the superior mesenteric artery is usually no more than 11 mm.[5] The renal arteries can be seen as lateral branches of the aorta (Figs. 6-3 and 6-4). The left renal artery goes directly to the left of the aorta to the renal hilum (Fig. 6-3). The right renal artery is seen posterior to the inferior vena cava (Fig. 6-3). It can be seen on transverse or longitudinal scans. On a longitudinal scan of the inferior vena cava, the right renal artery can be seen as a small anechoic structure posteriorly (Fig. 6-4).

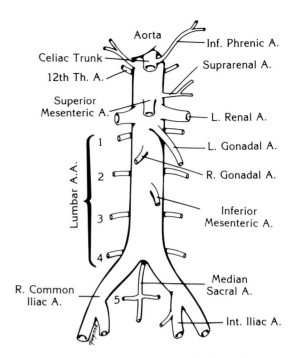

Fig. 6-8. Abdominal aorta and its branches.

Inferior Vena Cava

The inferior vena cava carries blood from the body below the diaphragm into the right atrium. It is formed to the right of the fifth lumbar vertebra by the junction of the two common iliac veins. Its longitudinal axis is anterior (superiorly) and posterior (inferiorly) (Fig. 6-7). It is related posteriorly to the right psoas muscle, right renal artery, right crus of the diaphragm, and the medial portion of the right adrenal gland. The head of the pancreas and second portion of the duodenum are located anterior to this structure. Branches include not only the two common iliacs, but also the lumbar veins (four on each side), gonadal veins, renal veins, right suprarenal and inferior phrenic veins, and hepatic veins.[6]

The inferior vena cava varies in its caliber. It is considered dilated if it is greater than 3.7 cm.[7] With inspiration and the Valsalva maneuver, it decreases in size (Figs. 6-9A and B), although in 50 percent of females in a study there was no decrease. With expiration, and maximum held inspiration, it normally increases in size[8] (Figs. 6-9C and D). The changes in caliber of the inferior vena cava are attributed to variations in blood flowing through the inferior vena cava in accordance with respiration and cardiac cycles. In inspiration, blood literally is sucked into the chest by negative pressure causing the vessel to collapse. Flow is high but pressure is decreased. During expiration and breath holding, the reverse is true; this causes ballooning of the inferior vena cava (Fig. 6-9C). With the Valsalva maneuver, the abdominal

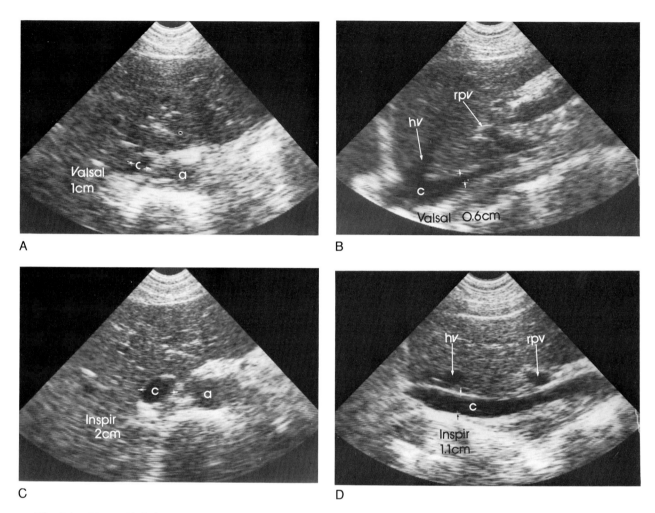

Fig. 6-9. Normal inferior vena cava. The inferior vena cava *(c)* is noted to be smaller in caliber on transverse (**A**) and longitudinal (**B**) scans with the Valsalva maneuver than with held inspiration on (**C**) and (**D**). (*a*, aorta; *hv*, hepatic vein; *rpv*, right portal vein.)

pressure is sufficient enough to force blood out of the inferior vena cava into the thorax.[8]

Inferior Vena Cava Branches

The inferior vena cava has numerous branches or tributaries (Fig. 6-10). Some are visualized with ultrasound; others are not seen. The right gonadal vein is seen lateral and below the level of the right renal vein. The left gonadal vein drains directly into the left renal vein (Fig. 6-11). The right renal vein and the right gonadal vein are best seen on the left lateral decubitus view using the kidney as a window. The right renal artery is posterior to the inferior vena cava and the right renal vein is seen anteriorly (Fig. 6-3). As the left renal vein courses between the aorta and superior mesenteric artery, it may be somewhat compressed over the aorta, resulting in the left

renal vein being larger near the renal hilum than the inferior vena cava[7,9] (Fig. 6-11). The left renal vein is considered distended only if the diameter lateral to the aorta is 50 percent greater than the diameter of the part directly in front of the aorta.[9] If the distance between the aorta and the superior mesenteric artery is 15 mm or less, then the left renal vein often appears distended.[9] The left renal vein may be dilated with portal venous hypertension owing to the development of gastrorenal or splenorenal collaterals.

The ascending lumbar veins are the abdominal analogues of the azygos-hemiazygos system and are branches of the common iliac veins (Figs. 6-12 and 6-13). The lumbar veins connect to the ascending lumbar vein, which ascends posterior to the psoas muscle, lateral to the spine and anterior to the transverse process (Fig. 6-13). Having passed deep to the crus, the veins ascend in the thorax as the azygous and hemiazygos.[6]

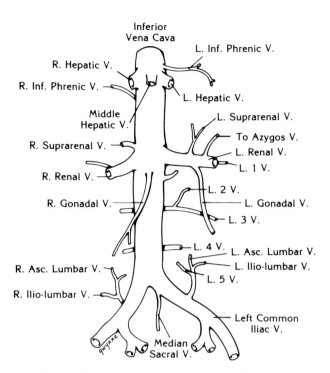

Fig. 6-10. Inferior vena cava and its tributaries.

The demonstration of a dilated right ascending lumbar vein at ultrasound may be a valuable indicator of congenital absence of the inferior vena cava. In cases of infrahepatic interruption of the inferior vena cava, the azygos vein, the cephalad continuation of the right lumbar vein, may be so enlarged as to present as a mediastinal mass. Other conditions causing compression or obstruction of the inferior vena cava would result in divergence of blood through the prevertebral venous system and will be apparrent on ultrasound.[10] As an important part of the abdominal prevertebral anastomotic network, the right ascending lumbar vein appears on ultrasound in 70 percent of patients as an anechoic tubular structure lying dorsal and parallel to the inferior vena cava in front of the roots of the transverse process of the lumbar vertebrae[6] (Fig. 6-13). It is seen between the aorta and inferior vena cava on a transverse scan; it is posterior to the right renal artery. Its mean diameter is 2.0 mm ± 0.8 (standard deviation). The normal lumbar veins, right adrenal vein and phrenic vein are not seen at ultrasound.[6]

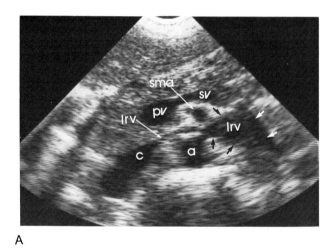

A

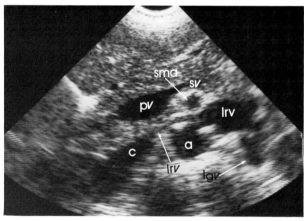

B

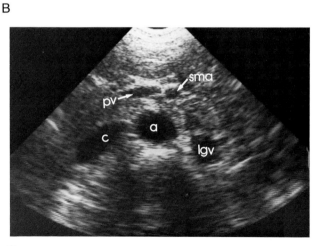

C

Fig. 6-11. Normal left renal vein. Transverse scans (A,B). The left renal vein (lrv) is seen passing between the superior mesenteric artery (sma) and aorta (a). It appears slightly dilated (arrows) just lateral to the aorta. The left gonadal vein (lgv) is seen draining into the left renal vein. (c, inferior vena cava; pv, portal vein; sv, splenic vein) (C) Transverse scan below level of (B). The left gonadal vein (lgv) is seen to the right of the aorta (a). (c, inferior vena cava; sma, superior mesenteric artery; pv, portal vein.)

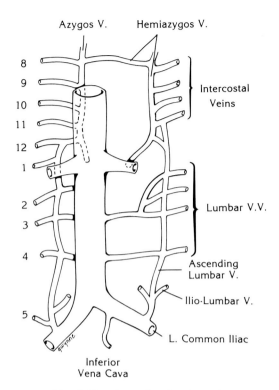

Fig. 6-12. Ascending lumbar vein.

Intravascular Echoes

There have been several explanations proposed for the mechanism of production of the echogenic particles seen in flowing blood at ultrasound. These echogenic particles are seen in the venous structures of the abdomen but not the arteries (Fig. 6-14).

Some investigators have felt these were due to red cell aggregation.[11] In one experiment, it was found there must be fibrinogen or its products plus red blood cells present to produce the echogenicity present. The echogenicity of blood during stasis that was detectable with real-time ultrasound was probably related to the physical layering of blood products. The disappearence of the reflective echoes was noted with agitation, suggesting that the layering effect was disrupted.[12] Some feel the echoes are simply produced by the red blood cells.[13] A red cell aggregation mechanism for blood-flow echogenicity would explain the increase prominence of internal echoes in lower shear rate venous blood flow compared with those of higher shear rate arterial blood flow.[14,15]

Others feel that interfaces between different fluids within a physiological range seem adequate to account for these intraluminal echoes. Laminar-flow echoes are seen downstream of junction sites where blood of different composition flows together notably at the renal and hepatic vein junction with the inferior vena cava but this phenomenon is not seen in arteries.[16]

AORTIC ABNORMALITIES

Aortic Aneurysm

An aneurysm is a localized abnormal dilatation of any vessel. There are three important factors predisposing to their formation: arteriosclerosis, syphilis, and cystic medial necrosis. Less commonly, aneurysms in smaller vessels are caused by polyarteritis nodosa; trauma that may lead to an arteriovenous aneurysm; congenital defect;

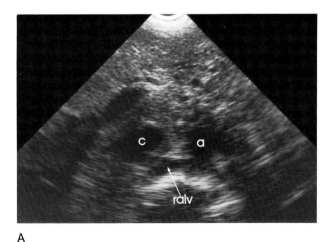

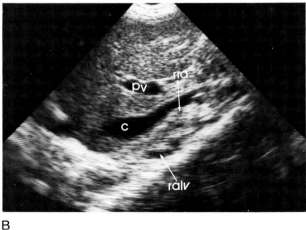

A   B

Fig. 6-13. Right ascending lumbar vein. Patient with mediastinal mass and superior vena caval syndrome. **(A)** Transverse scan. The right ascending lumbar vein *(ralv)* is seen between the aorta *(a)* and inferior vena cava *(c)*. **(B)** Longitudinal left lateral decubitus scan. The right ascending lumbar vein *(ralv)* is seen posterior to the inferior vena cava *(c)* and right renal artery *(rra)*. *(pv, portal vein.)*

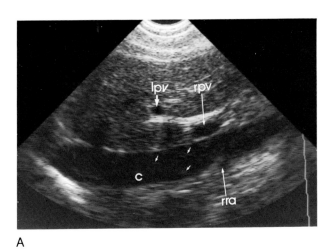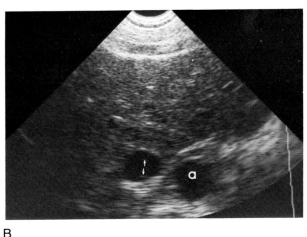

A   B

Fig. 6-14. Intravascular echoes. Longitudinal **(A)** and transverse **(B)** views of the inferior vena cava *(c)*. Small intravascular echoes (arrows) are seen on real-time flowing toward the heart. *(lpv,* left portal vein; *rpv,* right portal vein; *rra,* right renal artery)

and infection that significantly weakens the vascular wall (mycotic aneurysm).[17]

With decreasing incidence of tertiary syphilis, arteriosclerosis is the most common cause for aneurysms.[17] They are rare in individuals younger than 50 years, with a 5:1 ratio of men to women. There is usually involvement of the abdominal aorta, and/or common iliacs and sometimes associated involvement of the ascending aorta and descending thoracic aorta. Ninety-seven percent of abdominal aneurysms are arteriosclerotic. In general, they are fusiform, cylindroid, or saccular. Usually the aneurysm begins below the renals and extends down to the bifurcation. Not infrequently, there are smaller fusiform or saccular dilatations of the common iliacs.

There are several classifications of aneurysms. A berry aneurysm is a small spherical aneurysm of 1 to 1.5 cm. An aneurysm is called saccular if it is spherical and larger than a berry aneurysm — up to 5 to 10 cm. The aneurysmal sac in this case is connected to the vascular lumen by a mouth that varies in size but may be as large as the aneurysm. Characteristically, these are partially or completely filled with thrombus. The most common type, involving the abdominal aorta, would be the fusiform type with gradual dilatation of the vascular lumen. This spindle shaped aneurysm lumen is in direct continuity with the vascular lumen. Frequently, these are eccentric so that one aspect of the wall is more severely affected. They may be up to 20 cm with many involving the entire ascending and transverse aorta. Infrequently, there is dilatation longitudinally producing lengthening of the expanded vessel in a uniform diameter (cylindroid aneurysm).[17]

Symptoms of abdominal aortic aneurysms vary. They may produce symptoms by impinging upon adjacent structures. There may be occlusion of a vessel by either direct pressure or mural thrombus, particularly the vertebral branches that supply the spinal cord. Embolism may result from a mural thrombus. An aneurysm may rupture into the peritoneal cavity or retroperitoneum. The aneurysm may also present as an abdominal mass of unknown etiology.

The annual growth for a 3 to 5.9 cm abdominal aortic aneurysm is 0.23 to 0.28 cm for 1 year.[18] An abdominal aortic aneurysm 4 to 5 cm is followed unless symptomatic or increases in size 1 cm/yr.[18] For years, 6 cm has been considered maximum size for resection.[18] If the aneurysm is less than 6 cm, the patients rarely die from rupture, and also have a 75 percent rate of 1 year survival.[19] If it is greater than 6 cm, there is a 50 percent survival of 1 year.[19] If the aneurysm is greater than 7 cm, there is a greater than 75 percent risk of fatal rupture whereas if it is less than 5 cm, there is less than a 1 percent rupture rate.[19,20] The operative mortality before rupture is 5 percent but with emergency surgery for rupture the mortality increases to 50 percent.[17]

The ultrasound findings of an abdominal aortic aneurysm include increased aortic diameter (> 3 cm), focal dilatation, lack of normal tapering distally, presence of thrombus, and occasionally aortic dissection (Figs. 6-15 to 6-20). To make the aortic measurement, the outside diameter is measured, that is, the distance from the anterior margin or the strong echo defining the anterior wall to the posterior margin.[21] Thrombus is more commonly seen in large aneurysms but also occurs in smaller ones. In 69 percent of cases, intraluminal thrombus can be

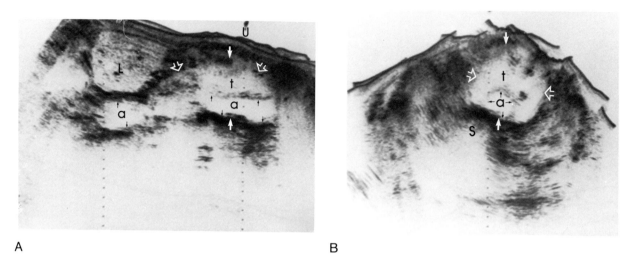

A   B

Fig. 6-15. Aortic aneurysm. Classic example. **(A)** Longitudinal scan in the midline. The distal aorta is dilated in a fusiform fashion. The lumen (*a*, small black arrows) of the aorta is seen as an anechoic area. The true size of the aorta exceeds 5 cm (solid arrows). Clot or thrombus (open arrows, *t*) is seen anteriorly. (*L*, liver; *U*, level of umbilicus.) **(B)** Transverse scan at 1 cm above the umbilicus. The lumen (*a*, small black arrows) of the aorta is seen surrounded by clot or thrombus (*t*, arrows). The anteroposterior dimension would be measured from the outside to the outside (solid arrows). (*S*, spine.)

revealed by a high-amplitude, linear echo along the lumen surface of the thrombus.[22] When thrombi are present, they are typically eccentric and usually along the anterior or anterolateral wall (Figs. 6-15 and 6-19). While a thrombus occupying the lumen of an aneurysm can usually be seen with a high-gain technique, there have been reports of ultrasound not detecting thrombi.[23]

Fresh clot is not as easily seen with ultrasound as old retracted clot, which is significantly greater in its echogenicity.[24] The major problems appear to be the inability to separate masses adherent to the aorta from the aortic wall and misleading measurements caused by the use of oblique scanning planes. The aortic wall as well as the layered intraluminal clot can usually be detected by ad-

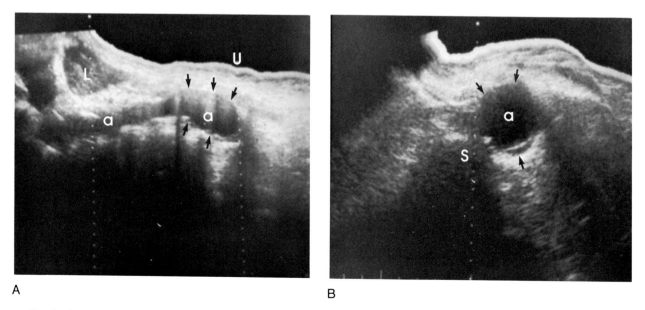

A   B

Fig. 6-16. Aortic aneurysm. Focal dilatation. **(A)** Midline longitudinal scan. The aorta *(a)* is focally dilated (arrows) at the level of the umbilicus *(U)*. (*L*, liver.) **(B)** Transverse scan just above the umbilicus. The distal aorta *(a)* is dilated. No definite thrombus or clot is seen. (*S*, spine.)

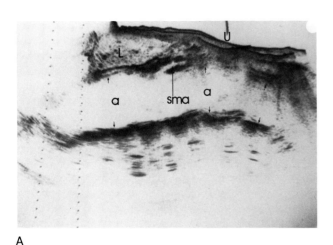
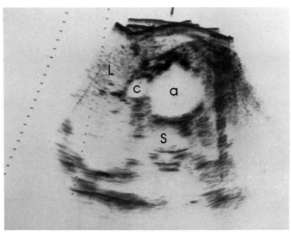

A   B

Fig. 6-17. Aortic aneurysm. Longitudinal (**A**) and transverse (**B**) scans at 9 cm above the umbilicus display aneurysmal dilatation of the entire aorta *(a,* arrows*)* (note cm marks on the scan). (*L,* liver; *c,* inferior vena cava; *sma,* superior mesenteric artery; *U,* level of umbilicus; *S,* spine.)

justing the sensitivity of the scanner.[23] Ultrasound can also readily detect calcification within the aortic wall, which appears as thick, high-amplitude, nonlinear echoes often with acoustic shadowing[22] (Fig. 6-18). Calcification is almost always present in the vascular wall; small flecks of calcification may occur within the thrombus.[22] Ultrasound has an accuracy of 98.8 percent in the detection of abdominal aortic aneurysms.[25,26]

The echo seen at the interface between flowing blood and thrombus is a specular reflection at an interface of two media of differing acoustic impedance (luminal blood and thrombus) that is produced when the incident beam is perpendicular to their interface. The absence of this echo at the lateral aspects of the thrombus tend to support this notion. This thin, nonshadowing, linear, high-amplitude echopattern should not be confused with aortic dissections. Dissections show a second recent channel with or without frank aneurysmal dilatation. An undulating motion may be seen to the intimal flap with real-time ultrasound.

Flowing arterial blood always appears echofree on conventional ultrasound. However, there have been reports of visualization of spontaneously echogenic arterial blood flow, probably due to clumping of red blood cells in an aortic aneurysm. It is postulated that the velocity of flow decreases significantly as the blood flows through an aneurysm resulting in agglutination of some red blood cells into relatively large clumps. These large clumps must have been of sufficient size to scatter the sound energy back to the scanhead. Alternately, the patients may have had some unrecognized abnormal coagulopathy that resulted in agglutination. Slow blood flow

may be the cause of the echogenicity of blood because the flow velocity for any given cardiac output decreases as the lumen diameter increases. Perhaps this phenomenon is a graphic display of the process of mural thrombus formation. Agglutination begins with the slowly moving red blood cells. In the usual small aneurysm, slow flow would be found in the thin layer of blood adjacent to the wall where the friction is the greatest. Adherence of agglutinating cells to the wall would result in the thrombus.

The echogenicity of arterial blood flow in these aneurysms is very different from the echogenicity of venous blood in the great veins and the right heart. It is also different from urine flow. These differing patterns of echogenicity of flowing fluids in the body suggest different mechanisms for their formation. Diffuse homogeneous echogenicity of a large volume of blood in these aneurysms implies clumping of red blood cells as a mechanism. Echogenicity of flowing venous blood appears as isolated discrete, rather then widely spaced, small foci. These venous echogenic foci may be microbubbles of absorbed gases, microemboli of blood elements, or possibly unusually large chylomicrons. Their relatively strong echogenicity for their small size favors the first possibility. Thus, they may represent transition of dissolved blood gas to a gaseous microbubble phase. Because of the slow rate of flow of venous blood, it seems unlikely that these microbubbles are caused by turbulence. Evanescent jet-like echogenicity of urine-flow into the bladder may be produced by such a mechanism; that is, the development of transitory microbubbles may be due to turbulence because turbulence is evident in the echopattern. Alternately, the echogenicity may be due to an impedance mismatch caused by a change of density of urine in the jet flowing into the bladder during diuresis, compared to the density of the urine in the bladder. In aortic aneurysms, microbubbles due to turbulence seem improbable. Echogenic foci are seen in more slowly flowing, less turbulent parts of the blood stream and seemed to increase in spatial density with flow decrease.[27]

Ultrasound measurements of aortic aneurysms are often compared to other techniques. The mean aneurysm diameter on the basis of physical examination overestimates the size by 1 cm. The lateral radiograph overestimates the aortic lumen by 1 cm. Ultrasound most closely approximates the operative true size with intraoperative measurements identical in 34 percent of cases in one study.[28] Ultrasound was within 0.5 cm in 75 percent of cases and within 1 cm in 92 percent of patients.[28] Another study found a problem in comparing

transverse measurements with ultrasound. They favored measuring the distance from the anterior wall of the aorta to the spine.[29] Calcification is seen on plain radiographs in 55 to 85 percent of cases.[19] One study found a closer correlation between aneurysmal size measured at surgery and CT.[30] In comparing ultrasound to digital subtraction angiography (DSA), it was found that DSA correctly identified all but one aneurysm but did not always correctly determine the size because of intraluminal clot.[31]

Pulsatile Abdominal Mass

Many patients are referred to ultrasound to evaluate a pulsatile abdominal mass that is suspected to be an aortic aneurysm. In one series, it was found that 12 percent of these patients had other pathologic abnormalities such as retroperitoneal tumor, fibroid, or paraortic nodes.[32] If

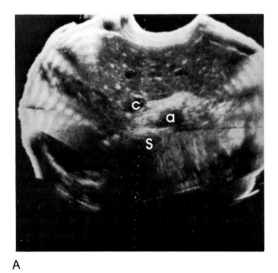

A

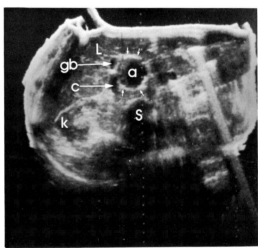

B

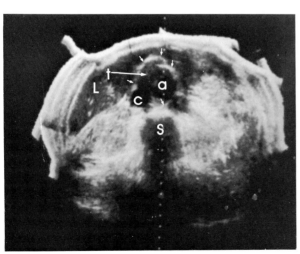

C

Fig. 6-18. Aortic aneurysm. Wall calcification. **(A)** Transverse scan at 12 cm above the umbilicus. The aorta *(a)* appears normal in caliber. (*c*, inferior vena cava; *S*, spine.) **(B)** Transverse scan 6 cm above the umbilicus. The dilated aorta *(a)* has a dense wall (arrows) due to calcification and is seen to the right of midline. (*c*, inferior vena cava; *L*, liver; *k*, right kidney; *gb*, gallbladder; *S*, spine.) **(C)** Transverse scan at 2 cm above the umbilicus. The aortic *(a)* wall is dense (arrows). The anterior right lumen contains low-level echoes representing thrombus *(t)*. The plane of separation between the aorta and inferior vena cava *(c)* is not clearly defined. (*S*, spine; *L*, liver) *(Figure continues.)*

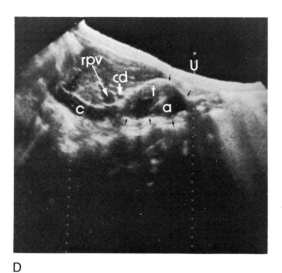

D

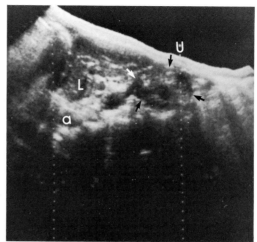

E

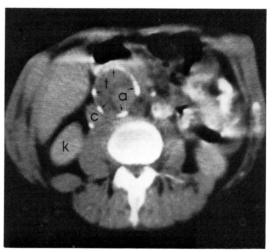

F

Fig. 6-18 *(Continued).* **(D)** Longitudinal scan 6 cm to the right of midline. The aortic aneurysm *(a,* arrows) containing anterior thrombus *(t)* projects to the right of midline compressing the inferior vena cava *(c). (rpv,* right portal vein; *cd,* common bile duct; *U,* level of the umbilicus.)) **(E)** Longitudinal scan in the midline. The lateral margin (arrows) of the aneurysm is seen. Its continuity with the upper aorta *(a)* could not be seen on this scan. *(L,* liver; *U,* level of umbilicus.) **(F)** CT scan similar to **(C).** The calcification (arrows) is seen as well as thrombus *(t)* in the right lateral wall. The lumen *(a)* is opacified. *(c,* inferior vena cava; *k,* right kidney.)

no aneurysm is found the pulsatile mass should be explained. It may be secondary to a tortuous aorta, but an extraaortic mass needs to be excluded. If the aorta is noted to be displaced anteriorly from the spine by more than 0.5 cm, a retroaortic mass must be suspected (Figs. 6-21A to C). Normally the distance from the anterior spinal body to the posterior aortic wall is 0 to 0.5 cm. Greater aortic displacement in the absence of hypertrophic spurs indicates retroaortic pathology[33] (Fig. 6-21D).

Next to aneurysm, the most common etiology for a pulsatile abdominal mass are nodes. These are usually due to lymphoma in the third and fourth decades. Often these patients have fever, weight loss, or generalized malaise. The pulse is a transmitted one due to the encirclement of the aorta by nodes. On ultrasound, these nodes appear as a lobulated, relatively echofree mass surrounding and elevating the aorta off the anterior vertebral bodies (Figs. 6-21A, 6-21B, and 6-22). The aortic

wall may be poorly defined. One should look for other nodes and splenomegaly. An ultrasound guided percutaneous biopsy may be performed to clinch the diagnosis.[34]

Pancreatic carcinoma may also present as a pulsatile abdominal mass. It too will appear on ultrasound as a hypoechoic mass, displacing the normal pancreas (Fig. 6-23). They are often associated with biliary system dilatation. This mass may also be biopsied with ultrasound guidance.[34]

Retroperitoneal sarcoma at times presents as a pulsatile abdominal mass. There can be a variety of presentations. It may extend into the root of the mesentery and give rise to a larger intraperitoneal component. The echodensity of the mass depends on the tissue type that predominates: fatty lesions are more echodense than predominately fibrous or myomatous lesions[34] (Fig. 6-24).

Less common causes for a pulsatile mass would be pancreatitis, pseudocyst, or pancreatic abscess. These are usually known to the clinician. Gastric dilatation and mesenteric hematoma are other possible etiologies.[34]

The evaluation of any pulsatile mass should begin with a good history and physical examination. Those patients who are noted on ultrasound to have an aneurysm, pancreatic carcinoma, nodes, or retroperitoneal tumor may be be referred for further studies. The solid masses may be biopsied with ultrasound guidance.[34]

Dissecting Aneurysm

A dissecting aneurysm is the most common catastrophic illness involving the aorta, occurring two to three times more frequently than ruptured aortic aneu-

rysm. There are 2,000 cases per year in the United States. Untreated, the risk of death is 35 percent 15 minutes after symptoms and 75 percent by the end of 1 week. The dissection of the blood is along the laminar planes of the aortic media with formation of a blood-filled channel within the aortic wall. It is not usually associated with marked dilatation of the aorta. "Acute aortic dissection" is a better term than dissecting aneurysm. The patients are in the 40 to 60-year-old range with 2 to 3 times more males than females. Hypertension is almost invariably antecedant (94 percent) and may play a role in the initiation of the intramural hemorrhage.[17]

The hemorrhage in a dissecting aneurysm occurs characteristically between the middle and outer thirds of the media. The intimal tear, presumably the origin of the dissection, is found in the ascending portion of the arch in 90 percent of cases, usually within 10 cm of the aortic

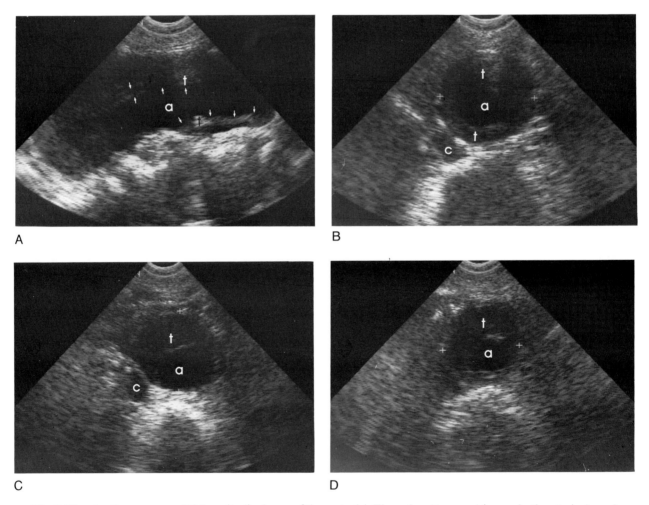

Fig. 6-19. Aortic aneurysm. **(A)** Longitudinal scan of the aorta *(a)*. Thrombus *(t,* arrows) is seen both anteriorly and posteriorly. The anterior wall is difficult to define on this view. Transverse scans **(B-D)** from superior to inferior demonstrate a dilated aorta *(a)*, which has a maximum anteroposterior dimension of 5.5 cm with a maximum transverse measurement of 5.2 cm. Thrombus *(t)* is seen as a hypoechoic area. *(c,* inferior vena cava.) *(Figure continues.)*

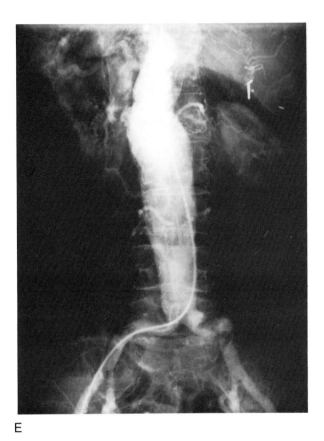

E

Fig. 6-19   *(Continued).*   **(E)** Aortogram confirming the aneurysm.

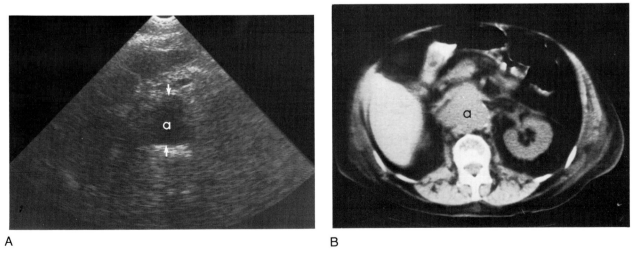

A   B

Fig. 6-20.   Mycotic aortic aneurysm. On transverse scan **(A)**, focal dilatation of only the upper aorta *(a)* is seen. There is irregularity to the lateral margins. This is an unusual location for an atherosclerotic aneurysm. **(B)** CT scan similarly displays only focal dilatation of the aorta *(a)* at this level. There are irregular margins to the aorta. A gallium scan demonstrated increased activity in the area of the dilatation.

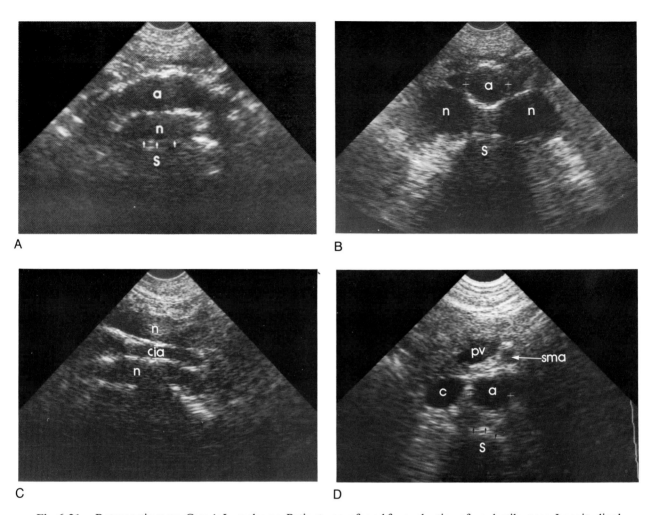

Fig. 6-21. Retroaortic mass. Case 1: Lymphoma. Patient was referred for evaluation of a pulsatile mass. Longitudinal **(A)** and transverse **(B)** scans demonstrate an aorta *(a)* with normal dimensions that is displaced from the spine (*S*, arrows) by enlarged retroaortic lymph nodes *(n)*. **(C)** There is also encasement of the common iliac artery *(cia)* by nodes *(n)* on this long axis view. Case 2: Hypertrophic spurs. This transverse **(D)** scan is similar to **(B)** but in this case the aorta *(a)* is displaced from the anterior surface of the spine *(S)* by hypertrophic spurs (arrows). (*c*, inferior vena cava; *sma*, superior mesenteric artery; *pv*, portal vein.)

valve. The dissection extends proximally toward the heart as well as distally, sometimes to the iliac and femoral arteries. Some blood reruptures into the lumen of the aorta, producing a second or distal intimal tear. The site of reentry most often is in the iliac, followed by the neck vessels. Five to 10 percent of dissecting aneurysms do not have an obvious intimal tear. Extravasation may completely encircle the aorta or extend along one segment of its circumference, or it may rupture into any of the body cavities. Quite rarely, there are cases in which a new vascular channel is formed within the media of the aortic wall that connects the intimal tear proximally and distally. These double-barrelled aortas with two tears permit establishment of through and through blood flow.[17]

There are two types of dissecting aneurysms. Type A involves the ascending aorta or the ascending and descending aorta. It is the most common and lethal type. Type B does not involve the ascending aorta and usually is located just distal to the subclavian artery, extending down into the descending and abdominal aorta.[17]

The pathogenesis of the dissecting aneurysm is not completely clear. Most exhibit media changes that weaken the wall. Most widely, there is cystic medial necrosis with accumulation of basophilic amorphous material in the media, often with the formation of mucoid cysts. The cause of cystic necrosis is unknown. There is a relatively high incidence of cystic changes and dissecting aneurysms in patients with the hereditary disorder of Marfan's syndrome. The hypothesis is that an intimal tear occurs due to hemodynamic factors accentuated by hypertension. The classic symptoms of dissecting aneurysm are excruciating pain in the anterior chest, with

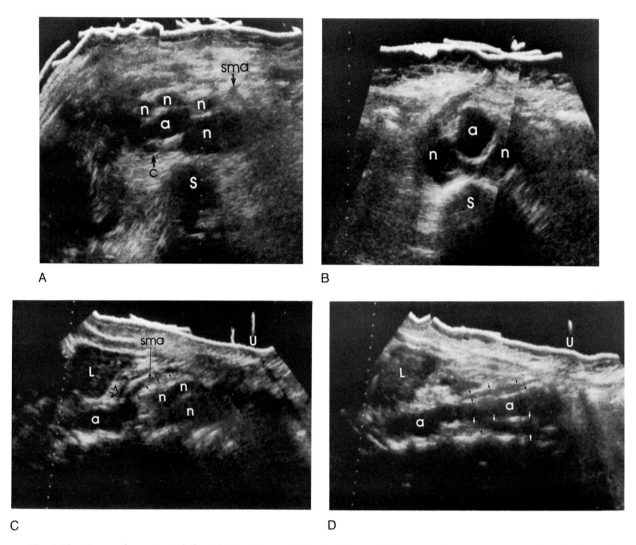

A

B

C

D

Fig. 6-22. Paraortic nodes: Histiocytic lymphoma. Patient with a pulsatile mass. Transverse scans at 9 cm **(A)** and 2 cm **(B)** above the umbilicus. Multiple hypoechoic nodes *(n)* are seen surrounding and displacing the aorta *(a)* to the right and anteriorly. The inferior vena cava *(c)* is compressed anteriorly and the superior mesenteric artery *(sma)* is displaced anteriorly and to the left. (*S*, spine.) **(C)** Longitudinal scan 0.5 cm to the left of midline. The superior mesenteric artery *(sma)* is displaced anteriorly (arrows) by the nodes *(n)*. The inferior aspect of the aorta *(a)* is not seen on this scan because it is displaced to the right. (open arrow, celiac artery; *L*, liver; *U*, umbilicus.) **(D)** Longitudinal scan 1.5 cm to the right of midline. A double-barrel effect (arrows) is seen surrounding the lower aorta *(a)*. Though this resembles the pattern seen with dissection, in this case it was produced by nodes. (*L*, liver; *U*, level of the umbilicus.)

radiation to the back, moving downward. Fifteen percent of patients may not have pain. Often the patients exhibit shock.[17]

Real-time ultrasound should be used to evaluate all aortas. In the case of a possible dissection, the examiner looks for an intimal flap.[18,35,36] This can be seen as an intraluminal, single linear collection of echoes moving with real-time scanning (Fig. 6-25). In addition, ultrasound can identify both the true and false lumens[36] (Figs. 6-26 and 6-27). The true lumen of the aorta may be markedly compressed by the intimal flap, which may

have a "pseudointraluminal" appearance[35] (Figs. 6-26, 6-27).

Ruptured Aortic Aneurysms

The classic symptoms for rupturing aneurysm include excruciating abdominal pain, shock, and an expanding abdominal mass.[18,37] Sometimes the clinical diagnosis is difficult. The operative mortality for a ruptured aortic aneurysm is 40 to 60 percent.[18,37,38] The mortality for

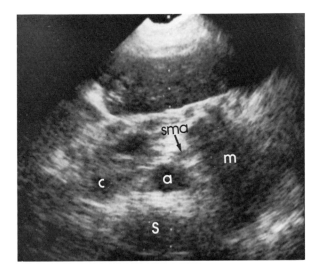

Fig. 6-23. Pancreatic carcinoma. Transverse scan demonstrates a hypoechoic mass *(m)* in the tail of the pancreas *(p)*. The aorta *(a)* is slightly displaced to the right. *(c*, inferior vena cava; *sma*, superior mesenteric artery; *S*, spine.)

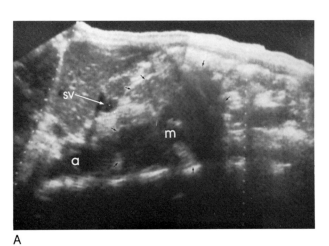

A

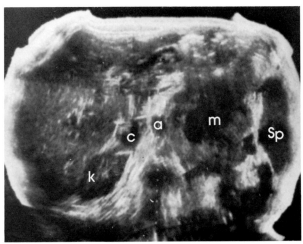

B

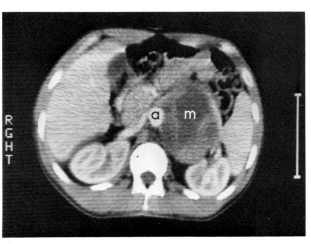

C

Fig. 6-24. Retroperitoneal tumor. Embryonal cell carcinoma. Longitudinal scan 2 cm to the left of midline **(A)** and transverse scan at 12 cm above the umbilicus **(B)** demonstrate a retroperitoneal mass *(m)* of mixed density. The aorta *(a)* is slightly displaced to the right. On the longitudinal scan **(A)**, only the upper aorta *(a)* is seen. The mass *(m)*, which is poorly defined (arrows), has displaced it to the right. *(c*, inferior vena cava; *k*, right kidney; *Sp*, spleen; *sv*, splenic vein.) **(C)** Enhanced CT scan similar in level to **(B)**. Again, the aorta *(a)* can be seen to be displaced to the right by the inhomogeneous mass *(m)*.

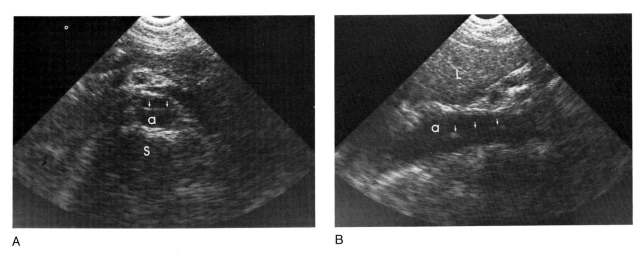

Fig. 6-25. Aortic dissection. Intimal flap. Transverse **(A)** and longitudinal **(B)** scans. A small linear echodensity (arrows) is seen within the aortic *(a)* lumen. This represented an intimal flap that moved at real-time. (*S*, spine; *L*, liver.)

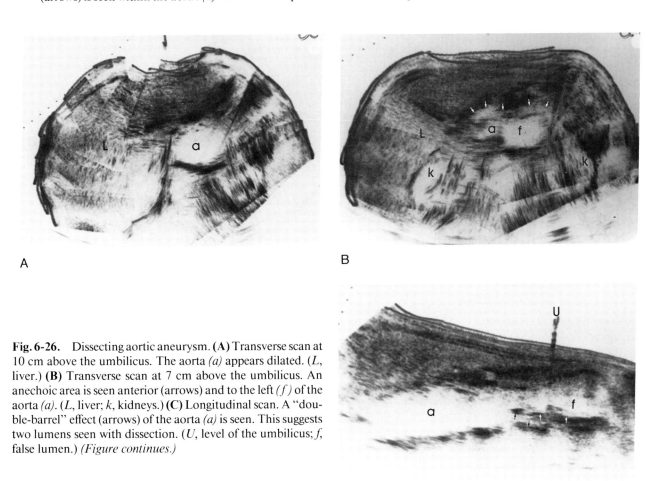

Fig. 6-26. Dissecting aortic aneurysm. **(A)** Transverse scan at 10 cm above the umbilicus. The aorta *(a)* appears dilated. (*L*, liver.) **(B)** Transverse scan at 7 cm above the umbilicus. An anechoic area is seen anterior (arrows) and to the left *(f)* of the aorta *(a)*. (*L*, liver; *k*, kidneys.) **(C)** Longitudinal scan. A "double-barrel" effect (arrows) of the aorta *(a)* is seen. This suggests two lumens seen with dissection. (*U*, level of the umbilicus; *f*, false lumen.) *(Figure continues.)*

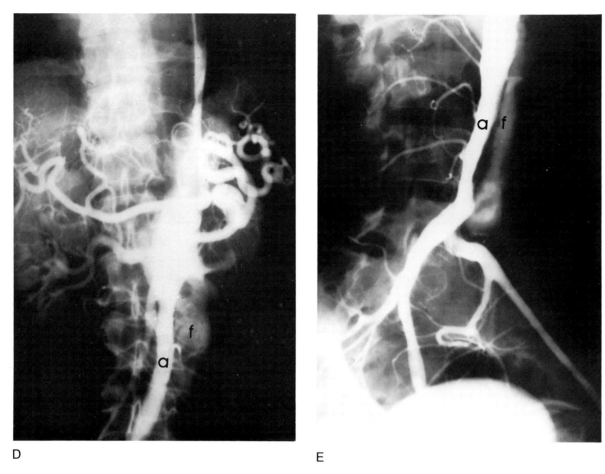

D   E

Fig. 6-26 *(Continued).* **(D,E)** Angiogram. Contrast is seen within the false lumen *(f)* corresponding to **(B,C)**. *(a,* aorta.)

patients with an untreated ruptured abdominoaortic aneurysm approaches 100 percent.[18,38] When the aneurysm ruptures, it may be into the perirenal space accounting for displacement of the renal hilar vessels, effacement of the aortic border, and silhouetting of the lateral psoas border at the level of the kidney (Fig. 6-28). The most common site of rupture is the lateral wall below the renals.[18,38,39] Hemorrhage into the posterior pararenal space accounts for loss of the lateral psoas merging inferior to the kidney and accounts for displacement of the kidney (Fig. 6-28). A perinephric hematoma may also account for renal displacement. As such, an aneurysm may rupture into several retroperitoneal compartments and the hematoma will collect at different levels along known anatomic pathways.[37]

A soft-tissue mass, silhouetting the psoas muscle, and renal displacement, associated with an abdominal aortic aneurysm, are the most important signs of a contained aortic rupture[37] (Fig. 6-29). Both ultrasound and CT can depict aortic aneurysms and hematomas. CT is superior in displaying the density, site, and extent of the retroperi-

toneal hematoma (Figs. 6-28 and 6-29). However, ultrasound may also demonstrate these signs.[37]

Angiographically there are several signs of rupture. Irregular collections of contrast outside the opacified aortic lumen or a calcified aneurysm that persists after the contrast is cleared from the aorta may be seen. There may be a localized saccular dilatation of the aorta in which contrast remains after being cleared from the aorta, or there may be an aortocaval fistula.[40]

Other Complications of Aortic Aneurysms

The aneurysms due to their size may compress neighboring structures. There has been a case of an aneurysm compressing the common bile duct producing biliary obstruction.[41] The aneurysm may compress a renal artery and produce hypertension and renal ischemia.[42] If a symptomatic patient with retroperitoneal fibrosis has an abdominal aortic aneurysm, ureteral involvement is

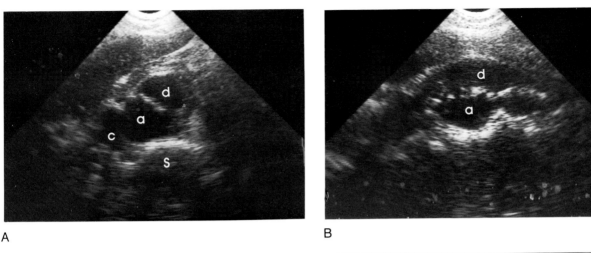

A   B

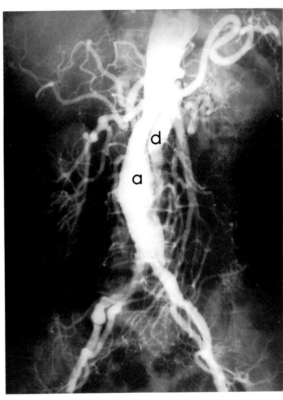

C

Fig. 6-27. Dissecting aortic aneurysm. False lumen. **(A)** Transverse real-time scan. The aorta *(a)* is displaced to the right by the false lumen *(d)* anterolaterally. The inferior vena cava *(c)* is compressed on this scan. Longitudinal scan **(B)**. Two lumens true *(a)* and false *(d)* are seen. (*S*, spine.) Angiogram **(C)** demonstrates the true *(a)* and false *(d)* lumens.

uniformly present.[43] In addition, if the aneurysm is quite high in the abdomen it may present on a chest radiograph as a chest mass[25] (Fig. 6-30). In such a case, ultrasound may be helpful in identifying the pathology and its abdominal location. A mycotic aneurysm may also develop, producing septic symptoms (Fig. 6-20). While ultrasound can identify the aneurysm, a gallium scan may localize to the aneurysm leading to the diagnosis of a mycotic aneurysm.[44]

Aortic Grafts

Ultrasound can be used to evaluate patients following prosthetic vascular grafts. There is a sharp demarcation between the native vessel and the graft. The grafts characteristically have distinct, clear-cut, straight borders and are transonic structures with a discrete border (Fig. 6-31). On longitudinal scan, the proximal anastomosis of the graft is often angled slightly downward into the

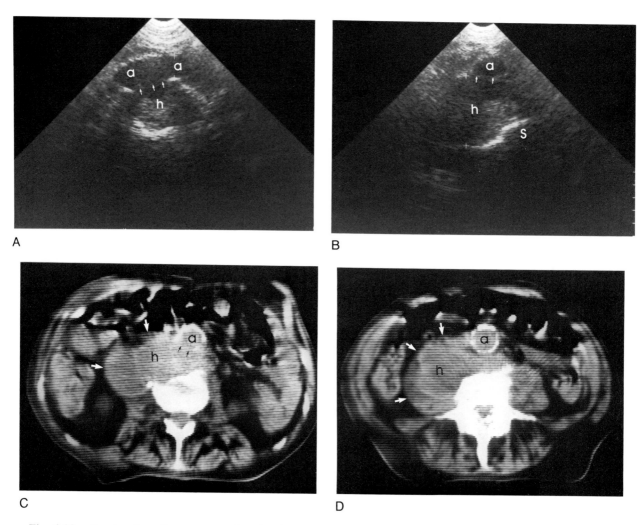

Fig. 6-28. Ruptured aortic aneurysm. Longitudinal **(A)** and transverse **(B)** real-time scans. There appears to be discontinuity in the posterior wall (arrows) of the aorta *(a)*. There is an echogenic mass representing hematoma *(h)* in that area posterior and to the right of midline. (*S*, spine.) **(C,D)** CT scans displaying the ruptured aortic wall (*a*, black arrows) with a hematoma *(h,* white arrows*)* seen as a soft tissue density mass in the right retroperitoneum.

pelvis at the level of the umbilicus.[45] On a transverse scan three vessels are seen: the inferior vena cava, the native aorta, and the graft straddling the other two structures with the graft anterior to the native aorta[45] (Fig. 6-31). Ultrasound can delineate the proximal anastomosis in 84 percent of patients and the iliac graft in 88 to 90 percent of patients.[46]

The normal appearance of an aortofemoral graft placed in an end-to-end fashion is that of a straightened discrete vascular channel with echogenic walls emanating anterior from the distal aorta (Fig. 6-32). The proximal anastomosis is characteristically widened. The limbs of the graft initially pass obliquely down into the groin. Discrete vascular channels with well-demarcated parallel echogenic walls are seen that merge anteriorly

with the native femoral artery at distal end-to-end anastomosis.[46]

The complications of prosthetic grafts include hematoma, infection, degeneration of the graft material, and false aneurysm formation at the graft anastomosis[18,45,47] (Figs. 6-33 to 6-37). Ultrasound is recommended as the initial method to evaluate suspected healing complications of arterial grafting and as a means for long-term follow-up.[46] The most common complication is the false aneurysm formation that occurs in slightly more than 1 percent of vascular anastomoses.[46] There may be no clinical manifestations. By defining vascular wall motion with real-time ultrasound, the examiner can differentiate static fluid adjacent to the graft from truly pulsating blood within a false aneurysm[46] (Figs. 6-33 to 6-35).

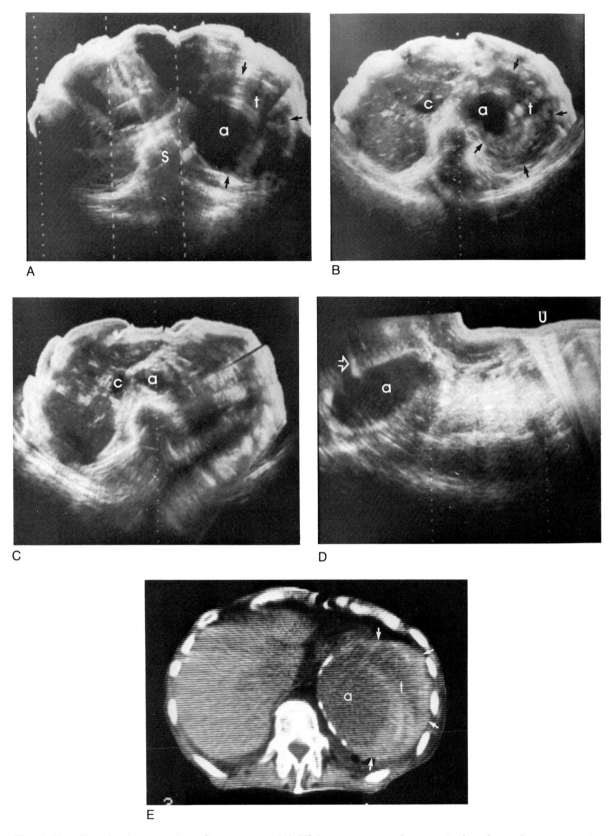

Fig. 6-29. Contained ruptured aortic aneurysm. **(A)** High transverse static scan. A gigantic aortic aneurysm (*a*, arrows) is seen in the high left upper quadrant with the lumen *(a)* and thrombus *(t)*. (*S*, spine.) **(B)** Transverse static scan at 10 cm above the umbilicus. The aneurysm (*a*, arrows) is smaller at this point. (*c*, inferior vena cava; *t*, thrombus.) **(C)** Transverse static scan at 8 cm above the umbilicus. The aorta *(a)* is much smaller. (*c*, inferior vena cava.) **(D)** Longitudinal static scan at 4 cm to the left of midline. A large aneurysm *(a)* is seen high in the epigastrum. (*U*, level of the umbilicus; open arrow, diaphragm.) **(E)** CT scan. Similar to **(A)** and **(B)**. The lumen *(a)* and thrombus *(t)* of the aneurysm (arrows) are identified.

466   ABDOMINAL ULTRASOUND

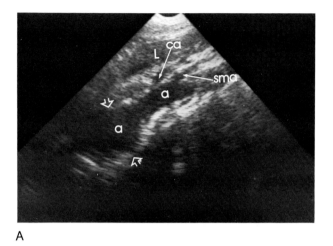

A

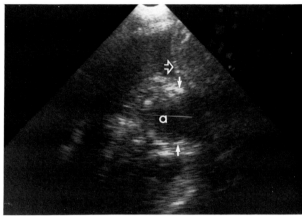

B

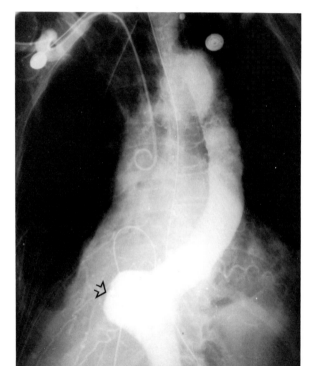

C

Fig. 6-30. Aortic aneurysm extending into the chest. **(A)** Longitudinal real-time scan of the abdominal aorta *(a)*. The lower aorta appears normal in caliber but the caliber near the diaphragm (arrows) appears dilated. (*L*, liver; *ca*, celiac artery; *sma*, superior mesenteric artery.) Longitudinal scan **(B)** through the right chest posteriorly. The dilated aorta (*a*, arrows) is seen as pulsatile anechoic area extending above the diaphragm (open arrow). **(C)** Angiogram displaying the aortic aneurysm (arrow) at the level of the diaphragm. The patient had a bloody pleural effusion; the aneurysm was leaking into her chest.

A pulsating hematoma connected to an arterial lumen may be seen with a false aneurysm or pseudoaneurysm.[45,47] These hematomas communicate with the lumen, commonly in the inguinal region. On ultrasound, an abrupt termination of the graft walls is seen within a fluid collection[47] (Figs. 6-33 and 6-34). Pseudoaneurysms caused by failure of the graft material are rare but are suggested if a dilated segment is delineated in a location remote from the anatomosis.[47] It is essential to

know the extent of the graft and the sites of anastomosis.[47]

Ultrasound can identify perigraft fluid collection secondary to hematoma, seroma and infection not detected by arteriography (Figs. 6-36 and 6-37). Hematomas that occur appear as hyperechoic or complex masses and tend to accumulate initially between the graft and residual aorta[45] (Fig. 6-36). The inguinal area is the most common site of infection with these vascular prosthe-

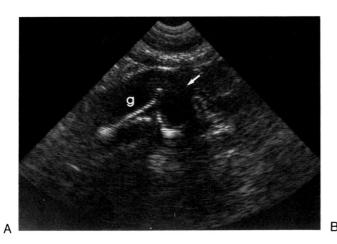
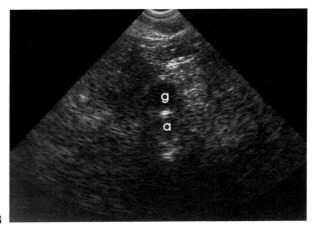

Fig. 6-31. Aortic graft. **(A)** Longitudinal scan. The aortic graft *(g)* has clear-cut straight serrated borders. The proximal graft is angled slightly downward (arrow) into the pelvis. **(B)** Transverse scan. The graft *(g)* is seen anterior to the native aorta *(a)*.

ses.[45] If perigraft fluid is seen and infection is a consideration, an aspiration can be performed. If the graft is completely occluded, the vessel may have a normal ultrasound appearance but demonstrate no pulsation on real-time ultrasound.[18,48] At times, with occlusion, no vascular channel may be demonstrated.[18,48]

Patients who have had grafts placed after aneurysmal rupture pose a dilemna. There is often extensive hematoma in the retroperitoneum and periaortic area commonly associated with rupture and these persist as a significant mass after surgery requiring months to finally resorb. It is important to try and differentiate an acute process that needs immediate attention from a chronic

problem associated with aortic rupture and repair. With rupture, an anechoic collection about the graft may not be acute.[38]

AORTIC BRANCH ABNORMALITIES

Celiac Artery Aneurysm

Any anechoic mass within the abdomen should be examined with real-time ultrasound as it could be an aneurysm. A celiac aneurysm may be mistaken for a pancreatic pseudocyst. It will appear anechoic and spherical on ultrasound and will be located anterior to

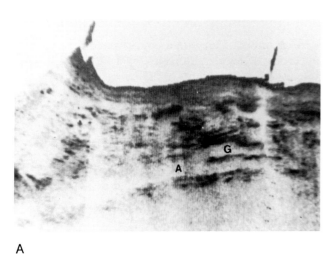
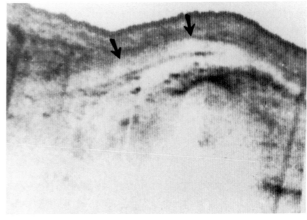

Fig. 6-32. Aortic graft. **(A)** Longitudinal scan of the proximal portion of a normal end-to-side aortofemoral graft *(G)*. *(A*, aorta) **(B)** Longitudinal scan of a normal distal end-to-side anastomosis of an aortofemoral graft. The graft (arrows) is anterior to the native vessel. (From Gooding GAW, Effeney DJ, Goldstone J: The aortofemoral graft: Detection and identification of healing complications by ultrasonography. Surgery 89:94, 1981.)

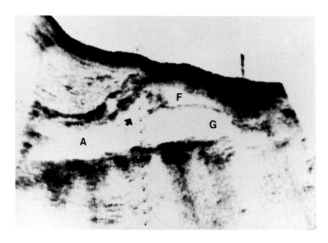

Fig. 6-33. Aortic graft, pseudoaneurysm. Longitudinal scan of a proximal false aneurysm (F) anterior to the vessel with disruption of the anterior wall of the anastomosis (arrow). (A, aorta; G, graft.) (From Gooding GAW, Effeney DJ, Goldstone J: The aortofemoral graft: Detection and identification of healing complications by ultrasonography. Surgery 89:94, 1981.)

the aorta just cephalad to the pancreas (Fig. 6-38). With real-time ultrasound, its continuity with the celiac artery may be demonstrated, which requires meticulous scanning technique. These lesions may be asymptomatic or present with vague epigastric pain prior to rupture. Rupture is a significant complication. A preoperative diagnosis of celiac aneurysm is infrequent.[49]

Superior Mesenteric Artery Aneurysm

Superior mesenteric artery aneurysmal production secondary to pancreatitis is an uncommon complication. The splenic artery is most commonly involved but other splanchnic vessels—celiac, common hepatic artery, gastric, and gastroduodenal may be involved. Intrinsic pulsations may or may not be seen with real-time ultrasound.[50] An aneurysm should be considered when a cystic area is seen in the region of the pancreas (see Fig. 3-26).

Splenic Artery Aneurysm

Splenic artery aneurysms are rare but potentially life-threatening lesions. They may be caused by atherosclerosis, infective emboli, infections, congenital factors, or trauma and seem particularly frequent in patients with portal hypertension and in females of childbearing years. Many are asymptomatic; if symptoms are present they are vague, with discomfort in the left upper quadrant,

pain to the shoulder, or nausea and vomiting. The incidence of rupture is 8 to 46 percent with a high mortality especially if the aneurysm ruptures into the stomach. On plain radiograph, a ring of calcification in the axis of the splenic artery may be seen.

Erosion of the splenic artery with pseudoaneurysm formation is a rare complication of pancreatitis and pseudocyst formation. Because the splenic capsule is continuous with the peritoneum enclosing the splenic vessels and covering the anterior surface of the pancreas, the splenic hilum is a natural pathway for an expanding pseudocyst near the pancreatic tail. Penetration into the spleen makes it more vulnerable to spontaneous rupture and invasion of the splenic artery may lead to pseudoaneurysm formation with major arterial hemorrhage. These two complications are uncommon.[51]

The splenic artery can be first identified at the bifurcation of the celiac artery. The splenic artery courses to the left in relation to the posterior and superior parts of the body and tail of the pancreas. This vessel can be followed with ultrasound (see Fig. 3-7). If a cystic mass is identified in the area of this vessel, the examiner needs to differentiate it from a pancreatic cyst, segmental dilatation of the pancreatic duct, ectasia of the splenic vein, lymphadenopathy, or gastric varices[52] (Fig. 6-39). On real-time ultrasound, a rounded hypoechoic mass is seen along the path of the splenic artery (Fig. 6-39). Pulsations may not be seen with real-time scanning. The combination of real-time scanning and Doppler effect provides precise anatomic location and the Doppler signals permit both detection of the presence of flow within deeply located structures and an analysis of its nature.[53]

Renal Artery Aneurysms

Renal artery aneurysms are relatively uncommon. In an autopsy series at random, a 9.7 percent incidence was noted with 17 percent of those being intrarenal.[54] Twenty percent are associated with rupture and death while 10 percent require nephrectomy for control of spontaneous hemorrhage.[54] It is recommended that there be removal of all noncalcified aneurysms, large calcified aneurysms, false aneurysms and any lesion associated with pain, bleeding, or hypertension. Only small calcified aneurysms (< 1.5 cm diameter) are felt to represent no danger to asymptomatic normotensive patients.[54]

Renal artery aneurysms may be true or false.[54] False ones arise from blunt or penetrating trauma including iatrogenic trauma (needle biopsy). One-third of true aneurysms are congenital with two-thirds acquired (atherosclerosis, polyarteritis nodosa).[54]

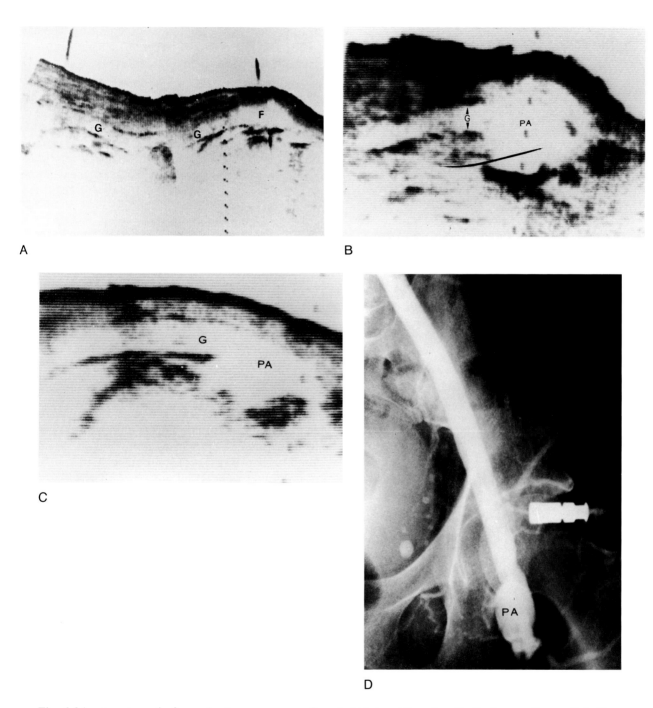

Fig. 6-34. Anastomotic femoral artery aneurysm. Case 1: **(A)** An oblique longitudinal scan of a small fusiform anastomotic femoral artery aneurysm *(F)*. (*G*, graft.) (From Gooding GAW, Effeney DJ, Goldstone J: The aortofemoral graft: Detection and identification of healing complications by ultrasonography. Surgery 89:94, 1981.) Case 2: **(B)** Longitudinal scan of a replacement graft *(G)* ending in a pseudoaneurysm *(PA)* in the left inguinal area. Case 3: **(C)** Long axis view of a left femoral graft. The graft *(G)* ends abruptly in a fluid collection *(PA)* representing a pseudoaneurysm. **(D)** Graft arteriogram. A small pseudoaneurysm *(PA)* is seen. (Figs. **B-D** from Wolson AH, Kaupp HA, McDonald K: Ultrasound of arterial graft surgery complications. AJR 133:869, © Am Roent Ray Soc, 1979.)

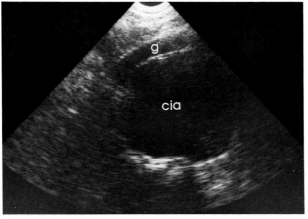

A

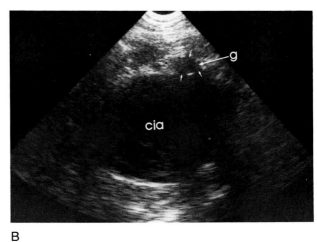

B

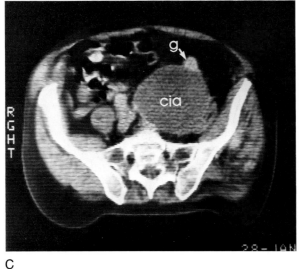

C

Fig. 6-35. Aortic graft, pseudoaneurysm? Patient with pulsatile mass postoperative for aortic graft. On real-time longitudinal **(A)** and transverse **(B)** scans of the left iliac graft *(g)* demonstrate a pulsatile tube anterior to a large hypoechoic mass *(cia)*. **(C)** Enhanced CT scan similar to **(B)**. (*g*, graft; *cia*, common iliac artery.) The mass was the large old (native) common iliac aneurysm.

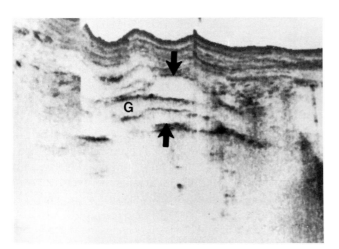

Fig. 6-36. Aortic graft, hematoma. Longitudinal scan of a perigraft hematoma surrounding the proximal portion of an end-to-end graft (arrows). (*G*, graft.) (From Gooding GAW, Effeney DJ, Goldstone J: The aortofemoral graft: Detection and identification of healing complications by ultrasonography. Surgery 89:94, 1981.)

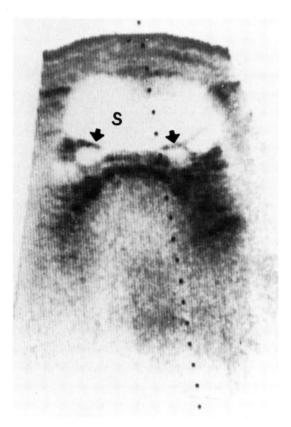

Fig. 6-37. Aortic graft, fluid. Transverse scan of a large seroma *(S)* above the iliac limbs of a graft (arrows). (From Gooding GAW, Effeney DJ, Goldstone J: The aortofemoral graft: Detection and identification of healing complications by ultrasonography. Surgery 89:94, 1981.)

Ultrasound is the screening test of choice in evaluating cystic or solid renal masses. Its accuracy approaches 90 to 96 percent.[54] All cystic appearing masses should be evaluated with real-time, especially before contemplating aspiration. A renal artery aneurysm would appear cystic but should be pulsatile on real-time ultrasound[54] (Fig. 6-40).

At times, a normal left renal vein may be mistaken for a renal artery aneurysm on ultrasound, especially in patients with a paucity of retroperitoneal fat[55] (Fig. 6-11). This false impression is produced by two factors: (1) the left renal vein unusually prominent from the hilus of the left kidney to the area between the superior mesenteric artery and aorta; and (2) part of the normal aortic wall adjacent to the left renal vein incompletely visualized.[55] This may be similar to superior mesenteric artery syndrome. In these individuals the left renal vein is compressed between the superior mesenteric artery and aorta

causing proximal enlargement. This "bulge" is felt to be physiologic.

Iliac Arteries

As has been stated earlier in this chapter, when evaluating the aorta the examiner should include the iliac arteries as part of the study. Iliac artery aneurysms are often asymptomatic and unsuspected. The majority are atherosclerotic with a less common etiology of trauma, pregnancy, congenital abnormality, abdominal or pelvic surgery, syphilis, and bacterial infection.[4,20] Ultrasound can detect and accurately size them, describing their extent and progression (Figs. 6-41 and 6-42). Left untreated, 50 percent of iliac artery aneurysms ultimately rupture. The incidence of internal iliac artery aneurysms is not known. It is one-tenth as common as aortic aneurysms. Greater than 70 percent of patients with aortic aneurysms present with symptoms. Internal iliac aneurysms rarely cause symptoms until they impinge on some structures. The most common complication of internal iliac artery aneurysm is death due to retroperitoneal or intraperitoneal hemorrhage. The natural history is one of progressive enlargement.[20]

Most of the aneurysms involving the internal iliac artery are found to be extensions of aortoiliac aneurysms. However, isolated common iliac aneurysms occur more often than initially suspected.[56] They are often bilateral. Isolated internal iliac aneurysms, a rare type of aneurysm, are located deep in the pelvis, do not often produce symptoms, and are difficult to detect clinically[56] (Fig. 6-43). Signs and symptoms may be urological, gastrointestinal, or neurologic and related to extrinsic pressure on the bladder or ureter, rectum or sigmoid or sacral plexus.[113] There may be a pulsatile mass revealed by abdominal, rectal, or vaginal examination or the mass may be nonpulsatile if filled with thrombus (Fig. 6-43). When there are bilateral internal iliac aneurysms, there may be colon ischemia, and vasculogenic impotence. Loss of both internal iliac arteries may interfere significantly with available collateral blood supply to colon.[57] They are usually 3 to 8 cm in diameter and occur predominantly in men older than 60 years.[56] As with abdominal aortic aneurysms, risk of rupture varies with size of the lesion.[56] Up to 5 percent of untreated isolated iliac (common and internal) aneurysms will eventually rupture with most going into the retroperitonium and rarely into the ureter or rectosigmoid.[56] Operative treatment is indicated because the natural course is one of progressive expansion and rupture. Elective surgical intervention has a mortality less 10 percent while a mortality of 80 percent has been reported with attempts at surgical repair after rupture.[56]

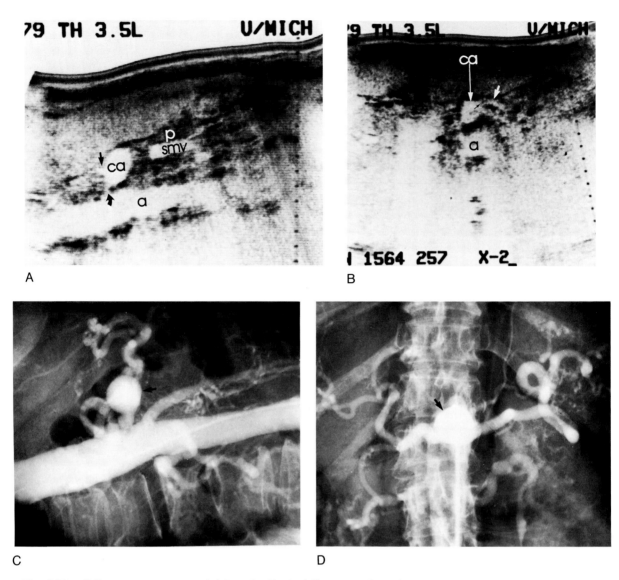

Fig. 6-38. Celiac artery aneurysm. **(A)** Longitudinal midline scan of a celiac artery aneurysm *(ca)* arising from the proximal celiac trunk (curved arrow). Note origin of left gastric artery (straight arrow) from the aneurysm. (*a*, aorta; *smv*, superior mesenteric vein; *p*, pancreas.) **(B)** Transverse scan 2 cm caudad to the xyphoid through the celiac aneurysm *(ca)*. Note origin (black arrow) and proximal portion (white arrow) of the splenic artery, arising from celiac artery *(ca)*. (*a*, aorta.) **(C)** Lateral and **(D)** anterior radiographs from an aortogram showing the celiac aneurysm (arrow). (From Herzler GM, Silver TM, Graham LM, Stanley JC: Celiac artery aneurysm: Ultrasonic diagnosis. J Clin Ultrasound 9:141, 1981.)

Arteriovenous Fistulas

The large majority of aorto-caval fistulas are acquired secondary to trauma, such as penetrating gunshot and stab injuries, and are reported postoperative to surgery for lumbar disc lesions.[58] Spontaneous aorto-caval fistulas may develop as a complication of arteriosclerotic aortic aneurysms. The clinical picture with a central arteriovenous fistula is distinctive: low back and abdominal pain, progressive cardiac decompensation, pulsatile abdominal mass associated with a bruit, and massive swelling of the lower trunk and lower extremities.[58] The clinical symptoms are explained on the basis of the altered hemodynamics produced by a high-velocity shunt leading to increased blood volume, increased venous pressure and cardiac output with cardiac failure and cardiomegaly.

When a dilated inferior vena cava is seen on ultrasound, the examiner should suspect an arteriovenous fistula, especially if there is lower trunk and leg edema (Fig.

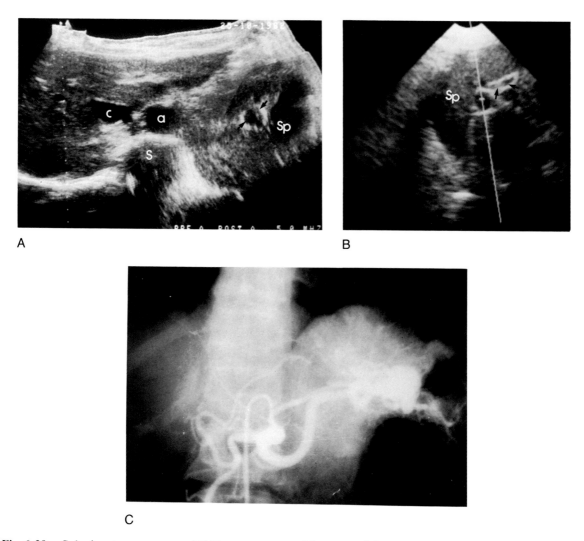

A

B

C

Fig. 6-39. Splenic artery aneurysm. **(A)** Transverse scan of the upper abdomen showing slight hepatosplenomegaly. At the splenic hilum, a hypoechoic rounded mass of about 1.5 cm is visible (arrows). (*Sp*, spleen; *a* aorta; *c*, inferior vena cava; *S*, spine.) **(B)** Longitudinal real-time scan of the left flank. The close relationship of the mass with the splenic vessels (small arrows) may be appreciated. The cursor indicating the pulsed Doppler sample volume has been positioned within the lesion. (*Sp*, spleen.) **(C)** Abdominal angiogram confirming the diagnosis of the splenic artery aneurysm. (From Derchi LE, Biggi E, Cicio GR et al: Aneurysms of the splenic artery: Noninvasive diagnosis by pulsed doppler sonography. J Ultrasound Med 3:41, 1984.)

6-44). If the fistula is large, the vein becomes markedly distended. A normal inferior vena cava is less than 2.5 cm with dilatation greater than 3.5 cm.[58] The inferior vena cava is rarely distended to a similar extent in long-standing cases of constrictive pericarditis, tricuspid incompetence, or cardiac failure.

Renal arteriovenous fistulas can be congenital or acquired.[59,60] The congenital type may be the crisoid type or the aneurysmal type.[60] The acquired ones are secondary to trauma, surgery, or may be secondary to inflammation or associated with neoplasm such as renal cell carcinoma.[59] With the increased frequency of renal biopsy, abdominal trauma, and certain types of urologic procedures, there is an increased number of acquired arteriovenous fistulas reported.[61] However, the incidence following renal biopsy is less than 15 percent.[61] With acquired arteriovenous fistulas three-fourths have a single arteriovenous communication. Renal arteriovenous fistulas present clinically with hypertension, cardiomegaly, heart failure, and an abdominal bruit. Such patients may also have abdominal pain and hematuria. There is usually conservative management of the patient with arteriovenous fistulas after trauma or renal biopsy. The lesion may close without surgical intervention. Ul-

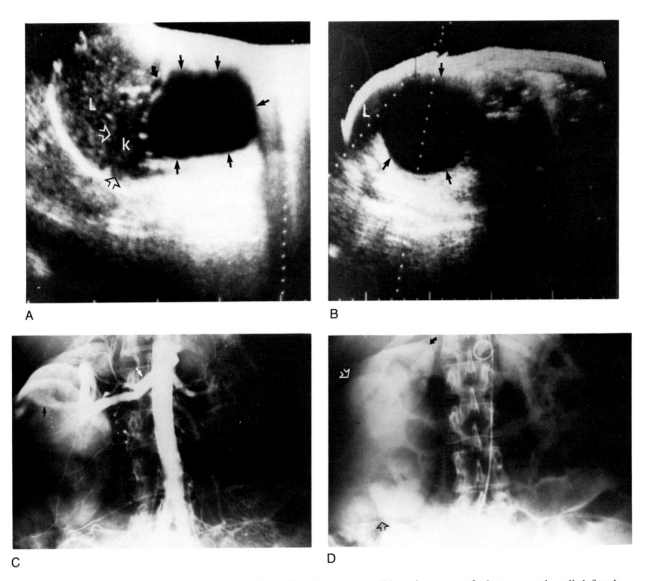

A

B

C

D

Fig. 6-40. Renal artery aneurysm. Longitudinal **(A)** and transverse **(B)** supine scans of a large, round, well-defined mass (black arrows) exhibiting anechoic and transonic characteristics plus strong back wall normally associated with simple cysts. The lesion occupies nearly all of the right kidney *(k)* except the apex (open arrows). Note the gallbladder (curved arrow) is displaced cephalad against the liver *(L)* edge. Early **(C)** and late **(D)** phases of a flush aortogram show progressive filling of a giant intrarenal artery aneurysm (open arrows). **(C)** Note changes of fibromuscular dysplasia within the lower pole branch and the "jet" phenomenon at the site of origin of the aneurysm (black arrow) that was also visible fluoroscopically during selective test injection. Although a normal upper pole branch feeds the right apex, the main right renal artery is twice as large as the left (white arrow). **(D)** The extent of the aneurysm (open arrows) matches the previous sonogram perfectly, occupying almost all of the right kidney except the apex (black arrow). (From Hantman SS, Barie JJ, Glendening TB et al: Giant renal artery aneurysm mimicking a simple cyst on ultrasound. J Clin Ultrasound 10:136, 1982.)

trasound is a noninvasive method for serial scans providing objective evidence of diminishment of the lesion.

The preoperative diagnosis of renal arteriovenous fistula generally involves angiography. At angiography, the crisoid type appears as multiple tortuous vascular channels supplied by segmental arterial branches associated with multiple arteriovenous communications, and arteriovenous shunting to a variable degree (Fig. 6-45C). The aneurysmal type is associated with a saccular aneurysm of variable size and is supplied by an enlarged renal artery or a segmental branch and is drained by an enlarged vein (Fig. 6-46).

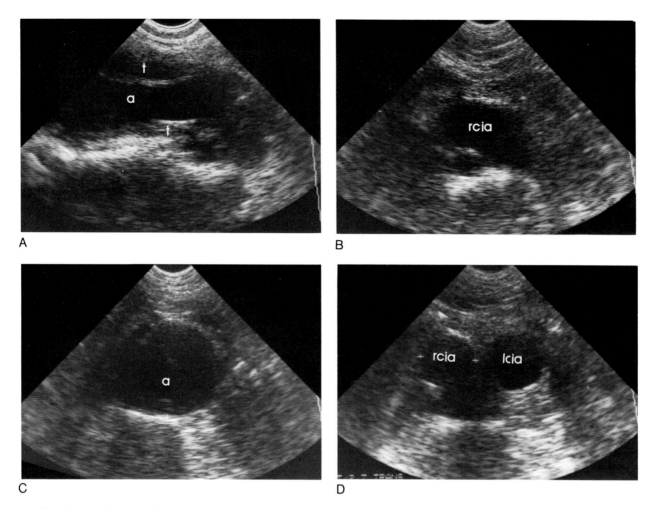

A

B

C

D

Fig. 6-41. Common iliac artery aneurysm. **(A)** Longitudinal scan of an aortic *(a)* aneurysm at the level of the umbilicus. There is thrombus *(t)* anterior and posteriorly. **(B)** Long axis view of the right iliac artery *(rcia)*, which is dilated (3 cm anteroposteriorly). **(C)** Transverse scan at 3 cm above the umbilicus. The aorta *(a)* measures 5.5 cm anteroposteriorly and 6.7 cm transversely. **(D)** Transverse scan at the umbilicus. The right *(rcia)* (2.7 cm transversely) and left *(lcia)* (2.6 cm transversely) are seen.

The ultrasound features of renal arteriovenous fistulas are representative of the angiography. The hallmark is the presence of multiple anechoic tubular structures feeding the malformation with an enlarged renal artery and vein, confirming increased blood flow to the kidney[60] (Figs. 6-45 and 6-46). The arteriovenous fistula may look like hydronephrosis or a parapelvic cyst in association with a dilated inferior vena cava.[60-62] The diagnosis is made by identifying one or more channels that enter the mass suggesting that the lesion is related to renal vasculature. Pulsatile motion may be seen with real-time ultrasound.[61] The crisoid type has a characteristic ultrasound appearance of a cluster of tubular anechoic structures within the kidney; it is supplied by an enlarged renal artery and drained by a dilated renal vein[60] (Fig. 6-45). The aneurysmal type is believed to be associated with a congenital arterial or venous aneurysm that may expand and eventually erode into the vein or artery, producing an arteriovenous fistula[60] (Fig. 6-46). The ultrasound features of the aneurysmal type are less characteristic. One should consider the possibility of a vascular lesion when the presence of thrombus is noted in the periphery of a mass with a tubular anechoic lumen with pulsations seen on real-time ultrasound (Fig. 6-46). Its appearance is identical to the typical aortic aneurysm (Fig. 6-46). In the proper clinical setting, the finding on ultrasound of a large cystic mass in the region of the kidney with marked inferior vena cava dilatation is highly suggestive if not diagnosis of arteriovenous fistula or malformation.[59]

On occasion, renal cell carcinoma may be associated with arteriovenous shunting due to invasion of the larger

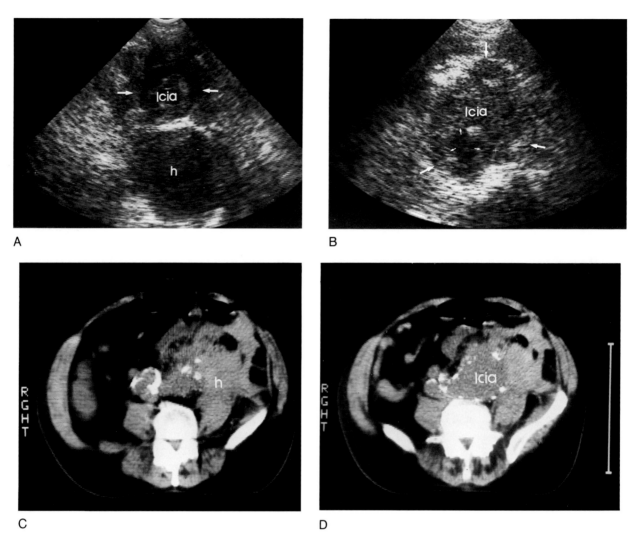

Fig. 6-42. Common iliac artery aneurysm. Transverse scans **(A,B)** reveal a large mass *(lcia,* arrows) in the left lower abdomen. A pulsatile lumen (small arrows) was seen. On the higher scan **(A)**, a mass *(h)* is seen posterior to the left common iliac artery. CT scans with **(C)** similar to **(A)** and **(D)** similar to **(B)**. A left common iliac aneurysm *(lcia)* is seen with a hematoma *(h)* from a leak posteriorly.

arteries and venous structures. With a neoplastic arteriovenous fistula, a lesion greater than 2 cm should be detected with ultrasound as an anechoic mass that may compress the renal pelvis producing calectasis and simulating hydronephrosis.[61] By identification of one or more channels entering the mass, the diagnosis of the lesion should be considered to be related to renal vasculature. The structure may be traced to aorta or inferior vena cava and may be pulsatile on real-time ultrasound. The ultrasound differentiation from a nonneoplastic fistula depends on detection of a solid mass in addition to the cluster of vascular structures.[60]

INFERIOR VENA CAVAL ABNORMALITIES

Congenital Abnormalities

The inferior vena cava is formed by three pairs of cardinal veins in the retroperitoneum; these undergo sequential development and regression (Fig. 6-47). Although appearing at about 6 weeks, the posterior cardinal veins form no part of the normal adult inferior vena cava but may be part of the anomalies. The subcardinal veins appearing at 7 weeks, produce the prerenal seg-

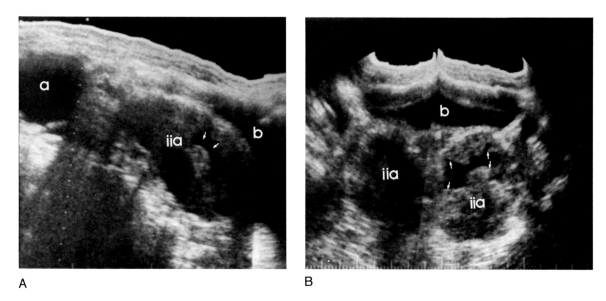

A   B

Fig. 6-43. Internal iliac aneurysms. **(A)** Longitudinal scan at 3 cm to the left of midline. The dilated distal aorta *(a)* at the level of the umbilicus is seen as well as a mass *(iia)* posterior to the bladder *(b)*. **(B)** Transverse scan through the bladder *(b)*. Bilateral internal iliac aneurysms *(iia)* are noted. The one on the right was clotted off and not pulsatile on real-time ultrasound. The lucency in the left one represents lumen (small arrows).

ment of the inferior vena cava. The supracardinal system, which becomes visible at 8 weeks, produces the postrenal segment of the inferior vena cava (Fig. 6-47). Above the diaphragm, the supracardinals form the azygos and hemiazygos. The anatomosis between the subcardinal and supracardinal systems form the renal veins (Fig. 6-47). The normal left cardinal system involutes and the right is composed of the posterior infrarenal, supracardinal vein, renal segment, anterior suprarenal subcardinal vein, and the confluence of hepatic veins.[6]

In double inferior vena cava, which has an incidence of 0.3 to 3 percent, the size of the two vessels can be the same or vary depending on the dominant side[6,63–65] (Fig. 6-48). The left inferior vena cava may mimic adenopathy. The commonest type is where the left inferior vena cava joins the left renal vein, which crosses the midline at its normal level to join the right inferior vena cava. With this there is no continuation of the left inferior vena cava above the left renal vein. Less commonly, the right inferior vena cava joins the azygos and the left inferior vena cava joins the hemiazygos. With a single left inferior vena cava (incidence 0.2 percent), it joins the left renal vein, which crosses the midline to join the right renal vein to form the right side of the inferior vena cava. The left inferior vena cava should not be confused with the left gonadal vein because both join the left renal vein. The left inferior vena cava is identified as arising from

the left common iliac, while the left gonadal vein exits from the abdomen in the inguinal area. The left inferior vena cava can persist above the level of the left renal vein, whereas the right inferior vena cava is not present above this point. In such a case the left inferior vena cava ascends the thorax by joining the hemiazygos. Recognition of caval duplication is important prior to surgical caval ligation, shunt procedure in renal venous hypertension, choosing renal transplant donors, umbrella placement, and repairing abdominal aortic aneurysm.[6,63]

With infrahepatic interruption of the inferior vena cava, there is failure of union of the hepatic veins and the right subcardinal vein and with it there can be azygos or, less commonly, hemiazygos continuation.[66,67] This is associated with acyanotic and cyanotic congenital heart disease, abnormalities of cardiac position, abdominal situs and with asplenia and polysplenia.[67] On ultrasound, the azygos vein continuation is identical to or larger than the inferior vena cava that passes along the aorta medial to the right crus.[67] The hepatic veins do not drain into it but drain into an independent confluence that passes through the diaphragm to enter the right atrium.[6,67]

The true position of the left renal vein is important in considering splenorenal shunts and prospective renal transplant donors. The incidence of a circumaortic renal vein is 1.5 to 8.7 percent and that of a retroaortic left renal vein 1.8 to 2.4 percent; both can be seen with

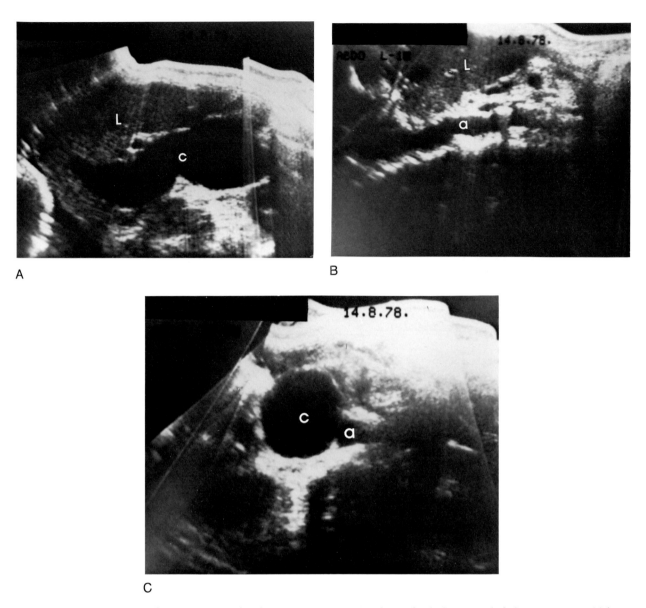

Fig. 6-44. Aorto-caval fistula. **(A)** Longitudinal scan 7 cm to the right of midline. The inferior vena cava *(c)* is markedly dilated. (*L*, liver.) **(B)** Longitudinal scan 1 cm to left of midline. The abdominal aorta *(a)* does not exhibit aneurysmal dilatation. (*L*, liver.) **(C)** Transverse scan 8 cm below the xyphoid. The markedly distended inferior vena cava *(c)* and normal aorta *(a)* are seen. At angiogram, the patient was found to have a right common iliac artery aneurysm with fistulous communication with the lower end of the inferior vena cava and a large left-to-right shunt through the fistula. (From Khoo HT: The large inferior vena cava—A sign in arteriovenous fistula between the right common iliac artery and the inferior vena cava. J Clin Ultrasound 10:291, 1982.)

ultrasound.[6,65] The posterior component crosses behind the aorta to join the right inferior vena cava at the level of 1 to 2 vertebral bodies below that of the preaortic segment[6] (Fig. 6-48).

Membranous obstruction of the inferior vena cava may simulate infrahepatic interruption of the inferior vena cava with azygos continuation. In this condition, a web or membrane obstructs the inferior vena cava at the level of the diaphragm and leads to chronic congestion of the liver with centrilobular and periportal fibrosis (Fig. 6-49). There are three types of obstructions: (1) a thin membrane at the level of the entrance to the right atrium; (2) an absent segment of the inferior vena cava (length varies), without characteristic conical narrow-

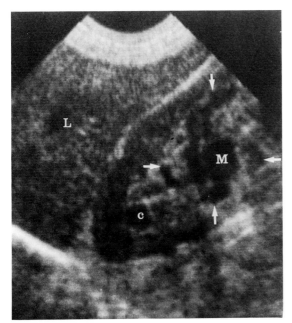

A

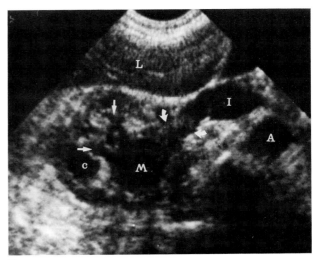

B

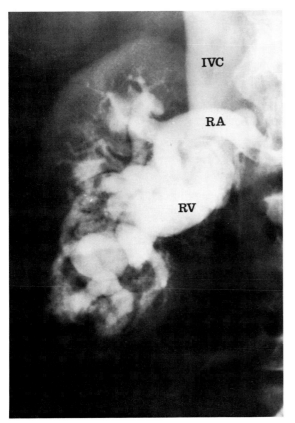

C

Fig. 6-45. Renal arteriovenous fistula. Crisoid type. **(A)** Longitudinal real-time scan through the liver *(L)* and right kidney reveals multiple anechoic tubular structures (arrows) ending in an anechoic mass *(M)* constituting a cirsoid arteriovenous malformation. (*c*, dilated upper pole calyx.) **(B)** Transverse real-time scan at the renal hilum. The arteriovenous malformation *(M)* is demonstrated supplied by multiple vessels (straight arrows) and drained by a dilated renal vein containing thrombus (curved arrows). (*c*, dilated calyx; *L*, liver; *I*, inferior vena cava; *A*, aorta.) **(C)** Selective renal angiogram reveals a hypertrophied renal artery *(RA)* supplying the malformation with arteriovenous shunting and early opacification of the renal vein *(RV)* and inferior vena cava *(IVC)*. (From Subramanyam BR, Lefleur RS, Bosniak MA: Renal arteriovenous fistulas and aneurysms: Sonographic findings. Radiology 149:261, 1983.)

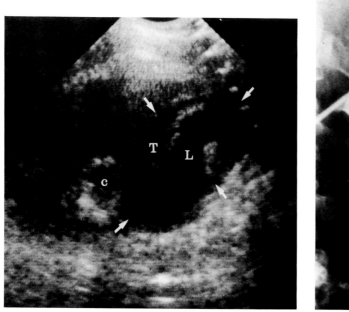

A

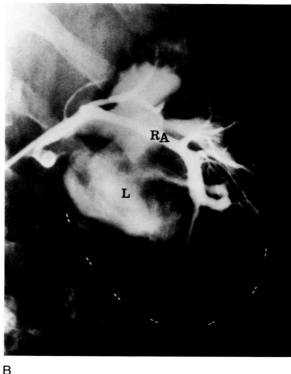

B

Fig. 6-46. Renal arteriovenous fistula. Aneurysmal type. **(A)** Longitudinal real-time scan revealing a large mass (arrows) involving the lower half of the kidney. Note the solid periphery representing thrombus *(T)* and a central hypoechoic tubular lumen *(L)*. (*c*, calyx.) **(B)** Left renal angiogram reveals an enlarged segmental renal artery *(RA)*, filling the lumen of the aneurysm *(L)*. The dotted lines represent the thrombosed segment of the aneurysm. (From Subramanyam BR, Lefleur RS, Bosniak MA: Renal arteriovenous fistulas and aneurysms: Sonographic findings. Radiology 149:261, 1983.)

ing; and (3) complete obstruction secondary to thrombosis.[68] Clinically, these patients are in the third to fourth decade with portal hypertension. The cause of membranous obstruction of the inferior vena cava is disputed; it may be congenital, acquired, or unknown.[6,68] On ultrasound, obstruction at the level of the diaphragm along with dilatation of the azygos system is seen (Fig. 6-49). An inferior vena cavagram shows conical obstruction of the inferior vena cava at the level of the diaphragm, with marked collateralization through the azygos and hemiazygos systems. Hepatic venography shows patency of the major intrahepatic veins, which can be seen on ultrasound.

Inferior Vena Caval Dilatation

Abnormal dilatation of the inferior vena cava may be seen with several abnormalities (Fig. 6-50). In normal individuals, the inferior vena cava collapses with expiration but in patients with right ventricular failure, the respiratory kinetics disappear and the inferior vena cava remains turgescent throughout the respiratory cycle.[69] Absence of inspiratory decrease in inferior vena caval size may be due to athersclerosis heart disease, pulmonary hypertension, pericardial tamponade, constrictive pericarditis, or atrial tumor.[6]

Inferior Vena Caval Tumor

Because the inferior venal cava is frequently involved in disease of the abdomen and retroperitoneum, it is critical to evaluate the inferior vena cava's entire course as it may help in determining the origin of an adjacent mass.[70] With ultrasound, the superior aspect of the inferior vena cava is successfully visualized; however, the distal portion is occasionally obscured by overlying bowel gas (Fig. 6-4 and 6-6). On longitudinal and transverse scans, the inferior vena cava can be identified along with its anatomic relationships (Fig. 6-51). In the longitudinal projection, the distal and midportion of the infe-

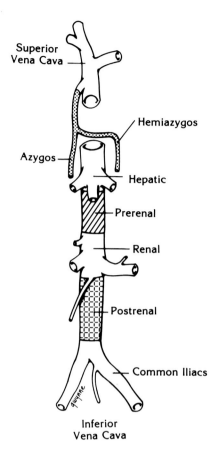

Fig. 6-47. Embryologic components of the inferior vena cava. (Modified from Hill MC, Sanders RC: Sonography of the upper abdominal venous system. p.271. In Sanders RC, Hill MC (eds): Ultrasound Annual 1983, Raven Press, New York, 1983.)

rior vena cava have a horizontal course while the more proximal portion is concave anteriorly (Fig. 6-4 and 6-6). The walls of the inferior vena cava are thin and prone to deformity by adjacent masses. Any displacement or change in shape of the inferior vena cava can be easily evaluated by either contrast or sonocavaography.[71]

The upper or hepatic portion of the inferior vena cava is that portion of the inferior vena cava from the diaphragm to the portal vein (Fig. 6-51). Expanding masses immediately posterior to this segment are most likely right adrenal, neurogenic, or hepatic in origin[72] (Fig. 6-52). With generalized enlargement of the liver, the inferior vena cava is compressed rather than displaced. A localized liver mass would produce posterior, lateral, or medial displacement of the inferior vena cava (Fig. 6-52A and B). A mass in the posterior caudate lobe and right lobe may elevate the inferior vena cava.[71]

The middle or pancreatic portion of the inferior vena cava is that region posterior to the pancreas extending from the portal vein to the extent of the pancreatic head (Fig. 6-51). Abnormalities of the right renal artery, right kidney, lumbar spine, and lymph nodes commonly elevate this segment (Figs. 6-53 and 6-54). A right renal artery aneurysm would displace the inferior vena cava anteriorly. The kidney may have middle and upper elevation of the vessel. Anterior changes in the lumbar vertebrae or interposed disc spaces may elevate the inferior vena cava with anterior osteophytes most common.[71]

The lower or small bowel segment is that portion of the inferior vena cava with the duodenum and jejunum anterior and extending from the pancreatic head to the bifurcation (Fig. 6-51). There are usually no major organs or blood vessels posterior to this segment and in general the only abnormalities are those of the lumbar spine and lymph nodes that elevate this portion of the inferior vena cava. Lymph node enlargement constitutes the majority of this group with retroperitoneal tumors and tortuous aorta as rarer causes (Fig. 6-54). The literature states that 20 percent of tortuous abdominal aortas curve convexly to the right impinging on the left side of the inferior vena cava (Fig. 6-18). Some extent posteriorly causing elevation of the inferior vena cava in its upper and cephalad portions of the middle division.[71]

With the knowledge of the masses that may affect the inferior vena cava posteriorly, the examiner can guess which ones might affect the vessel internally. Both thrombosis or tumor appear as single or multiple echogenic nodules along the wall on ultrasound and may extend into the lumen for varying length. At times, the inferior vena cava may be distended and full of echoes[6,73,75] (See Fig. 4-114). On sagittal scan, the anterior wall domes as it is stretched over the tumor thrombus. On real-time ultrasound, there may be a loss of normal venous pulsation.[73] Tumor tends to have a fine homogeneous echopattern, whereas blood clot alone has an inhomogeneous coarse echopattern.

The most common tumor to involve the inferior vena cava is renal cell carcinoma (9 to 33 percent), which is usually on the right because of the close proximity to the inferior vena cava.[6,70,76] The presence of venous tumor appears to be related to the size of the primary tumor. Venous tumor may be seen as intraluminal echogenic nodules or thrombi and can cause generalized inferior vena caval dilatation with innumerable diffuse, low-amplitude echoes emanating from lumen[76] (See Fig. 4-114). It may even extend to the right atrium. In children, Wilms' tumor may be similar to renal cell carcinoma.[6,77] Four to 10 percent of children with Wilms' tumor will have venous extension.[77] In addition, in renal tumor with arteriovenous shunting, the renal vein may be dilated in the absence of venous extension of the tumor. Other less common tumors involving the inferior vena cava are retroperitoneal liposarcoma, leiomyosarcoma,

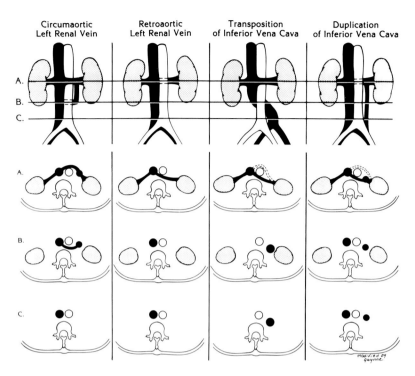

Fig. 6-48. Anomalies involving the inferior vena cava. Cross-sections of the aorta, inferior vena cava and left renal vein in anomalies of the inferior vena cava and left renal vein. In transposition and duplication, a venous structure may pass either anterior or posterior (dashed line) to the aorta at the level of the renal vein. (Modified from Royal SA, Callen PW: CT evaluation of anomalies of the inferior vena cava and left renal vein. AJR 132:759, © Am Roent Ray Soc, 1979.)

pheochromocytoma, osteosarcoma, and rhadomyosarcoma.[73,75] Benign tumors such as angiomyolipoma can also have venous involvement.[78] If there is no cause for the intraluminal mass, a primary vascular tumor, such as a leiomyosarcoma should be considered.[6]

Inferior Vena Caval Thrombosis

Inferior vena caval thrombosis is a potentially life-threatening condition of diverse etiology. Even with complete occlusion of the inferior vena cava, signs and

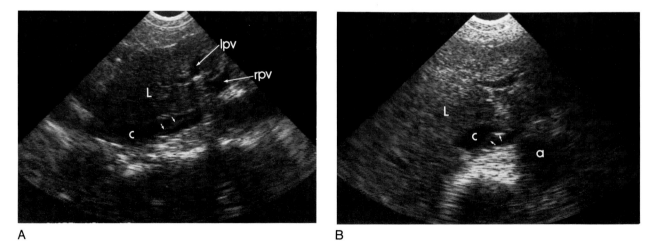

A   B

Fig. 6-49. Inferior vena caval web. Longitudinal (**A**) and transverse (**B**) real-time scans. A linear echodensity (arrows) is seen within the inferior vena cava *(c)*. This moved at real-time in the dilated inferior vena cava. (*a*, aorta; *lpv*, left portal vein; *rpv*, right portal vein; *L*, liver.)

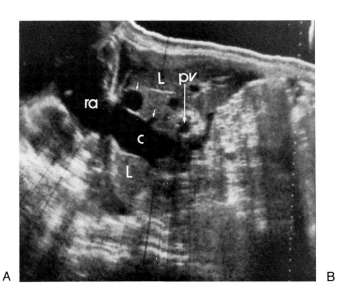
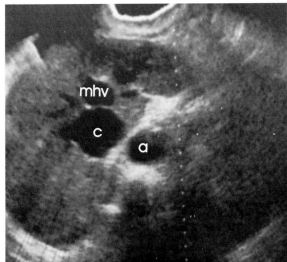
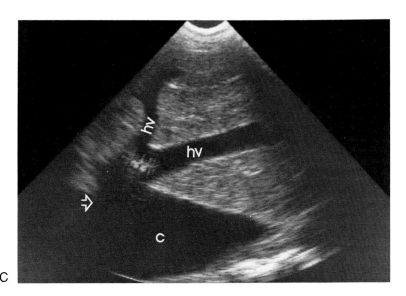

Fig. 6-50. Dilated inferior vena cava. Case 1: Congestive heart failure. Longitudinal **(A)** and transverse **(B)** scans. A markedly dilated inferior vena cava *(c)* is seen. Dilated hepatic veins (arrows) are seen draining into the inferior vena cava. (*L*, liver; *ra*, right atrium; *pv*, portal vein; *a*, aorta; *mhv*, middle hepatic vein.) Case 2: Congestive heart failure. Longitudinal **(C)** scan in this patient demonstrates dramatic enlargement of the hepatic veins *(hv)* and inferior vena cava *(c)*. (open arrow, level of the diaphragm.)

symptoms depend on the level of obstruction and include leg edema, low back pain, pelvic pain, gastrointestinal complaints, and renal and liver abnormalities.[79] Real-time ultrasound allows direct observation of the delicate pliable nature of the thrombus (Fig. 6-55). Its stretch and recoil with each cardiac cycle provides dramatic demonstration of the repetitive stress that may lead to fragmentation and embolization. The thrombus has a smoothly bordered uniform feature.[79]

Nontumoral clot usually results from extension from the iliac or renal vein. Extension from the iliacs is due to

an inflammatory process in the pelvis or due to thrombus in the deep venous system of the calf extending into the popliteal, femoral, and iliac.[6]

Inferior Vena Caval Filters

The commonest origin of pulmonary emboli is venous thrombosis from the lower extremities. This is usually treated with anticoagulant therapy unless there is

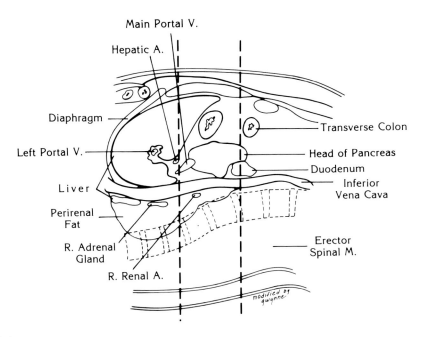

Fig. 6-51. Inferior vena cava segments. Longitudinal diagram of the inferior vena cava. Dashed lines divide the inferior vena cava into three segments: upper, middle, and lower. (Modified from Kurtz AB, Rubin C, Goldberg BB: Ultrasound diagnosis of masses elevating the inferior vena cava. AJR 132:401, © Am Roent Ray Soc, 1979)

contraindication. In recent years, transvenous insertion of filter devices into the inferior vena cava have been advocated to prevent recurrent embolization in patients who cannot tolerate anticoagulants.[6] These filters are associated with a low complication rate.[80]

The true position of the device can be followed with ultrasound to evaluate for complications. It is sometimes difficult to fully evaluate the inferior vena caval filter postoperatively without radiography and cavogram.[80] The preferred location of the filter is in the iliac bifurcation, preferably below the renal veins.[81] Some filters migrate cranially or caudally and can perforate the cava, producing a retroperitoneal bleed. They can perforate the duodenum, aorta, ureter, and hepatic vein as well as produce lower extremity thrombophlebitis with edema and stasis dermatitis. The filter itself may thrombose and become a source of recurrent pulmonary emboli. The overall morbidity related to the filter is 1 percent. The commonest used are the Mobin-Uddin (MU) and the Kimray-Greenfield (KG) filters. The KG filter is less thrombogenic and is less likely to perforate than the MU filter. Either can migrate caudally.[6]

Ultrasound can successfully identify the Kimray-Greenfield filter in 89 percent of cases.[80] By adding pulsed Doppler to the study, the investigator can evaluate flow above and below the filter in 76 percent, accurately predicting normal flow in most cases.[80] Doppler is 100 percent accurate in both detecting normal flow in patent vessels and determining thrombosis.[80] If there is

no flow shown by Doppler below the filter, then a contrast study may be done to confirm obstruction secondary to thrombosis. Ultrasound can be used to evaluate the inferior vena cava, renal vein, and bifurcation demonstrated on longitudinal and transverse scans (Fig. 6-56). The motion of the inferior vena cava with respiration can be studied as well as the renal veins. On longitudinal ultrasound scan the KG filter, which is a stainless steel wire cage, appears as a series of bright parallel lines. On transverse, scan a circle of bright, oblong echoes are seen[80] (Fig. 6-56).

INFERIOR VENA CAVAL BRANCH ABNORMALITIES

Renal Vein Thrombosis

Renal vein thrombosis is a serious complication seen in the dehydrated or septic infant.[82] It also may occur in adults with multiple renal abnormalities, notably nephrotic syndrome, shock, renal tumor, kidney transplant, and trauma.[83] The patient may present clinically with flank pain, hematuria, flank mass, and proteinuria. It is often associated with maternal diabetes and transient high blood pressure. There is usually faint or absent visualization of the affected kidney at excretory urogram. Prompt diagnosis of renal vein thrombosis is required in the affected child so proper therapy can be

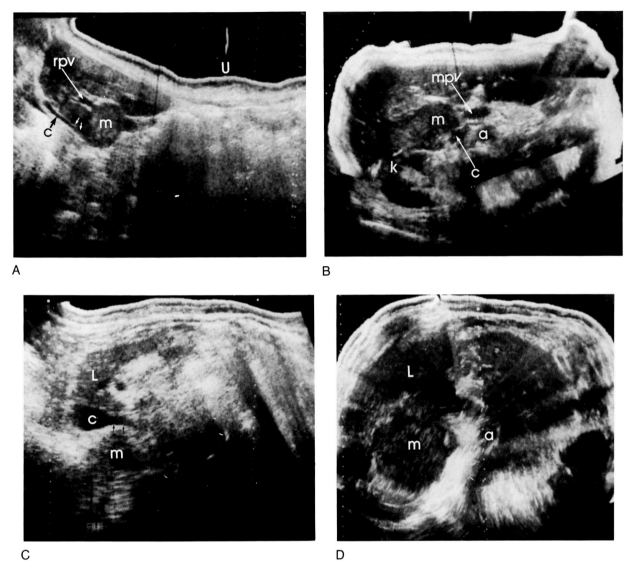

Fig. 6-52. Upper inferior vena caval compression. Case 1: Hepatic metastasis from carcinoma of the lung. Longitudinal scan at 4 cm to the right of midline **(A)** and transverse scan **(B)** at 2 cm above the umbilicus demonstrate compression (arrows) of the hepatic portion of the inferior vena cava *(c)* by the liver mass *(m)*. The lumen of the inferior vena cava could not be seen inferior to the mass. (*U*, level of the umbilicus; *rpv*, right portal vein; *mpv*, main portal vein; *k*, right kidney.) Case 2: Adrenal metastasis from carcinoma of the lung. Longitudinal scan at 5 **(C)** cm to the right of midline and transverse **(D)** scan 12 cm above the umbilicus show compression (arrows) of the inferior vena cava *(c)* by the adrenal tumor *(m)*. The inferior vena cava is not seen on **(D)**. (*L*, liver; *a*, aorta.)

instituted. While renal vein thrombosis may have a classic picture, the clinical diagnosis is often in doubt.[84] Renal vein thrombosis may develop when thrombi in the inferior vena cava extend into the renal vein, or thrombi begin in the arcuate and interlobular veins and spread to the main renal vein.

Ultrasound can be used to confirm that a palpable mass is kidney and to exclude hydronephosis and multicystic kidney as a cause of nonfunction (Fig. 6-57 and 6-58). Enlarged kidneys without cysts are seen in infants. Either medium level echoes distributed evenly throughout the kidney are seen or distinct clumps of echoes randomly scattered within the kidney with surrounding echofree spaces are visualized.[84] The parenchymal anechoic areas are due to hemorrhage and hemorrhagic infarcts (Fig. 6-58). As such, immediately after renal vein thrombosis, there is nephromegaly and decreased cortical echoes.[86] The ultrasound pattern of an enlarged

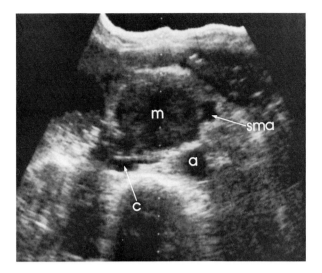

Fig. 6-53. Middle inferior vena caval compression. Pancreatic adenocarcinoma. Transverse scan demonstrates compression of the inferior vena cava *(c)* by the hypoechoic pancreatic head mass *(m)*. The superior mesenteric artery *(sma)* is displaced anteriorly and to the left. (*a*, aorta.)

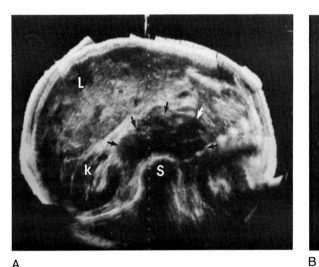

A

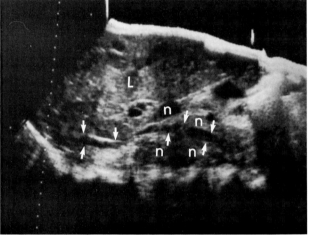

B

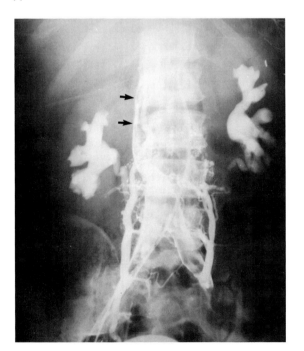

C

Fig. 6-54. Middle and lower inferior vena caval compression. Hairy cell leukemia (B-cell lymphoma). **(A)** Transverse scan. Multiple anechoic nodes (arrows) are seen in the paraortic and paracaval areas. The prevertebral vessels cannot be identified. There is also an inhomogeneous pattern in the liver *(L)*. (*k*, right kidney; *S*, spine.) **(B)** Longitudinal scan. The inferior vena cava (arrows) is compressed by nodes *(n)* anteriorly and posteriorly. (*L*, liver.) **(C)** Inferior vena cavagram. The cava is compressed (arrows).

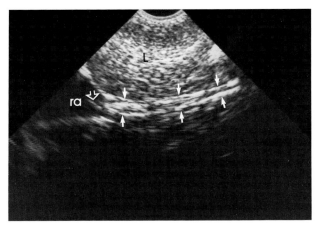

A

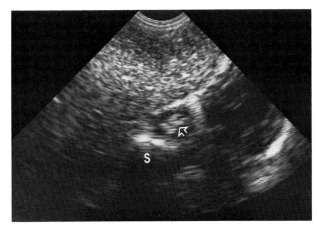

B

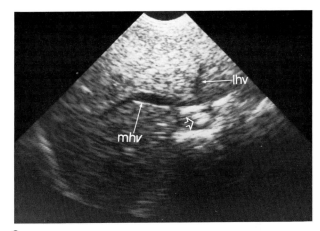

C

Fig. 6-55. Inferior vena caval thrombosis. **(A)** Longitudinal scan of the inferior vena reveals an echogenic "cast" (arrows) filling the lumen of the inferior vena cava. A portion of the thrombus (open arrow) projects into the right atrium *(ra)*. (*L*, liver) **(B)** High transverse scan. The thrombus (open arrow) is seen to be surrounded by the anechoic lumen of the inferior vena cava. (*S*, spine.) **(C)** Transverse scan at the level of the hepatic veins. Only the left *(lhv)* and middle *(mhv)* veins are demonstrated; the right hepatic vein was never seen. On this scan as well as those lower, no caval lumen was demonstrated. An echogenic thrombus (open arrows) is seen.

echogenic kidney with a distorted internal echopattern in association with the appropriate clinical finding should be sufficient to make the diagnosis of renal vein thrombosis without requiring invasive vascular studies[83,84] (Figs. 6-57 and 6-58). The increase in cortical echoes with preservation of the corticomedullary definition occurs within 2 weeks after renal vein thrombosis.[86] The renal pattern progresses to atrophy over a 2 month period.[83] The late findings include increased parenchymal echoes, loss of corticomedullary junction, and decreased renal size.[86] As such, ultrasound can yield a definite diagnosis of renal vein thrombosis if the following are present: (1) direct visualization of thrombi in the renal vein and inferior vena cava (Fig. 6-57); (2) demonstration of the renal vein dilated proximal to the point of occlusion; (3) loss of the normal renal structure (Fig. 6-58) and (4) increased renal size (acute phase).[83]

In a clinical and experimental study, it was found that renal vein thrombosis acutely led to decreased cortical echogenicity and nephromegaly.[85,86] Between 10 days and 3 weeks, there is increased cortical echogenicity with preservation of the corticomedullary definition. The late changes were decreased renal size, increased cortical echogenicity, and loss of the corticomedullary definition. On real-time ultrasound, there were decreased transmitted pulsations to the affected renal vein. On Doppler, there was absence of flow.[86]

Acute renal vein thrombosis patients may present with typical findings of pain, nephromegaly, hematuria, and evidence of thromboembolic phenomena elsewhere in the body. However, the findings in both acute and chronic renal vein thrombosis may be nonspecific. A variety of lesions may be associated with this abnormality. These include renal tumor, retroperitoneal tumor, phlebitis involving caval, and/or renal veins, trauma, dehydration, lymphoma, and a variety of primary renal diseases including membraneous glomerulonephritis and amyloidosis. The pathologic features include edema and hemorrhage which generally occur during the acute stage followed by cellular infiltration and fibrosis.[86]

On real-time ultrasound, the presence of normally transmitted pulsations to the renal vein is good evidence

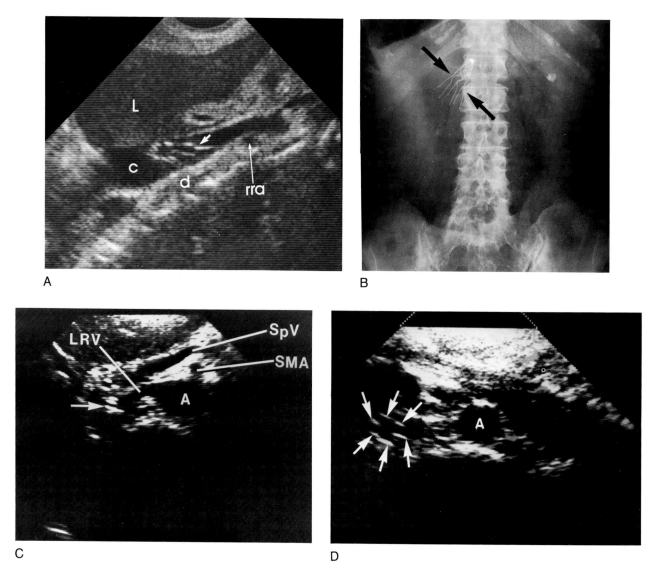

Fig. 6-56. Inferior vena caval filter. Kimray-Greenfield filter. Case 1: **(A)** Longitudinal scan with identification of the filter (arrow) in the inferior vena cava *(c)* superior to the right renal artery *(rra)*. (*L*, liver; *d*, right crus of the diaphragm.) **(B)** Radiograph of the filter device showing the metallic prongs (arrows) by which it attaches itself to the caval wall. (Figs. **A,B** from Hill MC, Sanders RC: Sonography of the upper abdominal venous system. p.271. In Ultrasound Annual 1983. Raven Press, New York, 1983.) Case 2: Transverse views of the inferior vena cava showing the filter (arrow) from the cephalad to caudad end. (*A*, aorta.) **(C)** Transverse scan at the level of the left renal vein *(LRV)*. Note the closely spaced bright dots that represent the cephalic portion (apex). (*SpV*, splenic vein; *SMA*, superior mesenteric artery.) **(D)** Transverse scan at the mid-portion of the filter. Note the six oblong echoes (arrows) arranged in a circle, representing the limbs of the filter within the *IVC*. (Figs. **C, D** from Pasto ME, Kurtz AB, Jarrell BE et al: The Kimray-Greenfield filter: Evaluation by duplex real-time/pulsed doppler ultrasound. Radiology 148:223, 1983.)

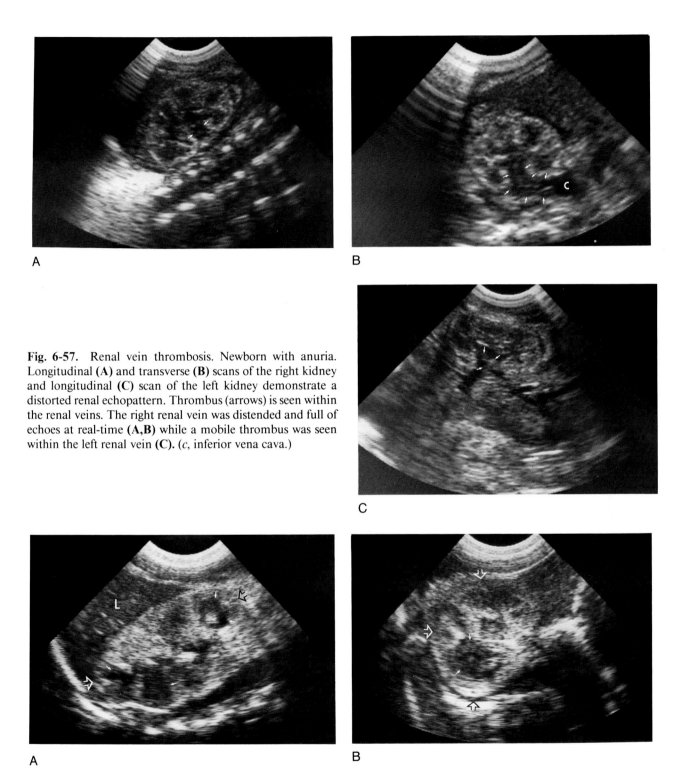

Fig. 6-57. Renal vein thrombosis. Newborn with anuria. Longitudinal **(A)** and transverse **(B)** scans of the right kidney and longitudinal **(C)** scan of the left kidney demonstrate a distorted renal echopattern. Thrombus (arrows) is seen within the renal veins. The right renal vein was distended and full of echoes at real-time **(A,B)** while a mobile thrombus was seen within the left renal vein **(C)**. (*c*, inferior vena cava.)

Fig. 6-58.   Acute renal vein thrombosis. Longitudinal **(A)** and transverse **(B)** scans of the right kidney (open arrows) in a newborn measuring 5.0 cm in length. The echopattern is very distorted with a mixed pattern in the area of the renal pyramids (arrows). (*L*, liver.) *(Figure continues.)*

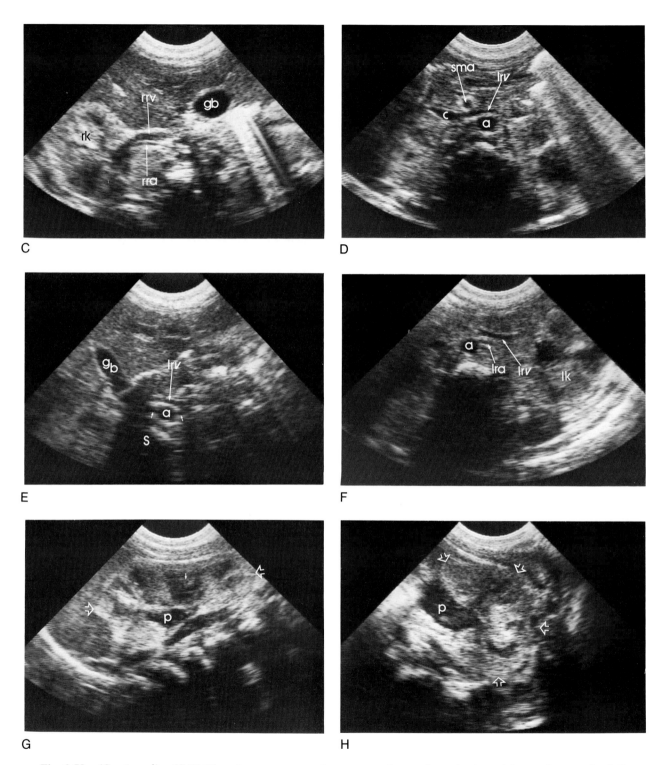

Fig. 6-58 *(Continued)*. **(C-F)** These transverse scans demonstrate the renal arteries (*rra*, right renal artery; *lra*, left renal artery; small arrows on **E**) and renal veins (*rrv*, right renal vein; *lrv*, left renal vein.) No definite venous thrombi were seen at real-time. (*gb*, gallbladder; *rk*, right kidney; *lk*, left kidney; *a*, aorta; *sma*, superior mesenteric artery; *c*, inferior vena cava; *S*, spine.) Longitudinal **(G)** and transverse **(H)** scans of the left kidney (open arrows). The renal pelvis *(p)* was dilated containing many echoes representing blood. The echopattern is very distorted, with a mixed pattern in the area of the pyramids (small arrow).

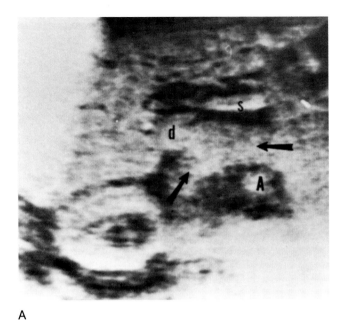

A

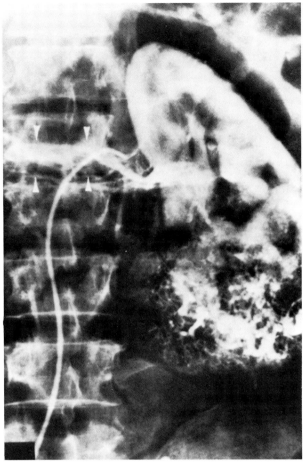

B

Fig. 6-59. Renal vein enlargement. Tumor. **(A)** Transverse scan. Tumor thrombus (arrows) in left renal vein and inferior vena cava. (*A*, aorta; *d*, duodenum; *S*, splenic vein.) **(B)** Selective renal angiogram. Hypervascular left lower pole mass and typical streaking associated with thrombus within renal veins (arrowheads.) (From Thomas JL, Bernardino ME: Neoplastic-induced renal vein enlargement: Sonographic detection. AJR 136:75, © American Roentgen Ray Society, 1981.)

against this abnormality. Absence may be valuable information but all normals do not have it. It is more significant if transmitted pulses are seen in one renal vein and not the other. Thus, the ultrasound evaluation of renal vein thrombosis is easier if it is a unilateral rather than bilateral process. The ability of pulsed Doppler to demonstrate flow within the normal renal vein and absence of flow in renal vein thrombosis indicates that Doppler complements real-time ultrasonography.[86] The direct ultrasound visualization of thrombus within the renal vein and inferior vena cava are of major importance in diagnosing renal vein thrombosis.[83,87]

Renal Vein Obstruction

Left renal vein obstruction may result from the spread of such nonrenal malignancies as carcinoma of the pancreas, lung, and lymphoma.[88] Retroperitoneal tumor (primary or secondary) can also occlude the left renal vein by direct extension into the vein lumen or compression of the lumen by contiguous mass. Renal vein ob-

struction can occur from thrombosis secondary to a hypercoagulable state that accompanies certain malignancies, especially colonic, pancreatic, and bronchogenic carcinoma. Ultrasound furnishes supportive evidence of venous occlusion with renal vein dilatation, increased renal size, and loss of normal renal echopattern.[88] Real-time ultrasound provides a rapid examination of vessels and, coupled with Doppler, can analyze blood flow in the renal vein.[88]

Renal Vein Enlargement

The etiology of renal vein enlargement is multiple. It could be secondary to tumor thrombus, neoplastic arteriovenous shunting, and portal systemic shunting into the left renal vein. With tumor thrombus there is echogenic enlargement of the renal vein (Fig. 6-59); with increased flow there is anechoic enlargement. The renal vein is considered dilated if it is greater than 1.5 cm. Abrupt enlargement of the inferior vena cava at the level of the renals is a better indicator of dilatation than abso-

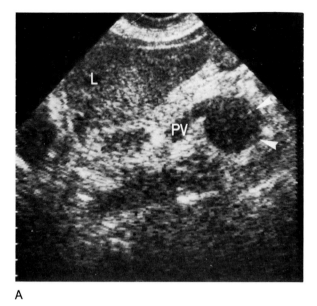

A

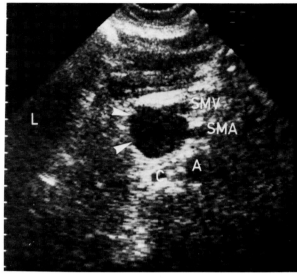

B

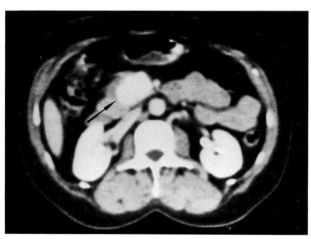

C

Fig. 6-60. Superior mesenteric vein aneurysm. Longitudinal (**A**) and transverse (**B**) scans of a cystic, compressible tumor (arrowheads) in the vicinity of the superior mesenteric vein *(SMV)*. (*L*, liver; *C*, inferior vena cava; *A*, aorta; *PV*, portal vein.) (**C**) CT scan with enhancement (arrow) during venous phase. (From Schild H, Schweden F, Braun B, Lang H: Aneurysms of the superior mesenteric vein. Radiology 145:641, 1982.)

lute measurement.[7] Since the Valsalva maneuver affects diameter, all measurements should be made in the same degree of inspiration. Congestive heart failure and obstruction of the inferior vena cava proximal to the renal vein are important causes of bilateral dilatation of the renal veins.

In an oncologic patient, unilateral dilatation of the renal vein is often associated with hypernephroma because it is a vascular tumor with propensity to invade the renal vein. Invasion of the renal vein may be associated with thrombus formation and/or arteriovenous shunting. Preoperative detection of tumor thrombus within the renal vein and inferior vena cava is important in surgical planning in hypernephroma patients. This type of tumor extension occurs in 21 to 55 percent of surgical specimens. Real-time ultrasound facilitates this detection.[7]

The presence of an arteriovenous fistula should be considered if ultrasound shows an enlarged renal vein with a dilated inferior vena cava above the abnormal vein.[7] Patients with portal venous hypertension may develop a spontaneous portosystemic shunt with increased flow and dilatation of the left renal vein that may present as a mass.[89] The left renal vein is a pathway for shunting through the gastrorenal or splenorenal circulation. If the patient has a normal blood pressure with a dilated left renal vein and normal left kidney, check the liver for portal venous hypertension because it can occur in cirrhosis and in neoplastic occlusion of the portal vein especially with hepatoma.[7] A left renal vein varix could ap-

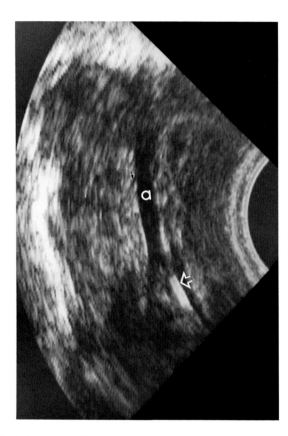

Fig. 6-61. Umbilical arterial catheter. Longitudinal (coronal) scan through the right flank. The abdominal aorta *(a)* is easily seen as are the renal arteries (arrows) and iliac vessels. The catheter tip (open arrow) can be seen within the right iliac artery.

pear similarly as a hypoechoic mass anterior to the kidney.[89] (See Fig. 3-40.)

It may be difficult to differentiate renal vein dilatation secondary to flow and tumor thrombus. Technical factors may result in low-level echoes within the renal vein and tumor may be anechoic. Large arteriovenous shunts should produce pulsatile motion of the venous walls on real-time ultrasound. Conceivably, Doppler could differentiate between renal vein enlargement due to flow or thrombus. Dilatation of the inferior vena cava inferior to the renal vein or abrupt narrowing of the dilated inferior vena cava between the renal vein and right atrium usually indicates obstruction while anechoic enlargement of the inferior vena cava above the renal vein is more compatible with increased flow due to shunting.[7]

The pitfall in this assessment is duplication of the inferior vena cava. The classic duplicated inferior vena cava lies to the left of the aorta and crosses to join the right sided inferior vena cava at the level of the renal vein.

Conceivably, the crossing left inferior vena cava to join the right may be mistaken for a dilated left renal vein. A transverse scan below the level of the renal vein should show a vessel to the left of the aorta to clarify this.[7]

Superior Mesenteric Vein Aneurysm

Venous aneurysms are rare compared to arterial aneurysms. They may involve the leg, neck, portal vein, or splenic vein. With a portal venous system aneurysm, if it is large, there are symptoms of duodenal compression, common bile duct obstruction, and chronic portal hypertension. With a superior mesenteric vein aneurysm, the theory of development is that one of the caudal components of the right vitelline vein does not obliterate all the way down to the ventral intervitelline anastomosis as normal but forms a small diverticulum at the junction with the ventral intervitelline anastomosis. Under the influence of mechanical forces like blood turbulence,

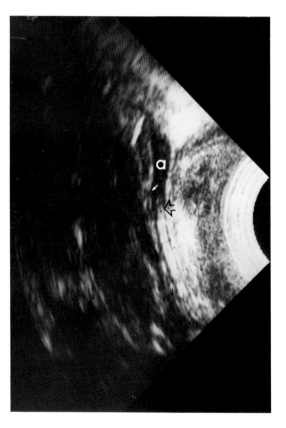

Fig. 6-62. Umbilical arterial catheter. Longitudinal scan through the left flank. The tip (open arrow) of the aortic *(a)* catheter is seen too high, just below the level of the renal arteries (arrow).

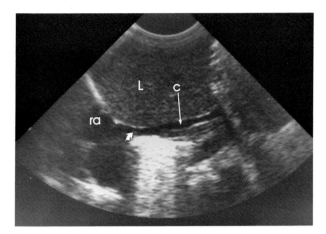

Fig. 6-63. Umbilical venous catheter. Longitudinal scan (coronal) through the right flank. The tip (curved arrow) of the catheter is seen near the entrance of the inferior vena cava *(c)* into the right atrium *(ra)*. (*L*, liver.)

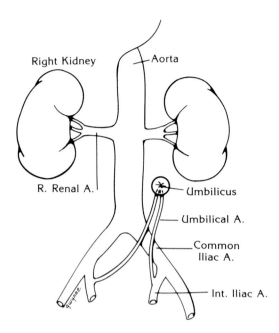

Fig. 6-65. Pathway of umbilical arterial catheter. The arterial catheter passes through either of the paired umbilical arteries traveling inferiorly toward the ipsilateral internal iliac artery. After entering the internal iliac artery, the catheter turns cephalad to pass up the common iliac artery and aorta.

this diverticulum could later enlarge and form an aneurysm[90] (Fig. 6-60).

INTERVENTIONAL

Umbilical Catheters

Umbilical arterial and venous catheters are an integral component of infant care in neonatal intensive care units. They provide ready diagnostic and therapeutic access to the neonatal central circulation. Thus, catheter position is critical. With incorrect location, there is in-

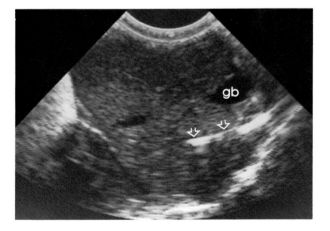

Fig. 6-64. Umbilical venous catheter. Longitudinal left lateral decubitus (coronal) scan through the right flank. The catheter is seen within the liver substance in the ductus venosus. (*gb*, gallbladder.)

creased incidence of complications and misleading pressure measurements. While most are radiopaque, their exact location in relation to vascular anatomic landmarks is not available from a radiograph but simply inferred from location. With ultrasound, by scanning through the flank (to avoid bowel gas), one can identify the catheter as a well-defined echogenic structure (Figs. 6-61 and 6-62). The arterial catheter should be above the aortic bifurcation but below the renal arteries[91] (Fig. 6-61 and 6-62). The venous catheter appears as either a parallel echogenic line or as a linear shadow[91,92] (Figs. 6-63 and 6-64). Direct visualization of the intrahepatic catheter is often not accomplished because the position of the catheter in the ductus venosus with a posterior angled course can not be positioned perpendicular to the axis of the sound beam.[91]

To understand the pathway of the umbilical catheters, one needs to be familiar with the anatomy (Figs. 6-65 and 6-66). The umbilical artery travels inferior toward the ipsilateral internal iliac artery. After entering the iliac, the catheter turns cephalad and passes retrograde up the internal iliac, and common iliac into the aorta. The optimal placement for the tip is below the origin of the renal artery and above the aorta bifurcation.[92] The venous catheter passes superiorly in the midline through the umbilical vein to the falciform ligament to enter the liver joining the left portal vein. A properly positioned

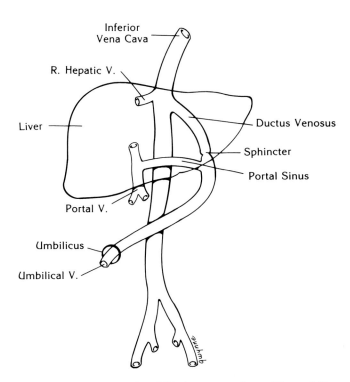

Fig. 6-66. Pathway of umbilical venous catheter. The umbilical venous catheter passes superiorly in the midline through the umbilical vein as it courses through the falciform ligament and enters the liver where the umbilical vein joins the left portal vein. Then the catheter ascends through the ductus venosus to enter an hepatic vein close to their confluence in the inferior vena cava.

catheter courses the left portal vein to enter the ductus venosus, which usually originates directly opposite the umbilical vein orifice. The catheter then ascends through the ductus to enter the left or middle hepatic vein close to the confluence of the inferior vena cava. The position for the tip of the venous catheter is in the intrathoracic inferior vena cava, although the right atrium is a suitable alternative.

Umbilical catheter tips must be checked immediately after their insertion to ensure the proper vessel is cannulated. The most commonly encountered incorrect catheter position in the umbilical artery is either above the renals or below the aortic bifurcation. The most common malposition of the umbilical vein catheter is the failure of the tip to pass through the liver substance into the central venous reservoir. Intrahepatic position increases the risk of portal venous thrombosis.[92]

In addition to the evaluation of umbilical catheter location, ultrasound can look for evidence of vascular compromise or catheter complications (Figs. 6-67 to 6-70). In one study, 17 percent of infants had clinically evident signs of vascular compromise. Of these, 83 per-

cent had abnormal intravascular echoes or lack of expansile pulsations at ultrasound (Figs. 6-67 and 6-69). Abnormal echogenic foci were consistent with thrombus and intimal dissection (Figs. 6-68 and 6-69). These abnormalities persisted from 2 to 70 days.[93]

Catheter Fragments

The intraluminal breaking of an angiographic catheter may be a serious complication with potential for significant morbidity or mortality. If the exact location of the catheter is known, the radiologist and surgeon can determine which method, percutaneous transcatheter retrieval or direct surgical extrication, is best for removal of the fragment. A 5F catheter can be seen routinely with ultrasound[94] (Fig. 6-71).

Complications of retained intravascular foreign bodies include sepsis, perforation, thrombosis, cardiac arrhythmia, and myocardial necrosis. With recent ad-

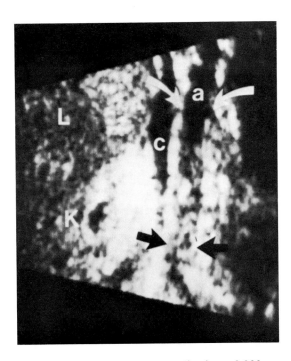

Fig. 6-67. Umbilical catheter complications. 3,033 g newborn with loss of femoral pulses and cyanotic legs. The catheter was removed immediately prior to examination. Coronal scan through the right flank demonstrates increased echogenicity within the infrarenal aorta *(a)* and bifurcation (black arrows). Real-time examination failed to reveal pulsation at this level. (curved arrows, renal arteries; *c,* inferior vena cava; *L,* liver; *K,* right kidney.) (From Oppenheimer DA, Carroll BA, Garth KE: Ultrasonic detection of complications following umbilical arterial catheterization in the neonate. Radiology 145:667, 1982.)

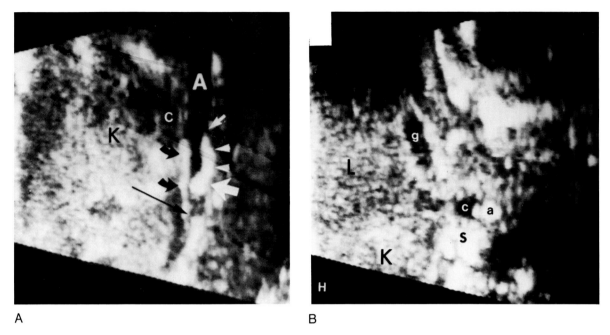

A   B

Fig. 6-68. Umbilical catheter complications. 700 g newborn with candida sepsis and leg swelling. The catheter was removed before the examination. The aortic abnormality was present at 70 days follow-up. **(A)** Coronal scan through right flank demonstrating a large echogenic plaque (arrowheads) along the aortic wall arising just below the left renal artery (small white arrow). A focal convex collection nearly fills the aortic lumen **(A)**, but a thin sonolucent zone is identified between it and the opposite aortic wall. The right infrarenal aortic wall is also of increased echogenicity (curved black arrows). Real-time demonstrated fixed abnormalities with pulsation identified in the aorta and common iliac arteries. (*C*, inferior vena cava; *K*, right kidney.) **(B)** A transverse scan through the right flank at the level of the focal convex echogenic collection in **(A)**. The collection appears to nearly fill the aortic lumen *(a)*. (*S*, spine; *L*, liver; *g*, gallbladder.) (From Oppenheimer DA, Carroll BA, Garth KE: Ultrasonic detection of complications following umbilical arterial catheterization in the neonate. Radiology 145:667, 1982.)

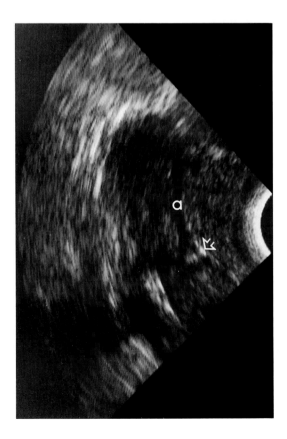

Fig. 6-69. Umbilical catheter complications. There were no femoral pulses palpable in this patient. At longitudinal real-time scan through the left flank, a nonpulsatile aorta *(a)* was seen. There was a dense echogenic (arrow) plaque in the left common iliac artery.

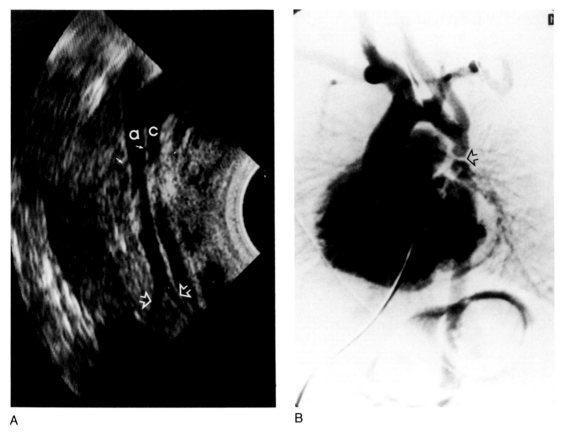

A   B

Fig. 6-70. Umbilical catheter complication? Coarctation of the aorta. Newborn with no palpable femoral pulses and a previous umbilical arterial catheter. **(A)** Coronal scan through the right flank revealed an echofree aorta *(a)* with no visible pulsations at real-time. No internal thrombus was seen on two examinations a week apart. (*c*, inferior vena cava; open arrows, iliacs; arrows, renal arteries.) **(B)** Digital Subtraction Angiogram. A coarctation of the aorta (arrow) is demonstrated, which accounted for the diminished pulses.

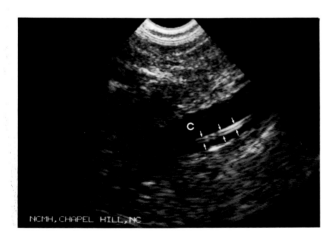

Fig. 6-71. Femoral catheter, adult. An inferior vena caval *(c)* catheter (arrows) inserted through the femoral vein in an adult can be seen in this longitudinal scan as a double echogenic line.

vances in real-time techniques, good quality images of the abdominal vessels are produced. The flexible mechanical sector scanner allows rapid localization of the area of interest. Catheter fragments, usually migrate to the superior or inferior vena cava, right side of the heart, or pulmonary arteries. Real-time ultrasound can be helpful in locating those nonopaque foreign bodies in the inferior vena cava or the right side of the heart. Because many of these patients are critically ill, percutaneous removal under real-time guidance should be attempted before subjecting the patient to major surgery.[95]

REFERENCES

1. Isikoff MB, Hill MC: Sonography of the renal arteries: Left lateral decubitus position. AJR 134:1177, 1980
2. Pardes JG, Kazam E, Kneeland JB et al: Sonography of the retroperitoneum: Value of oblique coronal view. Official

Proceedings of the American Institute of Ultrasound in Medicine. J Ultrasound Med 2:3, 1983

3. Athey PA, Tamez L: Lateral decubitus position for demonstration of the aortic bifurcation. J Clin Ultrasound 7:154, 1979
4. Gooding GAW: Ultrasonography of the iliac arteries. Radiology 135:161, 1980
5. Goldberg BB, Perlmutter G: Ultrasonic evaluation of the superior mesenteric artery. J Clin Ultrasound 5:185, 1977
6. Hill MC, Sanders RC: Sonography of the upper abdominal venous system. p.271. In Hill MC, Sanders RC (eds): Ultrasound Annual 1983. Raven Press, New York, 1983
7. Thomas JL, Bernardino ME: Neoplastic-induced renal vein enlargement: Sonographic detection. AJR 136:75, 1981
8. Grant E, Rendano F, Sevinc E et al: Normal inferior vena cava: Caliber changes observed by dynamic ultrasound. AJR 135:335, 1980
9. Buschi AJ, Harrison RB, Brenbridge ANAG et al: Distended left renal vein: CT/sonographic normal variant. AJR 135:339, 1980
10. Manor A, Itzchak Y, Strauss S, Graif M: Sonographic demonstration of right ascending lumbar vein. AJR 138:339, 1982
11. Beitler JC, Sigel B, Machi J, Justin JR: The effects of temperature on blood flow ultrasonic echogenicity in vitro. J Ultrasound Med 2:529, 1983
12. Sigel B, Coelho JCU, Spigos DG et al: Ultrasonography of blood during stasis and coagulation. Invest Radiol 16:71, 1981
13. Wolverson MX, Nouri S, Joist JH et al: The direct visualization of blood flow by real-time ultrasound: Clinical observations and underlying mechanisms. Radiology 140:443, 1981
14. Sigel B, Machi J, Beitler JC, Justin JR: Red cell aggregation as a cause of blood-flow echogenicity. Radiology 148:799, 1983
15. Machi J, Sigel B, Beitler JC et al: Relation of in vivo blood flow to ultrasound echogenicity. J Clin Ultrasound 11:3, 1983
16. Cosgrove DO, Arger PH: Intravenous echoes due to laminar flow: Experimental observation. AJR 139:953, 1982
17. Robbins SL, Cotran RS: Blood vessels p.593. In Pathologic Basis of Disease, WB Saunders, Philadelphia, 1979
18. Gomes MN: Clinical and Surgical aspects of abdominal aortic aneurysms. p. 156. In Raymond HW, Zwiebel WJ (eds): Seminars in Ultrasound. Vol. 3. Grune and Stratton, New York, 1982
19. Wheeler WE, Beachley MC, Ranniger K: Angiography and ultrasonography: A comparative study of abdominal aortic aneurysms. Am J Roentgenol 126:95, 1976
20. Marcus R, Edell SL: Sonographic evaluation of iliac artery aneurysms. Am J Surg 140:666, 1980
21. Hardy DC, Lee JKT, Weyman PJ, Melson GL: Measurement of the abdominal aortic aneurysms: Plain radiograph and ultrasonographic correlation. Radiology 141:821, 1981
22. Harter LP, Gross BH, Callen PW: Ultrasonic evaluation of abdominal aortic thrombus. J Ultrasound Med 1:315, 1982

23. Anderson JC, Baltaxe HA, Wolf GL: Inability to show clot: One limitation of ultrasonography of the abdominal aorta. Radiology 132:693, 1979
24. Gooding GAW: Aneurysms of the abdominal aorta, iliac and femoral arteries. p.170. In Raymond HW, Zwiebel WJ (eds): Seminars in Ultrasound. Vol. 3. Grune and Stratton, New York, 1982
25. Phillips G, Gordon D: Abdominal aortic aneurysm: Unusual cause for left hemidiaphragmatic elevation. AJR 136:1221, 1981
26. Goldberg BB: Aortosonography. Int Surg 62:294, 1977
27. King DL, Van Natta FC, Thorsen K, Lechich RL: Spontaneously echogenic arterial blood flow in abdominal aortic aneurysms. AJR 138:350, 1982
28. Hertzer NR, Beven EG: Ultrasound aortic measurement and elective aneurysmnectomy. JAMA 240:1966, 1978
29. Grueve AH, Carpenter CM, Wicks JD, Edwards WS: Discordance in the sizing of abdominal aortic aneurysm and its significance. Am J Surg 144:627, 1982
30. Gomes MN, Hakkal HG, Schellinger D: Ultrasonography and CT scanning: A comparative study of abdominal aortic aneurysms. Computed Tomography 2:99, 1978
31. Turnipseed WD, Acher CW, Detmer DE et al: Digital subtraction angiography and B-mode ultrasonography for abdominal and peripheral aneurysms. Surgery 92:619, 1982
32. Lee TG, Henderson SC: Ultrasonic aortography: Unexpected findings. Am J Roentgenol 128:273, 1977
33. Spirt BA, Skolnick ML, Carsky EW, Ticen K: Anterior displacement of the abdominal aorta: A radiographic and sonographic study. Radiology 111:399, 1974
34. Lyons EA, Barki Y: Ultrasound in the evaluation of the pulsatile epigastric mass. p.137. In Taylor KJW, Viscomi GN (eds): Clinics in Diagnostic Ultrasound: Ultrasound in Emergency Medicine. Churchill Livingstone, New York, 1981
35. Conrad MR, Davis GM, Green CE, Curry TS III: Real-time ultrasound in the diagnosis of acute dissecting aneurysms of the abdominal aorta. AJR 132:115, 1979
36. Kumari SS, Pillari G, Mandon V, Bank S: Occult aortic dissection and diagnosis by ultrasound. Br J Radiol 53:1093, 1980
37. Clayton MJ, Walsh JW, Brewer WH: Contained rupture of abdominal aortic aneurysms: Sonographic and CT diagnosis. AJR 138:154, 1982
38. Gooding GAW: Ruptured abdominal aorta: Postoperative ultrasound appearance. Radiology 145:781, 1982
39. McGregor JC: Unoperated ruptured abdominal aortic aneurysms: A retrospective clinicopathological study over a 10-year period. Br J Surg 63:113, 1976
40. Chisolm AJ, Sprayregen S: Angiographic manifestations of ruptured abdominal aortic aneurysms. Am J Roentgenol 127:769, 1976
41. Spinelli GD, Kleinclaus DH, Wenger JJ et al: Obstructive jaundice and abdominal aortic aneurysm: An ultrasonographic study. Radiology 144:872, 1982
42. Lepke RA, Pagani JJ: Renal artery compression by an aortic aneurysm: An unusual cause of hypertension. AJR 139:812, 1982
43. Henry LG, Donst B, Korns ME, Bernhard VM: Abdomi-

nal aortic aneurysm and retroperitoneal fibrosis: Ultrasonographic diagnosis and treatment. Arch Surg 113:1456, 1978

44. Michael JA III, Coleman RE: Localization of ^{67}Ga citrate in a mycotic aneurysm. Am J Roentgenol 129:1111, 1977

45. Gooding GAW, Herzog KA, Hedgcock MW, Eisenberg RL: B-mode ultrasonography of prosthetic vascular grafts. Radiology 127:763, 1978

46. Gooding GAW, Effeney DJ, Goldstone J: The aortofemoral graft: Detection and identification of healing complications by ultrasonography. Surgery 89:94, 1981

47. Wolson AH, Kaupp HA, McDonald K: Ultrasound of arterial graft surgery complications. AJR 133:869, 1979

48. Gooding GAW, Effeney DJ: Static and real-time B-mode sonography of arterial occlusions. AJR 139:949, 1982

49. Herzler GM, Silver TM, Graham LM, Stanley JC: Celiac artery aneurysm: Ultrasonic diagnosis. J Clin Ultrasound 9:141, 1981

50. Gooding GAW: Ultrasound of a superior mesenteric artery aneurysm secondary to pancreatitis: A plea for realtime ultrasound of sonolucent masses in pancreatitis. J Clin Ultrasound 9:255, 1981

51. Nino-Murcia M, Kurtz A, Brennan RE et al: CT diagnosis of a splenic artery pseudoaneurysm: A complication of chronic pancreatitis and pseudocyst formation. J Comput Assist Tomogr 7:527, 1983

52. Bolondi L, Casanova P, Arienti V et al: A case of aneurysm of the splenic artery visualized by dynamic ultrasonography. Br. J Radiol 54:1109, 1981

53. Derchi LE, Biggi E, Cicio GR et al: Aneurysm of the splenic artery: Noninvasive diagnosis by pulsed doppler sonography. J Ultrasound Med 3:41, 1984

54. Hantman SS, Barie JJ, Glendening TB et al: Giant renal artery aneurysm mimicking a single cyst on ultrasound. J Clin Ultrasound 10:136, 1982

55. Kurtz AB, Dubbins PA, Zegel HG et al: Normal left vein mimicking left renal artery aneurysm. J Clin Ultrasound 9:105, 1981

56. Baron RL, Banner MP, Pollack HM: Isolated internal iliac artery aneurysms presenting as giant pelvic masses. AJR 140:784, 1983

57. Perdue GD, Mittenthal MJ, Smith RB III, Salam AA: Aneurysm of the internal iliac artery. Surgery 93:243, 1983

58. Khoo HT: The large inferior vena cava—A sign in arteriovenous fistula between the right common iliac artery and the inferior vena cava. J Clin Ultrasound 10:291, 1982

59. Tepper JP, Udoff EJ, Minkin SD et al: Renal arteriovenous fistula—Angiographic and sonographic correlation. J Urol 127:106, 1982

60. Subramanyam BR, Lefleur RS, Bosniak MA: Renal arteriovenous fistulas and aneurysms: Sonographic findings. Radiology 149:261, 1983

61. Thomas JL, Lymberis MEB, Hunt TH: Ultrasonic features of acquired renal arteriovenous fistula. Am J Roentgenol 132:653, 1977

62. Rao AKR, Kimball WR: Ultrasonic appearance of an arteriovenous fistula of the kidney. J Clin Ultrasound 6:345, 1978

63. Richardson ML, Kinard RE, Levesque PH: Inferior vena cava duplication: Demonstration by sonography. J Clin Ultrasound 11:225, 1983

64. Hoffman JC, Morehouse HT, Koenigsberg M: Sonographic demonstration of an anatomic variant of the inferior vena cava. J Ultrasound Med 2:421, 1983

65. Royal SA, Callen PW: CT evaluation of anomalies of the inferior vena cava and left renal vein. AJR 132:759, 1979

66. Train JS, Henderson MR, Smith AP: Sonographic demonstration of left-sided inferior vena cava with hemiazygos continuation. AJR 134:1057, 1980

67. Garris JB, Kangarloo H, Sample WF: Ultrasonic diagnosis of infrahepatic interruption of the inferior vena cava with azygos (hemiazygos) continuation. Radiology 134:179, 1980

68. Huberman RP, Gomes AS: Membranous obstruction of the inferior vena cava. AJR 139:1215, 1982

69. Weill F, Maurat P: The sign of the vena cava: Echotomographic illustration of right cardiac insufficiency. J Clin Ultrasound 2:27, 1979

70. Gosink BB: The inferior vena cava: Mass effects. AJR 130:533, 1978

71. Kurtz AB, Rubin C, Goldberg BB: Ultrasound diagnosis of masses elevating the inferior vena cava. AJR 132:401, 1979

72. Bernardino ME, Libshitz HI, Green B, Goldstein HM: Ultrasonic demonstration of inferior vena caval involvement with right adrenal gland masses. J Clin Ultrasound 6:167, 1978

73. Pussell SJ, Cosgrove DO: Ultrasound features of tumour thrombus in the inferior vena cava in retroperitoneal tumors. Br J Radiol 54:866, 1981

74. Greene D, Steinback HL: Ultrasonic diagnosis of hypernephroma extending into inferior vena cava. Radiology 115:679, 1975

75. Hoffman JC, Weiner SN, Koenigsberg M et al: Pheochromocytoma invasion of the inferior vena cava: Sonographic evaluation. Radiology 149:793, 1983

76. Goldstein HM, Green B, Weaver RM Jr: Ultrasonic detection of renal tumor extension into inferior vena cava. AJR 130:1083, 1978

77. Slovis TL, Phillippart AL, Cushing B et al: Evaluation of the inferior vena cava by sonography and venography in children with renal and hepatic tumors. Radiology 140:767, 1981

78. Kutcher R, Rosenblatt R, Mitsudo SM et al: Renal angiomyolipoma with sonographic demonstration of extension into the inferior vena cava. Radiology 143:755, 1982

79. Sonnenfeld M, Finberg HJ: Ultrasonographic diagnosis of incomplete inferior vena cava thrombosis secondary to periphlebitis: The importance of a complete survey examination. Radiology 137:743, 1980

80. Pasto ME, Kurtz AB, Jarrell BE et al: The Kimray-Greenfield filter: Evaluation by duplex real-time/pulsed doppler ultrasound. Radiology 148:223, 1983

81. Dunne MG, Goldstein WZ: Computed tomography and ultrasound appearance of Kim-Ray Greenfield vena caval filters and potential for noninvasive localization. J Comput Tomogr 7:375, 1983

82. Metreweli C, Pearson R: Echographic diagnosis of neonatal renal venous thrombosis. Pediatr Radiol 14:105, 1984

83. Braun B, Weilemann LS, Weigand W: Ultrasonographic demonstration of renal vein thrombosis. Radiology 138:157, 1981

84. Rosenberg ER, Trought WS, Kirks DR et al: Ultrasonic diagnosis of renal vein thrombosis in neonates. AJR 134:35, 1980

85. Hricak H, Sandler MA, Madrazo BL et al: Sonographic manifestations of acute renal vein thrombosis: An experimental study. Invest Radiol 16:30, 1981

86. Rosenfield AT, Zeman RK, Cronan JJ, Taylor KJW: Ultrasound in experimental and clinical renal vein thrombosis. Radiology 137:735, 1980

87. Dowen AD, Smazal SF Jr: Ultrasound of coexisting right renal vein thrombosis and adrenal hemorrhage in a newborn. J Clin Ultrasound 9:511, 1981

88. Brennan RE, Kurtz AB, Curtis JA et al: Left renal vein obstruction associated with nonrenal malignancy: Detection by computed tomography and ultrasonography. Urology 6:329, 1982

89. Spira R, Kwan E, Gerzof SG, Widrich WC: Left renal vein varix simulating a pancreatic pseudocyst by sonography. AJR 138:149, 1982

90. Schild H, Schweden F, Braun B, Lang H: Aneurysms of the superior mesenteric vein. Radiology 145:641, 1982

91. Oppenheimer DA, Carroll BA: Ultrasonic localization of neonatal umbilical catheters. Radiology 142:781, 1982

92. Oppenheimer DA, Carroll BA, Garth KE, Parker BR: Sonographic localization of neonatal umbilical catheters. AJR 138:1025, 1982

93. Oppenheimer DA, Carroll BA, Garth KE: Ultrasonic detection of complications following umbilical arterial catheterization in the neonate. Radiology 145:667, 1982

94. Gooding GAW, Bank WO: Ultrasound visualization of 5-F catheter. Radiology 144:647, 1982

95. Woo VL, Gerber AM, Scheible W et al: Real-time ultrasound guidance for percutaneous transluminal retrieval of nonopaque intravascular catheter fragment. AJR 133:760, 1979

7

The Peritoneal Cavity and Abdominal Wall

Lawrence M. Vincent

Because the bulk of intraabdominal, extraorgan pathology consists of fluid or fluid-containing structures or is associated with intraperitoneal fluid, ultrasound is often an ideal diagnostic modality. In those disease entities perhaps better studied by other modalities, findings detected by ultrasound screening may play a pivotal role in directing speedy and cost-effective diagnostic management. With appropriate modifications in technique, ultrasound may also have a wide application in assessment of the abdominal wall and superficial soft tissues.

To realize the full diagnostic potential of ultrasound, the sonologist must combine a meticulous scanning technique with his or her knowledge of anatomic relationships—not always a simple task with certain pathologic states. In this chapter, technique and pertinent sonographic anatomy are reviewed. Sonographic appearances of a variety of intraperitoneal collections are detailed, including those representing ascites, pus or inflammatory fluid, blood, bile, and cerebrospinal fluid. Since a general overview of intraabdominal fluid collections is a major part of my intention, discussion is not strictly limited to the confines of the peritoneum. Thus, retroperitoneal collections of lymph and urine, as well as intraorgan and extraperitoneal cystic lesions and gynecologic pathology that may enter the differential diagnosis of intraperitoneal fluid collections, are highlighted. Finally, noncystic lesions involving the peritoneum, omentum, and mesentery, as well as abnormalities of the abdominal wall, are considered.

TECHNIQUE

As with all ultrasound imaging, strict adherence to appropriate transducer selection, correct gain and tissue attenuation compensation, and proper positioning of the patient is imperative. A systematic real-time survey or conventional transverse and longitudinal static imaging at 1-to-2-cm intervals may be initially performed, followed by further specific evaluation of regions of interest as determined by clinical presentation and sonographic findings. Abnormal collections should be characterized according to size, pattern of distribution, internal echo characteristics, and relationship to anatomic structures.

Optimal visualization of the superficial abdomen requires the use of a higher frequency transducer than is normally employed for routine intraabdominal work (i.e., 5 MHz short or medium focus), as depth of penetration may be sacrificed for increased resolution. Ideally, single-sweep static scanning with a slightly higher near gain and slightly lower overall gain than usual is complemented by the use of real-time ultrasound to select unorthodox scanning planes and demonstrate vascular pulsations or peristalsis (to identify a mass as bowel, distinguish a mass from bowel, or document adhesions). For specific evaluation of the inguinal and femoral region — principally for hernia detection — oblique static scanning from the anterior superior iliac spine to the pubis, at 0.5-cm intervals, is a recommended technique.[1]

Although real-time scanning is favored over static scanning by many because of general overall scan quality, ease of examination, and dynamic abilities, conventional static mode scanning offers certain advantages in evaluation of some intraabdominal extraorgan abnormalities and the superficial tissues of the abdominal wall, in particular. The primary disadvantage of real-time scanners in this specific setting is the relatively small field of view, which is especially limited in the near field with the use of sector scanners. With extensive fluid collections, for example, it may be difficult to precisely define anatomic relationships without the panoramic image obtained by conventional static or automated multitransducer scanners. Even in these instances, however, adjunctive real-time imaging may initially locate the region of interest or identify bowel loop peristalsis. Indeterminate real-time scanning planes may also occasionally hinder comparison with prior or subsequent ultrasound examinations or correlation with computed tomographic studies.

Another disadvantage of real-time scanning relates to detection of specular reflectors, such as membranes delimiting muscle groups or anatomic compartments, an ability dependent upon the orientation of the ultrasound beam relative to the reflecting surface. Because real-time scanners direct the sound beam from a single angle, and because specular reflectors are best seen when the beam is perpendicular to the surface, a slight change in ultrasound beam inclination to the planar surface of the reflector greatly reduces the intensity of the returning echo. This, in combination with the limited field of view, compromises the usefulness of real-time sonography in evaluation of the anterior peritoneum and the abdominal wall, for which identification of tissue layers is required for localization of pathology.[3]

Although examination with ultrasound is the preferred means of characterizing fluid-containing lesions, the "classic" sonographic findings of absence of internal echoes, smooth posterior wall margins, and distal acoustic enhancement are not necessarily reliable (or even primary) criteria for the diagnosis of these lesions. More specific criteria relating to the fluid nature of a mass, if present, include the presence of refraction shadows (acoustic shadowing occurring due to refraction of the sound beam at the boundary of a fluid and solid structure), internal septations, fluid-fluid levels, and anterior reverberation artifact.[4,5,6] Not only may homogeneous solid masses simulate cystic structures, but also complicated and even uncomplicated cystic masses may present with echopatterns that mimic solid lesions. Thus, even with careful technique, echopatterns may be misleading and technical pitfalls unavoidable, a limitation of which the sonologist must be ever mindful.

PERTINENT ANATOMY AND LOCALIZATION OF ABNORMALITIES

Determination of Intraperitoneal Location

The clinical importance of distinguishing intraperitoneal processes from pleural, subcapsular, retroperitoneal, and other extraperitoneal processes is obvious. Accurate sonographic localization may confirm or narrow the differential diagnosis and aid in decision-making regarding possible ultrasound guidance for diagnostic or therapeutic drainage. Awareness of patterns of distribution and recognition of normally placed and displaced

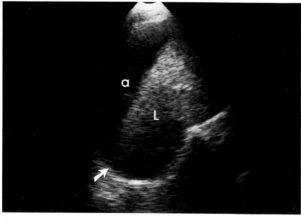
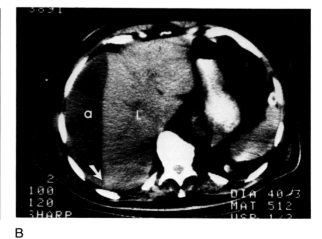

A   B

Fig. 7-1. Right subphrenic abscess. **(A)** Transverse ultrasound and **(B)** corresponding CT scan demonstrate clear demarcation of abscess *(a)* from adjacent liver *(L)*. Note that the collection does not extend medial to the attachment of the right superior coronary ligament, thus delineating the lateral margin of the bare area of the liver (arrow).

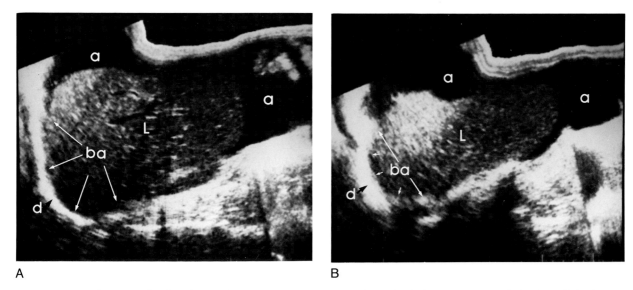

Fig. 7-2. Ascites. Longitudinal images 9 cm **(A)** and 12 cm **(B)** to right of midline demonstrate limitation of distribution of free intraperitoneal fluid *(a)* in the right upper quadrant by coronary ligamentous attachments. Note that the fluid does not extend between the bare area *(ba)* of the liver *(L)* and the diaphragm *(d)*.

anatomic structures is crucial for localization, particularly with large collections in the right upper quadrant posteriorly and in the lower abdomen/pelvis.

PLEURAL VERSUS SUBDIAPHRAGMATIC

Because of the coronary ligament attachments, collections in the right posterior subphrenic space cannot extend between the bare area of the liver and the dia-

phragm (Figs. 7-1 and 7-2). Conversely, because the right pleural space extends medially to the attachment of the right superior coronary ligament, pleural collections may appear in apposition to the bare area; in fact, unless loculated, pleural fluid will tend to distribute posteromedially (Fig. 7-3). Similarly, subcapsular collections need not be limited to the lateral aspect of the right upper quadrant. Transverse ultrasound images demonstrating perihepatic collections extending medially to the coro-

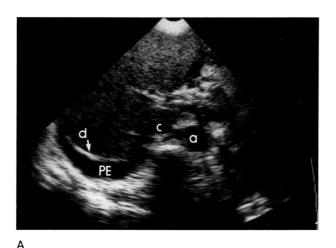
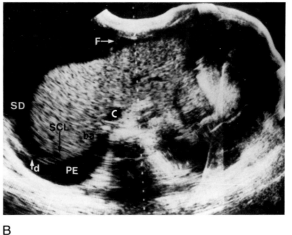

Fig. 7-3. Pleural effusion. **(A)** Transverse scan demonstrates a fluid collection *(PE)* posterior to the distinct curvilinear diaphragmatic echo complex *(d)*, extending posteromedially. *(a,* aorta; *c,* inferior vena cava.) **(B)** Transverse scan in a different patient with ascites in addition to pleural effusion *(PE)* demonstrates fluid outlining both sides of the diaphragm *(d)*. The ascites cannot extend medial to the attachment of the superior coronary ligament *(SCL)*, in contrast to the pleural effusion, which extends into the medial costophrenic angle. *(ba,* bare area of the liver; *c,* inferior vena cava; *SD,* subphrenic space; *F,* falciform ligament.) (Fig. B from Rubenstein WA, Auh YH, Whalen JP, Kazam E: The perihepatic spaces: computed tomographic and ultrasound imaging. Radiology 149:231, 1983.)

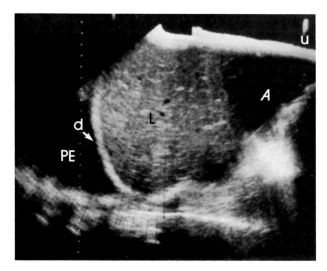

Fig. 7-4. Pleural effusion. Longitudinal scan demonstrates a fluid collection *(PE)* superior to the distinct curvalinear diaphragmatic echo complex *(d)*. Free intraperitoneal fluid *(A)* is also present in the right subhepatic space. (*L,* liver; *u,* level of umbilicus.)

nary ligamentous attachments must therefore represent either a pleural or subcapsular, rather than a subphrenic, process.[7,8]

Unfortunately, due to rib interference and obliquity of the sound beam to the dome of the liver, technically useful transverse scans of the high upper abdomen may sometimes be difficult to obtain. Differentiation of subpulmonic effusions from subphrenic fluid collections by ultrasound is more often determined by longitudinal imaging. Recognition of the distinct curvilinear echoes that form the diaphragmatic echo complex and identification of its relationship to the fluid allow compartmen-

talization (Fig. 7-4). Although a pleural effusion may produce a diminution in the diaphragmatic echo, the dome of the liver remains sharply marginated, whereas the well-defined liver border is generally lost with subphrenic collections[9] (Fig. 7-1A).

SUBCAPSULAR VERSUS INTRAPERITONEAL

Subcapsular liver and spleen collections are readily identified when demonstrated both as inferior to the diaphragmatic echo complex unilaterally and conforming to the shape of the organ capsule (see Figs. 1-103 and 8-28). Subcapsular liver collections will also be confined by the falciform ligament, and, unlike intraperitoneal fluid, may extend medially to the attachment of the superior coronary ligament. With respiration, there is characteristically a lack of change in the subcapsular collection relative to the organ.

RETROPERITONEAL VERSUS INTRAPERITONEAL

Retroperitoneal location of a mass is confirmed when anterior renal displacement (or anterior displacement of visualized, dilated ureters) can be documented sonographically (Fig. 7-5). A mass interposed anteriorly and/or superiorly to the kidneys, however, can be located either intraperitoneally or retroperitoneally (i.e., in the perirenal or anterior pararenal spaces). Determination of the anatomic origin of large masses in the posterior right upper quadrant may sometimes be possible on the basis of retroperitoneal fat displacement or vascular displacements.

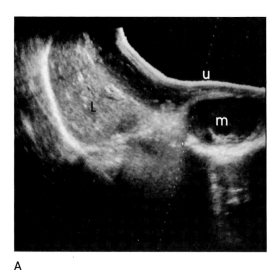

A

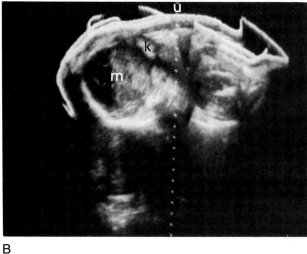

B

Fig. 7-5. Psoas hematoma. **(A)** Right longitudinal and **(B)** transverse scans demonstrate a large mass *(m)* of mixed echogenicity in the area of the psoas muscle. Retroperitoneal location is confirmed on the basis of anteromedial displacement of the right kidney *(k)*. (*u,* level of umbilicus; *L,* liver.)

Fatty and collagenous connective tissues in the perirenal (or anterior pararenal space) produce echoes that are best demonstrated on longitudinal scans. Since retroperitoneal lesions displace the echo ventrally and often cranially, while hepatic and subhepatic lesions produce inferior and posterior displacement, the vector of displacement of this retroperitoneal fat may permit diagnosis of the anatomic origin of right upper quadrant masses (see Figs. 1-52 and 1-53). However, since this sign is dependent upon adequate retroperitoneal fat, it is usually not present in children or in cachectic patients.[10]

Anterior displacement of the superior mesenteric vessels, splenic vein, renal vein, and inferior vena cava (except for the retrohepatic portion, which may be similarly displaced by posterior hepatic masses) excludes an intraperitoneal location. Large right-sided retroperitoneal masses distinctively rotate the intrahepatic portal veins to the left, such that the right portal vein is oriented in a posteroanterior direction instead of its normal left to right horizontal course. Similarly, the left portal vein may course horizontally from right to left, rather than the umbilical portion entering the liver in a posteroanterior direction. Right posterior hepatic masses of similar dimension produce only minor displacement of the intrahepatic portal vein.[11]

EXTRAPERITONEAL VERSUS INTRAPERITONEAL

Delineation of an undisrupted peritoneal line demarcates extraperitoneal from intraperitoneal locations. Although extraperitoneal fluid collections generally are lenticular with an acute superior angle (as commonly seen with fluid within the confines of the rectus sheath or in the prevesical space) (Fig. 7-6), collections caudal to the linea semicircularis may have a more variable configuration and be confused with pelvoabdominal pathology. Demonstration of posterior or lateral bladder displacement suggests an extraperitoneal (i.e., space of Retzius) or retroperitoneal location, respectively (see *Sonographic Evaluation of the Abdominal Wall* for further information).

Anatomy and Sonographic Identification of Intraperitoneal Compartments

Once the intraperitoneal location of a collection or mass is confirmed, further compartmentalization within the confines of the peritoneal cavity may suggest specific etiologies and thus also influence the direction of the subsequent diagnostic work-up. Accurate localization of abnormalities detected by ultrasound may be dependent to a large part on identification of ligaments and peritoneal attachments that are not visualized under normal circumstances (Fig. 7-7). The sonographic appearance of intraperitoneal ligaments and reflections, and the compartments they define, are described in this section. The visualization of this normal anatomy by ultrasound is, of course, dependent upon the pathologic presence of intraperitoneal fluid.

PERIHEPATIC AND UPPER ABDOMINAL COMPARTMENTS

The ligaments on the right side of the liver form the subphrenic and subhepatic spaces. The falciform ligament, which courses over the anterior surface of the liver

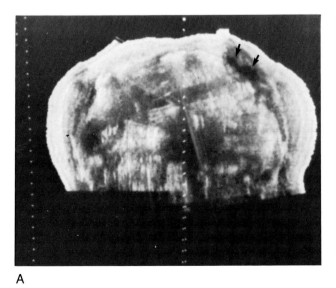
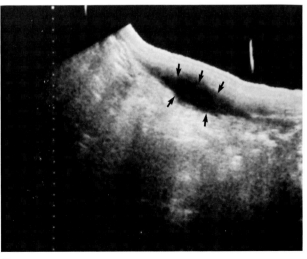

A   B

Fig. 7-6. Superficial abdominal wall hematoma. A lenticular extraabdominal anechoic collection (arrows) is seen in transverse **(A)** and left longitudinal **(B)** scans in a patient with a superficial abdominal stab wound.

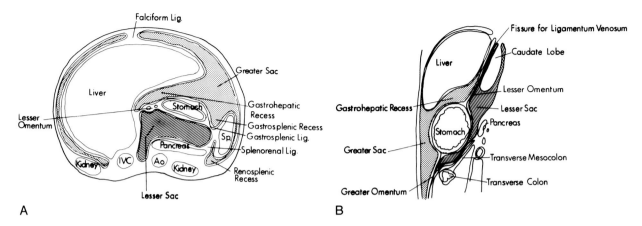

Fig. 7-7. Intraperitoneal compartments and their borders. **(A)** Transverse and **(B)** midline sagittal anatomic sections of the abdomen. Note that the lesser sac is separated from the more anterior gastrohepatic recess by the lesser omentum and stomach. The gastrosplenic ligament and splenorenal ligaments separate the gastrosplenic recess and the renosplenic recess from the lesser sac, respectively. Also note that the caudate lobe virtually projects into the lesser sac, which extends upward to the inferior surface of the diaphragm and then around the caudate lobe to the fissure for the ligamentum venosum.

and attaches to the lower surface of the diaphragm and the ventral abdominal wall, divides the subphrenic space into right and left components (Fig. 7-8). The ligamentum teres hepatis, the remnant of the umbilical vein, ascends from the umbilicus to the umbilical notch of the liver within the free margin of the falciform ligament prior to coursing within the liver (Fig. 7-9). The bare area of the liver is delineated by the right superior and inferior coronary ligaments, which separate the posterior subphrenic space from the right superior subhepatic space (Morison's pouch). Lateral to the bare area and the

right triangular ligament (formed by the fused right superior and inferior coronary ligaments), the posterior subphrenic and subhepatic spaces are continuous.

A single large and irregular perihepatic space surrounds the superior and lateral aspects of the left lobe of the liver, with the left coronary ligaments anatomically separating the subphrenic space into an anterior and a posterior compartment. The left subhepatic space is likewise divided into an anterior compartment (gastrohepatic recess) and a posterior compartment (lesser sac) by the lesser omentum and the stomach. Simplistically (and

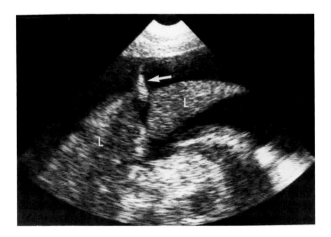

Fig. 7-8. Falciform ligament. Transverse image of a patient with ascites. The falciform ligament (arrow) courses over the anterior surface of the liver and attaches to the lower surface of the diaphragm and the ventral abdominal wall. It divides the anterior subphrenic space into right and left components. (*L*, liver.)

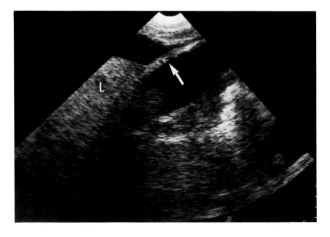

Fig. 7-9. Ligamentum teres hepatis. Longitudinal midline scan of a patient with ascites. The ligamentum teres hepatis (arrow) ascends from the umbilicus to the umbilical notch of the liver within the free margin of the falciform ligament. (*L*, liver.)

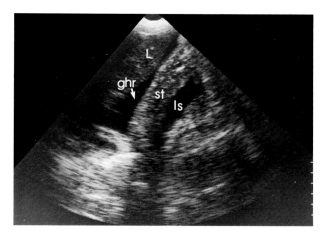

Fig. 7-10. Stomach. Identification of the stomach *(st)* and more posterior structures is dependent upon the presence of surrounding fluid and the absence of a significant amount of gastric air. In this longitudinal image to the left of midline, the stomach can be seen delineating the posterior lesser sac fluid *(ls)* from the more anteriorly located fluid in the gastrohepatic recess *(ghr)*. (*L,* liver.)

often misleadingly, as will be seen), the lesser sac lies anterior to the pancreas and posterior to the stomach. Definition of the stomach borders and more posterior structures by ultrasound is dependent upon the presence of surrounding fluid and the absence of a significant amount of gastric gas. If the stomach position is adequately localized, ultrasound enables the examiner to

distinguish fluid collections involving both the lesser and greater omental cavities (Fig. 7-10)

With fluid present in both the lesser and greater omental cavities, the lesser omentum may frequently be identified with real-time scanning (in both transverse and longitudinal planes) as a linear, undulating echodensity extending from the stomach to the porta hepatis (Fig. 7-11). Similarly, the gastrosplenic ligament, a left lateral extension of the greater omentum that connects the gastric greater curvature to the superior splenic hilum and forms a portion of the left lateral border of the lesser sac (demarcating it from the gastrosplenic recess of the greater sac), may be identified on transverse ultrasound images (Fig. 7-12). Thus, identification of the lesser omentum, stomach, and/or gastrosplenic ligament allows for accurate compartmentalization of the lesser sac (posteriorly) from the greater omental bursa (anteriorly).

Other boundaries of the lesser sac occasionally may be visualized by ultrasound in the presence of fluid. The splenorenal ligament, formed by the posterior reflection of peritoneum off the spleen and passing inferiorly to overlie the left kidney, forms the posterior portion of the left lateral border of the lesser sac and separates the lesser sac from the renosplenic recess (Fig. 7-13). The transverse mesocolon defines the inferoposterior extent of the lesser sac, and the greater omentum, which drapes from the greater curvature of the stomach and folds back on itself to attach to the transverse colon and mesocolon, forms the inferoanterior border (Fig. 7-14).

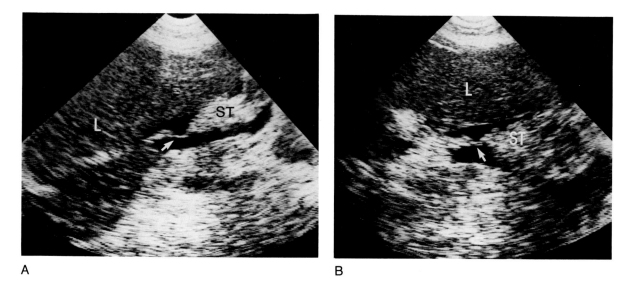

A   B

Fig. 7-11. Lesser omentum. **(A)** Longitudinal and **(B)** transverse images of a patient with ascites secondary to alcoholic liver disease demonstrate the lesser omentum (arrows) as a linear echodensity extending from the lesser curvature of the stomach *(ST)* to the porta hepatis. This landmark separates the fluid in the anterior gastrohepatic recess from that in the posterior lesser sac. (*L,* liver.)

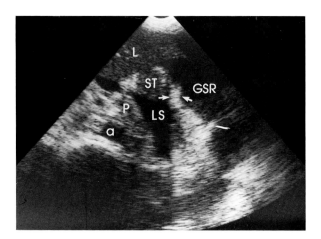

Fig. 7-12. Gastrosplenic ligament. Transverse oblique image of a patient with ascites and known metastatic adenocarcinoma demonstrates the gastrosplenic ligament (arrows) forming a portion of the left lateral border of the lesser sac. (*ST,* stomach; *P,* pancreas; *GSR,* gastrosplenic recess; *LS,* lesser sac; *L,* liver; *a,* aorta.)

THE LESSER OMENTAL BURSA

The lesser sac itself is partially subdivided into a larger lateroinferior space and a smaller mediosuperior recess by the gastropancreatic folds, which are produced by the left gastric and hepatic arteries. Superiorly and to both sides of midline, the lesser sac extends to the diaphragm. The superior recess of the bursa surrounds the anterior, medial, and posterior surfaces of the caudate lobe, mak-

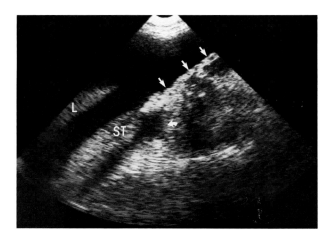

Fig. 7-14. Greater omentum. Left longitudinal image of a patient with intraperitoneal fluid in both the greater and lesser peritoneal cavities demonstrates the greater omentum (arrows) draping from the greater curvature of the stomach *(ST)* and folding back on itself to attach to the transverse colon and mesocolon. The greater omentum defines the inferoanterior extent of the lesser sac, while the transverse mesocolon (curved arrow) delimits the lesser sac inferiorly. (*L,* liver.)

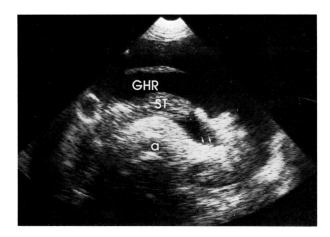

Fig. 7-13. Splenorenal ligament. Transverse scan in same patient as Figure 7-12 demonstrates the location of the splenorenal ligament (arrows), which forms the left posterolateral portion of the lesser sac, and separates the latter from the renosplenic recess. (*ST,* stomach; *GHR,* gastrohepatic recess; *a,* aorta.)

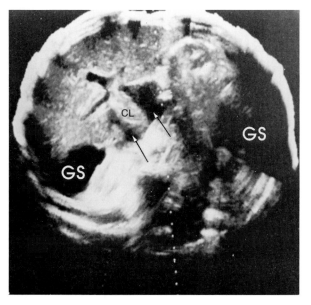

Fig. 7-15. Ascites, superior recess, lesser sac. Transverse scan of the upper abdomen in a peritoneal dialysis patient with both free and loculated upper abdominal fluid. In addition to the greater sac ascites *(GS),* fluid surrounds the caudate lobe (CL) both anteriorly and posteriorly (arrows). This "floating" caudate implies fluid within the superior recess of the lesser sac, because fluid strictly confined to the gastrohepatic recess will not be encountered in the posterior location. (From Vincent LM, Mittelstaedt CA, Mauro MA: The lesser sac and gastrohepatic recess: Sonographic appearance and differentiation. Radiology 150:515, 1984.)

ing the caudate essentially a lesser sac structure. Thus, the appearance of a caudate lobe that is "floating" in fluid confirms a lesser sac component, since fluid strictly confined to the gastrohepatic recess should not extend posterior to the caudate (Fig. 7-15).

Large upper abdominal fluid collections, particularly when loculated, may distort anatomic landmarks by displacing and compressing organs and vascular structures. Static transverse ultrasound images, permitting a larger field of view for establishing anatomic relationships, may be helpful as a supplement to real-time examination

in these instances, although compartmentalization of the fluid by ultrasound alone may be difficult or impossible. If the stomach is satisfactorily identified, the location of the fluid may be inferred by the manner of gastric displacement. Large lesser sac collections displace the lesser curvature of the stomach laterally and the posterior portion of the stomach anteriorly, while collections in the gastrohepatic recess displace the anterior portion of the stomach posteriorly[12] (Fig. 7-16 and 7-17).

Because of the anatomic boundaries of the lesser sac, large and/or loculated lesser sac fluid collections may

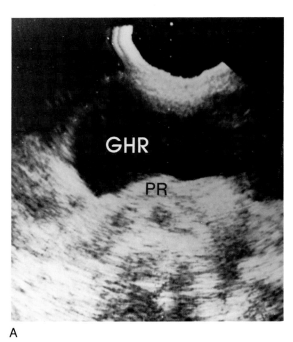

A

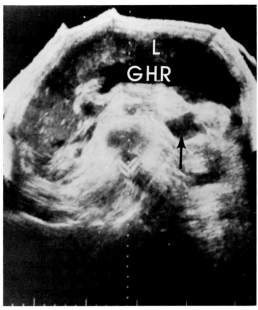

B

Fig. 7-16. Ascites, gastrohepatic recess. **(A)** Transverse scan of a patient with ovarian adenocarcinoma. A large fluid collection *(GHR)* is noted anterior to the pancreatic region *(PR)*. **(B)** Transverse scan at higher level than **(A)**. The previously seen collection appears in apposition to the left lobe of the liver *(L)* and represents the gastrohepatic recess *(GHR)*. A smaller amount of lesser sac ascites can be appreciated (arrow). **(C)** CT scan of approximately the same level as in **(B)**, documenting a large fluid collection in the gastrohepatic recess *(GHR)* with posterior stomach *(ST)* displacement. A small lesser sac collection was also identified on additional CT images (From Vincent LM, Mittelstaedt CA, Mauro MA: The lesser sac and gastrohepatic recess: sonographic appearance and differentiation. Radiology 150:515, 1984.)

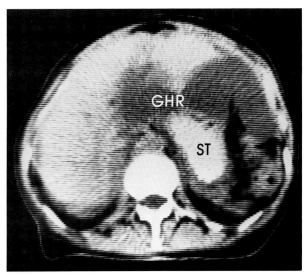

C

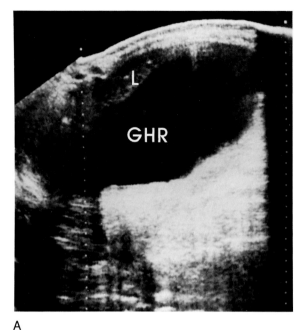

A

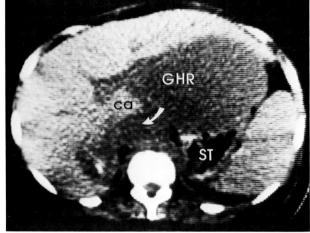

B

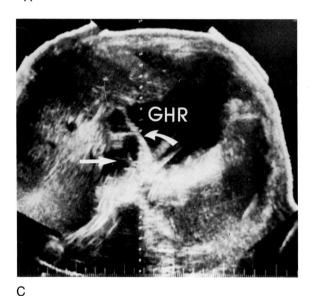

C

Fig. 7-17. Ascites, greater and lesser sacs. **(A)** Left longitudinal scan of a patient on chronic peritoneal dialysis demonstrates a large fluid collection *(GHR)* extending to the anterior abdominal wall. *(L, liver.)* **(B)** CT scan of the same patient documents a large collection in the gastrohepatic recess *(GHR),* with posterior displacement and compression of the stomach *(ST).* Note fluid (curved arrow) located posterior to the caudate lobe (*ca*). **(C)** Transverse ultrasound image at level of the previous CT image demonstrates the large gastrohepatic collection *(GHR).* In addition, fluid is seen in the superior recess of the lesser sac (straight arrow), posterior to the caudate lobe. The lesser omentum is seen as a linear echodensity separating these two collections (curved arrow). (From Vincent LM, Mittelstaedt CA, Mauro MA: The lesser sac and gastrohepatic recess: Sonographic appearance and differentiation. Radiology 150:515, 1984.)

appear more superiorly, anteriorly, or inferiorly than would be anticipated.[13] With lateral displacement of the stomach, lesser sac fluid may appear directly apposed to the ventral abdominal wall in the midline (Fig. 7-18). Although the caudal extent of the lowermost portion of the lesser sac is at the level of the transverse mesocolon, a well-defined inferior recess may persist between the anterior and posterior reflections of the greater omentum. Thus, lesser sac collections may extend a considerable distance below the plane of the pancreas by inferiorly displacing the transverse mesocolon or extending into the inferior recess of the greater omentum.[14]

LOWER ABDOMINAL/PELVIC COMPARTMENTS

With large fluid collections extending into the pelvis, the uterus and broad ligaments form a dividing septum between pelvic fluid in an anterior and a posterior compartment (the latter represented by the pouch of Douglas) (Fig. 7-19). The peritoneal reflection over the dome of the bladder may have an inferior recess extending anterior to the bladder (the cavum peritonei or the anterior paravesical fossa), and fluid contained within this space may appear rounded or ovoid when imaged trans-

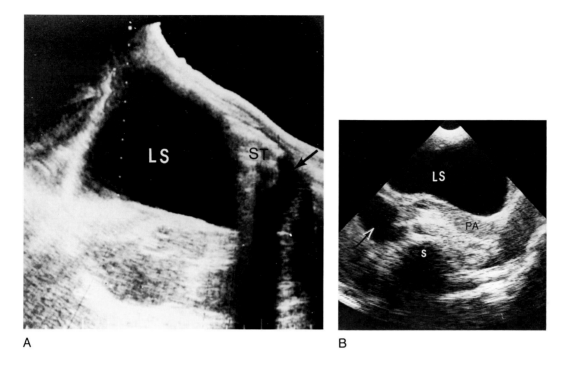

Fig. 7-18. Loculated lesser sac ascites. **(A)** Left longitudinal scan of a renal patient presenting with an epigastric mass. The large lesser sac fluid collection *(LS)* is noted to displace the stomach *(ST)* anteriorly, laterally, and inferiorly. Greater sac fluid is noted inferiorly to the displaced stomach (arrow). Note similarity in appearance of this image to Figure 7-17A. **(B)** Transverse ultrasound image of the same patient, demonstrating the apposition of the large fluid collection *(LS)* to the pancreas *(PA)*. A smaller subhepatic fluid collection is noted on the right (arrow). Note similarity in appearance to Figure 7-16A. (*s,* spine.) (From Vincent LM, Mittelstaedt CA, Mauro MA: The lesser sac and gastrohepatic recess: sonographic appearance and differentiation. Radiology 150:515, 1984.)

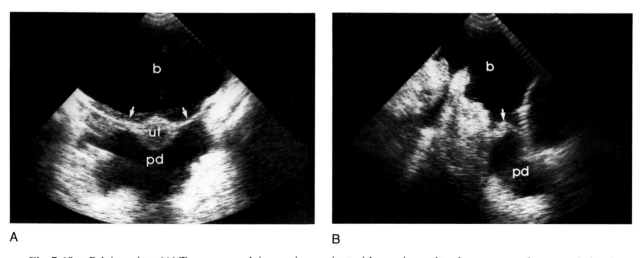

Fig. 7-19. Pelvic ascites. **(A)** Transverse pelvic scan in a patient with massive ascites demonstrates the uterus *(ut)* and broad ligaments (arrows) forming a dividing septum between pelvic fluid in the anterior and posterior compartments. (*pd,* pouch of Douglas.) **(B)** Right longitudinal image in the same patient again demonstrates the right broad ligament (arrow) separating anterior pelvic fluid from fluid in the pouch of Douglas *(pd)*. (*b,* bladder.)

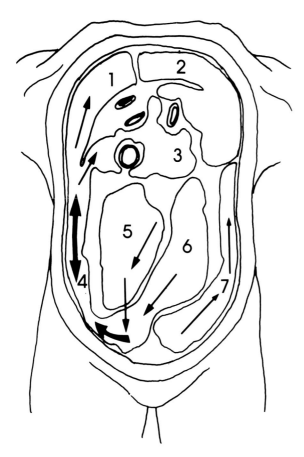

Fig. 7-20. Dynamic pathways of intraperitoneal fluid flow. Fluid from the inframesocolic compartments preferentially seeks the pelvic cavity. After filling the pouch of Douglas and the lateral paravesical recesses, fluid ascends both paracolic gutters. The right paracolic gutter, deeper than its left counterpart, serves as the main communication between the upper and lower abdominal compartments in both directions. (*1*, right subphrenic space; *2*, left subphrenic space; *3*, lesser sac; *4*, right paracolic gutter; *5*, right infracolic space; *6*, left infracolic space; *7*, left paracolic gutter.)

versely.[15] This relatively uncommon appearance of ascites can be differentiated from the extraperitoneal fluid within the prevesical fascial cleft (space of Retzius) by the acute superior angle of the extraperitoneal collection on longitudinal images.[16]

ABNORMALITIES OF THE PERITONEAL CAVITY: FLUID COLLECTIONS

Ascites

Typical serous ascites appears as echofree fluid regions indented and shaped by the organs and viscera it surrounds or is interposed between. In early experimental

cadaver work with A-mode ultrasound, a minimum of l00 ml of infused intraperitoneal fluid could be detected (in prone and right lateral decubitus positions).[17] With state of the art equipment, using volume estimates of the hepatorenal recess, as little as 30 to 40 ml of fluid in this particular location can be detected.[18] The amount of intraperitoneal fluid necessary for recognition by ultrasound is obviously dependent on fluid location as well as volume. Regardless, ultrasound is the primary imaging modality for the detection of intraabdominal fluid.

Factors other than fluid volume that affect the distribution of intraperitoneal fluid include the peritoneal pressure, patient position, area from which the fluid originates, the rapidity of fluid accumulation, the presence or absence of adhesions, the density of the fluid with respect to other abdominal organs, and the degree of bladder fullness.[19,20] The dynamic pathways of flow of intraperitoneal fluid in vivo have been established by peritoneography; they are pertinent not only for anatomic explanation of preferential location of ascitic fluid, but also directly relate to the intraperitoneal spread of exudates as well as intraperitoneal seeding of malignant disease. Briefly summarized, fluid in the inframesocolic compartments preferentially seeks the pelvic cavity; from the left infracolic space via the right side of the rectum and from the right infracolic space via the small bowel mesentery. After first filling the pouch of Douglas and then the lateral paravesical recesses, the fluid ascends both paracolic gutters. Since the left paracolic gutter is shallower than its counterpart, and since its cephalad extent is limited by the phrenicocolic ligament, the major flow from the pelvis is via the right paracolic gutter, which serves as the main communication between upper and lower abdominal compartments in both directions[21] (Fig. 7-20).

The smallest volumes of fluid in the patient in the supine position first appear around the inferior tip of the right lobe of the liver, in the superior portion of the right flank, and in the pelvic cul-de-sac, followed by collection in the paracolic gutters and lateral and anterior to the liver.[22] In a prospective study including 62 men with varying degrees of ascites secondary to liver disease, 92 percent had ascites around the liver, 77 percent in the pelvis, 69 percent in the paracolic gutters, and 63 percent in Morison's pouch. Of those with moderate or modest ascites, fluid was seen in Morison's pouch in 57 percent and 24 percent of patients respectively.[23]

Transudative ascites in Morison's pouch is less frequently encountered than might be expected, particularly since this recess is a preferential drainage site for contaminated collections. An explanation for this phenomenon is that the liver ordinarily sinks in ascitic fluid resulting in obliteration of this space in the supine position; with a large amount of ascites, the liver may be-

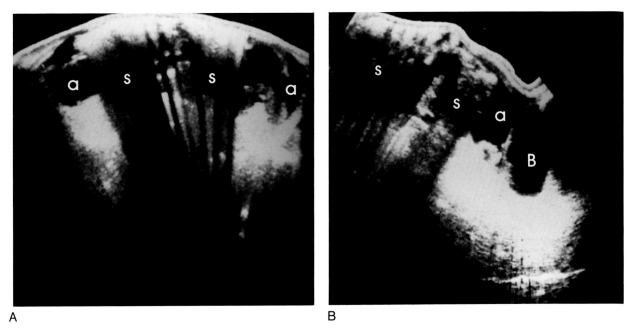

A   B

Fig. 7-21. Floating small bowel loops. **(A)** Transverse and **(B)** midline lower longitudinal ultrasound images demonstrate acoustic shadowing (*s*) from gas-filled small bowel loops which are floating to the anterior abdominal surface in a patient with ascites. (*a*, ascites; *b*, bladder.)

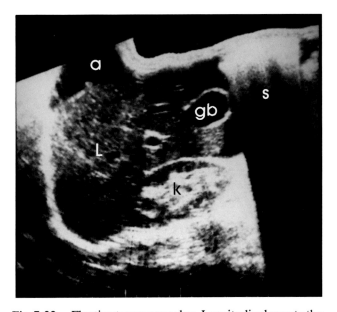

Fig. 7-22. Floating transverse colon. Longitudinal scan to the right of midline in a patient with ascites demonstrates bowel gas shadowing *(s)* from transverse colon floating on top of ascitic fluid. Ascending portions of the colon, fixed retroperitoneally, will remain in the normal location in the presence of ascites with or without intraluminal gas. (*L*, liver; *k*, right kidney; *gb*, gallbladder; *a*, ascites.)

come suspended under the distended abdominal wall by the falciform ligament, and the pouch may open up to accommodate fluid.[24] Similarly, relatively smaller amounts of fluid in the lesser sac are present with benign, transudative ascites, which suggests that the foramen of Winslow is normally more a potential than real communicating pathway in most adults.[25]

Small bowel loops will sink or float in surrounding ascitic fluid depending upon relative gas content and amount of fat in the mesentery (Fig. 7-21). The middle portion of the transverse colon usually floats on top of the fluid because of its gas content, whereas the ascending portions of the colon, which are fixed retroperitoneally, remain in their normal location with or without gas[26] (Fig. 7-22). Floating loops of small bowel, anchored posteriorly by mesentery and with fluid between the mesenteric folds, have a characteristic anterior convex fan shape or arcuate appearance (Fig. 7-23). In severely emaciated patients with little mesenteric fat, the entire small bowel mesentery complex may sink in ascitic fluid.[24] With "tense" ascites, bowel loops may be asymmetrically displaced and appear compressed (Fig. 7-24).

Although the pouch of Douglas is the most common site for intraperitoneal pelvic fluid accumulation, an overdistended bladder may entirely mask small quantities of such fluid. Partial bladder emptying during sonographic examination may thus permit detection of subtle cul-de-sac collections not initially appreciated.[20] Displaced cul-de-sac fluid from bladder overdistension, mi-

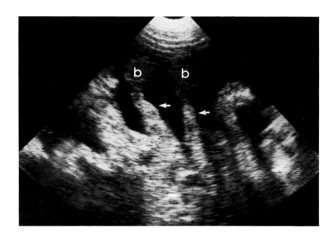

Fig. 7-23. Ascites in mesenteric folds. Longitudinal scan of the abdomen of a patient with ascites demonstrates floating small bowel *(b)* with fluid between the mesenteric folds (arrows), producing the characteristic fan-shaped appearance.

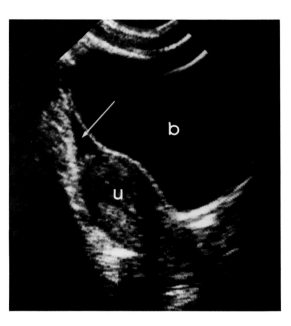

Fig. 7-25. Pelvic fluid, uterine fundal "cap". Longitudinal scan demonstrates a triangular fluid collection (arrow) at the interface of the uterine fundus (u) and the bladder (b) (From Nyberg DA, Laing FC, Jeffrey RB: Sonographic detection of subtle pelvic fluid collections. AJR 143:261, © Am. Roentgen Ray Society, 1984.)

grating to the peritoneal reflection adjacent to the anterior and superior aspect of the uterine fundus, may be visible as a well-defined triangular fluid "cap" on longitudinal sonograms[20] (Fig. 7-25). In one series of 146 patients with free pelvic fluid, a cul-de-sac location was initially detected by sonography in 122 patients (83.5 percent), although 32 patients in the latter group demon-

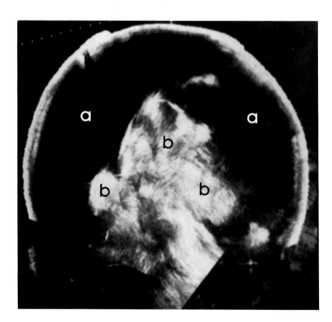

Fig. 7-24. Tense ascites. Transverse scan in a patient with pancreatic ascites demonstrates bowel loops *(b)* completely surrounded and compressed by the ascitic fluid *(a)* rather than floating. The presence of floating bowel loops in ascites is dependent upon relative gas content within the bowel, the amount of fat in the mesentery, and the degree of tenseness of the ascites.

strated a relatively more visible concurrent fundal cap (21.9 percent of the total study group). Of the 24 patients (16.5 percent) with no obvious cul-de-sac fluid, partial bladder emptying revealed cul-de-sac fluid in 14 cases (9.6 percent of total group), and a fundal cap provided the only sonographic evidence of fluid in the remaining 10 subjects (6.9 percent of total group).[20]

Certain deviations from the usual sonographic patterns associated with ascites suggest an exudative (i.e., inflammatory or malignant) rather than a transudative collection. These include fine or coarse internal echoes, loculation or unusual distribution, matting or clumping of bowel loops, and thickening of interfaces between the fluid and neighboring structures[27] (Fig. 7-26). In one series of 82 cases, the overall accuracy of ultrasound in differentiating transudates from exudates was approximately 82 percent. Absence of these findings, however, does not exclude exudative fluid, since approximately one fourth of exudates in the study just described demonstrated a transudative sonographic pattern.[22] Chylous ascites may also present with diffuse fine high-amplitude echoes.[28] Obviously the demonstration of sonographically visible liver metastases, abdominal masses, or adenopathy associated with intraperitoneal fluid is suggestive of malignant ascites regardless of its appearance.

Because disproportionate amounts of fluid within the lesser sac is not a typical manifestation of generalized

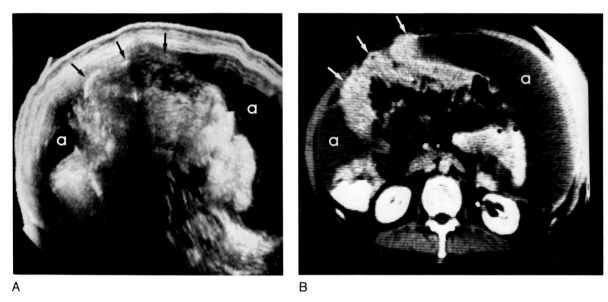

Fig. 7-26. Malignant ascites. **(A)** Transverse scan and **(B)** CT scan at comparable level in a patient with malignant ascites demonstrate adherence and clumping of bowel loops to a portion of the anterior abdominal wall (arrows), a pattern suggesting exudative ascites. (*a*, ascites.)

peritoneal ascites, its presence should direct a search for pathology in adjacent organs (e.g., acute pancreatitis and its complications or penetrating posterior gastric ulcer) or consideration of a malignant etiology, such as carcinoma of the pancreas or ovary.[25] Similarly, although fluid in the hepatorenal recess may be a manifestation of generalized ascites, its detection in the context of an acute abdomen may represent inflammatory fluid from acute cholecystitis, fluid due to pancreatic autolysis, or blood from a ruptured hepatic neoplasm or ectopic gestation[18] (Fig. 7-27).

Transudative ascites in association with preexisting bowel adhesions may simulate a pattern of malignant ascites. "Discordant" lesser sac fluid collections (i.e., an increased amount relative to fluid distribution in the greater omental bursa)—a pattern not typical of transudative ascites—have been demonstrated in renal failure patients on long-term intraperitoneal dialysis with prior episodes of peritonitis.[13] Localized intraabdominal fluid collections also may be commonly encountered in patients who have undergone recent abdominal surgery (in 19 percent of asymptomatic postoperative patients on the fourth day after surgery). Localized collections persisting as late as 12 days postoperatively, however, suggest abnormality (e.g., abscess).[29]

Transudative ascites, when exhibiting the typical sonographic characteristics as described above, is not likely to be confused with other entities. Nonetheless, bilious, chylous, urinary, or cerebrospinal fluid ascites may appear virtually indistinguishable, and fresh hematomas or inflammatory collections may occasionally pose similar

problems. Changing patient position may sometimes clarify matters, as in the case of transudative ascites in the pouch of Douglas emptying with a reverse Trendelenburg tilt, as opposed to persistence of an abscess collection in the region. Large cystic neoplasms, in particular cystadenocarcinoma of the ovary, may mimic ascites, although bowel loop displacement by tumor mass is clearly distinct from the central "floating" bowel loop

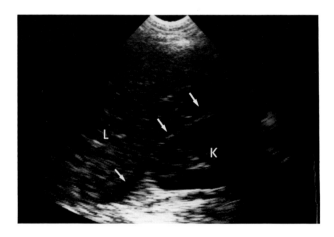

Fig. 7-27. Hemoperitoneum, hepatorenal recess. Right longitudinal upper abdominal scan in a patient with documented ruptured ectopic gestation and hemoperitoneum demonstrates fluid in the hepatorenal recess (arrows). Free intraperitoneal fluid was not identified elsewhere in the abdomen or pelvis. Fluid confined to the hepatorenal recess is not typical for transudative ascites. (*L*, liver; *K*, kidney.)

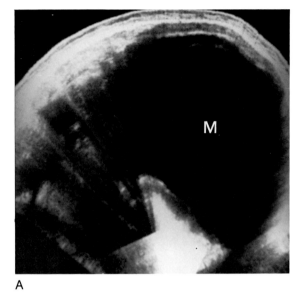
A

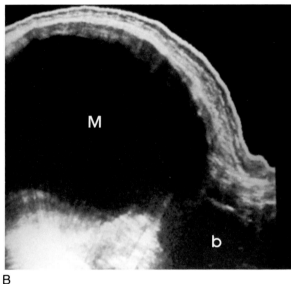
B

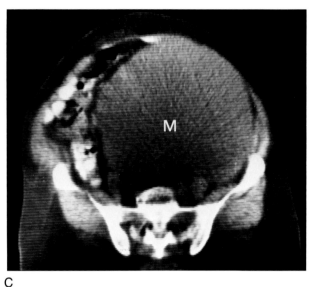
C

Fig. 7-28. Ovarian cystadenoma. **(A)** Transverse and **(B)** longitudinal midline scans demonstrate an enormous anechoic abdominopelvic mass *(M)*, correlating with CT scan findings. (*b*, bladder.) **(C).** Large cystic neoplasms of this nature may occasionally mimic ascites, although bowel loop displacement by the tumor mass is distinct from the floating bowel loop pattern that is more commonly seen with transudative ascites. Evaluation may be even more difficult when loculated ascitic fluid collections are present, or when cystic neoplasms exist concurrently with free or loculated ascites.

pattern commonly seen with transudative ascites (Fig. 7-28). Excess preperitoneal fat in the anterior abdominal wall may occasionally simulate a shallow collection of ascites, but its characteristic location (anterior to liver) and appearance (low-amplitude echoes and the lack of positional variation or interface with bowel) should obviate any possible confusion (Fig. 7-29).

Loculated or exudative collections of ascites may be more difficult to distinguish from other intraperitoneal cystic masses such as abscess, hematoma, lymphocele, pancreatic pseudocyst, or cystic neoplasm. Loculated ascitic collections incorporating bowel loops may add to the confusing sonographic picture, as will the coexistence of ascites and a large cystic neoplasm. Compared to cystic masses, loculated ascites tends to be more irregular in outline, generally shows less mass effect, and may

change shape slightly with positional variation.[22] This generalization need not hold true, however, since fluid confined within an anatomic compartment (such as the lesser sac) may appear regular in outline and produce significant displacement of stomach or bowel, mimicking a pancreatic pseudocyst or abscess. Pancreatic pseudocysts, when presenting in atypical locations, are especially likely to be confused with loculated ascites.

Abscesses

The gamut of the sonographic appearances of abscess collections ranges from a cyst-like, fluid appearance to a solid pattern, the variable appearances reflecting the physical characteristics of the collection at the time of

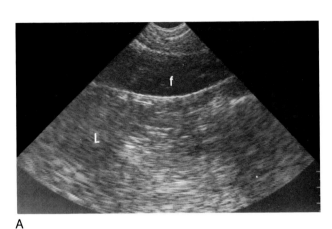

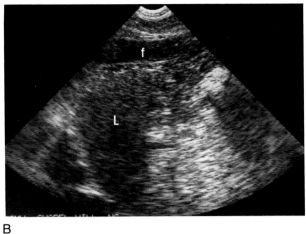

A   B

Fig. 7-29.   Preperitoneal fat. **(A)** Transverse and **(B)** longitudinal scan in different obese patients demonstrate excess preperitoneal fat *(f)*, which appears relatively hypoechoic and which may occasionally mimic a shallow collection of ascites. (*L,* liver.)

examination. In a large percentage of cases, weak echoes are dispersed throughout the collection, although well-defined fluid-debris levels may be seen. Large amounts of strongly echoing debris may also be encountered, often in the dependent portion of the collection, but occasionally creating a complex or solid echopattern. Septa or band-like internal echoing structures representing the walls of loculi may be demonstrated. Gas-containing abscesses may appear as densely echogenic

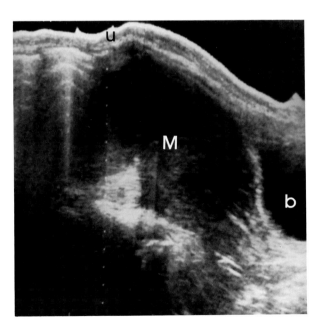

Fig. 7-30.   Postpartum pelvic abscess. Longitudinal midline scan in a postpartum female with fever demonstrates a large, complex, predominently anechoic pelvic mass *(M)*. (*b,* bladder; *u,* level of umbilicus.)

masses with acoustic shadowing, but may also be seen merely as regions of acoustic shadowing or as an echogenic mass, the last appearance presumably secondary to a "microbubble" contrast effect[30-33] (Figs. 7-30 to 7-34).

Although parenchymal abscesses are usually round or ellipsoidal, the configuration of intraperitoneal abscesses often varies depending upon the particular anatomic compartment in which the abscesses are localized (Figs. 7-35 and 7-36). Abscesses tend to hold their shape and displace or indent neighboring structures unless they meet with resistent boundaries such as the liver capsule or sacral promontory. Thus, a right-sided subphrenic abscess may have a curvilinear border and may mimic ascites; however, if under enough pressure, the collection may have convex rather than curvalinear margins[34,35] (Fig. 7-37). Nonsolid-appearing and nongas-containing abscesses generally transmit sound well, although the degree of potentiation of deep echoes is less than that of simple fluid collections. The walls of abscesses are typically finely irregular, although gross wall irregularity has been reported in 25 percent of abscesses in one series.[32] Abscesses involving retained surgical gauze are characterized by irregular, rough, and thick boundary echoes, and by internal echoes of irregular shape and high amplitude within an overall echofree mass.[36]

Potential difficulties with abscess searches using ultrasound include lack of specificity, the presence of incisions, drains, or ostomies, and obscuration by bowel gas. However, with meticulous examination and manipulation of patient position, the presence of bowel gas need not always severely limit ultrasound evaluation. Because the liver serves as a nearly constant window into both the right and left subhepatic spaces, as well as into the right subdiaphragmatic space, and since the bladder similarly

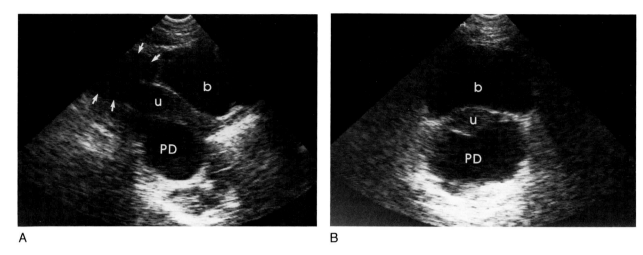

A   B

Fig. 7-31. Appendiceal abscess. **(A)** Longitudinal midline and **(B)** transverse scans of the pelvis in a septic 14-year-old female demonstrate ovoid hypoechoic collections anterosuperior to the uterus (arrows) and within the pouch of Douglas *(PD)*. Low-amplitude echoes are seen within both collections, along with slightly increased posterior acoustic enhancement. (*u,* uterus; *b,* bladder.)

provides a window into the pouch of Douglas and the supravesical pelvis, the right upper quadrant and pelvis are the anatomic regions best suited for ultrasound evaluation. With the spleen present, the left upper quadrant and left subphrenic region can frequently be evaluated by scanning intercostally or coronally with the patient in the right lateral decubitus position. Thus, many abscesses tend to occur in regions where obscuration by bowel gas is technically not a major factor. In certain intraabdominal locations, particularly in the anterior pararenal space, intervening bowel gas will preclude visualization of an abscess unless the collection is extensive enough to displace the interposed bowel loops. If the

patient is examined in the decubitus position, gas-distended bowel will usually not interfere with visualization of paracolic gutter abscesses. Similarly, the posterior pararenal space, the perirenal space, and the lesser sac may be demonstrated sonographically with the patient in the prone or decubitus position.[37]

When a large gas-containing abscess is examined with the transducer aimed posteriorly, beam reflection at the soft-tissue–gas interface will be indistinguishable from the acoustic shadowing and reverberation/ring down artifacts that would be encountered from an air-containing bowel loop. If the abscess is examined with the trans-

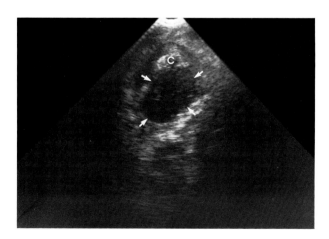

Fig. 7-32. Postappendectomy abscess. Longitudinal image of the right lower quadrant demonstrates a fairly well-delineated ovoid hypoechoic collection (arrows) adjacent to the cecum *(c),* with mild posterior acoustic enhancement.

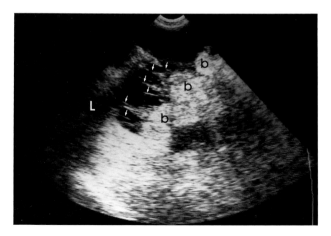

Fig. 7-33. Intraabdominal abscess. Longitudinal scan demonstrates strandy echodensities (arrows) within an anechoic collection surrounding bowel loops in the right upper abdomen of a patient following cecal perforation. (*L,* liver; *b,* bowel loops.)

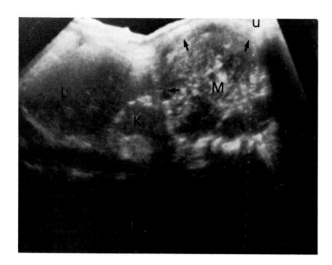

Fig. 7-34. Retroperitoneal abscess. Right longitudinal image demonstrates a large, solid-appearing hyperechoic complex mass (*M,* with arrows). A total of 13,000 ml of pus were ultimately removed from this large retroperitoneal abscess by needle aspiration as well as incisional drainage. (*L,* liver; *K,* kidney; *u,* level of umbilicus.)

ducer aimed anteromedially from the posterior aspect of the flank, the fluid portion of the abscess is first encountered, and at the fluid–gas interface, a dense echogenic line is produced due to the almost total reflection of the sound beam. Thus, a horizontal echogenic line representing an air-fluid level in a gas-containing abscess may be recognized when an abnormal fluid collection is viewed from a posterior position[38] (Fig. 7-38).

The overall accuracy of ultrasound in patients with a

suspected abscess has been reported to be as high as 96.8 percent, with a sensitivity of 93 percent, and a specificity of 98.6 percent.[39] Other investigators have reported sensitivities of less than 93 percent, although greater than 80 percent.[37,40–43] Nonetheless, there have been occasional jarring discrepancies in the literature, with one recent report of a 44 percent sensitivity for abscess detection using ultrasound.[44] This variance emphasizes the dependence of ultrasound upon the technique employed by the examiner, and perhaps to a lesser extent upon the equipment utilized. Real-time ultrasonography has the advantage of allowing complete sonofluoroscopy of the abdomen in a relatively short time, as well as the ability to distinguish fluid-filled loops of bowel by recognition of peristalsis or echodensities induced secondary to the oral or rectal administration of water. Static scanning provides a larger field of view and may provide better demonstration of superficial collections than real-time sector scanners. In a comparison of real-time and static scanning in suspected abscess patients, there was complete agreement with both methods, with an overall accuracy of 93 percent.[40]

It is apparent that a multiimaging approach to abscess detection is often superior to the use of any single modality. Computed tomography (CT) appears to have a well-documented advantage over ultrasound in the accuracy of abscess detection.[35,41–43] Ultrasound studies in the upper abdomen are generally more diagnostic than those in the lower abdomen, and the diagnostic rate is increased when there is a clinical direction to a specific location or quadrant.[43] Since ultrasound is a rapid and flexible modality, and because of its relative low cost and

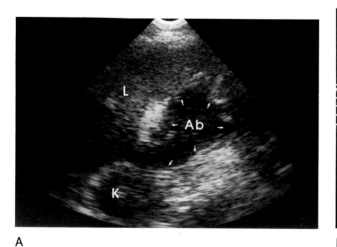

A

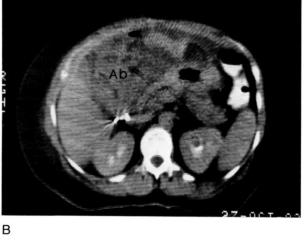

B

Fig. 7-35. Subhepatic abscess. **(A)** Transverse oblique scan of the right upper abdomen in a febrile patient following a gastrectomy demonstrates a homogeneous hypoechoic mass *(Ab)* occupying the right subhepatic space. **(B)** CT scan confirms abnormal soft tissue density *(Ab)* in the subhepatic region. Subsequent surgical drainage confirmed a large right subhepatic abscess. (*L,* liver; *K,* kidney.)

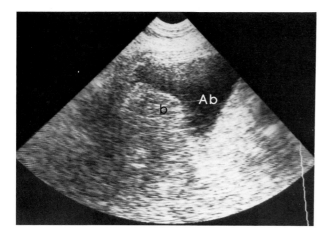

Fig. 7-36. Intraabdominal abscess. (Same patient as Figure 7-33). Longitudinal scan of the right lower abdomen in a patient following cecal perforation demonstrates a triangular-shaped collection with low-amplitude echoes *(Ab)* surrounding adjacent bowel *(b)*.

lack of ionizing radiation, it is often preferred as the initial screening examination for evaluation of a suspected abscess, particularly when there are localizing signs or symptoms. However, in some critically ill patients or patients with localized findings, CT may be the preferable initial modality depending upon such factors as patient habitus, suspected location of abnormality, presence of ileus, or presence of wounds and dressings. Despite demonstration of an abnormal collection by ul-

trasound, CT evaluation may still be desirable to further depict the extent of the process and relate it to surrounding structures, or to define a safe access route for aspiration biopsy or therapeutic drainage. A normal or equivocal ultrasound study may necessitate further evaluation, with nuclear imaging (gallium-67 citrate or indium-111 labeled white blood cells) often the next examination of choice. In the presence of marked symptoms or continued clinical suspicion, CT may be employed as an additional method of excluding abscess, or either CT or ultrasound may be used to subsequently evaluate abnormal areas detected by nuclear imaging. With nonlocalizing signs or symptoms in the nonemergent setting, nuclear medicine is often the initial modality of choice.[35,41,45]

Ultrasound directed needle aspiration of fluid collections will obviously enhance the specificity of sonography; it is also generally preferable to CT directed aspiration because of speed and cost advantages, although CT localization is advisable when precise anatomic detail is necessary with small or deep-seated lesions. Large superficial collections are ideal for ultrasound localization, but smaller collections may be aspirated successfully with the employment of transducer biopsy guides. With aspiration of fluid collections, transgression of bowel loops with the biopsy needle must be avoided, since an uninfected collection may become contaminated by the needle passage, and/or a false-positive diagnosis may be obtained with the culturing of inadvertant aspiration of bowel contents.[35]

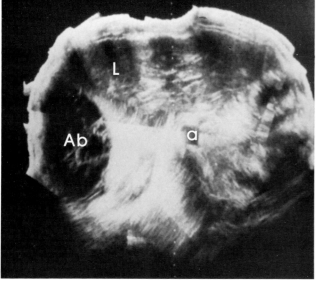

A

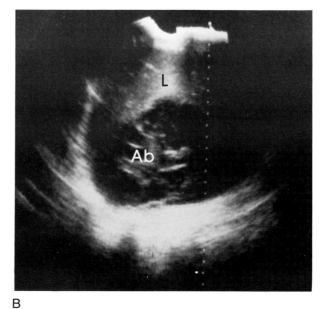

B

Fig. 7-37. Subphrenic abscess. **(A)** Transverse and **(B)** right longitudinal ultrasound scans in a patient with a documented right subphrenic abscess demonstrate a complex but largely anechoic mass *(Ab)* with a convex margin medially, indenting the liver parenchyma *(L)*. (*a*, aorta.)

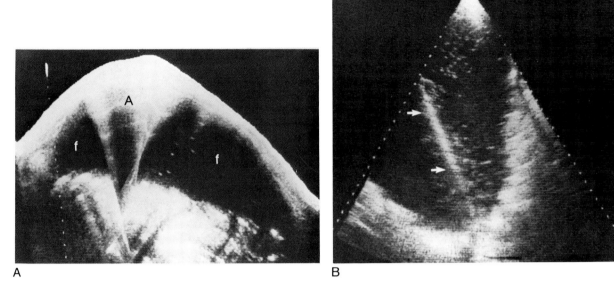

A   B

Fig. 7-38. Air-containing abscess. **(A)** Transverse scan of the upper abdomen demonstrates a large fluid collection *(f)*. Ring-down artifacts *(A)* seen anteriorly result from air in the nondependent portion of the cavity. **(B)** Real-time sector scan of the same patient, with the beam aimed anteromedially from a left posterolateral approach, demonstrates a linear echo (arrows) representing the air-fluid level. Since the position of the transducer corresponds to the top of the display, the entire image is rotated more than 90 degrees; thus, the echogenic line of the air-fluid level appears past the vertical rather than horizontal (From Golding RH, Li DKB, Cooperberg PL: Sonographic demonstration of air-fluid levels in abdominal abscesses. J Ultrasound Med 1:151, 1982.)

Hematomas

The echo characteristics of intraabdominal, extraorgan hematomas are highly variable and are dependent upon age of the collection and transducer frequency. In the acute phase of hemorrhage, hematomas imaged with abdominal transducer frequencies (2.25 to 3.0 MHz) typically exhibit a cystic ultrasound pattern, with absence of internal echoes and increased through transmission (Fig. 7-39). In vitro studies have shown, however, that fresh clot is highly echogenic when imaged with 5.0-, 7.5-, and 10.0-MHz transducers, despite an anechoic

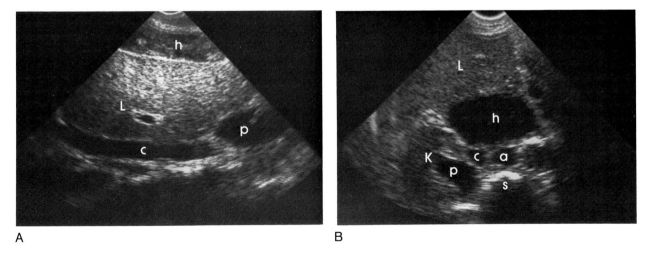

A   B

Fig. 7-39. Intraabdominal hematoma. Hematomas *(h)* are identified anterior to the liver on longitudinal scan **(A)** and in the right suphepatic region on transverse scan **(B).** Note that diffuse echoes are seen within both hematomas, although they appear somewhat more coarse in the former. Also noted incidentally is right hydronephrosis. (*L,* Liver; *K,* kidney; *p,* dilated renal pelvis; *c,* inferior vena cava; *a,* aorta; *s,* spine.)

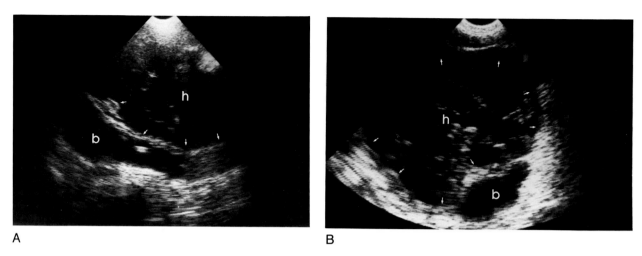

A   B

Fig. 7-40. Pelvic hematoma. **(A)** Longitudinal midline and **(B)** transverse pelvic scans in a young adult following a motor vehicle accident demonstrate bladder *(b)* compression by a large complex pelvic mass *(h)*. The coarse clumps of highly echogenic material as seen in this case are often a striking feature of chronic hematomas.

appearance with 2.25- and 3.0-MHz transducers. This echogenicity disappears within 96 hours following clotting; thus, hemolyzed clots are anechoic regardless of transducer frequency.[46]

Subsequent organization of a laminated clot or fragmentation of hemolyzed clot within a hematoma results in the generation of internal echoes, which most commonly disperse throughout the collection but may layer dependently. Coarse clumps of highly echogenic material may be a striking feature of chronic hematomas (Fig. 7-40). Because of continued clot lysis, late hematomas contain significantly fewer echoes than those less than 30 days old, and may eventually again become completely anechoic. Old hematomas, when anechoic, may contain either a thin serosanguinous fluid or a solid gelatinous material.[46-49]

The shape of hematomas appears determined primarily by location, with intraperitoneal collections generally ovoid or spherical and tending to displace rather than conform to adjacent structures.[34] A lenticular configuration, as well as conformity to surrounding organs, is more likely to be encountered in instances when hemorrhage dissects along well-defined tissue planes as with hematomas in the anterior abdominal wall or in a subcapsular location[49] (Fig. 7-6). The presence of wall irregularity and septations is variable and of no real diagnostic aid. The walls of fresh or older hematomas may be sharply defined; however, in one series (including intraorgan as well as intra- and extraperitoneal hematomas), 88 percent demonstrated irregularity of the wall by ultrasound at some time in their course.[49] The incidence of septations within hematomas ranges from 10 percent to 44 percent among separate series of hematomas in all locations.[32,49]

Intramural intestinal hemorrhage in hemophilia has been demonstrated sonographically as a tubular anechoic mass (hemorrhage) containing a core of strong echoes (bowel lumen), an appearance not unlike that of neoplastic or inflammatory diseases of bowel or other

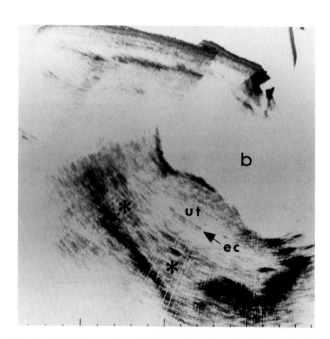

Fig. 7-41. Echogenic cul-de-sac clot. Longitudinal midline scan in patient with ruptured ectopic pregnancy reveals a fluid collection in the cul-de-sac *(*)* equal in echogenicity to that of the uterus *(ut)*. Water enema performed under real-time excluded echogenic bowel loops as a source of this echogenic lesion. (*ec,* endometrial cavity echo; *b,* bladder.) (From Jeffrey RB, Laing FC: Echogenic clot: A useful sign of pelvic hemoperitoneum. Radiology 145:139, 1982.)

causes of bowel wall thickening[50] (Fig. 9-56). Mesenteric hematomas arising spontaneously as a complication of long-term anticoagulent therapy or following trauma have also been documented by ultrasound as cystic masses containing internal echoes and/or septa.[51,52]

The sonographic appearance of hematomas is not specific; in particular, there may be considerable overlap with that of abscesses. Cystic masses containing clotted blood may appear indistinguishable from simple hematomas.[53] Nonetheless, the presence of a highly echogenic fluid collection in the pouch of Douglas may be of significant value in diagnosing pelvic hemoperitoneum, since most other fluid collections in the pelvis are predominantly anechoic with low-level echoes[54] (Fig. 7-41). Obviously, clinical correlation (i.e., history of trauma, bleeding diathesis, and/or drop in hematocrit) will permit sonographic diagnosis with a high degree of confidence in many cases.

Since there is no reliable means of detecting the presence of infection in a hematoma by ultrasound criteria, needle aspiration must be relied upon in certain clinical situations. Skinny-needle aspiration of a collection may be unsuccessful despite the "cystic" sonographic appearance if solid gelatinous material is contained within. In one series, however, all attempted aspirations of hematomas yielded a bloody aspirate when the collections contained echoes.[49]

Bilomas

Extrahepatic loculated collections of bile, termed bilomas, may develop as a complication of trauma, biliary surgery, or gallbladder neoplasm. Extravasated bile, by generating an intense inflammatory response, walls itself off with the formation of a sharply defined pseudocapsule. It is theorized that a secondary inflammatory reaction following the primary leak increases the original volume of fluid encapsulated.[55] On ultrasound, these collections characteristically are echofree with increased through transmission, sharply marginated, and located in the right or mid-upper abdomen in continuity with the liver or biliary structures (Fig. 7-42). They also tend to both surround and compress structures with which they come in contact.[55,56]

Bilomas may contain weak internal echoes or a fluid-debris level,[55] and those containing purulent bile have been noted to contain more internal echoes.[56] In one series, a surprisingly large percentage of patients (36 percent of 11) had bilomas that were localized in the left upper quadrant despite surgery on the right side,[57] while all but one of nine patients in another series had bilomas that were located in the right half of the abdomen.[56] Similarly, bilomas have been observed unrelated to the

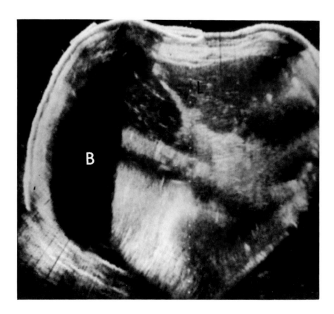

Fig. 7-42. Biloma. Large, primarily anechoic lenticular collection *(B)* is seen lateral to the liver *(L)* in a postcholecystectomy patient. (Transverse scan, 14 centimeters above the umbilicus.)

liver in the mid and lower abdomen of a postsurgical patient, presumably representing bile leakage early in the postsurgical course, when the patient was ambulatory.[55] Other unexpected clinical features reported in a series of 11 patients include presentation as a frank pyogenic subhepatic abscess in 36 percent of cases, and the presence of an active bile fistula in 45 percent of cases.[57]

As with other intraperitoneal cystic collections, the appearance of bilomas is relatively nonspecific, but a correct diagnosis may be suggested from the sonographic findings when they are correlated with the clinical history of recent trauma or biliary surgery. Needle aspiration is essential in confirming the diagnosis, and ultrasound directed guidance may be useful in this regard. Bilomas appear, in general, to be highly amenable to therapeutic catheter drainage, although failure of drainage appears more likely in patients with active leaks, particularly if the catheter tip cannot be placed in close proximity to the site of the leak. The initial appearance of the aspirate may be deceiving in those cases presenting as frank abscesses, with the purulent material not taking on a more bilious appearance until 24 to 48 hours of subsequent drainage.[57]

Inflammatory Fluid of Pancreatic Origin

Inflammatory fluid of pancreatic origin, including frank pancreatic pseudocysts, is perhaps the most variable in appearance of all intraabdominal fluid collec-

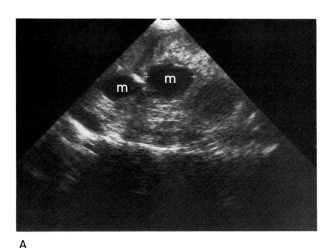

A

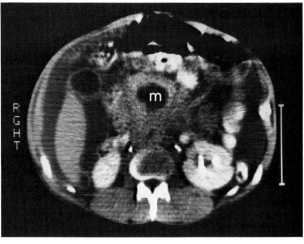

B

Fig. 7-43. Pancreatic pseudocysts. (A) Longitudinal midline scan demonstrates two relatively anechoic masses *(m)* with scattered low-amplitude echoes and increased through transmission. (B) CT scan through the lowermost lesion, revealing a somewhat irregular ovoid low-density area *(m)* within the body of the pancreas.

tions (see Chapter 3). They may be uni- or multilocular, ovoid or irregular in shape, and have smooth or ragged walls. They may be anechoic or contain a widely variable amount of debris, including the appearance of multiple septations or nondependent internal echoes due to contained and adherent inflammatory masses (Figs. 7-43 and 7-44); they may also mimic a solid mass, for example, when filled with organizing hematoma. Posterior acoustic enhancement is not necessarily present and, in

some instances, its absence has been explained by the presence of peripheral calcification. Differentiation from abscess and hematoma may be impossible based on ultrasound criteria alone, although pseudocysts are often accompanied by diffuse or focal pancreatic swelling. Change in internal echo characteristics with serial scanning may suggest intervening infection, hemorrhage, or rupture. In addition, evolution over a time interval may help to differentiate a left renal or adrenal cyst from a pancreatic tail mass.[31,32,34,58]

Extrapancreatic fluid collections (i.e., fluid that has tracked beyond the bounds of the pancreas into the surrounding tissues) need not be "cyst-like" or fixed by a dense fibrous capsule, particularly in the acute phase, when most distend an already existing anatomic space or conform to the borders of surrounding viscera. Extrapancreatic fluid collections may involve the lesser sac, the anterior and posterior pararenal spaces, or the perihepatic and juxtasplenic regions, or they may reside within the spleen itself or extend into the mediastinum.[59] This potential for a location remote from the pancreas clearly does not simplify sonographic diagnosis.

When hemorrhagic, pancreatic fluid collections vary in sonographic appearance depending upon age of hemorrhage. Acute hemorrhage may appear as well-defined masses with homogeneous echoes of medium intensity, with or without posterior enhancement. In the subacute phase (approximately one week after event), cystic structures containing clumps of internal echoes or septations may be seen, while remote hemorrhage may be visualized as a purely anechoic lesion.[60]

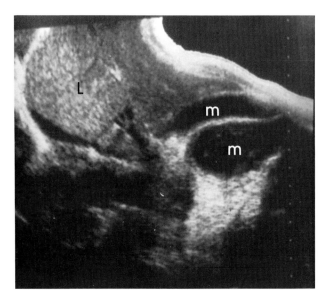

Fig. 7-44. Pancreatic pseudocysts. Longitudinal scan to the right of midline demonstrates adjacent, predominently anechoic masses in the right upper quadrant *(m)*. (*L,* liver.)

Omental and Mesenteric Cysts

Cystic lesions of the omentum and mesentery are uncommon lesions that do not share a single etiologic mechanism in their development. Abdominal cysts in general have been previously categorized as (1) embryologic and developmental, (2) traumatic or acquired, (3) neoplastic, and (4) infective and degenerative.[61] The first category includes lesions of lymphatic, enteric, or urogenital origin, as well as dermoid tumors, although some authors exclude dermoid as well as parasitic cysts in the classification of mesenteric cysts.[62] Other authors consider chylous cysts a separate entity, with "true" chylous cysts originating from the mesentery of the small bowel, and "false" chylous cysts originating from nonlymphatic sources or regional lymphatics.[63,64] In this sense, a lymphocele may be viewed as a variant form of the "false" variety of chylous cyst. Enterogenous cysts may be derived from intestinal diverticula or originate from short duplications, the lumens of which do not communicate with that of the main intestines.[65] In this latter instance, the duplication anomaly constitutes a variety of mesenteric cyst.

In broadest terms, any cystic structure that does not arise from a definitive organ of the body and yet resides in the mesentery is by definition a mesenteric cyst; specific identification as to etiology, if possible, lies in the domain of the pathologist. Histologically, the walls of mesenteric cysts are composed of fibrous tissue, and if present, an endothelial lining may suggest the derivation of the cyst.[66] Obviously, those of a traumatic or infectious etiology would not be expected to have an endothelial lining. Similarly, enterogenous cysts contain mucous membrane endothelium and layers of smooth muscle.

Omental cysts may differ from mesenteric cysts only by location, although the latter are more common and tend to be somewhat larger than the former. Mesenteric/omental cysts may range in size from small to large lesions virtually filling the entire abdominal cavity. The fluid contained may be serous, chylous, bloody, or mixed, or may be a thick "cheesy-white" material thought to be inspissated lymph fluid.[67] Mesenteric cysts may be found between the leaves of the mesentery anywhere from the duodenum to the rectum, with roughly half occurring in the small bowel mesentery, and half again of these in the ileomesentery. Only about 5 percent originate in the retroperitoneum.[68,69]

Ultrasound characteristically reveals a uni- or multilocular cystic structure with smooth walls and no internal echoes, unless there is superimposed hemorrhage or infection.[70-72] In these instances, mobile fluid-debris levels or solid components with grossly irregular contours have been indentified within the collections; a "honey-combed" appearance has also been de-

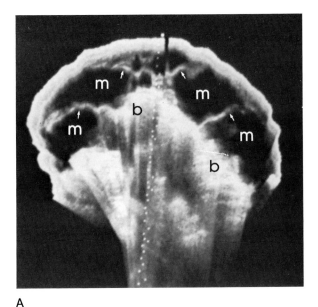

A

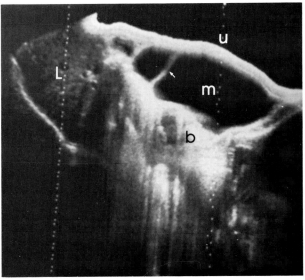

B

Fig. 7-45. Mesenteric cyst. Septated mesenteric cyst of the greater omentum appears on transverse (**A**) and right longitudinal (**B**) ultrasound scans as an extensive fluid-filled mass *(m)* closely conforming to the anterior abdominal wall. Note the presence of septations (arrows) as well as posterior displacement of bowel *(b)*.(*L,* liver; *u,* level of umbilicus.) (From Geer LL, Mittelstaedt CA, Staab EV, Gaisie G: Mesenteric cyst: Sonographic appearance with CT correlation. Pediatr Radiol 14:102, 1984.)

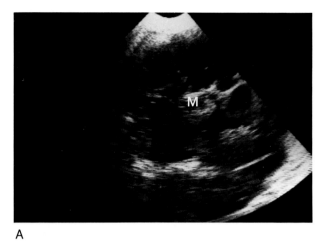

A

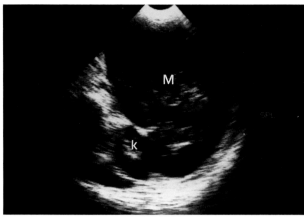

B

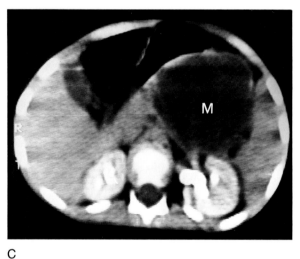

C

Fig. 7-46. Hemorrhagic mesenteric cyst. A complex left upper quadrant mass with a "honey-comb" appearance is seen in a 7-year-old male on left longitudinal (**A**) and left transverse oblique (**B**) scans. A corresponding CT scan at the level of the midkidneys (**C**) demonstrates a low-density intraabdominal mass with rim enhancement. (*k*, kidney.) (From Geer LL, Mittelstaedt CA, Staab EV, Gaisie G: Mesenteric cyst: sonographic appearance with CT correlation. Pediatr Radiol 14:102, 1984.)

scribed.[73-75] (Figs. 7-45 and 7-46). A fat-fluid level may also be identified, presumably representing a combination of inflammatory exudate with chyle.[76] Internal septations are not uncommonly present, and are more likely to be identified with ultrasound than by CT.[75,77] Rarely, mesenteric cysts may be calcified.[78,79]

Although mesenteric cysts may present as a discrete rounded mass, both mesenteric and particularly omental cysts may follow the contours of the underlying bowel and conform closely to the anterior abdominal wall rather than producing distention. In these instances, the collection may change configuration with changes in patient position.[73,80] Careful attention to distribution (e.g., anterior location of fluid with none posterior or between bowel loops) can help exclude free intraperitoneal fluid, but not necessarily a loculated collection of ascites. In summary, omental and mesenteric cysts may produce confusing mass effects or may mimic simple ascites. To even further muddle the diagnostic picture, hemorrhage into omental or mesenteric

cysts may cause rapid abdominal distention, and thus clinically mimic the sudden onset of ascites.[81]

Pseudomyxoma Peritonei

Pseudomyxoma peritonei, which arises from mucinous tumors of the appendix and ovary, is characterized by diffuse involvement of the peritoneal surfaces and omentum with gelatinous mucinous implants, often with massive gelatinous ascites.[82] Sonographically, the findings may suggest only an exudative ascites (i.e., with "non-floating" posterior position of bowel loops).[83] Ascites with numerous echoes or "ascites-like" masses may represent gelatinous ascites (Fig. 7-47) or a semisolid gelatinous mass.[84] Other reported appearances include highly echogenic masses containing scattered numerous cystic spaces[84] (Fig. 7-48), a large intraperitoneal multiseptated cystic-appearing mass,[83,85] numerous thick-walled multiseptate fluid-filled masses[86] (Fig.

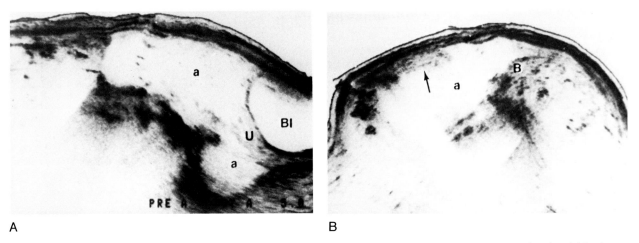

A   B

Fig. 7-47. Pseudomyxoma peritonei. **(A)** Longitudinal midline scan demonstrates a large amount of ascites *(a)* in the lower abdomen and pelvis. The numerous weak echoes within the ascites are due to gelatinous material. (*U*, uterus; *Bl*, bladder.) **(B)** transverse scan above the umbilicus again demonstrates the echogenic ascites *(a)*, as well as an echogenic peritoneal mass (arrow) in the anterior abdominal wall. (*B*, bowel.) (From Yeh H-C, Shafir MK, Slater G, et al: Ultrasonography and computed tomography in pseudomyxoma peritonei. Radiology 153:507, 1984.)

7-49), and multiple rounded echodense masses (amorphous calcification is present in the latter instances).[87] The appearance of widespread homogeneous masses surrounding echogenic bowel may suggest possible intraabdominal carcinomatosis or lymphomatous involvement.[88] Indentation of the liver edge by extrinsic pressure from implants, so-called "scalloping," may be identified sonographically, but this finding is more consistently demonstrated by CT.[83,85]

Cerebrospinal Fluid Pseudocysts/ Ascites

Cerebrospinal fluid (CSF) ascites and pseudocyst formation are rare complications of ventriculoperitoneal shunting. CSF ascites is a diffuse, nonloculated collection of cerebrospinal fluid that occurs secondary to a primary failure of the peritoneal cavity to absorb spinal fluid,[89] or possibly from lymphatic obstruction causing

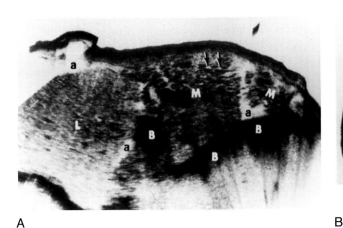
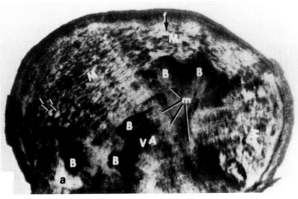

A   B

Fig. 7-48. Pseudomyxoma peritonei. **(A)** Longitudinal scan 6 cm to the right of midline demonstrates two large, highly echogenic masses *(M)* situated beneath the anterior abdominal wall and displacing the bowel *(B)* posteriorly. Numerous tiny cysts, and several larger ones (arrows) are scattered throughout the mass. Ascites *(a)* is present between the masses and adjacent to the liver *(L)*. **(B)** Transverse scan 5 cm above the umbilicus reveals multiple echogenic masses *(M)* and smaller masses *(m)* and cysts (arrows) beneath the anterior and lateral abdominal wall. (*v*, venal cava; *A*, aorta; *a*, ascites.) (From Yeh H-C, Shafir MK, Slater G et al: Ultrasonography and computed tomography in pseudomyxoma peritonei. Radiology 153:507, 1984.)

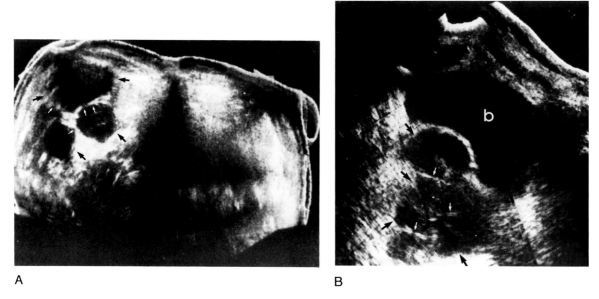

A   B

Fig. 7-49. Pseudomyxoma peritonei. **(A)** Transverse scan at the inferior margin of the liver demonstrates several thick wall cysts (black arrows) with the appearance of intervening septa (white arrows). On other scans, the inferior edge of the liver was indented by these cysts (peritoneal scalloping), although the liver itself appeared normal. **(B)** Longitudinal scan over bladder *(b)* in same patient demonstrates numerous retrovesical cysts (black arrows) with intervening septa (white arrows) (From Hopper KD: Ultrasonic findings in pseudomyxoma peritonei. Reprinted by permission from the Southern Medical Journal 76:1051, 1983.)

diminished return of the fluid to the vascular compartment.[90]

Encystation of CSF fluid complicating ventriculoperitoneal shunting has been reported more frequently in the literature, but still has a reported incidence of only 0.7 percent (11 occurrences in 1,585 shunt cases) in one large series.[91] The pathophysiology of the intraperitoneal pseudocyst apparently involves an inflammatory re-

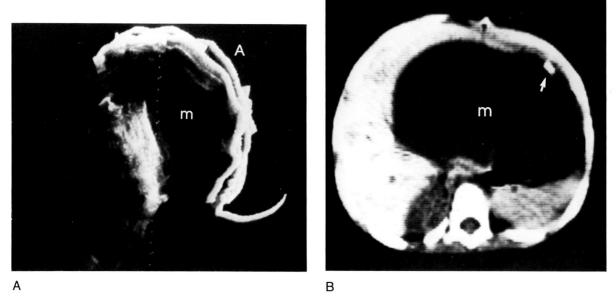

A   B

Fig. 7-50. Cerebrospinal fluid pseudocyst. **(A)** Transverse decubitus ultrasound and **(B)** corresponding abdominal CT scan demonstrate a large cystic intraabdominal mass *(m)* in a 4-year-old with a ventriculoperitoneal shunt and abdominal distension. The distal end of the shunt tube (arrow) is identified on CT scan. (*A,* anterior.)

sponse to either the catheter or some component of the draining CSF fluid. The inflammatory reaction around the catheter tip is speculated as secondary to a low-grade shunt infection and localized peritonitis,[92] although a possible common denominator may be a high concentration of a proteinaceous moiety in the peritoneal cavity associated with head injury, surgical procedures, or infection.[93,94] A small collection may form around the tip of the shunt tubing and preclude escape of the CSF fluid into the general peritoneal space, or a relatively large area of the peritoneal cavity may become isolated by dense adhesions that produce a multiloculated, poorly absorbing space.[95] The pseudocyst wall may be a thick fibrous capsule composed, for example, of intestinal loops matted together by connective tissue;[96] it also may be formed solely of inflamed serosal surfaces.[92]

Ultrasound demonstrates a typical intraabdominal cystic mass in association with the distal end of the shunt tube[95,97–100] (Figs. 7-50 and 7-51). Shunt tubing is identified as a linear echogenic structure from which acoustic shadowing may be produced, allowing differentiation from echoes arising from septa in a cystic mass. Demonstration of low-amplitude echogenic material contained within the cyst may be seen with superimposed infection.[101]

A small amount of free intraperitoneal CSF fluid is a normal concomitant of satisfactory ventriculoperitoneal shunt function, although its absence does not indicate shunt malfunction. A localized collection of fluid in association with the abdominal end of a ventriculoperitoneal shunt, however, is pathologic and indicates a malfunction in the system.[102] Nonloculated CSF ascites will be sonographically indistinguishable from transudative ascites, but the presence of generalized intraperitoneal

fluid in an infant with a ventriculoperitoneal shunt in place should suggest this rare entity. Although CSF pseudocysts may also be diagnosed by CT,[103] ultrasound is the initial modality of choice in the evaluation of shunt patients who present with abdominal symptoms or an abdominal mass, with or without associated neurological findings.

Differential Diagnostic Considerations

From the preceding discussion, the overlap of sonographic appearances of intraperitoneal extraorgan fluid-containing abnormalities is obvious, as is the need for clinical correlation and, in many instances, aspiration biopsy. Since a variety of other lesions, including retroperitoneal lymphoceles and urinomas, extraperitoneal urachal cysts, organ-associated cystic lesions, and primary gynecologic pathology may at times require consideration in the differential diagnosis, they are briefly discussed here, along with cystic-appearing solid lesions and pseudolesions.

LYMPHOCELES

Lymphocele, a lymph-filled space without a distinct epithelial lining, is a well-recognized complication of radical gynecologic procedures,[104] extensive pelvic urologic operations including staging lymphadenectomy for prostatic or bladder carcinoma,[105,106] and renal transplantation.[107,108] Although commonly located retroperitoneally in the pelvis, upper abdominal lymphoceles have been reported occurring secondary to aortofemoral bypass,[109] presumed simple nephrolithiasis,[110] and para-

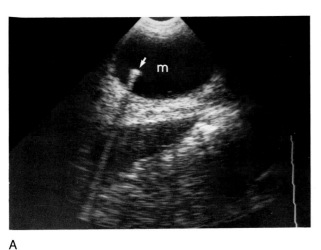

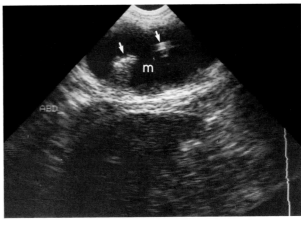

A   B

Fig. 7-51. Cerebrospinal fluid pseudocyst. Elderly patient following a ventriculoperitoneal shunt placement for normal pressure hydrocephalus, presenting with palpable abdominal mass. **(A)** Longitudinal and **(B)** transverse scans demonstrate an anechoic collection *(m)* associated with shunt tubing (arrows).

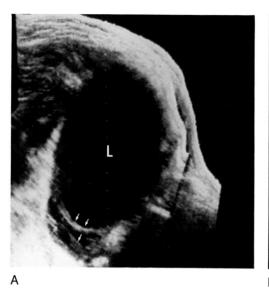
A

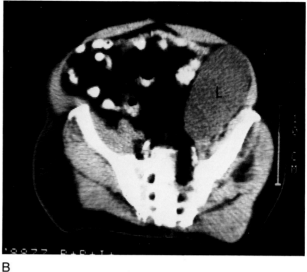
B

Fig. 7-52. Lymphocele. **(A)** Transverse scan of the left lower abdomen and **(B)** corresponding CT scan in a man following a radical prostatectomy. Ultrasound demonstrates the characteristic elliptical shape of the lymphocele *(L),* with sharp margins and slight wall irregularity, and with increased through transmission. Also noted are septations and internal echoes present posteriorly (arrows), a finding not appreciated on the CT scans.

aortic/renal hilar node dissections.[111] Lymphocele development usually results from surgical disruption of lymphatic channels, but in the case of renal transplants the lymph leakage may originate from the donor kidney itself, with episodes of rejection or prior perinephric hematoma as associated factors.[112] Lymphoceles may be unilateral or bilateral, but are most often unilocular.[105]

Sonographically, lymphoceles are generally elliptical, with sharp margins or varying degrees of wall irregularity. They are characterized by increased through transmission and no internal echoes, although thin septations have been seen in as many as 50 percent of cases in one reported series.[32] Since an uncomplicated lymphocele should not contain debris or internal echoes (other than thin septa, possibly), these findings suggest the presence of an abscess or hematoma, or a lymphocele complicated by infection. A pelvic lymphocele may markedly compress and displace the bladder to one side, but in general they displace organs to a lesser extent than the classic abscess, and may themselves be indented by adjacent solid organs[24,34] (Figs. 7-52 and 7-53).

Lymphoceles in the posterior pararenal compartment may be the result of cephalad spread from processes originating in the extraperitoneal pelvis, but the retroperitoneal location may be inferred by anterior kidney displacement. The retroperitoneal origin of the collection may be more difficult to ascertain sonographically if it occurs in an atypical location, such as a midlumbar lymphocele that is anteroinferior to the kidney rather than posterior to it.[111] When associated with renal trans-

plants, a lymphocele may occasionally produce deterioration of transplant function secondary to ureteral obstruction, thus mimicking rejection. Sonographically, they appear as an echofree region adjacent to the transplant kidney, extending in any direction[108,113] (see Figs. 4-140, 4-141 and 4-153).

The general differential diagnosis includes loculated

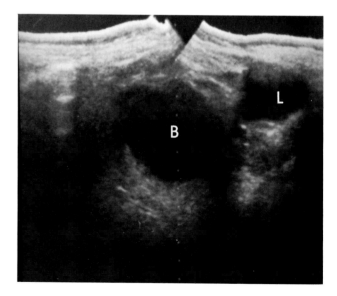

Fig. 7-53. Lymphocele. Transverse scan in a patient following radical hysterectomy demonstrates an anechoic mass (L) in the left groin region, adjacent to the bladder (B).

ascites, hematoma, abscess, and urinoma. The presence of internal echoes or debris may help to distinguish hematoma, abscess, or infected lymphocele from uncomplicated lymphocele. Distinction from loculated ascites may be possible if a definite retroperitoneal location can be established, such as with anterior renal or ureteral displacement by the collection. Urinomas and lymphoceles are likely to be indistinguishable by ultrasound.[34] As with all fluid collections demonstrated by ultrasound, correlation with history, physical examination, and available radiographic studies may suggest the origin of the collection, but needle aspiration of the visualized fluid may be the only way to establish a definitive diagnosis.

URINOMA

An encapsulated collection of urine, or urinoma, may result from closed renal injury or surgical intervention, or may arise spontaneously secondary to an obstructing lesion. Persistent leakage of urine from continued renal function stimulates an intense fibrous reaction and the formation of a characteristic thick wall that sometimes contains necrotic fat.[114]

Urine leakage tends to remain localized to the perinephric space, the obvious exceptions being in instances of renal trauma or after disruption of tissue boundaries by major surgery. However, collections under high enough pressure may potentially leak around the ureter,

where the perinephric fascia is the weakest, or even into adjoining fascial planes and the peritoneal cavity. Partially because of gravitation effect, these cystic masses are most often oriented inferomedially with upward and lateral displacement of the lower pole of the kidney along with medial displacement of the ureter, although in one large series this location represented only 25 percent of all collections.[114,115]

Sonographically, urinomas may be anechoic or contain low-level internal echoes, and have good increased through transmission. They characteristically have sharp margins and tend to be elliptical in shape, although they may be indented by adjacent solid organs[31] (Figs. 7-54 and 7-55). In one small series, thin septa were present in 60 percent.[32] Thus, by ultrasound criteria alone urinomas are virtually indistinguishable from lymphoceles, and needle aspiration may be essential for differentiation, particularly in the postrenal transplant patient.

URACHAL CYST

The adult urachus, the remnant of the embryologic connection between the ventral cloaca and the umbilicus, is normally a functionally closed fibrous cord located extraperitoneally in the midline between the peritoneum and the transversalis fascia. Incomplete regression of the urachus during development may result in various anomalies, including patent urachus, urachal

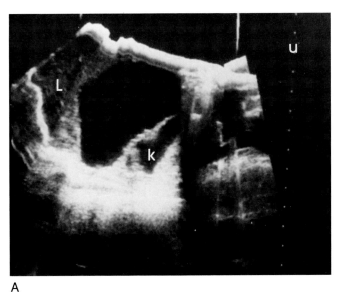

A

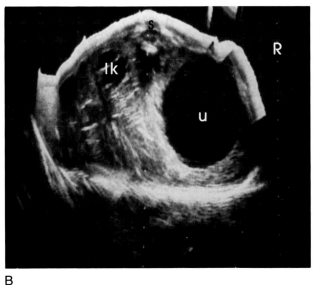

B

Fig. 7-54. Urinoma. **(A)** Right longitudinal supine and **(B)** transverse prone scans in a male newborn with posterior urethral valves demonstrate the encapsulated extravasated urine collection as a large anechoic intraabdominal mass *(u)* interposed between the hydronephrotic right kidney *(k)* and liver *(L)*. Left hydronephrosis is also apparent *(lk)*. *(s,* spine; *R,* right.)

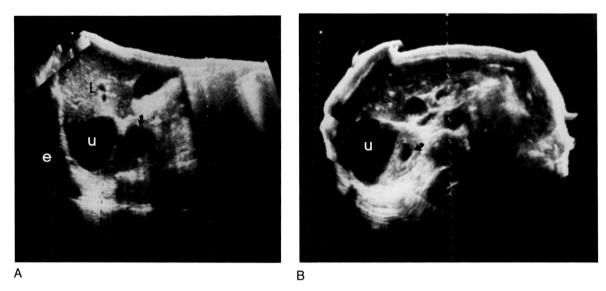

A   B

Fig. 7-55. Urinoma. **(A)** Right longitudinal and **(B)** transverse supine scans in a patient with hydronephrosis (arrow) and a right urinoma (*u*) secondary to obstructing lymph nodes from prostatic carcinoma. The anechoic mass is noted supralaterally to the kidney, producing compression on both the liver *(L)* and kidney. Incidentally noted on longitudinal images is a pleural effusion *(e)*.

diverticulum, urachal sinus, or urachal cyst.[116] (see Fig. 4-157). The latter entity, representing persistence of the urachal midportion with both cephalic and caudal ends closed, typically remains silent unless symptoms related to size or secondary infection supervene.[117]

The ultrasound appearance of urachal cysts ranges from a small cystic mass in the lower abdomen between the umbilicus and bladder[118,119] to a giant multiseptated cystic structure extending into the upper abdomen, with

compression and elongation of the bladder.[120] Mixed echogenicity may be encountered within the cyst when infection is present[121] (Fig. 7-56; see Fig. 4-158). Examination preferably should be performed with bladder distention to identify anatomic relationships. In the pediatric age group, change in configuration of the cystic mass post-voiding, with elongation and inferior extension of the caudal portion, suggests bladder communication (e.g., patent urachus instead of urachal cyst).[122]

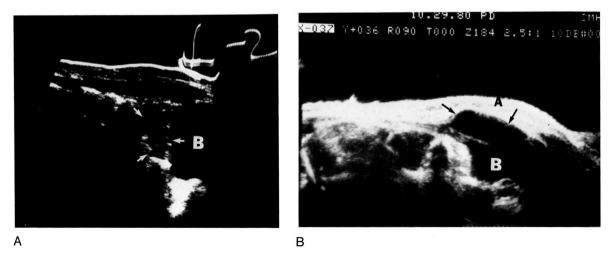

A   B

Fig. 7-56. Infected urachal cyst. **(A)** Infected urachal cyst is seen on a longitudinal scan as a mass of mixed echogenicity (arrow) adherent to and involving the dome of the bladder *(B)*. **(B)** Longitudinal scan in different patient shows apposition of an infected, abscess-forming urachal cyst (arrows) to the anterior wall of the bladder *(B)*. (*A*, anterior abdominal wall.) (From Spataro RF, Davis RS, McLachlan MSF, et al: Urachal abnormalities in the adult. Radiology 149:659, 1983.)

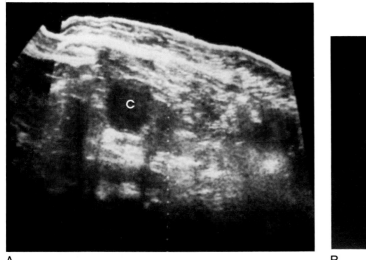

A   B

Fig. 7-57. Renal cyst in displaced kidney. **(A)** Longitudinal midline scan in a patient with a large adrenal mass (not shown) demonstrates a separate oval hypoechoic mass *(c)*. **(B)** Transverse real-time image reveals that this mass represents a large renal cyst emanating from the lower pole of the right kidney (*K* with arrows). Displacement of the kidney due to the large adrenal mass resulted in the unexpected midline location of this renal cyst (note longitudinal axis of kidney on transverse image).

ORGAN ASSOCIATED FLUID AND CYSTIC MASSES

Renal, hepatic, splenic, pancreatic, and adrenal cysts in adults usually can be easily localized to their respective organ with ultrasound, with certain exceptions (e.g., distinguishing left adrenal cyst or renal cyst from pancreatic tail lesion). Anatomic relationships may be less clearcut when cysts are associated with displaced or malpositioned organs (Fig. 7-57). Massive hydro- or pyonephrosis may initially be disorienting, but the diagnosis is suggested when an ipsilateral kidney cannot be visualized (Figs. 7-58 and 7-59). Extensive polycystic kidney/ liver disease (see Figs. 1-54, 4-20, and 4-21) and cystadenoma/adenocarcinoma of the biliary tree (see Figs. 2-78 and 2-79) or pancreas (see Figs. 3-49, 3-50, and 3-51) may also disorient the unwary or inexperienced sonologist.

A variety of nongynecologic cystic masses may be encountered in the pelvis in relation to the bladder, including obstructed pelvic kidney, bladder diverticula, ureterocele and hydroureter, seminal vesicle cysts (see Chapter 4), prostatic cysts, urachal cysts (Fig. 7-56; see 4-158), varices, and iliac artery aneurysms[123] (see Fig. 6-43).

Abnormalities that originate supradiaphragmatically may severely depress the diaphragm on sonographic examination; a large aneurysm involving the anteroinferior aspect of the left ventricle may present this way, for example.[124] The differential diagnosis of a cystic midepigastric or lower abdominal mass includes, of course, abdominal aortic aneurysm—demonstration of pulsa-

tions and continuity with vasculature structures is basic to diagnosis (see Chapter 6).

In the neonate, organ-associated fluid collections such as ovarian cyst (Fig. 7-60), choledochal cyst (see Fig. 2-90), hydrometrocolpos (Fig. 7-61), and even hydronephrosis secondary to ureteropelvic junction obstruction (see Figs. 4-28 to 4-30) may sometimes be difficult to localize with complete confidence. Bowel-associated cystic abdominal masses in the neonate include duplica-

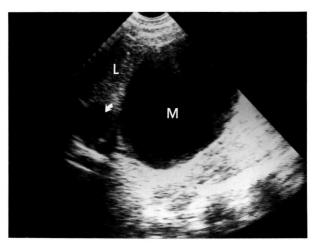

Fig. 7-58. Ureteropelvic junction obstruction. Transverse scan demonstrates a large cystic abdominal mass *(M)* adjacent to the right kidney. Right caliectasis is also seen (arrow). Left kidney was normal in appearance. (*L,* liver.)

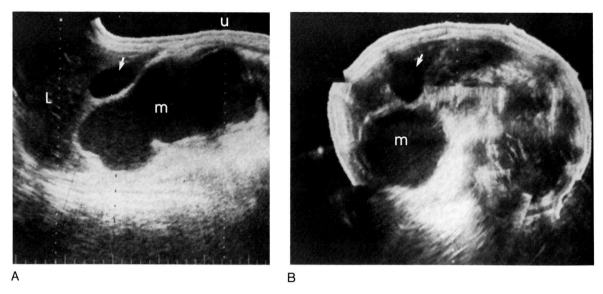

A   B

Fig. 7-59. Pyonephrosis. Massive pyonephrosis in a pregnant female with congenital right ureteropelvic junction obstruction is seen on right longitudinal (A) and transverse (B) scans as a large hypoechoic mass *(m)*. Diffuse low-amplitude echoes are seen within the mass, and are noted to be increased in amplitude in the more dependent portions of the dilated renal collecting system. (Arrow, gallbladder; *L,* liver; *u,* level of umbilicus.)

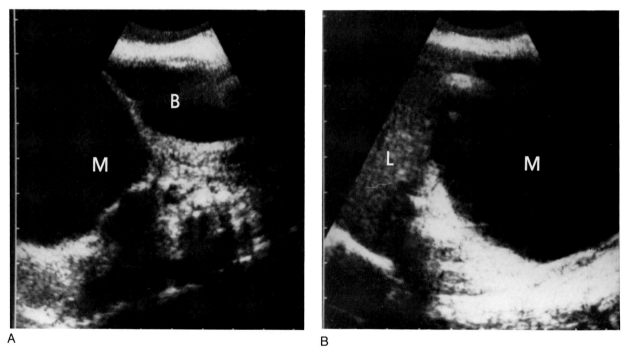

A   B

Fig. 7-60. Congenital ovarian cyst. Massive ovarian cyst in a 4-day-old infant presenting with an abdominal mass *(M)*. (A) Longitudinal midline pelvic image and (B) right longitudinal scan of the upper abdomen demonstrate the extensiveness of this lesion. (*L,* liver; *B,* bladder.) (Reprinted courtesy of the Department of Ultrasound, Moore Memorial Hospital, Pinehurst, North Carolina.)

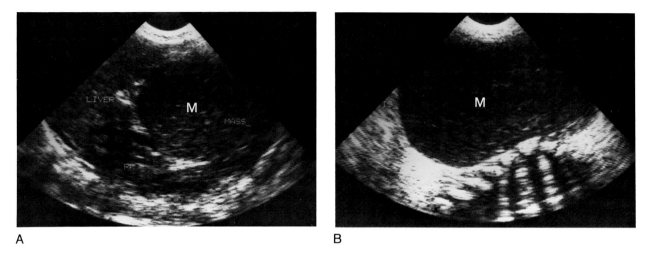

A   B

Fig. 7-61. Hydrometrocolpos. Right longitudinal scans of the upper (**A**) and lower (**B**) abdomen demonstrate the large abdominopelvic mass *(M)* containing diffuse low-amplitude echoes. (*RK,* right kidney.)

tion cysts, cystic meconium peritonitis/pseudocyst, segmental dilatation of bowel, and volvulus with peudocyst formation[125] (see Chapter 9).

CYSTIC-APPEARING SOLID LESIONS/NECROTIC LESIONS

Lymphomatous masses can at times appear extremely anechoic, exhibiting many features of fluid-filled or cystic masses (see Figs. 2-83, 4-130, and 5-52 to 5-57). In one series of patients with adenopathy, anechoic masses were observed in 83 percent of lymphoma cases and 53 percent of patients with metastatic lymph node involve-

ment. Of 23 patients with lymphoma, 5 exhibited nodes that were sonographically indistinguishable from cysts when the criteria of anechoicity, smooth walls, and increased through transmission were employed.[126] Other solid masses, including sarcomas, hypernephromas, and adenocarcinomas (such as metastatic breast lesions) may be diffusely hypoechoic or have localized areas of necrosis or fluid[4,6,34,127] (see Figs. 7-80 to 7-83). Uterine leiomyomas, particularly during pregnancy, may also appear hypoechoic or anechoic[6,34] (Fig. 7-62). Necrotic tumors typically contain an irregular cystic center surrounded by an echogenic rim of tissue that is distinct from adjacent soft tissues.[32]

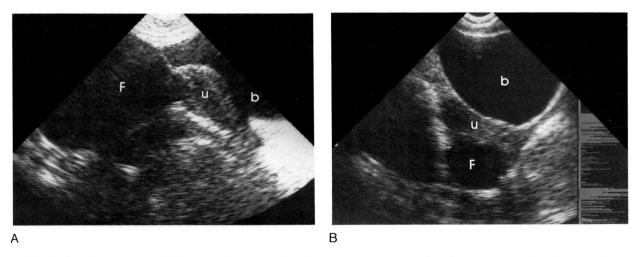

A   B

Fig. 7-62. Leiomyoma. (**A**) Longitudinal scan of the lower abdomen and pelvis demonstrates a large hypoechoic fibroid (*F*) emanating superiorly from the uterine fundus. (*u,* uterus; *b,* bladder). (**B**) Right longitudinal scan of the pelvis in a different patient reveals a cystic-appearing mass *(F)* in the cul-de-sac. At surgery, a pedunculated fibroid was removed. (*u,* uterus; *b* bladder.)

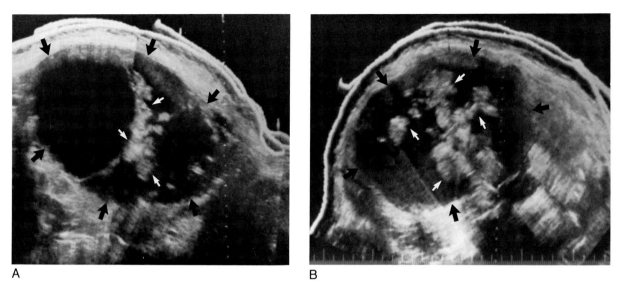

A   B

Fig. 7-63. Cystadenocarcinoma of the ovary. **(A)** Left longitudinal and **(B)** transverse scans demonstrate a large abdominopelvic mass (black arrows), characterized by large areas of anechoicity with intervening septa and irregular echodensities (white arrows).

GYNECOLOGIC PATHOLOGY

Gynecologic abnormalities that may present sonographically as abdominopelvic fluid-containing masses include ovarian epithelial neoplasms (Figs. 7-28 and 7-63), dermoid tumors (Fig. 7-64), endometriomas (Figs. 7-65 and 7-66), pyometra (Fig. 7-67), tubo-ovar-

ian abscesses (Fig. 7-68), hemato- or hydrosalpinges, ovarian or parovarian cysts (Figs. 7-69 and 7-70), leiomyoma/leiomyosarcoma (see Fig. 7-81), a variety of pelvic peritoneal cysts, and chronic ectopic pregnancy[128–136] (Fig. 7-71). Hemoperitoneum from ruptured ectopic gestation may appear as a typical fluid collection in the

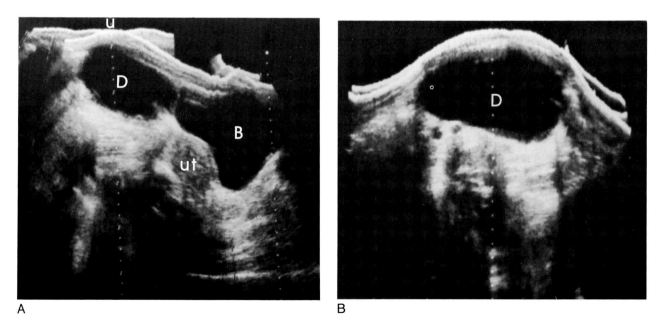

A   B

Fig. 7-64. Cystic dermoid. **(A)** Longitudinal midline and **(B)** transverse scans demonstrate an anechoic abdominopelvic mass *(D)*, with increased through transmission. No internal echoes are seen within this lesion. (*B,* bladder; *ut,* uterus; *u,* level of umbilicus.)

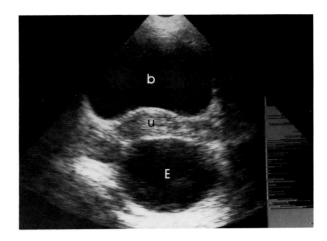

Fig. 7-65. Endometrioma. Transverse pelvic scan demonstrates an ovoid mass *(E)* to the left of midline, characterized by diffuse low-amplitude internal echoes. (*u,* uterus; *b,* bladder.)

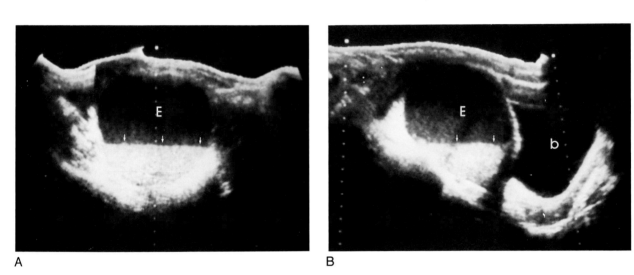

A   B

Fig. 7-66. Endometrioma. **(A)** Transverse and **(B)** longitudinal images demonstrate a midline pelvic mass *(E)* with a distinct fluid-fluid level *(arrows).* (*b,* bladder.)

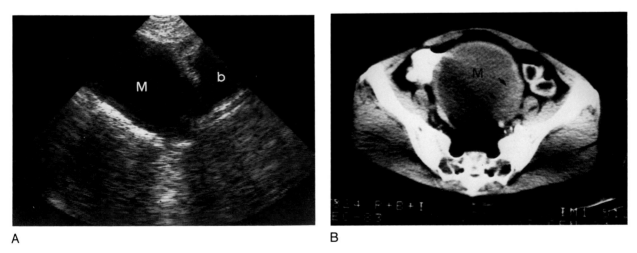

A   B

Fig. 7-67. Pyometra. **(A)** Midline longitudinal image demonstrates an irregular hypoechoic mass *(M).* No discrete uterus was identified separate from this lesion. (*b,* bladder.) **(B)** CT scan of the pelvis demonstrates a low-density mass *(M)* in the pelvis, with an asymmetrical rim of enhancing tissue (arrow).

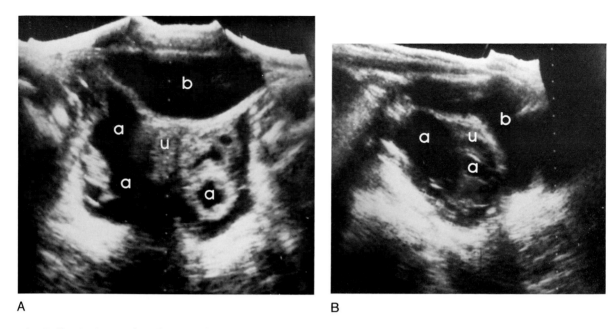

A   B

Fig. 7-68. Tubo-ovarian abscess. **(A)** Transverse and **(B)** longitudinal pelvic scans reveal multiple septated anechoic areas (a) surrounding the uterus *(u)*. (*b*, bladder.)

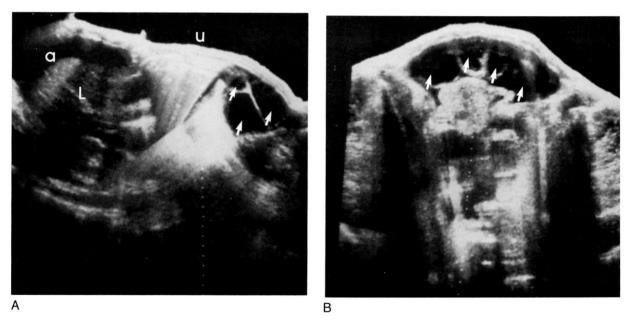

A   B

Fig. 7-69. Ovarian hyperstimulation. **(A)** Longitudinal midline and **(B)** transverse scans above the umbilicus demonstrate multiple septated cystic structures extending from the pelvis (arrows). The patient had received Pergonal for five days prior to admission with increased abdominal girth and bilateral pleural effusions. Ascites (a) is apparent in the upper abdomen. (*L*, liver; *u*, level of umbilicus.)

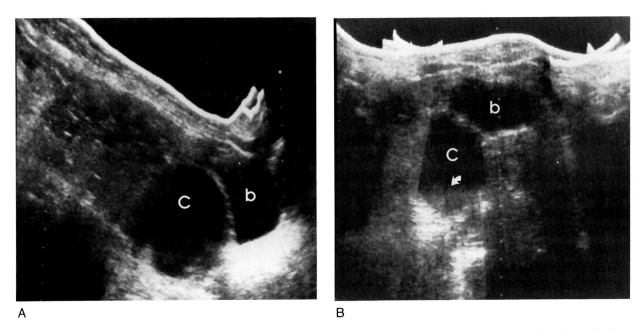

A   B

Fig. 7-70.   Right ovarian serous cyst. **(A)** Right longitudinal and **(B)** transverse scans reveal a predominantly anechoic mass *(C)* with some internal echoes, particularly dependently (arrow). (*b,* bladder.)

pelvis or elsewhere, but may also mimic a solid cul-de-sac mass[54] (Fig. 7-41).

PSEUDOLESIONS

Dilated and gas-free bowel may potentially be confused with an abnormal fluid collection by ultrasound, although in most instances bowel can be identified by contour, echo characteristics, and detection of peristalsis

with real-time sonography. Fluid-filled small bowel loops typically appear as cylindrical structures with a fine irregular wall and evenly distributed low-amplitude echoes. Differentiation may be considerably more difficult, however, if multiple loops of bowel are matted together in the shape of a mass by adhesions from prior surgery,[137] or if wads of omentum are involved in an inflammatory process or fill in prior surgical defects[138] (see Chapter 9).

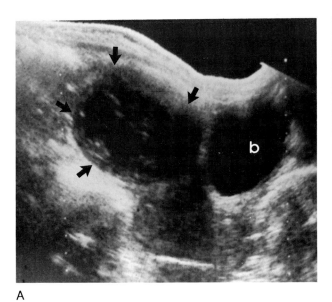

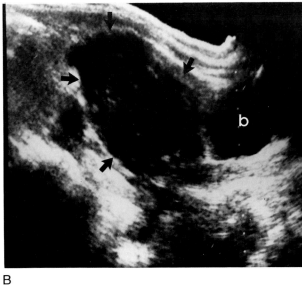

A   B

Fig. 7-71.   Chronic ectopic gestations. **(A,B)** Longitudinal midline images from two different patients with chronic ectopic gestation demonstrate large complex pelvic masses (arrows) with anechoic areas and increased through transmission. (*b,* bladder.)

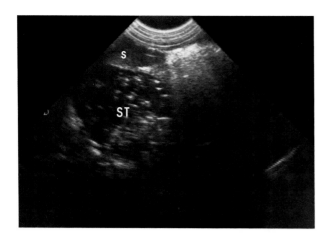

Fig. 7-72. Distended stomach. Left lateral decubitus longitudinal scan of neonate demonstrates a large complex mass *(ST)* in the left upper abdomen, representing normal stomach distended with infant formula. (*s*, spleen tip.)

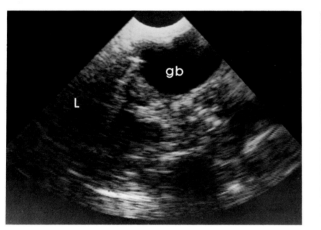

A

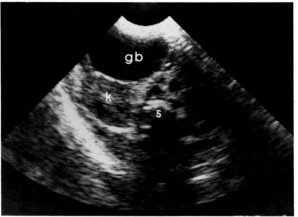

B

Fig. 7-73. Gallbladder pseudotumor. An abdominal mass was palpated in this two-day-old premature infant. **(A)** Longitudinal and **(B)** transverse scans identify the "mass" as a distended gallbladder (*L*, liver; *k*, kidney; *gb*, gallbladder; *s*, spine.) (From Durrell CA, Vincent LM, Mittelstaedt CA: Gallbladder ultrasonography in clinical context. Semin Ultrasound CT MR 5:315–332, 1984. By permission.)

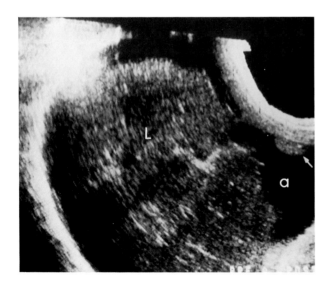

Fig. 7-74. Peritoneal metastasis. Longitudinal scan of right hypochondrium in patient with gastric antral carcinoma demonstrates a metastatic peritoneal implant (arrow) surrounded by ascitic fluid *(a)*. Metastatic liver disease is also present (*L*, liver.) (From Derchi LE, Biggi E, Rollandi GA et al: Sonographic staging of gastric carcinoma. AJR 140:273, ©Am Roentgen Ray Society, 1983.)

In the neonate, gastric distention may be mistaken for a cystic abdominal mass (Fig. 7-72); similarly, gallbladder distention secondary to parenteral hyperalimentation may be erroneously perceived as a cystic mass[139] (Fig. 7-73).

Excessive fat in the supradiaphragmatic region, appearing as a homogeneously echogenic well-defined area beneath the anterior abdominal wall, may simulate processes such as subdiaphragmatic abscess, subpulmonic effusion, ascites, or tumor[140] (Fig. 7-29).

tumors of childhood may secondarily involve the peritoneum.[141]

Sonographically, peritoneal metastases may exhibit a nodular, sheet-like, or irregular configuration, the last pattern resulting from irregular growth or consolidation of sheet-like masses (Figs. 7-74 and 7-75). Small nodules may appear attached to the peritoneal line, with the integrity of the line preserved, while larger masses will generally obliterate the line. Adhesion of bowel loops to the masses is not uncommon.[142]

NONCYSTIC INTRAPERITONEAL EXTRAORGAN LESIONS

Peritoneal Metastases

Peritoneal metastases usually develop from cellular implantation across the peritoneal cavity, although metastases may also be lymph or blood borne. The most common primary sites are the ovary, stomach, and colon. Other potential primary sites include the pancreas, biliary tract, kidneys, testicles, and uterus; similarly, sarcomas, melanomas, teratomas, and embryonic

Lymphoma of Omentum/Mesentery

Lymphomatous cellular infiltration of the greater omentum may be seen as a uniformly thick, hypoechoic band-shaped structure that follows the convexity of the anterior and lateral abdominal wall, the so-called omental band[143-145] (Fig. 7-76). Mesenteric lymphomatous involvement characteristically presents as a lobulated confluent anechoic mass surrounding a centrally positioned echogenic area. This appearance, the result of mass infiltrating the mesenteric leaves and encasing the superior mesenteric artery and veins, has been termed

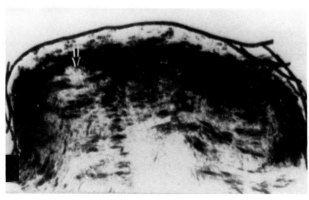

A

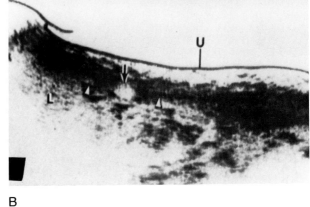

B

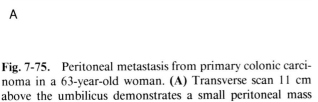

Fig. 7-75. Peritoneal metastasis from primary colonic carcinoma in a 63-year-old woman. **(A)** Transverse scan 11 cm above the umbilicus demonstrates a small peritoneal mass (arrow) in the right side of the abdomen. **(B)** Longitudinal scan 9 cm to the right of the midline in the same patient demonstrates interruption of the peritoneal line (arrowheads) by the mass. (*U,* level of umbilicus; *L,* liver.) **(C)** Eight months later, the peritoneal mass (arrow) appears much larger in size. A mesenteric mass (black arrowhead) has also developed. *(Figure continues.)*

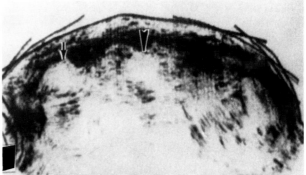

C

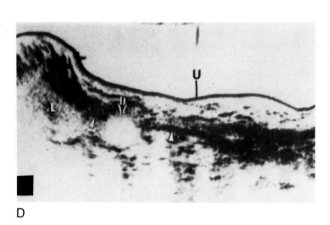

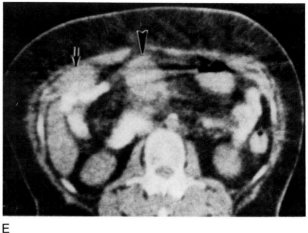

D

E

Fig. 7-75 *(Continued).* **(D)** Longitudinal scan demonstrating the enlarged mass (arrow) embedded in the abdominal wall and obliterating the peritoneal line (arrowheads). (*L,* liver; *U,* level of umbilicus.) **(E)** CT scan corresponding to **(C).** The internal oblique and transversus abdominis muscles are interrupted by the peritoneal mass (arrow). The mesenteric mass is also noted (arrowhead). (From Yeh H-C: Ultrasonography of peritoneal tumors. Radiology 133:419, 1979).

the "sandwich sign"[146] (Fig. 7-77). Since mesenteric involvement is seen in only 5 percent of Hodgkin's lymphoma[147] compared with 61 percent of non-Hodgkin's lymphoma,[148] documentation of this finding on ultrasound scans may be of clinical relevance.

Generally, mesenteric lymphomatous involvement is accompanied by paraortic or retroperitoneal adenopathy, although isolated mesenteric masses may occasionally be seen, as in cases of nodular undifferentiated lymphocytic lymphoma.[146,149] Isolated mesenteric involvement may be seen more commonly with metastatic

carcinoma. Also, despite the characteristic relatively or absolutely anechoic appearance of lymphoma (83 percent in one series of lymphoma patients), metastatic nodes may have a similar appearance (53 percent of soft tissue tumors in the same series), with a mixture of patterns in nearly one third of cases.[126] Thus, the presence of the sandwich sign is presumably more helpful in distinguishing lymphoma from metastatic carcinoma than is reliance upon the presence of associated adenopathy or the internal echo characteristics of the mesenteric masses.

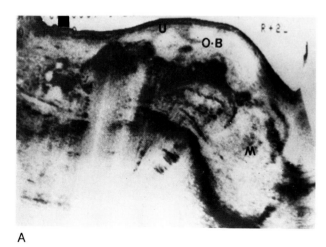

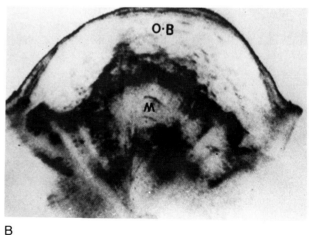

A

B

Fig. 7-76. Lymphoblastic lymphoma involving greater omentum. Omental band *(OB)* and solid pelvic mass *(M)* are demonstrated in longitudinal scan 2 cm to the right of midline **(A)** and transverse scan 8 cm above the symphysis pubis **(B).** (*U,* level of umbilicus.) (From Yaghoobian J, Demeter E, Colucci J: Ultrasound demonstration of lymphomatous infiltration of the greater omentum. Med Ultrasound 8:65, © 1984. Reprinted by permission of John Wiley & Sons, Inc.)

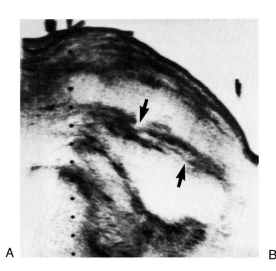

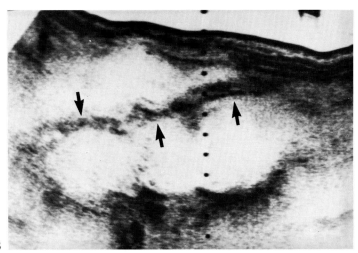

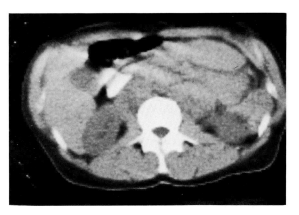

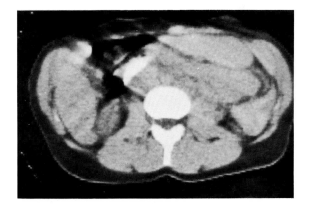

Fig. 7-77. Mesenteric lymphoma. **(A)** Transverse and **(B)** longitudinal scans demonstrate a homogeneous, anechoic mass surrounding a central area of linear echogenicity representing the mesentery (arrows). **(C)** CT scans reveal a solid mass encasing the mesenteric vessels. Retroperitoneal lymphadenopathy is apparent (From Mueller PR, Ferrucci JT Jr, Harbin WP et al: Appearance of lymphomatous involvement of the mesentery by ultrasonography and body computed tomography. Radiology 134:467, 1980.)

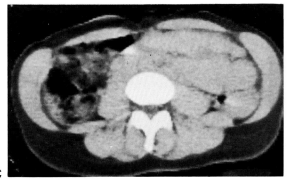

Primary Tumors of the Omentum/Mesentery

Secondary tumors and lymphoma are the neoplasms that most commonly involve the peritoneum and mesentery. Rarely, the peritoneum, mesentery, or omentum are the site for primary tumor involvement. In a review of forty-four such tumors (15 malignant, 29 benign) involving the mesentery, the histologic types identified included fibromatosis, xanthogranulomas, lipomatous tumors (lipomas/liposarcomas), smooth muscle tumors (leiomyomas/leiomyosarcomas), vascular tumors, neurofibromas, and mesenchymomas (including one rhabdomyosarcoma).[150] In a similar review of 24 primary solid tumors of the greater omentum, 8 small symptomless benign tumors were found by chance at laparotomy for some other disease; these tumors included lipomas, leiomyomas, and fibromatoses. Of 16 large and symptom-producing tumors (7 benign, 9 malignant), histologic types included leiomyoma/leiomyosarcoma, hemangiopericytoma (benign and malignant varieties), fibrosarcoma, liposarcoma, rhabdomyosarcoma, and myxoma.[151] Both series mentioned above excluded cases of peritoneal mesothelioma.

Fibrous tumors appear to represent the most common primary solid neoplasm of the mesentery, while smooth muscle tumors, which are also relatively frequent in the mesentery, are the most common lesions found in the greater omentum. Interestingly, lipomatous tumors are not dominant in either location and are relatively more common in the retroperitoneum. Also, almost the only important vascular tumor type in the mesentery/omentum is the uncommon hemangiopericytoma.[150,151] Whether benign or malignant, most of the primary tumors of the mesentery tend to grow to a large size. Just as in the omentum, where tumors can also reach massive proportions, the mobility of the mesentery often permits large growth before symptoms other than a palpable mass are produced. Mesenteric masses are often freely moveable, characteristically from side to side but not in the craniocaudad direction.[152]

FIBROMATOSES/FIBROSING MESENTERITIS

A fibromatosis is defined as an infiltrating fibroblastic proliferation showing none of the features of an inflammatory response and no features of unequivocal neoplasm.[153] Desmoids are a category of fibromatosis that arise from musculoaponeurotic structures in any area of the body, although they most frequently arise in the anterior abdominal wall. Fibroblastic masses that are localized intraabdominally may constitute an isolated abnormality or may be associated with subcutaneous soft tissue tumors and Gardner's syndrome. Fibromatoses

involving the mesentery and omentum most commonly arise in the mesentery of the small intestine.[153-155]

Reports of mesenteric desmoids with ultrasound correlation characterize these lesions as well-circumscribed and predominantly hypoechoic, containing scattered high-level echoes. With CT, dense reflected echoes have been shown to correspond to fat and mesenteric vessels[156] (Fig. 7-78). Depending upon the configuration of these echoes, mesenteric desmoids may mimic the sandwich sign of mesenteric lymphoma, although associated adenopathy would exclude the diagnosis of fibromatosis. Areas of acoustical shadowing arising from within the mass and not originating from echogenic foci have also been noted; they are believed to develop secondary to focal fibrotic areas with increased collagen content.[157]

Fibroinflammatory thickening of the mesentery, referred to by terms such as *fibrosing mesenteritis, sclerosing mesenteritis, retractile mesenteritis,* and *mesenteric*

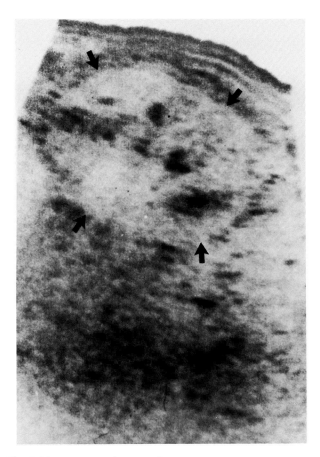

Fig. 7-78. Mesenteric desmoid. Transverse scan of the midabdomen with the patient supine demonstrates a well-circumscribed solid mass (arrows) containing scattered high amplitude echoes (Reprinted courtesy of RL Baron, MD, and JKT Lee, MD.)

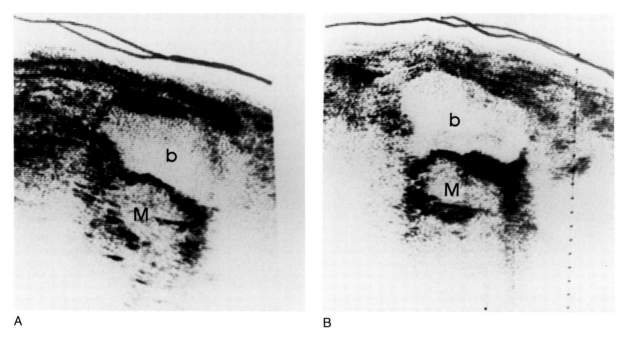

A   B

Fig. 7-79. Fibrosing mesenteritis. **(A)** Midline longitudinal and **(B)** transverse scans demonstrate a retrovesical mass *(M)* containing multiple internal echoes. The patient had a prior hysterectomy. (*b,* bladder.) (From Bendon JA, Poleynard GD, Bordin GM: Fibrosing mesenteritis simulating pelvic carcinomatosis. Gastrointest Radiol 4:195, 1979.)

panniculitis, probably represents a reparative process initiated by damage of mesenteric adipose tissue. Although the etiology of this grouping of abnormalities is unknown, as is its relationship to mesenteric desmoids, the presence of fatty and inflammatory changes of varying degrees warrants its consideration as a separate histopathologic entity from desmoids.[155,158] Involvement of the sigmoid mesentery by this process has been demonstrated sonographically as a lobulated retrovesical mass with multiple internal echoes[159] (Fig. 7-79).

SMOOTH MUSCLE, LIPOMATOUS, AND OTHER NONFIBROBLASTIC NEOPLASMS

As with all noncystic primary tumors involving the mesentery and omentum, sonographic descriptions in the literature are only infrequently encountered. This is particularly true of the nonfibroblastic lesions, which are rarer than other primary mesenteric neoplasms — uncommon themselves. Those entities more typically found in other locations, such as the retroperitoneum or in association with abdominal hollow viscera, are discussed in greater detail elsewhere in this text.

Four sonographic patterns have been observed in extra-hepatic mesenchymal sarcomas (including leiomyosarcoma, liposarcoma, fibrosarcoma, and rhabdomyosarcoma) involving mesentery, abdominal hollow viscera, and retroperitoneal areas: (1) hyperechoic masses intermixed with anechoic zones, (2) hyperechoic masses with central fluid-filled zones, (3) homogeneous hyperechoic masses, and (4) homogeneous hypoechoic masses[160] (Figs. 7-80 and 7-81). Because sarcomas have a tendency to central necrosis with cavitation and hemorrhage, the sonographic appearance of a large tumor mass with signs of necrosis should suggest the possibility of a

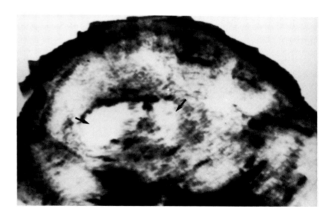

Fig. 7-80. Rhabdomyosarcoma. Transverse supine scan through midabdomen. A large hypoechoic mass fills the midabdomen. There are two irregular hypoechoic areas in the center of the mass representing areas of central necrosis without definite liquefaction (arrows). (From Bree RL, Green B: The gray scale sonographic appearance of intraabdominal mesenchymal sarcomas. Radiology 128:193, 1978.)

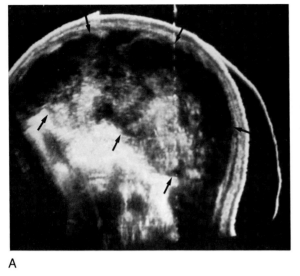

A

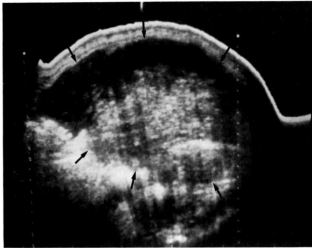

B

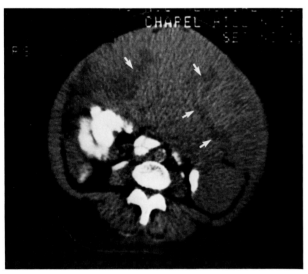

C

Fig. 7-81. Leiomyosarcoma. **(A)** Transverse and **(B)** left longitudinal scans of the abdomen demonstrate an extensive intraabdominal mass of mixed echogenicity (arrows). The more anterior portions of the mass are noted to be relatively hypo- and anechoic. **(C)** Corresponding CT scan of the abdomen demonstrates the extensive intraabdominal mass with scattered streaky areas of relatively low attenuation (arrows).

sarcoma, although in one series of 24 tumors, 54 percent of the sarcomas were classified as homogeneous sonographically.[160] When extensive necrosis is present, sarcomatous lesions may potentially mimic a benign fluid-filled mass such as a pancreatic pseudocyst.

Among the mesenchymal sarcomas in the series cited above, five liposarcomas were included and demonstrated a spectrum of ultrasound appearances, including homogeneously hypoechoic, homogeneously hyperechoic, and hyperechoic with hypoechoic zones[160] (Figs. 7-82 and 7-83). Since subcutaneous lipomas and adipose tissue may be either relatively echofree or echogenic, depending upon the ratio of lipid to aqueous constituents,[161] this variation in the echopattern of homogeneous lipomatous lesions is not surprising. It is also not surprising that ultrasound diagnoses of mesenteric or omental lipomas are lacking in the literature, as most are small and discovered only incidentally; in addition,

echogenic fat appears to be the most prevalent form in vitro, and with high-level internal echoes blending with the echopattern of bowel gas (or retroperitoneal fat), lipomatous abdominal masses may be easily overlooked.

PERITONEAL/OMENTAL MESOTHELIOMA

Mesotheliomas involve the peritoneum as a primary lesion much less commonly than the pleura, but the intraabdominal variety tends to follow a more virulent course. Regardless of the site of origin, mesotheliomas usually occur in middle-aged men; asbestos exposure is considered an etiologic factor. The most frequent initial symptom is abdominal pain, accompanied by significant weight loss and ascites. On gross examination, peritoneal mesotheliomas may present as a large tumor mass with discrete smaller nodules scattered over larger areas

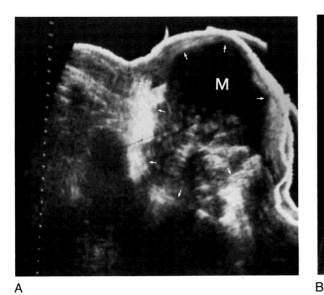 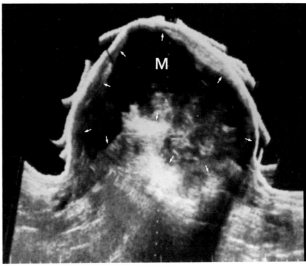

A   B

Fig. 7-82. Abdominal wall liposarcoma. **(A)** Longitudinal and **(B)** transverse scans of the lower abdomen demonstrate an extensive mass *(M)* with large anechoic components. The tumor was grossly necrotic and hemorrhagic at laparotomy.

of the visceral and parietal peritoneum, or as diffuse nodules and plaques that coat the abdominal cavity and envelop and matt together the abdominal viscera.[162,163]

Ultrasound typically demonstrates sheet-like or irregular masses of relatively low echogenicity contiguous with the anterior abdominal wall and usually accompanied by ascites (Fig. 7-84). A large nodular or globular mass, a pattern of presentation that may be encountered in carcinomatosis, is not likely to be seen with mesothelioma.[164] Scattered areas of bright reflections within the

mass may be present, representing entrapped intraabdominal and omental fat[165] (Fig. 7-85). Conversely, ascites may be mimicked by tumor, with an acoustically homogeneous anechoic echopattern surrounding the liver[166] (Fig. 7-86). Additional tumors may be seen as homogeneous masses attached to the abdominal mantle, separately attached to the peritoneal lining, or lying within mesenteric fat.[164] The inner surface of the mass is

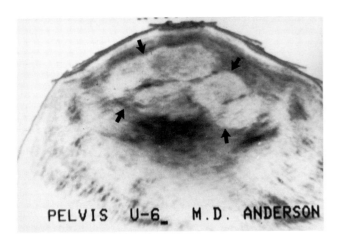

Fig. 7-83. Liposarcoma. Transverse supine scan through midpelvis demonstrates a large multilobulated hypoechoic mass in the pelvis (arrows). The mass is homogeneous without evidence of necrosis. (From Bree RL, Green B: The gray scale sonographic appearance of intraabdominal mesenchymal sarcomas. Radiology 128:193, 1978.)

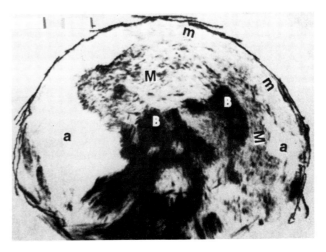

Fig. 7-84. Peritoneal mesothelioma. Transverse scan 6 cm above the umbilicus demonstrates an omental mass (M) fusing with a diffuse peritoneal mass *(m)*. Bowel loops *(B)* are displaced posteriorly by the abdominal mass. Ascites *(a)* is also present (From Yeh H-C, Chahinian AP: Ultrasonography and computed tomography of peritoneal mesothelioma. Radiology 135:705, 1980.)

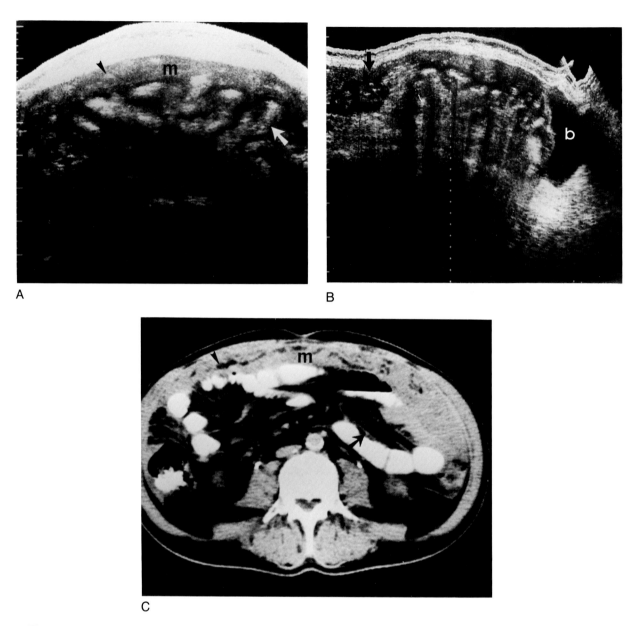

Fig. 7-85. Peritoneal mesothelioma, mantle-like omental mass. **(A)** Transverse scan demonstrates bright echoes representing entrapped omental fat (arrowhead) within the peritoneal mass *(m)*. (white arrow, mesentery/bowel.) **(B)** Longitudinal midline scan on the same patient. Note origin of mass (arrow) below the hepatic margin, representing the origin of omentum. *(b,* bladder) **(C)** Transverse CT scan corresponding to **(A)**. "Woven" pattern of mass *(m)* is caused by entrapped omental fat (arrowhead). (arrow, thickened mesentery.) (From Reuter K, Raptopoulos V, Reale F, et al: Diagnosis of peritoneal mesothelioma: computed tomography, sonography, and fine-needle aspiration biopsy. AJR 140:1189, © Am. Roentgen Ray Society, 1983.)

characteristically lobular and may either encase small bowel loops or be separated from them by a hypoechoic line representing ascitic fluid or thickening of the bowel wall.[165,167] Mesenteric involvement is common, resulting in adhesions, bowel fixation, and an ultrasound pattern that has been described as pleated or fan-like.[165]

Although CT may have advantages over ultrasound in its ability to detect small nodules, pleural plaques, and mesenteric and peritoneal thickening, ultrasound may be preferable for evaluation of the pelvis, directing needle biopsy, and detecting bowel fixation with the use of real-time sonography.[165]

SONOGRAPHIC EVALUATION OF THE ABDOMINAL WALL

Superficial abdominal lesions are readily evaluated with ultrasound. In addition to characterizing and localizing clinically palpable abnormalities, ultrasound may be useful in the patient who has undiagnosed abdominal complaints, suspected hernia, or postoperative incisional complaints.

As mentioned previously, real-time scanners may be at a disadvantage in screening for, and completely assessing, superficial abnormalities due to limitations in the field of view (particularly with sector scanners) and a dependency upon transducer orientation for specular reflectors. Although a palpable mass may be satisfactorily characterized, localization relative to muscular layers or the peritoneum may not be clear-cut with sector real-time scanning alone. Nonetheless, the dynamic capabilities of real-time ultrasound are indispensable in the identification of bowel peristalsis and vascular pulsations.

Normal Sonographic Anatomy

The paired rectus abdominis muscles are delineated medially in the midline of the body by the linea alba, while laterally, the aponeuroses of the external oblique, internal oblique, and transversus abdominis muscles unite to form a band-like vertical fibrous groove called the linea semilunaris, or Spigelian fascia. Through the upper two thirds of the anterior abdominal wall, the aponeurotic sheath of the three anterolateral abdominal muscles invests the rectus both anteriorly and posteriorly. Approximately midway between the umbilicus and the symphysis pubis, at the linea semicircularis (or arcuate line of Douglas), the entire aponeurotic sheath passes anteriorly to the rectus only. Thus, while the pos-

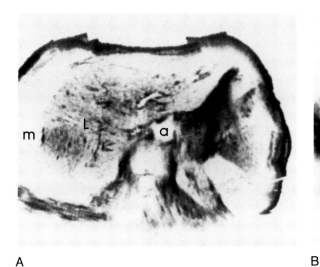

A

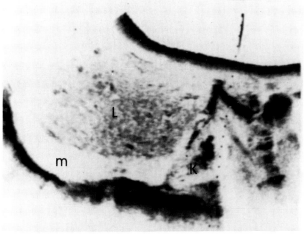

B

Fig. 7-86. Peritoneal mesothelioma. **(A)** Transverse scan 12 cm above the umbilicus. Anechoic tumor mass *(m)* surrounding liver *(L)* mimicking ascites. No acoustic enhancement is present. *(a,* aorta.) **(B)** Sagittal scan 6 cm to right of midline again demonstrates the diffusely encasing tumor *(m). (K,* right kidney; *L,* liver.) **(C)** Transverse CT scan 13 cm above umbilicus after ingestion of oral contrast. Low-density tumor mass *(m)* surrounds the liver *(L)* (From Dach J, Patel N, Patel S, Petasnick J: Peritoneal mesothelioma: CT, sonography, and gallium-67 scan. AJR 135:614, © Am. Roentgen Ray Society, 1980.)

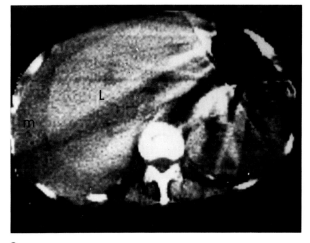

C

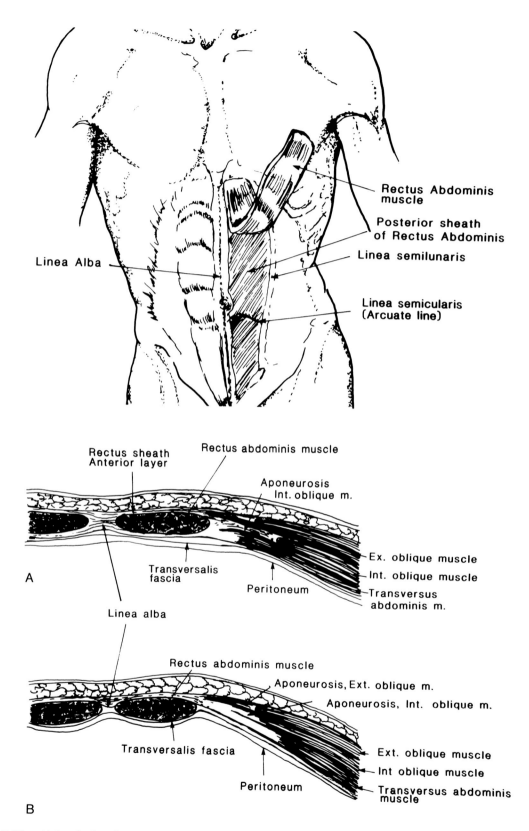

Fig. 7-87. Abdominal wall anatomy. Above the level of the arcuate line **(A)**, the rectus muscle is enveloped by its sheath both anteriorly and posteriorly, while more caudally **(B)** the muscle is separated from the anterior abdominal contents only by the transversalis fascia and the peritoneum.

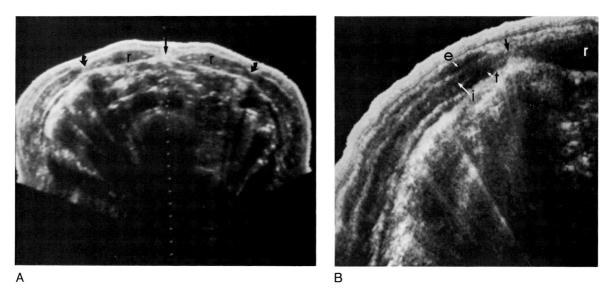

A   B

Fig. 7-88. Abdominal wall anatomy. **(A)** Transverse scan 1 cm above the umbilicus demonstrates the paired rectus abdominis muscles *(r)* delineated by the midline linea alba (straight arrow) and the linea semilunaris (curved arrows). **(B)** Magnified view again demonstrates the rectus muscle group *(r)*, the linea semilunaris (arrow), and the anterolateral muscle groups. (*e,* external oblique; *i,* internal oblique; *t,* transversus abdominis.)

terior rectus sheath is composed of aponeuroses from both the internal oblique and transversus abdominis muscles above the arcuate line, below the line the rectus muscle is separated from the intraabdominal contents only by the transversalis fascia and the peritoneum (Fig. 7-87).

With a high-frequency, short-focused transducer, the midline and anterolateral muscle groups can be identified by ultrasound beneath the superficial fascia and subcutaneous tissue; the distinctness of the individual muscle groups is largely dependent upon the degree of patient muscular development (Fig. 7-88). On trans-

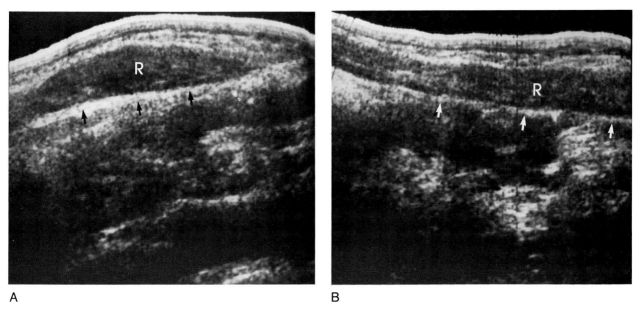

A   B

Fig. 7-89. Rectus abdominis muscle. **(A)** Right transverse and **(B)** right longitudinal scans demonstrate a normal rectus abdominis muscle *(R)*. The peritoneal line can be seen in both transverse and longitudinal images as a discrete linear echogenicity in the deepest layer of the abdominal wall (arrows). Echogenic subcutaneous tissues are noted anteriorly to the muscle group.

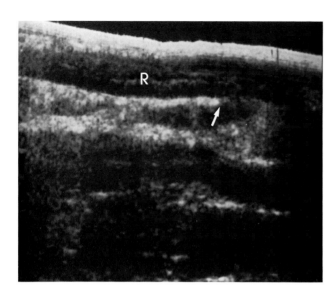

Fig. 7-90. Rectus abdominis muscle. Longitudinal scan to the right of midline, at a lower level than in Figure 7-89B again demonstrates a distinct peritoneal line, which becomes less distinct sonographically at the level of the arcuate line of Douglas (arrow). (*R*, rectus abdominis.)

verse images, the rectus muscles can be visualized as a biconvex muscle group delimited by the linea alba and the linea semilunaris. On both longitudinal and transverse images, the peritoneal line is seen as a discrete linear echogenicity in the deepest layer of the abdominal wall (Fig. 7-89). Although this line usually represents a combination of the peritoneum and the deep abdominal fascia, with abundant extraperitoneal fat the peritoneum and deep fascia may be appreciated as two separate linear echodensities.[168] On longitudinal images on either side of the midline linea alba, the region of the arcuate line can be identified at the zone of transition in which the peritoneal line becomes somewhat less distinct sonographically (Fig. 7-90).

Pathology of the Abdominal Wall

The basic categories of disease processes involving the abdominal wall include hematoma, inflammatory lesions, neoplasm, hernia, and postsurgical lesions. Other abnormalities that may present in the anterior abdominal wall include endometriosis and venous collaterals. Regardless of the amount of fat or muscle present, the left and right sides of the abdominal wall should appear symmetrical, with asymmetry representing an important clue to superficial disease.

RECTUS SHEATH HEMATOMAS

Rectus sheath hematomas are acute or chronic collections of blood lying either within the rectus muscle or between the muscle and its sheath. Vascular disruption and hemorrhage may be the result of direct trauma, pregnancy, cardiovascular diseases, degenerative muscle diseases, surgical injury, anticoagulation therapy, long-term steroid therapy, extremes of certain types of physical exercise, or sudden vigorous uncoordinated muscular contraction (e.g., in association with an episode of coughing or sneezing). Onset is often acute, usually with a sharp, persistent nonradiating pain that may mimic intraabdominal pathology, particularly if the hemorrhage is below the arcuate line, where peritoneal irritation is more likely. When occurring above the arcuate line, a mass may be palpable within the confines of the rectus sheath.[169-174]

With ultrasound, rectus sheath hematomas typically appear largely anechoic, with scattered internal echoes dependent upon the stage of clot breakdown (Figs. 7-91 and 7-92). Above the arcuate line, the hematoma is limited laterally by the linea semilunaris and medially by the linea alba. Confined also by the rectus sheath anteriorly and posteriorly, these hematomas characteristically are biconvex in shape, appearing spindle-like on longitudinal images and ovoid when demonstrated transversely.[175,176] Below the linea semicircularis, where there is no posterior fascial sheath and the retrorectus space communicates with the prevesicular space of Retzius, hematomas can expand extensively into the extraperitoneal space passing inferiorly, laterally, and posteriorly to impinge upon the bladder and potentially mimic primary pelvic pathology[177,178] (Fig. 7-93).

INFLAMMATORY LESIONS

Abdominal wall abscesses may appear anechoic or demonstrate a variable amount of internal echoes, depending upon the extent of cellular debris, and usually exhibit good through transmission. Gas bubbles producing strong echoes and acoustic shadowing are highly suggestive of abscess, but, when present, the abnormality must be distinguished from a hernia on the basis of presence or absence of peristalsis, abdominal wall defect, or accompanying swelling/pus. Although the margins are usually irregular due to the dissecting nature of the infectious process, an abscess is usually more well-defined when compared with the more diffuse, ill-defined lateral margins of cellulitis or a phlegmon. With phlegmon involving different layers of the abdominal wall, the boundaries between the layers remain intact[168,176] (Fig. 7-94).

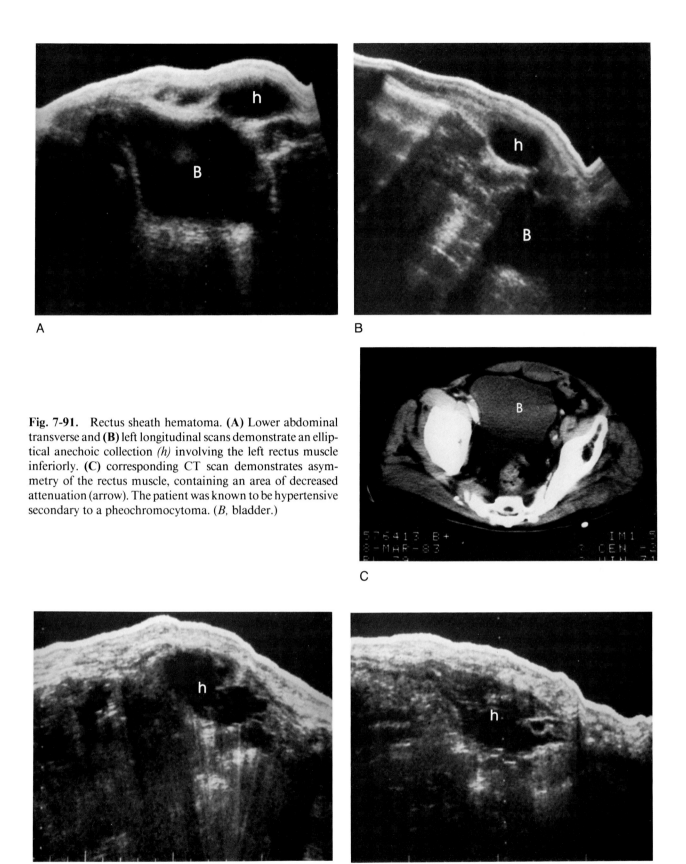

Fig. 7-91. Rectus sheath hematoma. **(A)** Lower abdominal transverse and **(B)** left longitudinal scans demonstrate an elliptical anechoic collection *(h)* involving the left rectus muscle inferiorly. **(C)** corresponding CT scan demonstrates asymmetry of the rectus muscle, containing an area of decreased attenuation (arrow). The patient was known to be hypertensive secondary to a pheochromocytoma. *(B,* bladder.)

Fig. 7-92. Abdominal wall hematoma. **(A)** Transverse and **(B)** left longitudinal scans of the lower abdomen and pelvis in this woman receiving subcutaneous heparin demonstrate an anechoic abdominal wall collection *(h)* containing areas of increased echogenicity.

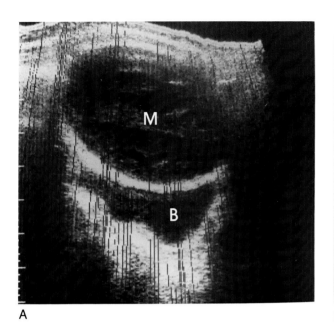

A

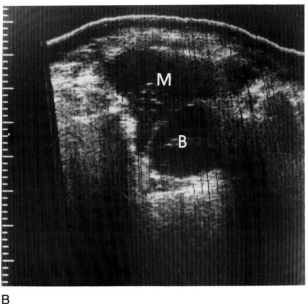

B

Fig. 7-93. Rectus sheath hematoma. **(A)** Midline longitudinal scan demonstrates a large, relatively well-defined hypoechoic mass arising out of the pelvis, containing multiple low-level internal echoes. (*M,* mass; *B,* bladder.) **(B)** Transverse scan in a different patient demonstrates an irregular fluid mass *(M),* containing some internal echoes, to the right and anterior to the bladder *(B).* Rectus hematomas arising inferior to the arcuate line may occur to both sides of midline and simulate pelvic pathology. (From Benson M: Rectus sheath haematomas simulating pelvic pathology: the ultrasound appearances. Clin Radiol 33:651, 1982.)

Abscesses are usually flat, spindle-shaped, or ovoid in shape, with configuration depending upon size, location, and extension. For example, they may appear flat or spindle-shaped when widely spread, ovoid when dis-

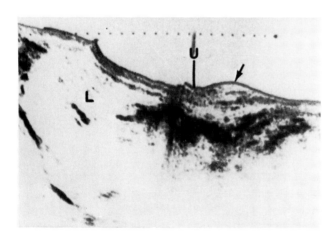

Fig. 7-94. Abdominal wall phlegmon. Longitudinal scan 6 cm to the right of midline demonstrating a phlegmon of the abdominal wall (arrow) at the surgical wound 12 days following appendectomy. Note that there is swelling of all layers of the abdominal wall. (*L,* liver; *U,* level of umbilicus.) (From Yeh H-C, Rabinowitz JG: Ultrasonography and computed tomography of inflammatory abdominal wall lesions. Radiology 144:859, 1982.)

tended with pus, and bonnet-shaped when an intramuscular or subcutaneous collection has a wider extension into the extraperitoneal fat space[168] (Figs. 7-95 and 7-96). When large, abscesses involving the extraperitoneal fat may appear intraperitoneal, but delineation of the peritoneal line will avoid misdiagnosis. When in the pelvoabdominal region, where the peritoneal line may be harder to document, posterior displacement of the bladder suggests involvement of the space of Retzius.

INCISION-RELATED ABNORMALITIES

When evaluating for subincisional fluid collections, the greatest care possible must be taken to remove bandages and surgical appliances. When indicated, the ultrasound transducer can be sterilely draped and a sterile conducting medium utilized. Incisional abscesses typically present as a clearly defined fluid collection associated with the incisional line.[179,180] Although irregular margins or internal echoes might suggest infection, absence of these findings does not permit unequivocal differention from hematomas or wound seromas, the latter appearing characteristically anechoic with smooth margins, superficial and intimately related to the wound, and associated with a localized mass effect[176] (Fig. 7-97).

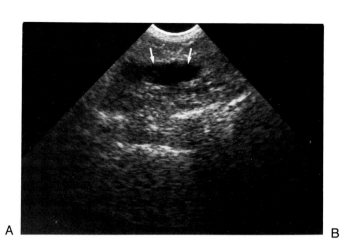
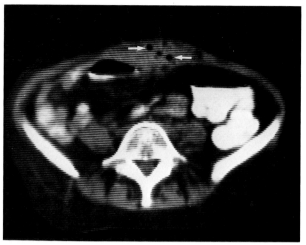

Fig. 7-95. Abdominal wall abscess. **(A)** Transverse midline scan in the lower abdomen of a patient with Crohn's disease demonstrates an elliptical anechoic collection within the abdominal wall (arrows). **(B)** CT scan in same patient at corresponding level demonstrates abnormal soft tissue density within the anterior abdominal wall, containing multiple air lucencies (arrows). Gas within this abscess is much more clearly delineated on CT than with ultrasound.

Fig. 7-96. Abdominal wall abscess. Midline longitudinal scan demonstrates a huge bonnet-shaped abscess causing marked protrusion of the abdomen in a patient with Crohn's disease. The abscess extends through a defect (small arrowheads) in the abdominal wall muscle into the extraperitoneal fat space, which is markedly distended with pus (large arrowhead). The huge abscess in the extraperitoneal fat space was shown to produce compression (arrow) on the liver *(L)*. Numerous echoes within the abscess are due to necrotic tissue debris. (*A,* aorta.) (From Yeh H-C, Rabinowitz JG: Ultrasonography and computed tomography of inflammatory abdominal wall lesions. Radiology 144:859, 1982.)

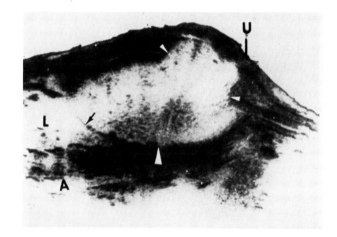

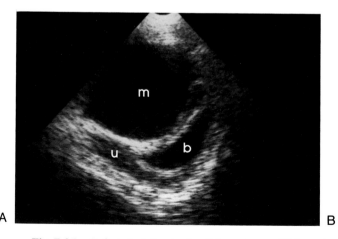
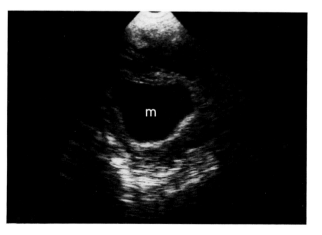

Fig. 7-97.   Infected abdominal wall hematoma. **(A)** Longitudinal and **(B)** transverse scans demonstrate a well-defined hypoechoic mass *(m)* characterized by diffuse low-amplitude echoes. These scans were obtained after a right salpingo-oophorectomy for benign cystic teratoma, the patient subsequently presenting with fever and lower abdominal pain. (*b,* bladder; *u,* uterus.)

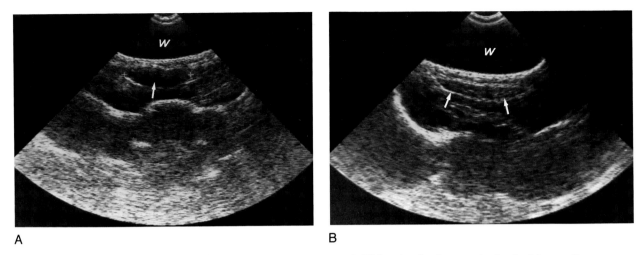

A   B

Fig. 7-98. Abdominal wall desmoid tumor. **(A)** Transverse and **(B)** longitudinal scans obtained with use of a water bath *(W)* demonstrate an ellipsoid hypoechoic mass within the abdominal wall (arrows). Posterior transmission of sound appears diminished.

ABDOMINAL WALL NEOPLASMS

Neoplasms of the abdominal wall include lipomas, desmoid tumors, and, rarely, malignant tumors arising from muscle or fat. Omental tumors or peritoneal metastases may involve the anterior abdominal wall and appear sonographically inseparable from it, but the relative extent of involvement demonstrated by ultrasound may be helpful in determining site of origin. Tumors of

the abdominal wall as a rule are hypoechoic, even cystic in appearance; the exception being lipomas, which may be difficult to separate from adjacent subcutaneous tissues because of their echogenic nature.[180-182]

One of the more likely primary tumors to be encountered in the anterior abdominal wall is the desmoid tumor, a benign fibrous neoplasm of aponeurotic structures, which most commonly arises in relation to the rectus abdominis and its sheath. In a series of 38 patients

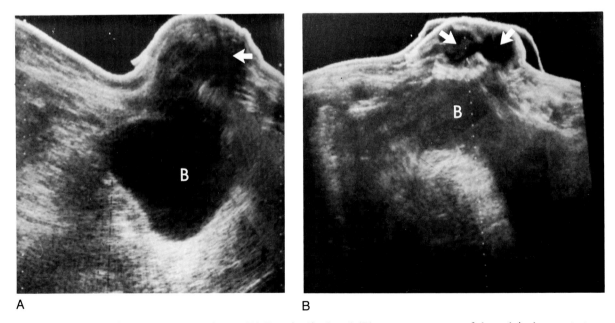

A   B

Fig. 7-99. Abdominal wall endometrioma. **(A)** Longitudinal and **(B)** transverse scans of the pelvis demonstrate a bilobed anechoic mass (arrows) within the superficial tissues adjacent to the bladder *(B)*. Patient had undergone a cesarean section 8 years prior to the examination and first noticed the midline mass 4 years later (From Vincent LM, Mittelstaedt CA: Scar endometrioma: sonographic demonstration. J Ultrasound Med 4:437, 1985.)

with abdominal wall desmoids, the overwhelming sex preponderance was female (76 percent), with roughly 16 percent directly related to pregnancy. One fifth of cases involved the linea alba, and approximately 16 percent were associated with surgical scars.[183] The generally accepted etiologic factors are trauma (including injury during pregnancy) and, occasionally, hormonal disturbances, in addition to the known association with familial intestinal polyposis.[183]

Abdominal desmoid tumors appear anechoic or hypoechoic sonographically, typically with smooth and sharply defined margins, although lateral borders may appear somewhat ill defined or irregular. Posterior transmission of sound may be poor, although in many instances posterior acoustic enhancement is present[184-186] (Fig. 7-98).

ABDOMINAL WALL ENDOMETRIOSIS

Endometriosis in the superficial soft tissues is an uncommon occurrence, usually developing within the umbilicus or in surgical incisions and scars. Possible mechanisms of development include proliferation of endometrial cells transported to an abnormal location, metaplasia of endometrial tissue at an ectopic site, or an interdependent mechanism in which endometrial cells, when transmitted by any means to a susceptible tissue, themselves stimulate imitative metaplasia.[187] In a review of 82 patients with cutaneous endometriosis in all locations, 54 percent had pain or tenderness, 40 percent demonstrated exascerbation of symptoms during menstruation, and 12 percent manifested cyclical bleeding. Nearly one third of cases arose in scars from Caesarian section, and all but 5 cases arose either in surgical wounds or in the physiologic scar of the umbilicus.[187] Since abdominal wall endometriosis can apparently arise after saline abortion along the track of the needle that entered the uterus, it may potentially represent a late complication of amniocentesis.[188]

Superficial endometriomas may appear sonographically as anechoic masses (Fig. 7-99), although a solid-type echopattern with an echotexture similar to adjacent muscle has been reported in a case involving the posterior rectus sheath in an unscarred right upper abdomen.[189] When associated with a surgical scar or the umbilicus, and combined with a suggestive clinical history, the diagnosis of superficial endometriosis should be seriously entertained regardless of sonographic appearance.

HERNIA

Ultrasound is of established value in hernia detection, especially in the patient in whom definitive clinical evidence is lacking or ambiguous[190-194] (Figs. 7-100 and 7-101). Although real-time identification of peristalsing bowel within a palpable mass presents no diagnostic dilemma, peristalsis may be absent with incarceration, and herniation may involve the omentum only. In addition, because the echopattern of bowel may suggest a solid, fluid-filled, and/or gas-containing structure, hernia may potentially mimic other superficial masses such as cysts, hematomas, abscesses, metastases, or desmoid tumors. Thus, care must be taken to sonographically document fascial disruption for definitive diagnosis. Meticulous scanning technique is particularly important for abdominal wall sonographic screening in the patient with abdominal or groin pain of unknown etiology, especially in the obese patient in whom no mass is palpable.

Herniation of deep tissues through a defect in the linea semilunaris, or spigelian hernia, is often difficult to appreciate clinically, as classic findings are frequently lacking. Most commonly originating near the junction of the linea semilunaris and the arcuate line, the spigelian hernia sac itself may dissect between the muscle layers or subcutaneous tissues to move elsewhere. The hernia is often tiny, with only a small tag of omentum intermittently trapped within the peritoneal defect. Careful sonographic imaging, particularly using transverse images, may demonstrate the fascial disruption and the hernial contents limited ventrally by the external oblique aponeurosis[176,190,195-198] (Fig. 7-102).

Evaluation of the inguinal and femoral regions is best performed by oblique scanning between the anterior su-

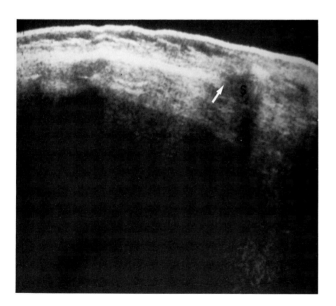

Fig. 7-100. Ventral hernia. Right longitudinal scan directly over a large palpable ventral hernia demonstrates disruption of the peritoneal line (arrow) and echodensity within the mass with distal air shadowing (s). Peristalsis within bowel loops was identified during real-time examination.

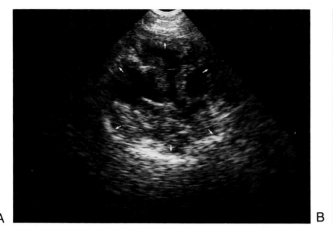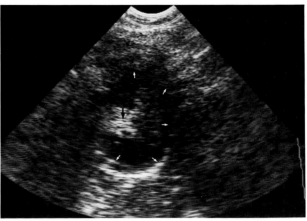

A   B

Fig. 7-101. Ventral hernia. **(A)** Transverse and **(B)** longitudinal real-time images in a patient with a tender right lower quadrant mass (white arrows). No peristalsis was identified within the abnormality, but the region of the mass contained a mixed echo pattern. In the longitudinal image, the mass appeared tubular in configuration and was associated with adjacent increased echoes (black arrow); the latter was felt to represent omentum. The hernia was clinically reduced, and the patient returned later for elective hernia repair. Note that on these real-time sector images, delineation of the peritoneal line is difficult, as is definite compartmentalization of the mass.

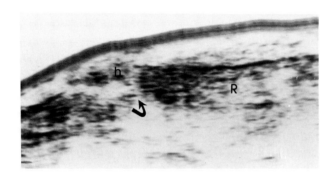

Fig. 7-102. Spigelian hernia. Transverse scan of the right lateral abdomen demonstrates a defect in the anterior abdominal wall in the region of the spigelian fascia (arrow), with interposed bowel contents *(h)* penetrating the aponeuroses of the internal oblique and transversus abdominis muscle but restricted by the external oblique aponeurosis. *(R,* rectus abdominis.) (From Engel JM, Deitch EE: Sonography of the anterior abdominal wall. AJR 137:73, © Am. Roentgen Ray Society, 1981.)

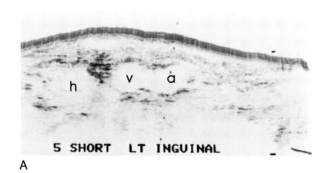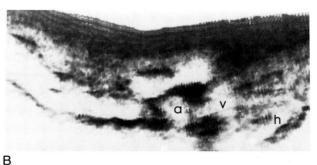

A   B

Fig. 7-103. Femoral hernia. **(A)** Left femoral scan demonstrating femoral hernia *(h)* seen as an anechoic mass medial to the femoral artery *(a),* and femoral vein *(v)* (From Deitch EA, Soncrant MC: The value of ultrasound in the diagnosis of nonpalpable femoral hernias. Arch Surg 116:185, 1981.) **(B)** In a different patient, right femoral scan demonstrates similar findings. *(a,* femoral artery; *v,* femoral vein; *h,* hernia.) (Reprinted courtesy of Edwin A. Deitch, M.D.)

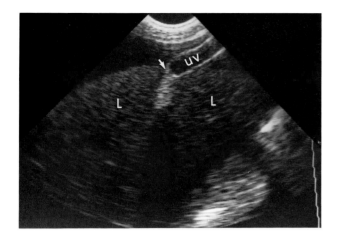

Fig. 7-104. Venous collateral. Transverse scan of the upper abdomen in a chronic alcoholic with portal hypertension demonstrates a tubular anechoic structure (*uv*, umbilical vein) anterior to the liver *(L)*. The structure could be followed along the anterior abdominal wall, and is seen to enter the liver in the region of the ligamentum teres (arrow). Ascites is also present.

perior iliac spine and the pubic crest, along the course of the inguinal ligament. Normal soft tissue structures are related to the anterior superior iliac spine, the iliopubic junction, and the pubic crest. The femoral artery and vein are identified just anterior to the iliopubic junction; the femoral vein is located more medially and will be shown to distend with the Valsalva maneuver. Supplemental real-time evaluation may be helpful in identifying this respiratory variation as well as femoral artery

pulsations. The psoas muscle and lymphatic channels occupy the space between the anterior superior iliac spine and the iliopubic junction.[1]

Masses arising in relation to the femoral vessels and beneath the inguinal ligament include femoral hernias (located medial to the femoral vein, as the latter represents the lateral border of the femoral canal), lipomas, soft tissue sarcomas, and lymph nodes. Abnormalities arising superior to the femoral vessels and inguinal ligament (in the region of the deep inguinal ring) include direct and indirect inguinal hernias, ectopic testicles, and extension of femoral hernias. Extensions of inguinal hernias, ectopic testicles, varicoceles, and other cord masses can be identified sonographically in the region of the superficial ring or in the area extending from the deep ring medially and inferiorly toward the pubic crest[1,199] (Fig. 7-103).

Because the patient is examined in the supine position and a small nonpalpable hernia may not be identifiable even with straining, sonography appears more reliable in the diagnosis of occult disease in the femoral than in the inguinal region.[200]

VENOUS COLLATERALS

In portal hypertension, recanalization of the umbilical vein may provide a collateral pathway between the left portal vein and the superficial epigastric veins. Sonographically, the vein appears as a tubular anechoic structure coursing beneath the anterior abdominal wall in the

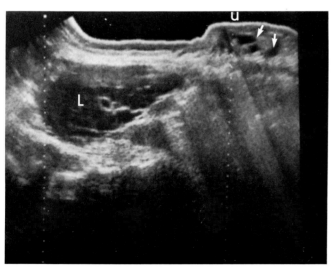
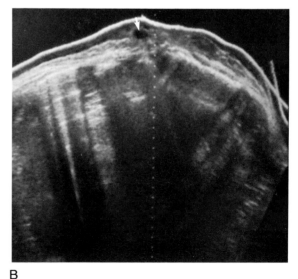

A   B

Fig. 7-105. Venous collaterals (superficial epigastrics). **(A)** Midline longitudinal and **(B)** transverse scans at the level of the umbilicus (*u*) demonstrate multiple tubular anechoic structures within the superficial soft tissues (arrows). No patent umbilical vein or connection with the left portal vein could be demonstrated. The patient was known to have a long-standing occlusion of the inferior vena cava secondary to deep venous thrombosis. (*L*, left lobe of liver.)

midline, extending from the region of the umbilicus to the expected location of the ligamentum teres[201,202] (Fig. 7-104). With periumbilical epigastric varices (caput medusae), the vessel may be seen entering a conglomerate of round and oval anechoicities distally.[203] The sonographic appearance of these portosystemic collaterals and their obvious connection with the liver, in the clinical setting of portal hypertension, should preclude confusion of these structures with the other abdominal wall abnormalities described earlier.

Superficial collateral vessels need not imply portal hypertension, as they may also be associated with obstruction of the inferior vena cava. When present under these circumstances, however, the pathways do not involve the umbilical vein—in general, the inferior and superficial epigastric veins drain into the internal mammary and thoracoabdominal veins, respectively[204] (Fig. 7-105).

REFERENCES

1. Engel JM, Deitch EE: Sonography of the anterior abdominal wall. AJR 137:73, 1981
2. Hunter TB, Haber K: A comparison of real-time scanning with conventional static B-mode scanning. J Ultrasound Med 2:363, 1983
3. Slasky BS, Lenkey JL, Skolnick ML et al: Sonography of soft tissues of extremities and trunk. Semin Ultrasound 3:288, 1982
4. Callen PW, Marks WM: Lymphomatous masses simulating cysts by ultrasonography. J Can Assoc Radiol 30:244, 1979
5. Sommer FG, Filly RA, Minton MJ: Acoustic shadowing due to refractive and reflective effects. AJR 132:973, 1979
6. Bree RL, Silver TM: Differential diagnosis of hypoechoic and anechoic masses with gray scale sonography: New observations. J Clin Ultrasound 7:249, 1979
7. Rubenstein WA, Auh YH, Whalen JP, Kazam E: The perihepatic spaces: Computed tomographic and ultrasound imaging. Radiology 149:231, 1983
8. Griffin DJ, Gross BH, McCracken S, Glazer GM: Observations on CT differentiation of pleural and peritoneal fluid. J Comput Assist Tomogr 8:24, 1984
9. Landay M, Harless W: Ultrasonic differentiation of right pleural effusion from subphrenic fluid on longitudinal scans of the right upper quadrant: importance of recognizing the diaphragm. Radiology 123:155, 1977
10. Gore RM, Callen PW, Filly RA: Displaced retroperitoneal fat: sonographic guide to right upper quadrant mass localization. Radiology 142:701, 1982
11. Engel IA, Auh YH, Rubenstein WA, et al: Large posterior abdominal masses: Computed tomographic localization. Radiology 149:203, 1983
12. Whalen JP: Radiology of the Abdomen: Anatomic Basis. Lea and Febiger, Philadelphia, 1976
13. Vincent LM, Mauro MA, Mittelstaedt CA: The lesser sac and gastrohepatic recess: sonographic appearance and differentiation. Radiology 150:515, 1984
14. Jeffrey RB, Federle MP, Goodman PC: Computed tomography of the lesser peritoneal sac. Radiology 141:117, 1981
15. Callen PW, Filly RA, Korobkin M: Ascitic fluid in the anterior paravesical fossa: Misleading appearance on CT scans. Am J Roentgenol 130:1176, 1978
16. Spring DB, Deshon GE Jr, Babu S: The sonographic appearance of fluid in the prevesical space. Radiology 147:205, 1983
17. Goldberg BB, Goodman GA, Clearfield HR: Evaluation of ascites by ultrasound. Radiology 96:15, 1970
18. Weill F, LeMouel A, Bihr E et al: Ultrasonic diagnosis of intraperitoneal fluid in Morrison's pouch (and in the splenoperitoneal recess): The moon crescent sign. J Radiol 61:251, 1980
19. Proto AV, Lane EJ, Marangola JP: A new concept of ascitic fluid distribution. Am J Roentgenol 126:974, 1976
20. Nyberg DA, Laing FC, Jeffrey RB: Sonographic detection of subtle pelvic fluid collections. AJR 143:261, 1984
21. Meyers MA: Intraperitoneal spread of infections. p. 1. In Meyers MA (ed): Dynamic Radiology of the Abdomen. Springer-Verlag, New York, 1976
22. Gefter WB, Arger PH, Edell SL: Sonographic patterns of ascites. Semin Ultrasound 2:226, 1981
23. Gooding GAW, Cummings SR: Sonographic detection of ascites in liver disease. J Ultrasound Med 3:169, 1984
24. Yeh H-C, Wolf BS: Ultrasonography in ascites. Radiology 124:783, 1977
25. Gore RM, Callen PW, Filly RA: Lesser sac fluid in predicting the etiology of ascites: CT findings. AJR 139-71, 1982
26. Jolles H, Coulam CM: CT of ascites: Differential diagnosis. AJR 135:315, 1980
27. Edell SL, Gefter WB: Ultrasonic differentiation of types of ascitic fluid. AJR 133:111, 1979
28. Franklin JT, Azose AA: Sonographic appearance of chylous ascites. J Clin Ultrasound 12:239, 1984
29. Neff CC, Simeone JF, Ferrucci JT Jr, et al: The occurrence of fluid collections following routine abdominal surgical procedures: sonographic survey in asymptomatic postoperative patients. Radiology 146:463, 1983
30. Schwerk WB, Dürr HK: Ultrasound gray-scale pattern and guided aspiration puncture of abdominal abscesses. J Clin Ultrasound 9:389, 1981
31. Doust BD, Quiroz F, Stewart JM: Ultrasonic distinction of abscesses from other intra-abdominal fluid collections. Radiology 125:213, 1977
32. Hill M, Sanders RC: Gray scale B scan characteristics of intra-abdominal cystic masses. J Clin Ultrasound 6:217, 1978
33. Kressel HY, Filly RA: Ultrasonographic appearance of gas-containing abscesses in the abdomen. Am J Roentgenol 130:71, 1978
34. Doust BD, Thompson R: Ultrasonography of abdominal fluid collections. Gastrointest Radiol 3:273, 1978

35. Mueller PR, Simeone JF: Intraabdominal abscesses: diagnosis by sonography and computed tomography. p. 425. In Federle MP (ed): Symposium on CT and Ultrasonography in the Acutely Ill Patient. Vol. 21. W.B. Saunders, Philadelphia, 1983

36. Sekiba K, Akamatsu N, Niwa K: Ultrasound characteristics of abdominal abscesses involving foreign bodies (gauze). J Clin Ultrasound 7:284, 1979

37. Filly RA: Annual oration: Detection of abdominal abscesses: A combined approach employing ultrasonography, computed tomography and gallium-67 scanning. J Can Assoc Radiol 30:202, 1979

38. Golding RH, Li DKB, Cooperberg PL: Sonographic demonstration of air-fluid levels in abdominal abscesses. J Ultrasound Med 1:151, 1982

39. Taylor KJW, Wasson JFM, deGraaff C, et al: Accuracy of grey-scale ultrasound diagnosis of abdominal and pelvic abscesses in 220 patients. Lancet 1:83, 1978

40. Gross BH, Chinn DH, Callen PW, Filly RA: Real-time vs. static scanning in the diagnosis of abdominal and pelvic abscesses. J Ultrasound Med 2:223, 1983

41. Carroll B, Silverman PM, Goodwin DA, McDougall IR: Ultrasonography and indium 111 white blood cell scanning for the detection of intraabdominal abscesses. Radiology 140:155, 1981

42. Knochel JQ, Koehler PR, Lee TG, Welch DM: Diagnosis of abdominal abscesses with computed tomography, ultrasound, and ¹¹¹In leukocyte scans. Radiology 137:425, 1980

43. Moir C, Robins RE: Role of ultrasonography, gallium scanning, and computed tomography in the diagnosis of intraabdominal abscess. Am J Surg 143:582, 1982

44. Lundstedt C, Hederström E, Holmin T et al: Radiological diagnosis in proven intraabdominal abscess formation: a comparison between plain films of the abdomen, ultrasonography and computerized tomography. Gastrointest Radiol 8:261, 1983

45. Biello DR, Levitt RG, Melson GL: The roles of gallium-67 scintigraphy, ultrasonography, and computed tomography in the detection of abdominal abscesses. Semin Nucl Med 9:58, 1979

46. Coelho JCU, Sigel B, Ryva JC et al: B-mode sonography of blood clots. J Clin Ultrasound 10:323, 1982

47. Kaplan GN, Sanders RC: B-scan ultrasound in the management of patients with occult abdominal hematomas. J Clin Ultrasound 1:5, 1973

48. Goldberg BB: Ultrasound in the diagnosis of intraabdominal hemorrhage and pseudocyst. p. 275. In Clearfield HR, Dinoso VP Jr (eds): Gastrointestinal Emergencies. Grune and Stratton, New York, 1976

49. Wicks JD, Silver TM, Bree RL: Gray scale features of hematomas: an ultrasonic spectrum. Am J Roentgenol 131:977, 1978

50. Lee TG, Brickman FE, Avecilla LS: Ultrasound diagnosis of intramural intestinal hematoma. J Clin Ultrasound 5:423, 1977.

51. Fon GT, Hunter TB, Haber K: Utility of ultrasound for diagnosis of mesenteric hematoma. AJR 134:381, 1980

52. Raghavendra BN, Grieco AJ, Balthazar EJ, et al: Diag-

nostic utility of sonography and computed tomography in spontaneous mesenteric hematoma. Am J Gastroenterol 77:570, 1982

53. Frank B, Bolich P, Reichert J: Sonographic appearance of organized blood within a cyst: 2 case reports. J Clin Ultrasound 3:233, 1975

54. Jeffrey RB, Laing FC: Echogenic clot: a useful sign of pelvic hemoperitoneum. Radiology 145:139, 1982

55. Zegel HG, Kurtz AB, Perlmutter GS, Goldberg BB: Ultrasonic characteristics of bilomas. J Clin Ultrasound 9:21, 1981

56. Kuligowska E, Schlesinger A, Miller KB et al: Bilomas: a new approach to the diagnosis and treatment. Gastrointest Radiol 8:237, 1983

57. Mueller PR, Ferrucci JT Jr, Simeone JF, et al: Detection and drainage of bilomas: Special considerations. AJR 140:715, 1983

58. Laing FC, Gooding GAW, Brown T, Leopold GR: Atypical pseudocysts of the pancreas: An ultrasonographic evaluation. J Clin Ultrasound 7:27, 1979

59. Siegelman SS, Copeland BE, Saba GP, et al: CT of fluid collections associated with pancreatitis. AJR 134: 1121, 1980

60. Hashimoto BE, Laing FC, Jeffrey RB Jr, Federle MP: Hemorrhagic pancreatic fluid collections examined by ultrasound. Radiology 150:803, 1984

61. Beahrs OH, Judd ES Jr, Dockerty MB: Chylous cysts of the abdomen. Surg Clin North Am 30:1081, 1950

62. Baker AH: Developmental mesenteric cysts. Br J Surg 48:534, 1961

63. Rifkin MD, Kurtz AB, Pasto ME: Mesenteric chylous (lymph-containing) cyst. Gastrointest Radiol 8:267, 1983

64. Oh C, Danese CA, Dreiling DA: Chylous cysts of mesentery. Arch Surg 94:790, 1967

65. Bremer JL: Diverticula and duplications of the intestinal tract. Arch Pathol 38:132, 1944

66. Robbins SL, Cotran RS, Kumar V (eds): Pathologic Basis of Disease. Third Edition. p. 879. W.B. Saunders, Philadelphia, 1984

67. Walker AR, Putnam TC: Omental, mesenteric, and retroperitoneal cysts: a clinical study of 33 new cases. Ann Surg 178:13, 1973

68. Caropreso PR: Mesenteric cysts. Arch Surg 108:242, 1974

69. Chirathivat S, Shermeta D: Recurrent retroperitoneal mesenteric cyst. Gastrointest Radiol 4:191, 1979

70. Takeuchi S, Yamaguchi M, Sakurai M, et al: A case of mesenteric cyst diagnosed by ultrasound examination and a review of Japanese literatures. Jpn J Surg 9:359, 1979

71. Mittelstaedt C: Ultrasonic diagnosis of omental cysts. Radiology 117:673, 1975

72. Nordshus T, Løtveit T: Multiple mesenteric cysts diagnosed by ultrasound. Ann Chir Gynaecol 65:234, 1976

73. Haller JO, Schneider M, Kassner EG, et al: Sonographic evaluation of mesenteric and omental masses in children. Am J Roentgenol 130:269, 1978

74. Nicolet V, Grignon A, Filiatrault D, Boisvert J: Sono-

graphic appearance of an abdominal cystic lymphangioma. J Ultrasound Med 3:85, 1984

75. Geer LL, Mittelstaedt CA, Staab EV, Gaisie G: Mesenteric cyst: Sonographic appearance with CT correlation. Pediatr Radiol 14:102, 1984

76. van Mil JBC, Laméris JS: Unusual appearance of a mesenteric cyst. Diagn Imaging 52:28, 1983

77. Araki I, Ohtomo K, Itai Y, Iio M: Demonstration of septa in cystic lesions: comparison study by computed tomography and ultrasound. Clin Radiol 33:325, 1982

78. Burnett WE, Rosemond GP, Bucher RM: Mesenteric cysts: Report of three cases, in one of which a calcified cyst was present. Arch Surg 60:699, 1950

79. Hardin WJ, Hardy JD: Mesenteric cysts. Am J Surg 119:640, 1970

80. Wicks JD, Silver TM, Bree RL: Giant abdominal masses in children and adolescents: ultrasonic differential diagnosis. Am J Roentgenol 130:853, 1978

81. Gordon MJ, Sumner TE: Abdominal ultrasonography in a mesenteric cyst presenting as ascites. Gastroenterology 69:761, 1975

82. Fernandez RN, Daly JM: Pseudomyxoma peritonei. Arch Surg 115:409, 1980

83. Seshul MB, Coulam CM: Pseudomyxoma peritonei: Computed tomography and sonography. AJR 136:803, 1981

84. Yeh H-C, Shafir MK, Slater G, et al: Ultrasonography and computed tomography in pseudomyxoma peritonei. Radiology 153:507, 1984

85. Hann L, Love S, Goldberg RP: Pseudomyxoma peritonei: preoperative diagnosis by ultrasound and computed tomography. Cancer 52:642, 1983

86. Hopper KD: Ultrasonic findings in pseudomyxoma peritonei. South Med J 76:1051, 1983

87. Seale WB: Sonographic findings in a patient with pseudomyxoma peritonei. J Clin Ultrasound 10:441, 1982

88. Merritt CB, Williams SM: Ultrasound findings in a patient with pseudomyxoma peritonei. J Clin Ultrasound 6:4l7, 1978

89. Davidson RI: Peritoneal bypass in the treatment of hydrocephalus: historical review and abdominal complications. J Neurol Neurosurg Psychiatry 39:640, 1976

90. Weidman MJ: Ascites from a ventriculoperitoneal shunt. J Neurosurg 43:233, 1975

91. Gutierrez FA, Raimondi AJ: Peritoneal cysts: a complication of ventriculoperitoneal shunts. Surgery 79:188, 1976

92. Parry SW, Schuhmacher JF, Llewellyn RC: Abdominal pseudocysts and ascites formation after ventriculoperitoneal shunt procedures. Report of four cases. J Neurosurg 43:476, 1975

93. Fischer EG, Shillito J Jr: Large abdominal cysts: a complication of peritoneal shunts. Report of three cases. J Neurosurg 31:441, 1969

94. Davidson RI, Lingley JF: Intraperitoneal pseudocyst: Treatment by aspiration. Surg Neurol 4:33, 1975

95. Cunningham JJ: Evaluation of malfunctioning ventriculoperitoneal shunts with gray scale echography. J Clin Ultrasound 4:369, 1976

96. Nakagaki H, Matsunaga M, Maeyama R, Mizoguchi R: Intraperitoneal pseudocyst after ventriculoperitoneal shunt. Surg Neurol 11:447, 1979

97. Goldfine SL, Turetz F, Beck AR, Eiger M: Cerebrospinal fluid intraperitoneal cyst: an unusual abdominal mass. Am J Roentgenol 130:568, 1978

98. Raghavendra BN, Epstein FJ, Subramanyam BP, Becker MH: Ultrasonographic evaluation of intraperitoneal CSF pseudocyst. Report of three cases. Childs Brain 8:39, 1981

99. Price HI, Rosenthal SJ, Batnitzky S, et al: Abdominal pseudocysts as a complication of ventriculoperitoneal shunt. A report of two cases. Neuroradiology 21:273, 1981

100. Lee TG, Parsons PM: Ultrasound diagnosis of cerebrospinal fluid abdominal cyst. Radiology 127:220, 1978

101. Brenbridge ANAG, Buschi AJ, Lees RF, Sims T: Sonography of CSF pseudocyst. Am J Dis Child 133:646, 1979

102. Fried AM, Adams WE Jr, Ellis GT et al: Ventriculoperitoneal shunt function: Evaluation by sonography. AJR 134:967, 1980

103. Chuang VP, Fried AM, Oliff M et al: Abdominal CSF pseudocyst secondary to ventriculoperitoneal shunt: diagnosis by computed tomography in two cases. J Comput Assist Tomogr 2:88, 1978

104. Dodd GD, Rutledge F, Wallace S: Postoperative pelvic lymphocysts. Am J Roentgenol 108:312, 1970

105. Basinger GT, Gittes RF: Lymphocyst: ultrasound diagnosis and urologic management. J Urol 114:740, 1975

106. Morin ME, Baker DA: Lymphocele: a complication of surgical staging of carcinoma of the prostate. Am J Roentgenol 129:333, 1977

107. Starzl TE, Groth CG, Putnam CW et al: Urological complications in 216 human recipients of renal transplants. Ann Surg 172:1, 1970

108. Phillips JF, Neiman HL, Brown TL: Ultrasound diagnosis of posttransplant renal lymphocele. Am J Roentgenol 126:1194, 1976

109. Fitzer PM, Sallade RL, Graham WH: Computed tomography and the diagnosis of giant abdominal lymphocele. Va Med 107:448, 1980

110. Hyson EA, Belleza NA, Lowman RM: A nontraumatic para-aortic lymphocele complicating nephrolithiasis. Radiology 124:648, 1977

111. Fried AM, Williams CB, Litvak AS: High retroperitoneal lymphocele: unusual clinical presentation and diagnosis by ultrasonography. J Urol 123:583, 1980

112. Rashid A, Posen G, Couture R, Wellington J: Accumulation of lymph around the transplanted kidney (lymphocele) mimicking renal allograft rejection. J Urol 111:145, 1974

113. Koehler PR, Kanemoto HH, Maxwell JG: Ultrasonic "B" scanning in the diagnosis of complications in renal transplant patients. Radiology 119:661, 1976

114. McInerney D, Jones A, Roylance J: Urinoma. Clin Radiol 28:345, 1977

115. Cricco RP, Lindert DJ, McCuskey B: Urinoma formation secondary to tumor obstruction of the ureter. W Va Med J 76:311, 1980

116. Blichert-Toft M, Nielsen OV: Congenital patent urachus and acquired variants. Acta Chir Scand 137:807, 1971

117. Bauer SB, Retik AB: Urachal anomalies and related umbilical disorders. p. 195. In Jeffs RD (ed): Symposium on Congenital Anomalies of the Lower Genitourinary Tract (Urol Clin North Am, Volume 5). W.B. Saunders, Philadelphia, 1978

118. Morin ME, Tan A, Baker DA, Sue HK: Urachal cyst in the adult: ultrasound diagnosis. AJR 132:831, 1979

119. Bouvier J-F, Pascaud E, Mailhes F et al: Urachal cyst in the adult: ultrasound diagnosis. J Clin Ultrasound 12:48, 1984

120. Williams BD, Fisk JD: Sonographic diagnosis of giant urachal cyst in the adult. AJR 136:417, 1981

121. Spataro RF, Davis RS, McLachlan MSF et al: Urachal abnormalities in the adult. Radiology 149:659, 1983

122. Anderson ML, Miller JH, Reid BS, Gilsanz V: "How's urachus." Proceedings from American Institute of Ultrasound in Medicine, (Abstract 723) p. 221, 1983

123. Rifkin MD, Needleman L, Kurtz AB et al: Sonography of nongynecologic cystic masses of the pelvis. AJR 142:1169, 1984

124. Hansen GR, Laing FC: Sonographic evaluation of a left ventricular aneurysm presenting as an upper abdominal mass. J Clin Ultrasound 8:151, 1980

125. Effman EL, Griscom NT, Colodny AH, Vawter GF: Neonatal gastrointestinal masses arising late in gestation. AJR 135:681, 1980

126. Hillman BJ, Haber K: Echographic characteristics of malignant lymph nodes. J Clin Ultrasound 8:213, 1980

127. Yeh H-C, Wolf BS: Ultrasonography and computed tomography in the diagnosis of homogeneous masses. Radiology 123:425, 1977

128. Ouimette MV, Bree RL: Sonography of pelvoabdominal cystic masses in children and adolescents. J Ultrasound Med 3:149, 1984

129. Walsh JW, Taylor KJW, Rosenfield AT: Gray scale ultrasonography in the diagnosis of endometriosis and adenomyosis. AJR 132:87, 1979

130. Swayne LC, Love MB, Karasick SR: Pelvic inflammatory disease: Sonographic-pathologic correlation. Radiology 151:751, 1984

131. Alpern MB, Sandler MA, Madrazo BL: Sonographic features of parovarian cysts and their complications. AJR 143:157, 1984

132. Nocera RM, Fagan CJ, Hernandez JC: Cystic parametrial fibroids mimicking ovarian cystadenoma. J Ultrasound Med 3:183, 1984

133. Lees RF, Feldman PS, Brenbridge ANAG et al: Inflammatory cysts of the pelvic peritoneum. Am J Roentgenol 131:633, 1978

134. Cancelmo RP: Sonographic demonstration of multilocular peritoneal inclusion cyst. J Clin Ultrasound 11:334, 1983

135. Kutcher R, Rosenblatt R: A sonographic survey of benign fluid collections in the abdomen and pelvis—Review and presentation of new findings. Proceedings from American Institute of Ultrasound in Medicine, p. 243, 1983

136. Bedi DG, Fagan CJ, Nocera RM: Chronic ectopic pregnancy. J Ultrasound Med 3:347, 1984

137. Cunningham JJ: False-positive gray-scale ultrasonography for intra-abdominal abscesses. Arch Surg 111:810, 1976

138. Engel JM, Deitch EA: Omentum mimicking cystic masses in the pelvis. J Clin Ultrasound 8:31, 1980

139. Barth RA, Brasch RC, Filly RA: Abdominal pseudotumor in childhood: distended gallbladder with parenteral hyperalimentation. AJR 136:341, 1981

140. Rao KG, Woodlief RM: Excessive right subdiaphragmatic fat: A potential diagnostic pitfall. Radiology 138:15, 1981

141. Daniel O: The differential diagnosis of malignant disease of the peritoneum. Br J Surg 39:147, 1951

142. Yeh H-C: Ultrasonography of peritoneal tumors. Radiology 133:419, 1979

143. Stein MA: Omental band: new sign of metastasis. J Clin Ultrasound 5:410, 1977

144. D'amico RJ: The omental band sign in reticulum cell sarcoma. J Med Soc NJ 76:441, 1979

145. Yaghoobian J, Demeter E, Colucci J: Ultrasonic demonstration of lymphomatous infiltration of the greater omentum. Med Ultrasound 8:65, 1984

146. Mueller PR, Ferrucci JT Jr., Harbin WP et al: Appearance of lymphomatous involvement of the mesentery by ultrasonography and body computed tomography: the "sandwich sign." Radiology 134:467, 1980

147. Kadin ME, Glatstein E, Dorfman RF: Clinicopathologic studies of 117 untreated patients subjected to laparotomy for the staging of Hodgkin's disease. Cancer 27:1277, 1971

148. Goffinet DR, Castellino RA, Kim H et al: Staging laparotomies in unselected previously untreated patients with non-Hodgkin's lymphomas. Cancer 32:672, 1973

149. Bernardino ME, Jing BS, Wallace S: Computed tomography diagnosis of mesenteric masses. AJR 132:33, 1979

150. Yannopoulos K, Stout AP: Primary solid tumors of the mesentery. Cancer 16:914, 1963

151. Stout AP, Hendry J, Purdie FJ: Primary solid tumors of the great omentum. Cancer 16:231, 1963

152. Weinberger HA, Ahmed MS: Mesenchymal solid tumors of the omentum and mesentery: report of four cases. Surgery 82:754, 1977

153. MacKenzie DH: The fibromatoses: a clinicopathological concept. Br Med J 4:277, 1972

154. DasGupta TK, Brasfield RD, O'Hara J: Extra-abdominal desmoids: A clinicopathological study. Ann Surg 170:109, 1969

155. Sacks B, Joffe N, Harris N: Isolated mesenteric desmoids (mesenteric fibromatosis). Clin Radiol 29:95, 1978

156. Baron RL, Lee JKT: Mesenteric desmoid tumors. Radiology 140:777, 1981

157. Sampliner JE, Paruleker S, Jain B et al: Intra-abdominal mesenteric desmoid tumors. Am Surg 48:316, 1982

158. Reske M, Namiki H: Sclerosing mesenteritis. Report of two cases. Am J Clin Pathol 64:661, 1975

159. Bendon JA, Poleynard GD, Bordin GM: Fibrosing mesenteritis simulating pelvic carcinomatosis. Gastrointest Radiol 4:195, 1979

160. Bree RL, Green B: The gray scale sonographic appear-

ance of intraabdominal mesenchymal sarcomas. Radiology 128:193, 1978

161. Behan M, Kazam E: The echographic characteristics of fatty tissues and tumors. Radiology 129:143, 1978

162. Moertel CG: Peritoneal mesothelioma. Gastroenterology 63:346, 1972

163. Banner MP, Gohel VK: Peritoneal mesothelioma. Radiology 129:637, 1978

164. Yeh H-C, Chahinian AP: Ultrasonography and computed tomography of peritoneal mesothelioma. Radiology 135:705, 1980

165. Reuter K, Raptopoulos V, Reale F et al: Diagnosis of peritoneal mesothelioma: computed tomography, sonography, and fine-needle aspiration biopsy. AJR 140:1189, 1983

166. Dach J, Patel N, Patel S, Petasnick J: Peritoneal mesothelioma: CT, sonography, and gallium-67 scan. AJR 135:614, 1980

167. Shah JM, King DL: Gray scale sonographic presentation of a mesothelioma of the greater omentum. J Clin Ultrasound 7:147, 1979.

168. Yeh H-C, Rabinowitz JG: Ultrasonography and computed tomography of inflammatory abdominal wall lesions. Radiology 144:859, 1982

169. Lee PWR, Bark M, Macfie J, Pratt D: The ultrasound diagnosis of rectus sheath haematoma. Br J Surg 64:633, 1977

170. Manier JW: Rectus sheath hematoma. Six case reports and a literature review. Am J Gastroenterol 54:443, 1972

171. Hopper KD, Smazal SF Jr, Ghaed N: CT and ultrasonic evaluation of rectus sheath hematoma: a complication of anticoagulant therapy. Milit Med 148:447, 1983

172. Trias A, Boctor M, Echave V: Ultrasonography in the diagnosis of rectus abdominus hematoma. Can J Surg 24:524, 1981

173. Tromans A, Campbell N, Sykes P: Rectus sheath haematoma: Diagnosis by ultrasound. Br J Surg 68:518, 1981

174. Spitz HB, Wyatt GM: Rectus sheath hematoma. J Clin Ultrasound 5:413, 1977

175. Kaftori JK, Rosenberger A, Pollack S, Fish JH: Rectus sheath hematoma: Ultrasonographic diagnosis. Am J Roentgenol 128:283, 1977

176. Fried AM, Meeker WR: Incarcerated spigelian hernia: Ultrasonic differential diagnosis. AJR 133:107, 1979

177. Wyatt GM, Spitz HB: Ultrasound in the diagnosis of rectus sheath hematoma. JAMA 241:1499, 1979

178. Benson M: Rectus sheath haematomas simulating pelvic pathology: The ultrasound appearances. Clin Radiol 33:651, 1982

179. Cunningham J, Thomas JL: Detection and localization of subincisional abscesses with gray scale echography. Am Surg 45:388, 1979

180. Goldberg BB: Ultrasonic evaluation of superficial masses. J Clin Ultrasound 3:91, 1975

181. Miller EI, Rogers A: Sonography of the anterior abdominal wall. Semin Ultrasound 3:278, 1982

182. O'Malley BP, Qizilbash AH: Mesenchymal chondrosarcoma of the rectus sheath. Case report with ultrasonic findings. J Clin Ultrasound 5:348, 1977

183. Brasfield RD, DasGupta TK: Desmoid tumors of the anterior abdominal wall. Surgery 65:241, 1969

184. Hanson RD, Hunter TB, Haber K: Ultrasonographic appearance of anterior abdominal wall desmoid tumors. J Ultrasound Med 2:141, 1983

185. Wallace JHK: Ultrasonic diagnosis of abdominal wall desmoid tumor. J Can Assoc Radiol 31:120, 1980

186. Yeh H-C, Rabinowitz JG, Rosenblum M: Complementary role of CT and ultrasonography in the diagnosis of desmoid tumor of abdominal wall. Comput Radiol 6:275, 1982

187. Steck WD, Helwig EB: Cutaneous endometriosis. Clin Obstet Gynecol 9:373, 1966

188. Ferrari BT, Shollenbarger DR: Abdominal wall endometriosis following hypertonic saline abortion. JAMA 238:56, 1977

189. Miller WB Jr, Melson GL: Abdominal wall endometrioma. AJR 132:467, 1979

190. Spangen L: Ultrasound as a diagnostic aid in ventral abdominal hernia. J Clin Ultrasound 3:211, 1975

191. Lineaweaver W, Vlasak M, Muyshondt E: Ultrasonic examination of abdominal wall and groin masses. South Med J 76:590, 1983

192. Deitch EA, Engel JM: Ultrasonic diagnosis of surgical diseases of the anterior abdominal wall. Surg Gynecol Obstet 151:484, 1980

193. Thomas JL, Cunningham JJ: Ultrasonic evaluation of ventral hernias disguised as intraabdominal neoplasms. Arch Surg 113:589, 1978

194. Yeh H-C, Lehr-Janus C, Cohen BA, Rabinowitz JG: Ultrasonography and CT of abdominal and inguinal hernias. J Clin Ultrasound 12:479, 1984

195. Sutphen JH, Hitchcock DA, King DC: Ultrasonic demonstration of spigelian hernia. AJR 134:174, 1980

196. Deitch EA, Engel JM: Spigelian hernia: an ultrasonic diagnosis. Arch Surg 115:93, 1980

197. Nelson RL, Renigers SA, Nyhus LM et al: Ultrasonography of the abdominal wall in the diagnosis of spigelian hernia. Am Surg 46:373, 1980

198. Balthazar EJ, Subramanyam BR, Megibow A: Spigelian hernia: CT and ultrasonography diagnosis. Gastrointest Radiol 9:81, 1984

199. Deitch EA, Soncrant MC: The value of ultrasound in the diagnosis of nonpalpable femoral hernias. Arch Surg 116:185, 1981

200. Deitch EA, Soncrant MC: Ultrasonic diagnosis of surgical disease in the inguinal-femoral region. Surg Gynecol Obstet 152:319, 1981

201. Glazer GM, Laing FC, Brown TW, Gooding GAW: Sonographic demonstration of portal hypertension: the patent umbilical vein. Radiology 136:161, 1980

202. Subramanyam BR, Balthazar EJ, Madamba MR et al: Sonography of portosystemic venous collateral in portal hypertension. Radiology 146:161, 1983

203. Jüttner H-U, Jenney JM, Ralls PW et al: Ultrasound demonstration of portosystemic collaterals in cirrhosis and portal hypertension. Radiology 142:459, 1982

204. Ferris EJ, Vittimberga FJ, Byrne JJ et al: The inferior vena cava after ligation and plication. Radiology 89:1, 1967

8

The Spleen

On abdominal sonograms, the liver, spleen, gallbladder, pancreas, aorta, kidneys, and other abdominal structures are easily identified, and many abnormalities are diagnosed. As a rule, the only remark concerning the spleen is splenomegaly, otherwise, no statement is made.

The spleen is often ignored on ultrasound because it is difficult to visualize at times. In the supine position, a normal-sized spleen lies high under the rib cage and posterior to the stomach, a strong reflective structure. In addition, ultrasound is a relative newcomer to the diagnostic armentarium for evaluation of the spleen. Its potential, restrictions, and diagnostic capabilities have not been fully ascertained. Some investigators have described the variability of ultrasonic patterns,[1-3] and have analyzed amplitude histograms of splenic texture or consistency.[4] Still, ultrasound can often be useful in evaluating disease processes of the spleen. Most abnormalities involving the spleen produce enlargement, which permits excellent sonographic visualization.

TECHNIQUE

Preparation

There is no special patient preparation prior to an ultrasound of the spleen.

Ultrasound Technique

The spleen can be scanned with the patient in various positions. If the spleen is quite large, it can be adequately evaluated with the patient supine, employing both longitudinal and transverse planes (Fig. 8-1). Although the normal-sized spleen can be visualized in the supine position, the minimally enlarged to normal-sized spleen is best examined with the patient in the right-lateral decubitus or prone position[2] (Fig. 8-2). Both longitudinal and transverse scans are obtained during held inspiration. The right-lateral decubitus position is my preferred position for evaluating the spleen because in this position the spleen is closest to the near field of the transducer and the best detail of the splenic architecture is obtained (Fig. 8-2D to E). Careful attention should be paid to the time gain compensation (TGC) and transducer characteristics because incorrect use of either can produce misleading artifacts.[5] The normal splenic echopattern should be homogeneous with the internal echoes slightly less[5] or equal to the liver.[2,3]

Most studies can be adequately done with real-time ultrasound. If the spleen is quite large and a comparison needs to be made between the spleen and liver echopattern, then static scans should be performed (Fig. 8-1), or, if the spleen is being followed for size change, then static scans will need to be performed. If the spleen is minimally enlarged or normal-sized, it is easier to scan with real-time than static systems.

NORMAL ANATOMY

The spleen, the largest unit of the reticuloendothelial system, plays an important role in the defense mechanism of the body and is involved in pigment and lipid metabolism. With its architecture consisting of the white pulp (lymphoid tissue) and the intervening red pulp (red blood cells and reticulum cells), the spleen is normally devoid of hematopoietic activity.[6] Rarely the primary site of disease, the spleen is often affected by systemic disease processes.

The spleen is an intraperitoneal structure lying between the left hemidiaphragm and stomach. It is related to the 8th, 9th, 10th, and 11th ribs. Its superior surface is in contact with the left hemidiaphragm; its medial sur-

face is related to the stomach, tail of pancreas, left kidney, and splenic flexure of the colon (Fig. 8-3). The left hemidiaphragm is seen as a bright curvilinear echogenic structure that is close to the proximal superior lateral surface of the spleen (Figs. 8-1D, 8-2C, 8-2E, and 8-2G). The spleen is covered with peritoneum except for its hilum. It is held in position by the lienorenal, gastrosplenic, and phrenicocolic ligaments.[5] These ligaments

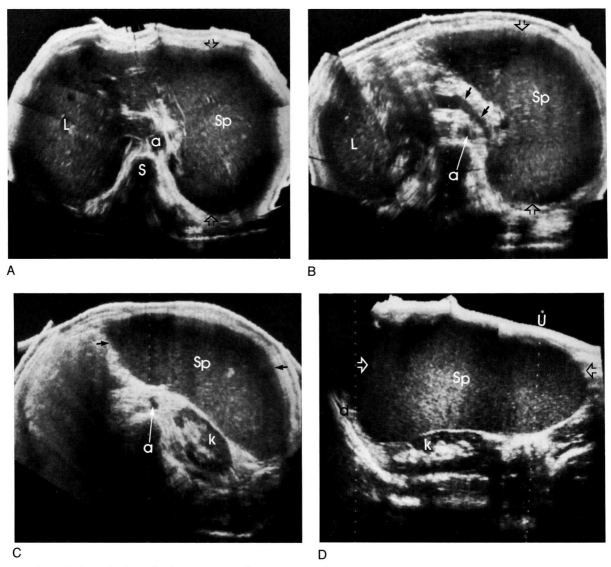

Fig. 8-1. Enlarged spleen. Supine transverse views at 18 cm **(A)**, 10 cm **(B)** and 2 cm **(C)** above the umbilicus as well as a longitudinal scan **(D)** at 8 cm to the left of midline demonstrate a markedly enlarged spleen *(Sp)* with an isoechoic (same density as liver *(L)* parenchyma) echopattern in this patient with non-Hodgkin's lymphoma. To determine the splenic volumetric index (SVI), the splenic width (black arrows) can be measured on **(C)** with the anteroposterior (open arrows) dimension measured on **(A)** or **(B)**. The length (open arrows) can be measured on **(D)**. The values obtained are multiplied and the product is divided by 27. In this case, the SVI is 156 with normal being 8 to 34. (*a*, aorta; solid black arrows, splenic vein; *k*, left kidney; *S*, spine; *Ant*, anterior; *d*, diaphragm; *U*, level of the umbilicus.) *(Figure continues.)*

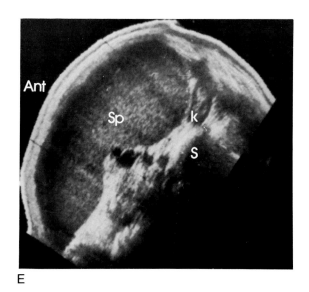

E

Fig. 8-1. *(Continued).* This transverse right lateral decubitus view **(E)** does not add additional information in this case.

are derived from layers of the peritoneum that form the greater and lesser sac. The spleen's close proximity to left kidney, pancreas, and the gastrointestinal tract facilitate the extension of inflammatory processes.[5]

Various studies have been performed to evaluate splenic size. One investigation has determined a splenic volumetric index.[7] The breadth, thickness, and height are obtained on a compound scan with each measurement taken at the largest point (Figs. 8-1 and 8-2). The breadth (width) and thickness (AP) may be measured on a transverse, supine scan at the level of the xyphoid in a normal to minimally enlarged spleen or at the widest portion in an enlarged spleen. On a longitudinal scan in the mid-axillary line in the normal to minimally enlarged spleen, the height (length) is measured (Fig. 8-2E). In the enlarged spleen, the longest length is obtained on a supine scan (Fig. 8-1D). The values obtained are multiplied by each other and the product is divided by 27 (the cube of the three values). The splenic volumetric index (SVI) was found to be 8 to 34 in 95 percent of normals.[7] There were no statistically significant differences related

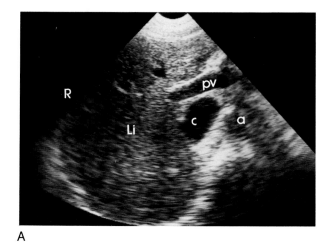

A

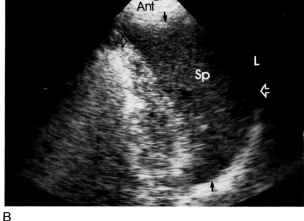

B

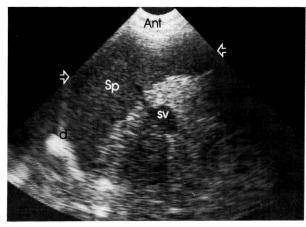

C

Fig. 8-2. Normal spleen. **(A)** Supine transverse scan of the liver *(Li).* (*c,* inferior vena cava; *pv,* portal vein; *a,* aorta; *R,* right.) Transverse **(B)** and longitudinal **(C)** supine views of the spleen *(Sp).* It is isoechoic (same density as the liver in **(A)**). (*sv,* splenic vein; *L,* left; *d,* diaphragm; *Ant,* anterior.) *(Figure continues.)*

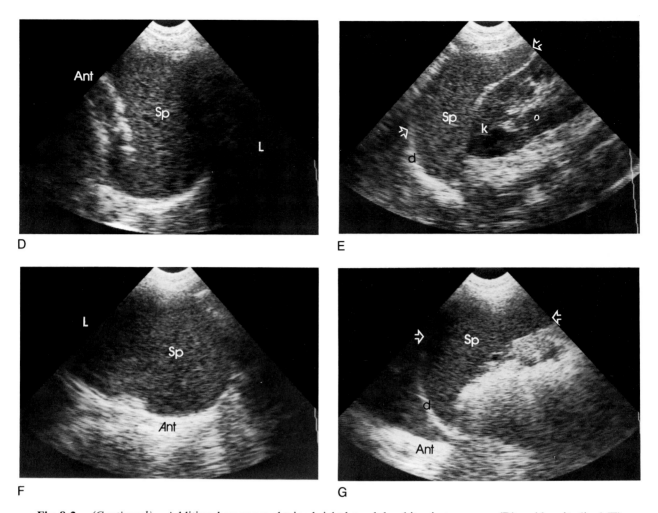

D   E

F   G

Fig. 8-2. *(Continued).* Additional scans are obtained right lateral decubitus in transverse (**D**) and longitudinal (**E**) planes as well as prone transverse (**F**) and longitudinal (**G**). (*d*, diaphragm; *k*, left kidney; *L*, left; *Ant*, anterior.) To determine the splenic volumetric index (SVI), the splenic width (open arrows) can be measured on (**B**), the anteroposterior dimension (black arrows) on (**B**) and the length (open arrows) on (**C**),(**E**) or (**G**). The dimensions are determined on the views that give the sharpest definition to the splenic margins and largest measurements; this is most often the supine view for the width, and anteroposterior measurements with the longitudinal scan in the right lateral decubitus position for the length. The values obtained are multiplied and the product is divided by 27. In this normal case, the SVI was 24.4 with 95 percent of normals 8 to 34.

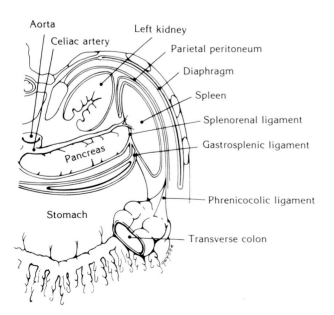

Aorta
Celiac artery
Left kidney
Parietal peritoneum
Diaphragm
Spleen
Splenorenal ligament
Gastrosplenic ligament
Pancreas
Phrenicocolic ligament
Stomach
Transverse colon

Fig. 8-3. Normal spleen. The spleen is related to the left hemidiaphragm superiorly and the stomach, pancreatic tail and splenic flexure of the colon medially. It is covered with peritoneum except for its hilum and is held in position by the splenorenal, gastrosplenic, and phrenicocolic ligaments.

to age, sex, or morphology. From this study, it was felt a distinction could be made between normal and abnormal on the basis of the SVI.

Depending on patient position and machine control settings, the normal splenic echopattern can vary considerably. It may be weakly echogenic (hypoechoic), homogeneous, and transonic or strongly echogenic (hyperechoic), similar in echodensity to the liver. The gain and time-gain compensation controls are usually set in order to obtain adequate echoes within the liver when the patient is supine. The normal spleen appears to have the same relative echodensity as the liver in the supine position (Fig. 8-2). The same spleen that appeared echodense in the supine position may appear hypoechoic when the patient is scanned in the right-lateral decubitus or prone positions. This is felt to be secondary to scanner technique.

In order for a standard technique for the spleen and other organs to be established, a gray-scale phantom is needed. Without such a phantom at this time, the next best way for establishing standard technique is internal control within each patient. Amplitude histograms of splenic texture or consistency have been analyzed by some investigators[8] and the variability of gray-scale ultrasonic patterns have been reported.[1] It has been my experience in determining the echodensity of the spleen that the liver echodensity in the supine position serves as an adequate standard provided the liver is normal (no hepatocellular or metastatic disease). The splenic pattern is described as isoechoic, if the spleen and liver have the same relative echodensity (Figs. 8-1 and 8-2). It is listed as hypoechoic, if the echopattern within the spleen is relatively less echogenic than the liver (Fig. 8-4). Focal lesions within the spleen are described as hypoechoic or hyperechoic depending on their relationship to the rest of the splenic echodensity. Perisplenic lesions, are also described as hypoechoic or hyperechoic depending on their comparative echodensity to the spleen.

By comparing the echodensity of the liver and spleen on supine, transverse, compound scans, there is some inherent error in the technique described. This technique described may not be as reproducible in other laboratories as it has been in my experience, because there are some inaccuracies in compound scanning. A constant sonographic standard is needed.

FOCAL DISEASE

Focal defects in the spleen may be single or multiple, and may be found in normal-sized or enlarged spleens. The major nontraumatic causes for focal splenic defects include tumors (benign and malignant), infarction, abscesses, and cysts. Detection of focal splenic defects may

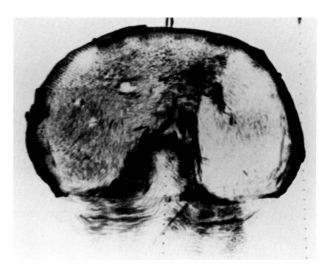

Fig. 8-4. Lymphopoietic abnormality of the spleen. Chronic lymphocytic leukemia. This is a transverse static scan at 13 cm above the umbilicus. The spleen is hypoechoic or less echodense than liver. (From Mittelstaedt CA, McCartney WH, Mauro MA et al: Spleen. p.235. In Simeone J (ed): Clinics in Diagnostic Ultrasound: Coordinated Diagnostic Imaging. Churchill Livingstone, New York, 1984.)

be incidental (e.g., unsuspected splenic defect demonstrated as part of a technetium sulfur colloid (TcSC) study of the liver), or may be encountered in the evaluation of clinically suspected splenic disease (e.g., splenic infarct or abscess).[9]

Ultrasound not only allows differentiation between solid and cystic lesions but also permits evaluation of adjacent abdominal structures. However, examination of the spleen by ultrasound may be hampered by rib artifact or excessive bowel gas in the left upper quadrant. In addition, ultrasound is less sensitive for detection of focal abnormalities in patients without splenomegaly and, therefore, is usually not the primary screening procedure for possible focal splenic lesions.

Tumors of the Spleen

BENIGN PRIMARY NEOPLASMS (RARE)

Hamartomas, cavernous hemangiomas, and cystic lymphangiomas are the most common benign neoplasms involving the spleen. Typically, splenic hamartomas have both solid and cystic components, with the solid portion appearing hyperechoic on ultrasound[10] (Fig. 8-5). These lesions are usually discovered as incidental findings at autopsy as they usually cause no symptoms. The importance in recognizing these benign neoplasms rests in differentiating them from other lesions. Splenic hamartomas may be solitary or multiple

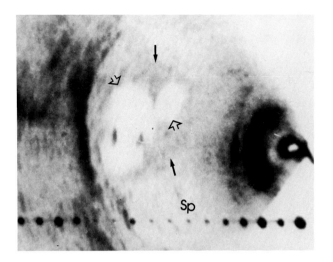

Fig. 8-5. Splenic hamartoma. Transverse scan, right lateral decubitus position. A mass (arrows) is seen within the spleen, which is more dense than spleen (Sp). Note the cystic component (open arrows) within the mass. (From Brinkley AA, Lee JKT: Cystic hamartoma of the spleen: CT and sonographic findings. J Clin Ultrasound 9:136, 1981.)

and are well defined but not encapsulated.[10] They are composed either of lymphoid tissue or a combination of sinuses and structures that are equivalent to the pulp cords of normal splenic tissue.

A splenic hemangioma has been described as a large inhomogeneously echogenic mass on ultrasound with multiple small hypoechoic areas[11] (Figs. 8-6 and 8-7). Most splenic hemangiomas are small and usually the

patients are asymptomatic.[12] The incidence is 1 in 600 cases based on an autopsy series.[12] When patients are symptomatic, the symptoms are related to either the size of the spleen that compresses neighboring organs, sometimes anemia, or low-grade infection with fever and malaise.[12] Splenic rupture with peritoneal symptoms can occur in up to 25 percent of cavernous hemangiomas. A mixed ultrasound appearance can be accounted for by

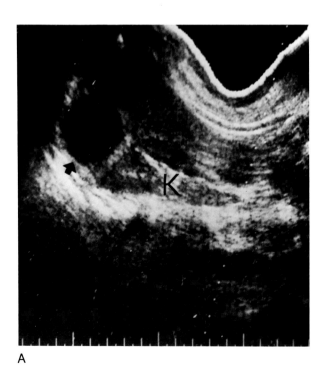

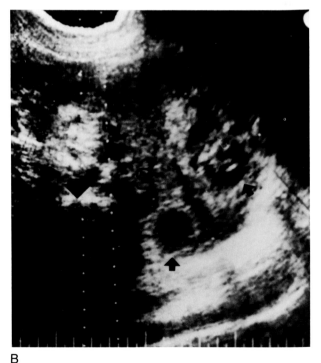

A   B

Fig. 8-6. Splenic hemangioma. **(A)** Longitudinal coronal scan. A large cystic lesion (arrow) is seen within the spleen *(S)* with acoustic enhancement. (*K*, kidney.) **(B)** Transverse scan demonstrating a mixed lesion in the spleen *(S)*. Hypoechoic areas are seen (arrows). (Large arrow, spine.) *(Figure continues.)*

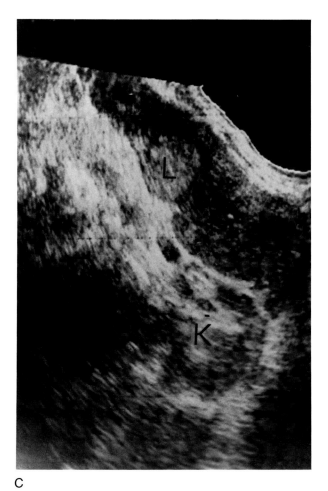

C

Fig. 8-6. *(Continued).* **(C)** Transverse scan of the spleen *(S)* with a well-circumscribed echodense lesion *(L)*. *(K,* kidney.) (From Manor A, Starinsky R, Garfinkel D et al: Ultrasound features of a symptomatic splenic hemangioma. J Clin Ultrasound 12:95, 1984.)

Fig. 8-7. Splenic hemangioma. Coronal scan of a cavernous hemangioma. The enlarged spleen contains areas of increased echoes and a few small hypoechoic areas. (From Solbiati L, Bossi MC, Bellotti E et al: Focal lesions in the spleen: Sonographic patterns and guided biopsy. AJR 140:59, © American Roentgen Ray Society, 1983.)

infarction with coagulated blood or fibrin in the cavities. The ultrasound features are not specific and as such lesions such as hydatid cyst, abscess, dermoid, or metastasis cannot be excluded.[12]

Cystic lymphangiomatosis, a benign malformation of the lymphatics composed of endothelium-lined cystic spaces, appears as a mass with extensive cystic replacement of the splenic parenchyma[2,3,13,14] (Fig. 8-8). Lymphangiomatosis affects predominately the somatic soft tissue and is found in the neck, axilla, mediastinum, retroperitoneum, and soft tissues of the extremities.[13] The process may diffusely involve multiple organ systems or may be confined to a solitary organ such as liver, spleen, kidney, or colon. Splenic involvement is rare.[13] The multicystic appearance is fairly characteristic.

MALIGNANT PRIMARY NEOPLASM (RARE)

Hemangiosarcoma is a rare malignant neoplasm arising from the vascular endothelium of the spleen. Findings with ultrasound have been scantily reported.[11] These lesions may, however, look similar to cavernous hemangiomas on ultrasound with a mixed to cystic pattern (Figs. 8-9 and 8-10). The one reported case[11] appeared as a large mass with a nonhomogeneous, mainly hyperechoic pattern; it was similar to that observed with hemangiomas apart from the lack of hypoechoic areas.

LYMPHOMA (COMMON)

The spleen is commonly involved in lymphoma, with involvement at initial presentation in 32 percent of patients with non-Hodgkin's lymphoma[15] and 39 percent

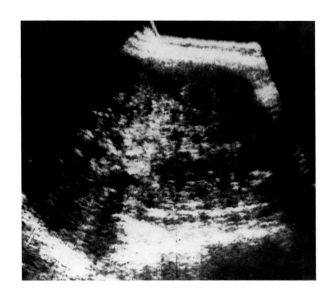

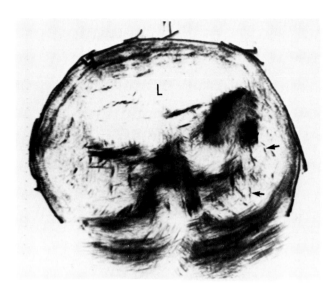

Fig. 8-8. Cystic lymphangiomatosis. Supine transverse scan at 12 cm above the umbilicus demonstrating a cystic, anterior, mid-abdominal lymphangioma (L) with multiple cystic areas (arrows) of involvement within the spleen. (From Mittelstaedt CA, Partain CL: Ultrasonic-pathologic classification of splenic abnormalities: Gray-scale patterns. Radiology 134:697, 1980.)

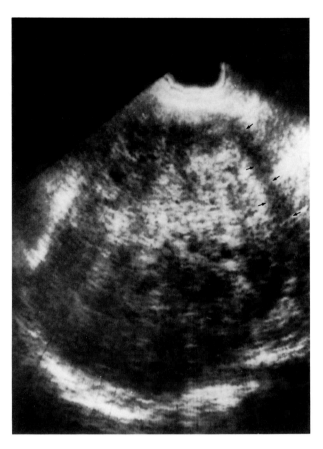

Fig. 8-9. Splenic hemangiosarcoma. Coronal scan with a large, inhomogeneous, mainly echogenic spleen with a pattern similar to Figure 8-7. A rim of normal splenic tissue (arrows) is seen in the lower pole. (From Solbiati L, Bossi MC, Bellotti E et al: Focal lesions in the spleen: Sonographic patterns and guided biopsy. AJR 140:59, © Am Roentgen Ray Society, 1983.)

of patients with Hodgkin's disease.[16] In one series, 4 of 12 patients with Hodgkin's disease and 9 of 12 patients with histiocytic lymphoma had discrete masses in the spleen, while such focal "tumorous" involvement was not found in any of 24 other cases of non-Hodgkin's lymphoma.[17]

Unfortunately, detection of splenic lymphoma is quite difficult. A sensitivity of 22 percent has been reported for detection of lymphomatous involvement of the spleen with either TcSC or contrast-enhanced CT.[18] Previous studies utilizing TcSC scanning were also discouraging, with only 10 percent sensitivity in detection of splenic lymphoma.[19] Similarly disappointing was Gallium citrate imaging with only 41 percent of splenic sites of lymphoma detected in one large series with both Hodgkin's disease and non-Hodgkin's lymphoma patients[20], and 26 percent sensitivity for detection of splenic sites in a series of non-Hodgkin's lymphoma patients.[21] Nonenhanced CT studies detected lymphomatous involvement of the spleen in only 5 of 11 proven cases. (45 percent).[22] There has been a recent report of similar sensitivity results for contrast-enhanced CT examinations—45 percent for non-Hodgkin's lymphoma and 61 percent for Hodgkin's disease of the spleen.[23]

Although focal splenic lesions in lymphoma are typically hypoechoic at ultrasound[2,3,14] (Fig. 8-11), focal echogenic areas have also been described[11] (Fig. 8-12).

One investigator claimed a 78 percent sensitivity for ultrasound in the detection of splenic lymphoma; splenomegaly and low-level echoes were the criteria employed, not focal abnormality.[24]

METASTASES (UNCOMMON)

Splenic metastases are generally regarded as the result of hematogenous spread.[25,26] In a postmortem study, the spleen was the 10th most common site of metastatic disease, with the most common sites of origin being breast (21 percent), lung (18 percent), ovary (8 percent), stomach (7 percent), melanoma (6 percent), and prostate (6 percent). Frequency of splenic involvement, expressed as the percentage of each primary tumor that had splenic metastases, was melanoma (34 percent), breast (12 percent), ovary (12 percent), lung (9 percent), prostate (6 percent), and stomach (4 percent).[25]

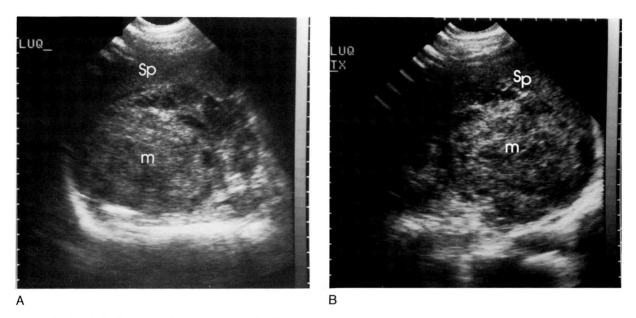

A   B

Fig. 8-10. Splenic hemangiosarcoma. Longitudinal **(A)** and transverse **(B)** scans of the spleen *(Sp)* demonstrating a poorly defined hyperechoic mass *(m)*. The mass is inhomogeneously echogenic. (Courtesy of Jerome J. Cunningham, M.D., Department of Radiology, Ohio State University, Columbus, Ohio.)

In most instances, splenic metastases are associated with metastatic involvement of other organs.[26] Despite the presumed rarity of isolated splenic metastases, one group found liver metastases to be absent in 70 percent of cases of splenic metastases.[27] Frequently these metastatic deposits are only microscopically evident (32 per-

cent of cases in one series).[25] As a result, splenic metastases are only rarely symptomatic, though splenic infarction with associated perisplenitis has been attributed to tumor emboli.[28]

Ultrasound may delineate focal metastases as either hypoechoic or hyperechoic lesions[2,3,14,29-31] (Fig. 8-13).

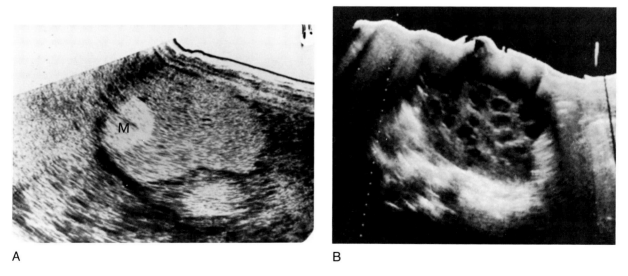

A   B

Fig. 8-11. Splenic lymphoma. **(A)** Case 1: Histiocytic lymphoma. Longitudinal supine scan with a hypoechoic lymphomatous mass **(M)** in the superior aspect of the spleen. (From Mittelstaedt CA, Partain CL: Ultrasonic-pathologic classification of splenic abnormalities: Gray-scale patterns. Radiology 134:697, 1980.) **(B)** Case 2: Mixed lymphocytic-histiocytic lymphoma. Prone, longitudinal view with multiple hypoechoic areas seen within the spleen. (From Mittelstaedt CA, McCartney WH, Mauro MA et al: Spleen. p.235. In Simeone J (ed): Clinics in Diagnostic Ultrasound: Coordinated Diagnostic Imaging. Churchill Livingstone, New York, 1984)

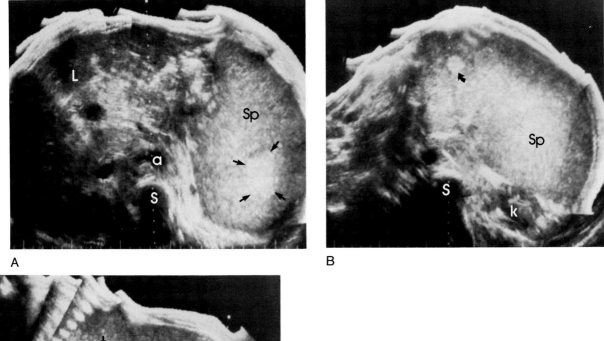

A

B

C

Fig. 8-12. Hairy cell leukemia of the spleen (B-cell lymphoma). Transverse supine scans at 14 cm **(A)** and 2 cm **(B)** above the umbilicus and a longitudinal scan **(C)** in the left midaxillary line demonstrate multiple focal echogenic areas (arrows) within an enlarged and echodense spleen *(Sp)*. (*a,* aorta; *L,* liver; *S,* spine; *k* left kidney.)

Melanoma deposits appear as hypoechoic lesions, but of higher echo amplitude than lymphoma; some are echodense.[11] There has been one case report of splenic plasmacytoma in which the lesion appeared as hyperechoic.[31]

CORRELATIVE IMAGING

All the standard noninvasive imaging modalities (TcSC, ultrasound, and CT) have been shown to be effective in the detection of focal splenic lesions.[9] TcSC, though quite sensitive in the detection of focal defects, is nonspecific and only evaluates the spleen and liver. Because CT requires intravenous contrast injection for optimal detection of focal disease, the utility of this modality may be limited in patients with contrast allergy.

Systematic comparisons of the relative effectiveness of imaging modalities (TcSC, ultrasound, and CT) for the

detection of focal splenic lesions are lacking. However, comparative imaging studies evaluating suspected liver metastases may serve as a basis for modality selection for splenic imaging.[32-35] Most studies have shown TcSC and CT to have similar sensitivities for the detection of hepatic lesions but with CT having a greater specificity.[32-35] In the one series including ultrasound as well as TcSC and CT, ultrasound had the lowest sensitivity.[34]

Infarction (Common)

Infarction of the spleen occurs due to septic emboli and local thromboses in patients with pancreatitis, subacute bacterial endocarditis, leukemia, lymphomatous disorders, sickle cell anemia, sarcoidosis, or polyarteritis nodosa.[11,36] Ultrasound characteristics of infarcts have not been widely described, although in one case, a local-

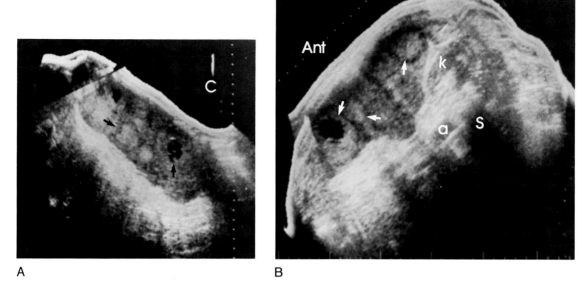

A   B

Fig. 8-13. Splenic metastases. Carcinoma of the lung. Longitudinal **(A)** and transverse **(B)** scans in the right lateral decubitus position demonstrate multiple hyperechoic lesions (arrows) within the spleen. Some have a bull's-eye pattern and some have necrotic (hypoechoic) centers. (*C*, level of the iliac crest; *a*, aorta; *S*, spine; *Ant*, anterior.) (From Mittelstaedt CA: Ultrasound of the spleen. p.233. In Raymond HW, Zwiebel WJ (eds): Seminars in Ultrasound. Vol. 2. Grune and Stratton, New York, 1981. By permission.)

ized hypoechoic area was noted[3] (Fig. 8-14). The sonographic appearances vary according to the time since onset.[11] A fresh hemorrhagic infarct appears hypoechoic (Figs. 8-14A and C) while a healed infarction, because of scar tissue formation, appears as echogenic wedge-shaped lesions with their base toward the subcapsular surface on the spleen[11] (Fig. 8-14B). One group of investigators has used ultrasound to evaluate the spleen for infarcts following splenic embolization.[37] They found that ultrasound was able to detect wedge-shaped defects with well-demarcated borders. While both abscesses and infarcts are hypoechoic, these lesions could be distinguished. Abscesses as a rule were poorly defined, irregular with variable shape, and may have thick and/or shaggy walls. Infarcts were seen as wedge-shaped hypoechoic lesions with well-demarcated borders. With follow-up, these investigators found the infarcts became smaller and increasingly echogenic but retained their triangular shape[37] (Fig. 8-14B).

Abscess (Uncommon)

Splenic abscesses are relatively uncommon; an incidence of only 0.14 to 0.22 percent was reported in a large autopsy series.[5,38,39] The infrequency of splenic abscess is probably related to the phagocytic activity of its efficient reticuloendothelial system and leukocytes. This effective defense system may be breached in several manners.

There may be overwhelming hematogenous seeding from bacterial endocarditis, septicemia, depressed immunological states, or intravenous drug abuse.[38-41] In 75 percent of cases there is hematogenous spread from distant foci.[5] Infective endocarditis is the most common single source of splenic abscesses and is seen in up to 40 percent of cases.[42] *Streptococcus* is the most common etiologic organism with *Staphylococcus, Salmonella* and *E.coli* following.[5,39] Nidus formation from underlying splenic damage (traumatic hematoma or infarction in sickle cell disease, leukemia, other hemaglobinopathies, or other conditions) may be the cause.[38-42] In 15 percent of cases, there is an association with a history of trauma.[5] Invasion by an extrinsic process (perinephric or subphrenic abscess, perforated gastric or colonic lesions, or pancreatic abscess) may occur.[38-42] Direct extension of inflammatory processes from adjacent organs occurs in 10 percent of cases.[5]

The high mortality associated with delay in diagnosis of splenic abscess emphasizes the need for prompt detection and therapy.[5,41-44] Despite antibiotic therapy, the mortality is high.[42] The overall mortality for splenic abscess is 41 percent.[5] TcSC will show a splenic abscess as a nonspecific focal defect. Gallium scanning may add specificity by showing a rim of increased activity around the splenic lesion, but this approach may delay diagnosis by 48 hours.[43,45]

Patients with splenic abscesses may be confusing in their presentation. Their clinical findings may be subtle.

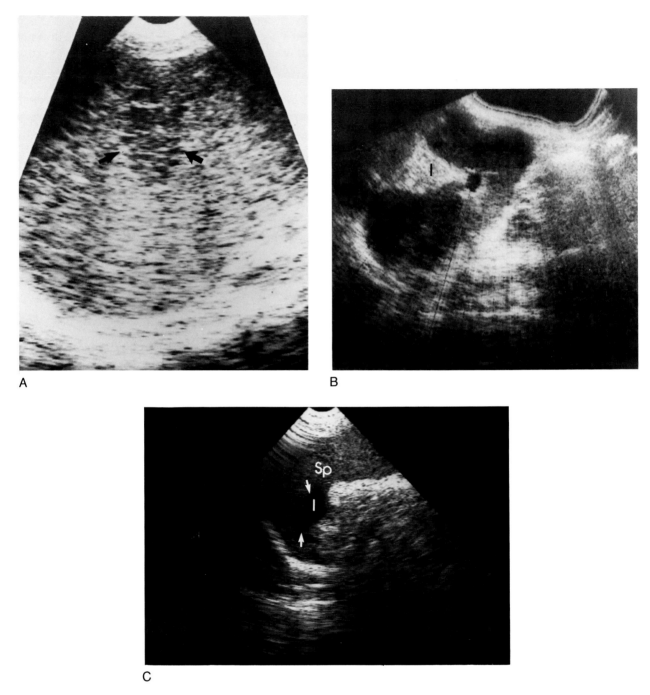

Fig. 8-14.   Splenic infarction. Case 1: **(A)** Longitudinal scan of a patient after embolization of the splenic artery. A wedge-shaped hypoechoic area (arrows) is seen. (From Weingarten MJ, Fakhry J, McCarthy J et al: Sonography after splenic embolization: The wedge-shaped acute infarct. AJR 141:957, © Am Roentgen Ray Society, 1984.) Case 2: **(B)** Longitudinal scan with a triangular, highly echogenic area *(I)* seen due to a scar. (From Solbiati L, Bossi MC, Bellotti E et al: Focal lesions in the spleen: Sonographic patterns and guided biopsy. AJR 140:59, © Am Roentgen Ray Society, 1983.) Case 3: Longitudinal **(C)** supine view demonstrating a hypoechoic area (*I*, arrows), which appears round on transverse scan and somewhat triangular on longitudinal view. (*Sp*, spleen.)

In one series, 95 percent of the patients had fever while 42 percent had left upper quadrant tenderness.[42] One-third of the patients had an elevated left hemidiaphragm or pleural effusion.[42] Fever (fever and tachycardia 90 percent), abdominal pain (60 percent), left chest pain, and left shoulder and flank pain are most common.[5,39] Splenomegaly (40 percent), a vague mass, and/or left upper quadrant tenderness may be found.[5,39]

Ultrasound has proven quite effective in the detection of splenic abscess. These lesions generally exhibit mixed echopatterns—predominately hypoechoic but often containing hyperechoic foci that represent debri or gas[5,39,41,44,46] (Figs. 8-15 and 8-16). Some investigators describe anechoic lesions.[39,42] The definition of these lesions is usually poor and they may have thick and/or shaggy walls.[37,39,44] As a rule, there is no increased through-transmission associated with these lesions.[44] Some investigators describe a variable amount of associated acoustic enhancement.[5] Gas within an abscess appears as scattered hyperechoic areas with acoustic shadowing or reverberation artifact[5,42] (Fig. 8-16). In contrast to the echofree acoustic shadow caused by foci of calcium, the shadow caused by gas contains ill-defined low-level echoes and has poorly defined margins.[5] The ultrasound appearance of abscess is not entirely characteristic and as such, the lesion cannot be totally differentiated from infarct, neoplasm, or hematoma on the basis of the ultrasound pattern alone.[5,42] Ultrasound also has the advantage of delineating abnormalities in the adjacent left subphrenic and perinephric spaces. Ultrasound has been reported to have an accuracy of 96 percent in detecting abscesses and is 99 percent accurate in correctly excluding abscesses.[5] CT's accuracy varies from 75 to 100 percent with that of gallium scanning 60 to 82 percent with a higher false positive rate.[5] Ultrasound is the method of choice for the early diagnosis of patients with suspected splenic abscess and represents a good screen in patients with fever and nonspecific abdominal symptoms.[5]

CT shows splenic abscesses as focal areas of decreased attenuation, best demonstrated when intravenous contrast is used to enhance the normal splenic parenchyma.[46-48] An abscess may appear loculated or may contain fluid layers with different attenuation.[47,48] Due to its sensitivity for detection of air, CT provides a more specific diagnosis in the case of air-containing abscesses.[46,48]

Cysts (Uncommon)

Splenic cysts that are relatively rare have been classified as parasitic or nonparasitic in origin.[49] *Echinococcus* is the only parasite that forms splenic cysts. While such hydatid cysts are the most common world-wide cause of splenic cysts, they are uncommon in our country.[50,51]

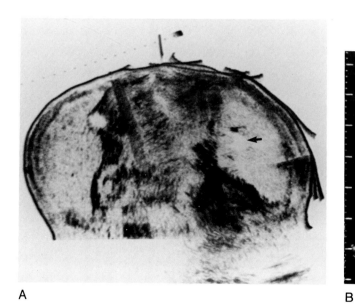

A

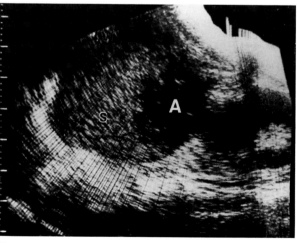

B

Fig. 8-15. Splenic abscess. *(A)* Case 1: Transverse scan 12 cm above the umbilicus in a patient with Felty's syndrome. A poorly defined hypoechoic area (arrow) is seen in the inferior aspect of the spleen. (From Mittelstaedt CA, Partain CL: Ultrasonic-pathologic classification of splenic abnormalities: Gray-scale patterns. Radiology 134:697, 1980.) **(B)** Case 2: Coronal scan with a large anechoic mass *(A)* in the inferior aspect of the spleen *(S)*. The mass contains scattered echoes due to debris. (From Pawar S, Kay CJ, Gonzalez R et al: Sonography of splenic abscess. AJR 138:259, © Am Roentgen Ray Society, 1982.)

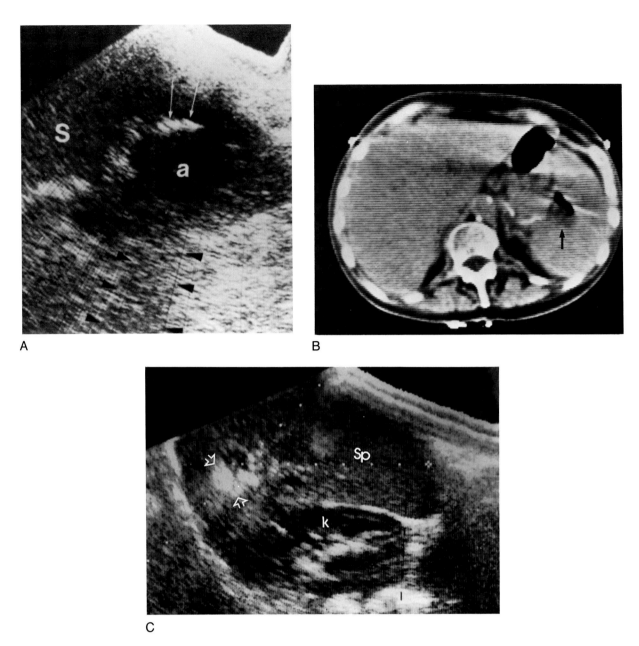

Fig. 8-16. Splenic abscess. Case 1: **(A)** Coronal scan of the spleen *(S)* with a large relatively anechoic abscess *(a)* with scattered internal echoes. Increased echogenicity (arrows) and acoustic shadowing (arrowheads) are due to the gas within the abscess. This was confirmed on CT **(B)** as an area of diminished attenuation (arrow) with a collection of gas in its anterior aspect. (From Pawar S, Kay CJ, Gonzalez R et al: Sonography of splenic abscess. AJR 138:259, © Am Roentgen Ray Soc, 1982.) Case 2: **(C)** Longitudinal scan with an abscess with increased echogenicity of the walls (arrows). (*k*, left kidney; *Sp*, spleen.) (From Kay CJ, Pawar S, Rosenfield AT: Sonography of splenic abscesses. p. 91. In Raymond HW, Zwiebel WJ (eds): Seminars in Ultrasound: Abscesses. Vol. 4, Grune and Stratton, New York, 1983. By permission.)

Parasitic cysts appear as anechoic lesions with possible daughter cysts and calcifications or as solid masses with fine internal echoes and poor distal enhancement.[11] Nonparasitic cysts of the spleen have been categorized as either (1) true or "primary" cysts (epidermoid cysts) containing an epithelial lining and considered to be of congenital origin, or (2) false or "secondary" cysts lacking a cellular lining, probably developing as a result of prior trauma to the spleen and accounting for approximately 80 percent of nonparasitic splenic cysts.[51]

Epithelial lined cysts or epidermoid cysts are lined by cells thought to arise from mesothelial cells that migrate during embryogenesis from the primitive coelomic cavity into the splenic analge.[52] These cysts are usually solitary, unilocular, and rarely contain calcification. The internal surface of the cyst may be smooth or trabecu-

lated. The fluid within the cyst may be clear or turbid and may contain protein, iron, bilirubin, fat, and cholesterol crystals.[52]

The epidermoid cysts occur more commonly in females, with 50 percent in patients less than 15 years old.[52] Although most patients present with an asympto-

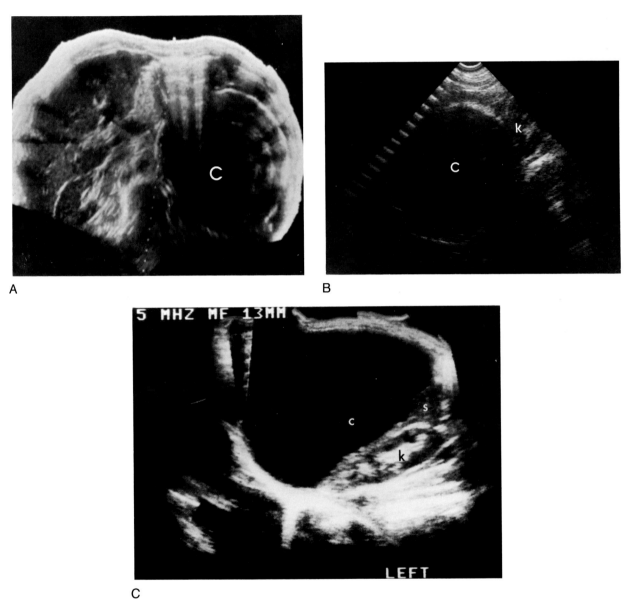

A

B

C

Fig. 8-17. Splenic cyst. Simple. Case 1: Supine transverse scan **(A)** at 12 cm above the umbilicus and prone longitudinal scan **(B)** demonstrating an anechoic mass *(C)* with dense borders in the area of the spleen. The wall of the cyst was calcified. (*k*, left kidney.) (Fig. **A** from Mittelstaedt CA, McCartney WH, Mauro MA et al: Spleen. p.235. In Simeone J (ed): Clinics in Diagnostic Ultrasound: Coordinated Diagnostic Imaging. Churchill Livingstone, New York, 1984) Case 2: **(C)** Longitudinal scan showing a large rounded echofree cyst *(c)* with surrounding margin of normal splenic tissue *(s)* inferiorly and posteriorly. The left kidney *(k)* is pushed inferiorly and the upper pole is squashed anteroposteriorly. (From Daneman A, Martin DJ: Congenital epithelial splenic cysts in children: Emphasis on sonographic appearances and some unusual features. Pediatr Radiol 12:119, 1982.)

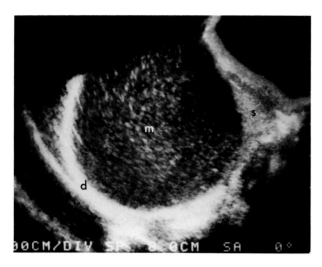

Fig. 8-18. Splenic cyst. Echogenic. Longitudinal scan demonstrating a large rounded echogenic mass *(m)* surrounded by normal splenic tissue *(s)* inferiorly. *(d,* diaphragm.) Echoes within the cyst were due to the high content of fat droplets within the cyst fluid. (From Daneman A, Martin DJ: Congenital epithelial splenic cysts in children: Emphasis on sonographic appearances and some unusual features. Pediatr Radiol 12:119, 1982.)

matic left upper quadrant mass, symptoms, when present, include mild left-sided abdominal discomfort or pain, and postprandial fullness.

Ultrasound findings are distinctive: hypoechoic or anechoic foci with well-defined walls and increased through-transmission (Figs. 8-17 to 8-19). The sonographic appearance of epidermoid cysts may include in-

creased internal echoes at higher gain settings, although even at these settings posttraumatic cysts tend to remain echofree.[52,53] Their complex pattern with irregularities and thickness of the posterior wall may be due to epithelial trabeculations and internal echoes from blood clots.[11] There has been a report of a case of a splenic cyst that was homogeneously echogenic[52] (Fig. 8-18). There have also been reports of cysts with internal hemorrhage producing a fluid-fluid level[54] (Fig. 8-19).

Biopsy

In many cases, an imaging technique used may only lead to a differential, not a specific diagnosis. For a definitive diagnosis and as a possible alternate to laparotomy, a fine-needle biopsy may be undertaken with a high degree of safety.[11,55,56] One investigator has performed more than 1,000 splenic punctures without complication.[55,56] Others have performed needle biopsies in 45 cases of diffuse and focal splenic disease without immediate or subsequent adverse reactions.[11] No intrasplenic hematomas, or lesions along the needle path were seen in the 23 patients who underwent splenectomy soon after fine-needle aspirations biopsy. Real-time ultrasound guidance was used in eight cases of splenic masses in which the final diagnoses without surgery were made in five cases. Two of these were cysts that were drained percutaneously and were not seen to recur on follow-up examination. Fine-needle aspiration should be considered as major diagnostic tool in evaluation of focal splenic lesions of unknown etiology.

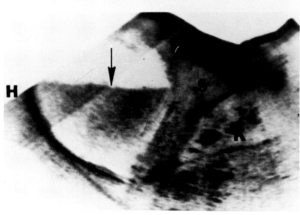

A

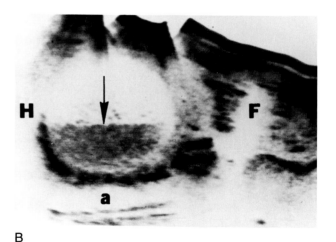

B

Fig. 8-19. Splenic cyst. Fluid-fluid level. Longitudinal scans **(A,B)** through the spleen *(S)* demonstrating a fluid interface (arrow) in a hemorrhagic cyst. *(K,* kidney.) The fluid interface, shifted with change in position **(B)**. *(a,* aorta; *H,* direction of patient's head; *F,* direction of patient's feet.) (From Propper RA, Weinstein BJ, Skolnick ML, Kisloff B: Ultrasonography of hemorrhagic splenic cysts. J Clin Ultrasound 7:18, 1979.)

DIFFUSE DISEASE

Hematopoietic Abnormalities

Hematopoietic abnormalities include those disease processes affecting erythropoiesis, granulocytopoiesis, and lymphopoiesis.[57] The myeloproliferative disorders are classified as abnormalities of both erythropoiesis and granulocytopoiesis.[57]

ERYTHROPOIETIC ABNORMALITIES

The erythropoietic abnormalities include sickle cell disease, hereditary spherocytosis, hemolytic anemias, chronic anemias, polycythemia vera, thalassemia, and the myeloproliferative disorders. Congestion of the red pulp and reticuloendothelial cell hypertrophy are often seen pathologically.[6,57]

Erythropoietic abnormalities generally produce an isoechoic splenic pattern on ultrasound (same density as the liver)[2,3] (Fig. 8-20). One author has described an isoechoic splenic pattern in a case of hereditary spherocytosis.[58]

GRANULOCYTOPOIETIC ABNORMALITIES

Cases of reactive hyperplasia due to acute and chronic infection, as well as splenitis associated with chronic granulomatous disease (sarcoid, tuberculosis, etc.), are

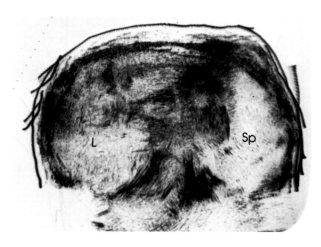

Fig. 8-21. Granulocytopoietic abnormality. Noncaseous granulomatous disease. The spleen *(Sp)* is noted to be less echodense than the liver *(L)* in this static scan 12 cm above the umbilicus. (From Mittelstaedt CA, Partain CL: Ultrasonic-pathologic classification of splenic abnormalities: Gray-scale patterns. Radiology 134:697, 1980.)

included in this category. Pathologically, these spleens demonstrate lymphoid hyperplasia of the white pulp and lymphocytes, neutrophils and/or phagocytic cells in the red pulp.[6,57]

Other than splenomegaly, no definite abnormalities are usually demonstrated on TcSC or CT scans. In contrast, ultrasound has been shown to exhibit a specific pattern—a spleen that is diffusely hypoechoic (less dense than liver)[2,3] (Fig. 8-21).

MYELOPROLIFERATIVE DISORDERS

The diseases in this category include acute and chronic myelogenous (granulocytic or myelocytic) leukemias, polycythemia vera, myelofibrosis, megakaryocytic leukemia, or erythroleukemia. All of these appear to have a common myeloproliferative stimulus.[57] Extramedullary hematopoiesis may replace the normal splenic architecture. In the myelogenous leukemias, the spleen is infiltrated by leukemic cells of the granulocytic series.[6]

In acute and chronic myelogenous leukemia, the spleen exhibits an isoechoic ultrasound pattern similar to that seen with the erythropoietic abnormalities[2,3] (Fig. 8-22). A case has been described in which the red pulp was dominant with infiltration by the hematopoietic elements pathologically.[59] Although other authors describe cases of chronic myelogenous leukemia and myelofibrosis as having an increased splenic echopattern, their examples appear to demonstrate a hypoechoic pattern when splenic echogenicity is compared to that of the liver.[58] Still others have illustrated a case of chronic mye-

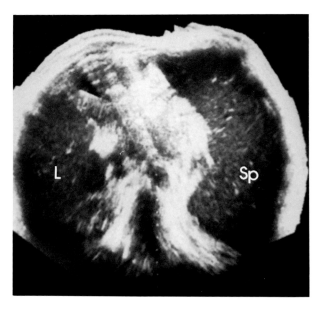

Fig. 8-20. Erythropoietic abnormality. Diffuse disease. Polycythemia Vera. Transverse supine scan shows an enlarged spleen *(Sp)* with an echopattern similar to liver *(L)*.

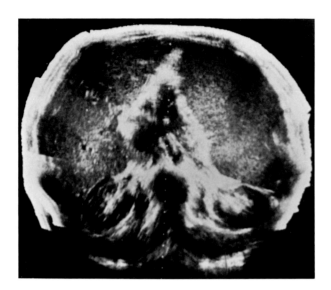

Fig. 8-22. Myeloproliferative disorder. Chronic myelogenous leukemia. Supine transverse view at 10 cm above the umbilicus. The liver and spleen are isosonic. (From Mittelstaedt CA, McCartney WH, Mauro MA et al: Spleen. p.235. In Simeone J (ed): Clinics in Diagnostic Ultrasound: Coordinated Diagnostic Imaging. Churchill Livingstone, New York, 1984.)

logenous leukemia that appeared to have an isoechoic splenic pattern.[60]

LYMPHOPOIETIC ABNORMALITIES

Pathologically, spleens involved by these disease processes demonstrate infiltration of the normal splenic architecture by cells of lymphoietic origin.[6] This category includes the lymphocytic leukemias, lymphoma, and Hodgkin's disease.

On ultrasound, most spleens affected with lymphocytic leukemia, lymphoma, and Hodgkin's disease demonstrate a diffusely hypoechoic splenic pattern[2,3,8,24,58,60,61] (Fig. 8-4). Focal hypoechoic lesions may also be present in both Hodgkin's and non-Hodgkin's lymphoma[2,3] (Fig. 8-11). Non-Hodgkin's lymphoma and "lymphoid malignancy" have also been reported as having an isoechoic echopattern (Fig. 8-1).

Reticuloendothelial Disorders

Diseases having reticuloendothelial hyperactivity and varying degrees of lipid storage in phagocytes are included in this category.[57] Examples would include Wilson's disease, Felty's syndrome, Still's disease, and reticulum cell sarcoma. On ultrasound scan, the splenic pattern appears isoechoic[2,3] (similar to Figures 8-1, 8-20, and 8-22).

Congestion

There is thickening of the trabeculae, fibrosis of the red pulp, and atrophy of lymphoid tissue with chronic passive congestion.[57] In most cases, the congestion is secondary to hepatocellular disease.

In the majority of cases of congestive splenomegaly due to cirrhosis, there is increased uptake of the radionuclide in the spleen relative to the liver and increased uptake in the bone marrow.[62] Some patients may have normal splenic uptake with increased marrow uptake.[62]

On ultrasound scan, the spleen may either demonstrate an isoechoic or hypoechoic pattern.[2,3] Because the liver is abnormal in these cases, it cannot be used as an internal standard for comparison.

TRAUMA

The spleen is the intraabdominal organ most commonly injured as a result of blunt abdominal trauma.[63] Automobile accidents are responsible for most of these injuries. Splenic trauma is often associated with injuries of other structures including (in decreasing order of incidence) chest wall (rib fractures), left kidney, spinal cord, liver, lung, craniocerebral structures, small intestines, large intestines, pancreas, and stomach.[64]

Trauma to the spleen may result in linear or stellate lacerations, capsular tears secondary to traction from adhesions or suspensary ligaments, puncture wounds from foreign bodies or rib fractures, subcapsular hematomas, avulsion of the vascular pedicle, and laceration of the short gastric vessels. Free intraperitoneal blood is most often seen acutely, that is, immediately after injury. However, delayed rupture occurring days to weeks following the traumatic event occurs in 10 to 15 percent of patients with free intraperitoneal blood. Delayed ruptures are probably related to a slowly enlarging subcapsular hematoma with subsequent rupture or a small splenic laceration that was temporarily tamponaded. Occult splenic rupture is a term applied to a posttraumatic pseudocyst, generally secondary to an organized intrasplenic or parasplenic hematoma.[64] Splenic trauma may result in autotransplantation of splenic tissue on to peritoneal surfaces, a condition termed splenosis. Patients with splenosis may subsequently develop adhesions leading to intestinal obstruction.[65]

Clinically, 10 to 20 percent of splenic lacerations are not clinically obvious.[66] The main presenting symptoms include left upper quadrant pain (100 percent), left shoulder pain (50 percent), left flank pain (36 percent) and postural dizziness (21 percent).[67] The most frequent clinical signs are left upper quadrant tenderness (100

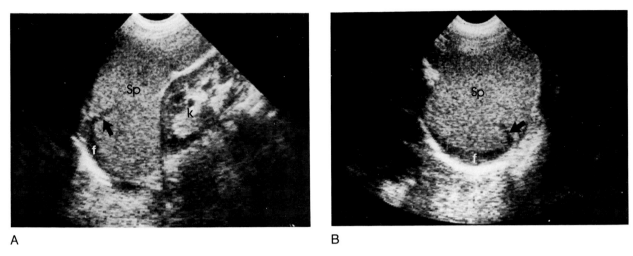

Fig. 8-23. Splenic laceration. **(A)** Coronal scan 4 days after injury demonstrating a small peripheral splenic laceration (arrow) in continuity with a perisplenic fluid collection *(f)*. *(Sp,* spleen; *k,* kidney.) **(B)** Transverse scan showing the laceration (arrow) and the perisplenic fluid collection *(f)*. *(Sp,* spleen.) (From Lupien C, Sauerbrei EE: Healing in the traumatized spleen: Sonographic investigation. Radiology 151:181, 1984.)

percent), hypotension (36 percent) and decreased hemaglobin level (43 percent).[67] Peritoneal lavage is a sensitive technique for the detection of intraperitoneal bleeding but is invasive, may be falsely positive, and will not detect either retroperitoneal hemorrhage or a subcapsular splenic hematoma without free intraperitoneal blood. Although splenectomy is the most common treatment for splenic trauma, simple observation, splenorrhaphy (suture repair of laceration), partial splenectomy, and percutaneous aspiration are now being performed for some cases of subcapsular hematoma and small lacerations.[68-70] Splenectomy may predispose patients to subsequent septicemia and therefore should not be performed unnecessarily. It is clear, therefore, that splenic trauma must be detected as well as characterized in an attempt to define those patients who can receive conservative management.

Because plain films are most often normal or equivocal in cases of subcapsular hematoma, imaging modalities may assume great importance in the evaluation of

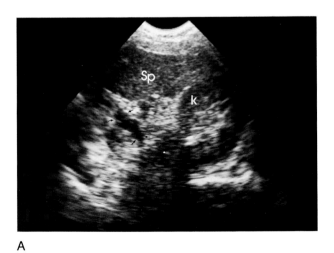

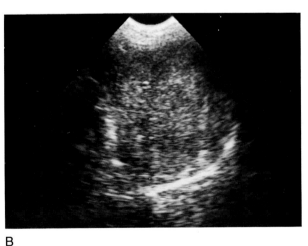

Fig. 8-24. Splenic transection. Right lateral decubitus longitudinal **(A)** and transverse **(B)** scans in a 7-year-old child on the same day as his trauma. A dilated splenic vein (arrows) is seen in **(A)** in the region of the splenic hilum. *(Sp,* spleen; *k,* left kidney) On the transverse view **(B)** no focal defect was seen but the echopattern is inhomogeneous. As seen on Figure 8-30, there was peritoneal fluid. At surgery, the spleen was found to be transected in the area of the splenic hilum.

splenic trauma. Selection of the proper examinations can help expedite the patient's diagnostic workup in achieving an accurate appraisal of the spleen and other intraabdominal structures.

Ultrasound has not been shown to be as reliable as either TcSC or CT in the evaluation of splenic trauma. Technically inadequate examinations have been shown to occur in as many as 20 percent of cases secondary to accompanying rib fractures and contusions of chest tubes.[71] With the advent of the new high-resolution sector real-time systems, ultrasound has become a rapid, accurate examination in many cases. Ultrasonic signs of splenic trauma include splenomegaly or progressive splenic enlargement, an irregular splenic border, intrasplenic fluid (hematoma), splenic inhomogeneity (contusion), subcapsular and pericapsular fluid collections (subcapsular hematoma), free intraperitoneal blood, and left pleural effusion[67,69,72] (Figs. 8-23 to 8-30). A small peripheral laceration appears as a linear echopoor defect (Fig. 8-23). With transection, a more extensive plane of fluid may be seen transversing the entire thick-

ness of the splenic pulp or the spleen may have an inhomogeneous echopattern (Fig. 8-24). Focal hematomas are represented by intrasplenic fluid collections (Figs. 8-25 and 8-26). With a subcapsular hematoma, perisplenic fluid is seen (Figs. 8-27 to 8-29).

The findings with splenic trauma can change considerably in a short period of time. Blood exhibits varying echopatterns depending on the age of the trauma. In less than 24 hours, intraparenchymal hemorrhage may appear hyperechoic.[67] As such a fresh hematoma may be indistinguishable from normal splenic tissue, giving only the appearance of splenomegaly or a double contour to the spleen[69] (Fig. 8-27). As the protein and cells resorb and the hematoma becomes organized, the fluid collection becomes hyperechoic. Focal areas of inhomogeneity probably represent tiny splenic lacerations that give rise to small collections of blood interspersed with disrupted splenic pulp (contusion). With time, the hematoma will become more fluid or lucent appearing (Figs. 8-25, 8-26, 8-28, and 8-29). Echofree intraperitoneal fluid probably represents blood, perhaps intermixed

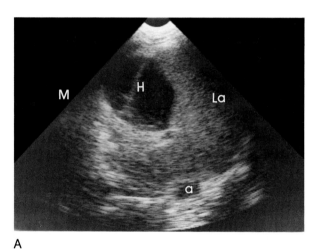

A

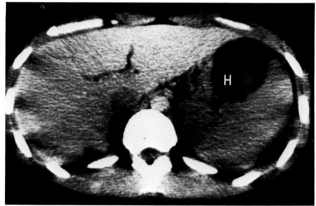

B

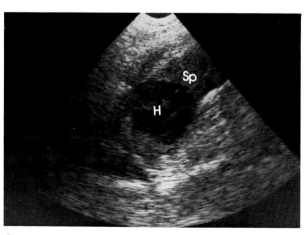

C

Fig. 8-25. Intrasplenic hematoma. Case 1: (A) Transverse, supine real-time scan. There is a hypoechoic mass *(H)* in the region of the splenic hilum. (*M*, medial; *La*, lateral; *a*, aorta.) (B) CT scan, enhanced, demonstrating the hematoma *(H)* in the area of the splenic hilum. (From Mittelstaedt CA, McCartney WH, Mauro MA et al: Spleen. p.235. In Simeone J (ed): Clinics in Diagnostic Ultrasound: Coordinated Diagnostic Imaging. Churchill Livingstone, New York, 1984.) Case 2: Longitudinal right lateral decubitus (C) scan. A poorly defined hypoechoic area *(H)* is seen within the spleen *(Sp)*.

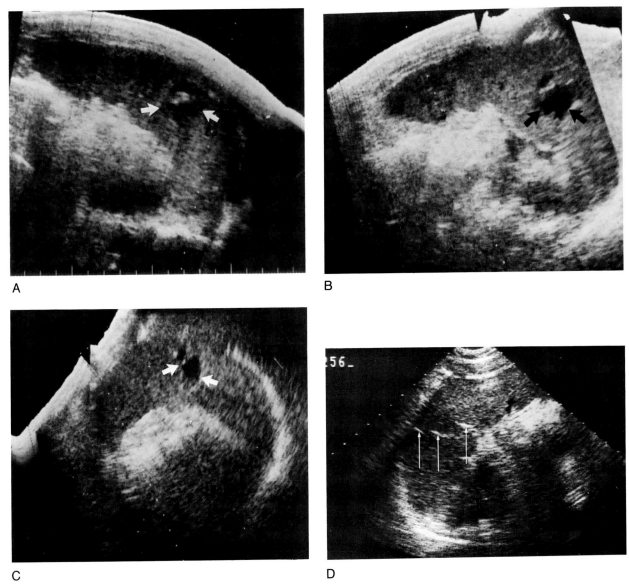

Fig. 8-26. Intrasplenic hematoma — Healing. **(A)** Scan demonstrating a focal area of inhomogenicity (arrows) 3 days after initial injury. **(B)** Ten days later the lesion has become echofree (arrows). **(C)** Two weeks after **(B)** shows a decrease in the size of the intrasplenic fluid collection (arrows). **(D)** Sixteen months after the initial trauma, only small echogenic lines (arrows) are seen in the area of the previous splenic lesion. These are likely fibrous scars. (From Lupien C, Sauerbrei EE: Healing in the traumatized spleen: Sonographic investigation. Radiology 151:181, 1984.)

with peritoneal transudate due to the presence of blood within the cavity[67] (Fig. 8-30).

The pattern of splenic healing and the time it takes depends on the nature and size of the initial lesion[67] (Fig. 8-26). Small peripheral lacerations tend to disappear several weeks after the injury but intrasplenic hematomas and contusion take months to resolve (7 to 66 weeks).[67] Large lesions persist for longer periods of time. Free fluid collections disappear more quickly because fluid is transported across pleural and peritoneal membrane

rapidly. Pleural effusion and intraperitoneal fluid disappears quickly (2 and 4 weeks respectively) while intrasplenic hematoma and contusion usually resorb over a period of a month (up to year). Intrasplenic hematomas and contusions take so much longer likely because the fluid, protein, and necrotic debris must be resorbed from within a solid organ in which the blood supply is already been focally disrupted.[67] When followed to complete resolution, the spleen may become normal, or small irregular foci may be present that are echogenic, probably rep-

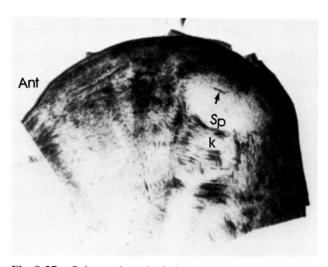

Fig. 8-27. Subcapsular splenic hematoma. This patient was in a motorcycle accident 24 hours prior to the scan. This transverse scan in the right lateral decubitus position demonstrates a very subtle double contour (arrow) to the spleen *(Sp)*. This was produced by a "fresh" hematoma that was similar in echodensity to the remainder of the spleen. (*k*, left kidney; *Ant*, anterior.) (From Mittelstaedt CA, Partain CL: Ultrasonic-pathologic classification of splenic abnormalities: Gray-scale patterns. Radiology 134:697, 1980.)

resenting scar[67] (Fig. 8-26). As a rapid, noninvasive diagnostic technique, ultrasound can be used for multiple follow-up examinations if the clinical condition warrants.

Because of the reduction in immunologic competence and the increased risk of sepsis in patients who have undergone splenectomy, clinicians now adapt a nonsurgical approach in patients with an injured spleen.[67] The nonoperative management requires careful clinical observation, bed rest and serial hematocrit.[73] Patients are selected for nonoperative management on the basis of a stable clinical status and laboratory evidence of cessation of bleeding.[73] An initial ultrasound might be valuable to serve as a baseline for those with repeated trauma and/or new symptoms.[67] The decision to operate should be based on a combination of clinical and ultrasound findings.[67]

Percutaneous Aspiration

In recent years nonoperative management of splenic rupture has been recommended and used increasingly because postsplenectomy patients have been shown to have an increased susceptibility to overwhelming infection.[70] With ultrasound guidance, fine needle aspiration of the perisplenic or subcapsular fluid can confirm the

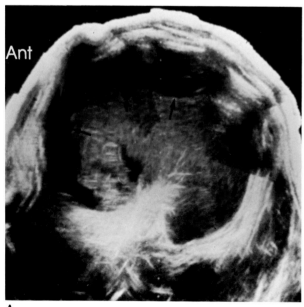

A

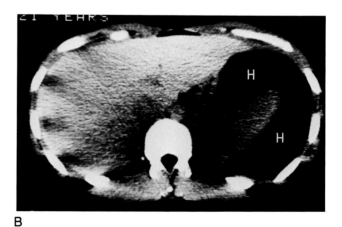

B

Fig. 8-28. Subcapsular splenic hematoma, same patient as Fig. 8-25A and B. **(A)** Transverse static scan in the right lateral decubitus position at 15 cm above the iliac crest. A perisplenic fluid collection (arrows) is seen. (*Ant*, anterior.) **(B)** CT scan, enhanced, with the perisplenic hematoma *(H)* demonstrated. (From Mittelstaedt CA, McCartney WH, Mauro MA et al: Spleen. p.235. In Simeone J (ed): Clinics in Diagnostic Ultrasound: Coordinated Diagnostic Imaging. Churchill Livingstone, New York, 1984.)

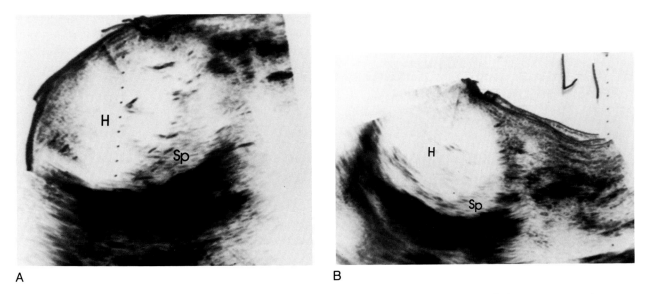

Fig. 8-29. Subcapsular splenic hematoma. This patient had been kicked by a horse on the left side three years prior to this examination. Prone transverse **(A)** and longitudinal **(B)** scans demonstrate a cystic mass *(H)* within the spleen *(Sp)*. It does contain a few internal echoes but demonstrates acoustic enhancement. This represented an old hematoma.

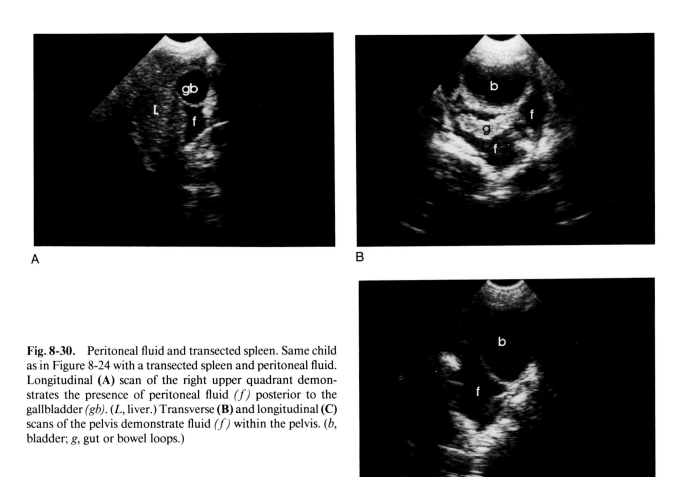

Fig. 8-30. Peritoneal fluid and transected spleen. Same child as in Figure 8-24 with a transected spleen and peritoneal fluid. Longitudinal **(A)** scan of the right upper quadrant demonstrates the presence of peritoneal fluid *(f)* posterior to the gallbladder *(gb)*. (*L*, liver.) Transverse **(B)** and longitudinal **(C)** scans of the pelvis demonstrate fluid *(f)* within the pelvis. (*b*, bladder; *g*, gut or bowel loops.)

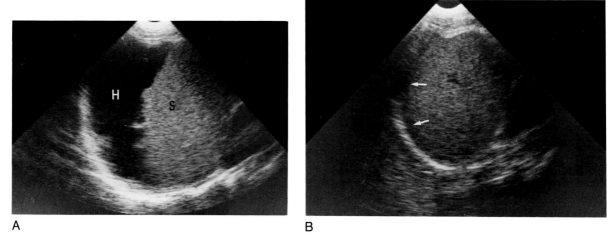

A   B

Fig. 8-31.   Splenic hematoma aspiration. **(A)** Longitudinal prone scan for localization of the subcapsular hematoma *(H)* for drainage. *(Sp,* spleen.) (Same patient as Figures 8-25A, 8-25B and 8-28). **(B)** Longitudinal scan after the removal of 625cc of old blood. A very small amount of remaining subcapsular fluid (arrows) is seen on this scan. No reaccumulation was seen on follow-up examination. The intrasplenic hematoma (Figure 8-25A, 8-25B) remained unchanged in size. (From Mittelstaedt CA, McCartney WH, Mauro MA et al: Spleen. p.235. In Simeone J (ed): Clinics in Diagnostic Ultrasound: Coordinated Diagnostic Imaging. Churchill Livingstone, New York, 1984.)

diagnosis and often be therapeutic[69] (Fig. 8-31). One author reports three patients with infectious mononucleosis and splenic rupture diagnosed and followed as outpatients by ultrasound; laparotomy was avoided in these cases. One of the hematomas was aspirated percutaneously with ultrasound guidance, and did not recur on the follow-up examination.

OTHER

Variant Orientation and Contour

The normal spleen is highly variable in both contour and orientation. These variations are generally without clinical significance and are commonly noted as incidental findings during imaging procedures. Nonetheless, unusual splenic configurations and positions may mimic pathologic entities and may complicate, or even precipitate, diagnostic workups. Appropriate imaging procedures and a knowledge of these variations may easily obviate this confusion and eliminate the necessity of further unwarranted or invasive procedures.

Three major splenic configurations have been described: orange-segment (44 percent), tetrahedral (42 percent), and triangular (14 percent) (Fig. 8-32). Additionally, splenic configuration has been categorized into two major types: (a) a compact spleen, with a narrow hilus, and even borders; and (2) a distributed spleen, with

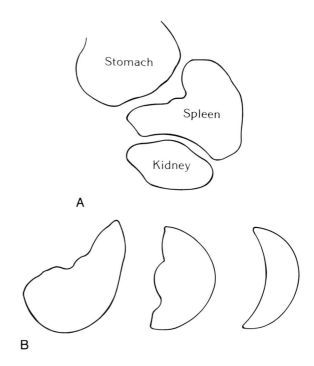

A

B

Fig. 8-32.   Splenic configurations. Note the variable splenic contours (A,B) on cross section at the splenic hilum where a prominent ridge or lobulation may be seen. (Modified from Piekarski J, Federle MP, Moss AA, London SS: Computed tomography of the spleen. Radiology 135:683, 1980.)

widespread hilus, a notched anterior border, a thumb-like lobe at the inferior pole, and an expanded portion or "tubercle" at the upper medial pole[74] (Fig. 8-33). In most individuals there is good splenic contact with the diaphragm and the lateral abdominal wall; poor contact can often be accounted for by enlargement of the left lobe of the liver, ascites, deformity of the left hemidiaphragm, or a small, horizontally positioned spleen.[75] Left upper quadrant masses, or even gastric dilatation, may displace the spleen inferiorly, producing "pseudosplenomegaly."[76] Caudad displacement may also be secondary to subdiaphragmatic abscesses, splenic cysts or abscesses, left pleural effusion, or marked cardiomegaly; cephalad displacement may be caused by left lung volume loss, left pneumonectomy, paralysis of the left hemidiaphragm, or a large intraabdominal mass.[77] In patients whose status is postrepair of congenital ventral hernia, the spleen and the liver may have an abnormal shape and be ventrally located.[78]

The so-called upside-down spleen is most likely due to developmental rotation of the spleen on its longitudinal-anteroposterior axis, causing the hilus to be directed cephalad or laterally[79] (Fig. 8-34). The typical scintigraphic pattern — a spleen with its hilus oriented superiorly, a concave superior and a convex inferior margin — should not be confused with splenic trauma or infarction. On abdominal radiographs or ultrasound, the upside-down spleen can mimic a left suprarenal mass.[80]

Other splenic variations may simulate renal or suprarenal masses on routine radiographic studies. Although downward and/or medial displacement of the entire left kidney by an enlarged spleen is common and easily recognized, localized flattening of the upper pole of the left kidney can be the result of a "distributed" spleen with a "lumpy" contour, a transverse spleen, a rotated and ptotic spleen, or an accessory spleen[81] (Fig. 8-35). Similarly, variant splenic configurations may suggest a retrogastric mass or a fundal lesion on barium study.[82,83] A

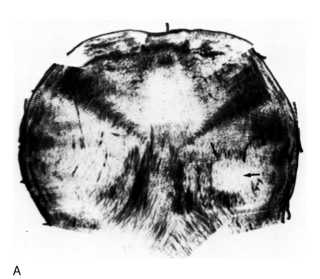

A

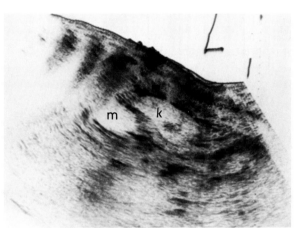

B

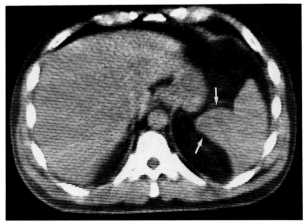

C

Fig. 8-33. Normal splenic variant. Medial tubercle. **(A)** Transverse scan at 20 cm above the umbilicus. A hypoechoic mass (arrows) is seen medial to the area of the spleen. **(B)** Prone longitudinal scan demonstrating a hypoechoic mass *(m)* anterior to the left kidney *(k)*. On TcSC liver/spleen scan functional tissue was demonstrated in the area of the mass seen on ultrasound. **(C)** CT scan confirms the medial tubercle (arrows) as being part of the spleen. (Figs. **A** and **C** from Mittelstaedt CA, McCartney WH, Mauro MA et al: Spleen. p.235. In Simeone J (ed): Clinics in Diagnostic Ultrasound: Coordinated Diagnostic Imaging. Churchill Livingstone, New York, 1984.)

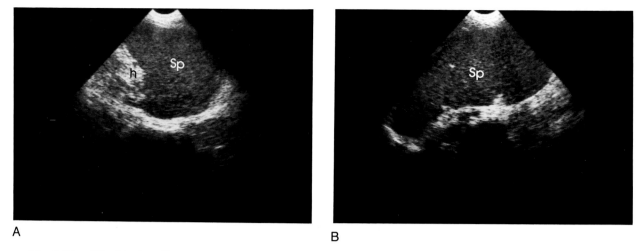

A

B

Fig. 8-34. "Upside-down" spleen. Longitudinal **(A)** and transverse **(B)** scans of the spleen *(Sp)*. Note that the splenic hilum *(h)* is directed superiorly on the longitudinal scan **(A)**. (Fig. **A** from Mittelstaedt CA, McCartney WH, Mauro MA et al: Spleen. p.235. In Simeone J (ed): Clinics in Diagnostic Ultrasound: Coordinated Diagnostic Imaging. Churchill Livingstone, New York, 1984.)

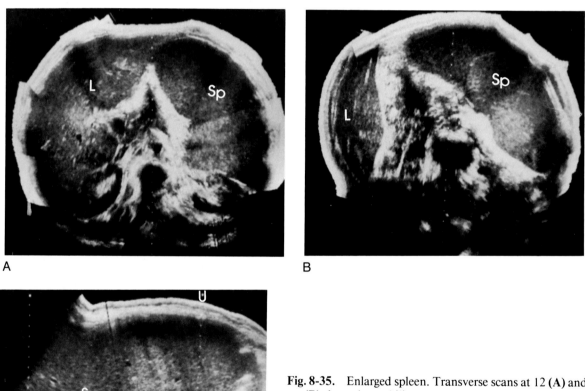

A

B

C

Fig. 8-35. Enlarged spleen. Transverse scans at 12 **(A)** and 4 cm **(B)** above the umbilicus as well as a longitudinal scan 10 cm to the left of midline **(C)** demonstrate that the palpable mass is spleen *(Sp)*. It extends well below the level of the umbilicus *(U)*, to the right of midline, and displaces the left kidney *(k)* inferiorly. The patient was found to have chronic myelogenous leukemia.

normal sized spleen with a medial lobulation projecting between the pancreatic tail and the left kidney may be confused with a cystic mass in the tail of the pancreas on prone ultrasound examination[84] (Figs. 8-33 and 8-36).

Documentation of the fact that splenic variation is to blame for suspected left upper quadrant mass can often be provided by ultrasound or TcSC (Figs. 8-33 to 8-36). Satisfactory ultrasound evaluation, however, can be dif-

ficult in an obese or gaseous patient. In addition, upper quadrant examination in the prone position is not without pitfalls. Although TcSC will delineate splenic variation, relationships between splenic tissue and adjacent structures is not always clear-cut, and anomalous bulges of splenic tissue are not necessarily seen to best advantage in standard views. In many instances, CT scanning with oral contrast administration is the most successful

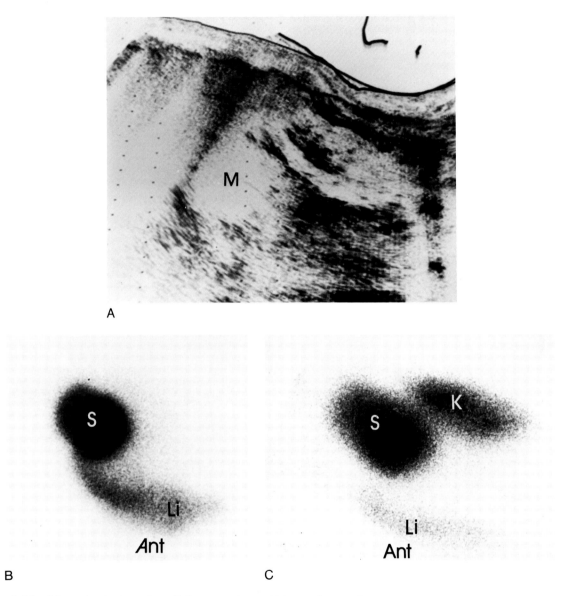

Fig. 8-36. Normal splenic variant. Spleen anterior to kidney mistaken for pseudocyst. (A) Prone longitudinal scan demonstrating a hypoechoic mass *(M)* anterior to the kidney in a patient with a past history of pancreatic pseudocysts. (B) TcSC: Left lateral view with uptake in the liver *(Li)* and spleen *(S)*. *(Ant,* anterior.) (C) ^{99m}Tc-glucohepatonate scan performed after the TcSC scan in (B). This lateral view confirms that the mass seen on ultrasound was the spleen *(S)* because it is maintaining the same relationship to the kidney *(K)* as seen in (A). *(Ant,* anterior; *Li,* liver.) (Figs. A and C from Shirkhoda A, McCartney WH, Staab EV et al: Imaging of the spleen: A proposed algorithm. AJR 135:195, © Am Roentgen Ray Society, 1980.) (Fig. B from Mittelstaedt CA, McCartney WH, Mauro MA et al: Spleen. p.235. In Simeone J (ed): Clinics in Diagnostic Ultrasound: Coordinated Diagnostic Imaging. Churchill Livingstone, New York, 1984.)

imaging modality in clarifying splenic configuration and orientation as it relates to adjacent organs, i.e., as the cause of a retrogastric or suprarenal mass effect.

Wandering Spleen/Splenic Torsion

"Wandering spleen," (also known as "ectopic spleen," "aberrant spleen," "floating spleen," and "splenic ptosis") refers to migration of the spleen from its normal location in the left upper quadrant. This relatively rare variant is most probably the result of embryologic anomaly of the supporting ligaments of the spleen, although splenomegaly and abdominal laxity (the latter sometimes associated with multiparity and hormonal effects

of pregnancy) have been considered predisposing factors.[85,86]

Clinical presentations include an asymptomatic abdominal or pelvic mass, mild discomfort (from splenic congestion and perhaps ligamentous/visceral pressure), intermittent abdominal pain (attributed to spontaneous torsion and detorsion of the splenic pedicle), and abdominal catastrophe (resulting from splenic volvulus).[87] Bleeding gastric varices have been reported as presenting findings, presumed secondary to splenic vein occlusion associated with chronic torsion of the vascular pedicle.[88]

Ultrasound is often the preliminary study for evaluation of abdominal pain or mass, and sonographic imaging should strongly suggest the diagnosis of wandering spleen when a solid "mass" is demonstrated and splenic

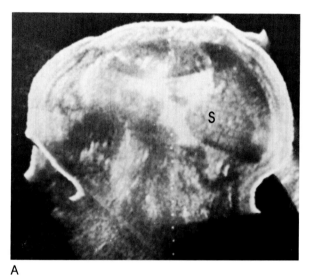

A

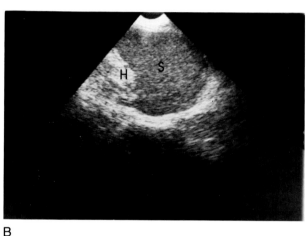

B

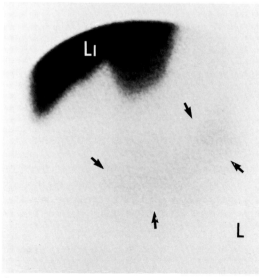

C

Fig. 8-37. Wandering spleen with torsion. Patient with pain and an abdominal mass. **(A)** Supine, transverse scan at the level of the umbilicus. The spleen *(S)* is seen at this level instead of in the left upper quadrant. **(B)** Supine, longitudinal real-time image of the spleen. The image appears to be reversed because the splenic hilum *(H)* is superior to the spleen *(S)*. The patient was referred for ^{99m}Tc-sulfur colloid radionuclide splenic scintigraphy (TcSC) to confirm the diagnosis and evaluate splenic vascularity. **(C)** Anterior view of TcSC scan with the camera centered over the spleen located at the level of the umbilicus. Uptake in the spleen (arrows) is barely visible when scans are taken for a predetermined count. (*L*, left; *Li*, liver.) *(Figure continues.)*

Fig. 8-37. *(Continued).* **(D)** Anterior view of a TcSC scan centered over the spleen with the scan taken for a predetermined time instead of for counts. The liver *(Li)* is shielded. The spleen *(S)* appears reversed from its normal orientation. The decreased activity in the spleen is compatible with vascular compromise. (*L*, left.) **(E)** CT scan confirms the presence of a rotated spleen *(S)* in the lower abdomen. **(F)** CT scan at a higher level in the abdomen than the CT in **(E)**. The dilated splenic vessels *(SV)* are noted in the splenic hilum. Angiography demonstrated a 720° torsion. (From Mittelstaedt CA, McCartney WH, Mauro MA et al: Spleen. p.235. In Simeone J (ed): Clinics in Diagnostic Ultrasound: Coordinated Diagnostic Imaging. Churchill Livingstone, New York, 1984.)

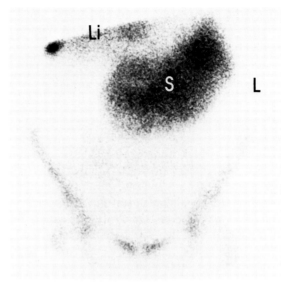

D

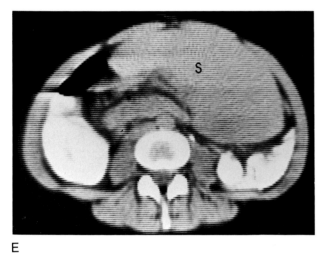

E

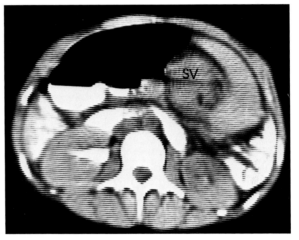

F

echoes are absent from their normal location[89] (Figs. 8-34 and 8-37). Demonstration of a "feeding vessel" associated with the mass should heighten suspicion further.[90]

In the case of uncomplicated splenic displacement, TcSC or ultrasound will confirm the abnormal spleen location.[91] However, as the spleen moves into and out of normal position, sequential TcSC or ultrasound scanning may be required for documentation. Obviously, in the case of a "transient" abdominal mass, scans must be wisely timed to coincide with the mass being palpable.[92] If torsion has occurred, the spleen may not be visualized by scintigraphy, or splenic uptake may be relatively diminished, dependent upon the degree of vascular supply compromise.[93] Absence of splenic visualization with TcSC is not entirely specific, because non-visualization may be secondary to acquired functional asplenia.[94]

Nonetheless, in the absence of preexisting disease (most commonly, sickle cell anemia), splenic nonvisualization in the face of an abdominal mass or an acute abdomen should provide a key clue to the diagnosis of splenic volvulus.

Accessory Spleens/Splenosis

Accessory spleens, resulting from failure of fusion of the separate splenic masses forming on the dorsal mesogastrium, are most commonly located in the splenic hilum or along splenic vessels or associated ligaments. Their occurrence has also been reported from the diaphragm to the scrotum.[95] They are solitary in 88 percent of cases, double in 9 percent and greater than two in 3 percent.[96] Despite a reported autopsy incidence of 10 to

31 percent, accessory spleens are detected incidentally in only about 0.05 percent of routine TcSC scans.[97] This discrepancy may be explained by the difficulty in visualizing accessory splenic tissue owing to obscuration by surrounding splenic radionuclide accumulation or relatively low tracer accumulation in the accessory tissue. Additionally, the field of view in routine TcSC scanning will not include less characteristic locations.[98]

Customarily, accessory spleens remain small and do not present as clinical problems. Rarely, torsion and infarction of an accessory spleen may present as an acute abdomen.[99,100] Accessory spleens may also simulate pancreatic, suprarenal, and retroperitoneal tumors[101,102], and may even be mistaken as such at arteriography[103] or mimic an intragastric neoplasm on upper GI examination.[104] An accessory spleen that has undergone compensatory hypertrophy after splenectomy may present as an abdominal mass. Although the appearance of a well-defined, almost spherical or uniform soft tissue density in the region of the splenectomy bed should be suggestive of the diagnosis on CT, this appearance is not specific, and could be produced by primary or secondary retroperitoneal neoplasms.[105] Similarly, accessory splenic tissue may resemble recurrent renal tumor after nephrectomy.[106]

Ultrasound has been found to be able to identify and document accessory spleens based on their appearance, location and most importantly blood supply.[96] They are round or oval solid structures with echogenicity similar to that of the main spleen[96] (Figs. 8-38 to 8-40). They are surrounded by high amplitude interfaces that separate them from adjacent parenchymal organs. In one series, most were found in the splenic hilum, with a smaller number in the splenocolic ligament and anterior to the tail of the pancreas. In 90 percent, the blood supply of the accessory spleen can be identified with ultrasound[96] (Figs. 8-38 and 8-39). In 34 percent, the arterial supply from the splenic artery can be seen as a single tortuous arterial branch originating from the splenic artery near the splenic hilum[96] (Fig. 8-38). In 66 percent, a single straight vein is seen originating from the accessory spleen and draining into the splenic vein[96] (Fig. 8-39).

Scintigraphy is the most sensitive modality for the detection and localization of functional accessory splenic tissue. Aside from its utility in instances of simulated mass lesions, detection of residual splenic tissue may have important clinical implications in postsplenectomy patients with autoimmune hemolytic anemias, idiopathic thrombocytopenic purpura, and hereditary spherocytosis. A possible cause of relapsing disease after splenectomy in these patients is recurrent splenic function, be it from hypertrophy of a previous small accessory spleen or the growth of new tissue from seeded spleen tissue.[107,108] Scanning may initially be performed with a radiocolloid, but because hepatic uptake may obscure small amounts of splenic tissue, repeat scanning may be performed with a spleen-specific agent, such as chemical or heat denatured ^{99m}Tc labelled red blood cells[109] (Fig. 8-40B).

Splenosis, or posttraumatic autotransplantation of splenic tissue in the pleural or peritoneal cavities, may also be diagnosed by TcSC.[110,111] Unlike accessory

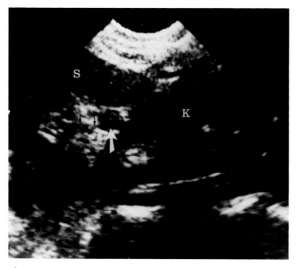
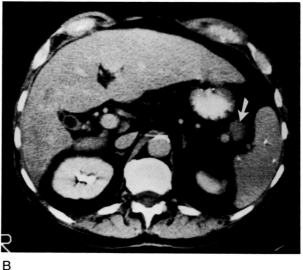

A   B

Fig. 8-38. Accessory spleen. **(A)** Longitudinal scan with accessory spleen (white arrow) separated from main spleen *(S)* and left kidney *(K)* by high-amplitude interface. The blood supply (black arrows) is from the splenic artery. **(B)** CT, enhanced, with accessory spleen (arrow) isodense to main spleen. (From Subramanyam BR, Balthazar EJ, Horii SC: Sonography of the accessory spleen. AJR 143:47, © Am Roentgen Ray Society, 1984.)

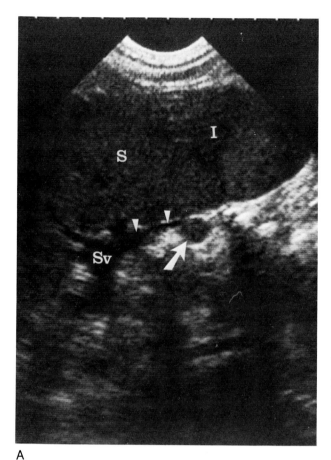

A

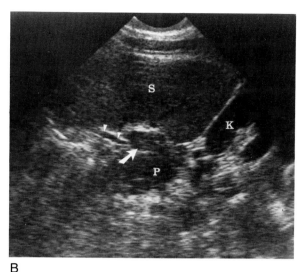

B

Fig. 8-39. Accessory spleen. **(A)** Longitudinal scan in a patient with splenomegaly *(S)* and an area of infarct *(I)*. The accessory spleen (arrow) is drained by a branch (arrowheads) of the splenic vein *(Sv)*. **(B)** Oblique scan demonstrating an oval accessory spleen (arrow) with venous drainage (arrowheads). Note its relationship to spleen *(S)*, tail of pancreas *(P)* and left kidney *(K)*. (From Subramanyam BR, Balthazar EJ, Horii SC: Sonography of the accessory spleen. AJR 143:47, © Am Roentgen Ray Society, 1984.)

spleens, the functioning tissue in splenosis does not follow the pattern of splenic embryologic development and is often more numerous and widespread. Recent evidence suggests that splenosis is a frequent occurrence after splenectomy for trauma.[112] Although the diagnosis is usually made incidentally at surgery for obstruction or abdominal pain, the history of prior trauma, with or without splenectomy, may provide the clue for appropriate imaging and a correct preoperative diagnosis.[113] Multiple splenic foci may not be visualized routinely on liver-spleen scanning without modification of the technique, in particular, the use of a higher intensity setting on the gamma camera.[114]

The Spleen and Congenital Heart Disease

The infrequent asplenia/polysplenia syndromes occur in association with a variable constellation of complex cardiac malformations, bronchopulmonary abnormalities, and visceral heterotaxia (anomalous placement of organs or major blood vessels). The latter includes a horizontal liver, malrotation of the gut, and interruption

of the inferior vena cava with azygous continuation.[115] Although CT has recently been employed to demonstrate various components of polysplenia in a relatively older patient,[116] nuclear medicine techniques offer the most assistance in evaluation of these syndromes. Ultrasound, as a rule, is not used for evaluation in these instances.

TcSC may be the initial imaging agent utilized; however this agent may be unable to definitely establish the presence or absence of splenic tissue, owing to superimposition of a midline liver or inadequate resolution. In these instances, selective imaging of the spleen with heat-natured red blood cells labeled with ^{99m}Tc appears to be a complementary and superior technique.[117] Comparison of TcSC scans with scans employing hepatobiliary agents may be of use in suspected asplenia — a discrepancy in organ morphology between the two studies indicates the presence of the spleen, wheras similarity of the image suggests asplenia.[118]

Following injection of radionuclide agents into the foot veins, it is possible to image the inferior vena cava and, thus demonstrate inferior vena cava anomalies, including absence of the renal-to-hepatic portion with azygous extension, left-sided inferior vena cava, and double

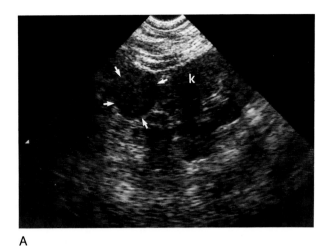

A

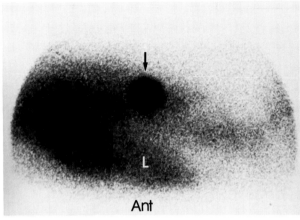

B

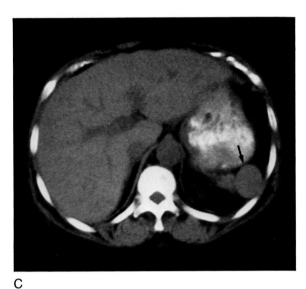

C

Fig. 8-40. Accessory spleen. Patient with idiopathic thrombocytopenic purpura and prior splenectomy. On longitudinal (A) right-lateral decubitus scan, a round echodense mass (arrows) is seen in the area of the splenic bed. The left kidney *(k)* is separate from the mass. Left lateral (B) view of a scan with ^{99m}Tc heat damaged red blood cells demonstrates a round area (arrow) of increased activity in the area of the spleen. (*L*, liver; *Ant*, anterior.) (C) Unenhanced CT scan demonstrating the accessory spleen (arrow).

inferior vena cava.[119] Because the location of the inferior vena cava has great significance in establishing situs or abdominal heterotaxia, such radionuclide venography in conjunction with TcSC studies may obviate the need for arteriography in some instances. Similarly, this technique may be of considerable aid in the selection of the appropriate approach for cardiac catheterization in those patients who will undergo palliative or corrective surgery.

PERISPLENIC ABNORMALITIES

Lesions of the pancreas, left kidney, left adrenal, and left lobe of the liver may impinge upon the spleen and mimic primary splenic disease.[120] Ultrasound, is a valuable technique in differentiating primary splenic disease from perisplenic abnormalities.

Pancreatic Disease

Lesions of the body and tail of the pancreas can mimic a primary splenic process when extension of the inflammatory or neoplastic lesion occurs by direct extension or by extension along the splenorenal ligament (Figs. 8-41 and 8-42). This ligament attaches the tail of the pancreas to the visceral parietal covering of the spleen. Exudation of pancreatic fluid in the anterior pararenal space from acute pancreatitis may track along this ligament to produce a perisplenic or intrasplenic fluid accumulation that may mimic a splenic cyst or perisplenic abscess or hematoma[121,122] (Fig. 8-42).

TcSC scanning typically demonstrates an extrinsic impression upon the spleen in the case of perisplenic abnormalities, whereas an intrasplenic lesion often shows a rim of functioning tissue around the photon deficient area. However, the TcSC scan is frequently unable to differentiate primary splenic lesions from peri-

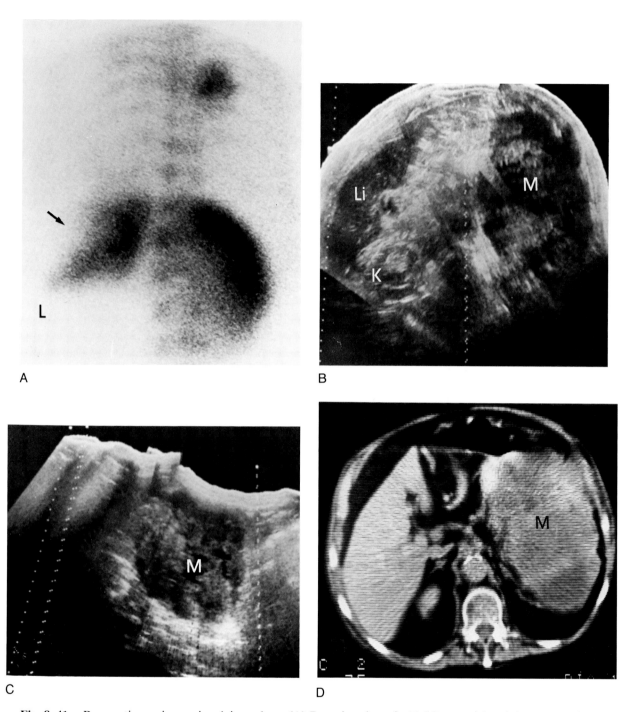

Fig. 8-41. Pancreatic carcinoma involving spleen. **(A)** Posterior view of a TcSC scan with a defect (arrow) in the superior lateral margin of the spleen. (*L*, left.) **(B)** Supine, transverse scan at 12 cm above the umbilicus. An echodense mass *(M)* is seen in the left upper quadrant. (*Li*, liver; *K*, right kidney.) **(C)** Right lateral decubitus, longitudinal view through the area of the spleen. A predominately echodense mass *(M)* is seen and is not separable from the spleen. **(D)** Enhanced CT scan. A large mass *(M)* is seen in the area of the spleen with inhomogeneous enhancement. Pancreatic origin could not be established from the CT scan. (From Mittelstaedt CA, McCartney WH, Mauro MA et al: Spleen. p.235. In Simeone J (ed): Clinics in Diagnostic Ultrasound: Coordinated Diagnostic Imaging. Churchill Livingstone, New York, 1984.)

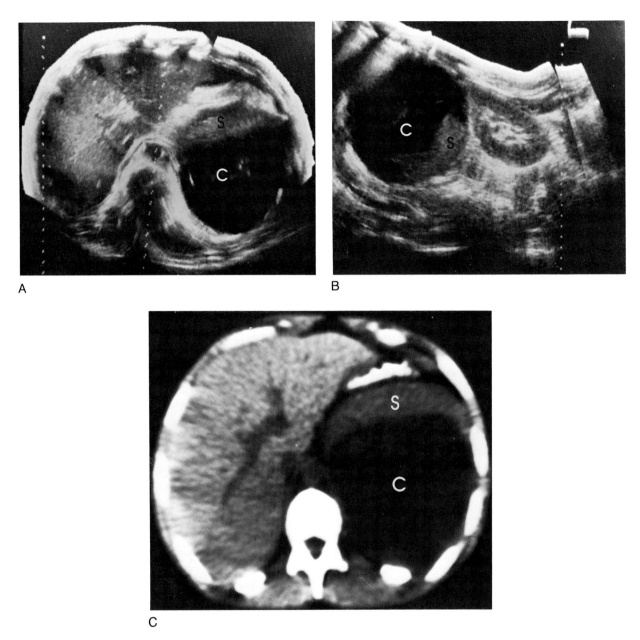

Fig. 8-42. Pancreatic pseudocyst involving spleen. **(A)** Supine, transverse scan at 16 cm above the umbilicus. A cystic mass *(C)* is seen in the left upper quadrant posterior to the spleen *(S)*. **(B)** Prone, longitudinal scan demonstrating the relationship of the pseudocyst *(C)* to the spleen *(S)* and the left kidney. On ultrasound alone, this pseudocyst could not be differentiated from a splenic hematoma. (Fig. **B** from Mittelstaedt CA: Ultrasound of the spleen. p.233. In Raymond HW, Zwiebel WJ (eds): Seminars in Ultrasound. Vol. 2. Grune and Stratton, New York, 1981. By permission.) **(C)** Enhanced CT scan. A large low-density area (pseudocyst, *C*) is seen posterior to the spleen *(S)*. As with ultrasound, the relationship to pancreas could not be established and a splenic hematoma could not be excluded. (Fig. **A** and **C** from Mittelstaedt CA, McCartney WH, Mauro MA et al: Spleen. p.235. In Simeone J (ed): Clinics in Diagnostic Ultrasound: Coordinated Diagnostic Imaging. Churchill Livingstone, New York, 1984.)

splenic abnormalities such as pancreatic disease, although it does provide a sensitive method for initial detection of such abnormalities.

Ultrasound examination may show a relatively anechoic fluid collection located posterior and lateral to the spleen, which is often anteromedially displaced (Fig. 8-42). Differentiation between an intrasplenic cyst, splenic hematoma, and an anechoic intrasplenic pancreatic pseudocyst may be extremely difficult unless the radiologist is aware of this uncommon entity and the clinical situation is appropriate. If the pseudocyst contains debris that produced internal echoes, it may be difficult to exclude necrotic tumor or abscess on the basis of the ultrasound appearance alone.

CT may help differentiate an intrasplenic pseudocyst from a primary splenic cyst by showing secondary signs of pancreatitis, thereby suggesting a pancreatic etiology. Secondary signs detected by CT include loss of the fat planes separating the pancreas from adjacent organs and thickening of Gerota's fascia lateral to the left kidney in the left paracolic gutter.[121]

The optimal radiographic assessment of a splenic defect or perisplenic fluid collection seen on TcSC or ultrasound includes confirmation of associated secondary findings of pancreatitis by CT scan. Needle aspiration of the perisplenic fluid collection using ultrasound or CT guidance may confirm an inflammatory pancreatic etiology by showing an elevated amylase. The aspirate may also be positive for carcinoma by cytology or demonstrate an unsuspected perisplenic abscess or hematoma.

Renal Disease

The upper pole of the left kidney impinges upon the splenic hilum and the medial surface of the spleen is cupped around the lateral border of the left kidney. The splenorenal ligament provides the attachment between the left kidney's perirenal space and the visceral parietal coat of the spleen.

A peripheral renal cyst that is situated in the lateral or superior left kidney may indent the splenic parenchyma and produce an impression on TcSC scan or ultrasound that is difficult to differentiate from a splenic cyst (Figs. 8-43 and 8-44). If an extrinsic impression in the spleen is detected by TcSC scan, ultrasound of the spleen may demonstrate both the cyst and a "beak" of renal parenchyma surrounding it (Fig. 8-44). This "beak" sign, as with excretory urography, is helpful in both CT and ultrasound demonstration of cysts. Used in conjunction, the ultrasound examination may confirm the cystic nature of the lesion and the CT scan with contrast enhancement may demonstrate the "beak" sign of renal parenchyma surrounding the cyst. CT alone is not entirely reliable in detection of benign cystic renal disease versus solid low-density neoplasm.

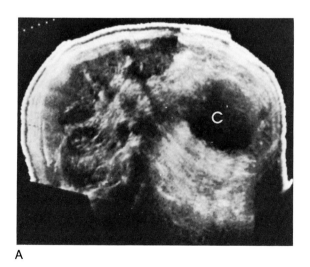
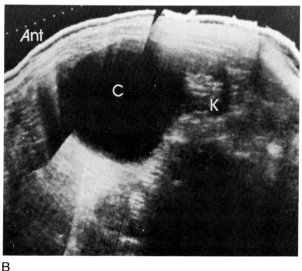

A   B

Fig. 8-43. Renal cyst. **(A)** Supine, transverse scan at 14 cm above the umbilicus. A cystic area *(C)* is seen in the left upper quadrant. **(B)** Right lateral decubitus, transverse scan at 7 cm above the iliac crest. This clearly established the renal origin of the mass *(C)*. (*K*, left kidney; *Ant*, anterior.) (From Mittelstaedt CA, McCartney WH, Mauro MA et al: Spleen. p.235. In Simeone J (ed): Clinics in Diagnostic Ultrasound: Coordinated Diagnostic Imaging. Churchill Livingstone, New York, 1984.)

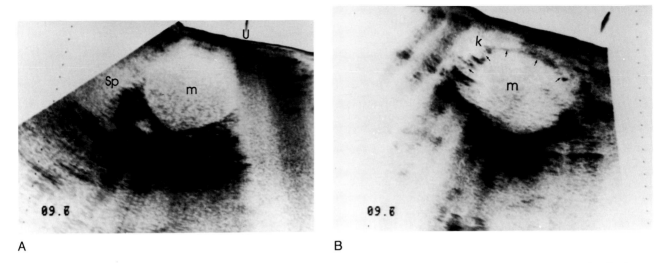

A   B

Fig. 8-44. Hemorrhagic renal cyst. This 4-year-old child was referred for evaluation of splenomegaly. On longitudinal supine view (**A**), a cystic mass *(m)* is seen separate from the spleen *(Sp)*. Although it contains internal echoes, it exhibits acoustic enhancement. (*U*, level of the umbilicus.) On a prone longitudinal (**B**) scan, the mass *(m)* can be seen originating from the left kidney (*k*, arrows).

Neoplastic or inflammatory involvement of the kidney may extend retroperitoneally along the splenorenal ligament or directly into the spleen's medial surface (Fig. 8-45). Again, in confusing cases, needle aspiration may reveal the primary site of a neoplastic lesion or lead to percutaneous catheter drainage of a perisplenic or renal abscess.

Adrenal Lesions

The left adrenal gland may be the source of tumors or cysts that extrinsically compress the spleen (Fig. 8-46). Hemorrhage of the adrenal or adrenal cysts is usually confined to the perirenal space. If a cyst, tumor, or hematoma is not large enough to impinge upon the spleen's

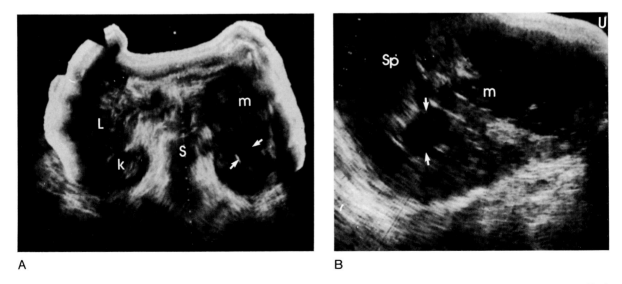

A   B

Fig. 8-45. Renal neoplasm. Transverse scan 12 cm above the iliac crest (**A**) and longitudinal scan (more magnified than the transverse) 8 cm to the left of midline (**B**) demonstrate a mass *(m)* of mixed density inseparable from spleen *(Sp)* or left kidney. The kidney as such is not identified. The mass, although solid, contains anechoic areas (arrows) representing regions of tumor necrosis. (*L*, liver; *k*, right kidney; *S*, spine.)

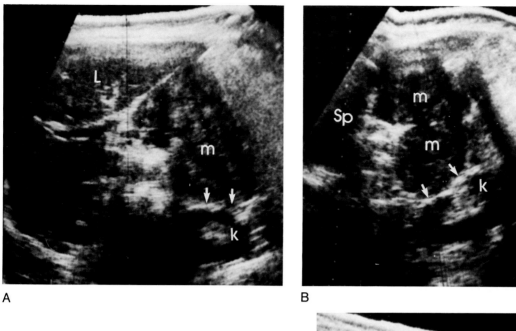

A

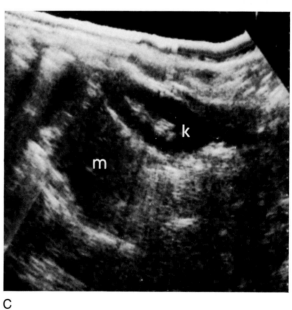

B

C

Fig. 8-46. Adrenal neoplasm. Ganglioneuroma in a child. A large solid, echodense mass *(m)* is seen in the left upper quadrant on a transverse scan **(A)** at 3 cm below the xyphoid and on longitudinal **(B)** scan 4 cm to the left of midline. It cannot be entirely separated from spleen *(Sp)* although it seems to be separate (arrows) from the left kidney *(k)*. (*L*, liver; *U*, level of the umbilicus.) On a prone longitudinal scan **(C)** at 4 cm to the left, the mass *(m)* appears separate from the left kidney *(k)*. Spleen as such is not identified on this scan.

medial border and be detected on TcSC scan, CT or ultrasound may suggest the adrenal etiology of this finding.

With the advent of high-resolution CT scanning using 1.5 mm, 2 mm, or 4 mm slice thickness, the adrenals can be reliably imaged in nearly all patients. However, if an adrenal neoplasm is large enough to impress upon the spleen, there may be some difficulty differentiating adrenal from renal primary, especially with tumor invasion of the left kidney on CT or ultrasound.

CONCLUSION

In general, screening for lesions suspected in the spleen can be done with TcSC techniques. Lesions in the left upper quadrant, whether they are within the spleen and adjacent organs or structures such as the kidney or diaphragm can be nicely investigated with ultrasound. When localization is less certain, evaluation of the patient should probably be initiated with CT.

REFERENCES

1. Taylor KJW: Atlas of Gray Scale Ultrasonography. Churchill Livingstone, New York, 1978
2. Mittelstaedt CA: Ultrasound of the spleen. p.233. In Raymond HW, Zwiebel WJ (eds): Seminars in Ultrasound. Vol.2. Grune and Stratton, New York, 1981
3. Mittelstaedt CA, Partain CL: Ultrasonic-pathologic classification of splenic abnormalities: Gray-scale patterns. Radiology 134:697, 1980
4. Taylor KJW, Milan J: Differential diagnosis of chronic splenomegaly by gray-scale ultrasonography: Clinical observations and digital A-scan analysis. Br J Radiol 49:519, 1976
5. Kay CJ, Pawar S, Rosenfield AT: Sonography of splenic abscesses. p.91. In Raymond HW, Zwiebel WJ (eds): Seminars in Ultrasound: Abscesses. Vol. 4. Grune and Stratton, New York, 1983
6. Robbins S, Cotran RS: Spleen. p.803. In Pathologic Basis of Disease. Saunders, Philadelphia, 1979
7. Pietri H, Boscaini M: Determination of a splenic volumetric index by ultrasonic scanning. J Ultrasound Med 3:19, 1984
8. Vicary FR, Souhami RL: Case reports: Ultrasound and Hodgkin's disease of the spleen. Br J Radiol 50:521, 1977
9. Mittelstaedt CA, McCartney WH, Mauro MA et al: Spleen. p.235. In Simeone J (ed): Clinics in Diagnostic Ultrasound: Coordinated Diagnostic Imaging. Churchill Livingstone, New York, 1984
10. Brinkley AA, Lee JKT: Cystic hamartoma of the spleen: CT and sonographic findings. J Clin Ultrasound 9:136, 1981
11. Solbiati L, Bossi MC, Bellotti E et al: Focal lesions in the spleen: Sonographic patterns and guided biopsy. AJR 140:59, 1983
12. Manor A, Starinsky R, Garfinkel D et al: Ultrasound features of a symptomatic splenic hemangioma. J Clin Ultrasound 12:95, 1984
13. Rao BK, AuBuchon J, Lieberman LM et al: Cystic lymphangiomatosis of the spleen: A radiologic-pathologic correlation. Radiology 141:781, 1981
14. Shirkhoda A, McCartney WH, Staab EV et al: Imaging of the spleen: A proposed algorithm. AJR 135:195, 1980
15. Stein RS: Saturday conference: Non-Hodgkin's lymphoma. South Med J 71:1261, 1978
16. Kaplan HS: Hodgkin's Disease. Harvard University Press, Cambridge, 1980
17. Ahmann DL, Kiely JM, Harrison EG, Payne WS: Malignant lymphoma of the spleen. Cancer 19:461, 1966
18. Zornoza J, Ginaldi S: Computed tomography in hepatic lymphoma. Radiology 138:405, 1981
19. Silverman S, DeNardo GL, Glatstein E, Lipton MJ: Evaluation of the liver and spleen in Hodgkin's disease. Am J Med 52:362, 1972
20. McCaffrey JA, Rudders RA, Kahn PC et al: Clinical usefulness of Gallium-67 scanning in the malignant lymphomas. Am J Med 60:523, 1976
21. Longo DL, Schilsky RL, Blei L et al: Gallium-67 scanning: Limited usefulness in staging patients with non-Hodgkin's lymphoma. Am J Med 68:695, 1980
22. Breiman RS, Castellino RA, Harell GS et al: CT-pathologic correlations in Hodgkin's disease and non-Hodgkin's lymphoma. Radiology 126:159, 1978
23. Castellino RA: Noninvasive evaluation of lymphoma. Radiologic techniques. Presented at The 68th Annual Meeting of the Radiological Society of North America, Chicago, 1982
24. Glees JP, Taylor KJW, Gazet JC et al: Accuracy of gray-scale ultrasonography of liver and spleen in Hodgkin's disease and other lymphomas compared with isotope scans. Clin Radiol 28:233, 1977
25. Berge T: Splenic metastases: Frequencies and patterns. Acta Path Microbiol Scand 82:499, 1974
26. Marymont JH, Gross S: Patterns of metastatic cancer in the spleen. Am J Clin Path 40:58, 1963
27. Piekarski J, Federle MP, Moss AA, London SS: Computed tomography of the spleen. Radiology 135:683, 1980
28. Verheyden CN, Van Heerden JA, Carney JA: Symptomatic metastatic melanoma of the spleen. Minn Med 57:693, 1974
29. Murphy JF, Bernardino ME: The sonographic findings of splenic metastases. J Clin Ultrasound 7:195, 1979
30. Paling MR, Shawker TH, Love IL: The sonographic appearance of metastatic malignant melanoma. J Ultrasound Med 1:75, 1982
31. Adler DD, Silver TM, Abrams GD: The sonographic appearance of splenic plasmacytoma. J Ultrasound Med 1:323, 1982
32. MacCarty RL, Wanner HW, Stephens DH et al: Retrospective comparison of radionuclide scans and computed tomography of the liver and pancreas. Am J Roentgenol 129:23, 1977
33. Biello DR, Levitt RG, Siegel BA et al: Computed tomography and radionuclide imaging of the liver: A comparative evaluation. Radiology 127:159, 1978
34. Snow JH, Goldstein HM, Wallace S: Comparison of scintigraphy, sonography, and computed tomography in the evaluation of hepatic neoplasm. AJR 132:915, 1979
35. Knopf DR, Torres WE, Fajman WJ, Sones PF: Liver lesions: Comparative accuracy of scintigraphy and computed tomography. AJR 138:623, 1982
36. Kim EE: Focal splenic defect. Semin Nucl Med 9:320, 1979
37. Weingarten MJ, Fakhry J, McCarthy J et al: Sonography after splenic embolization: The wedge-shaped acute infarct. AJR 141:957, 1984
38. Lawhorne TW, Zuidema GD: Splenic abscess. Surgery 79:686, 1976
39. Hertzanu Y, Mendelsohn DB, Goudie E, Butterworth A: Splenic abscess: A review with the value of ultrasound. Clinical Radiol 34:661, 1983
40. Gadacz T, Way LW, Dunphy JE: Changing clinical spectrum of splenic abscess. Am J Surg 128:182, 1974
41. Ralls PW, Quinn MF, Colletti P et al: Sonography of pyogenic splenic abscess. AJR 138:523, 1982

42. Rudick MG, Wood BP, Lerner RM: Splenic abscess diagnosed by ultrasound in the pediatric patient: Report of three cases. Pediatr Radiol 13:269, 1983

43. Chulay JD, Landerani MR: Splenic abscess: Report of ten cases and review of the literature. Am J Med 61:513, 1976

44. Laurin S, Kaude JV: Diagnosis of liver-spleen abscesses in children — with emphasis on ultrasound for the initial and followup examinations. Pediatr Radiol 14:198, 1984

45. Brown JJ, Sumner TE, Crowe JE, Staffner LD: Preoperative diagnosis of splenic abscess by ultrasonography and radionuclide scanning. South Med J 72:575, 1979

46. Pawar S, Kay CJ, Gonzalez R et al: Sonography of splenic abscess. AJR 138:259, 1982

47. Grant E, Mertens MA, Mascatello VJ: Splenic abscess: Comparison of four imaging methods. AJR 132:465, 1979

48. Moss ML, Kirschner LP, Peereboom G, Fereis RA: CT demonstration of a splenic abscess not evident at surgery. AJR 135:159, 1980

49. Fowler RH: Non-parasitic benign cystic tumors of the spleen. Internat Abstr Surg 96:209, 1953

50. Volpe JA, DeNardo GL: The preoperative diagnosis of spleen cysts by scintiscanning. Am J Roentgenol 94:839, 1965

51. Shanser JD, Moss AA, Clark RE, Palubinskas AJ: Angiographic evaluation of cystic lesions of the spleen. Am J Roentgenol 119:166, 1973

52. Daneman A, Martin DJ: Congenital epithelial splenic cysts in children. Emphasis on sonographic appearances and some unusual features. Pediatr Radiol 12:119, 1982

53. Moran C, Geisse G: Epidermoid cysts of the spleen. J Can Assoc Radiol 28:150, 1977

54. Propper RA, Weinstein BJ, Skolnick ML, Kisloff B: Ultrasonography of hemorrhagic splenic cysts. J Clin Ultrasound 7:18, 1979

55. Soderstrom N: How to use cytodiagnostic spleen puncture. Acta Med Scand 199:1, 1976

56. Soderstrom N: Cytology of the spleen. p. 229. In Zajicek J (ed): Aspiration Biopsy Cytology, Part 2 Cytology of Infradiaphragmatic Organs. Basel, Karger, 1979

57. Anderson WAD: Pathology. Mosby, St. Louis, 1971

58. Siler J, Hunter TB, Weiss J, Haber K: Increased echogenicity of the spleen in benign and malignant disease. AJR 134:1011, 1980

59. Hunter TB, Haber K: Unusual sonographic appearance of the spleen in a case of myelofibrosis. Am J Roentgenol 128:138, 1977

60. Cooperberg P: Ultrasonography of the spleen. p. 244. In Sarti DA, Sample WF (eds): Diagnostic Ultrasound: Text and Cases. GK Hall, Boston, 1980

61. Cunningham JJ: Ultrasonic findings in isolated lymphoma of the spleen simulating splenic abscess. J Clin Ultrasound 6:412, 1978

62. Beckerman C, Gottschalk A: Diagnostic significance of the relative uptake of liver compared with spleen in 99m Tc sulfur colloid scintiphotography. J Nucl Med 12:237, 1971

63. Stivelman RL, Glaubitz JP, Crampton RS: Laceration of the spleen due to nonpenetrating trauma: One hundred cases. Am J Surg 106:888, 1963

64. Schwartz SI: Spleen. p. 1285. In Schwartz SI, Hume DM, Lillenei RC et al (eds): Principles of Surgery. McGraw-Hill, New York, 1974

65. Gentry LR, Brown JM, Lindren RD: Splenosis: CT demonstration of heterotopic autotransplantation of splenic tissue. J Comput Assist Tomogr 6:1184, 1982

66. Villarreal-Rios A, Mays ET: Efficacy of clinical evaluation and selective splenic arteriography in splenic trauma. Am J Surg 127:310, 1974

67. Lupien C, Sauerbrei EE: Healing in the traumatized spleen: Sonographic investigation. Radiology 151:181, 1984

68. Goodman PC, Federle MP: Splenorrgraphy: CT appearance. J Comput Assist Tomogr 4:251, 1980

69. Johnson MA, Cooperberg PL, Boisvert J et al: Spontaneous splenic rupture in infectious mononucleosis: Sonographic diagnosis and followup. AJR 136:111, 1981

70. Ein SH, Shandling B, Simpson JS, Stephens CA: Nonoperative management of traumatic spleen in children: How and why. J Pediatr Surg 113:117, 1978

71. Froelich JW, Simeone JF, McKusick KA et al: Radionuclide imaging and ultrasound in liver/spleen trauma: A prospective comparison. Radiology 145:457, 1982

72. Asher WM, Parvin S, Virgillio RW, Haber K: Echographic evaluation of splenic injury after blunt trauma. Radiology 118:411, 1976

73. Morgenstern L, Uyeda RY: Nonoperative management of injuries of the spleen in adults. Surgery 157:513, 1983

74. Michels NA: The variational anatomy of the spleen and splenic artery. Am J Anat 70:21, 1942

75. Kreel L, Mindel S: The radiographic position of the spleen. Br J Radiol 42:830, 1969

76. Landgarten S, Spencer RP: Splenic displacement due to gastric dilatation. J Nucl Med 13:223, 1971

77. Go RT, Tonami N, Schapiro RL, Christie JH: The manifestations of diaphragmatic and juxta-diaphragmatic diseases in the liver-spleen scintigraph. Radiology 115:119, 1975

78. Viamonte M, Sheldon JJ: Computed Tomography. p.320. In Margulis AR, Burhenne HJ (eds): Alimentary Tract Radiology (Abdominal Imaging) Vol. III. CV Mosby Company, St. Louis, 1979

79. Westcott JL, Krufky EL: The upside-down spleen. Radiology 105:517, 1972

80. D'Altorio RA, Cano JY: Upside-down spleen as cause of suprarenal mass. Urology 11:422, 1978

81. Madayag M, Bosniak MA, Beranbaum E, Becker J: Renal and suprarenal pseudotumors caused by variations of the spleen. Radiology 105:43, 1972

82. Brown RB, Dobbie RP: Splenic indentation of the gastric fundus resembling gastric neoplasm. Am J Roentgenol 81:599, 1959

83. Font RG, Sparks RD, Herbert GA: Ectopic spleen mimicking an intrinsic fundal lesion of the stomach. Am J Digest Dis 15:49, 1970

84. Gooding GAW: The ultrasonic and computed tomographic appearance of splenic lobulations: A consideration in the ultrasonic differential of masses adjacent to the left kidney. Radiology 126:719, 1978

85. Abell I: Wandering spleen with torsion of the pedicle. Ann Surg 98:722, 1933

86. Woodward DAK: Torsion of the spleen. Am J Surg 114:953, 1967

87. Gordon DH, Burrell MI, Levin DC et al: Wandering spleen—The radiological and clinical spectrum. Radiology 125:39, 1977

88. Sorgen RA, Robbins DI: Bleeding gastric varices secondary to wandering spleen. Gastrointest Radiol 5:25, 1980

89. Hunter TB, Haber KK: Sonographic diagnosis of a wandering spleen. Am J Roentgenol 129:925, 1977

90. Setiawan H, Harrell RS, Perret RS: Ectopic spleen. A sonographic diagnosis. Pediatr Radiol 12:152, 1982

91. Isikoff MB, White DW, Diaconis JN: Torsion of the wandering spleen, seen as a migratory abdominal mass. Radiology 123:36, 1977

92. Barnett SM, Poole JR, Briggs RC: Sequential liver-spleen scanning for documentation of wandering spleen. Clin Nuc Med 6:528, 1981

93. Broker FHL, Khettry J, Filler RM, Treves S: Splenic torsion and accessory spleen: A scintigraphic demonstration. J Pediatr Surg 10:913, 1975

94. Spencer RP, Dhawan V, Suresh K et al: Causes and temporal sequence of onset of functional asplenia in adults. Clin Nucl Med 3:17, 1978

95. Curtis GM, Movitz D: The surgical significance of the accessory spleen. Ann Surg 123:276, 1946

96. Subramanyam BR, Balthazar EJ, Horii SC: Sonography of the accessory spleen. AJR 143:47, 1984

97. Spencer RP, Wasserman I, Dhawan V, Suresh K: Incidence of functional splenic tissue after surgical splenectomy. Clin Nucl Med 2:63, 1977

98. Wahner-Roedler DL, Hoagland HC, Wahner HW: Idiopathic thrombocytopenic purpura: Detection of accessory splenic tissue. Clin Nucl Med 6:141, 1981

99. Babcock TL, Coker DD, Haynes JL, Conklin HB: Infarction of an accessory spleen causing an acute abdomen. Am J Surg 127:336, 1974

100. Bass RT, Yao ST, Freeark RJ: Torsion of an accessory spleen of the cecum presenting as acute appendicitis. N Eng J Med 277:1190, 1967

101. Stiris MG: Accessory spleen versus left adrenal tumor: Computed tomographic and abdominal angiographic evaluation. J Comput Assist Tomogr 4:543, 1980

102. Rosenkranz W, Kamhi B, Horowitz M: Retroperitoneal accessory spleen simulating a suprarenal mass. Br J Radiol 42:939, 1969

103. Clark RE, Korobkin M, Palubinskas AJ: Angiography of accessory spleens. Radiology 102:41, 1972

104. DasGupta TK, Busch RC: Accessory splenic tissue producing indentation of the gastric fundus resembling gastric neoplasm. N Engl J Med 263:1360, 1960

105. Beahrs JR, Stephens DH: Enlarged accessory spleens: CT appearance in post-splenectomy patients. AJR 135:483, 1980

106. Alter AJ, Uehling DT, Zwiebel WJ: Computed tomography of the retroperitoneum following nephrectomy. Radiology 133:663, 1979

107. Spencer RP: Accessory splenic tissue and recurrence of idiopathic thrombocytopenic purpura or other hematologic disorders. Clin Nucl Med 1:62, 1976

108. Verheyden CN, Beart RW, Clifton MD, Phyliky RL: Accessory splenectomy in management of recurrent idiopathic thrombocytopenic purpura. Mayo Clin Proc 53:442, 1978

109. Atkins HL, Goldman AG, Fairchild RG et al: Splenic sequestration of 99m-Tc labeled, heat treated red blood cells. Radiology 136:501, 1980

110. Moinuddin M: Splenosis: First scintigraphic demonstration of extension splenic implants. Clin Nuc Med 7:67, 1982

111. Jacobson SJ, DeNardo GL: Splenosis demonstrated by splenic scan. J Nucl Med 12:570, 1971

112. Pearson HA, Johnston D, Smith KA, Touloukian RJ: The born-again spleen: Return of splenic function after splenectomy for trauma. N Engl J Med 298:1389, 1978

113. Fitzer PM: Preoperative diagnosis of splenosis by 99m-Tc sulfur colloid scanning. Clin Nucl Med 2:348, 1977

114. Andrus MS, Johnston GS: Visualization of residual splenic tissue: A high intensity technique. Clin Nucl Med 6:577, 1981

115. Randall PA, Moller JH, Amplatz K: The spleen and congenital heart disease. AJR 119:551, 1973

116. DeMaeyer P, Wilms G, Baert AL: Polysplenia. J Comput Assist Tomogr 5:104, 1981

117. Ehrlich CP, Papanicolaou N, Treves S et al: Splenic scintigraphy using Tc-99m labeled heat-denatured red blood cells in pediatric patients: Concise communication. J Nucl Med 23:209, 1982

118. Rao BK, Shore RM, Lieberman LM, Polcyn RE: Dual radiopharmaceutical imaging in congenital asplenia syndrome. Radiology 145:805, 1982

119. Freedom RM, Treves S: Splenic scintigraphy and radionuclide venography in the heterotaxy syndrome. Radiology 107:381, 1973

120. Raymond HW, Zwiebel WJ, Gaumut: Fluid filled left upper quadrant masses. p.151. In Raymond HW, Zwiebel WJ (eds): Seminars in Ultrasound. Vol 1. Grune and Stratton, New York, 1980

121. Vick CW, Simeone JF, Ferrucci JT et al: Pancreatitis associated fluid collections involving the spleen: Sonographic and computed tomographic appearance. Gastrointest Radiol 6:247, 1981

122. Okuda K, Taguchit, Tshinara K, Kono A: Intrasplenic pseudocyst of the pancreas. Clin Gastroenterol 3:37, 1981

9

The Gastrointestinal Tract

For years, the gastrointestinal (GI) tract has created problems for ultrasound. If it is not full of fluid simulating a cyst, then it is full of stool causing a pseudotumor, or gas that creates artifacts and prevents visualization of many of the abdominal anatomic structures. The development of real-time ultrasound has greatly improved this situation by making it easier to identify the GI tract, especially by observing peristalsis. Today, evaluation of the GI tract is the "last frontier" for the sonologist/sonographer who really enjoys a challenge.

TECHNIQUE

Preparation

Ultrasonographic evaluation of the GI tract is tailored to the portion of the tract being examined, as is the prior preparation. If the upper GI tract (UGI, stomach and duodenum) is being examined, the patient is scanned prior to the oral ingestion of tap water. The patient may drink 10 to 40 oz of water through a straw, providing he or she is not scheduled for an UGI series the same day or is not prohibited from taking fluids by mouth. For evaluation of the lower GI tract (LGI, small bowel and colon), there is usually no preparation. Occasionally there may be the need for a water enema when evaluating a pelvic mass.

Scan Technique

Real-time ultrasound adds significantly to the recognition and evaluation of the GI tract by displaying characteristic changes in configuration of the tract produced by peristaltic contraction or motion of the intraluminal contents. While static scanning may identify the GI tract as a structure, it simply is not as informative as real-time scanning. Static scanning is similar to overhead films in an UGI series, and these are not as informative as fluoroscopy (real-time scanning) and spot films (freeze-frame images).

As a rule, patients are not referred to ultrasound for evaluation of the GI tract; they are referred because of nonspecific complaints or an abdominal mass. Usually, they have not as yet had barium studies. As such, it is important for the sonographer and sonologist to recognize a GI tract lesion when visualized and to evaluate it as completely as possible.

STOMACH

Sometimes a cystic mass may be identified in the left upper quadrant (Fig. 9-1). Is this stomach or a cystic mass of other origin? In past days, without real-time ultrasound, the examiner would give such a patient a substance to drink that produced carbonation, such as "sparkles" (Fig. 9-1D). The patient would be scanned before and after drinking to evaluate the mass for change. As a rule, a dramatic change would occur once air had entered the "mass." It is easier to observe air within the stomach than to try and denote a change in fluid amount, such as would be seen after drinking large amounts of fluid or nasogastric tube suction. Also prior to real-time ultrasound, the examiner could scan the patient on another day to look for a change in the mass; however, the entire study is greatly simplified with real-time ultrasound. By viewing the cystic "mass" with real-time scanning, one can observe characteristic peristalsis. If no motion is visible, the patient can be asked to drink 10 to 40 oz of tap water while erect, which will permit the examiner to monitor the change on real-time ultrasound. If the "mass" is indeed fluid-filled stomach, real-time ultrasound will determine it as such, since a swirling motion and many microbubbles of air will be seen. (Fig. 9-2).

Although the most common evaluation of the stomach is to differentiate it from a cystic mass, there may occasionally be a solid mass in the left upper quadrant and a question concerning its relationship to stomach. Once again, the patient is scanned with real-time ultrasound prior to water ingestion. Then the patient drinks 10 to 40 oz of tap water through a straw. The straw is used to diminish the amount of air ingested. The scanning begins with the patient erect and continues in the left lateral decubitus position, supine, and right lateral decubitus positions, much like a barium UGI series. By

moving patients through these various maneuvers, the examiner takes advantage of the fluid in the stomach as an acoustic window, which displaces the air to the nondependent location. With transverse, longitudinal, and sometimes oblique scans, it is usually easy to identify the stomach and its relationship to the mass in question.[1] The only real limitation of this entire technique is an uncooperative patient or one unable to move, which is infrequent.

To specifically scan the stomach for intraluminal mass or masses, a different method would need to be employed.[2] Some investigators give 1 mg of hyposcin-N-butylbromide (Busopan), a smooth muscle relaxant, intramuscularly before giving fluid. Then, 1,000 ml of tea are given in 3 to 5 minutes, using a straw. The patient is scanned in a half-sitting or shallow left posterior position.[2] Others recommend 1 mg of intravenous Glucagon before oral water for gastric distension.[3] This method produces gastric dilatation for 30 to 60 minutes.

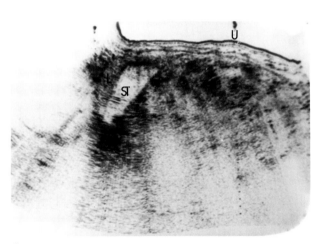

A

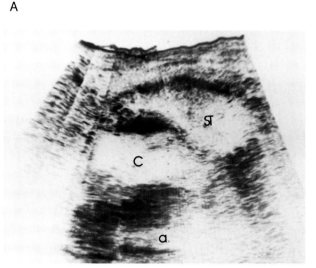

C

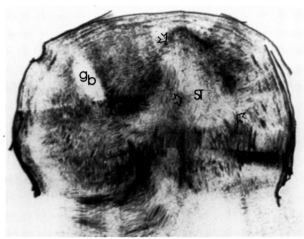

B

Fig. 9-1. Fluid-filled stomach and mass. **(A)** Longitudinal static scan to the left of midline. A fluid-filled mass *(ST)* is seen inferior to the left lobe of the liver *(L)*. (*U*, level of the umbilicus.) **(B)** Transverse static scan. A hypoechoic mass *(ST)* with poorly defined margins (arrows) is seen in the left upper quadrant. (*gb*, gallbladder.) **(C)** Transverse static, cone-down view of the mass. The cystic mass *(ST)* is seen to be comma-shaped and is anterior to an anechoic mass (*C*, pseudocyst) in the area of the pancreas. (*a*, aorta.) *(Figure continues.)*

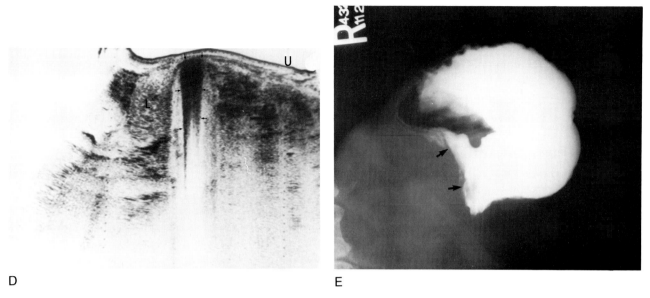

D

E

Fig. 9-1 *(Continued).* **(D)** Longitudinal static scan at the same location as Figure **(A)** taken after oral ingestion of "sparkles" which produces carbonation. In the area of the previous mass there is a reflective pattern (reverberation artifacts, arrows) produced by the air in the stomach. (*L*, liver; *U*, level of the umbilicus.) **(E)** Upper GI series, lateral view. The gastric antrum is noted to be compressed (arrows). The pseudocyst produced partial gastric outlet obstruction.

When specifically examining for hypertrophic pyloric stenosis, the procedure is begun with the patient in a supine position. No fluid is needed, except at times to quiet the patient. Fluid intake is minimized, since the stomach is often already filled with fluid owing to the obstructive effect of the stenosis. The examination by real-time ultrasound evaluates the stomach and identifies the region of the pylorus. This region should be scanned in the longitudinal and transverse planes to obtain views of the wall from which measurements can be taken. The transverse plane should be 90° to the long axis of this channel for the most accurate measurement. By obtaining long-axis views, the examiner can often see the radiologic "string sign" so characteristic of pyloric stenosis. With the patient drinking fluid, the lumen is often nicely outlined.

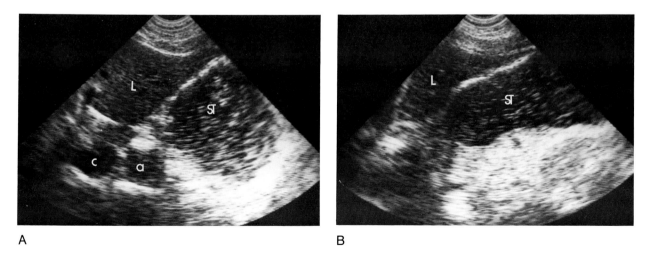

A

B

Fig. 9-2. Microbubbles in stomach. Transverse **(A)** and longitudinal **(B)** scans of a fluid-filled stomach *(ST)*. Note all the small linear echodensities representing microbubbles of air within the ingested fluid. (*L*, liver; *a*, aorta; *c*, inferior vena cava.)

DUODENUM

The duodenum may cause problems at times either owing to its air interfering with visualization of the head of the pancreas or its fluid content stimulating a mass (Fig. 9-3). The duodenum can be evaluated by the same techniques used in gastric scanning: a scan is made before the patient's ingestion of water, then another after ingestion of 10 to 40 oz of tap water and while the patient is erect. By placing the patient in the right lateral decubitus position, the duodenum is nicely outlined with fluid. This entire technique of fluid distension of the stomach and duodenum can be used to evaluate the pancreas and other prevertebral structures.

SMALL BOWEL

For evaluation of the small bowel, no special water technique is employed. If fluid-filled structures are seen and their bowel origin is in question, the examiner simply scans with real-time ultrasound, looking for peristal-

sis, air movement, or movement of the intraluminal fluid contents. In most cases, some peristalsis is seen. If not, bowel can usually be identified by its characteristic appearance; it is tubular in long axis and round in transverse. Often the valvulae conniventes may be seen within the small bowel that is distended with fluid.

COLON

Ultrasound is usually not used to evaluate the colon. Occasionally, the colon may be fluid-filled (usually in diarrhea or obstruction) and present as a mass. In such case, ultrasound scanning visualizes a fluid-filled tubular structure in the characteristic location of colon and often the haustral markings in the ascending and transverse colon are seen. When a solid mass is present, it may be difficult to identify its colonic origin unless the bowel wall can be seen as well as the echogenic air-filled lumen.

The water-enema technique is generally reserved for evaluation of pelvic masses.[4] When there is a question as

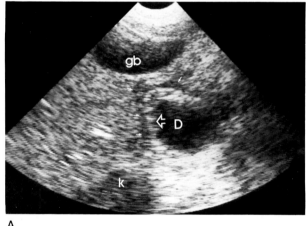

A

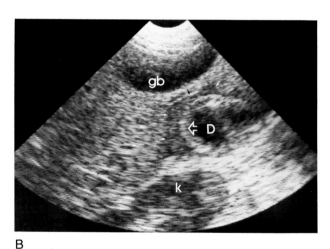

B

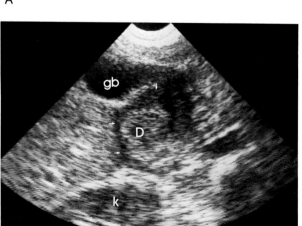

C

Fig. 9-3. Fluid-filled duodenum. Longitudinal real-time scans through a distended (**A**), partially contracted (**B**), and contracted (**C**) second portion of the duodenum *(D)*. Note that the duodenal wall (hypoechoic areas, arrows) is thickened. The patient had pancreatitis with inflammation of the bowel wall. The duodenum was identified on real-time scans by its location and peristalsis. (*gb*, gallbladder; *k*, right kidney).

to whether a mass is colonic or pelvic, a water enema may be used (Fig. 9-4). In this procedure the patient is first scanned with his or her bladder full. Then a barium enema bag is filled half full with lukewarm water or isotonic saline. A Bortex enema tip is inserted into the rectum, and instillation of the water is controlled, with the patient initially in the left lateral decubitus position. The examiner can follow the rectum and rectosigmoid colon with real-time scanning, similarly to how fluoroscopy is used in a barium enema. As a rule, this technique is only used for evaluation of the rectum and rectosigmoid colon to differentiate a questioned pelvic mass. The well-defined fluid-filled bowel provides a soft tissue interface and establishes a boundary between various pelvic structures, which permits assessment of tumor extension.[4] It also defines the relationship to the sacrum. This technique is not routinely used, since the patient often experiences discomfort with distention and the pelvic mass origin can usually be sorted out without this technique.

Future

Some investigators have evaluated the use of a high-frequency transducer mounted to a gastroscope.[5] This technique visualizes small hepatic and pancreatic tumors as well as intrinsic bowel wall lesions. Although the procedure is technically more difficult than conventional ultrasound, it appears to provide information not currently available.

Others have evaluated the use of an endoluminal ultrasound scan to evaluate the degree of tumor infiltration in the muscular wall and perirectal tissue.[6] With further development this equipment may also be a valuable additional diagnostic tool in evaluation of GI tract tumors.

NORMAL ANATOMY

There are certain patterns which help to identify the GI tract on ultrasound, and these are related to gas, mucus, and fluid within the tract. Intraluminal air is

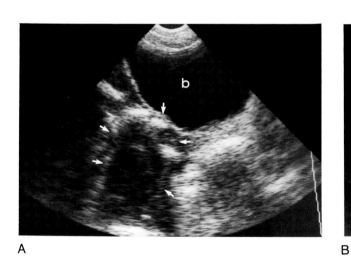

A

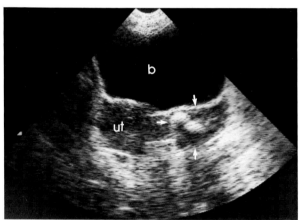

B

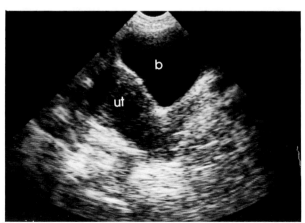

C

Fig. 9-4. Colon—Water enema technique. This patient was referred for evaluation of a possible pelvic mass. A mass effect (arrows) was seen within the left pelvis on longitudinal (**A**) and transverse (**B**) scans. The uterus *(ut)* was noted to be separate from the "mass" on transverse (**B**) and right longitudinal scans (**C**) (*b*, bladder.) To differentiate the "mass" from colon, a water enema was performed under real-time visualization. *(Figure continues.)*

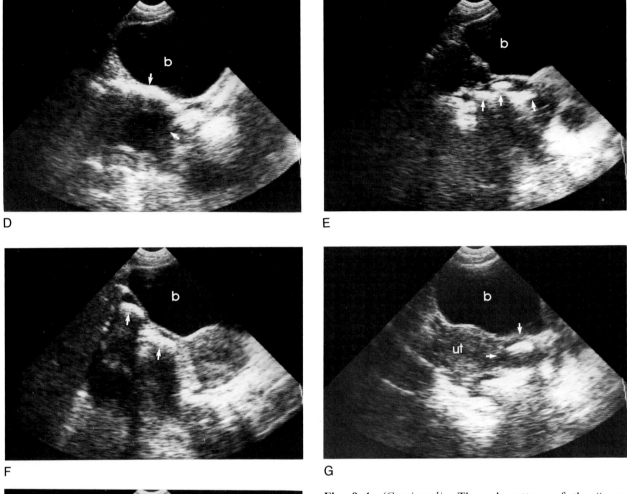

D

E

F

G

H

Fig. 9-4 *(Continued).* The echopattern of the "mass" (arrows) was seen to change during the water enema on sequential longitudinal (**D,E,F**) and transverse (**G,H**) scans. The dense echoes (arrows), due to the air, were seen to move. The "mass" seen on ultrasound was colon. (*ut*, uterus; *b*, bladder.)

echogenic and is usually associated with an incomplete or mottled distal acoustic shadow produced by the scattering effect of gas contained within the tract.[7-11] This shadow may appear similar to that produced by stones.[11] The mucus pattern is an intraluminal echogenicity but is not associated with an acoustic shadow.[8-14] The rim of lucency represents the wall (intima, media, and serosa),

and its periserosal fat produces the outer echogenic border of the tract wall[12,13] (Fig. 9-5). This rim should not measure greater than 5 mm even when that portion of the tract is contracted.[11] If that portion of the tract is distended, it should not measure more than 3 mm.[15] The thickness is measured from the edge of the echogenic core (intraluminal gas) to the outer border of the anechoic halo (bowel wall)[15] (Fig. 9-5). If the segment is dilated, the measurement is taken from the fluid to the outside of the wall. Distension is considered adequate if the stomach is greater than 8 cm, the small bowel is greater than 3 cm, and the lower bowel is greater than 5 cm.[15] The entire halo should measure less than 2 cm.[10] When this abnormal pattern is present, it is pathologically significant in greater than 90 percent of patients.[14] However, it is seen in benign disease in greater than 50 percent of cases.[14] As such, the GI tract in cross-section

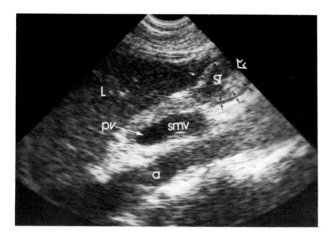

Fig. 9-5. Target pattern. Longitudinal midline scan through the contracted stomach. By the level and location, it can be surmised that the target (open arrow) represents gastric antrum. The wall is the hypoechoic area (arrows) around the lumen *(ST)*, the echogenic center. The thickness of the wall is determined by measuring from the edge of the echogenic center to the outer border of the halo. (*L*, liver; *a*, aorta; *smv*, superior mesenteric vein; *pv*, main portal vein.)

looks much like a target, while in long axis, it looks much like a kidney.[9,11,14]

When fluid is within the tract, it gives intraluminal transonicity, with motion of tiny particles seen within the fluid in a linear pattern.[10,11] These particles represent trapped intraluminal gas and/or food particles. The direction of the bubbly motion characteristically depends on the segment of the tract being scanned.[11]

Stomach

On the usual ultrasound scan of the upper abdomen, the stomach as a whole is not visualized. There are, however, portions which can be frequently identified even without gastric distension. The esophagogastric (EG) junction can be seen on a longitudinal scan to the left of midline as a "bull's-eye" or "target" structure anterior to the aorta and posterior to the left lobe of the liver, next to the hemidiaphragm (Fig. 9-6). Visualization of the EG junction depends on the left lobe of the liver being large enough to project anterior to it. Without the left lobe in this location, the EG junction is not usually identified. It is important to be familiar with this structure, as at times it can be misinterpreted as an abnormality.

The gastrum antrum can also be seen as a "target" sign in the midline (Fig. 9-5). This configuration can be seen on longitudinal scanning just inferior to the liver. Air is often seen within the lumen.

The remainder of the stomach is not usually visualized without water distension. With distension, the majority of the stomach can usually be visualized, provided the patient drinks at least 40 oz and the stomach does not rapidly empty into the duodenum and small bowel (Figs. 9-2 and 9-7). To promote nonemptying, the patient may be asked to drink while in the left lateral decubitus position. The patient is then scanned, first in this position, then in the supine, and right lateral decubitus positions. The wall of the stomach is thin and uniform. There should be no intraluminal masses, provided the patient has not eaten and there is no gastric outlet obstruction. Peristalsis occurs with a swirling fashion, much like a tornado.

Duodenum

As a rule, only the gas filled duodenal cap is seen in its characteristic location to the right of the pancreas (Fig. 9-8). Sometimes fluid may be seen within the second portion of the duodenum (Figs. 9-3 and 9-9). In either case, the duodenum is identified by its characteristic location and contiguity with the stomach.

The duodenum may be divided into four portions.[16] The first portion is superior and courses anteroposteriorly from the pylorus to the level of the neck of the gallbladder. At the level of the gallbladder, the duodenum takes a sharp bend into the second or descending portion, which runs along the right side of the inferior

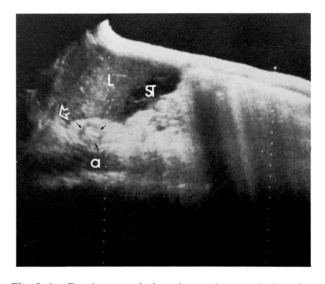

Fig. 9-6. Esophagogastric junction and stomach. Longitudinal static scan to the left of midline. The EG junction (arrows) is seen as a target lesion anterior to the aorta *(a)*, inferior to the diaphragm (open arrow), and posterior to the left lobe of the liver *(L)*. (*ST*, fluid-filled stomach.)

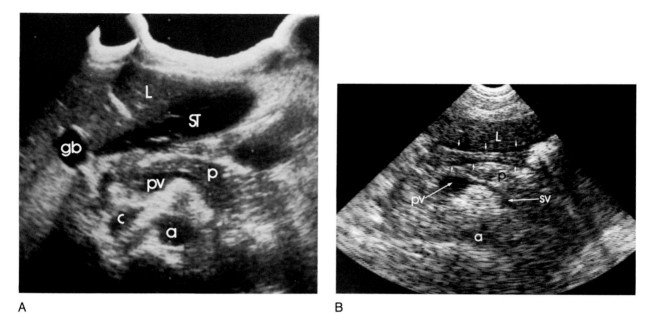

A   B

Fig. 9-7. Gastric antrum. **(A)** Transverse scan. The fluid-filled gastric antrum *(ST)* is seen at the midline anterior to the pancreas *(p)*. (*gb*, gallbladder; *c*, inferior vena cava; *a*, aorta; *L*, liver.) **(B)** Transverse scan of the contracted antrum. The anterior and posterior walls (arrows) are seen as lucent areas with the lumen echodense. (*pv*, main portal vein; *sv*, splenic vein; *a*, aorta; *L*, liver; *p*, pancreas.)

vena cava approximately at the level of L4 (Figs. 9-3 and 9-9). The transverse portion passes right to left with slight inclination upward in front of the great vessels and crura (Fig. 9-9B). The fourth or ascending portion rises to the right of the aorta, reaches the upper border of L2 where

at the duodenojejunal flexure, it turns forward to become the jejunum (Fig. 9-9C). This portion is usually not seen with ultrasound.

Small Bowel

Most of the small bowel, other than duodenum, normally can not be visualized by ultrasound. One might see air moving within the abdomen with real-time ultrasound and not be able to identify the structure. Occasionally, fluid may be within the lumen. If there is adequate fluid, the valvulae conniventes may be seen as linear echodensities spaced 3 to 5 mm apart, a configuration referred to as the "keyboard" sign[10,17] (Fig. 9-10). The valvulae conniventes are seen in the duodenum and jejunum. The ileum appears with smooth featureless walls. The small bowel wall is less than 3 mm.[18]

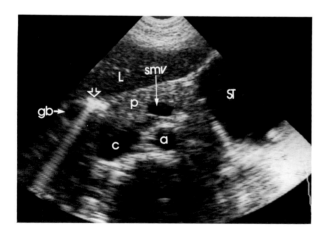

Fig. 9-8. Duodenum cap. On this transverse scan through the pancreas, the gas-filled second portion of the duodenum (open arrow) is identified by its location lateral to the head of the pancreas *(p)* and its reflective pattern (reverberation artifacts). Often on real-time, peristalsis may be seen. (*ST*, fluid-filled stomach; *smv*, superior mesenteric vein; *a*, aorta; *c*, inferior vena cava; *gb*, gallbladder; *L*, liver.)

Colon

Much like the small bowel, the colon is not usually visualized well enough on real-time ultrasound to be identified as such. Occasionally when filled with fluid, the colon can be identified by its haustral markings,

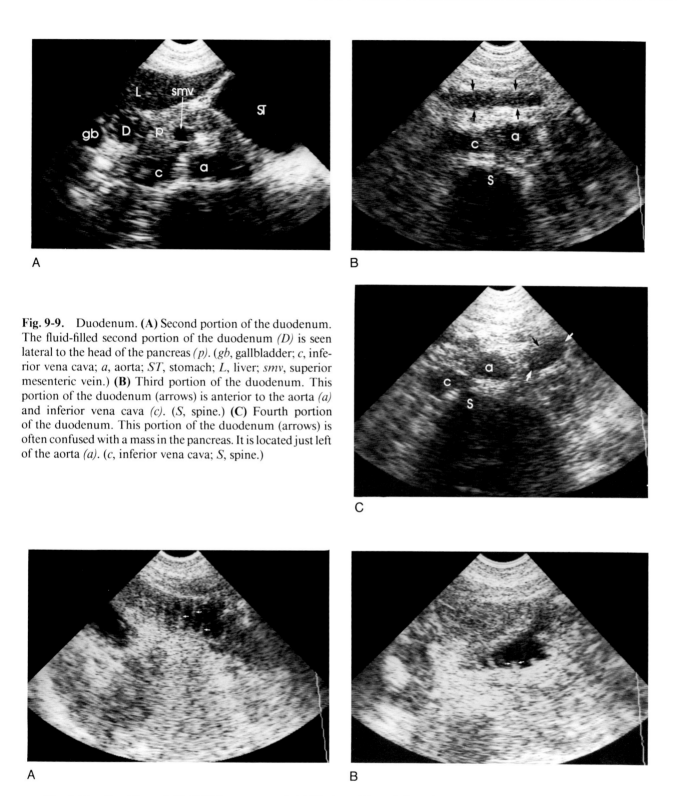

Fig. 9-9. Duodenum. **(A)** Second portion of the duodenum. The fluid-filled second portion of the duodenum *(D)* is seen lateral to the head of the pancreas *(p)*. (*gb*, gallbladder; *c*, inferior vena cava; *a*, aorta; *ST*, stomach; *L*, liver; *smv*, superior mesenteric vein.) **(B)** Third portion of the duodenum. This portion of the duodenum (arrows) is anterior to the aorta *(a)* and inferior vena cava *(c)*. (*S*, spine.) **(C)** Fourth portion of the duodenum. This portion of the duodenum (arrows) is often confused with a mass in the pancreas. It is located just left of the aorta *(a)*. (*c*, inferior vena cava; *S*, spine.)

Fig. 9-10. Small bowel. **(A,B)** This represents fluid-filled small bowel since the valvulae conniventes are identified as linear echogenic structures (arrows) approximately 3 to 5 mm apart within the fluid-filled bowel lumen.

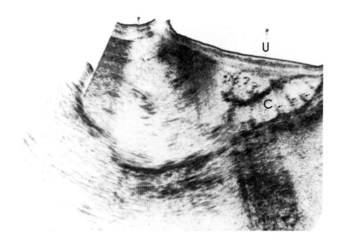

Fig. 9-11. Colon. This fluid-filled tubular structure on a right longitudinal scan is identified as colon *(C)* on the basis of the haustral marking (arrows) spaced 3 to 5 cm apart. (*U*, level of the umbilicus.)

which are 3 to 5 cm apart[10,17] (Fig. 9-11). While the ascending and transverse colon are seen to have haustral markings, the descending colon is seen as a tubular structure with an echogenic border.[10] At times, it may appear as a mass but can be identified as a tubular structure in its characteristic location.

ABNORMALITIES OF THE STOMACH

Gastric Dilatation

At times, a large fluid-filled stomach may present as an abdominal mass (Figs. 9-12 and 9-13). The fluid-filled stomach may be secondary to pylorospasm, inflammation, intrinsic or extrinsic tumor, electrolyte imbalance, diabetes, amyloidosis, neurologic disease, and medication.[19] Such a stomach is seen as a pear-shaped cystic structure that may fill the left upper quadrant, and sometimes even extend into the pelvis. The stomach is easily recognized with real-time ultrasound by its characteristic configuration, discrete thin walls, movement of strong echoes (food particles) when light pressure is applied, gas-fluid-food level, and compressibility.[18]

Gastric Duplication

Duplication cysts are embryologic mistakes and may or may not cause symptoms, depending on their location, size, and histology.[20] Gastric duplication is rare and may arise from the duodenum or pancreas; occasionally it arises without communication with the gastrointestinal tract.[21] These cysts occur more frequently in females

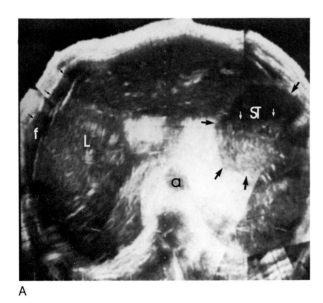

A

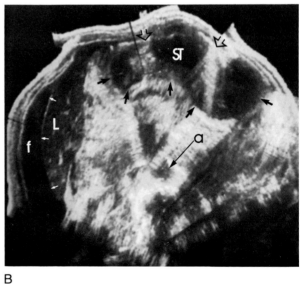

B

Fig. 9-12. Mass—Gastric dilatation. This patient, with a history of amyloidosis, presented with a left upper quadrant mass. **(A)** On this static transverse scan 14 cm above the umbilicus, a round cystic mass *(ST*, black arrows) with a fluid-fluid level (white arrows) is seen. (*a*, aorta; *L*, liver; *f*, small black arrows, ascites bordering the liver.) **(B)** At 11 cm above the umbilicus, the mass (*ST*, black arrows) is seen to be more anteriorly located than in **(A)** and extends across the midline. A reflective echopattern (reverberation artifacts, open arrows) due to air is seen anteriorly within the mass. (*L*, liver; *f*, white arrows, ascites; *a*, aorta.) *(Figure continues.)*

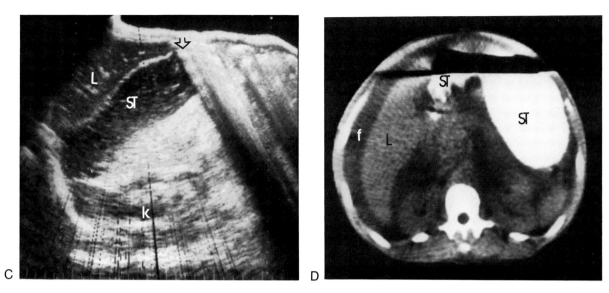

Fig. 9-12 *(Continued).* **(C)** On this longitudinal scan 6 cm to left of midline, the "mass" *(ST)* is seen to be inferior to liver *(L)* in the characteristic location for stomach. It contains many small linear echodensities that have a very reflective pattern (open arrows) due to air at its most anterior inferior border. (*k*, left kidney.) **(D)** CT scan, similar to **(B)**, which substantiates that the mass is stomach *(ST)*. (*L*, liver; *f*, ascites.)

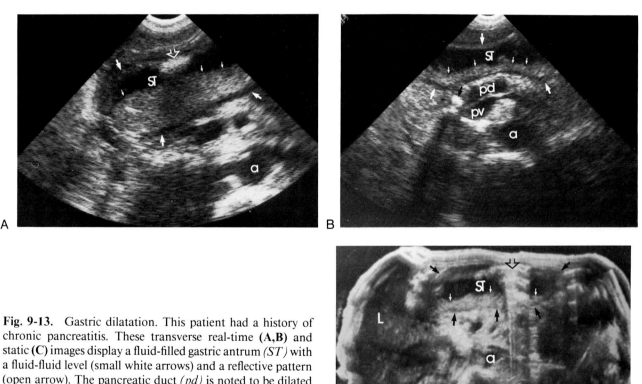

Fig. 9-13. Gastric dilatation. This patient had a history of chronic pancreatitis. These transverse real-time **(A,B)** and static **(C)** images display a fluid-filled gastric antrum *(ST)* with a fluid-fluid level (small white arrows) and a reflective pattern (open arrow). The pancreatic duct *(pd)* is noted to be dilated on **(B)** with an internal calculus (black arrow). (*a*, aorta; *pv*, main portal vein; *L*, liver.)

(2:1) and are usually on the greater curvature of the stomach.[20,23] Once cysts are identified, a search should be made for other duplications along the alimentary tract. Although duplications are usually epigastric, intrathoracic occurrences have been reported. Such a patient usually presents in infancy with symptoms of high intestinal obstruction including distension, vomiting, and abdominal pain. Duplications may also be associated with complications such as abdominal pain, vomiting, hemorrhage, and fistula formation.[21] The solid component of the mass is apparently caused by hemorrhage and inspissated material within the cyst.[23]

On ultrasound, such a cyst appears as an anechoic mass with a thin inner echogenic (mucosa) rim and a wider outer hypoechoic rim (muscle layer) (Fig. 9-14). This pattern should suggest an enteric cyst.[21,23]

The criteria for the diagnosis of gastric duplication include: cyst lined by alimentary tract epithelium; well-developed muscular wall; and contiguity with stomach. On ultrasound, the differential diagnosis for such a lesion would have to include mesenteric or omental cyst, pancreatic cyst or pseudocyst, enteric cyst, renal cyst, splenic cyst, congenital cyst of the left lobe of the liver, and gastric distension.[22]

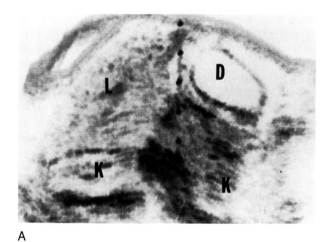

A

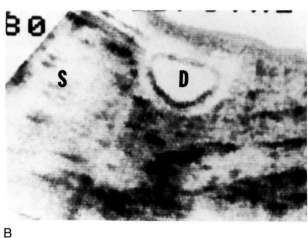

B

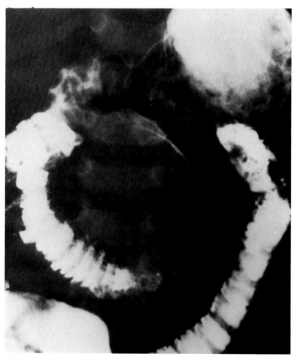

C

Fig. 9-14. Gastric duplication. A mass *(D)* is seen anteriorly within the left upper quadrant on transverse (**A**) and longitudinal (**B**) scans. It is anechoic with a thin echogenic inner lining. The outer anechoic wall is about 10 mm wide. (*L*, liver; *K*, kidneys; *S*, stomach.) (**C**) UGI. The epigastric mass compresses and displaces the antrum, duodenum and transverse colon. (From Moccia WA, Astacio JE, Kaude JV: Ultrasonographic demonstration of gastric duplication in infancy. Pediatr Radiol 11:52, 1981.)

Hypertrophic Pyloric Stenosis

Hypertrophic pyloric stenosis is familial, with a 4:1 male-to-female ratio. It is characterized by hypertrophy and hyperplasia of the circular muscle, which result in elongation of the pylorus and constriction of the canal.[24] The narrowing may lead to edema or inflammatory changes. The typical patient presents with projectile vomiting in the second or third week of life. An abdominal mass that is detected by palpation in 40 to 100 percent of cases is the hypertrophied muscle.[25,26]

The diagnosis of pyloric stenosis is usually based on medical history.[27] In the hands of the experienced clinician, the diagnosis is usually straightforward. With a

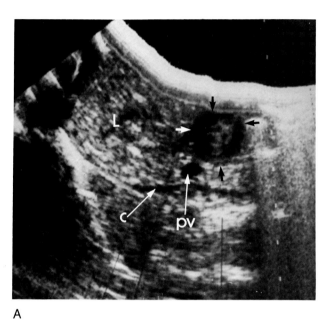

A

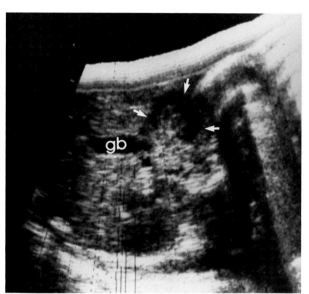

B

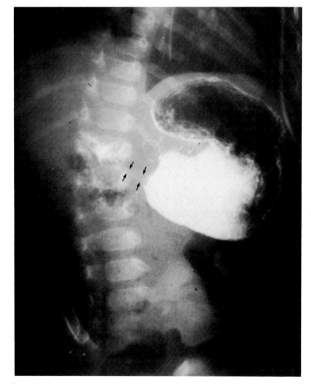

C

Fig. 9-15. Hypertrophic pyloric stenosis. **(A)** Longitudinal scan to the right of midline. In the location of the pylorus, a bull's-eye patterned mass (arrows) is seen. The wall (the lucent rim) is greater than 4 mm thick. (c, inferior vena cava; pv, portal vein; L, liver.) **(B)** Transverse scan with the bull's eye lesion (arrows) seen to the left of the gallbladder (gb). **(C)** UGI with typical narrowing (arrows) of the pyloric channel.

patient of the appropriate age, history of projectile vomiting, observation of peristaltic wave crossing the anterior abdominal wall, and palpation of the pyloric "olive," there is sufficient indication for surgery. When some of the clinical findings are unclear, imaging studies are necessary for the diagnosis. If there is a question, the UGI series is the diagnostic imaging procedure of choice, although there is a reported error rate of 4.5 to 11.1 percent. Such a series also involves ionizing radiation and introduces additional fluid into an obstructed stomach.[25,27]

Some authors advocate real-time ultrasound as the initial imaging procedure of choice, as it has the advantage of visualizing the hypertrophied muscle directly.[27–29] The lesion is seen as a target medial to the gallbladder, anterior and caudal to the portal vein, anterior to the kidney, and lateral to the head of the pancreas (Fig. 9-15). The wall or hypoechoic rim represents the hypertrophied muscle.[30,31] Normally, the wall thickness is less than 4 mm, with a diameter of less than 10 mm.[24,27–29] If the rim measures greater than 4 to 4.5 mm, and/or the diameter is greater than or equal to 13 to 13.4 mm, a diagnosis of pyloric stenosis can be made.[18,24,28,29,32] One series reported a 72 percent accuracy in diagnosing hypertrophic pyloric stenosis using an anteroposterior diameter of 1.5 cm or greater; a 92 percent accuracy was achieved using a wall thickness of 4 mm or greater.[33]

The target lesion associated with pyloric stenosis is located by orienting the transducer in a longitudinal plane. By aligning the transducer with the long axis of the pyloric channel, the most diagnostic images are obtained. This alignment displays the continuity of the mucosal and muscle layers between the stomach and pylorus and depicts the characteristic elongated pyloric channel as a mucosal double-track sign, such as described on barium studies[28,29,33] (Fig. 9-16). The length of the thickened segment is usually equal to or greater than 19 to 20 mm, with normal being less than 15 mm.[24] Using a range of 2 cm or greater for target lesion size, one study reports a 100 percent accuracy in diagnosing pyloric stenosis.[33] Indirect signs of pyloric stenosis on ultrasound include obstructed fluid-filled stomach, exaggerated peristaltic waves, failure of fluid to pass from the stomach into the duodenum, and failure to image the descending duodenum.[25,27] Known morphologic changes associated with pyloric stenosis include: impingment on the fluid-filled antrum, prepyloric antral thickening, extensive fluid in the proximal portion of the pyloric canal, and the angle formed between the antral peristaltic wave and the pyloric mass.[32] Since ultrasound scanning results in no false-positive diagnoses of pyloric

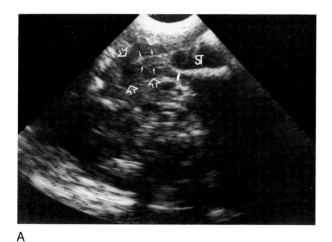

A

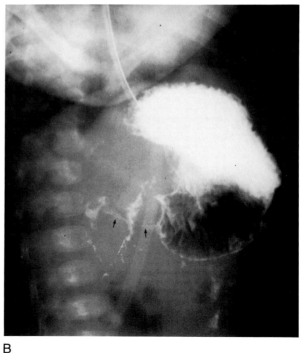

B

Fig. 9-16. Hypertrophic pyloric stenosis. **(A)** This is an oblique transverse view demonstrating the pyloric channel (small arrows) in long axis. The contracted echogenic lumen is seen, as well as the thickened wall (open arrows). (*ST*, fluid-filled stomach.) **(B)** UGI with the typical narrowing (arrows) of the pyloric channel.

stenosis, it is recommended as the initial diagnostic imaging procedure in a patient suspected of pyloric stenosis. If the ultrasound scan is positive, no other exam is needed. If ultrasound is negative, or equivocal, then UGI series may be performed.[27] Some believe that nonvisualization of the pylorus is strong evidence against pyloric stenosis.[33]

Besides evaluating patients for hypertrophic pyloric stenosis, ultrasound can be used to monitor patients after surgery. In one series, the pyloric wall was found to return to normal (4 mm) within 6 weeks of surgery.[24]

Gastritis and Ulcer Disease

Chronic gastritis may cause diffuse or localized thickening of the gastric wall, whereas localized thickening is seen with benign gastric ulcer disease. This thickening

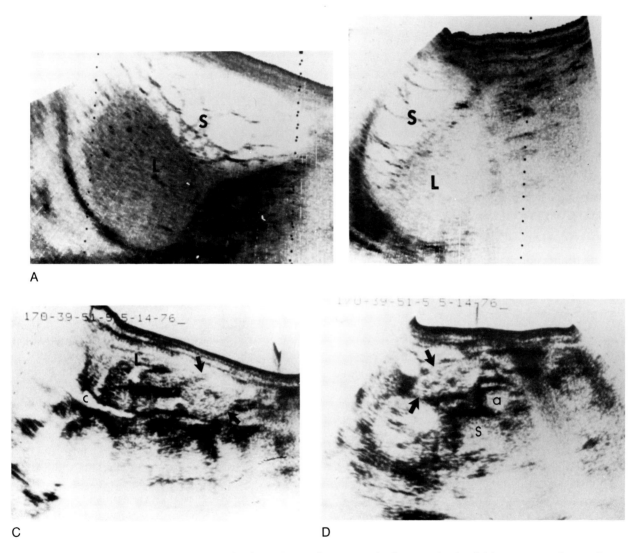

Fig. 9-17. Peptic ulcer disease—Complications. Case 1. Scans 1 week after an episode of right upper quadrant pain. **(A)** Longitudinal scan demonstrating a large predominately anechoic fluid collection along the anterior and diaphragmatic surfaces of the liver *(L)*, which displace it posteriorly. There are septa *(S)* within the fluid. **(B)** Transverse scan with the septa *(S)* seen within the fluid as well as the separation of the liver *(L)* from the rib cage. The patient had an UGI series demonstrating an 8-mm ulcer that was projecting from the anterosuperior aspect of the pylorus. Case 2. Duodenal ulcer penetrating into the pancreas. **(C)** Longitudinal scan 2 cm to the right of midline with a solid mass in the pancreatic head (arrows). *(L,* liver; *c,* inferior vena cava.) **(D)** Transverse scan with a solid mass (arrows) that involves the pancreatic head. *(a,* aorta; *S,* spine.) (From Madrazo BL, Hricak H, Sandler MA, Eyler WR: Sonographic findings in complicated peptic ulcer disease. Radiology 140:457, 1981.)

can not be distinguished from tumor by ultrasound alone.[18] Ultrasound is not routinely used to evaluate ulcer disease, and there have been no reports of ulcer craters identified by this modality.

Ultrasound may be helpful in evaluating complications of peptic ulcer disease[34] (Fig. 9-17). The most common complications of peptic ulcer disease in decreasing order of frequency are obstruction, hemorrhage, penetration, and perforation.[24] Perforation occurs in 3 to 13 percent of patients with benign peptic ulcer disease. Thirty percent of patients with perforation do not exhibit air on a radiograph. In addition, penetration into adjacent structures may not be apparent on an abdominal radiograph or contrast study. The passage of food and digestive juices through the perforation incite peritoneal response and production of an exudate. On ultrasound the exudate may appear fluid-filled, mixed, or solid (Fig. 9-17).

Since the distal stomach and proximal duodenum are the most frequent sites of peptic ulcer disease, focal peritonitis due to perforation usually is located in the right upper quadrant, which is accessible to ultrasound scanning. This characteristic peritoneal exudate surrounds the perforated ulcer and can vary depending on the elapsed time between the perforation and surgery. In its early stage the exudate is fibrinous and in its later stage becomes viscous. Unlike free peritoneal fluid, this localized exudate does not change shape or location when the patient's position is altered.[34]

Chronic Granulomatous Disease

Chronic granulomatous disease is a X-linked recessive disorder that results from a defect in the bactericidal activity of the polymorphonuclear leukocytes.[35] Stomach involvement is not common but may be underdiagnosed owing to incomplete obstruction and spontaneous resolution. On ultrasound, circumferential antral thickening causes a target lesion.[35] Such thickening can not be differentiated on ultrasound from malignancy, inflammation such as Crohn's disease, peptic ulcer disease, and post-radiation changes.

Benign Tumors

Small benign polypoid lesions are usually not seen with ultrasound; however, one study reports identification of polypoid gastric lesions.[2] These lesions could only be seen with fluid distension of the stomach and appeared as solid masses adherent to the gastric wall.[2] The differential diagnosis of such polypoid lesions would have to include hyperplastic polyps, pseudopolypoid lesions, polypoid infiltration, or gastric mucosal lymphoma.[2]

Leiomyoma, the most common tumor of the stomach, can be seen as a mass similar to carcinoma and is usually small and asymptomatic.[18,36] It is four times more frequent than sarcoma, its patient population having a mean age of 41 years. Even when the leiomyoma is large and symptomatic, it is rarely palpable.[36] An exogastric pedunculated configuration, though sometimes seen, is uncommon. It may appear as a solid mass with cystic areas that represent necrosis[36] (Fig. 9-18).

Malignant Tumors

GASTRIC CARCINOMA

Ninety to 95 percent of malignant tumors of the stomach are carcinomas, with 3 percent being lymphoma and 2 percent leiomyosarcomas. Gastric carcinoma is the sixth leading cause of cancer death in the United States and occurs more frequently in males (2:1). One half of these tumors occur in the pylorus and one fourth occur in the body and fundus. The lesions may be fungating, ulcerated, diffuse, polypoid, and/or superficial. Three fourths of these tumors occur in patients greater than 50 years. The clinical manifestations are nonspecific, with 25 percent of patients presenting with a palpable mass.[26]

On ultrasound, the examiner looks for the typical target or pseudo-kidney ascribed to GI lesions[18,19,37] (Figs. 9-19 to 9-20). While the target lesion may be seen with tumor, it also may be secondary to lymphoma, metastatic disease, caustic gastritis, pancreatitis involving the stomach, and chronic granulomatous disease of childhood[38] (Fig. 9-21). Identification depends on the type of tumor, its location, and extent. It may be seen as a large mass in the left upper quadrant or as gastric wall thickening; the latter is due to tumor infiltration of the wall and may or may not exhibit surrounding inflammatory changes.[39] This wall thickening may be localized or diffuse.[18,37,40] With localized thickening, the wall is eccentrically thickened (Figs. 9-19 and 9-20). The wall may have a C-shaped appearance when only the involved wall is delineated.[18,39] When ultrasound demonstrates a mass, it usually indicates significant infiltration of the mucosa and muscularis and/or exogastric extension. An antral carcinoma may present with gastric dilatation due to obstruction. This gastric dilatation may also be secondary to pylorospasm, inflammation, intrinsic or extrinsic tumor, electrolyte imbalance, diabetes, neurologic disease, or medication.[19]

Besides identifying the gastric primary tumor, ultrasound may be used for staging.[41] When such a patient is referred for evaluation of liver metastases (Fig. 9-22), it is

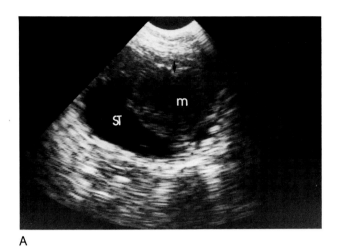

A

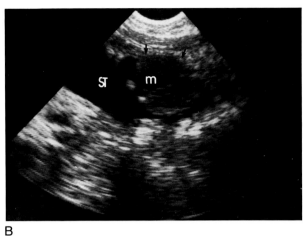

B

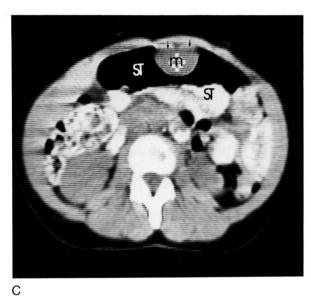

C

Fig. 9-18. Gastric leiomyoma. Transverse **(A)** and longitudinal **(B)** real-time scans of the fluid-filled stomach *(ST)*. An echodense mass *(m)*, the leiomyoma, is seen projecting from the anterior surface of the stomach (arrows). **(C)** CT image further confirming the presence of a soft-tissue density intraluminal gastric *(ST)* mass *(m)*.

worthwhile to gather additional information about extent of the tumor. This is done by performing a complete sonographic examination of the abdomen and pelvis and by attempting to visualize the primary neoplasm and its relationship to surrounding organs (Fig. 9-22). Ultrasound has a sensitivity of 71.4 percent and a specificity of 85.7 percent for evaluation of lymph node metastases.[41] For direct invasion, it has a sensitivity of 75 percent and a specificity of 100 percent.[41] This carcinoma may spread to the surrounding gastric wall and adjacent organs and structures directly, or it may spread via lymphatics to perigastric lymph nodes. There is hematogenous spread to the liver and distant organs. In addition, there is peritoneal seeding to the omentum, parietal peritoneum, ovary, and pelvic cul-de-sac (Fig. 9-22F). Since the only effective therapy at the present time is surgical resection, tumor type and extent are based on its location and on its exogastric spread. Preoperative

knowledge of local and distant tumor extent greatly help the surgeon to plan the therapeutic approach more accurately. Such knowledge may even obviate a laparotomy in patients with far advanced disease. Such patients may instead receive other types of treatment and undergo surgery only if and when palliative procedure for relief of obstruction and/or hemorrhage are needed.[41]

LYMPHOMA

Lymphoma can occur as a primary tumor of the GI tract. As a primary tumor, it most often affects the stomach and ileum and, less frequently, the colon and rectum. In disseminated lymphoma, the primary tumor occurs as multifocal lesions in the GI tract. Presumably, gastric lymphoma arises within lymphoid aggregates and represents 1 to 5 percent of gastric neoplasms.[42] In the small bowel and colon, lymphoma originates in normal

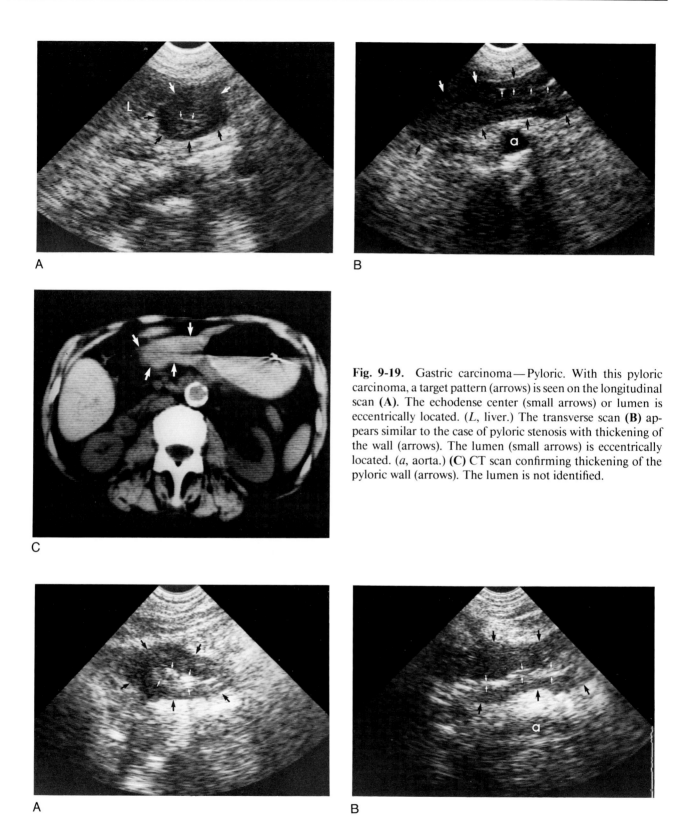

Fig. 9-19. Gastric carcinoma—Pyloric. With this pyloric carcinoma, a target pattern (arrows) is seen on the longitudinal scan **(A)**. The echodense center (small arrows) or lumen is eccentrically located. (*L*, liver.) The transverse scan **(B)** appears similar to the case of pyloric stenosis with thickening of the wall (arrows). The lumen (small arrows) is eccentrically located. (*a*, aorta.) **(C)** CT scan confirming thickening of the pyloric wall (arrows). The lumen is not identified.

Fig. 9-20. Gastric carcinoma—Pyloric. On longitudinal **(A)** and transverse **(B)** scans, there is thickening of the gastric wall (black arrows). The lumen is echogenic (white arrows). (*a*, aorta.)

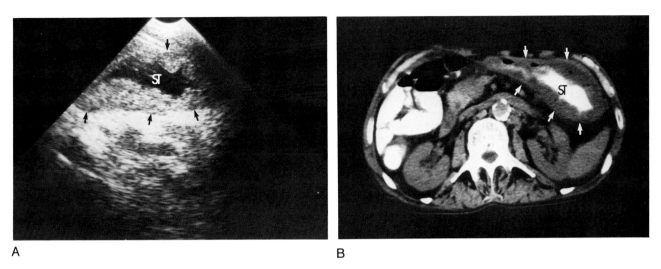

A   B

Fig. 9-21. Gastric wall thickening—Pancreatitis. This patient had pancreatitis and pseudocysts within the tail of the pancreas. The gastric wall (arrows) is noted to be thickened on transverse real-time scan **(A)** and CT scan **(B)**. (*ST*, fluid-filled stomach.)

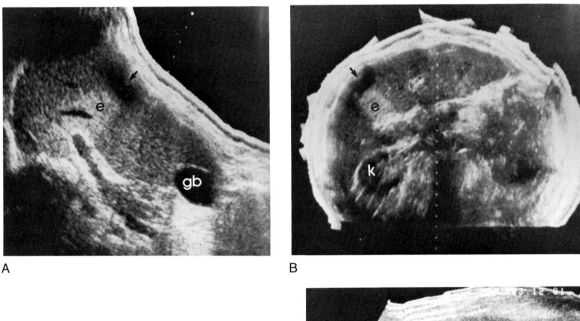

A   B

Fig. 9-22. Gastric metastases. Left lateral decubitus longitudinal **(A)** and transverse **(B)** scans of the liver in a patient with gastric carcinoma. An anechoic lesion (arrow) proved to be a metastasis. Note the posterior acoustic enhancement *(e)*. (*k*, right kidney; *gb*, gallbladder.) **(C)** Transverse scan of the right kidney in a patient with tumor recurrence. A rounded 2 cm hypoechoic metastasis is seen in the posterior kidney (arrow). (*L*, liver.) *(Figure continues.)*

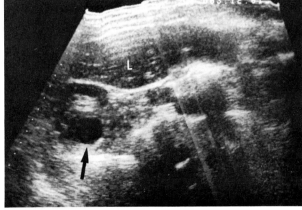

C

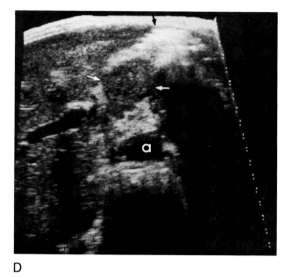

D

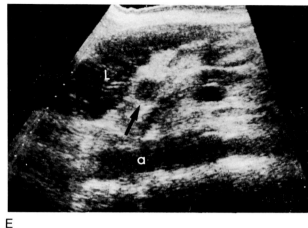

E

F

Fig. 9-22 *(Continued).* **(D)** Transverse scan in a patient with tumor of the gastric fundus. A rounded solid mass, which has medium-level echoes (white arrows) due to lymph node metastasis, is seen along the lesser curvature, medial to the acoustic shadow that is caused by air within the body of the stomach (black arrows). (*a,* aorta.) **(E)** Longitudinal scan along the aorta *(a)* in a patient with an ulcerated tumor of the lesser curvature. In the celiac region, an enlarged lymph node is seen as a relatively small (1.5 cm) rounded solid mass with medium-level echoes (arrow). (*L,* liver.) **(F)** Longitudinal scan demonstrating an echodense mass *(m)* that is separate from the uterus *(ut).* This represents metastatic disease to the ovary or Kruckenberg's tumor. (*b,* bladder; *U,* level of the umbilicus.) (Figs. C–E from Derchi LE, Biggi E, Rollandi GA et al: Sonographic staging of gastric cancer. AJR 140:273, © Am Roentgen Ray Society, 1983)

mucosal lymphoid aggregates. Gastric lymphoma has a number of gross anatomic findings including enlarged and thickened mucosal folds, multiple submucosal nodules, ulceration, a large predominately extraluminal mass, or a combination of two or more of these features.[42] Patients with gastric lymphoma present with similar symptoms to those with gastric carcinoma. Ninety percent of lymphoma patients complain of pain,[26] and in 25 percent there is an abdominal mass.[42]

On ultrasound, gastric lymphoma is usually seen as a relatively large and poorly echogenic (hypoechoic) mass[18,39,42–44] (Fig. 9-23). There may be marked thickening of the gastric walls due to tumor infiltration.[18] One group of investigators have reported two features helpful in the diagnosis of gastric lymphoma.[42] The first is a characteristic spoke-wheel pattern within the target-like lymphomatous mass. The spoke-wheel pattern is produced by the marked increase in thickness and height of the mucosal folds. The echogenic spokes are produced by the mucosal surfaces dividing the folds. The other pattern with lymphoma is the thickened gastric wall, which is hypoechoic. The pattern is homogeneous with an absence of induced fibroblastic reaction within the infiltrated wall. When an exophytic lesion is present, it may be difficult to differentiate lymphoma and leiomyosarcoma. Leiomyosarcoma is usually a complex mass having both solid hyperechoic tissue and areas of liquefactive necrosis.[42]

LEIOMYOSARCOMA

Leiomyosarcoma, the second most common gastric sarcoma, is usually a large bulky intramural or subserosal mass and represents 1 to 5 percent of gastric tumors.[26,45–47] These lesions occur in the fifth to sixth

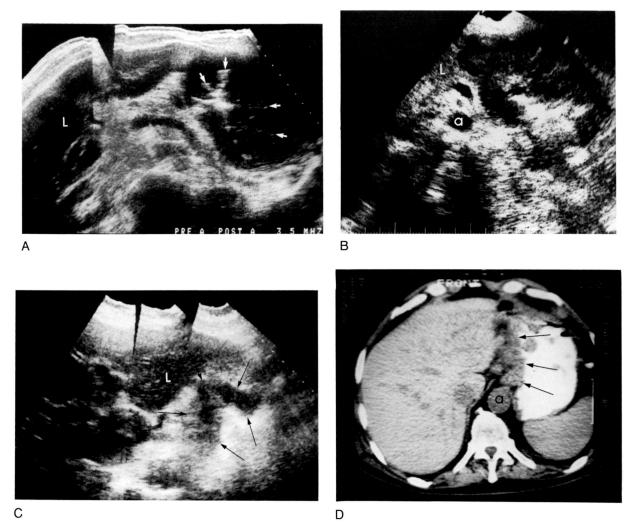

Fig. 9-23. Gastric lymphoma. Case 1. **(A)** Transverse scan with a large target-like mass occupying most of the left epigastrium. The thickened gastric wall has a hypoechoic, almost echofree structure. High and thick mucosal folds may be seen within the mass outlined by the strong luminal echoes (arrows) that radiate from an echogenic core towards the periphery like the spokes of the wheel. (*L*, liver.) Case 2. **(B)** Transverse scan with a large gastric mass. The thickened gastric wall is less echogenic than liver *(L)* parenchyma; the luminal echoes are distorted and irregular without a radial pattern. (*a*, aorta.) Case 3. **(C)** Transverse scan demonstrating thickening of only the lesser curvature and anterior wall of the stomach (arrows). (*L*, liver.) **(D)** CT scan shows both thickening (arrows) of the gastric wall and polypoid gastric lesions. (*a*, aorta.) (From Derchi LE, Banderali A, Bossi MC et al: The sonographic appearance of gastric lymphoma. J Ultrasound Med 3:251, 1984.)

decade of life.[46] They are generally globular or irregular and may attain a huge size, outstripping their blood supply with subsequent central necrosis leading to cystic degeneration and cavitation. This cavity may connect with the GI tract.[46]

On ultrasound, a typical target lesion may be identified, but the pattern is variable. If there is necrosis without liquefaction, the mass may appear without enhancement as a echofree zone.[45] With liquefactive necrosis, there will be fluid-containing spaces.[45] Hemorrhage and necrosis may occur causing irregular echoes or a cystic

cavity.[39] With a pattern of a solid mass anteriorly located outside a solid viscus, presence of necrosis, and intestinal lumen and/or air in close relation to the mass, a leiomyosarcoma is highly suggestive[45] (Fig. 9-24).

METASTATIC DISEASE

Metastatic carcinoma to the stomach is rare. The most common form is generalized lymphoma or leukemia, with most multiple growths primarily affecting the submucosa and muscularis.[26] If the lesion is aggressive, such

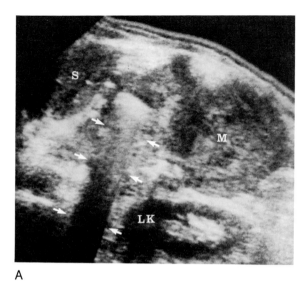
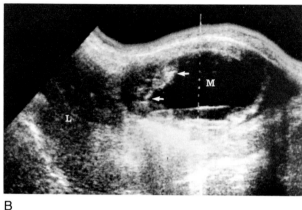

A   B

Fig. 9-24.   Gastric leiomyosarcoma. **(A)** Case 1. Longitudinal scan in the right lateral decubitus position showing a leiomyosarcoma along the greater curvature. A hyperechoic mass *(M)* is seen in the left upper quadrant, separate from spleen *(S)* and anterior to the left kidney *(LK)*. There is acoustic shadowing (arrows) from air in the gastric lumen following ingestion of water. **(B)** Case 2. Longitudinal scan with leiomyosarcoma within the anterior wall of the body of the stomach. A large mass *(M)* is seen that is hyperechoic at the periphery (arrows) and has a central fluid level due to liquefaction necrosis. *(L,* liver.) (From Subramanyam BR, Balthazar EJ, Raghavendra BN, Madamba MR: Sonography of exophytic gastrointestinal leiomyosarcoma. Gastrointest Radiol 7:47, 1982.)

as with anaplastic bronchogenic carcinoma, the mass may infiltrate the wall.[18] A target pattern would again be identified.[37]

ABNORMALITIES OF THE SMALL BOWEL

Obstruction and/or Dilatation

Small bowel obstruction is associated with dilatation of the bowel loops proximal to the site of the obstruction; radiography is usually more useful in this situation than ultrasound. The dilated loops are usually filled with gas, which impedes the transmission of the sound beam. In 6 percent of cases though, the dilated loops are filled with fluid and can easily be mistaken for a soft tissue mass on radiographs.[18] The hallmark of intestinal obstruction on ultrasound, whether due to mechanical cause or absence of peristalsis, is intraluminal accumulation of fluid.[48] The dilated fluid-filled loops can be identified by their tubular (long axis) and oval or round (cross-section) echofree appearance[11,18,48–50] (Figs. 9-25 and 9-26). In adynamic ileus, dilated bowel loops have normal to somewhat increased peristaltic activity.[51] There is generally less distension than with dynamic ileus. In dynamic ileus (obstructive), the fluid-filled loops are almost per-

fectly round with minimal deformity at the interfaces with adjacent loops of distended bowel.[51] Often the valvulae conniventes can be seen as well as peristalsis.[17,18,48,50] Peristaltic motion is demonstrated by a "bubble-like" pattern.[17] The level of the obstruction may be judged by the distribution of the distended fluid-filled loops.[11] If fluid-filled loops are only in the upper abdomen, the examiner should suspect obstruction of the distal small bowel.

Fluid-filled loops of bowel are not always associated with obstruction.[48] They occur with gastroenteritis and with paralytic ileus. If no peristalsis is seen, pressure applied with the transducer can often demonstrate pliability and compressibility of the bowel wall, as well as induce movement of echoes.[18]

CLOSED LOOP OBSTRUCTION OR VOLVULUS

Sometimes a single dilated aperistaltic loop of bowel is observed, such as with a closed loop obstruction or volvulus.[18,49] With this problem, air cannot enter the involved bowel loop, and ultrasound provides important information.[48] With volvulus, the involved loop is doubled back on itself abruptly, so that a "U" appearance is seen on a longitudinal scan and a C-shaped anechoic area with a dense center is seen on transverse scan[51] (Fig.

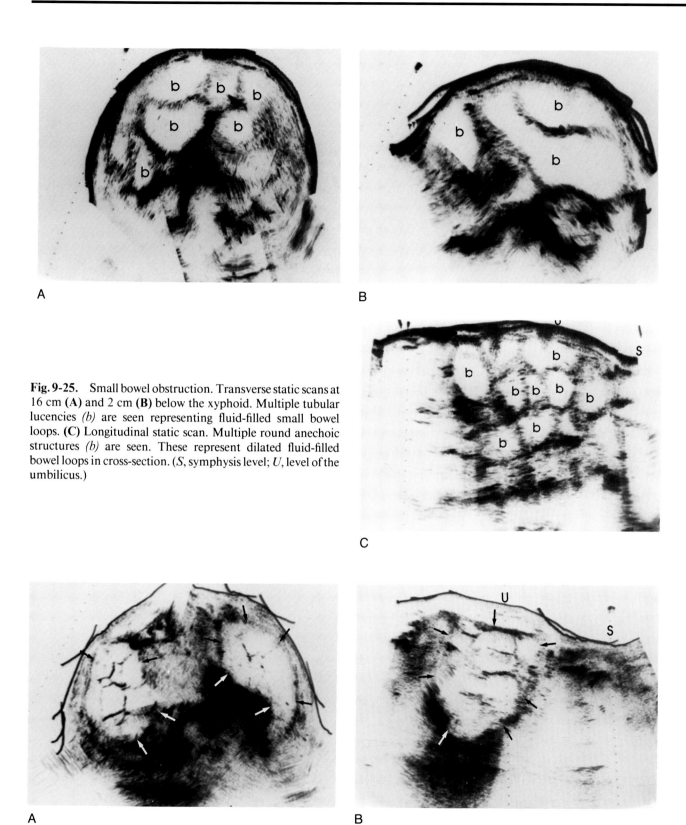

Fig. 9-25. Small bowel obstruction. Transverse static scans at 16 cm **(A)** and 2 cm **(B)** below the xyphoid. Multiple tubular lucencies *(b)* are seen representing fluid-filled small bowel loops. **(C)** Longitudinal static scan. Multiple round anechoic structures *(b)* are seen. These represent dilated fluid-filled bowel loops in cross-section. (*S*, symphysis level; *U*, level of the umbilicus.)

Fig. 9-26. Small bowel obstruction. In this postoperative patient, the fluid-filled small bowel loops (arrows) give the appearance of masses on transverse scan 15 cm above the symphysis **(A)** and longitudinal scan **(B)** 8 cm to the right of midline. Peristalsis was seen within the anechoic "masses" at real-time. (*S*, level of the symphysis; *U*, level of the umbilicus.)

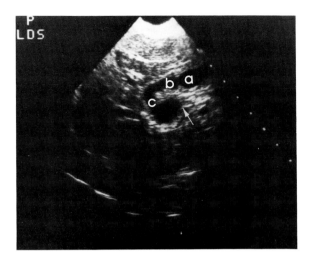

Fig. 9-27. Duodenal obstruction—Midgut volvulus. Longitudinal real-time scan. There is distension of the fluid-filled antropylorus *(a)*, duodenal bulb *(b)*, and duodenal C loop *(c)*. Tapering of the distal obstructed duodenum (arrow) is seen. (From Hayden CK Jr, Boulden RF, Swischuk LE, Lobe TE: Sonographic demonstration of duodenal obstruction with midgut volvulus. AJR 143:9, © Am Roentgen Ray Soc, 1984)

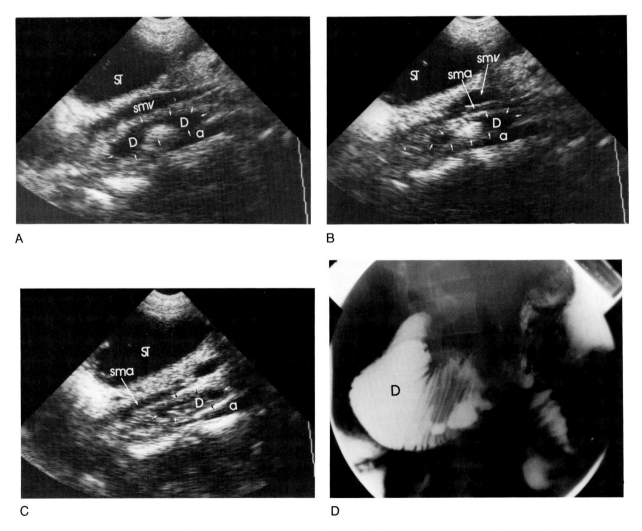

Fig. 9-28. Superior mesenteric artery syndrome. Sequential longitudinal right lateral decubitus scans from the long axis of the superior mesenteric vein *(smv)* to that of the superior mesenteric artery *(sma)* **(A,B,C)**. The fluid-filled stomach *(ST)* is seen anteriorly. The dilated third portion of the duodenum *(D)* is seen posterior to the *smv* on **(A)**. By scanning from the *smv* to the *sma*, the duodenal lumen is greatly decreased in size posterior to the *sma* **(B,C)**. (*a*, aorta.) **(D)** Cone-down view from an UGI study. The dilated duodenum *(D)* is seen to be compressed in its third portion.

9-27). The dense center represents the medial bowel wall and mesentery.

Midgut volvulus is an acute medical emergency that often occurs during the neonatal period.[52] The infant usually presents with an acute onset of vomiting that contains bile. The radiograph may be normal or have the classical signs of intestinal obstruction; only when a distended descending duodenum is seen is the diagnosis made with certainty. Once duodenal obstruction is demonstrated, a presumptive diagnosis of duodenal bands, malrotation, and potential midgut volvulus can be made. Ultrasound may suggest the diagnosis if to-and-fro hyperperistaltic motion is observed in an obstructed duodenal loop[52] (Fig. 9-27).

SUPERIOR MESENTERIC ARTERY SYNDROME

In superior mesenteric artery syndrome, the stomach and duodenum may be dilated to the point in the third portion of the duodenum where the superior mesenteric vessels indent the duodenum. The pathogenesis of the syndrome is controversial, but mechanical factors appear to be important in the production of this entity. As a rule, these findings are seen with the patient supine and disappear when the patient is prone. This condition is more common in extremely thin patients (especially females with anorexia nervosa), patients with extensive burns, and those with rapid weight loss, acute pancreatitis, severe trauma, or a body cast.

In most cases of superior mesenteric artery syndrome, no finding may be seen on ultrasound. However, one may see a dilated fluid-filled second portion of the duodenum that exhibits a to-and-fro peristaltic motion on real-time ultrasound (Fig. 9-28). On a longitudinal scan, the dilated duodenum can be followed to the point where the superior mesenteric artery crosses the duodenum and the duodenum becomes nondilated (Fig. 9-28).

MATTED BOWEL LOOPS

At times, matted loops of bowel may present a confusing picture on ultrasound (Fig. 9-26). Matted loops may be caused by adhesions, peritoneal implants, or intraperitoneal inflammatory processes. These loops assume a variety of appearances such as a group of tortuous, echofree tubular structures; a complex of mass-like lesions with echofree areas and areas with weak or strong echoes; or an irregular lesion with weak echoes similar to a solid mass[18] (Fig. 9-26).

AFFERENT LOOP OBSTRUCTION

Afferent loop obstruction usually occurs after a subtotal gastrectomy in which a Billroth II anastomosis is performed for ulcer disease. In these instances, the obstruction most often is due to internal herniation or a kink of the afferent loop.[53] Less often the afferent loop is obstructed secondary to recurrent pancreatic tumor following a Whipple operation, or to recurrent gastric carcinoma.[53] Patients with afferent loop obstruction may present as an abdominal emergency that mimicks acute pancreatitis, both chemically and biochemically. The more chronic or intermittent form presents with bouts of abdominal pain due to distension of the loop from pancreatic and biliary secretions. The symptoms are alleviated by copious bilious emesis, which relieves distension.[53]

Afferent loop obstruction is difficult to diagnose confidently before surgery. On barium studies, there is nonfilling of the loops, which is not helpful in making the diagnosis. On endoscopy, successful visualization of the afferent loop is accomplished in only 75 to 80 percent of patients.[53] When visualized on ultrasound, this entity typically appears as a large cystic structure in the upper abdomen and may have echogenic debris in its dependent part[54] (Fig. 9-29). On coronal plane, a U-shaped configuration of an obstructed afferent duodenal loop is helpful in making a diagnosis. Some peristalsis may be seen within the loop.[53]

ILEOVESICAL ANATOMOSIS

Occasionally a dilated ileal loop associated with an ileovesical anastomosis may be mistaken for an abscess.[55] The curved tubular nature of the ileal loop becomes apparent with serial scans. Peristalsis may or may not be seen on real-time ultrasound; it is sometimes absent owing to marked long-standing dilatation.[55]

Hematoma

Recognition of an intestinal hematoma has important bearing on therapy and prognosis. Intramural hemorrhage may occur from complex causes, with or without trauma. Such causes include bleeding diatheses, hemophilia, anticoagulant therapy, blunt trauma, leukemia, lymphoma, Henoch-Schonlein anaphylactoid purpura, and thrombocytopenic purpura.[56] When the duodenum is affected, there may be secondary effects of gastric outlet obstruction, obstruction of the biliary tree, and extrinsic compression on the inferior vena cava.[57] Since the duodenum is fixed in position, it is more often affected by trauma than is the remainder of the GI tract. Because a lesion in the duodenum produces thickening of the wall, the target sign or possibly an echogenic mass (extramural and intramural) will be visible[51,56,57] (Fig. 9-30). A hematoma usually produces eccentric thickening of the bowel wall.[51]

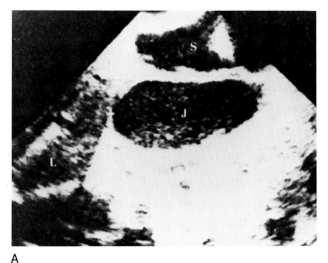

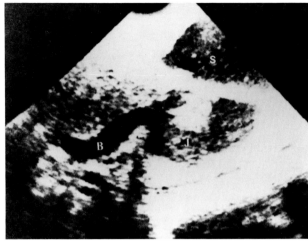

A

B

C

Fig. 9-29. Afferent loop obstruction. **(A)** Midline longitudinal scan. Fluid-filled jejunum *(J)* is seen posterior to the distended gastric remnant *(S)* and caudal to the liver *(L)*. **(B)** Oblique scan of the right upper quadrant. The dilated common bile duct *(B)* is seen entering the afferent jejunal segment *(J)*. *(S,* gastric remnant.) **(C)** Delayed film from a percutaneous transhepatic cholangiogram. The biliary tree drains into the markedly enlarged afferent loop (arrows), corresponding to the soft-tissue mass seen on plain film of the abdomen. (From Hopens T, Coggs GC, Goldstein HM, Smith BD: Sonographic diagnosis of afferent loop obstruction. AJR 138:967, © Am Roentgen Ray Soc, 1982)

Duplication

The etiology of duplication cysts is most commonly thought to be errors of canalization. The solid GI tract at 6 weeks of intrauterine life becomes a hollow tube by the eighth week, as multiple vacuoles coalesce. If there are two channels rather than one running through part of the solid cord, a duplication cyst occurs parallel to the normal lumen. Diagnosis of such a lesion is usually made in the first year of life, often within the first week. Obstruction is the most common symptom, with the ileum being the most common site.

Ultrasound evaluation of a suspected abdominal mass in the child has become routine. Identifying the rare congenital anomaly, such as duplication of the GI tract,

can aid in diagnosis and obviate extensive workup. Lesions can have a varying appearance, ranging from anechoic cyst to echogenic mass[30] (Figs. 9-31 and 9-32). An echogenic inner rim is highly suggestive of the diagnosis.[23] If the cyst contains clear fluid, the lucent mass will have strong posterior wall echoes and acoustic enhancement. An echogenic mass may be seen, which is the result of hemorrhage and inspissated material.[23] The site of the cyst cannot be predicted from the location of the cyst on ultrasound.[20]

Cystic duplication of the duodenum is an uncommon entity that manifests most often in the pediatric age group. An abdominal mass is the most common clinical finding, accompanied by varying degrees of nausea, vomiting, and high intestinal obstruction. The radio-

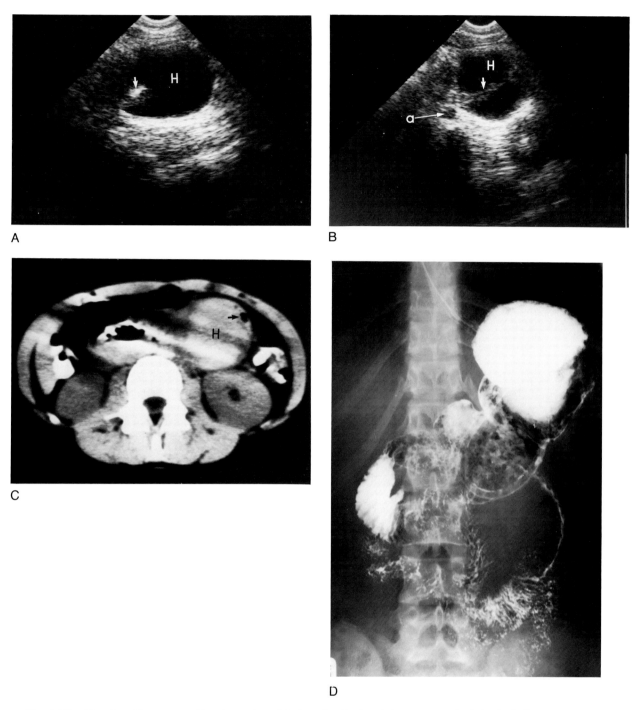

Fig. 9-30. Duodenal hematoma fourth portion. **(A)** Longitudinal real-time scan to the left of midline. An anechoic mass *(H)* is seen with an echodense area (arrow) at its apex. This represented duodenal lumen. **(B)** Transverse real-time scan. Again, the duodenal lumen is seen as an echodense area (arrow) more medial with the anechoic area *(H)* the hematoma. *(a,* aorta.) **(C)** CT similar to **(B)**. The hematoma *(H)* appears dense with air (arrow) in the bowel lumen. **(D)** UGI with displacement of bowel loops (arrows) by the mass.

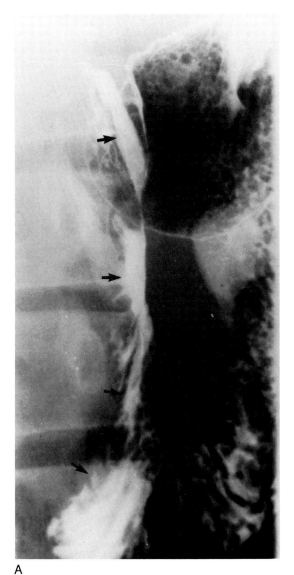

A

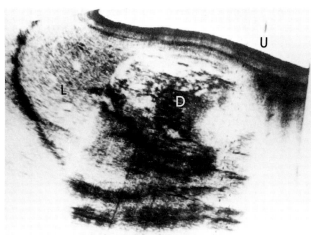

B

Fig. 9-31. Duodenal duplication cyst. **(A)** UGI with external compression (arrows) by a large mass on the second portion of the duodenum. **(B)** Longitudinal scan with an echogenic duplication *(D)* cyst separate from gallbladder. (*L*, liver; *U*, level of the umbilicus.) The cyst was filled with hemorrhagic fluid. (From Kangarloo H, Sample WF, Hansen G et al: Ultrasonic evaluation of abdominal gastrointestinal tract duplication in children. Radiology 131:191, 1979.)

graphic diagnosis is limited to the extrinsic pressure defect produced by the cyst, since only 10 to 20 percent of duplications communicate with the duodenal lumen. On ultrasound, a cystic right upper quadrant mass is seen.[58] The differential diagnosis would include gallbladder, choledochal cyst, and pseudocyst.

Intussusception

Intussusception is the most common cause of obstruction in the child, but it is fairly uncommon in the adult.[18,59] In 75 to 85 percent of adult cases, there is an identifiable bowel lesion at the leading point.[18,60] When located in the colon, 50 percent of such lesions prove to

be malignant, whereas in the small bowel the majority are benign.[60]

The clinical presentation of intussusception is varied and nonspecific. It may have a protracted course, with symptoms present for 3 or more months. As the intussusceptum progresses into the intussuscipiens, the bowel wall becomes edematous.[60] The intussusceptum is telescoped into the intussuscipiens until it can go no further owing to traction on the mesentery, which is dragged between the entering and returning walls of the intussusceptum. Venous obstruction ensues with exudation of fluid and resultant wall edema. The edema is greatest at the apex of the intussusceptum, but extends to involve the entering and returning intussusceptum walls.[61] If intussusception is acute, the patient may present with abdominal pain, vomiting, and rectal passage of blood and mucus or "current jelly" stools.[62] If chronic, which is the more common variety in adults, the patient may have minimal pain, diarrhea, and, less frequently, vomiting. An abdominal mass is present in 63 to 85 percent of cases.[59]

The barium enema is indicated to confirm the diagnosis and, in acute cases, to reduce it hydrostatically.[62] When the presentation is atypical, ultrasound can be helpful. A variation in the typical target-like or bull's-eye pattern is seen[37] (Fig. 9-33). The thickened hypoechoic rim represents the edematous intussuscipiens that surrounds the hyperechoic center, which is due to multiple interfaces of compressed mucosal and serosal surfaces of the intussusceptum.[62]

The target lesion seen on ultrasound is nonspecific and can appear following primary or secondary cancer, lymphoma, Crohn's disease, inflammation due to pan-

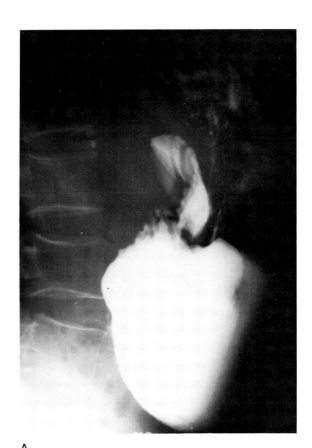

A

Fig. 9-32. Duodenal duplication cyst. **(A)** Lateral view of an UGI. Extrinsic compression is seen on the posteromedial aspect on the duodenal bulb. **(B)** Longitudinal scan 5 cm to the right of midline showing cystic duplication of the duodenum *(c)* superior to the fluid-filled duodenal bulb *(d)*, and posterior to the gallbladder *(gb)*. (*L*, liver; *U*, level of the umbilicus.) **(C)** Transverse scan 4 cm below the xyphoid. The cystic *(c)* duplication is seen lateral to the pancreas *(p)*. (*a*, aorta; *S*, spine; *L*, liver; *k*, right kidney.) (From Fried AM, Pulmano CM, Mostowycz L: Duodenal duplication cyst: Sonographic and angiographic features. Am J Roentgenol 128:863, © Am Roentgen Ray Soc, 1977.)

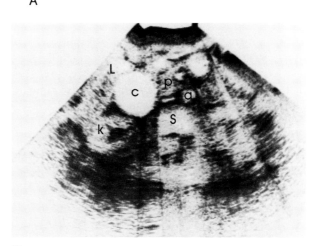

B   C

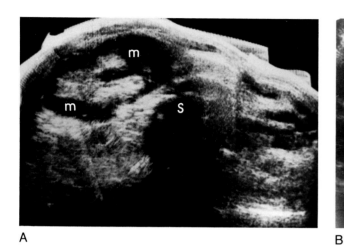

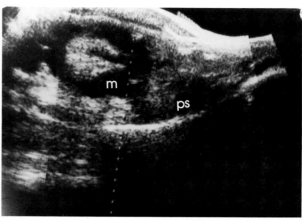

A   B

Fig. 9-33. Intussusception. **(A)** Transverse scan 4 cm above the umbilicus. A large intraabdominal mass *(m)*, having a target pattern, is shown to the right of midline. The hypoechoic rim represents the edematous intussucipiens that surrounds the hyperechoic center; this is owing to multiple interfaces of compressed mucosal and serosal surfaces of the intussusceptum. (*s,* spine.) **(B)** Longitudinal scan to the right of midline shows a mass *(m)* sitting on the anterior margin of the psoas muscle *(ps).* (From Weissberg DL, Scheible W, Leopold GR: Ultrasonographic appearance of adult intussusception. Radiology 124:791, 1977.)

creatitis, bowel infarction, radiation ileitis, and hematoma. A scan of the long axis helps to make a more definite diagnosis of intussusception (Fig. 9-34). On a cross-section through the apex of the intussusceptum, the more common target lesion is seen with a very thick hypoechoic rim due to the severe edema of the entering and returning intussusceptum walls and resultant obliteration of the interface between them.[63] When scanning through the more proximal portion where the parietal edema is less severe, an image of two concentric rings and an inner circular area is seen.[61,63,64] The outer and inner rings represent the returning and entering walls of the intussusceptum; the intermediate hyperreflective ring separates the walls, due to changes in the interface between them. When the long axis is scanned, three parallel stripes of low echogenicity are delineated as well as two reflective areas.[63]

Intussusception may be a complication in jejunoileal bypass surgery to correct obesity; it occurs secondary to inadequate fixation of the free end of the defunctionalized loop. After surgical bypass, a large percentage of small bowel cannot be visualized with conventional radiographic techniques.[65] Intussusception is thus difficult to diagnose and is confused with colonic pseudo-obstruction because it has the same symptoms of crampy abdominal pain.[65] It is a potentially catastrophic complication and may occur in 0.5 to 3.5 percent of bypass patients.[66] As with the usual type of intussusception, the ultrasound pattern is that of a large target: a hypoechoic or anechoic mass with a hyperechoic center is seen.[66]

Granulomatous Enterocolitis

Crohn's disease or regional enteritis represents a recurrent granulomatous inflammatory disease that affects the terminal ileum and/or colon at any level. This granulomatous inflammatory reaction involves the entire thickness of the bowel wall. These patients present with diarrhea, fever, and right lower quadrant pain. The complications of this disease include fibrosing strictures and fistulas to another loop of bowel, bladder, perineum, or peritoneal abscess.[26]

As might be expected, Crohn's disease is associated with a target lesion due to the thickened bowel wall[18] (Figs. 9-35, 9-36). However, it may also be associated with abscess formation seen as irregular or ill-defined, poorly echogenic masses (Fig. 9-37). These abscesses can extend into the iliopsoas muscle, or anteriorly into the rectus muscle, or may even compress the bladder.[18]

Serial ultrasound is ideal for demonstrating progression or regression of the inflamed bowel loops as well as abscesses; bowel is identified by visualizing peristalsis.[67] Real-time ultrasound helps to differentiate fluid-filled or matted, inflamed bowel loops from abscess. Static scanning is better suited for delineation of the abdominal wall abscess, which is the most common abscess associated with this disease. The incidence of external fistula is 8.7 to 21 percent.[67] Intraperitoneal abscesses frequently surround matted, inflamed bowel. On ultrasound, matted bowel loops produce a large mass having irregular internal echoes; these conditions may simulate

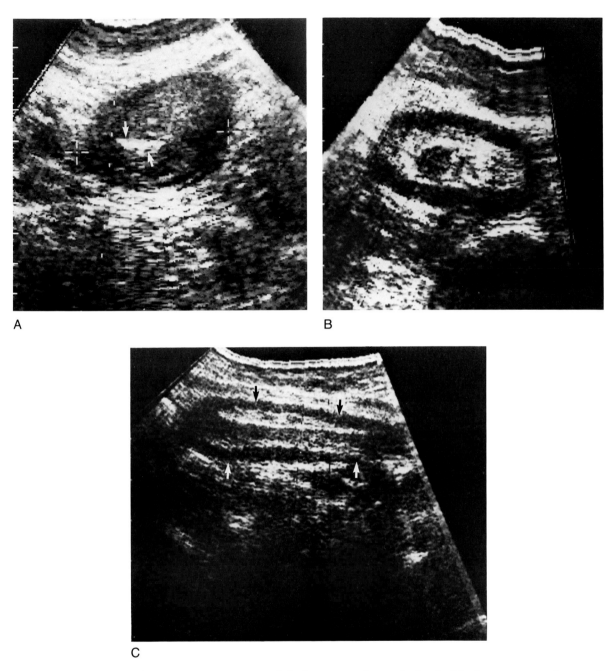

A

B

C

Fig. 9-34. Intussusception. **(A)** Transverse scan of the intussusception at the level of the intussusceptum's apex. A target-like pattern is seen; the central echogenic lumen (arrow) is surrounded by a very thick hypoechoic rim. The thick hypoechoic rim is due to severe edema of the entering and returning intussusceptum walls and the resultant obliteration of interface between them. **(B)** Cross-section of the intussusception at a more proximal level. A hypoechoic outer ring surrounds a highly reflective area with an echopoor center. The outer and inner hypoechoic areas represent the returning and the entering wall of the intussusceptum respectively. The echogenic area is the interface between the walls. **(C)** Longitudinal view of the intussusception (arrows) obtained with a scan through its long axis. There are three hypoechoic stripes delineating two echogenic areas. (From Montali G, Croce F, De Pra L, Solbiati L: Intussusception of the bowel: A new sonographic pattern. Br J Radiol 56:621, 1983).

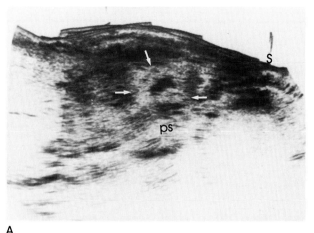

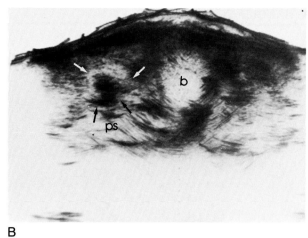

A

B

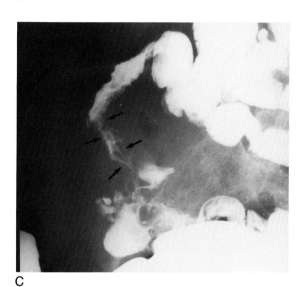

C

Fig. 9-35. Crohn's disease—Target pattern. (A) Longitudinal scan to the right of midline. A bull's-eye pattern (arrows) is seen anterior to the psoas muscle *(ps)*. (*S*, symphysis level.) (B) Transverse scan with a bull's-eye pattern (arrows) seen within the right lower quadrant. The thickened wall of the ileum produces this pattern. (*b*, bladder; *ps*, psoas muscle). (C) On the GI series the ileal channel is narrowed (arrows). On a gallium scan, an area of increased activity was seen in the right lower quadrant, corresponding to the bowel involvement.

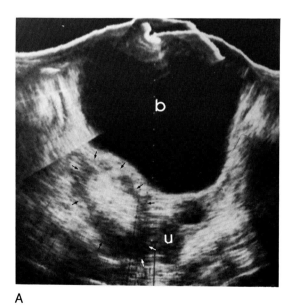

A

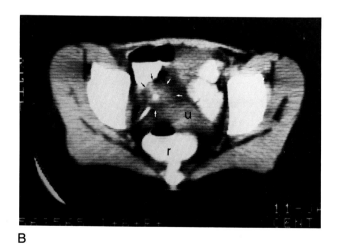

B

Fig. 9-36. Crohn's disease—Pelvic mass. (A) Transverse scan of the pelvis demonstrating a target lesion (arrows) within the right pelvis. The dense center is bowel lumen. (*u*, uterus; *b*, bladder). (B) CT scan with oral and rectal barium. A soft tissue density mass (arrows) is seen in the right pelvis. There is barium seen within the center lumen of the mass. (*u*, uterus; *r*, rectum.)

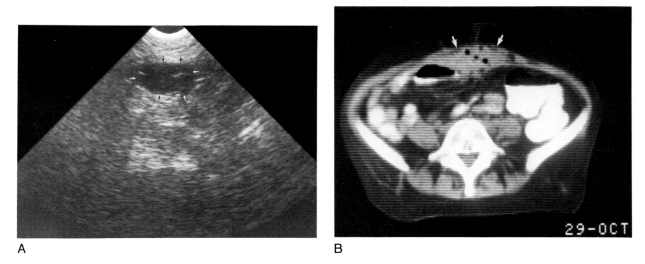

A   B

Fig. 9-37.   Crohn's disease—Fistula. **(A)** Transverse real-time scan. A hypoechoic superficial mass (arrows) is seen anteriorly within the abdomen. **(B)** CT scan. A soft-tissue density mass (arrows) is seen within the abdominal wall, having internal air consistent with abdominal wall abscess and fistula formation.

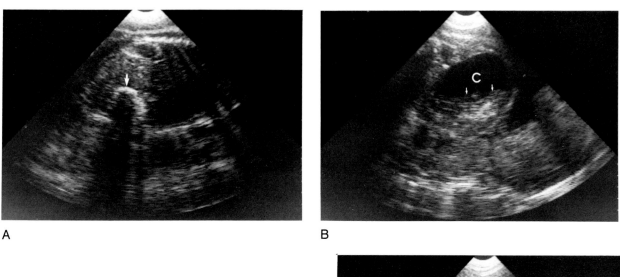

A   B

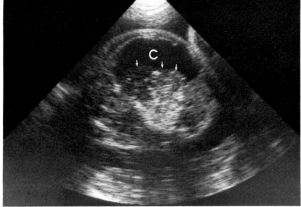

Fig. 9-38.   Meconium cyst—In utero. **(A)** Longitudinal scan of the fetal abdomen. Several echogenic areas (arrow), which represent calcifications are seen within the fetal abdomen. Transverse scans with patient supine **(B)** and in the right lateral decubitus position **(C)**. A rounded cystic mass *(C)* contains a fluid-fluid level (arrows). The fluid-fluid level shifted with change in maternal position.

C

a large abscess.[67] An associated abscess may contain gas bubbles if bowel gas enters these fistulae or if gas-containing bacteria are present. These may be difficult to see on ultrasound.[67]

Meconium Peritonitis and Cyst

Meconium peritonitis is a sterile chemical peritonitis resulting from extrusion of meconium from the fetal gut into the peritoneal cavity.[67,69] In utero, it is possible to see polyhydramnios, fetal ascites, and echogenic calcific foci with shadowing[70] (Fig. 9-38). The causes for these conditions include bowel perforation proximal to obstruction, meconium ileus, volvulus, hernia, and atresia (Figs. 9-39 and 9-40). Intestinal stenosis or atresia and meconium ileus accompany 65 percent of cases.[72] This irritant me-

conium causes peritonitis, which frequently localizes and results in formation of a sterile abscess (Fig. 9-40). With healing, calcification takes place and scattered plaques form on the peritoneal surface.[68]

There are three clinical forms of meconium peritonitis: cystic, fibroadhesive, and generalized.[73] A meconium cyst is formed when bowel perforates in utero (oc-

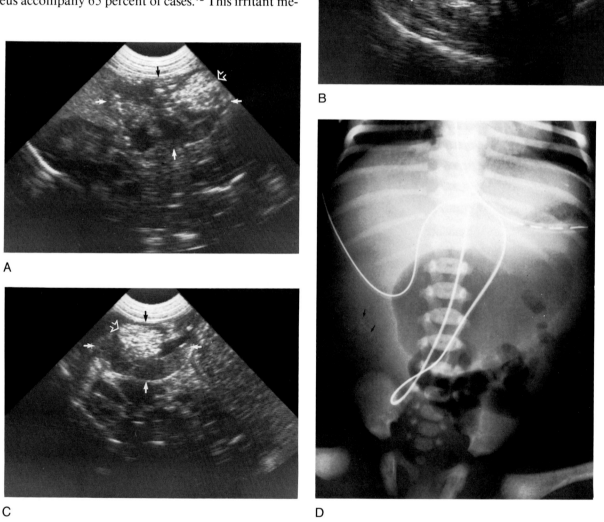

A

B

C

D

Fig. 9-39. Meconium ileus. Ileoatresia. A complex mass (*m*, arrows) is seen on longitudinal (**A**) and transverse scans from (**B**) superior to (**C**) inferior. There is one large, dense area (open arrow) with multiple lucent areas in a radial pattern. At surgery, these were found to be necrotic bowel loops arranged in a spiral fashion, with a large proximal ileal segment. (**D**) Plain film shows some calcifications (arrows).

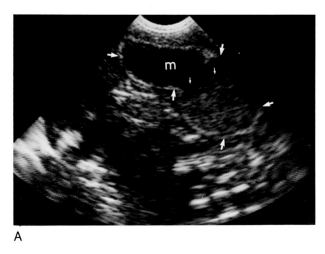

A

Fig. 9-40. Meconium ileus. Cystic fibrosis with a sterile abscess. **(A)** A "figure 8" configuration mass *(m)* representing the abscess is seen within the right abdomen with a fluid-fluid level (small arrows). **(B)** Plain film. A mass effect is noted within the right abdomen with meconium (arrows).

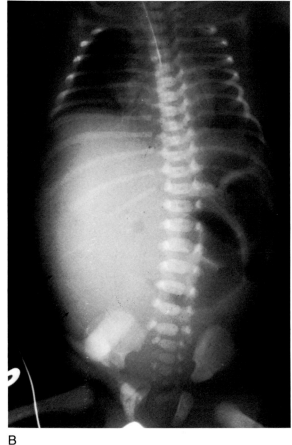

B

curing in 17 to 60 percent of patients with meconium peritonitis) and meconium is extruded into the peritoneal cavity, which becomes walled off by fibrous adhesions (Fig. 9-38). Ultimately, a well-defined capsule of fibrous granulomatous tissue is formed. The cyst may contain only spilled meconium or may encase bowel loops. If the perforation remains open, the meconium cyst is in communication with the bowel at the site of perforation. This cyst is relatively uncommon and is lined by thick membrane that contains thick plaque and scattered calcific deposits. On ultrasound, the following pattern has been described: an inhomogeneous mass with several central areas of increased echogenicity, faint posterior shadowing, and a highly echogenic, thick peripheral rim[73-75] (Fig. 9-41). Such a mass could represent an omental or mesenteric cyst, a GI tract duplication cyst, choledochal cyst, or ovarian cyst; the thick, well-circumscribed echogenic cyst wall, which contains areas of focal calcification, should be compatible with meconium cyst association with meconium peritonitis.[75]

Meconium peritonitis may be characterized by a chemical peritonitis that has intense fibroplastic reaction to digestive enzymes contained in the meconium. Bowel obstruction does not have to be present, although it is usually combined with perforation as the most frequent cause of meconium peritonitis. If the bowel perforation closes before birth, fibroadhesion occurs and meconium peritonitis usually results. Perforation may persist postnatally, or a dense adherent membrane may be formed on the peritonal surface, which effectively seals off the site of perforation and leads to fibroadhesive meconium peritonitis. If perforation occurs late during the perinatal period, bowel contents escape freely into the peritoneal cavity, and a generalized pattern is produced.

Tumors

LYMPHOMA

Neoplastic disease, except for lymphoma, is rare in the small bowel.[18] Lymphoma of the GI tract most frequently occurs around age 65, but it is the most common tumor of the GI tract in the child, especially under 10 years of age.[76] This lymphoma is usually part of a systemic involvement and presents with multiple nodules, although lymphoma may originate in the GI tract in 10

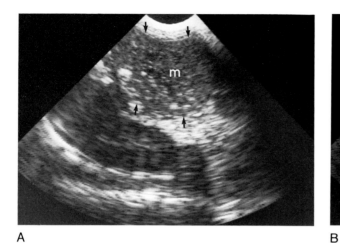

A

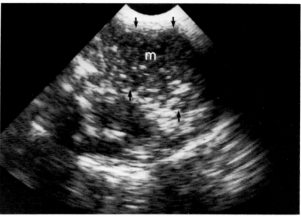

B

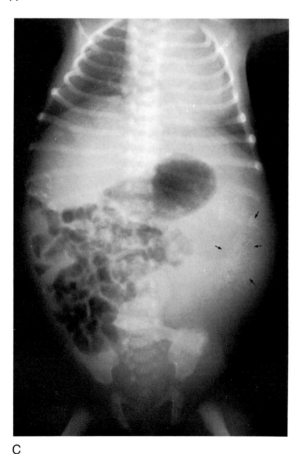

C

Fig. 9-41. Meconium cyst. Scan of the patient in Fig. 9-38, following birth. No longer is a cystic mass seen. Instead, a poorly defined echogenic mass (arrows, *m*) is seen on longitudinal (**A**) and transverse (**B**) scans. The mass contained many internal echoes and exhibited acoustic enhancement. Its borders were difficult to discern. (**C**) Plain radiograph. A mass effect is noted in the left abdomen containing meconium (arrows). At surgery, a large cyst filled with meconium-stained fluid was found in the left upper quadrant. Calcification was seen within the cyst and the right upper quadrant.

to 20 percent.[76] Intraperitoneal masses frequently involve the mesenteric vessels which encase them.[18]

Patients with small bowel lymphoma may present with intestinal blood loss, weight loss, and anorexia. Abdominal pain is frequent with a sprue-like syndrome. There is a variable degree of intestinal obstruction, which may be related to encroachment on the bowel lumen. More than 50 percent of children have a palpable mass.[76]

The most frequent histologic type that involves bowel is non-Hodgkin's lymphoma, which includes Burkitt's, undifferentiated, and histiocytic lymphoma. Burkitt's lymphoma has a particular tendency to involve loops of bowel in a rapidly growing mass[30] (see Fig. 5-58). Hodgkin's disease almost never presents as an isolated GI process, although it eventually involves the GI tract in 50 percent of cases. Lymphoma in the child starts as a unifocal lesion, usually in the terminal ileum in the lymphoid follicles, and spreads circumferentially throughout the submucosa, gradually involving the muscular coat to present as a subserosal tumor.

Primary lymphoma of the small bowel usually presents as a large irregular mass that has internal echoes due to necrosis. In most cases, the lymphoma mass is complex, with completely anechoic areas and central densely reflective areas indicative of GI mucosa and/or mucus[76] (Fig. 9-42). This pattern reflects the thickening of the bowel wall. The polypoid type of lymphoma tends to extend into the mesentery in a predominately exoenteric manner. Ultrasound is able to detect a mass having either an eccentric or exoenteric growth pattern.[76] The patterns that have been described include: a large discrete mass (5 to 11 cm in diameter) with a target pattern, an exoenteric pattern with a large mass on the mesenteric surface of bowel, and a small anechoic mass (1 to

2 cm) representing subserosal nodes or mesenteric nodal involvement.

LEIOMYOSARCOMA

Leiomyosarcoma represents 10 percent of the primary small bowel tumors.[45,46] Ten to 30 percent of these occur in the duodenum, 30 to 45 percent in the jejunum, and 35 to 55 percent in the ileum. Most occur in the fifth to sixth decade of life.[45,46] On ultrasound, diagnosis may be suggested if a large solid mass containing necrotic areas, is seen anterior to a solid viscus, and if intestinal lumen and/or air is in close relation to the mass[45] (Fig. 9-43).

CARCINOID

Carcinoids (Argentaffinomas) can arise anywhere in the GI tract, bronchi, biliary tree, pancreas, or wherever enterochromaffin cells are normally found.[26] In decreasing order of frequency, they are found in the appendix (35 to 45 percent), small bowel (20 to 25 percent), rec-

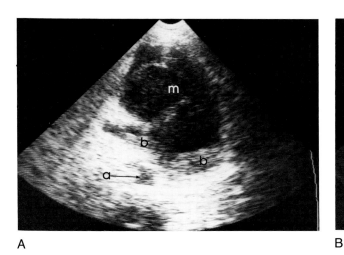

A

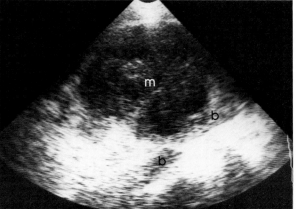

B

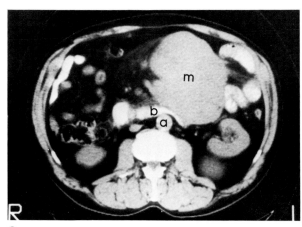

C

Fig. 9-42. Non-Hodgkin's lymphoma, small bowel. Transverse (A) and longitudinal (B) scans demonstrate a mass *(m)* of mixed density involving the small bowel *(b)* and extending into the mesentery. (*a*, aorta.) (C) CT scan similarly shows a soft tissue density mass *(m)* and bowel *(b)* involvement. (*a*, aorta.)

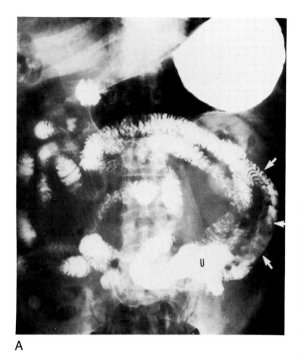

A

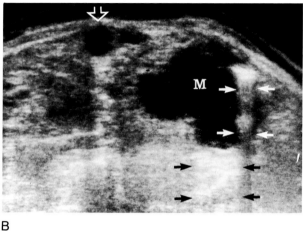

B

Fig. 9-43. Small bowel—Leiomyosarcoma. (A) Small bowel series. There is extrinsic pressure (arrows) on jejunal loops and an ulceration *(U)*. (B) Transverse scan of the lower abdomen. A hypoechoic mass *(M)* with enhanced transmission (black arrows) suggests liquefaction necrosis. Note the eccentric location of the acoustic shadow (white arrows) adjacent to the mass *(M)*. Omental metastasis (open arrow) has a similar appearance. (From Subramanyam BR, Balthazar EJ, Raghavendra BN, Madamba MR: Sonography of exophytic gastrointestinal leiomyosarcoma. Gastrointest Radiol 7:47, 1982.)

tum (15 percent) and lower bowel (excluding rectum, 10 percent). Detection of carcinoid tumors at a resectable stage is important, since the 5-year survival rate is up to 90 percent when there is complete excision of the lesion.[77] Over 73 percent of the lesions are less than 1.5 cm and thus are difficult to see. The intraluminal component of a symptomatic malignant carcinoid tumor is typically small in relation to the extension into the mesentery, and the barium enema is occasionally normal.[77] On ultrasound, a carcinoid tumor has been described as a sharply marginated hypoechoic mass with a strong back wall and as a lobulated contour with a lack of acoustic enhancement, all of which are nonspecific.

PEUTZ-JEGHERS SYNDROME

Peutz-Jeghers syndrome is characterized by polyps found throughout the GI tract, particularly the small bowel, and is associated with melanin pigmentation of the buccal mucosa, lips, and digits.[26] These polyps represent hamartomatous overgrowths rather than true neoplasms but have a slight (3 percent) increased incidence of malignancy of the GI tract.[78] If the patient presents with symptoms of intussusception, and an UGI with

barium is temporarily contraindicated, ultrasound may be helpful. If there is distension of the small bowel loops, large intraluminal oval structures (polyps) may be seen.

ABNORMALITIES OF THE APPENDIX

Acute Appendicitis

Acute appendicitis can occur at any age but is more prevalent in the young adult.[26] As a rule, there are no findings associated with appendicitis that can be seen on ultrasound[18]; however, the typical target lesion has been reported in the right lower quadrant with this disease.[79,80] Thickening of the bowel wall in this instance is due to edema, and the echogenic core is due to the necrotic appendix or appendiceal lumen.[79] The complications of this disease include peritonitis, localized periappendical abscess, pylephlebitis with thrombosis of the portal venous drainage, liver abscess, and septicemia.[26]

Appendiceal calculus within the abscess can be recognized as an hyperechoic structure that has an acoustic shadow[79] (Fig. 9-44). These calculi or fecaliths result from accumulation and inspissation of fecal material

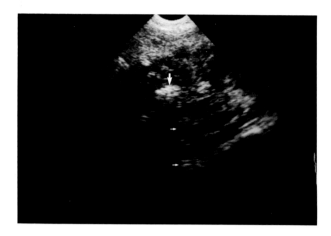

Fig. 9-44. Appendiceal calculus. A persistent echogenic structure (large arrow) with shadowing (small arrows) is seen in the right lower quadrant on longitudinal scan. A mass was not seen.

around vegetable fiber. When present, they may obstruct the appendiceal lumen, frequently resulting in acute appendicitis. These calculi are also associated with a high incidence of acute complications such as perforation.

Appendiceal Abscess

With an abscess, ultrasound may demonstrate an echofree or poorly echogenic lesion in which irregular or ill-defined borders are restricted to the right lower quadrant[79] (Figs. 9-45 and 9-46). This abscess may extend.[18] With a retrocecal appendiceal abscess, the mass may be seen as a complex cystic mass posterior to the kidney.[69]

Periappendiceal abscess or peritonitis does not necessarily mean perforation, as the organism may permeate the wall.[26] In the female it may be difficult to differentiate an appendiceal abscess from a tubo-ovarian abscess, twisted ovarian cyst, ruptured tubal pregnancy, or ruptured follicular or luteal ovarian cyst.[79] Ultrasound may be used to evaluate postoperative patients for appendicitis or abscess. At times, a postoperative abscess may be found (Fig. 9-47, see Fig. 5-25). Care should be taken not to mistake colon for abscess (Fig. 9-48). If such a question exists, a water enema may be performed and monitored on real-time ultrasound.

Mucocele

A mucocele is a relatively rare lesion occurring in 0.25 to 0.3 percent of a series of 43,000 appendectomies.[81,82] It is usually a benign condition that obliterates the lumen of the appendix by inflammatory scarring or fecalith, with accumulation of sterile mucus in the isolated segment. The term "mucocele" implies a distention of the appendix by mucus and does not convey its true pathologic nature.[82] Postappendiceal scarring is the most common cause of mucocele, with others including fecaliths, appendiceal polyps, cecal carcinoma, cecal diaphragm, carcinoma of the ascending colon, and appendiceal valve. There is progressive cystic dilatation up to 4

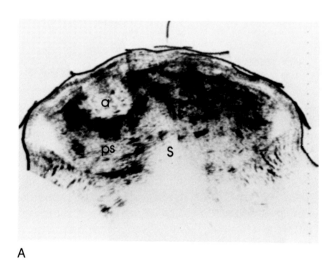

A

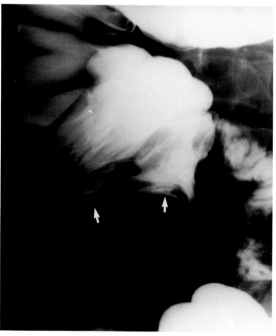

B

Fig. 9-45. Appendiceal abscess. **(A)** Transverse scan at 9 cm above the symphysis, which demonstrates a hypoechoic mass *(a)* anterior to the psoas muscle *(ps)*. (*S*, spine.) **(B)** Barium enema. A mass effect (arrows) is seen on the cecum.

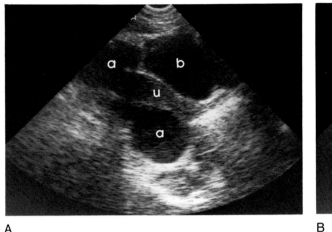

A

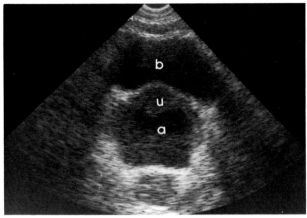

B

C

Fig. 9-46. Appendiceal abscess. **(A)** A poorly defined hypoechoic mass *(a)* surrounds the uterus *(u)* on this longitudinal scan. (*b*, bladder.) **(B)** Transversely, the mass *(a)* is seen posteriorly. (*b*, bladder; *u*, uterus.) **(C)** Barium enema demonstrating a mass effect (arrows) on the cecum.

to 6 cm.[26] Patients are generally older than 50 years of age and may be asymptomatic or present with a palpable right lower quadrant mass and/or pain.[83] In one series, 64 percent of patients experienced right lower quadrant pain while 23 percent were asymptomatic.[82] The disease's clinical significance lies in its complications: rupture, leakage of the mucocele with development of pseudomyxoma peritonei, torsion with gangrene, hem-

orrhage, and herniation into the cecum which causes varying degrees of bowel obstruction. The pseudomyxoma peritonei assumes a malignant potential only when epthelial cells occur within the gelatinous peritoneal fluid in association with carcinoma.[82]

There are two principal theories for causation of the mucocele.[79,84] The obstruction theory asserts that the distal mucosa of the appendix is stimulated to produce

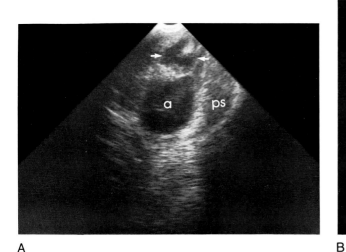

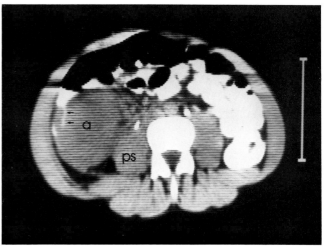

A   B

Fig. 9-47. Appendicitis, postoperative abscess. This patient was postoperative for appendicitis. **(A)** On a longitudinal real-time scan, a hypoechoic mass *(a)* was seen anterior to the psoas *(ps)* muscle. A target pattern with a thickened wall and dense center was seen anterior to the mass representing cecum (arrows). **(B)** CT scan at a similar level to **(A)**. A soft tissue density mass *(a)* is seen anterior to the psoas *(ps)* muscle. Contrast (arrows) can be seen entering the mass. This mass represented a postoperative abscess.

excessive secretion of mucin as a result of proximal obstruction of the lumen by feces, inflammatory fibrosis, or presence of a neoplasm. In the second theory, it is felt the mucosa of the obstructed appendix undergoes an ill-defined neoplastic change. Either way, the appendix progressively distends owing to the accumulation of mucus. On ultrasound, a well-defined predominately cystic or hypoechoic mass, which may contain an echogenic solid area, is seen in the right lower quadrant[79,81-84] (Fig.

9-49). This mass has an irregular inner wall caused by mucinous debris with varying degrees of epithelial hyperplasia.[82]

There are several classifications of mucoceles. If the tumor remains encapsulated and there are no malignant cells, the lesion should be called a mucocele.[83] If the mucus spreads through the abdominal cavity without evidence of malignant cells, the condition is called pseudomyxoma peritonei. If the pseudomyxoma peritonei

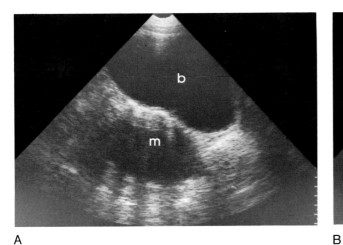

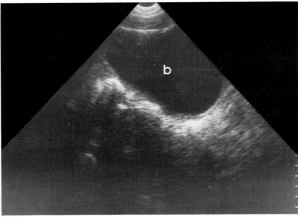

A   B

Fig. 9-48. Appendicitis, postoperative mass. This male patient was febrile, and question arose concerning a postoperative abscess. Longitudinal **(A)** scan of the pelvis demonstrates a hypoechoic mass *(m)* posterior to the bladder *(b)*. It has poorly defined margins. **(B)** Longitudinal scan of the pelvis, similar to **(A)**, after a bowel movement. No mass is seen; The mass, as such, represented rectosigmoid colon.

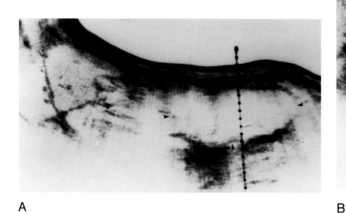

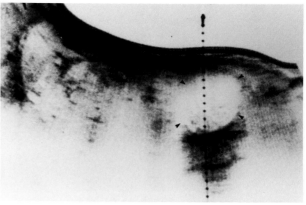

A   B

Fig. 9-49. Mucocele of the appendix. **(A)** Longitudinal scan 3 cm to the right of midline with a fluid-filled right lower quadrant mass (arrowheads) containing thin septae. **(B)** A scan farther to the right of the mass (arrowheads) exhibits some dependent layering of internal echoes. (From Athey PA, Hacken JB, Estrada R: Sonographic appearance of mucocele of the appendix. J Clin Ultrasound 12:333, 1984.)

results from rupture of a benign mucocele, the procedure is to simply remove the mucocele and the collection of fluid; it carries a good prognosis. If the pseudomyxoma peritonei is due to a primary mucinous cystoadenocarcinoma of the appendix in which mucus containing malignant cells has spread diffusely throughout the abdominal cavity, the prognosis is worse, since the mucocele behaves like an invasive neoplasm. One fourth of these mucoceles rupture, causing peritoneal seeding.[26]

Crohn's Disease

The appendix may become involved in Crohn's disease, usually secondary to cecal or terminal ileal granulomatous disease and local extension. The Crohn's disease may be limited to the appendix without involvement of the colon or small bowel but is much rarer. In isolated cases in which Crohn's disease involves only the appendix, the patient presents with clinical manifesta-

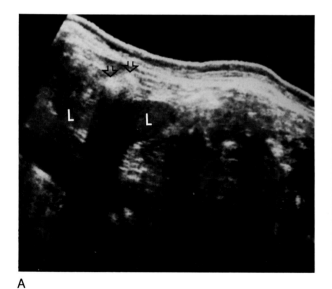

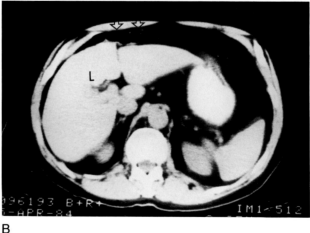

A   B

Fig. 9-50. Colon interposition. This patient presented with vague abdominal pain. **(A)** A longitudinal scan demonstrates a reflective pattern (open arrows) with shadowing produced by air in the bowel anterior to the liver *(L)*. Peristalsis was seen within this area with real-time ultrasound. **(B)** CT scan documentating air-filled transverse colon (open arrows) anterior to liver *(L)*.

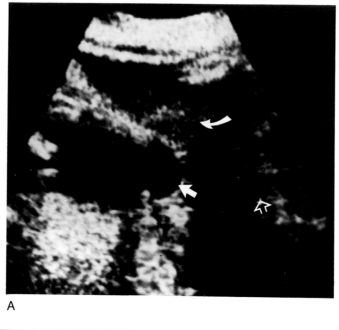

A

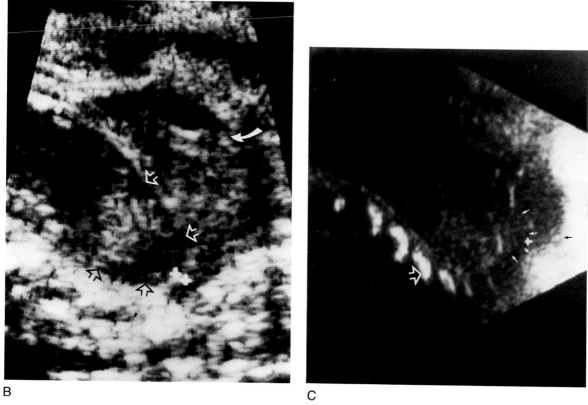

B   C

Fig. 9-51. Imperforate anus. **(A)** Longitudinal transabdominal scan demonstrates the distal rectal pouch (arrow) terminating above the base of the bladder (curved arrow). The examiner's finger, which is echogenic, is seen at the anal dimple (open arrow). **(B)** Longitudinal transabdominal scan demonstrates the distal rectal pouch (+ +, open arrows) terminating cephalad to the base of the bladder (curved arrow) in an infant with a high imperforate anus. **(C)** Longitudinal transperineal scan shows the distal rectal pouch (white +, arrows) and the perineal surface (black arrow). The open arrow indicates the sacrum. The pouch-skin distance (between + and black arrow) was less than 1.1 cm. (From Oppenheimer DA, Carroll BA, Shochat SJ: Sonography of imperforate anus. Radiology 148:127, 1983.)

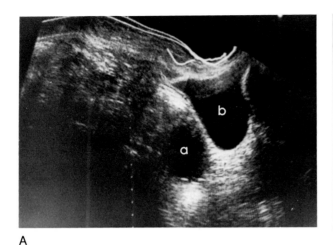

A

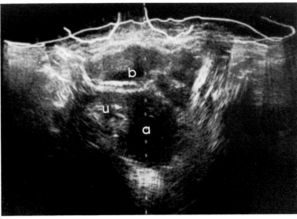

B

C

Fig. 9-52. Diverticular abscess. **(A)** Longitudinal scan at 1 cm to the left of midline. A poorly defined hypoechoic mass *(a)* is seen posterior to the bladder *(b)*. **(B)** Transverse scan. The abscess *(a)* is seen to the left of the uterus *(u)*. *(b,* bladder.) **(C)** CT scan. A soft-tissue mass *(a)* containing air (arrows) is seen to the left of the uterus *(u)*. *(b,* bladder; *rs,* rectosigmoid colon.)

tions of acute appendicitis. These two entities cannot be differentiated by ultrasound.[79]

Tumor

Primary adenocarcinoma of the appendix is very uncommon. Carcinoid accounts for 88.2 percent of carcinomas of the appendix and mucinous adenocarcinoma for 8.3 percent.[85] The majority of patients with primary appendiceal carcinoma present clinically as acute appendicitis. Due to the obstruction of the appendix by carcinoma, appendicitis or perforation results. Ultrasound visualizes the condition as an asymmetric central echogenic core originating from the collapsed lumen, and having an irregular and lobulated anatomy with greater than 2 cm thickness of the wall secondary to tumor.[85]

ABNORMALITIES OF THE COLON

Normally, the colon is not usually identified as a structure as such on ultrasound, since it usually contains gas bubbles that produce acoustic shadows[18] (Fig. 9-50).

Imperforate Anus

Real-time ultrasound provides a noninvasive method to determine the level of obstruction in a patient with an imperforate anus. This is a common congenital anomaly that requires rapid evaluation and possible early surgery. The appropriate surgery depends on the position of the distal rectal pouch and its relationship to the puborectalis portion of the levator sling. If the pouch is identified less than 1.5 cm from the perineum, it is consistent with

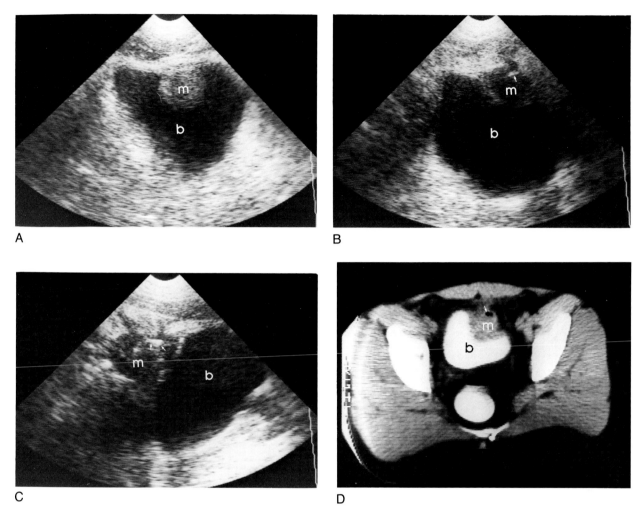

Fig. 9-53. Diverticular abscess. This patient presented with suprapubic pain. At cystoscopy, a bladder wall mass was visualized; a biopsy revealed inflammation. Transverse scans (**A,B**) through the bladder *(b)*, from inferior to superior views, reveal an echodense mass *(m)* projecting into the bladder. On (**B**), there was a linear echodensity (arrow) within the mass. Peristalsis was seen there with real-time scanning. (**C**) Longitudinal scan demonstrates a mass *(m)* superior to the bladder *(b)*. Like (**B**) peristalsis was seen in the area of the linear echodensity (arrows). As such, this mass was felt to be related to bowel. (**D**) CT scan similar to (**B**). A soft tissue density mass *(m)* is seen projecting into the bladder *(b)*. Air (arrow) is seen within the mass. On CT scan at a higher level than in (**D**) air was seen within many diverticuli. At surgery, the patient was found to have a diverticular abscess involving the bladder wall.

a low lesion that can be passed through the puborectalis portion of the levator sling.[86,87] If the pouch terminates above the base of the bladder, it is indicative of a high lesion.[86]

To evaluate the rectal pouch, the patient, with a full bladder, is scanned supinely in the lithotomy position with either an anterior or longitudinal midline transperineal approach.[87] The examiner places a finger in the pouch to measure the distance from the perineum[86] (Fig. 9-51).

Diverticular Disease

The term "diverticular disease" includes both diverticulosis and diverticulitis, both of which are characterized by numerous saccular outpouchings in the colon.[26] Most often diverticulosis may be asymptomatic, but at times it can produce symptoms. Both forms of diverticular disease can produce generalized lower abdominal discomfort with intermittent or continuous pain.[26] Constipation, which is frequent, sometimes alternates with

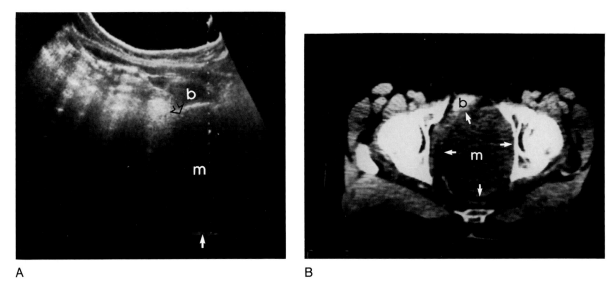

A   B

Fig. 9-54. Colon carcinoma. Rectal carcinoma. A hypoechoic mass (*m*, arrows) is seen posterior to the bladder *(b)* on longitudinal **(A)** scan. **(B)** CT scan. A large soft tissue mass (*m*, arrows) is seen posterior to the bladder *(b)* in the area of the rectum.

diarrhea. Diverticular disease is quite common in western societies, occurring in about one third of people over the age of 60.[26] In most cases, the condition is found incidently during a barium enema exam. The sigmoid colon is the most often involved segment of colon (in 95 percent of cases) but the descending and entire colon may be affected.[26]

Diverticula represent herniations of the mucosa through the muscle coat at points of weakness, such as between the longitudinal teniae and where the circular muscle is weakened by the segmental blood vessels that pierce it in two rows on each side of the colon. The mechanical force creating these herniations at points of

weakness is provided by elevated intracolonic pressure. The increased pressure is attributed to changes in the quantity and character of the stools, which in turn alter the force and mechanical characteristics of the peristaltic contractions.[26]

While colonic diverticuli are not identified on ultrasound, if perforation of an inflammatory diverticulum or spread of a peridiverticulitis gives rise to a paracolic abscess, a hypoechoic-to-anechoic mass may be identified within the pelvis (Figs. 9-52 and 9-53). If a hypoechoic mass is seen, when the patient is known to have diverticular disease and is symptomatic an abscess should be suspected. A CT scan may be performed to

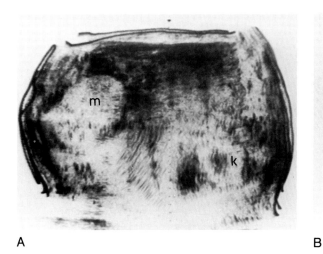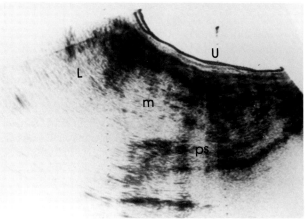

A   B

Fig. 9-55. Colon carcinoma. Hepatic flexure carcinoma. Transverse scan **(A)** at 9 cm above the umbilicus (below level of the liver) and longitudinal scan **(B)**. A poorly defined hypoechoic, solid mass *(m)* is seen on the right. The mass had no relationship to any anatomic structure. (*U*, umbilicus level; *ps*, psoas muscle; *k*, left kidney; *L*, liver.)

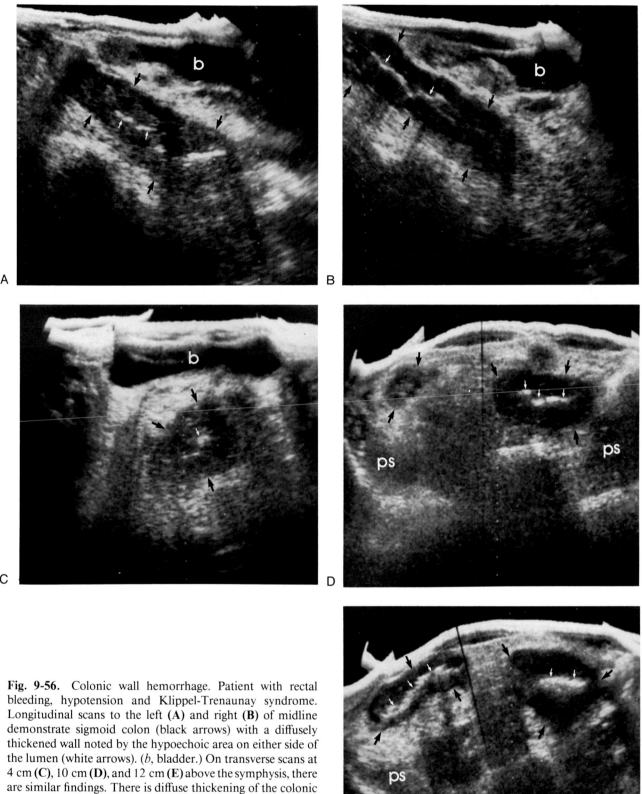

Fig. 9-56. Colonic wall hemorrhage. Patient with rectal bleeding, hypotension and Klippel-Trenaunay syndrome. Longitudinal scans to the left (**A**) and right (**B**) of midline demonstrate sigmoid colon (black arrows) with a diffusely thickened wall noted by the hypoechoic area on either side of the lumen (white arrows). (*b*, bladder.) On transverse scans at 4 cm (**C**), 10 cm (**D**), and 12 cm (**E**) above the symphysis, there are similar findings. There is diffuse thickening of the colonic wall due to hemorrhage. (*b*, bladder; *ps*, psoas muscle.)

confirm the diagnosis, since the ultrasound usually does not define the relationship of the abscess to bowel.

Tumor

CARCINOMA

It is a prime challenge for the medical profession to identify cancer of the colon, since this lesion produces symptoms early and is potentially curable by resection.

Eighty percent of cases occur in the rectum, rectosigmoid, or sigmoid colon, with 2.6 to 5 percent being multiple.[26,8] Peak incidence occurs in the seventh decade, with less than 20 percent of patients diagnosed under 50 years of age. Lesions of the left colon tend to grow in an annular encircling fashion, while those on the right tend to be polypoid and fungating masses. The patient most commonly presents with rectal bleeding and/or a change in bowel habit.[26]

While these lesions are usually diagnosed by barium

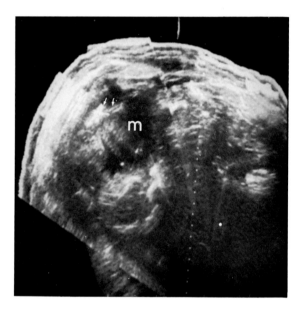
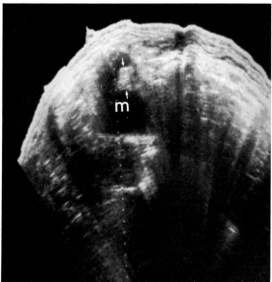
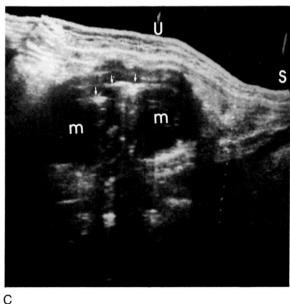
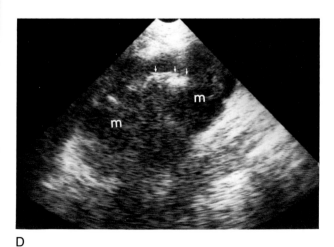

C

D

Fig. 9-57. Colon—Non-Hodgkin's lymphoma. Transverse scans at 3 cm above the umbilicus **(A)** and 6 cm above the symphysis **(B)** and longitudinal static scan 3 cm to the right of midline **(C)** and longitudinal real-time ultrasound **(D)** demonstrate a large, lobulated hypoechoic mass *(m)*. A reflective pattern (arrows), which represents air in the bowel lumen, is seen. (*U*, level of the umbilicus; *S*, level of the symphysis.) *(Figure continues.)*

THE GASTROINTESTINAL TRACT

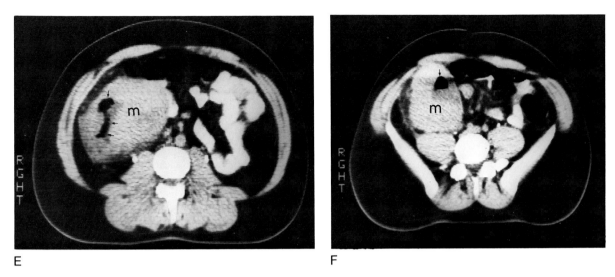

E   F

Fig. 9-57 *(Continued).* **(E)** CT scan similar to **(A)**, and **(F)** CT scan similar to **(B)** demonstrate a soft tissue density mass *(m)* that encases the colon. Air (arrows) is seen within the bowel lumen.

enema, rectal exam, or sigmoidoscopy, ultrasound can sometimes detect such tumors. Limited by intraluminal gas, ultrasound only occasionally is able to see either mural or intramural lesions (Figs. 9-54 and 9-55). With a high degree of obstruction and a fluid-filled proximal bowel, the obstructive lesion may be visible as in hypertrophic pyloric stenosis.[89] If the bowel wall is thickened and compressed or obliterated, a tumor should be suspected.[89] A bull's-eye pattern is generally seen, with wall thickening producing the hypoechoic oval-shaped mass and a central echogenic area produced by luminal air.[18,88,90] The more the wall is infiltrated, the broader the

hypoechoic area[88] (Fig. 9-54). If this mass is in the right lower quadrant, the examiner should suspect a cecal origin; with a right upper quadrant target lesion, hepatic flexure tumor should be suspected (Fig. 9-55). The differential diagnosis for the target pattern would have to include tuberculosis and amebiasis as well as tumor.[90] (Fig. 9-56)

LYMPHOMA

Colonic lymphomas are infrequent relative to their occurrence in the stomach and small intestine. These

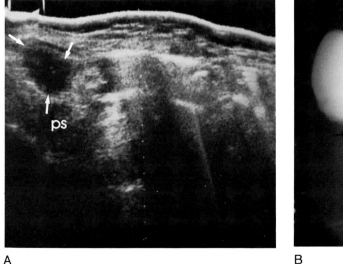

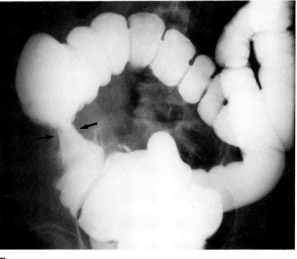

A   B

Fig. 9-58. Colon—Metastatic ovarian carcinoma. **(A)** Transverse static scan at 7 cm above the umbilicus. A hypoechoic mass (arrows) is seen in the right abdomen anterior to the psoas muscle *(ps).* **(B)** Barium enema. An apple-core type lesion (arrows) involves the ascending colon in the region of the mass on ultrasound.

tumors have the same morphologic and clinical characteristics as those in the upper segments of the bowel, which were described earlier. On ultrasound, a target pattern may be seen or simply a hypoechoic mass (Fig. 9-57). If on real-time scanning a reflective pattern (due to bowel gas) or peristalsis is seen within the mass, the examiner should suspect bowel involvement. Colonic involvement is suspected if such a mass is in the area of the colon.

METASTATIC DISEASE

Metastatic disease to the colon is uncommon. Such lesions could produce a target pattern or a solid mass (Fig. 9-58).

CONCLUSION

It is not suggested that ultrasound should replace the barium study and gastroscopy in the diagnosis of GI disease. Since ultrasound scanning is usually made prior to these procedures, it is important to recognize features of GI lesions on ultrasound in order to streamline the patient's workup.[91] The pattern caused by concentric thickening of the infiltrated bowel wall holds true for lesions involving the wall of any portion of the alimentary tract.[7] While inflammation and neoplastic infiltration of the wall are primary considerations when bowel thickening is demonstrated, other possible diagnoses should include Crohn's disease, ileocecal tuberculosis, periappendiceal tumor, extensive ulcerative or hyperplastic coarse giant folds in Menetrier's disease, and edema of the intestinal wall in thrombosis of the mesenteric veins.[92] Ultrasound is usually performed as the first diagnostic measure in cases of palpable abdominal masses and can usually differentiate whether the mass originates from a parenchymal organ or the GI tract.[9] Ultrasound is not suitable for diagnosing the early stage of GI tumors confined to the mucosa and submucosa, or for definitive exclusion of advanced-stage tumors.[92]

REFERENCES

1. Gooding GAW, Laing FC: Rapid water infusion: A technique in the ultrasonic discrimination of the gas-free stomach from mass in the pancreatic tail. Gastrointest Radiol 4:139, 1979
2. Kremer H, Grobner W: Sonography of polypoid gastric lesions by the fluid-filled stomach method. J Clin Ultrasound 9:51, 1981
3. Weighall SL, Wolfman NT, Watson N: The fluid-filled stomach: A new sonic window. J Clin Ultrasound 7:353, 1979
4. Rubin C, Kurtz AB, Goldberg BB: Water enema: A new ultrasound technique in defining pelvic anatomy. J Clin Ultrasound 6:28, 1978
5. Rifkin MD, Gordon SJ, Goldberg BB: Sonographic examination of the mediastinum and upper abdomen by fiberoptic gastroscope. Radiology 151:175, 1984
6. Drugsted J, Gammelgaard J: Endoluminal ultrasonic scanning in the evaluation of rectal cancer: A preliminary report of 13 cases. Gastrointest Radiol 8:367, 1983
7. Peterson LR, Cooperberg PL: Ultrasound demonstration of lesions of the gastrointestinal tract. Gastrointest Radiol 3:303, 1978
8. Fleischer AC, Muhletaler CA, James AE Jr: Detection of bowel lesions during abdominal and pelvic sonography. JAMA 244:2096, 1980
9. Fakhry JR, Berk RN: The "target" pattern: Characteristic sonographic feature of stomach and bowel abnormalities. AJR 137:969, 1981
10. Fleischer AC, Muhletaler CA, James AE Jr: Sonographic patterns arising from normal and abnormal bowel. Radiol Clin North Am 18:145, 1980
11. Fleischer AC, Muhletaler CA, Kurtz AB, James AE Jr: Real-time sonography of bowel. p.117. In Winsberg F, Cooperberg PL (eds): Clinics in Diagnostic Ultrasound: Real-Time Ultrasonography. Churchill Livingstone, New York, 1982
12. Torp-Pedersen S, Gronvall S, Holm HH: Ultrasonically guided fine-needle aspiration biopsy of gastrointestinal mass lesions. J Ultrasound Med 3:65, 1984
13. Ennis MG, MacErlean DP: Biopsy of bowel wall pathology under ultrasound control. Gastrointest Radiol 6:17, 1981
14. Bluth EI, Merritt CRB, Sullivan MA: Ultrasonic evaluation of the stomach, small bowel and colon. Radiology 133:677, 1979
15. Fleischer AC, Muhletaler CA, James AE Jr: Sonographic assessment of the bowel wall. AJR 136:887, 1981
16. Oliva L, Biggi E, Derchi LE, Cicio GR: Ultrasonic anatomy of the fluid-filled duodenum. J Clin Ultrasound 9:245, 1981
17. Fleischer AC, Dowling AD, Weinstein ML, James AE Jr: Sonographic patterns of distended, fluid filled bowel. Radiology 133:681, 1979
18. Yeh H-C, Rabinowitz JG: Ultrasonography of gastrointestinal tract. p.331. In Raymond HW, Zweibel WJ (eds): Seminars in Ultrasound: Potpourri. Vol. 3, No. 4. Grune & Stratton, New York, 1982
19. Komaiko MS: Gastric neoplasms: Ultrasound and CT evaluation. Gastrointest Radiol 4:131, 1979
20. Teele RL, Henschke CI, Tapper D: The radiographic and ultrasonographic evaluation of enteric duplication cysts. Pediatr Radiol 10:9, 1980
21. Moccia WA, Astacio JE, Kaude JV: Ultrasonographic demonstration of gastric duplication in infancy. Pediatr Radiol 11:52, 1981
22. Gorelik I, Goldman SM, Minkin SD et al: Gastric duplica-

tion originating from the tail of the pancreas — ultrasonically demonstrated. J Clin Ultrasound 4:429, 1976

23. Kangarloo H, Sample WF, Hansen G et al: Ultrasonic evaluation of abdominal gastrointestinal tract duplication in children. Radiology 131:191, 1979

24. Sauerbrei EE, Paloschi GGB: The ultrasonic features of hypertrophic pyloric stenosis with emphasis on the postoperative appearance. Radiology 147:503, 1983

25. Strauss S, Itzchak Y, Manor A et al: Sonography of hypertrophic pyloric stenosis. AJR 136:1057, 1981

26. Robbins SL, Cotran RS: The gastrointestinal tract. p.918. In Pathologic Basis of Disease, WB Saunders, Philadelphia, 1979

27. Ball TI, Atkinson GO Jr, Gay BB Jr: Ultrasound diagnosis of hypertrophic pyloric stenosis: Real-time application and the demonstration of a new sonographic sign. Radiology 147:499, 1983

28. Blumhagen JD, Noble HGS: Muscle thickness in hypertrophic pyloric stenosis: Sonographic determination. AJR 140:221, 1983

29. Blumhagen JD, Coombs JB: Ultrasound in the diagnosis of hypertrophic pyloric stenosis. J Clin Ultrasound 9:289, 1981

30. Teele RL: The pancreas, spleen, mesentery and gastrointestinal tract. p. 104. In Haller JO, Shkolnik A (eds): Clinics in Diagnostic Ultrasound: Ultrasound in Pediatrics. Churchill Livingstone, New York, 1981

31. Teele RL, Smith EH: Ultrasound in the diagnosis of idiopathic hypertrophic pyloric stenosis. N Engl J Med 296:1149, 1977

32. Graif M, Itzchak Y, Avigad I et al: The pylorus in infancy: Overall sonographic assessment. Pediatr Radiol 14:14, 1984

33. Wilson DA, Vanhoutte JJ: The reliable sonographic diagnosis of hypertrophic pyloric stenosis. J Clin Ultrasound 12:201, 1984

34. Madrazo BL, Hricak H, Sandler MA, Eyler WR: Sonographic findings in complicated peptic ulcer disease. Radiology 140:457, 1981

35. Kopen PA, McAlister WH: Upper gastrointestinal and ultrasound examinations of gastric antral involvement in chronic granulomatous disease. Pediatr Radiol 14:91, 1984

36. Schabel SI, Rittenberg GM, Bubanj R, Warren E: Pedunculated gastric leiomyoma: A wandering abdominal mass demonstrated by ultrasound. J Clin Ultrasound 7:211, 1979

37. Morgan CL, Trought WS, Oddson TA et al: Ultrasound patterns of disorders affecting the gastrointestinal tract. Radiology 135:129, 1980

38. Mascatello VJ, Carrera GF, Telle RL et al: The ultrasonic demonstration of gastric lesions. J Clin Ultrasound 5:383, 1977

39. Yeh H-C, Rabinowitz JG: Ultrasonography and computed tomography of gastric wall lesions. Radiology 141:147, 1981

40. Walls WJ: The evaluation of malignant gastric neoplasms by ultrasonic B-scanning. Radiology 118:159, 1976

41. Derchi LE, Biggi E, Rollandi GA, et al: Sonographic staging of gastric cancer. AJR 140:273, 1983

42. Derchi LE, Banderali A, Bossi MC, et al: The sonographic appearance of gastric lymphoma. J Ultrasound Med 3:251, 1984

43. Salem S, Hiltz CW: Ultrasonographic appearance of gastric lymphosarcoma. J Clin Ultrasound 6:429, 1978

44. Carroll BA, Ta HN: The ultrasonic appearance of extranodal abdominal lymphoma. Radiology 136:419, 1980

45. Subramanyam BR, Balthazar EJ, Raghavendra BN, Madamba MR: Sonography of exophytic gastrointestinal leiomyosarcoma. Gastrointest Radiol 7:47, 1982

46. Kaftori JK, Aharon M, Kleinhaus U: Sonography features of gastrointestinal leiomyosarcoma. J Clin Ultrasound 9:11, 1981

47. Sandler MA, Ratanaprakarn S, Madrazo BL: Ultrasonic findings in intramural exogastric lesions. Radiology 128:189, 1978

48. Scheible W, Goldberger LE: Diagnosis of small bowel obstruction: The contribution of diagnostic ultrasound. AJR 133:685, 1979

49. Pozderac RV, Doust BD: Confusing appearance of a dilated jejunal loop. J Clin Ultrasound 6:165, 1978

50. Pon MS, Scudamore C, Harrison RC, Cooperberg PL: Ultrasound demonstration of radiographically obscure small bowel obstruction. AJR 133:145, 1979

51. Miller JH, Kemberling CR: Ultrasound scanning of the gastrointestinal tract in children: Subject review. Radiology 152:671, 1984

52. Hayden CK Jr, Boulden TF, Swischuk LE, Lobe TE: Sonographic demonstration of duodenal obstruction with midgut volvulus. AJR 143:9, 1984

53. Hopens T, Coggs GC, Goldstein HM, Smith BD: Sonographic diagnosis of afferent loop obstruction. AJR 138:967, 1982

54. Hauser JB, Stanley RJ, Geisse G: The ultrasound findings in an obstructed afferent loop. J Clin Ultrasound 2:287, 1974

55. Yeh H-C, Rose J, Rabinowitz, JG: Sonography of an obstructive ileovesical anastomosis. J Clin Ultrasound 8:160, 1980

56. Lee TG, Brickman FE, Avecilla LS: Ultrasound diagnosis of intramural intestinal hematoma. J Clin Ultrasound 5:423, 1977

57. Foley LC, Teele RL: Ultrasound of epigastric injuries after blunt trauma. AJR 132:593, 1979

58. Fried AM, Pulmano CM, Mostowycz L: Duodenal duplication cyst: Sonographic and angiographic features. Am J Roentgenol 128:863, 1977

59. Burke LF, Clark E: Ileocolic intussusception — A case report. J Clin Ultrasound 5:346, 1977

60. Weissberg DL, Scheible W, Leopold GR: Ultrasonographic appearance of adult intussusception. Radiology 124:791, 1977

61. Morton ME, Blumenthal DH, Tan A, Li YP: The ultrasonic appearance of ileocolic intussusception. J Clin Ultrasound 9:516, 1981

62. Bowerman RA, Silver TM, Jaffe MH: Real-time ultra-

sound diagnosis of intussusception in children. Radiology 143:527, 1982

63. Montali G, Croce F, De Pra L, Solbiati L: Intussusception of the bowel: A new sonographic pattern. Br J Radiol 56:621, 1983

64. Holt S, Samuel E: Multiple concentric ring sign in the ultrasonographic diagnosis of intussusception. Gastrointest Radiol 3:307, 1978

65. Sarti DA, Zablen MA: The ultrasonic findings in intussusception of the blind loop in a jejunoileal bypass for obesity. J Clin Ultrasound 7:50, 1979

66. Kaude JV, McDowall JD, Neustein CL et al: Intussusception after jejunoileal bypass as diagnosed by ultrasound. Gastrointest Radiol 6:135, 1981

67. Yeh H-C, Rabinowitz JC: Granulomatous enterocolitis: Findings by ultrasonography and computed tomography. Radiology 149:253, 1983

68. Garb M, Risenborough J: Meconium peritonitis presenting as fetal ascites on ultrasound. Br J Radiol 53:602, 1980

69. Gonzalez AC, Hanes JD: Retrorenal abscess secondary to a ruptured retrocecal appendix diagnosed by ultrasound B scan and ^{67}Ga radionuclide scan. J Clin Ultrasound 5:114, 1977

70. Dunne M, Haney P, Sun C-CJ: Sonographic features of bowel perforation and calcific meconium peritonitis in utero. Pediatr Radiol 13:231, 1983

71. Brugman SM, Bjelland JJ, Thomasson JE et al: Sonographic findings with radiologic correlation in meconium peritonitis. J Clin Ultrasound 7:305, 1979

72. Blumenthal DH, Rushovich AM, Williams RK, Rochester D: Prenatal sonographic findings of meconium peritonitis with pathologic correlations. J Clin Ultrasound 10:350, 1982

73. Bowen A, Mazer J, Zarabi M, Fujioka M: Cystic meconium peritonitis: Ultrasonographic features. Pediatr Radiol 14:18, 1984

74. Silverbach S: Antenatal real-time investigation of meconium cyst. J Clin Ultrasound 11:455, 1983

75. Carroll BA, Moskowitz PS: Sonographic diagnosis of neonatal meconium cyst. AJR 137:1262, 1981

76. Miller JH, Hindman BW, Lam AH: Ultrasound in the evaluation of small bowel lymphoma in children. Radiology 135:409, 1980

77. Morin ME, Panella J, Baker DA, Engle J: Ultrasound detection of a carcinoid tumor. Gastrointest Radiol 4:359, 1979

78. Walecki JK, Hales ED, Chung EB, Laster HD: Ultrasound contribution to diagnosis of Peutz-Jeghers syndrome. Pediatr Radiol 14:62, 1984

79. Parulekar SG: Ultrasonographic findings in diseases of the appendix. J Ultrasound Med 2:59, 1983

80. Deutsch A, Leopold GR: Ultrasonic demonstration of the inflamed appendix: Case Report. Radiology 140:163, 1981

81. Sandler MA, Pearlberg JL, Madrazo BL: Ultrasonic and computed tomographic features of mucocele of the appendix. J Ultrasound Med 3:97, 1984

82. Horgan JG, Chow PP, Richter JO, Rosenfield AT, Taylor KJW: CT and sonography in the recognition of mucocele of the appendix. AJR 143:959, 1984

83. Athey PA, Hacken JB, Estrada R: Sonographic appearance of mucocele of the appendix. J Clin Ultrasound 12:333, 1984

84. Li YP, Morin ME, Tan A: Ultrasound findings in mucocele of the appendix. J Clin Ultrasound 9:406, 1981

85. Tan A, Lau PH: Sonography of primary adenocarcinoma of the appendix with pathological correlation. Am J Gastroenterol 78:488, 1983

86. Oppenheimer DA, Carroll BA, Shochat SJ: Sonography of imperforate anus. Radiology 148:127, 1983

87. Schuster SR, Teele RL: An analysis of ultrasound scanning as a guide in determination of "high" or "low" imperforate anus. J Pediatr Surg 14:798, 1979

88. Kremer H, Lohmoeller G, Zollner N: Primary ultrasonic detection of a double carcinoma of the colon. Radiology 124:481, 1977

89. Schabel SI, Rittenberg GM, Johnson EG III: Carcinoma of the colon demonstrated by ultrasound. J Clin Ultrasound 6:436, 1978

90. Gooding GAW: Ultrasonography of the cecum. Gastrointest Radiol 6:243, 1981

91. Salem S, O'Malley BP, Hiltz CW: Ultrasonographic appearance of gastrointestinal masses. J Can Assoc Radiol 31:163, 1980

92. Schwerk W, Braun B, Dombrowski H: Real-time ultrasound examination in the diagnosis of gastrointestinal tumors. J Clin Ultrasound 7:425, 1979

10

Interventional Ultrasound

Ultrasound has made a major contribution not only to diagnosis but also to biopsy and aspiration or drainage procedures. Many procedures that were once considered difficult and time consuming are now done quickly and simply with ultrasound and CT guidance.

BIOPSY

Percutaneous biopsy has become the most frequently performed interventional radiologic procedure. Its increased use is related to the newer imaging techniques that facilitate needle placement, the greater safety of small needles, and the advances in cytology. Both ultrasound and CT allow tissue sampling, with considerable safety, from areas that previously could not be visualized with fluoroscopy. Thus, the accuracy and safety of the biopsy procedure has increased its acceptance by clinicians. While the accuracy rate varies among institutions and depending on which organ is biopsied, it generally depends on operator expertise, patient cooperation, number of samples obtained, and close cooperation with the pathologist.[1] The contribution of percutaneous biopsy has led to more efficient diagnosis and therapy planning, which indicates it will be used increasingly in the future.

Ultrasound Technique

A biopsy of a target structure may be performed with direct ultrasound visualization or ultrasound may be used for localization of a structure and the biopsy performed without direct ultrasound visualization or "blindly." With either technique, the structure to be biopsied is scanned, taking into account the most suitable skin entry site, depth, angle, and phase of respiration.[2] One should choose the most direct approach, using the least angle possible and the shortest distance to the target. It is best to advance the needle in a quick thrust, as a slow advancement of the needle often results in displacement of the target lesion without penetration.

There are several sonographic methods of guiding a biopsy. Firstly, the target may be localized using static ultrasound and marking the point of entry on the patient's skin. This technique is fine for larger, more superficial targets. The operator may also use static ultrasound with an aspiration/biopsy transducer (Fig. 10-1). This is a specialized transducer with a central channel for the needle.[3] The transducer can be sterilized and as such used in a sterile fashion. As the transducer passes over the target, the needle is quickly thrust. This type of transducer has several disadvantages. The presence of the needle channel may degrade the image to a varying extent.[2,3] Either more gain or output energy is required than with the standard transducer.[2] In addition, the size of the needle is limited, and at times the procedure may be cumbersome.[2]

With real-time ultrasound, it is possible to localize a target or monitor the entire procedure.[4] The transducer may or may not be in the sterile field. The disadvantage of a linear array transducer is its difficulty in scanning over a target that lies deep to a rib interspace. The angle of the puncture is also limited. Most sector transducers are mechanical sectors consisting of rotating or oscillating crystals, or acoustic reflectors. With this type of sys-

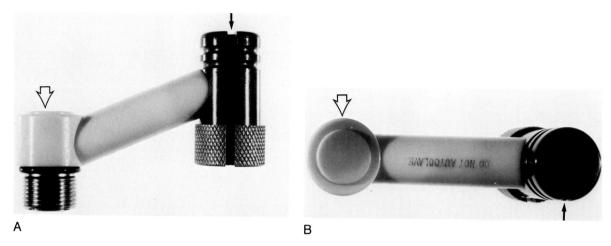

A   B

Fig. 10-1. Static biopsy transducer. **(A)** Side and **(B)** top views. Using this transducer, the biopsy needle is inserted through the center (arrow) hole of the transducer while watching on the A-mode. (open arrow, portion of transducer screwed into the static scanning arm.)

tem, it is more practical to design a needle attachment than to modify the transducer itself for biopsy purposes[2,3,5-12] (Fig. 10-2). Like CT, ultrasound scans represent a slice thickness. The purpose of the needle guide is to ensure that the needle remains within the scan thickness when advanced to the target.[2] This can be tested in a water bath prior to instituting a procedure. The needle guide is designed so that the needle path lies in the center of the scan thickness. With proper placement, the length of the needle is visualized when the needle is placed in the guide in a water bath (Fig. 10-3).

This needle guide is sterilized and usually attached to the scanhead by a baseplate. The sector transducer cannot be sterilized, so gel is placed on the scanning surface and the scanhead is placed either in a sterile glove or bag (Fig.10-4A–F). Then, the needle guide is "popped" onto

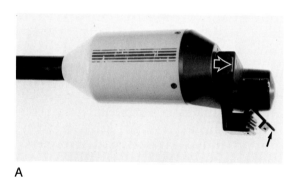

A   B

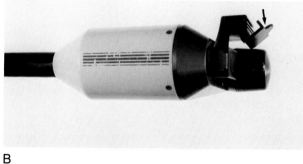

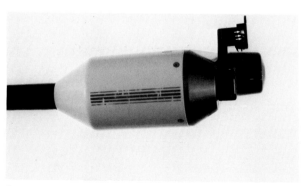

Fig. 10-2. Real-time biopsy guide. This commercially available needle guide can be attached or "popped" on to a baseplate (open arrow) on either the right **(A)** or left **(B,C)** side of the scanning surface. A needle is inserted through the guide grooves (small arrows on **(C)**) depending on the size of the needle. The guide can be detached from the needle by opening (black arrow) the guide.

C

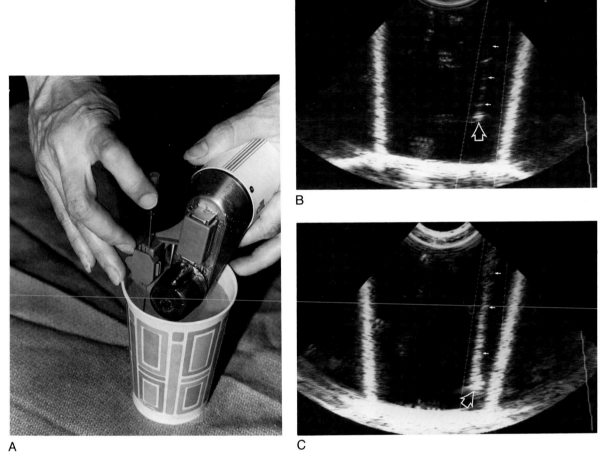

Fig. 10-3. Real-time biopsy guide and water bath. **(A)** The needle can be seen within the guide extending into the water. **(B,C)** On the screen, the echoes returning from the needle (small arrows) can be seen within the path marked by the computer software. The proper depth to the needle tip (open arrow) can be measured. (Fig. B, 22-gauge spinal needle; Fig. C, 20-gauge Teflon-coated Cook needle.)

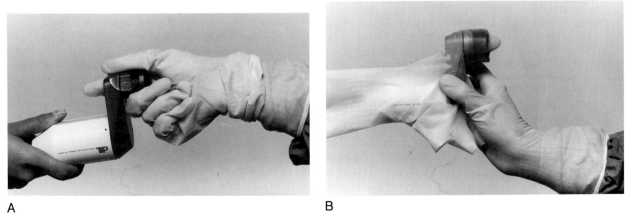

Fig. 10-4. Preparation for biopsy procedure. **(A)** After placing gel on the scanning surface of the transducer and placing a second sterile glove on the right hand (size 8), the transducer is grasped with the thumb on the scanning surface. **(B)** The second glove is inverted over the transducer so that the scanning surface is in the thumb of the glove. Tape is placed around the cuff of the glove. *(Figure continues.)*

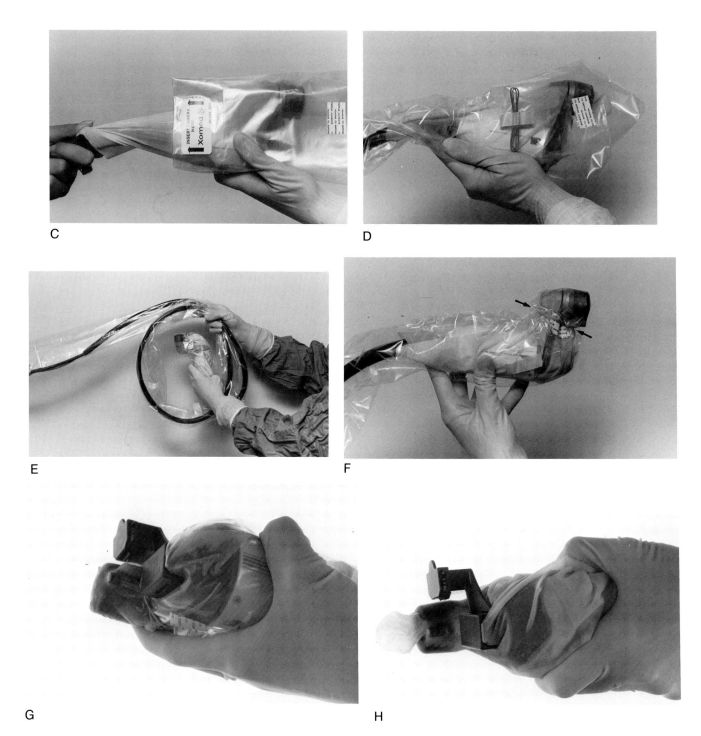

Fig. 10-4 *(Continued).* **(C–E)** If the transducer cable needs to be covered, a sterile drape is passed over the gloved transducer and its cable. **(F)** The corner of the bag is removed so that the scanning surface (in the glove thumb) is exposed and a sterile rubberband (arrows) is placed around the neck of the scanhead. The biopsy guide is "popped" onto the baseplate over the bag and glove **(G)** or over just the glove **(H)**.

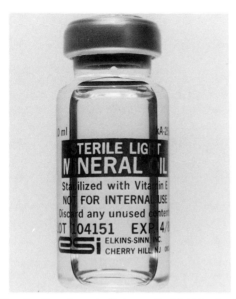

Fig. 10-5. Sterile mineral oil. A small vial (10 ml) of sterile mineral oil that is commercially available. This amount of oil is generally more than is needed for any one biopsy/aspiration procedure.

the baseplate (Fig. 10-4G,H). The entire procedure may then be performed sterilely, using sterile mineral oil (Fig. 10-5). By far, the larger needles (18 gauge) are easier to see than the smaller (22–23 gauge). With the larger ones, the entire needle may be visualized, but with the smaller only the tip is seen as a strong reflective echo.[13] For proper positioning of the transducer, most real-time systems have a soft-ware program that shows the course of the needle path (Fig. 10-6).

If the biopsy is performed without continuous real-time visualization, air can be used to "mark" the site of the biopsy.[14,15] After the biopsy needle is inserted into the target lesion, 0.3 to 0.5 ml of air can be introduced via a tuberculin syringe. After completion of the biopsy, a scan is obtained to document the biopsy site.

As has been stated, real-time ultrasound may be used for continuous visualization of the procedure but can also be used simply to localize a target much like static ultrasound. The real-time guide is usually reserved for the following: (1) puncture of a small fluid collection, (2) complete aspiration of a fluid collection, (3) when other methods fail to obtain fluid or tissue, (4) aspiration of fluid adjacent to or surrounded by other similar fluid or vascular structures, and (5) complex procedures requiring localization and fluoroscopy such as nephrostomy tube placement, abscess drainage, or biliary drainage.[2]

Choice of Needle

There are numerous needles available for use in biopsies[2,16,17] (Fig. 10-7). The Chiba 22-gauge needle, or the spinal needle, has a beveled tip, while the Greene needle

and the Madayag have a pencil-point-type stylet with an outer cutting needle (Fig. 10-7). For deeper lesions, the cutting needle is more likely to result in a core of tissue. The beveled tips tend to be displaced in the direction opposite to the bevel face, as a result of increased resistance of the tissue during advancement.[2]

In one study, the Turner (20-gauge) needle biopsies were compared to the Chiba (22-gauge.)[16] The Turner needle had a positive reading for histology alone in 83 percent of cases; while in 90 percent of cases, there was a positive reading for both histology and cytology. The histology yielded a positive diagnosis in most patients with a false-negative cytology. The histology provided the cell type or tissue of origin in most cases. Raising the bevel angle to 45° produces the tissue core. The Chiba needle has a 25° bevel. Obtaining the histology is especially valuable in lymphoma.[16]

Another group evaluated the Madayag (22-gauge), the Menghini (18-gauge) and the Tru-cut (14-gauge) needles. The Madayag had a high recovery rate and provided adequate histologic information in a large percent of cases. The larger needles more consistently demonstrated a higher recovery rate and diagnostic specimen than the Madayag. The specimen obtained from the Madayag needle was correct for malignancy (including histology and cytology) in 78 percent of cases. With the larger core biopsy, there was a positive diagnosis in 92 percent of cases. The large-core needles were more informative in 54 percent of cases. The larger amount of tissue obtained and the better preservation of the tissue architecture improved the pathologic evaluation. They recommended using the Madayag needle to confirm recurrence or spread of disease, while the larger needles were used for a lesion with unknown origin.[17]

At our institution, we use the spinal needle, Surecut, or E-Z-EM cutting needles most frequently with real-time guidance. The Teflon-coated needles by Cook are more readily visible on real-time ultrasound than the other needles, especially when using small gauges (Figs. 10-3B,C). In addition, if there is a problem in visualizing the needle tip, the stylet may be pulled back.

Patient Preparation

In most cases there is no special preparation. Some radiologists use mild sedation for their patients.[18]

Contraindications

There are only a few contraindications to the percutaneous aspiration biopsy procedure, among them is uncontrollable bleeding diathesis.[18] Caution is recom-

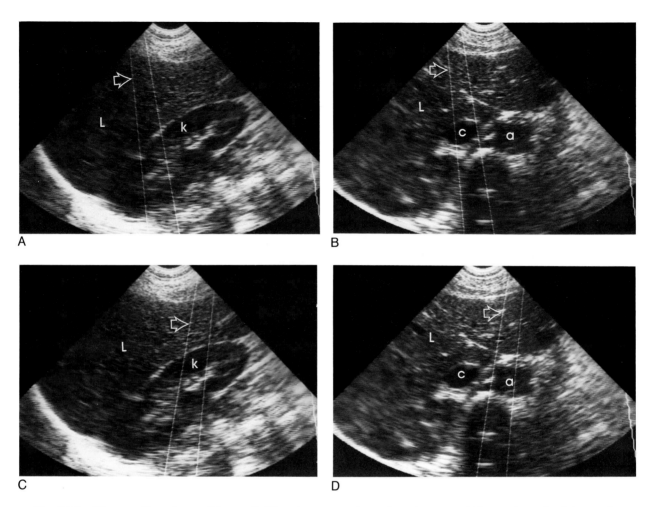

Fig. 10-6. Biopsy guide-software. The parallel lines (open arrow) noted on the screen delineate the path of the needle when performing a biopsy/aspiration using a left- **(A,B)** or right- **(C,D)** sided guide in longitudinal **(A,C)** or transverse **(B,D)** planes. (*c*, inferior vena cava; *a*, aorta; *k*, right kidney; *L*, liver.)

mended when taking biopsies of suspected highly vascular primary liver neoplasms, such as hepatocellular carcinoma and hemangioma; however, these can usually be biopsied safely. Patient inability to cooperate is a relative contraindication.

Biopsy Technique

After the target is localized, the area is prepped and draped. Local anesthesia is instilled in the area marked on the skin. If the procedure is performed "blind," the appropriate needle is inserted to the predetermined depth with a quick thrust, using care to maintain the angle and phase of respiration used during localization. Often there is a gritty feeling when the needle enters the target. Once the desired depth is reached, the needle stylet is removed and the needle is attached to a 6 to

20 ml syringe.[18,19] With continuous suction, the needle is advanced within the lesion in short up-and-down rotary movements, through a 1 cm path.[2,15,18-23] The suction is released prior to withdrawing the needle. Some investigators use Aspir-gun (gas-sterile, plastic holder for a syringe) or other syringe designs that rapidly produce or release suction within the syringe[24] (Fig. 10-8). Three to four passes are made. A greater number of passes is associated with increased risk of complications; less passes may not yield adequate material. After each pass, the tissue is processed according to the method determined by the pathologist responsible for examining the tissue. This varies from institution to institution.[2]

A "tandem" needle placement may be used.[18,19] Once the first needle is placed in the target, several other needles are placed at similar depths next to the first needle. Then, the aspiration/biopsies are performed. When appropriate, guided multiquadrant biopsies of the periph-

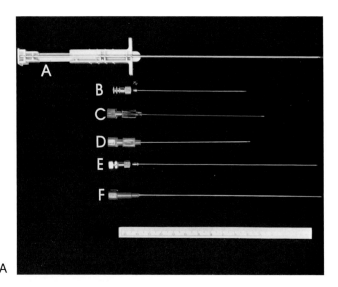

Fig. 10-7. Biopsy needles. These are several of the needles available for use. (*A*, 14-gauge Trucut; *B*, 22-gauge spinal; *C*, 20-gauge teflon-coated spinal; *D*, 20-gauge Turner; *E*, 22-gauge Chiba; and *F*, 18g E-Z-EM cutting needle. Notice length (**A**), needle tips (**B**), and bevel angle (**C**).

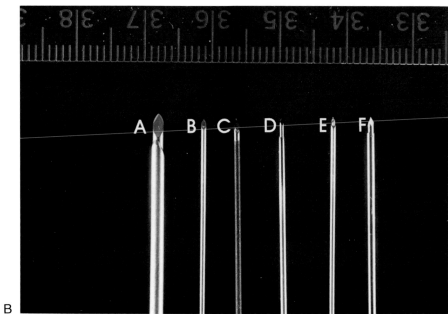

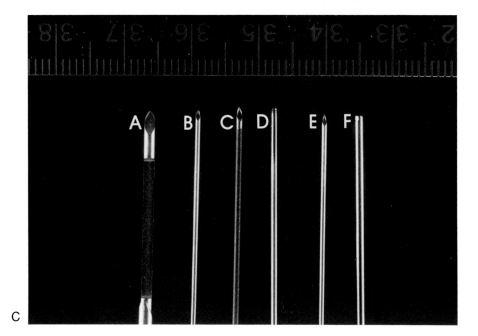

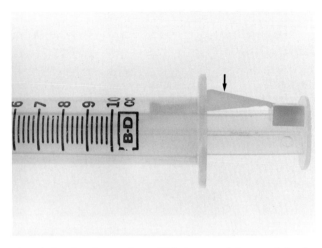

Fig. 10-8. Suction syringe. This is one of the specially designed syringes that provide automatic suction when performing a biopsy due to the attached notched lever (arrow).

ery of a target may be used to minimize the likelihood of a false-negative specimen from a necrotic area.[18]

If the biopsy is done with real-time visualization using the needle guide, the procedure is slightly different (Fig.

10-9). After the area is prepped and draped, the target is scanned by means of sterile oil and a transducer that is draped with a sterile glove or bag. Since the needle guide is offset, it is necessary to administer the local anesthesia directly under the guide (Fig. 10-9A). After this point is localized and the area infiltrated, the biopsy procedure begins. The needle is placed into the skin, sterile oil is placed on the skin, and the needle guide is opened so that the needle may be placed within it (Figs. 10-9B – E). The target is scanned. The needle is thrust within the target under real-time visualization. Once the tip of needle is seen within the lesion (Fig. 10-10), the transducer and guide are removed from the field, and the biopsy is performed "free-hand," much as described above. This is repeated for each needle pass. With this technique, there is verification and documentation (film) of the location of the biopsy (Fig. 10-10).

Complications

Adverse effects of fine-needle aspiration/biopsy procedure are infrequent despite assumed occasional penetration of bowel and blood vessels.[18] The size of the nee-

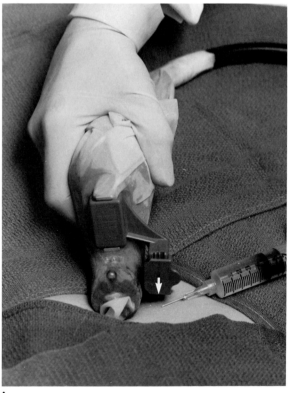

A

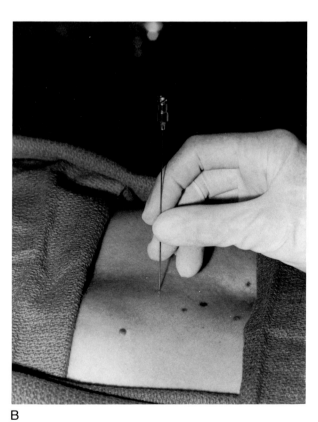

B

Fig. 10-9. Biopsy procedure. **(A)** The site for the biopsy is noted under the needle guide and local anesthesia is given (arrow). **(B)** The needle is inserted into the skin at the localized spot and sterile oil is placed on the skin. *(Figure continues.)*

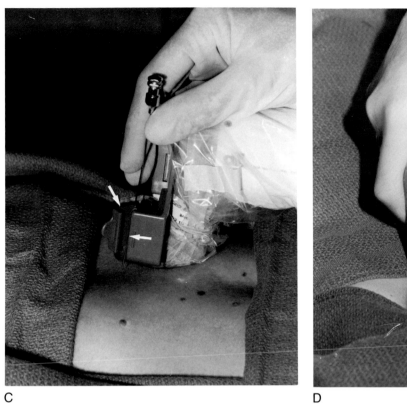

C

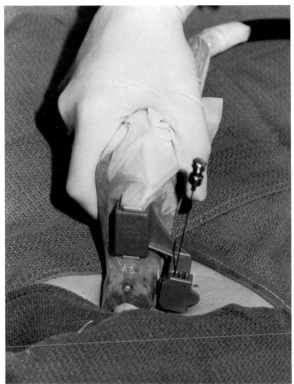

D

Fig. 10-9 *(Continued).* The needle guide is opened (arrows) **(C)** and closed (arrows) **(D,E)** over the needle. The excursion of the needle is watched with real-time until the tip is within the target lesion. The transducer and guide are then removed from the biopsy needle and the biopsy is performed "free-hand" with a syringe attached to the needle.

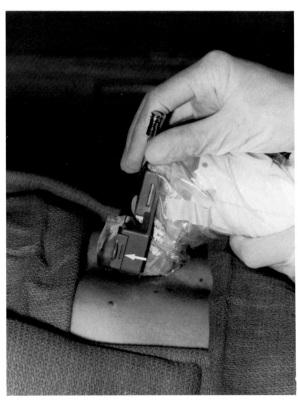

E

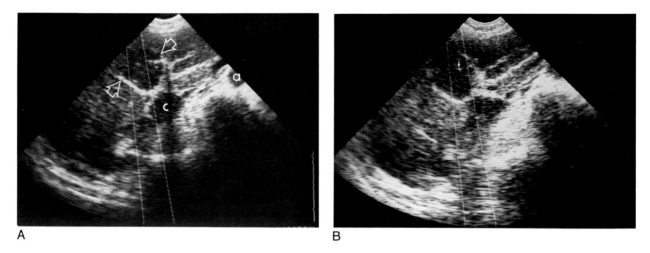

A   B

Fig. 10-10.   Liver biopsy. Patient with a known primary tumor. **(A)** A lesion (open arrows) is noted within the liver in the porta hepatis region. It is hypoechoic compared to liver parenchyma with fairly well defined margins. The lesion was localized using a biopsy guide in a somewhat oblique projection. The depth to the middle of the lesion is measured (+). (*a*, aorta; *c*, inferior vena cava.) **(B)** A 22-gauge spinal needle was inserted into the lesion using real-time visualization. The needle tip (small arrow) can be seen within the lesion. This biopsy was positive for recurrent tumor.

dle and the vascularity of the punctured lesion invariably influence the potential for bleeding complication. Reports list a complication rate of 2.2 to 3.0 percent.[18,25]

dependent on the operator's expertise, patient cooperation, number of samples obtained, and close cooperation with the pathologist.

Organ Application

A percutaneous biopsy is indicated when distinguishing (1) cyst versus solid mass, (2) benign versus malignant disease, and (3) abscess versus tumor.[1,26] The accuracy rate of this procedure varies among institutions and according to the organ being biopsied, but in general is

LIVER

The primary indication for a needle biopsy of the liver is to document the presence of malignancy in order to avoid a diagnostic laparotomy[27] (Figs. 10-10 and 10-11). A needle biopsy may also be performed to identify whether a lesion is benign or malignant. This procedure

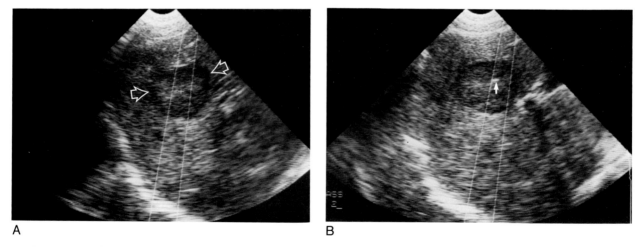

A   B

Fig. 10-11.   Liver biopsy. Patient with known malignant melanoma. **(A)** On longitudinal scan, a well-defined lesion (open arrows) is localized and the depth is measured (+). **(B)** Similar scan to **(A)** with the needle tip (arrow) within the lesion. The cytology was consistent with malignant melanoma.

is similar to the procedure described for biopsy technique. If the lesion is large, a blind biopsy may be done; if the lesion is small, the biopsy should be done with real-time guidance. The needle used is usually a 22-gauge. In recent years, the larger 18-gauge needle has been advocated in order to obtain a tissue core and provide more information.[1] An accuracy of 83 to 98 percent has been reported.[1,26-29] Others report a rate of positive diagnosis in guided liver biopsies of 97 percent,[30] while others report an overall accuracy of 91.6 percent, with a sensitivity of 92.2 percent and a specificity of 88.9 percent.[31]

Some complications reported with liver biopsy include retroperitoneal bleed, subcapsular hematoma, septic shock, and fistula formation between various arteries, veins, or biliary channels.[1] These occur rarely when small needles are used; it is inadvisable to use larger needles in vascular masses.[1] A relative contraindication to this procedure would be bowel dilatation and abnormal bleeding; ascites and obstructive jaundice are not regarded as contraindications.[27]

SPLEEN

There are few reports of fine-needle biopsies of the spleen, but these have shown that this procedure may be undertaken with a high degree of safety.[32-34] One group has performed needle biopsies in 45 cases of diffuse and focal splenic disease without immediate or subsequent adverse reactions.[32] No intrasplenic hematomas or lesions along the needle path were seen in the 23 patients who underwent splenectomy soon after fine-needle aspiration biopsy. Fine-needle aspiration should be considered a major diagnostic tool in the evaluation of focal splenic lesions of unknown etiology.

PANCREAS

One of the difficulties in obtaining positive tissue from the pancreas is that cancer incites an inflammatory response.[1,19,22] This requires tissue sampling from various areas.[1] Fine-needle pancreatic biopsy is indicated in order to (1) avoid surgery by obtaining histologic diagnosis, (2) determine staging of a neoplastic disease process, and (3) facilitate therapy planning.[35] There is a positive yield of 88 percent for cytologic diagnosis compared to 27 percent for core biopsy.[19] There is an 80 percent accuracy reported in differentiating benign from malignant disease.[36] Others report an accuracy of 60 to 93 percent.[1,18,26,35,37-39] Some investigators report the predictive value of a positive test to be 100 percent, with that of a negative test to be 77.7 percent.[40]

Reported complications include focal pancreatitis, hemorrhage, fistula formation, and bile peritonitis.[1]

There has also been a report of needle tract seeding from a biopsy of an unresectable pancreatic carcinoma.[41] Because of the difficulty in obtaining a specimen and the risk of complication, it may be more appropriate to biopsy an associated abdominal mass in the patient with the pancreatic lesion than to sample the pancreatic lesion directly.[1]

In contrast to the liver and spleen, there are more failures in visualization of the target lesion with ultrasound. If the pancreas is not seen or the mass is not visualized, then the biopsy should not be performed with ultrasound guidance. Larger patients and those with lots of bowel gas are more often biopsied with CT guidance, while patients who are thin and less gaseous are biopsied with ultrasound (Fig. 10-12).

ADRENAL AND RENAL

An adrenal mass in a patient with a known oncologic process should be biopsied to determine whether the lesion is a metastasis or a nonfunctioning adenoma (Fig. 10-13). If the lesion is found serendipitous (no known malignancy) and it is less than 3 to 4 cm, then it can be followed.[1] Adrenal adenomas 0.5 to 3.0 cm in diameter have been found slightly more commonly, with a 1.5 to 8.0 percent incidence at autopsy.[42] If the mass is 3 to 4 cm or greater, there is a greater chance for malignancy.[42]

The chance of obtaining a positive tissue diagnosis of the adrenal has greatly increased with CT; the accuracy is in the range of 90 to 93 percent.[1,43] Ultrasound has been reported to have a diagnostic accuracy of 80 to 90 percent with regard to fine-needle adrenal aspiration biopsies.[42] CT is the guidance method of choice for adrenal biopsies if the gland is normal size or small, or if the procedure would be technically difficult with ultrasound.[42] Ultrasound guidance may be used if the lesion is visualized and the biopsy approach is technically feasible. Ultrasound is more flexible than CT, since it allows many different approaches. Some investigators recommend a posterior approach that provides access to most adrenals, and utilizes the space between the spine and kidney, which is free of overlying blood vessels, bowel, or other abdominal organs.[43] Others recommend a flexible approach: (1) right adrenal—biopsied either from a lateral approach through the intercostal spaces or from an anterior approach (liver may be crossed but kidney avoided); and (2) left adrenal—biopsied from a posterior paraspinal approach with patient prone, lateral approach with needle between kidney and spleen or an anterior approach with patient's back extended by a pillow in order to push the mass toward the anterior abdominal wall.[42]

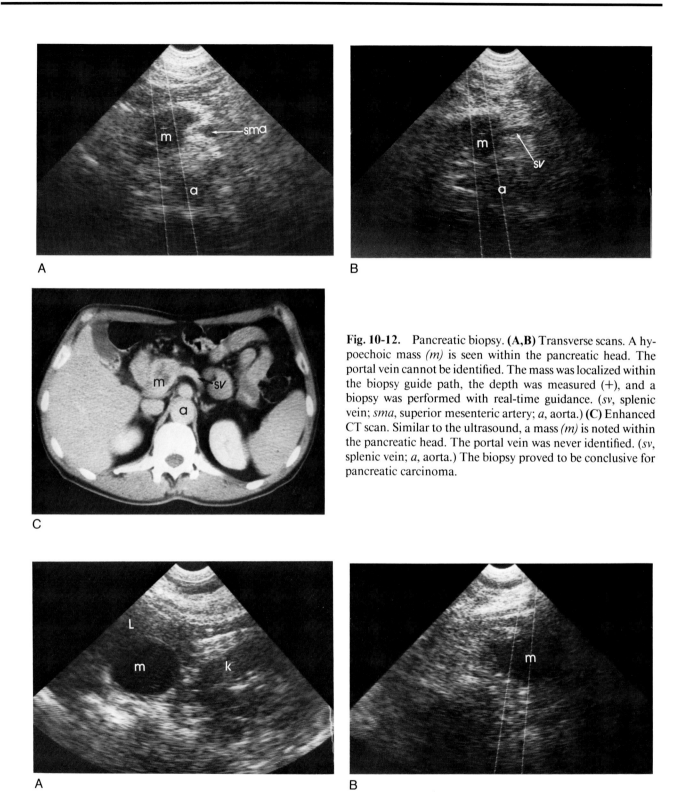

Fig. 10-12. Pancreatic biopsy. **(A,B)** Transverse scans. A hypoechoic mass *(m)* is seen within the pancreatic head. The portal vein cannot be identified. The mass was localized within the biopsy guide path, the depth was measured (+), and a biopsy was performed with real-time guidance. (*sv*, splenic vein; *sma*, superior mesenteric artery; *a*, aorta.) **(C)** Enhanced CT scan. Similar to the ultrasound, a mass *(m)* is noted within the pancreatic head. The portal vein was never identified. (*sv*, splenic vein; *a*, aorta.) The biopsy proved to be conclusive for pancreatic carcinoma.

Fig. 10-13. Adrenal biopsy. Patient with known primary tumor and adrenal mass. **(A)** A right hypoechoic adrenal mass *(m)* is seen on longitudinal scan in the left lateral decubitus position. (*k*, right kidney; *L*, liver.) **(B)** This mass *(m)* was localized for biopsy with the patient in the left lateral decubitus position using a transverse scan plane and a posterior approach. It proved to be an adrenal cyst.

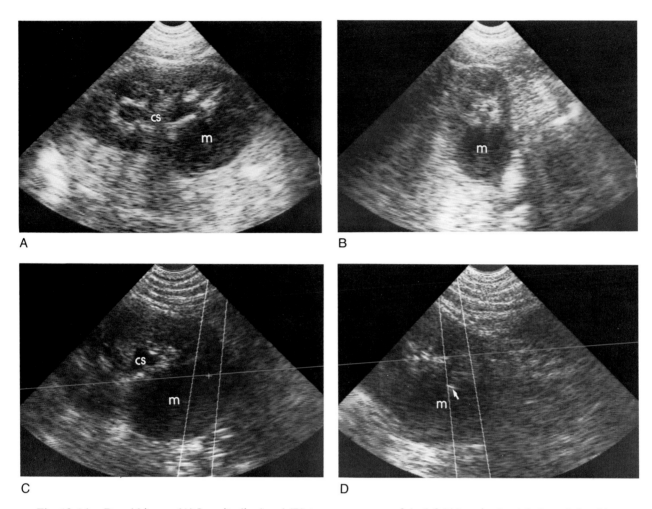

A

B

C

D

Fig. 10-14. Renal biopsy. **(A)** Longitudinal and **(B)** transverse scans of the left kidney in the right lateral decubitus position. A hypoechoic mass *(m)* is seen in the lower pole of the kidney. This patient had a similar mass in the pancreas (see Fig. 3-62) and was febrile. (*cs*, collecting system.) **(C)** This hypoechoic mass *(m)* was localized for biopsy with the patient prone. (*cs*, collecting system.) **(D)** The needle tip (arrow) is seen within the mass *(m)* as an echodense dot. This proved to be histiocytic lymphoma.

Cysts and tumors of the kidney can be easily biopsied with CT, ultrasound, or angiography (Fig. 10-14). There is little risk in tumor seeding along the needle tract.[1] With ultrasound guidance, there has been a reported accuracy of 96 percent.[26]

In patients with renal disease ultrasound may also be used to guide a large needle in the biopsy of the native kidney or renal transplant.[44-50] The success rates in obtaining adequate tissue have been reported to be 82.5 to 96.0 percent.[44,45,50] The lower pole of the left kidney is localized while the patient is lying prone on a rolled sheet or pillow[51] (Fig. 10-15). With static ultrasound, a square is marked on the patient's back, noting the lower pole, medial, and lateral borders of the kidney and the lower end of the collecting system (Fig. 10-15B).

Real-time guidance using the needle guide has greatly improved the success of this procedure at our institution (Fig. 10-16). Other investigators report a 96 percent success rate in obtaining adequate tissue employing a needle guide with a real-time system.[50] The nephrologist generally performs the biopsy using a Tru-cut needle, while the sonologist handles the ultrasound guidance. Using the needle guide has decreased the time required for the procedure and decreased the number of passes made to obtain adequate tissue. This same procedure may be employed in biopsying the transplanted kidney. In this instance, the superior-lateral pole of the kidney is usually chosen as the target site; with the patient supine a transverse scan plane is employed (Fig. 10-17).

Complications with adrenal and renal biopsies are

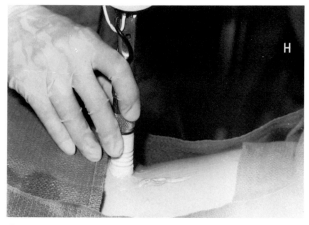

A

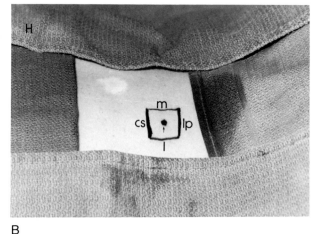

B

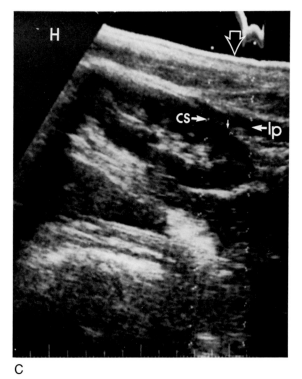

C

Fig. 10-15. Renal biopsy—Static guidance. **(A)** The patient is scanned in the prone position in longitudinal and transverse planes. (*H*, patient's head.) **(B)** The medial *(m)* and lateral *(l)* borders of the kidney, the inferior aspect of the collecting system *(cs)* and the lower pole *(lp)* are marked on the patient's skin forming a square. A point (arrow) is localized in the center of the square within the center of the lower pole. (*H*, patient's head.) **(C)** Longitudinal scan showing where the center point (open arrow) was marked. The depth was measured from the skin to renal capsule (small arrow) and to the midpoint of the lower pole. The biopsy was performed "free-hand". (*cs*, lower margin of the collecting system; *lp*, end of lower pole; *H*, patient's head.)

minimal with proper patient selection, choice of needle, and technique. Hemorrhage is most often noted with renal biopsy (Fig. 10-18). Another frequent complication is gross hematuria occurring in 12 percent of cases.[46] Some patients with biopsied adrenals (particularly on the left) have shown an increased incidence of pneumothorax if a posterior approach is used.[1]

RETROPERITONEAL

One of the greatest difficulties in the management of lymphoma is the detection of involvement of inaccessible nodes. While lymphangiography is useful for visual-izing pelvic and retroperitoneal nodes, splenic and mesenteric nodes and nodes totally replaced by tumor are not visualized. Lymphangiography is useful for detecting involved nonenlarged nodes and for very precise fluoroscopic biopsies. The newer imaging modalities of CT and ultrasound have greatly improved the staging and identification of nodal involvement; however, the diagnosis of lymphoma is based predominately on cytology, with the pattern of involvement of nodes, spleen, or other organs being important in determining the final diagnosis.

Lymphoma requires a large tissue sample for accurate diagnosis because it is important to type the cell pattern

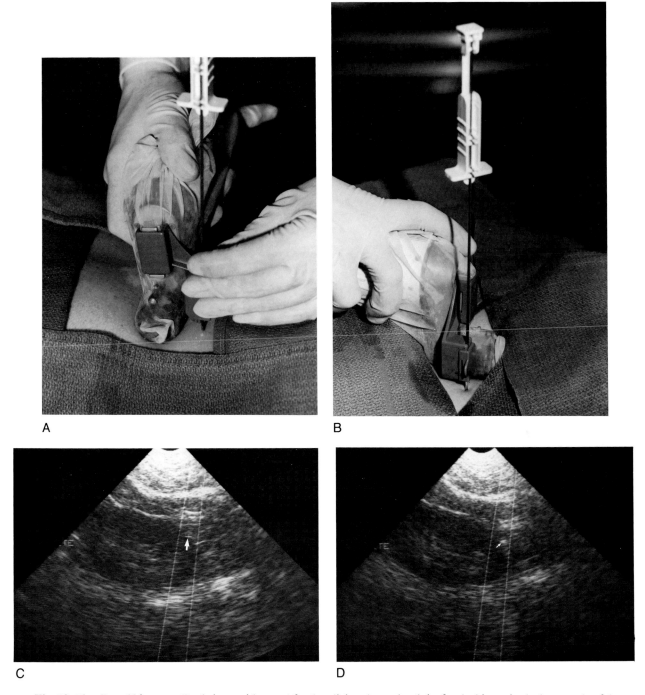

A   B   C   D

Fig. 10-16. Renal biopsy — Real-time guidance. After localizing the optimal site for the biopsy in the lower pole of the kidney with the patient prone, the skin is infiltrated with local anesthesia under the needle guide. The biopsy needle is inserted into the skin, and sterile oil is placed on the skin. **(A,B)** The needle is inserted into the needle guide and the procedure is performed with real-time guidance. **(C)** A depth (arrow) is measured from the skin to the renal capsule within the guide path. **(D)** Once the needle tip (arrow) reaches the renal capsule the guide and transducer are removed. The biopsy is performed "free-hand".

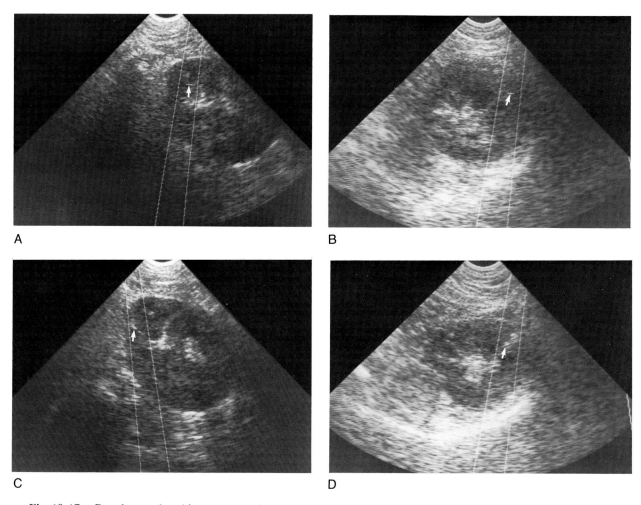

Fig. 10-17. Renal transplant biopsy—Real-time guidance. The superior pole or lateral pole (if kidney in transverse lie) is localized in a longitudinal plane **(A)** or a transverse plane **(B)** and local anesthesia is placed under the needle guide. A depth (arrow) is measured to the renal capsule or within the parenchyma. The needle is inserted into the skin and the needle is popped into the needle guide with the transducer in a **(C)** longitudinal or **(D)** transverse operation. The needle is inserted into the kidney under real-time guidance until the needle (arrow on C and D) reaches the desired depth. The guide is then removed.

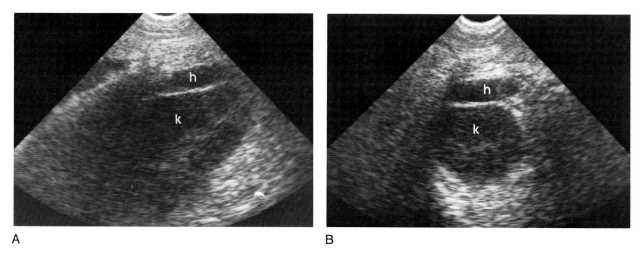

Fig. 10-18. Renal transplant biopsy. Postbiopsy hematoma. In this patient, a point was localized with real-time guidance and the biopsy was performed without direct real-time guidance and the needle guide. Following the procedure, a hypoechoic mass *(h)* or hematoma was seen on longitudinal **(A)** and transverse **(B)** scans of the kidney *(k)*.

in the lymphoma classification.[19,56] The initial diagnosis should be made from a larger amount of tissue than provided by the 22-gauge aspiration needle. If lymphoma is suspected, a large needle such as a Tru-cut is usually needed to obtain enough tissue for proper cell classification. The complications reported are small. Nodes are smaller and moveable, and thus more difficult to hit. A smaller gauge aspiration needle (22-gauge) is recommended for nodal biopsy, since these nodes are usually close to vascular structures.[52] Care should be taken to avoid the aorta or inferior vena cava. Masses between the aorta and inferior vena cava should be biopsied using an anterior approach, while those lateral to the aorta or inferior vena cava should be biopsied from a posterior access.[1]

Correct diagnosis based on nodal biopsy can be achieved in 54 percent of cases, while that in masses or organs is 76 percent.[52] The accuracy of a nodal biopsy for carcinoma is 20 percent greater than that for lymphoma.[1] Others report an accuracy for lymphoma biopsy of 65 to 90 percent.[1,52,53] It is important to differentiate nodal metastases or lymphoma.

Other retroperitoneal masses and primary or metastatic tumor may be biopsied with ultrasound guidance (Figs. 10-19 to 10-21) provided they are adequately visualized and the approach is technically feasible.

GASTROINTESTINAL TRACT

Although a target lesion does not provide an accurate diagnosis on conventional imaging studies, ultrasound allows accurate localization of a site for the purpose of biopsy. This is of particular benefit in the lesion, which has an infiltration or exophytic-type growth pattern and minimal mucosal involvement. The lesion can be biopsied using a 22-gauge needle and following the described procedure.[54,55]

Pathologist's Role

The role of the pathologist cannot be overemphasized. It is the single most important factor in obtaining an accurate diagnosis, and cooperation with the pathologist should be sought and maintained. The methods of tissue sampling, tissue fixation, and sample handling in the pathology department vary from institution to institution. It is important to deliver the tissue sample to the pathologist in the manner he or she prefers.[1]

Summary

What is the preferred method for percutaneous aspiration biopsy? It is the simplest imaging procedure that provides sufficient delineation of the target to monitor needle insertion.[18] In one series, CT was reported to have an accuracy of 91 percent, while ultrasound was 76 percent.[18] Since that 1980 study, other authors have reported an ultrasound ability to accurately diagnose or exclude malignancy of 81 percent.[24] Still others report an accuracy of 90 to 93 percent using the needle guide.[11,23]

In the past, only the larger, more superficial lesions were biopsied with ultrasound guidance. The high-reso-

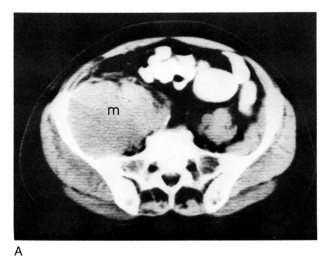

A

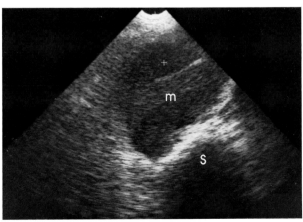

B

Fig. 10-19. Retroperitoneal biopsy. This patient was known to have multiple myeloma and developed leg swelling and pain. (A) CT scan. A large soft-tissue density mass (m) is seen on the right involving the iliac bone. (B) With real-time guidance, the solid hypoechoic mass (m) was localized. (S, spine.) The biopsy was consistent with large cell lymphoma.

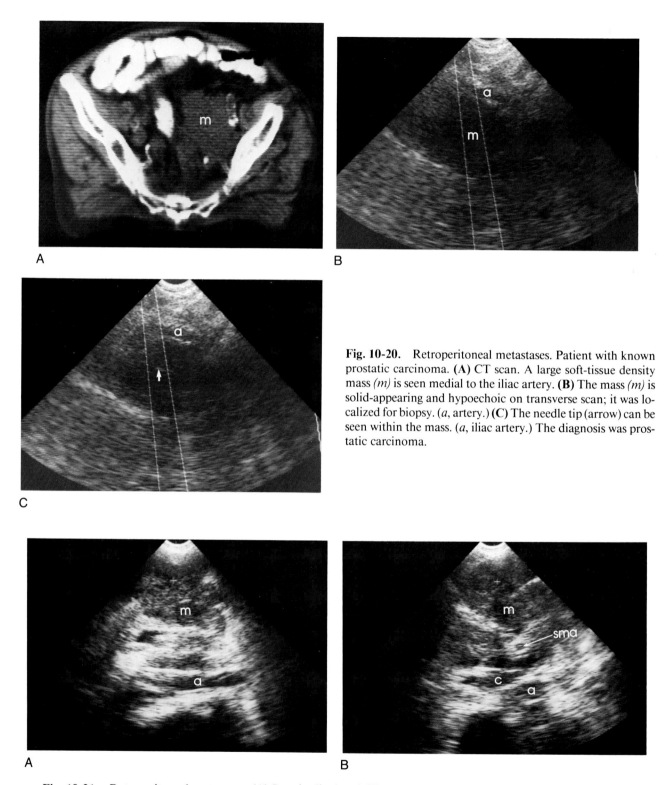

Fig. 10-20. Retroperitoneal metastases. Patient with known prostatic carcinoma. **(A)** CT scan. A large soft-tissue density mass *(m)* is seen medial to the iliac artery. **(B)** The mass *(m)* is solid-appearing and hypoechoic on transverse scan; it was localized for biopsy. (*a*, artery.) **(C)** The needle tip (arrow) can be seen within the mass. (*a*, iliac artery.) The diagnosis was prostatic carcinoma.

Fig. 10-21. Retroperitoneal metastases. **(A)** Longitudinal and **(B)** transverse scans demonstrate a large echodense mass *(m)* anterior to the aorta *(a)*. It is difficult to define the vascular anatomy. The mass is localized measuring a depth *(+)* to the center. (*a*, aorta; *sma*, superior mesenteric artery; *c*, inferior vena cava.) This proved to be undifferentiated carcinoma consistent with pancreatic carcinoma.

lution real-time systems that use needle guides show great promise for increased use. The exceptions might be very small (<2 cm) lesions, lesions high near the diaphragm, and small lesions (<3 cm) deep in the pelvis, which are not usually seen with ultrasound. When possible, ultrasound is the preferred method because of its simplicity of performance, lack of ionizing radiation, and cost. It does have disadvantages: (1) inability to constantly observe the exact needle localization when biopsing smaller solid lesions, which is much improved with needle guides, (2) potentially technically unsatisfactory exam due to overlying intestinal gas, and (3) inability to perform the exam due to skin access problems from incision, ostomies and the like.[18]

Ultrasound has distinct advantages over CT.[56] By using constant real-time visualization, movement of the target during needle introduction is easily seen. The needle tip can be continually visualized as the tip is advanced. Alteration of size, shape, and orientation of a fluid-filled structure can be monitored while emptying or injecting contrast.

Many sites that are routinely biopsied today could not be biopsied in the past. More liberal percutaneous biopsy has significantly decreased the cost and length of a hospital stay. Even if the biopsy is guided with CT, it still costs much less than surgery. The cost-effectiveness of the procedure, its safety and accuracy make it an important diagnostic tool that will be used increasingly over the next decade.[1]

ASPIRATION

Patient Preparation

No specific patient preparation is needed.

Contraindications

The contraindications for an aspiration procedure are the same as those for the biopsy and drainage procedures.

Procedure

The basic aspiration procedure is very similar to the procedure described for biopsy technique. This procedure is used for diagnostic aspiration of fluid or for needle drainage of a fluid-containing structure.[57,58] It begins by the localization of the target fluid, whether it is in the liver, kidney, or abdomen. The approach is planned so that the most direct route is used. If the area to be aspir-

ated is large, the examiner simply localizes the target with static or real-time ultrasound and needles it "blindly." If the fluid collection is small or needs to be totally evacuated, real-time guidance should be undertaken.

Once the field is prepped and draped, local anesthesia is administered. When using real-time guidance, it is necessary to anesthesize under the needle guide (Fig. 10-9A). As with the biopsy procedure, the transducer is placed in a sterile glove or bag after gel is applied to the scanning surface (see Fig. 10-4). Sterile mineral oil is used on the patient's skin. With real-time guidance, a 22-gauge needle is inserted within the skin and then placed within the needle guide attachment (see Fig. 10-9). With direct visualization, the needle is thrust into the fluid collection. A "pop" is usually felt when the needle enters the fluid collection. Once in, the needle is detached from the needle guide, and fluid is aspirated using a 20 cc syringe. If no fluid is obtained and the needle is definitely within the lesion, (demonstrated on real-time ultrasound) the procedure may be repeated using a larger gauge needle, since the fluid may be viscous. If no fluid is obtained with an 18-gauge needle, and the needle tip is definitely within the lesion, then it is unlikely there is drainable fluid.[59] If the procedure is being done to evacuate the fluid totally, the needle remains attached to the transducer or is reattached intermittently to evaluate the amount of remaining fluid[60] (Fig. 10-22). Some prefer to use an angiocath-type system when complete evacuation of a fluid collection is desired. As the fluid collection decreases in amount, the needle tip or angiocath may need to be repositioned under real-time scanning.

A needle aspiration of a suspected abscess serves several purposes.[59] First, it confirms the presence of fluid. Not all fluid collections look cystic on imaging studies; some may appear echodense on ultrasound. Secondly, by performing a gram stain on the aspirated fluid, it is possible to determine whether the fluid collection is infected. If there is a fluid-fluid or fluid-debris level demonstrated, care should be taken to aspirate fluid from the dependent portion of the fluid, as the supernatant may give a false-negative test for infection. Lastly, the aspiration procedure determines if the material is liquified enough to be drainable.[59]

Specific Applications

LIVER

Aspiration of a cystic liver lesion is indicated when (1) distinguishing a cyst from a solid lesion, (2) determining, in the case of diagnostic aspiration, if a lesion is an abscess, and (3) aspirating liver cysts when they are symptomatic. Since a metastatic lesion may look very similar to a cyst on ultrasound (particularly gastric carcinoma), a biopsy or aspiration of the lesion needs to be undertaken for diagnostic purposes. If fluid is obtained, it is sent for cytologic evaluation. Percutaneous aspiration appears to lack permanent therapeutic benefit in hepatic cysts.[61] Definitive therapy requires the surgical removal of the cyst lining or internal drainage by marsupialization.[61] When an abscess is suspected, a small amount of fluid is aspirated for a gram stain. If pus is obtained, the patient is usually referred for catheter drainage[62,63] (Fig. 10-23). Some patients with multiple hepatic cysts experience pain, which may be due to hemorrhage within the cysts or distension of the liver capsule. By aspirating multiple cysts, the patient's symptomatology may improve (Fig.

10-24). A suspected echinococcal cyst should not be punctured, since anaphylaxis is known to be a potential complication of the spread of the scolices into the peritoneal cavity.[64] A travel history should be obtained before puncture.

SPLEEN

In recent years, nonoperative management of splenic rupture has been recommended and used increasingly, since post-splenectomy patients have been shown to have an increased susceptibility to overwhelming infection.[65] With ultrasound guidance, fine-needle aspiration of the perisplenic or subcapsular fluid can confirm the diagnosis and often be therapeutic[66] (see Figs. 8-31A and B).

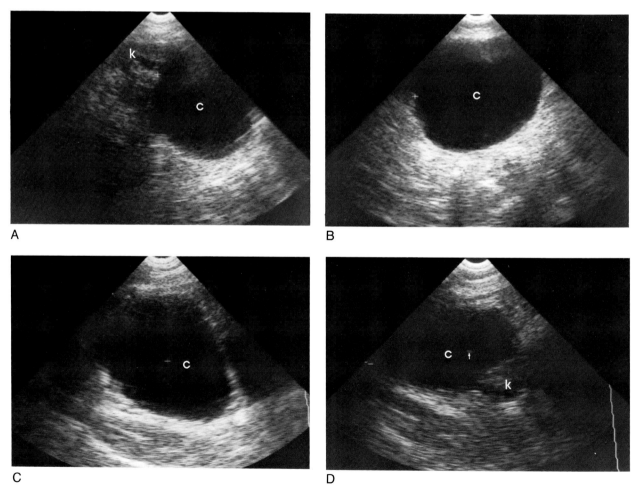

Fig. 10-22. Fluid aspiration. Renal cyst. On longitudinal **(A)** and transverse **(B)** prone scans of the left kidney *(k)*, a gigantic (11.4 × 11.6 cm) anechoic mass *(c)* is seen in the lower pole. Because the patient was experiencing pain and discomfort relative to this, a drainage procedure was undertaken. On prone longitudinal scan **(C)**, the mass *(c)* and depth *(+)* were determined. **(D)** After draining 300 ml of fluid, the cyst *(c)* was checked transversely. The needle tip (arrow) is seen. (k, kidney.) *(Figure continues.)*

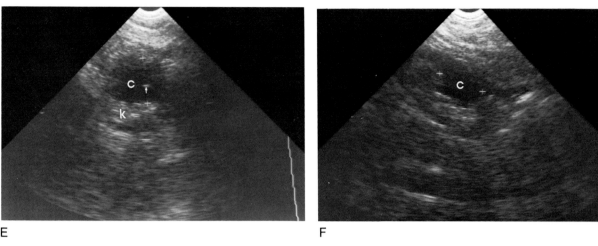

E   F

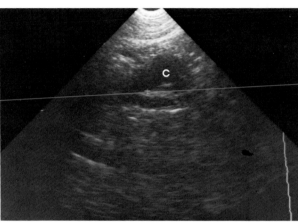

G

Fig. 10-22 *(Continued).* **(E)** After 700 ml were drained, the cyst *(c)* had greatly diminished in size. (*k*, kidney; arrow, needle tip.) **(F,G)** The procedure was discontinued after draining 900 ml. Only a small (4.2 × 3.4 cm) mass *(c)* remains on longitudinal **(F)** and transverse **(G)** scans.

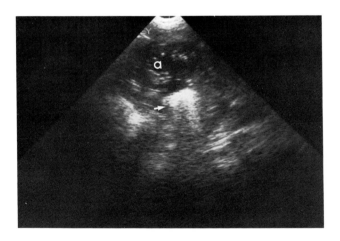

Fig. 10-23. Liver abscess. Longitudinal scan of liver abscess. This hypoechoic lesion *(a)*, which contains air (arrow), was localized and the depth was measured to the midpoint (6 cm). A needle was inserted and pus was obtained. The patient was sent for catheter drainage.

BILIARY

Ultrasound may be used for localization of dilated ducts for a percutaneous cholangiogram.[67-71] This is particularly true if mainly the left ducts are dilated[2] (see Fig. 2-93). In fact, some authors prefer the left duct approach.[2,71] The left is the largest of the hepatic ducts in most cases, and is nearest to the body surface. In addition, the entire biliary system can be opacified when the patient is supine because contrast is heavier than bile. With a right duct injection, the patient must be turned on the left side to fill the left ducts.[2] The ultrasound technique can be used to localize and mark a spot on the patient's skin or to guide the needle in with a real-time needle guide. If the ducts are quite large, guidance is not needed. If there is minimal ductal dilatation, real-time guidance is very helpful. This procedure is best done in the fluoroscopy/special procedure room so that a single puncture can be performed. Once the needle is in the

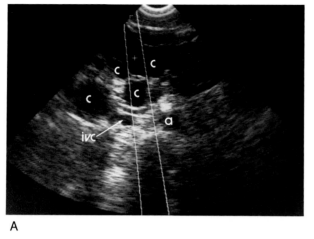

A

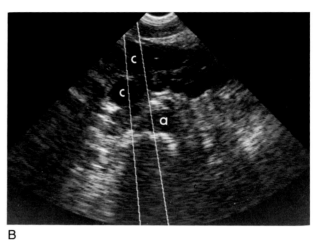

B

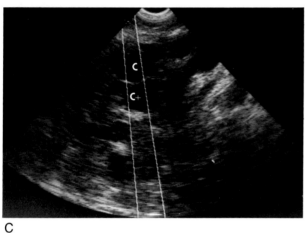

C

Fig. 10-24. Polycystic liver. This patient was experiencing pain due to liver capsule distension by the multiple hepatic cysts *(c)*. To relieve pain, real-time aspiration of several cysts was undertaken. **(A)** Transverse scan, localizing and measuring a depth *(+)* of an anterior cyst in the left lobe. (*a*, aorta; *ivc*, inferior vena cava.) **(B)** Upon rescanning, the anterior cyst *(c)* had decreased somewhat in size with drainage. Several other cysts *(c)* at a different level in the liver were subsequently localized **(C)** and drained.

duct, the ultrasound system can be returned to the ultrasound laboratory.

Ultrasound may be used to guide a puncture of the gallbladder in an antegrade study of the gallbladder and common bile duct.[72] An antegrade study may be used for diagnosis and as a therapeutic approach to treat biliary disease; it can be used to successfully treat the severely ill. It allows another method of evaluating the gallbladder lumen, aspiration of bile, and evaluation of the common bile duct.

PANCREAS

Ultrasound-guided percutaneous puncture of a pseudocyst appears to be an easy and simple procedure that carries little risk and causes little discomfort to the patient (Fig. 10-25). It can be used for verification of the diagnosis, for definitive therapy, for decompression in case of a threatening rupture, and for allowance of time for maturation of the cyst membrane before surgical intervention.[73]

Surgery for acute pseudocysts is postponed or eliminated with this technique. Relief of pain and obstructive symptoms, as well as time gained for maturation of the cyst wall, can be achieved by this procedure. The management of acutely developed pancreatic pseudocysts is unsatisfactory because of the high mortality and morbidity associated with surgery in this serious illness. When surgery is necessary for severe symptoms or for sepsis, external drainage is essential, but there is often a risk of pancreatic fistula with prolonged drainage. A 22-gauge needle can usually be used for aspiration of such a lesion. If the material is viscous, an 18-gauge needle is used. Following the aspiration, total collapse of the cyst can be documented on ultrasound.[74]

Aspiration of pancreatic/peripancreatic fluid should be performed if an abscess is suspected.[75] A gram stain of the fluid is important in order to make an immediate diagnosis. Percutaneous aspiration reduces the high mortality associated with pancreatic abscess by positive identification and avoids surgery in those with sterile fluid collections. Complications reported with this pro-

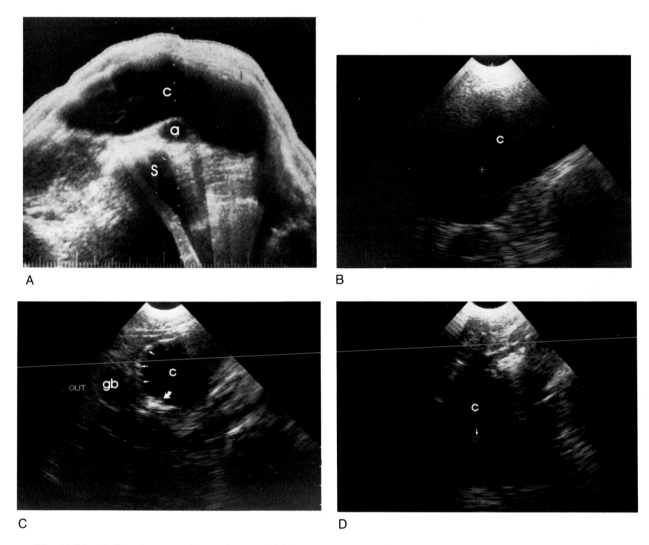

Fig. 10-25. Infected pancreatic pseudocyst. **(A)** Transverse scan at 12 cm below the xyphoid. A very large pancreatic pseudocyst *(c)*, which is seen as an anechoic mass, extended low within the abdomen from the pancreatic area. Since the patient was septic, he underwent percutaneous catheter drainage. (*a*, aorta; *S*, spine.) **(B)** On longitudinal scan, a depth *(+)* was localized for drainage of the pseudocyst *(c)*. Transverse **(C)** and longitudinal **(D)** scans after some drainage of the cyst *(c)* with the catheter (small arrows) seen curled along the right lateral margin of the cyst on **(C)**. The catheter (arrow) can be seen in cross-section on **(D)**. Its tip (curved arrow) is seen on **(C)**. (*gb*, gallbladder.)

cedure include superinfection of pseudocyst and hemoperitoneum.

Ultrasound may also be used to guide percutaneous pancreatography.[76-78] A good pancreatogram provides valuable information for planning surgery or in follow-up of pancreatojejunostomy for chronic pancreatitis with or without pancreatic surgery.[77] A preoperative study is usually obtained by endoscopic retrograde cannulation of the duct. A needle aspiration of an obstructed duct may cause pancreatitis, and as in percutaneous transhepatic cholangiography of an obstructed biliary tree, it should be followed by surgical decompres-sion within 24 to 48 hours. A 23-gauge needle may be used with removal of 5 cc of fluid and the injection of 15 cc of 60 percent sodium diatriozoate.[78]

ADRENAL AND RENAL

As a rule, there is no need for aspiration of a cystic adrenal lesion. Cysts are frequently encountered incidently and are rarely symptomatic, so a conservative approach is recommended.[79] If the patient is symptomatic because of the lesion, or if there is some question concerning the etiology of the lesion, an ultrasound aspiration may be performed (see Fig. 10-13). As a rule, this would be performed from a posterior approach. Again, if the lesion is not well seen or is very small, CT guidance should be employed.

The indications for renal cyst aspiration have decreased over the years with improved resolution of ultrasound equipment. It has been shown that if a renal lesion meets all the criteria for a cyst (echofree, well-defined borders and acoustic enhancement), then the accuracy for diagnosing a cyst approaches 100 percent.[80] If the lesion is indeterminate (does not meet all the criteria), then it is aspirated to determine if it is a cyst or neoplasm. There is usually no real need to aspirate a clear-cut cyst. Sometimes, though, a patient may experience pain because of the lesion and show improvement in symptomatology after aspiration (see Fig. 10-22). When performing a renal cyst aspiration, a 22-gauge needle is used. If the cyst is large, an area is localized with ultrasound and the puncture is performed in a "blind" fashion. If the lesion is small, needs to be drained completely, or is in the upper pole near the diaphragm, then the procedure is performed with direct real-time guidance. A "pop" is usually felt when the needle enters the cyst. Generally, 20 cc are withdrawn for cytology. If the cyst or cysts are to be completely evacuated, real-time visualization is maintained throughout the procedure (see Fig. 10-22).

There are very few complications reported in association with renal cyst aspiration. In fact in many institutions this procedure is performed on an outpatient basis. Of the major complications that do occur, perirenal hemorrhage is the most common. The frequency of major complications is 0.75 percent.[81] Pneumothorax, arteriovenous fistulae, infection, pericystic hemorrhage, intracystic hemorrhage, and traumatic urinoma are others reported.[82] The most common minor complication is microscopic hematuria.[80,81] The frequency of minor complications is 10 percent.[81]

Besides guiding the puncture of renal cysts, ultrasound may localize and guide the aspiration of suspected abscesses. If a patient is febrile and has a lesion that meets most of the criteria for a cyst or an apparent solid renal lesion, an abscess should be suspected, and a diagnostic needle aspiration is performed (Fig. 10-26, see also Figs. 10-14 and 4-67). If there is a very high suspicion of an abscess, this diagnostic tap may be performed in the special fluoroscopy laboratory in order to decrease the number of needle passes and lessen the need to move the patient. If the procedure is performed in ultrasound, after removing 5 to 10 cc of pus, a similar amount of contrast may be injected to facilitate the percutaneous catheter drainage. Or, the needle may be left in place and the patient transported to fluoroscopy. The sonologist should not always depend on the appearance of the fluid to diagnose an abscess. A gram stain should be per-

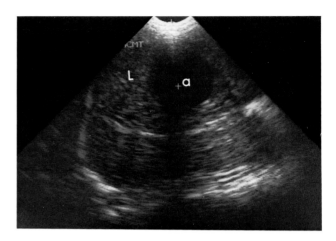

Fig. 10-26. Renal abscess aspiration. The right hypoechoic renal abscess *(a)* (seen also in Figure 4-67) is localized in the upper pole of this kidney with the patient prone in the transverse plane. The depth of the lesion to its midpoint is measured (+). Pus was obtained and the patient obtained catheter drainage of the lesion. (*L*, liver.)

formed before beginning percutaneous catheter drainage.

LYMPHOCELE

Lymphoceles may be safely aspirated with ultrasound guidance (see Fig. 10-27). However, the aspiration often does not lead to resolution.[83,84] Some lymphoceles may be drained with a percutaneous catheter.

ABSCESS DRAINAGE

Despite availability of advanced surgical techniques and current medical therapy intraabdominal abscesses remain a common diagnostic and therapeutic problem.[85] Percutaneous abscess drainage via a catheter method has emerged during the past few years as an important option in the management of selected patients with infected or sterile fluid collections. The benefits of the procedure include the avoidance of general anesthesia, laparotomy, and prolonged hospitalization, and in gravely ill patients, its resuscitative temporizing benefits can reverse a potentially fatal situation.[86] Percutaneous drainage has a high success rate and relatively low number of complications, which makes this procedure an attractive alternative to surgery in the individual (adult or child) at high risk for operation and general anesthesia, or even in the healthy patient who may benefit from a simple, less morbid percutaneous drainage.[87-89]

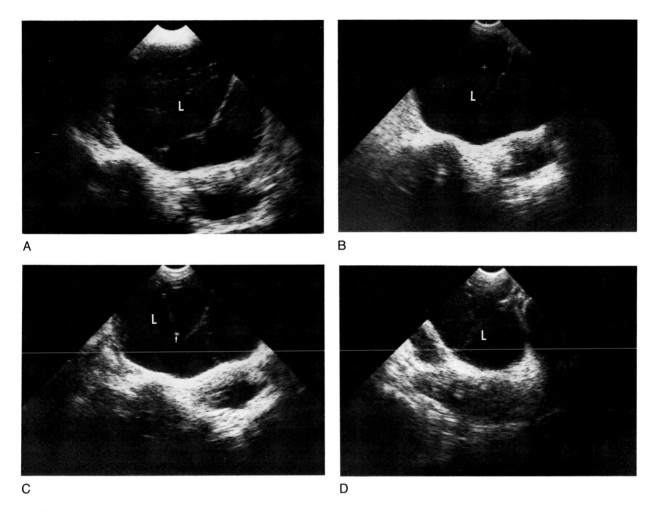

A

B

C

D

Fig. 10-27. Lymphocele. This pelvic lymphocele developed in association with a renal transplant. **(A)** On longitudinal scan of the pelvis, a large multiseptated cystic mass *(L)* is seen. The kidney is seen more lateral and superior to the mass. Because the patient had hydronephrosis, a percutaneous aspiration was undertaken. **(B)** The cystic mass *(L)* was localized in longitudinal plane. A depth (+) was measured. **(C)** On this longitudinal scan, the needle tip (arrow) can be seen within the mass *(L)*. This was done following drainage of 92 ml of fluid. **(D)** After drainage of 252 ml, the mass *(L)* was rescanned. No more fluid could be obtained. Because the mass reoccurred in a short period of time, the patient had percutaneous catheter drainage. Ultimately, the patient required surgical drainage.

On ultrasound, a typical abscess appears as a round or oval-shaped fluid collection that often contains internal echoes.[85] It may have irregular walls and be slightly echogenic. An abscess in a parenchymal organ is usually spherical (Figs. 10-23, 10-26, and see Figs. 4-67 and 4-68) while intraperitoneal abscesses can have multiple configurations.

Indications

There are several distinct indications for abscess drainage. They include: (1) demonstration of discretely loculated, preferably unilocular collections, (2) estab-

lishment of a safe access route, (3) agreement between surgeon and radiologist as to the risks and benefits, and (4) availability of the operating room in the unlikely event of serious complication or failure of the radiologic procedure.[88,90-94] Phlegmons, abscesses containing very thick debris, and multiloculated collections may not be amenable to successful percutaneous drainage.[88] Ultrasound-guided abscess drainage may also be performed at the bedside in the desperately ill patient.[95] Patients who are at high risk for a surgical procedure may undergo an initial catheter drainage as a temporizing procedure.[96] As such, the procedure may be performed in critically ill patients who have a complicated abscess that is poorly defined, multiloculated, phlegmonous, and associated with fistulas.[86] While the percutaneous procedure may not be a cure in some, patients dramatically improve and become fit for surgery.[96]

Patient Preparation

The coagulation studies of the patient should be within the acceptable range. The prothrombin (PT) time should be within 33 sec of control. The partial thromboplastin (PPT) should be no greater than 45 sec, and the platelet count should be greater than 50,000 per cm^3. These values should be recent, preferably within a week. A bleeding time should be performed if a patient has been on salicylates or has other reasons for thrombocytopenia.[88]

Antibiotic therapy should be instituted in the patient.[87,88,90,93] A broad spectrum antibiotic is given intravenously, using a combination of cephalosporin, clindamycin, or chloramphenicol along with an aminoglycoside.[88]

In addition, it is important to administer satisfactory analgesia throughout the procedure. The patient may be premedicated with intramuscular or intravenous meperidine hydrochloride (Demerol) or Diazepam (Valium). During the procedure, more medication should be given as necessary.[88]

Contraindications

There are several instances in which percutaneous drainage should not be used.[87] A pancreatic phlegmon, which is largely inflammatory granulation tissue, is not amenable to drainage. Congenital hepatic cysts usually fail to collapse with drainage. Amebic abscesses are best treated with Flagyl alone. Other lesions that are better treated surgically include: (1) abscess in the pelvis adjacent to the rectum, (2) tuboovarian abscess, and (3) Echinococcal cyst. However, our interventional group has successfully drained pelvic abscesses with transrectal catheter drainage. Some patients are poor candidates but respond well; these include patients with interloop abscesses and GI or GU fistula.[87] In addition, the procedure is not recommended if there is absence of a safe or appropriate access, internal septation, or loculation and/or primary or secondary coagulopathy.[92]

Procedure

If there is a question of infection or abscess, a diagnostic needle aspiration is performed using an 18- to 22-gauge needle. The area of concern is localized; if the area is large, the aspiration is performed "blindly." If the lesion is small, then real-time guidance is used. If pus is obtained on aspiration, a small amount is removed for gram stain, bacteriology, chemistry, and hematology. The aspirate appearance may be misleading. Even if the fluid "looks" negative for abscess, a gram stain should be performed and examined for white blood cells and organisms. If no white blood cells are found but the fluid is positive for organisms, this would indicate that there had been inadvertent bowel aspiration. However, sterile abscesses can occur.[88] The needle may be left in place for catheter placement, or a small amount of contrast may be injected and the needle removed. This is the case if the diagnostic procedure is performed in ultrasound. If the procedure is performed in the special procedure suite where fluoroscopy is available, an 18-gauge needle may be inserted, pus obtained, and using the same needle, a catheter placed. Using the two-needle placement, a 22-gauge needle is used for diagnosis, and an 18-gauge is inserted right next to the 22-gauge for catheter exchange.

In contrast to solid tumors, transgression of bowel should be avoided, even to the extent of not performing the procedure. If the abscess is large and/or superficial, it may be localized with ultrasound. CT is frequently required to provide anatomic detail necessary for locating a safe access route, particularly in smaller collections or those contiguous with bowel. Sterile fluid collections, such as pseudocyst, seroma, biloma, or hematoma, can be infected inadvertently. The exception has been the safe aspiration and drainage of pancreatic pseudocysts through the stomach, which is relatively bacteria free.[88]

SELDINGER TECHNIQUE

Using this method, a 19-gauge needle is inserted at a predetermined depth, parallel or tandem to the course of the first diagnostic needle. The insertion is performed under suspended respiration and with fluoroscopy. Aspiration of fluid is obtained to verify the position of the needle. A 0.035- or 0.038-inch J-shaped or torque guide wire is introduced through the sheath, advanced, and coiled.[87,88] Care is taken not to penetrate the wall. It is frequently necessary to dilate the skin and subcutaneous tissue by introduction of a series of dilators up to 12 to 14 French (F). Then the appropriate catheter is selected, depending on the size of the cavity and the character of the contents. There is better drainage with a larger catheter. A smaller catheter can be used for thin, nonviscous fluid. The advantage of the Seldinger technique is that with fluoroscopy guidance, the wire can be used to delineate the full extent of the lesion.[88,92] There are numerous catheter kits commercially available (Fig. 10-28).

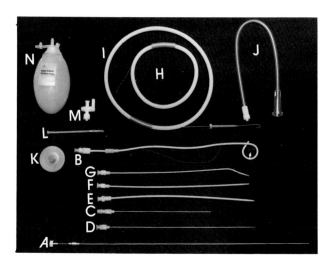

Fig. 10-28. Cook-Cope type loop nephrostomy set. This system consists of *(A)* catheter introduction stiffening cannula; *(B)* 8.2F catheter; *(C)* 21-gauge, 15-cm long needle; *(D)* stiffening cannula 20-gauge, 22 cm long; *(E,F)* vessel dilators, 20-cm long (*E,* 4F; *F,* 7.5F); *(G)* introducing catheter (6.3F, 22 cm long); *(H)* wire guide for introduction system (0.018 in diameter, stainless steel, extra stiff, 60 cm long with a flexible curved tip); *(I)* wire guide for catheter (0.038 in, 100 cm long, 3 mm "J" tip); *(J)* connecting tube, 14F, 30 cm long; *(K)* molnar disc; *(L)* pull tie; and *(M)* one-way stopcock. A suction apparatus (Heyer-Schulte) *(N)* is also displayed. A drawstring (arrow) is attached to the tip of the catheter for forming a loop after insertion. The latex ring secures and prevents leakage around the drawstring.

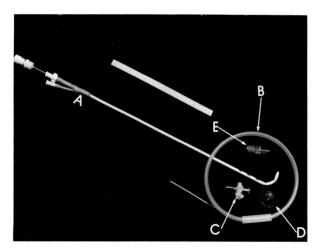

Fig. 10-29. VanSonnenberg sump kit. This kit consists of *(A)* 12F sump catheter; *(B)* 0.038 in guidewire; *(C)* 3-way stopcock; *(D)* microbial filter; *(E)* suction adapter; and adhesive pads. The catheter *(A)* has a 30-cm working length with a 7-cm flexible tip. The sump catheter has a double lumen, the larger of which has five large oval side holes and a distal hole at the tip for fluid drainage. The smaller lumen serves as an ingress sump acting as an air vent. The vent is capped with the microbial filter *(D)* to maintain sterility. A removeable internal cannula provides support for introduction of the sump catheter. A 19-gauge trocar stylet is inserted within the cannula if direct puncture is to be performed.

TROCAR TECHNIQUE

This is initially similar to the Seldinger technique but instead of using the guide wire followed by a catheter, the catheter is inserted by a "single-stick" method.[88] The trocar catheter consists of a multihole catheter and an internal hollow-metal introducer or stiffener within which there is a sharp pointed stylet (12 or 16F) for the introduction (Fig. 10-29). The stiffness by the introducer supports the catheter and allows direct introduction into the cavity with thick or fibrous walls. It is important to avoid perforating the far wall of the cavity during trocar catheter introduction, since substantial effort is required to advance the catheter through the soft tissue. With the central stylet maintained in a fixed position, the catheter is carefully advanced into the cavity until the tip engages the distal wall of the abscess. To ensure correct position, the stylet is removed and the catheter is injected through the introducer. The central stylet is removed and the cavity aspirated.[88]

CATHETER SELECTION

There is a wide selection of catheters commercially available. The choice of the catheter and technique of insertion depends on the depth, size, access route, and location of the fluid collection. Generally the catheters that are used range from 7 to 14F; selection of the catheter depends on the size of the internal lumen and the number and size of side holes (Figs. 10-28 and 10-30). Smaller catheters are usually adequate for a nonviscous collection, but larger "sump" catheters are required for thick purulent collection[88] (Fig. 10-29).

The choice of the drainage catheter depends on the size, depth, ease of access, and location of the abscess.[90] The small lumen capacity and side hole caliber of the medium bore nonsump catheters limit their effectiveness in patients who have thick pus or necrotic debris, but are useful for drainage of nonviscous fluid such as loculated ascites, bilomas, and seromas.[59] Contents of many abscesses have such a low viscosity that adequate drainage may be obtained through an angiocatheter of the 8F caliber.[87] The smaller, less traumatic 8F pigtail catheter can be used for small, deep abscesses having a

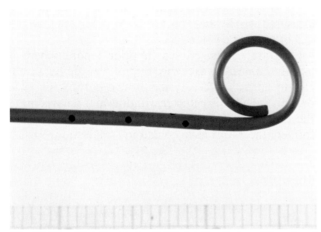

Fig. 10-30. Pigtail catheter. 7.1F pigtail catheter with end and side holes.

narrow window, for abscesses in intimate relation to bowel, and for parenchymal abscesses.[90,94] A pigtail catheter or a nephrostomy catheter may be used for small abscesses. Larger more superficial nonparenchymal abscesses may be drained with a 12 or 16F trocar catheter.[90,94] The use of a trocar catheter is avoided in vascular parenchymal organs because of the danger of laceration and hemorrhage.

Some radiologists use the double-lumen sump catheter system[59,87,97,98] (Fig. 10-29). Since the single most important step for successful percutaneous drainage is complete aspiration of the cavity contents, some radiologists prefer the large-bore sump catheter for drainage of pus if the estimated volume is greater than 100 ml.[59] The multiple-side-hole sump catheter can be inserted either with the trocar technique or over a guide wire. This system is available in 12 and 14F sizes, with a larger side hole that ensures good drainage. The large lumen caliber and large side-hole aperatures assure ready flow of thick purulent material.[59] The sump system allows simultaneous injection and aspiration.

Multiple loculations or multiple abscesses may require several catheters.[87] More than two are seldom used, and two are often helpful in an abscess of any length.

FOLLOWING CATHETER PLACEMENT

Following catheter placement with either method, the fluid contents of the cavity are aspirated completely. To ensure total evacuation of the cavity, liberal irrigation of the cavity is undertaken by injection of the abscess catheter, using normal saline.[59,88,99] Some find irrigation inadviseable because it might disseminate the infection.[92] By performing saline irrigation of the catheter only after all freely drained purulent material is evacuated, the risk of blood-stream contamination by infected detritus and bacterial toxins is minimized.[59] Small aliquots (20 to 50 cc) of saline are hand injected and aspirated from the cavity while the patient changes position on the fluoroscopy table.[88] In this way necrotic material and debris are completely broken down and evacuated. Usually a total of 200 to 300 cc of saline are required.[88] The endpoint is not reached until the return irrigant is clear. This irrigation eliminates occlusion of the catheter by debris and often permits drainage of locules and septations.[59] After total evacuation, a sinogram may be performed to delineate the size of the cavity.[87,88,91]

After securely suturing the catheter to the patient, the catheter is connected to a suction system like the Heyer-Schulte suction apparatus (Fig. 10-31). This facilitates irrigation of the catheter throughout the drainage.[88] At the onset, irrigation is performed every 3 to 4 hours. This irrigation with 10 to 25 ml of saline maintains catheter

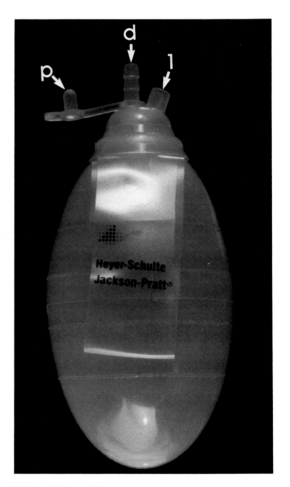

Fig. 10-31. Heyer-Schu
suction reservoir. This is
inlet port; *p*, drainage p

patency and is a simple bedside nursing maneuver.[59] The intervals gradually lengthen, and the volume of the cavity closes.[91,99]

At times, it may be necessary to change catheters.[91] Initially, it is preferable to use the smallest catheter (8.3 or 10F). If the drainage is not continuing, then the catheter may be exchanged for a 12 to 14F.[91]

POSTINSERTION CARE

The criteria for successful catheter drainage is monitored by clinical, radiologic, and catheter follow-up. Clinically, the temperature should return to normal within 24 to 48 hours. The white blood count may take several days to show substantial reduction. If the temperature does not fall, the possibility of multiple abscesses should be considered.[88]

Radiologically, there should be a decrease in size of the cavity throughout the course of drainage. The size of the cavity may be monitored with ultrasound, CT, or sinogram.[87,88] The sinogram is not helpful unless a fistula is present.

It is the responsibility of the radiologist to follow the clinical course of the patient while on catheter drainage. The catheter should be watched for patency and may require irrigation to prevent clogging.[88]

CATHETER REMOVAL

The removal of the catheter is based on several criteria.[87] The fever must have decreased to normal for a minimum of 2 to 3 days prior to removal. The white blood count should have decreased and there should be improvement in the patient's general clinical status. The abscess cavity should be nearly collapsed, and there should be marked decrease in drainage. A final exam with CT should demonstrate resolution of the cavity as well as absence of other disease. The actual drainage time is 10 to 20 days on the average, with the catheter left in 2 to 3 days longer than is felt necessary to avoid potential recurrence due to premature removal.[90,92]

Some investigators base catheter removal on clinical analysis of catheter output feeling it is a better indicator than CT or ultrasound.[59] Guidelines for withdrawal are based on analysis of the amount and character of the drainage along with observation of change in character of contents. In cases of parenchymal abscesses of the liver or perihepatic location, the fluid drainage usually decreases over 5 to 7 days. Abscesses in potential spaces, such as intraperitoneal or pericolic areas, yield larger amounts of fluid over longer periods of time. In the presence of an open fistula, the drainage may continue

for 3 to 4 weeks. The relative amount of drainage is measured serially and appears more important than actual quantitative volume data.[59]

Contrary to suggestions in prior reports, there is usually no need to exchange a multiple-side-hole catheter to an end-hole catheter for the purpose of withdrawal.[59] Since the catheter withdrawal is delayed until the drainage is minimal and a well-matured track is formed, the risk of local contamination is minimized.[59]

RESULTS

The success of the procedure is determined mainly by significant clinical improvement and avoidance of surgery. It is more often related to the characteristics of the abscess than the location. Those associated with fistulae, viscous debris, extension, or multiple cavities have a poor prognosis. The single most frequently reported failure is the drainage of a pancreatic abscess.[87] The overall success has been reported to be 80 to 90 percent.[86-88,92,93,99,100] There is a 4 percent mortality with a 6 to 10.4 percent complication rate.[86,87] Causes for catheter failures include multiloculation, phlegmon, abscess associated with fistula, thick hematoma or organized tissue, tumor mistaken for abscess, and improper catheter position.[86] The most frequent causes for recurrence include an abnormal communication or leak with the GU, GI, biliary, or lymphatic system.[86] A recurrence is defined as initial evacuation and clinical improvement but eventual reaccumulation of fluid.[86]

COMPLICATIONS

Serious complications of percutaneous abscess drainage are relatively uncommon. Hemorrhage, empyema, sinus tract or fistula formation, peritonitis, and septicemia have been reported.[88,92,101] There is a 4 to 10.4 percent complication rate reported.[86,88,102] The low complication rate supports the contention that the most difficult aspect of the percutaneous abscess drainage remains finding an appropriate access route.[88]

Area Application

LIVER

Liver abscesses are usually successfully drained with percutaneously catheters[63] (see Figs. 10-23; 1-65 to 1-68). The route is transperitoneal and transhepatic via a posterolateral skin entry site. Multiple lesions can be drained using multiple catheters.[92] If surgery should be needed, the catheter defines the surgical approach.[103]

SUBPHRENIC OR SUBHEPATIC

Subphrenic or subhepatic fluid collections are best drained via a posterior subcostal extraperitoneal approach. A "triangulation" technique of angled needle and catheter placement, with CT guidance, is used to avoid pleura. The needle guide is used with real-time guidance. Catheters are advanced as superiorly as possible in the subphrenic space for adequate drainage. Subhepatic collections are usually posterior and intraperitoneal, so a subhepatic posterior entry site is used with an cephalic angulation.[92] The postoperative subphrenic abscess mortality is reported to be 7.5 to 43.0 percent, with a recurrence rate of up to 47 percent when drained surgically.[104]

LESSER SAC

Entry into the lesser sac is made using a left lateral approach, usually intercostal. The angle of the entry is posterior to the midcoronal plane, with the needle anterior and ventral to the tip of the spleen and posterior to the stomach.[92]

INTERLOOP AND PELVIC ABSCESS

Interloop abscesses are the most difficult to drain. CT is mandatory. Some consider this abscess undrainable percutaneously.[92]

As a rule, there is no safe approach for drainage of a pelvic abscess unless it is quite large.[92] At times, such an abscess may be drained by a transrectal catheter.

PANCREAS

Supervening sepsis with a preexisting pancreatic pseudocyst is quite different from infected pancreatic phlegmon in its response to percutaneous drainage[90] (Fig. 10-25). With a pseudocyst, there may be complete aspiration of the fluid and rapid resolution without recurrence. With a phlegmon, percutaneous catheter drainage may only be a temporary measure.

RENAL AND PERINEPHRIC

Combined with appropriate antibiotic coverage, percutaneous drainage is an effective nonsurgical treatment for unilocular intrarenal abscesses[105] (see Figs. 10-26; 4-61, 4-67, and 4-68). The choice of the catheter is determined by the location and size of the lesion. If the lesion is large a 8F or 12F trocar may be used. If the lesion is small and less accessible, a pigtail catheter is used.[100,105,106] A posterior and/or angled approach is used.[106]

In a perinephric abscess, pus is in the space between the kidney and Gerota's fascia.[107,108] These abscesses appear more lobular in contour and have irregular walls and internal echoes[109] (see Fig. 5-41). Most originate within the renal parenchyma as a renal abscess, which then ruptures perinephrically. This abscess is usually confined to Gerota's fascia and may extend cephalad and caudad for a considerable distance within this fascial plane.[109] As such, catheters may need to be placed within the kidney as well as the perinephric space.[108]

OTHER FLUID COLLECTIONS

Bilomas

Percutaneous catheter drainage provides adequate therapeutic drainage in most patients.[110,111]

Cholecystostomy

A percutaneous route can be used for biliary drainage when a transhepatic approach is not possible. A gallbladder catheter drainage can also be used for gallbladder empyema or acute cholecystitis.[112,113] The gallbladder can be entered by a single direct insertion. The advantage of the direct catheter cholecystostomy under ultrasound control is the precise localization of the gallbladder and the ease with which the gallbladder can be directly catheterized in the seriously ill patient.[112,114,115]

One group of investigators have reported life-threatening vagal reactions associated with percutaneous cholecystostomy.[116] This occurred in 4 out of 5 patients who underwent cholecystostomy for septicemia, due to suspected cystic duct obstruction and hydrops of the gallbladder. The patients suffered profound vagal reactions with severe hypotension and bradycardia. One patient had a cardiac arrest. Atropine given prior to the procedure appeared to blunt the reaction in one patient. It is recommended that caution be used in selecting patients for this procedure. The adverse effects could be minimized by limiting manipulation of the guide wire and catheter, with removal of bile in small aliquots and the administration of atropine.[116]

Nephrostomy

INDICATIONS

The indications for percutaneous nephrostomy tube placement include: (1) malignant obstruction of the urinary tract, (2) infection, (3) obstruction by renal calculus, (4) nonobstructive renal stone, (5) stone extraction or infusion for stone lysis, (6) traumatic or iatrogenic ureteric tear, (7) pyonephrosis, (8) percutaneous nephroscopy, (9) biopsy of collecting system, and (10) for ureteral fistula[2,119-125] (see Figs. 4-30, 4-54). In neonates, infants, and children, the indications for percutaneous nephrostomy include: (1) preservation of renal function while awaiting growth of the infant, (2) preservation of renal function in anticipation of relief of transient obstruction, (3) drainage, (4) pyonephrosis, and (5) assessment of reversibility of impaired renal function.[124]

PATIENT PREPARATION

The patient should be adequately premedicated prior to the procedure. Some authors recommend the use of 0.6 to 1 mg of intramuscular or intravenous atropine for prophylaxis of vasovagal hypotension which occurs. In addition, strong acting analagesics such as intravenous Sublimaze (Fentamyl) or intramuscular or intravenous Demerol should be administered. Intravenous antibiotics should be given prior to the procedure if there is any suggestion of infection of the urinary tract.[2] In a child under 1 year of age, 50 to 75 mg/kg of chloral hydrate can be administered. If the child is older than 1 year, Demerol 25 mg, Phenergan 6.25 mg, Thorazine 6.25 mg are given intramuscular in the amount of 1 cc/10 kg to a maximum of 2 cc.[125]

CONTRAINDICATIONS

There are only a few contraindications. These include severe obesity, patient inability to cooperate, bleeding diatheses or anticoagulant therapy, suspected tumor or severe hypertension.[122,126]

CATHETER SYSTEMS

There are numerous nephrostomy catheter systems available (Fig. 10-28). The Vance system (8.3 or 10F) provides needles, guide wire, dilators, and pigtail catheter. The Cystocatheter system provides a large trocar and cannula, as well as a soft flexible catheter. In this system, the trocar and cannula are thrust into the collecting system, and once urine is obtained, the trocar is removed. The smaller catheter is fed through the cannula and then the cannula is removed.[2] The Cook pigtail percutaneous nephrostomy set contains a 8.3 or 10F catheter. The Ingram trocar catheter system is a 14 or 16F.[122]

In the child less than 2 years of age, serial dilators are used up to 7F, followed by a 6F pigtail catheter. If the child is greater than 2 years of age, a 8.3F pigtail catheter is used with dilatation up to 9F.[125]

PROCEDURE

The procedure is modified with each patient. If the collecting system is visualized after contrast injection, ultrasound guidance is not needed. In some cases, the

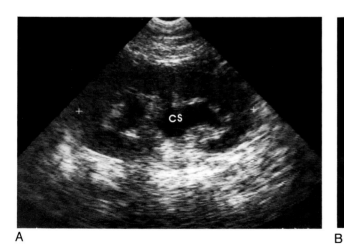

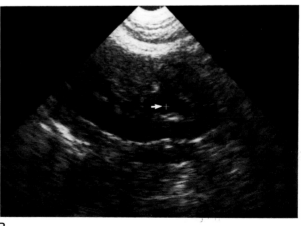

A   B

Fig. 10-32. Nephrostomy procedure. **(A)** Longitudinal scan. The dilated collecting system *(cs)* is demonstrated. **(B)** The depth (+, arrow) to the collecting system is localized. After local anesthesia, a needle is inserted with real-time guidance into the collecting system. Once the needle tip is seen within the collecting system, the transducer and guide are removed. A guide wire is inserted through the needle, and after the needle is removed a catheter is passed over the guide wire.

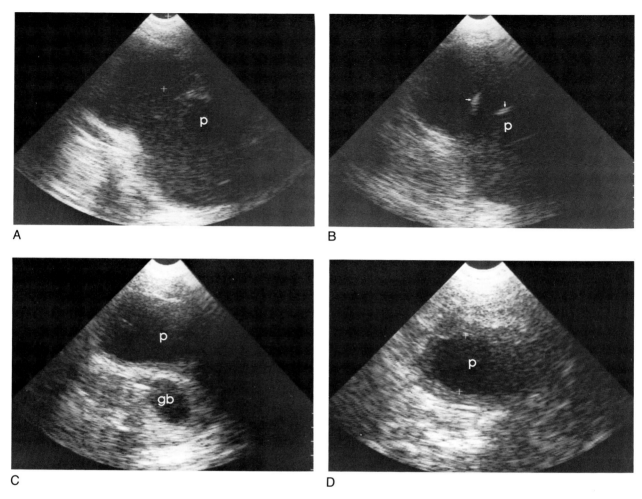

Fig. 10-33. Pyonephrosis. This patient was 8 weeks' pregnant with a congenital ureteropelvic junction obstruction on the right, which became infected. (See Figs. 4-30 and 4-54.) **(A)** On longitudinal scan, an area (+) within the dilated renal pelvis *(p)* was localized for puncture with the patient prone. The procedure was done with real-time sonography alone. **(B)** On longitudinal scan, the catheter (arrows) is seen within the renal pelvis *(p)*. **(C)** After draining 630 ml, the size of the fluid collection *(p)* is greatly decreased on this transverse scan. (*gb*, gallbladder.) **(D)** After draining 876 ml, the collection *(p)* is quite small on transverse scan. A catheter was left for drainage and the patient did well.

renal pelvis is punctured with ultrasound guidance using a 22-gauge needle, then contrast is injected, and the patient is transferred to fluoroscopy for catheter placement.[2] The use of ultrasound for the initial puncture has significantly decreased the number of puncture attempts and potential iatrogenic risks; it has also eliminated need for intravenous contrast, allowed safe introduction of a large caliber needle, and decreased length of time needed to perform the procedure.[127,128]

A direct posterior approach is avoided, since this may cause injury to the vessels. With a lateral puncture, there is a lower risk of vascular injury.[119,129] In addition, with the greater thickness of renal cortex, there is better fixation or stabilization of both the puncture and final catheter, and the renal pelvis is at a greater depth[129,130] (Fig.

10-32). With the catheter in the posterolateral position, the patient is comfortable in both the supine and decubitus positions. In this position, if a ureteral stint needs to be placed, there is a more direct course from the renal pelvis to the ureter for guide wire placement when the puncture is in the posterior axillary line.[2] Lasix augmentation for renal pelvis size may be used when appropriate.[129]

The procedure may be done with one or two needles. With one needle, ultrasound guidance is used with an 18-gauge needle. With two, a 22-gauge needle is placed within the collecting system and the system is opacified. A larger needle is placed under fluoroscopy. The choice is determined by the position of the kidney in relation to the patient's ribs. When using real-time in fluoroscopy, the procedure may be done with one needle. It is particularly helpful to have ultrasound guidance if there is minimal hydronephrosis.[2,130] The remainder of the procedure is done similarly to the abscess drainage procedure.

COMPLICATIONS

There are relatively few complications reported. The incidence of major complications is 4 percent for nephrostomy tube placement.[2,121] If the patient is infected, it is essential that he or she receive a full dose of intravenous antibiotics because the injection and needle/catheter manipulation of the collecting system frequently is accompanied by transient septicemia. Transient hematuria is almost invariable as an immediate result but clears within 1 to 2 days and is not regarded as a complication.[2,121,122] Small perinephric hematomas occur in 8 percent and usually resorb unless infected.[2]

SUCCESS RATE

The success rate for this procedure is 97 to 100 percent. Placement failure probably occurs only in slightly dilated systems. The success depends on the placement and maintenance of adequate drainage.[121]

PYONEPHROSIS

Ultrasound offers prompt diagnosis of hydronephrosis, and if the needle puncture yields pus, the diagnosis can be made for pyonephrosis (Fig. 10-33; see 4-30 and 4-54). A percutaneous catheter may be inserted for drainage of the infected urine as well as evaluation of the residual kidney function before surgery. The catheter is used for diagnostic nephrostogram, ureteral perfusion, therapeutic dissolution of stones, and indefinite drainage. The procedure is performed similarly to that described for the percutaneous nephrostomy. In fact, in a series of nephrostomies, 15 percent had pyonephrosis.[131] The complications of percutaneous nephrostomy placement in the septic patient is high, but in one series there were no reported deaths.[131] Intravenous aminoglycosides should be given before urinary tract manipulation, since there is a danger of gram-negative shock.[131]

REFERENCES

1. Bernardino ME: Percutaneous biopsy. AJR 142:41, 1984
2. Chang R: Ultrasonic puncture techniques: A practical guide. p. 241. In Sanders RC (ed): Ultrasound Annual 1982. Raven Press, New York, 1982
3. Goldberg BB, Pollack HM: Ultrasonic aspiration-biopsy transducer. Radiology 108:667, 1973
4. Goldberg BB, Cole-Beuglet C, Kurtz AB, Rubin CS: Real-time aspiration-biopsy transducer. J Clin Ultrasound 8:107, 1980
5. Pedersen JR: Percutaneous puncture guided by ultrasonic multi-transducer scanning. J Clin Ultrasound 5:175, 1977
6. Yeh E-L: An ultrasonic deflector for aspiration and biopsy. J Clin Ultrasound 3:125, 1975
7. Yeh H-C, Mitty HA, Wolf BS: A simple ultrasonic guide for needle puncture. J Clin Ultrasound 4:53, 1976
8. Saitoh M, Watanabe H, Ohe H et al: Ultrasonic real-time guidance for percutaneous puncture. J Clin Ultrasound 7:269, 1979
9. Reid MH: Real-time sonographic needle biopsy guide. AJR 140:162, 1983
10. Grant EG, Richardson JD, Smirniotopoulos JG, Jacobs NM: Fine-needle biopsy directed by real-time sonography: technique and accuracy. AJR 141:29, 1983
11. Bree RL, Schwab RE, Barrett RE, McCarroll KA: Effectiveness of real-time sector guides for abdominal mass biopsies: comparison with CT. Proceedings 28th American Institute of Ultrasound in Medicine, J Ultrasound Med 2:15, 1983
12. Buonocore E, Skipper GJ: Steerable real-time sonographically guided needle biopsy. AJR 136:387, 1981
13. Ohto M, Karasawa E, Tsuchiya Y et al: Ultrasonically guided percutaneous contrast medium injection and aspiration biopsy with real-time puncture transducer. Radiology 136:171, 1980
14. Lee TG, Knochel JQ: Air as an ultrasound contrast marker for accurate determination of needle placement: Tumor biopsy localization and other application. Radiology 143:787, 1982
15. Ferrucci JT Jr, Wittenberg J: CT biopsy of abdominal tumors: Aids for lesion localization. Radiology 129:739, 1978
16. Lieberman RP, Hafez GR, Crummy AB: Histology from aspiration biopsy: Turner needle experience. AJR 138:561, 1982
17. Haaga JR, LiPuma JP, Bryan PJ et al: Clinical comparison of small and large caliber cutting needles for biopsy. Radiology 146:665, 1983
18. Ferrucci JT Jr, Wittenberg J, Mueller PR et al: Diagnosis of abdominal malignancy by radiologic fine-needle aspiration biopsy. AJR 134:323, 1980
19. Isler RJ, Ferrucci JT Jr, Wittenberg J et al: Tissue core biopsy of abdominal tumors with a 22 gauge cutting needle. AJR 136:725, 1981
20. Itoh K, Yamanaka T, Kasahara K et al: Definite diagnosis of pancreatic carcinoma with percutaneous fine needle aspiration biopsy under ultrasound guidance. Am J Gastroenterol 71:469, 1979
21. Cohen MM: Early diagnosis of pancreatic cancer using ultrasound and fine needle aspiration cytology. Am Surg 45:715, 1979
22. Goldman ML, Naib ZM, Galambos JT et al: Preopera-

tive diagnosis of pancreatic carcinoma by percutaneous aspiration biopsy. Digestive Disease 22:1076, 1977

23. Phillips G, Schneider M: Ultrasonically guided percutaneous fine needle aspiration biopsy of solid masses. Cardiovasc Intervent Radiol 4:33, 1981

24. Skolnick ML, Dekker A, Weinstein BJ: Ultrasound guided fine-needle aspiration biopsy of abdominal masses. Gastrointest Radiol 3:295, 1978

25. Pelaez JC, Hill MC, Dach JL et al: Abdominal aspiration biopsies: sonographic vs computed tomographic guidance. JAMA 250:2663, 1983

26. Yeh H-C: Percutaneous fine needle aspiration biopsy of intra-abdominal lesions with ultrasound guidance. Am J Gastroenterol 75:148, 1981

27. Zornoza J, Wallace S, Ordonez N, Lukeman J: Fine-needle aspiration biopsy of the liver. AJR 134:331, 1980

28. Nosher JL, Plafker J: Fine-needle aspiration of the liver with ultrasound guidance. Radiology 136:177, 1980

29. Pagani JJ: Biopsy of focal hepatic lesions: Comparison of 18 and 22 gauge needle. Radiology 147:673, 1983

30. Elyaderani MK: Ultrasonic guidance of liver biopsy and fine-needle aspiration in difficult cases. South Med J 76:850, 1983

31. Schwerk WB, Schmitz-Moormann P: Ultrasonically guided fine-needle biopsies in neoplastic liver disease: cytohistologic diagnoses and echo pattern of lesions. Cancer 48:1469, 1981

32. Solbiati L, Bossi MC, Bellotti E et al: Focal lesions in the spleen: sonographic patterns and guided biopsy. AJR 140:59, 1983

33. Soderstrom N: How to use cytodiagnostic spleen puncture. Acta Med Scand 199:1, 1976

34. Soderstrom N: Cytology of the spleen. p. 229. In Zajicek J (ed): Aspiration Biopsy Cytology. II. Cytology of Infradiaphragmatic Organs. Basel, Karger, 1979

35. Goldstein HM, Zornoza J, Wallace S et al: Percutaneous fine-needle aspiration biopsy of pancreatic and other abdominal masses. Radiology 123:319, 1977

36. Lieberman RP, Crummy AB, Matallana RH: Invasive procedures in pancreatic disease. p. 192. In Raymond HW, Zwiebel WJ (eds): Seminars in Ultrasound. Vol. 1. Grune & Stratton, New York, 1980

37. Tatsuta M, Yamamoto R, Yamamura H et al: Cytologic examination and CEA measurement in aspirated pancreatic material collected by percutaneous fine-needle aspiration biopsy under ultrasonic guidance for diagnosis of pancreatic carcinoma. Cancer 52:693, 1983

38. Ho C-S, McLoughlin MJ, McHattie JD, Laing-Che T: Percutaneous fine-needle aspiration biopsy of the pancreas following endoscopic retrograde cholangiopancreatography. Radiology 125:351, 1977

39. Mitty HA, Efremidis SC, Yeh H-C: Impact of fine-needle biopsy on management of patients with carcinoma of the pancreas. AJR 137:1119, 1981

40. Holm HH, Als O, Gammelgaard J: Percutaneous aspiration and biopsy procedures under ultrasound visualization. p. 137. In Taylor KJW (ed): Clinics in Diagnostic Ultrasound: Diagnostic Ultrasound in Gastrointestinal Disease. Vol. 1. Churchill Livingstone, New York, 1979

41. Ferrucci JT Jr, Wittenberg J, Margolies MN, Carey RW: Malignant seeding of the tract after thin needle aspiration biopsy. Radiology 130:345, 1979

42. Montali G, Solbiati L, Bossi MC et al: Sonographically guided fine-needle aspiration biopsy of adrenal masses. AJR 143:1081, 1984

43. Heaston DK, Handel DB, Ashton PR, Korobin M: Narrow gauge needle aspiration of solid adrenal masses. AJR 138:1143, 1982

44. Bolton WK, Vaughan ED Jr: A comparative study of open surgical and percutaneous renal biopsies. J Urol 117:696, 1977

45. Goldberg BB, Pollack HM, Kellerman E: Ultrasonic localization of renal biopsy. Radiology 115:167, 1975

46. Chan JCM, Brewer WH, Still WJ: Renal biopsies under ultrasound guidance: 100 consecutive biopsies in children. J Urol 129:103, 1983

47. Mets T, Lameire N, Matthys E, Afschrift M: Sonically guided renal biopsy. J Clin Ultrasound 7:190, 1979

48. Parker RA, Elliott WC, Muther RS et al: Percutaneous aspiration biopsy of renal allografts using ultrasound localization. Urology 15:534, 1980

49. Spigos D, Capek V, Jonasson O: Percutaneous biopsy of renal transplants using ultrasonographic guidance. J Urol 117:699, 1977

50. Saitoh M: Selective renal biopsy under ultrasonic real-time guidance. Urol Radiology 6:30, 1984

51. Maxwell DR, Asher WM: Ultrasound localization of the kidneys for closed renal biopsy. J Clin Ultrasound 2:279, 1974

52. Zornoza J, Cabanillas FF, Altoff TM et al: Percutaneous needle biopsy in abdominal lymphoma. AJR 136:97, 1981

53. Zornoza J, Jonsson K, Wallace S, Lukeman JM: Fine needle aspiration biopsy of retroperitoneal lymph nodes and abdominal masses: An updated report. Radiology 125:87, 1977

54. Torp-Pedersen S, Gronvall S, Holm HH: Ultrasonically guided fine-needle aspiration biopsy of gastrointestinal mass lesions. J Ultrasound Med 3:65, 1984

55. Ennis MG, MacErlean DP: Biopsy of bowel wall pathology under ultrasound control. Gastrointest Radiol 6:17, 1981

56. Holm HH: Real-time biopsy techniques. p. 137. In Winsberg F, Cooperberg PL (eds): Clinics in Diagnostic Ultrasound: Real-time Ultrasonography. Vol. 10. Churchill Livingstone, New York, 1982

57. Schwerk WB, Durr HK: Ultrasound gray-scale pattern and guided aspiration puncture of abdominal abscesses. J Clin Ultrasound 9:389, 1981

58. Gronvall J, Gronvall S, Hegedus V: Ultrasound-guided drainage of fluid-containing masses using angiographic catheterization techniques. Am J Roentgenol 129:997, 1977

59. Mueller PR, VanSonnenberg E, Ferrucci JT Jr: Percutaneous drainage of 250 abdominal abscesses and fluid collections. Radiology 151:343, 1984

60. Otto R, Deyhle P: Guided puncture under real-time sonographic control. Radiology 134:784, 1980

61. Saini S, Mueller PR, Ferrucci JT Jr et al: Percutaneous aspiration of hepatic cysts does not provide definitive therapy. AJR 141:559, 1983

62. Kimura M, Tsuchiya Y, Ohto M et al: Ultrasonically guided percutaneous drainage of solitary liver abscess: Successful treatment in four cases. J Clin Gastroenterol 3:61, 1981

63. Kuligowska E, Conners SK, Shapiro JH: Liver abscess: Sonography in diagnosis and treatment. AJR 138:253, 1982

64. Roemer CE, Ferrucci JT Jr, Mueller PR et al: Hepatic cysts: Diagnosis and therapy by sonographic needle aspiration. AJR 136:1065, 1981

65. Ein SH, Shandling B, Simpson JS, Stephens CA: Nonoperative management of traumatic spleen in children: how and why. J Pediatr Surg 113:117, 1978

66. Johnson MA, Cooperberg PL, Boisvert J et al: Spontaneous splenic rupture in infectious mononucleosis: sonographic diagnosis and follow-up. AJR 136:111, 1981

67. Ohto M, Karasawa E, Tsuchiya Y, et al: Ultrasonically guided percutaneous contrast medium injection and aspiration biopsy using a real-time puncture transducer. Radiology 136:171, 1980

68. Mueller PR, Ferrucci JT Jr, vanSonnenberg E et al: Obstruction of the left hepatic duct: Diagnosis and treatment by selective fine-needle cholangiography and percutaneous biliary drainage. Radiology 145:297, 1982

69. Makuuchi M, Bandai Y, Ito T et al: Ultrasonically guided percutaneous transhepatic bile drainage. Radiology 136:165, 1980

70. Douillet P, Brunelle F, Chaumont P et al: Ultrasonography and percutaneous cholangiography in children with dilated bile ducts. Am J Dis Child 135:131, 1981

71. Makuuchi M, Bandai Y, Ito T, Wanda T: Ultrasonically guided percutaneous transhepatic cholangiography and percutaneous pancreatography. Radiology 134:767, 1980

72. Phillips G, Bank S, Kumari-Subaiya S, Kurtz LM: Percutaneous ultrasound-guided puncture of the gallbladder. (PUPG) Radiology 145:769, 1982

73. Hancke S, Pedersen JF: Percutaneous puncture of pancreatic cysts guided by ultrasound. Surg Gynecol and Obstet 142:551, 1976

74. MacErlean DP, Bryan PJ, Murphy JJ: Pancreatic pseudocyst: management by ultrasonically guided aspiration. Gastrointest Radiol 5:255, 1980

75. Hill MC, Dach JL, Barkin J et al: The role of percutaneous aspiration in the diagnosis of pancreatic abscess. AJR 141:1035, 1983

76. Ohto M, Saotome N, Saisho H et al: Real-time sonography of the pancreatic duct: application to percutaneous pancreatic ductography. AJR 134:647, 1980

77. Matter D, Adloff M, Warter P: Ultrasonically guided percutaneous opacification of a pancreatojejunostomy. Radiology 148:218, 1983

78. Cooperberg PL, Cohen MM, Graham M: Ultrasonographically guided percutaneous pancreatography: report of two cases. AJR 132:662, 1979

79. Scheible W, Coel M, Siemers PT, Siegel H: Percutaneous aspiration of adrenal cysts. Am J Roentgenol 128:1013, 1977

80. Thompson IM Jr, Kovac A, Geshner J: Ultrasound follow-up of renal cyst puncture. J Urol 124:175, 1980

81. Lang EK: Renal cyst puncture and aspiration: A survey of complications. Am J Roentgenol 128:723, 1977

82. Silver TM, Thornburg JR: Pneumothorax: A complication of percutaneous aspiration of upper pole renal masses. Am J Roentgenol 128:451, 1977

83. Brockis JG, Hulbert JC, Patel AS et al: The diagnosis and treatment of lymphoceles associated with renal transplantation. Br J Urol 50:307, 1978

84. Spigos D, Capek V: Ultrasonically guided percutaneous aspiration of lymphoceles following renal transplantation: A diagnostic and therapeutic method. J Clin Ultrasound 4:45, 1976

85. Mueller PR, Simeone JF: Intraabdominal abscess: diagnosis by sonography and computed tompography. Radiol Clin North Am 21:425, 1983

86. vanSonnenberg E, Mueller PR, Ferrucci JT Jr: Percutaneous drainage of 250 abdominal abscesses and fluid collection. Part I. Results, failures and complications. Radiology 151:337, 1984

87. Sones PJ: Percutaneous drainage of abdominal abscesses. AJR 142:35, 1984

88. Papanicolaou N, Butch RJ, Mueller PR: Percutaneous abscess drainage. p. 117. In Raymond HW, Zwiebel WJ (eds): Seminars in Ultrasound: Abscesses. Vol. 3. Grune & Stratton, New York, 1983

89. Stanley P, Atkinson JB, Reid BS, Gilsanz V: Percutaneous drainage of abdominal fluid collections in children. AJR 142:813, 1984

90. Gerzof SG, Robbins AH, Birkett DH et al: Percutaneous catheter drainage of abdominal abscesses guided by ultrasound and computed tomography. AJR 133:1, 1979

91. vanSonnenberg E, Ferrucci JT Jr, Mueller PR et al: Percutaneous drainage of abscesses and fluid collections: Technique, results and application. Radiology 142:1, 1982

92. Clark RA, Towlin R: Abscess drainage with CT and ultrasound guidance. Radiol Clin North Am 21:445, 1983

93. Gerzof SG, Robbins AH, Johnson WC et al: Percutaneous catheter drainage of abdominal abscesses. N Engl J Med 305:653, 1981

94. Aeder MI, Wellman JL, Haaga JR, Hau T: Role of surgical and percutaneous drainage in the treatment of abdominal abscesses. Arch Surg 118:273, 1983

95. Crass JR, Karl R: Bedside drainage of abscesses with sonographic guidance in the desperately ill. AJR 139:183, 1982

96. vanSonnenberg E, Wing VW, Casola G, et al: Temporizing affect of percutaneous drainage of complicated abscesses in critically ill patients. AJR 142:821, 1984

97. vanSonnenberg E, Mueller PR, Ferrucci JT Jr et al: Sump catheter for percutaneous abscess and fluid drainage by trocar or Seldinger technique. AJR 139:613, 1982

98. Martin EC, Karlson KB, Fankuchen EI et al: Percutaneous drainage of postoperative intraabdominal abscesses. AJR 138:13, 1982

99. vanSonnenberg E, Ferrucci JT Jr, Mueller PR, et al: Percutaneous radiographically guided catheter drainage of abdominal abscesses. JAMA 247:190, 1982

100. Gronvall S, Gammelgaard J, Haubek A, Holm HH: Drainage of abdominal abscesses guided by sonography. AJR 138:527, 1982

101. Schnyder PA, Candardjis G, Anderegg A: Peritonitis after thin-needle aspiration biopsy of an abscess. AJR 137:1271, 1981

102. Johnson WC, Gerzof SG, Robbins AH, Nabseth DC: Treatment of abdominal abscesses: comparative evaluation of operative drainage versus percutaneous catheter drainage guided by computed tomography or ultrasound. Ann Surg 194:510, 1981

103. Yaremchuk MJ, Kane R, Cady B: Ultrasound-guided catheter localization of intrahepatic abscesses—An aid in open surgical drainage. Surgery 91:482, 1982

104. MacErlean DP, Owens AP, Hourihane JB: Ultrasound guided percutaneous abdominal abscess drainage. Br J Radiol 54:394, 1981

105. Cronan JJ, Amis ES Jr, Dorfman GS: Percutaneous drainage of renal abscesses. AJR 142:351, 1984

106. Kuligowska E, Newman B, White SJ, Caldarone A: Interventional ultrasound in detection and treatment of renal inflammatory disease. Radiology 147:521, 1983

107. Conrad MR, Sanders RC, Mascardo AD: Perinephric abscess aspiration using ultrasound guidance. Am J Roentgenol 128:459, 1977

108. Gerzof SG: Percutaneous drainage of renal and perinephric abscess. Urol Radiol 2:171, 1981

109. Gerzof SG, Gale ME: Computed tomography and ultrasonography for diagnosis and treatment of renal and retroperitoneal abscesses. Urol Clin North Am 9:185, 1982

110. Hillman BJ, Smith EH, Holm HH: Ultrasound diagnosis and treatment of gallbladder fossa collections following biliary tract surgery. Br J Radiol 52:390, 1979

111. Mueller PR, Ferrucci JT Jr, Simeone JF et al: Detection and drainage of bilomas: special considerations. AJR 140:715, 1983

112. Radder RW: Ultrasonically guided percutaneous catheter drainage for gallbladder empyema. Diagn Imaging 49:330, 1980

113. Shaver RW, Hawkins IF, Soong J: Percutaneous cholecystostomy. AJR 138:1133, 1982

114. Elyaderani MK, McDowell DE, Gabriele OF: A preliminary report of percutaneous cholecystostomy under ultrasonography and fluroscopy guidance. J Clin Gastroenterol 5:277, 1983

115. Salerno NR: Percutaneous aspiration and drainage of gallbladder. J Ultrasound Med 1:129, 1982

116. vanSonnenberg E, Wing VW, Pollard JW, Casola G: Life-threatening vagal reactions associated with percutaneous cholecystostomy. Radiology 151:377, 1984

117. Sumner TE, Crowe JE, Resnick MI: Ultrasonically guided antegrade pyelography of an obstructed solitary pelvic kidney. J Clin Ultrasound 6:262, 1978

118. Saitoh M, Watanabe H: Ultrasonically guided percutaneous pyeloscopy. Urology 17:457, 1981

119. Pedersen JF, Cowan DF, Kristensen JK et al: Ultrasonically-guided percutaneous nephrostomy: report of 24 cases. Radiology 119:429, 1976

120. Barbaric ZL, Wood BP: Emergency percutaneous nephropyelostomy: Experience with 34 patients and review of the literature. Am J Roentgenol 128:453, 1977

121. Stables DP, Johnson ML: Percutaneous nephrostomy: The role of ultrasound. p. 73. In Rosenfield AT (ed): Clinics in Diagnostic Ultrasound: Genitourinary Ultrasonography. Vol. 2. Churchill Livingstone, New York, 1979

122. Alter AJ: Percutaneous nephropyelostomy. p. 61. In Raymond HW, Zwiebel WJ (eds): Seminars in Ultrasound, Vol. 2. Grune & Stratton, New York, 1981

123. Bush WH, Crane RE, Brannen GE: Steerable loop snare for percutaneous retrieval of renal calyx calculi. AJR 142:367, 1984

124. Winfield AC, Kirchner SG, Brun ME et al: Percutaneous nephrostomy in neonates, infants and children. Radiology 151:617, 1984

125. Stanley P, Bear JW, Reid BS: Percutaneous nephrostomy in infants and children. AJR 141:473, 1983

126. Sadlowski RW, Finney RP, Branch WT et al: New technique for percutaneous nephrostomy under ultrasound guidance. J Urol 121:559, 1979

127. Zegal HG, Pollack HM, Banner MP et al: Percutaneous nephrostomy: comparison of sonographic and fluoroscopic guidance. AJR 137:925, 1981

128. Dubuisson RL, Eichelberger RP, Jones JB: A simple modification of real-time sector sonography to monitor percutaneous nephrostomy. Radiology 146:232, 1983

129. Burnett KR, Handler SJ, Conroy RM et al: Percutaneous nephrostomy utilizing B-mode and real-time ultrasound guidance: The lateral approach and puncture facilitation with furosemide. J Clin Ultrasound 10:252, 1982

130. Baron RL, Lee JKT, McClennan BL, Melson GL: Percutaneous nephrostomy using real-time sonographic guidance. AJR 136:1018, 1981

131. Yoder IC, Pfister RC, Lindfors KK, Newhouse JH: Pyonephrosis: Imaging and intervention. AJR 141:735, 1983

11

Intraoperative Abdominal Real-Time Ultrasound

With the development of high-resolution real-time sector systems, a new application of ultrasound has evolved: intraoperative (OR) evaluation. Tissue dissection and manipulation are required in order to obtain information at exploratory surgery. The morbidity and time for exploratory operation may be significantly reduced by the use of imaging modalities during the surgical procedure. The major advantages of real-time ultrasound are its ability to precisely localize structures, its three-dimensional capability, its noninvasiveness without radiation or the administration of contrast, and its ability to be used repeatedly. Scans are instantaneous, repeatable, multidimensional and magnified at will.[1] Abnormalities can be localized and characterized, calculi can be detected regardless of chemical composition, and guidance can be provided for drainage, stone extraction, or biopsy.[1] In most cases, real-time sonography has the potential of assisting the surgeon in improving patient care.

TECHNIQUE

Transducer

Those involved in intraoperative abdominal ultrasound have described various transducers that are used.[1-23] As with any ultrasound procedure, the highest frequency transducer that allows adequate penetration of the organ or structure to be scanned should be used. High-frequency, real-time transducers with frequencies of 7.5 to 10 MHz, which are capable of providing resolu-

tion in the range of 1 mm, may be used because the depth of penetration for intraoperative ultrasound is generally less than 3 to 4 cm[4-19,22] (Fig. 11-1). Nonetheless, 5 MHz short-focused transducers have been routinely used by some investigators; these are more available than the higher frequency transducers for ophthalmologic work[2,3,23,24] (Fig. 11-2). Unlike the all-purpose units designed mainly for abdominal and obstetrical work, ophthalmologic units are calibrated for a different velocity of sound. Although most structures can be adequately scanned with the short-focused, high-frequency transducers, a low-frequency scanhead, such as a 3 MHz head, must be employed for evaluation of deep structures like the liver.

Newer transducers designed specifically for OR work are capable of variable frequencies; this allows flexibility in depth of penetration without requiring substitution of the scanhead. Sequenced linear array scanners may be too bulky to be suitable for OR work because of the large size of the scanning surfaces[20,21] (Fig. 11-3). Most commercially available scanheads with an L-shape (Fig. 11-2) are less unwieldly but not ideal for all OR situations. They generally do have a faster frame rate and a significantly larger sector viewing angle than the ophthalmologic units. The scanheads designed like a "big pencil" with variable frequency selections have limitations (Fig. 11-4). They tend to have a slower frame rate, are more difficult to orient than the L-shaped transducers, and are limited by their shape in various scanning situations. The future may see the development of newer transducers; in the meantime the sonologist and surgeon can use the commercially available equipment and still derive some benefit from ultrasound in the OR.

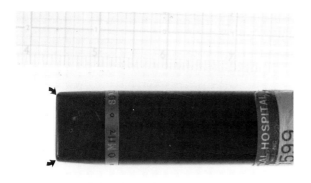

Fig. 11-1. Ophthalmologic transducer. Note the size of the scanning surface (between arrows) of this 10 MHz transducer.

Sterilization

While some scanheads can be sterilized by gas, most of the latest mechanical devices cannot be sterilized by any means. Some surgeons prefer the sterilized devices because there is less risk of contamination of the operating field. The major disadvantages of this method include (1) time—sterilization takes 12 hours; (2) transducer—the number of studies performed depends on the number of transducers available; and (3) advance time—scans must be prescheduled. The use of a sterile glove and a sterile camera drape, arthroscope bag or a sterile disposable cover is a very successful alternative[1–4,23] (Fig. 11-5). Such a disposable cover may be 3 inches in diameter, 6 feet in length and closed at one end, composed of a double layer of 1-mil polyethelene fused together.[4] The bags rarely break, if handled carefully; and by using the bag, many more operative ultrasounds can be performed in one day than when the transducer is gas sterilized.

The technique for "sterilizing" the transducer using a bag is as follows:[2,3,23]

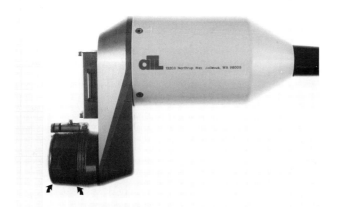

Fig. 11-2. L-shaped sector transducer. This is the shape of a common commercially available transducer. Note the size of the scanning surface (between arrows).

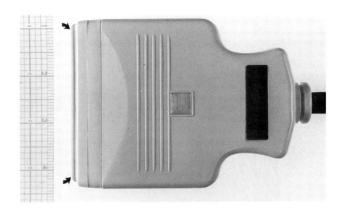

Fig. 11-3. Linear array transducer. Note the length of the scanning surface (between arrows) of this 5 MHz linear array transducer.

1. After placing gel on the scanhead of a sector real-time transducer, and with a second sterile glove (size 8) on the right hand, the transducer scanhead is grasped with the thumb on the scanning surface (see Fig. 10-4A).
2. The second glove is inverted over the transducer until the scanhead is in the thumb of the glove (see Fig. 10-4B).
3. The cuff of the glove is held while a sterile camera drape (Tekna Med Corp., 4½″ × 80″ or Xomed Arthroscope camera drape, 5″ × 96″) is fed over the gloved transducer scanhead and its cable (See Figs. 10-4C to E).
4. The corner of the bag is removed so that only the sterile gloved scanning surface (in glove thumb) is exposed and a rubber band is placed around the neck of the scanhead (See Fig. 10-4F).
5. The surface of the thumb of the glove is wiped with a wet 4 × 4 sponge to remove any powder on the glove surface.
6. Following the procedure, the glove and the sterile bag are carefully removed to check the scanhead for blood, which would indicate contamination.

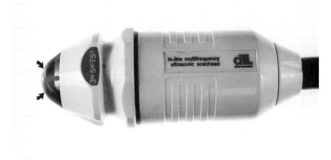

Fig. 11-4. "Big-pencil" transducer. This is a multifrequency transducer that is held like a pencil. It has a small scanning surface (between arrows).

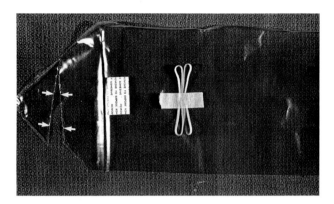

Fig. 11-5. Sterile transducer drape. This is a sterile arthroscope bag that is commercially available and comes in various sizes. The corner (between arrows) can be removed for the scanning surface.

Scanning Technique

The scanning technique intraoperatively is very similar to that extraoperatively. When scanning, care should be taken to maintain correct orientation as to right/left, anterior/posterior, cephalad/caudad or longitudinal/transverse. The appropriate transducer position should always be noted on the screen along with any other pertinent localizing data. The ceiling lights need to be turned off in order to eliminate the glare on the monitor while the surgical field lights may be left on. Besides videotaping the procedure, freeze-frame images should be taken. These may be photographed on film at the time of the procedure or taken from the videotape at a later time.

Although not always necessary, warm sterile saline may be used in the surgical field as an acoustic coupling agent. By producing a 5 to 10 mm probe-to-surface distance, an intervening saline bath may correct the deficiency of poor resolution in the near field in some instances.[13,21]

The person to scan intraoperatively should be the person most experienced in scanning and interpretation whether it be a radiologist (sonologist), or surgeon. In our institution, intraoperative ultrasound is a team approach. The radiologist (sonologist) scans while the surgeon performs the operative procedure under real-time guidance; the experienced sonographer (technologist) handles the machine settings, recordings, measurements, and photography. Generally, it is difficult to interpret an intraoperative ultrasound without having one's hand on the transducer. While it is the surgeon who has the greatest knowledge of the intraoperative anatomy, it is generally the sonologist who has the greatest understanding and experience in ultrasound. The intraoperative ultrasound is often best served by the combined efforts of these two specialists.

Successful utilization of OR ultrasound requires close cooperation between the surgeon and sonologist, which may present a logistical problem. A relatively inexperienced surgeon necessitates the sonologist's physical presence in the OR for each examination, whereas a more experienced surgeon might use a sonologist as a back-up consultant (as with intraoperative cholangiography). For this latter setting to occur, though, the surgeon must have both technical and interpretative skill.[1]

Modifications of the General Technique

RENAL

Several modifications of the standard technique are used for renal calculi removal. In cases of single or multiple stone, the kidney is mobilized and scanned systematically. The stone or stones are localized. If possible, the stone or stones are removed under direct real-time visualization using curved forceps inserted through the renal pelvis. If this is not successful, then a 22-gauge needle is inserted along either side of the scanhead until the tip of the needle is in contact with the stone (as seen on real-time)[3,13,23] (Fig. 11-6). The depth to the stone is measured. After removing the scanhead, an incision is made between the two needles, and the stone is extracted. The procedure is repeated as needed for other stones. Other investigators have reported the use of Doppler ultrasound for localization of intrarenal arteries with real-time localization of stones so as to have an avascular atraumatic nephrotomy; that way, clamping the renal artery and the cooling process are not necessary.[25] An operative radiograph is obtained to document complete removal of stones.

In cases of staghorn calculi, the real-time ultrasound is performed following the removal of all visible stones. Ultrasound is used to document the absence of retained fragments[2,13,23] (Fig. 11-7). If a stone is found, the procedure described for single or multiple stones is repeated. An operative radiograph is obtained following removal of all stones located by ultrasound.

HEPATOBILIARY

In hepatobiliary scanning, the gloved transducer is placed directly on the gallbladder, liver, or extrahepatic ducts after a saline wash of the operative field (Fig. 11-8). The organ/structure to be examined is scanned with direct contact. The gallbladder is scanned systematically in both transverse and longitudinal planes. Care is taken to scan all portions of the common bile duct, including the retroduodenal portion. The bile duct is immobile, while the hepatic artery pulsates, and the portal vein moves

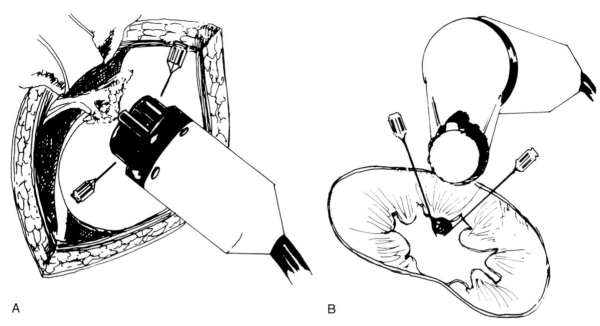

A   B

Fig. 11-6. Renal technique. **(A)** Diagram demonstrating the placement of needles on either side of the scanhead in the real-time localization of a stone. With direct real-time visualization, the needles are placed so that they come in contact with the stone. **(B)** Cross-section showing the relationship of the scanhead and needles to the stone. (From Vincent LM, Mittelstaedt CA: Intraoperative abdominal ultrasound. p.95. In Sanders RC, Hill M (eds): Ultrasound Annual 1984. Raven Press, New York, 1984.)

with respiration.[19] As a rule, the intrahepatic ducts need not be scanned unless stones are found elsewhere.

Although longitudinal and transverse projections are required, the extrahepatic biliary tree is scanned predominately with the longitudinal axis. The supraduodenal segment of the bile duct is scanned through the free edge of the gastrohepatic ligament, while the retroduodenal segment is scanned transduodenally. The inferior portion of the duct is evaluated by directing the scanhead into the pancreaticoduodenal groove; the retroduodenal segment and the termination of the duct are scanned from its posterior aspect after anteromedial mobilization of the duodenum.[18,19]

PANCREAS

After transection of the gastrocolic omentum, the pancreas is scanned transversely and longitudinally with the scanhead directly on the surface of the pancreas. If inflammation does not allow this access to the lesser sac, the evaluation can be performed through adjacent structures such as the lesser and greater omentum, transverse mesocolon and duodenum.[15,19] Both the parenchyma and ducts should be assessed and landmarks such as the superior mesenteric artery, superior mesenteric vein, and common bile duct should be identified.

Beginning with the duct, the common bile duct can be identified by scanning transversely in the pancreatico-

duodenal groove and followed to its termination at the sphincter of Oddi. The portal vein can be traced to the superior mesenteric vein and uncinate process, again with transverse scans in the pancreaticoduodenal groove. In the transverse projection, the entire pancreas can be examined with the pancreatic duct and splenic vein in cross-section. Scanning along the long axis of the pancreas demonstrates the common bile duct, superior mesenteric vein and portal vein in cross-section, and the splenic vein and pancreatic duct in long axis.[16]

APPLICATIONS

Since the development of diagnostic ultrasound, multiple uses have evolved. All have suffered from the usual difficulties related to bowel gas and patient body habitus. One of ultrasound's newest applications, intraoperative ultrasound, does not have these same limitations. Unlike extraoperative ultrasound, the transducer with operative real-time is in direct contact with the organ or structure to be examined. Because a high-frequency, short-focused transducer is used and there is little intervening tissue to attenuate and scatter the incident sound energy, the resolution of the scan on the whole is greatly improved. This allows high-resolution scanning of multiple structures such as the kidney, hepatobiliary system, pancreas, and others.

Renal

Most large series reporting experience with surgery for multiple or staghorn calculi indicate that the incidence for retained stones is approximately 10 percent. Surgical removal is either straight forward or difficult.[26] Reports of the fate of the retained stones following nephrolithotomy show that over 60 percent of these patients have progression of their disease. Radiologic techniques for detecting stones at surgery have improved but still are associated with excessive time and technically poor results. Percutaneous endoscopic examination of the upper urinary tract allows direct removal of renal calculi.[26] Stones too large to remove have been fragmented or destroyed by ultrasonic or electrohydraulic lithotrite.[26] Intraoperative real-time ultrasound has added immensely to this procedure. Following an initial evaluation in a procine kidney model, we have used intraoperative real-time ultrasound to aid the urologist in removing stones.[27]

Although operative radiography has proved to be a significant advance in renal calculi localization, there are problems. The image is often suboptimal because portable equipment is used. There are many artifacts and many times the film must be repeated, necessitating more radiation exposure. The advantages of this technique include visualization of radiopaque calculi and detection of stones as small as 2.0 mm. The disadvan-

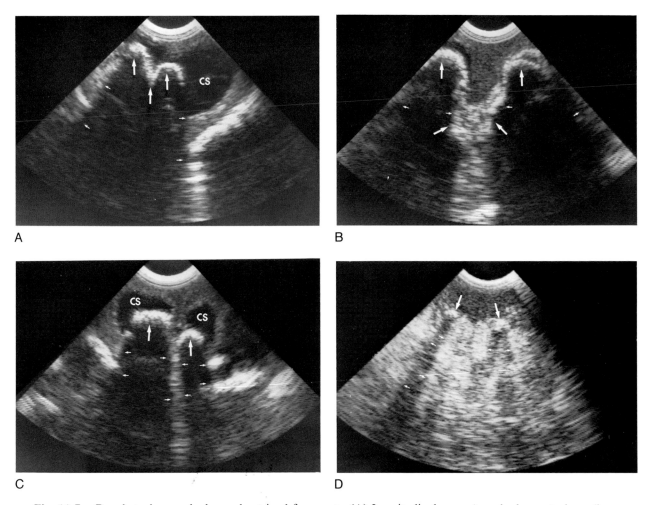

A

B

C

D

Fig. 11-7. Renal staghorn calculus and retained fragments. **(A)** Longitudinal scan. An echodense staghorn (long arrows) is seen within a dilated collecting system *(cs)*. Posterior acoustic shadowing is seen (small arrows). **(B,C)** Transverse scans. An echodense staghorn (long arrows) is seen with posterior acoustic shadowing (small arrows). The dilated collecting system *(cs)* is seen around the stone on **(C)**. (Figs. A-C from Mittelstaedt CA, Staab EV, Drobnes WE et al: The intraoperative uses of real-time ultrasound. Radiographics 4:267, 1984.) **(D)** This scan was performed following the removal of a staghorn. Several retained stone fragments (long arrows) are noted on this longitudinal scan with associated shadowing (small arrows). (Fig. D from Vincent LM, Mittelstaedt CA: Intraoperative abdominal ultrasound. p.95. In Sanders RC, Hill M (eds): Ultrasound Annual 1984. Raven Press, New York, 1984.)

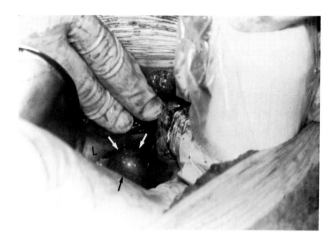

Fig. 11-8. Gallbladder scan. The draped scanhead is seen in contact with the gallbladder (arrows). (*L*, liver.) (From Mittelstaedt CA, Staab EV, Drobnes WE et al: The intraoperative uses of real-time ultrasound. Radiographics 4:267, 1984.)

tages include radiation, many artifacts, time consumption, and film of variable quality.

Ultrasound provides a three-dimensional picture with a dynamic capability. The ultrasound appearance of the normal kidney is known: the renal cortex is moderately echogenic (similar in density to liver parenchyma); the pyramids are hypoechoic; and the renal sinus is highly echogenic. There is a highly reflective pattern between the cortex and the renal sinus fat. The collecting system, if fluid-filled, will appear as an anechoic area contained by the surrounding echogenicity. Despite knowledge of this appearance, the inexperienced OR sonologist might find the intrarenal anatomy initially unfamiliar because

of the size discrepancy between the greatly magnified display image and the corresponding limited field of view.

The intraoperative indications for renal ultrasound would include all of the following:[3,23]

1. Documentation of complete removal of staghorn calculi.
2. Localization of solitary or multiple stones.
3. Evaluation of unsuspected renal mass.
4. Evaluation of radiolucent defects within the collecting system.

Ultrasound has been used as a diagnostic tool for evaluation of the kidney for the past 15 years. Established uses include the distinction between renal cyst and tumor, the detection of hydronephrosis, and the determination of renal size. OR ultrasound is useful in locating and removing small renal stones broken from larger stones during extraction, stones in calyces proximal to narrowed infundibuli, and parenchymal calculi that should be removed.[28] As noted in our experience as well as by others, real-time ultrasound can accurately localize stones as small as 1 to 2 mm in size.[20,21,29] These stones, regardless of composition, appear echodense and cast an accoustic shadow[3,21,23,26] (Fig. 11-9). If the overall gain of the system is diminished, the brighter stone echoes should persist. This technique requires a certain familiarity with the equipment and experience in interpretation.[8]

Although ultrasound appears to be an accurate procedure, there are problems. After the kidney is incised down to a calyx, air enters the collecting system. This

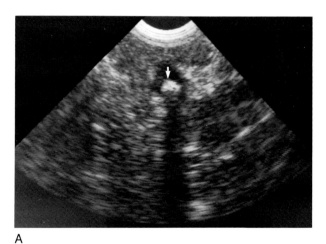

A

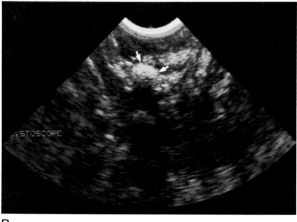

B

Fig. 11-9. Renal calculus. OR scans with several calculi. On (**A**), the calculus is seen as an echodensity (arrow) with shadowing surrounded by a dilated calyx. On (**B**), the other calculus (arrow) is not encompassed by fluid in its calyx. (Fig. **A**, from Vincent LM, Mittelstaedt CA: Intraoperative abdominal ultrasound. p. 95. In Sanders RC, Hill MA (eds): Ultrasound Annual 1984. Raven Press, New York, 1984.)

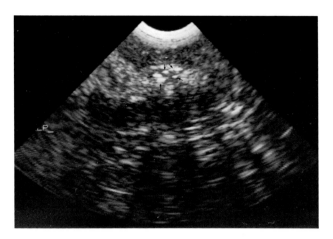

Fig. 11-10. Renal collecting system air. Following the removal of a calculus, this kidney was scanning to evaluate for stone fragments. Linear echodensities (arrows) without associated shadowing were seen within a calyx. These moved freely with motion of the kidney. (From Vincent LM, Mittelstaedt CA: Intraoperative abdominal ultrasound. p.95. In Sanders RC, Hill MA (eds): Ultrasound Annual 1984. Raven Press, New York, 1984.)

produces a dense pattern with shadowing much like a calculus (Fig. 11-10). In these instances, it is helpful to fill the kidney with sterile saline and/or immerse it in fluid. Stones as a rule tend to cast an acoustic shadow with sharper margins than air (Fig. 11-9). In addition, by slightly moving the kidney, air bubbles tend to move and present a continually changing gaseous interface. Another potential source of confusion are areas of calyceal calcification that are also echodense with good shadows.[29] A scar or thrombus can be mistaken for a neoplasm initially, although exclusion of a stone is straightforward due to the absence of shadowing distal to either of these entities. Also, a transitional cell carcinoma must be questioned when a nonopaque (on radiography) calyceal filling defect without distal shadowing is demonstrated by ultrasound.

Operative real-time ultrasound and radiography can be combined leading to decreased operating time, and less maceration of the kidney, lessening the likelihood of stone retention. Besides the obvious advantage of three dimensional capability and dynamic imaging, ultrasound is particularly beneficial in identifying calculi regardless of composition, migrating stones, localization of small, nonpalpable calculi, and rapid assessment after removal of staghorn calculi.[13] It is a rapid procedure with instant results ultimately leading to less trauma to the kidney than "blind" exploration. Prior to nephrotomy or pyelotomy, scanning is recommended; it should also be used following stone extraction. To document the absence of stones, an operative radiograph is obtained

following the procedure. Disadvantages include air in collecting system, which produces artifact, dependence on the experience of operator, and dependence on the resolution of equipment. One series found ultrasound to be helpful in 70 percent of cases.[8]

Occasionally, a surgeon may encounter an unsuspected renal mass when operating for nephrolithiasis or for some other reason. Ultrasound has the capability of characterizing the lesion as solid or cystic and directing a biopsy if needed[23,28] (Figs. 11-11 and 11-12). It may also influence the need for further exploration.

Hepatobiliary

INDICATIONS

The indications for hepatobiliary intraoperative ultrasound might include the following:[2,4,5,8,10,18,20]

1. Detection of gallbladder calculi when the diagnosis is questioned by the surgeon, especially in the morbidly obese patient who cannot be evaluated preoperatively.
2. Location of the common bile duct, which is especially important in cases where the anatomy is distorted.
3. Evaluation for choledocholithiasis.
4. Localization of liver lesion(s) for biopsy, aspiration, or removal.
5. Characterization of unsuspected liver lesion(s) found at surgery.
6. Evaluation of liver lesion for extension through the hepatic and portal veins, which would change surgical protocols.

GALLBLADDER

Ordinarily, it is extremely difficult to evaluate the gallbladder of the morbidly obese patient radiographically or with ultrasound. Because these patients are at an increased risk of gallbladder disease following a gastric bariatric procedure (gastrogastrostomy or gastric bypass Roux-en-Y), it is important to know at the time of surgery whether the gallbladder is abnormal so it can be electively removed.[2,23]

Various abnormalities of the gallbladder can be detected intraoperatively. The normal gallbladder is anechoic with a wall of less than 2 to 3 mm in thickness. Gallstones appear much like they do extraoperatively; they are echodense structures that generally cast an acoustic shadow (Fig. 11-13). They are located in the dependent portion of the gallbladder and move with movement of the gallbladder. Small (3 mm or less) intraluminal nonshadowing densities have also been described (Figs. 11-13 and 11-14). These have proven to be

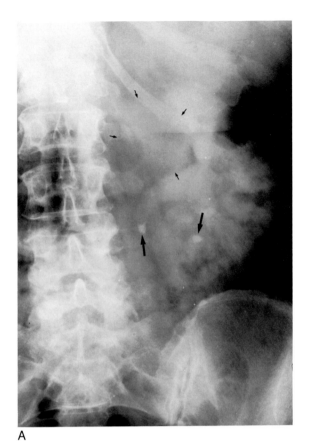

A

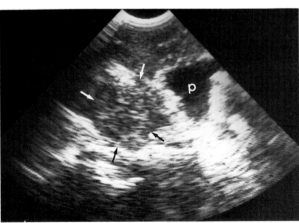

B

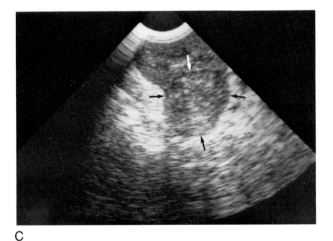

C

Fig. 11-11. Renal cell carcinoma. **(A)** Intravenous pyelogram. Although the left lower pole calculi (long arrows) were seen, the upper pole mass (small arrows) was not appreciated preoperatively. Longitudinal **(B)** and transverse **(C)** scans demonstrate a solid mass (arrows) in the upper pole. (*p*, pelvis.) (Figs. **B** and **C** from Vincent LM, Mittelstaedt CA: Intraoperative abdominal ultrasound. p.95. In Sanders RC, Hill M (eds): Ultrasound Annual 1984. Raven Press, New York 1984.)

cholesterol crystals in most cases, but clumped white blood cells in some[2,23] (Fig. 11-14). In cholesterolosis, often small densities (nonshadowing) adherant to the gallbladder wall have been seen (Fig. 11-15). In addition, there are often small intraluminal densities (cholesterol crystals) in cholesterolosis[2,23] (Fig. 11-13).

Ultrasound has been shown to be more accurate than surgical palpation by some investigators.[2,4] In one series, surgical palpation failed to reveal the presence of stones in 18 percent of instances in which they were correctly documented by ultrasound.[4] In a series of gallbladder operations performed on obese patients, only 50 percent of abnormal examinations were felt abnormal by palpation during surgery.[2]

At times, when surgery is performed for some other indication, an abnormal gallbladder may be questioned at the time of operation.[18] Ultrasound can quickly assess the gallbladder in question and assist the surgeon in determining whether to perform a cholecystectomy in those cases.

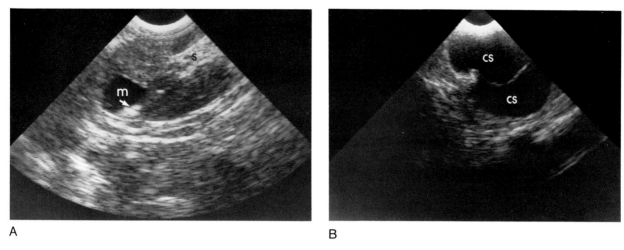

A   B

Fig. 11-12. Unsuspected renal mass. **(A)** Hemorrhagic renal cyst in a patient with known adrenal neoplasm in whom an unsuspected renal mass was identified. An anechoic mass *(m)* with a density (arrow) along its medial border is demonstrated on this transverse scan. (*s*, renal sinus) (Fig. **A**, from Vincent LM, Mittelstaedt CA: Intraoperative abdominal ultrasound. p. 95. In Sanders RC, Hill M (eds): Ultrasound Annual 1984. Raven Press, New York, 1984.) **(B)** Hydronephrosis in a patient undergoing a radical hysterectomy and node dissection for cervical carcinoma. A renal mass was palpated at surgery. A markedly dilated collecting system *(cs)* is seen producing the mass on this transverse scan.

EXTRAHEPATIC DUCTS

The operative evaluation of the common bile duct is the most important application of ultrasound imaging in the biliary tree.[10] Ultrasound is useful in localizing the common bile duct in the presence of acute inflammation and other abnormal anatomy, measuring the caliber of the common bile duct, identifying calculi in the com-

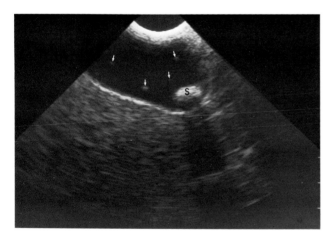

Fig. 11-13. Gallstone and cholesterol crystals. Longitudinal scan of the gallbladder with an echodense gallstone *(s)* and its associated acoustic shadowing. Note there are small linear echodensities (arrows) within the gallbladder lumen. These represented cholesteral crystals. (From Mittelstaedt CA, Staab EV, Drobnes WE et al: The intraoperative uses of real-time ultrasound. Radiographics 4:267, 1984.)

mon bile duct, and is a useful adjunct to the preoperative cholangiogram.[10] Intraoperative ultrasound can permit earlier and more precise appraisal of operative findings and decrease the operating time. Surgery for removal of biliary tract calculi is facilitated by OR radiography. To decide on the need for common bile duct exploration is probably the most frequent reason to perform an operative cholangiogram.[11] With wider experience, the question is raised about the cost effectiveness of using radiography as a screening procedure for common bile duct exploration in view of the relatively small yield of positive findings.[11]

Clinical comparisons between OR ultrasound and OR radiography have documented comparable accuracies.[16-19] Lane and Sigel have shown the accuracy that is possible in this area. Lane reported a sensitivity/specificity for ultrasound of 96 percent/93 percent, while cholangiography in the same cases had a sensitivity/specificity of 96 percent/96 percent.[16] Neither ultrasound or cholangiography detected all stones, but ultrasound demonstrated a greater number of stones.[19] Ultrasound was more accurate in cases with dilated ducts but less accurate in detecting stones at the ampulla.[19] Sigel reported a sensitivity/specificity of ultrasound to be 89 percent/96 percent and radiography to be 91 percent/73 percent. He found that both cholangiography and cholangiosonography were comparable in sensitivity, specificity, efficiency, and predictability of a negative test.[17] Ultrasound does have an inherent advantage over cholangiography: the quality of the image is not time-depen-

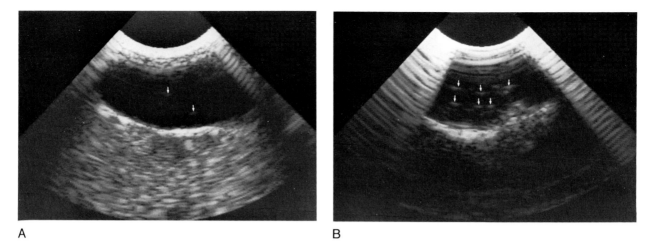

A   B

Fig. 11-14. Clumped white blood cells. **(A)** Transverse scan of the gallbladder. Multiple small echodensities (arrows) are seen within the gallbladder lumen. These moved with movement of the gallbladder and were more readily identified at real-time. **(B)** Scan of the bile from the gallbladder in **(A)**. The bile was placed in a cup to scan. Multiple small echodensities (arrows) are seen. These proved to be clumped white blood cells.

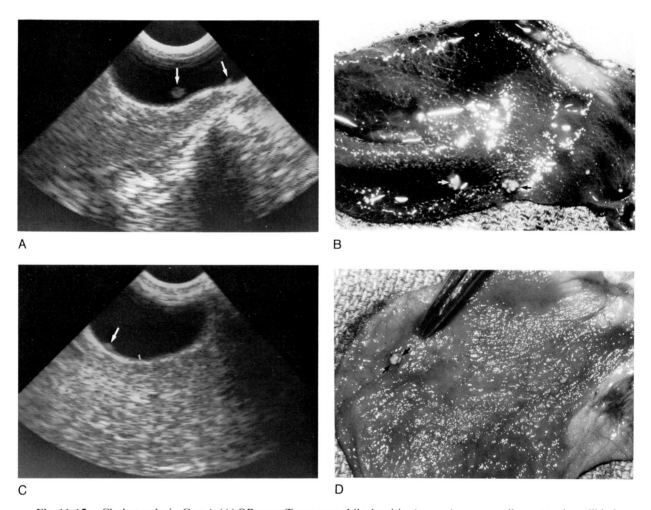

A   B

C   D

Fig. 11-15. Cholesterolosis. Case 1: **(A)** OR scan. Two nonmobile densities (arrows) are seen adherent to the gallbladder wall. **(B)** Gross specimen. Two cholesterol polyps (arrows) are seen in a gallbladder that exhibited diffuse cholesterolosis. (Figs. **A** and **B** from Mittelstaedt CA, Staab EV, Drobnes WE et al: The intraoperative uses of real-time ultrasound. Radiographics 4:267, 1984.) Case 2: **(C)** Longitudinal scan of the gallbladder with a nonshadowing echodense lesion (arrow) that is adherent to the gallbladder wall. **(D)** Gross specimen. A cholesterol polyp (arrow) is seen. (Fig. **C** from Vincent LM, Mittelstaedt CA: Intraoperative abdominal ultrasound. p.95. In Sanders RC (eds): Ultrasound Annual 1984. Raven Press, New York, 1984.)

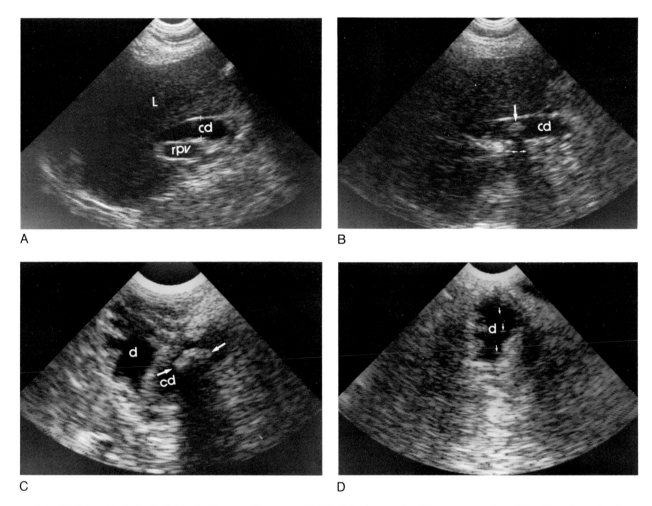

A   B

C   D

Fig. 11-16. Choledocholithiasis. Preoperative scans **(A,B)** of the long axis of the common duct. The dilated proximal duct *(cd)* is seen on **(A)**. An echodense stone (long arrow) is seen within the distal dilated common duct *(cd)* on **(B)** along with its shadow (small arrows). (*rpv*, right portal vein.) **(C)** Intraoperative transverse scan demonstrating the stone as an echodensity (arrow) in the distal end of the common duct *(cd)*. There is fluid within the second portion of the duodenum *(d)*. **(D)** Intraoperative transverse scan of the fluid-filled second portion of the duodenum *(d)*. Sterile fluid was injected into the duct to evaluate for patency. Small microbubbles seen as linear echodensities (arrows) were noted to flow into the duodenum on real-time. (Figs. **B-D** from Vincent LM, Mittelstaedt CA: Intraoperative abdominal ultrasound. p.95. In Sanders RC, Hill M (eds): Ultrasound Annual 1984. Raven Press, New York, 1984.)

dent upon contrast injection.[12] Both investigators felt that ultrasound was very desirable due to its rapidity, its noninvasive nature, and safety to patient and operating room personnel.[22] The use of ultrasound led to decreased operating time, radiation, and contrast exposure to the patient. It appeared to reduce the number of negative surgical explorations of the common bile duct. Ultrasound has been found to have a higher predictability of a positive test than radiography with 86 percent for ultrasound and 74 percent for radiography.[17] Ultrasound is reported to have a false positive rate of 9 percent while that of radiography is 16 to 29 percent.[30,31]

The ultrasound signs of biliary calculi include (1) echodense structure, (2) persistent sonic density after

"low gain" results in lucency surrounding the structure, (3) acoustic shadow, and (4) convex meniscus (with shadow) at the lower end of the bile duct, as opposed to concavity (without shadow) of the empty duct[16,19,22] (Fig. 11-16). Air bubbles can be distinguished from calculi by movement, and irregular edges.[22] The posterior acoustic shadow while not dependent upon shape, surface characteristics, or calcium content does relate to the angle of scanning as well as the size of the calculus relative to the transducer frequency.[32] At times an echogenic defect in the duct need not be appreciated but the presence of shadowing by itself, breaking the linear continuity of the back wall of the duct usually indicates the presence of stone.[16]

Although many authors report success in evaluating the extrahepatic ducts, we have not been successful in evaluating the nondilated common bile duct using the currently available sector transducers. This is largely due to the fact that the duct is too near to the transducer to visualize. Despite a "water bath" technique, visualization of the normal-sized duct has been a major problem in our hands. On the other hand, it is generally easy to visualize the dilated common bile duct. Flow through the ampulla can be checked by instilling fluid into the T-tube (in place in the common duct) and watching for microbubbles of air in the duodenum (Fig. 11-16D).

OR ultrasound does have limitations. Stones at the distal end of the duct may be missed because of poor shadowing or due to the inability to document functional presence of flow.[19] Stones located high in the intrahepatic ducts may also be overlooked due to inadequate depth penetration by the transducer. Another restriction of ultrasound may be seen in patients with biliary-enteric fistulae or post-ERCP papillotomy, secondary to a large amount of air in the biliary tree. Lastly, ultrasound evaluation of the common duct may be hampered by small ductal diameter or difficult access because of the size discrepancy between the transducer and the duct, particularly when the general purpose transducer is employed in this situation.

LIVER

There are numerous applications of intraoperative ultrasound of the liver. It is useful in characterizing unsuspected lesions palpated at surgery[20] (Figs. 11-17 and 11-18). Ultrasound can localize these lesions for biopsy

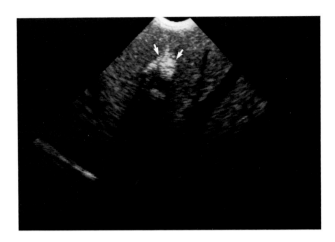

Fig. 11-18. Bile duct hamartoma. On this longitudinal scan, a well-defined echodense mass (arrows) is seen with associated acoustical shadowing. (From Mittelstaedt CA, Staab EV, Drobnes WE et al: The intraoperative uses of real-time ultrasound. Radiographics 4:267, 1984.)

or drainage. In cases of tumor, this modality can evaluate extension through the hepatic and portal vein, which would change the surgical protocols.[20]

Pancreas

OR ultrasound has been shown to significantly assist in the operative management of both tumor and inflammatory disease of the pancreas. Sigel has described the application of ultrasound in evaluating the pancreas in the operating room.[14,15,30] This modality can assist in establishing a diagnosis not made during the preoperative testing; more precisely, it can localize pancreatic abnormalities in relation to visible anatomic landmarks, exclude the presence of pseudocyst, abscess cavity and dilated ducts, and it can define precise location of tumor and evaluate the tumor for spread.[7,15,18,20,30]

The intraoperative sonographic findings of pancreatic inflammatory disease are similar to extraoperative findings. The appearance of pancreatitis is highly variable, and may range from a diffusely hypoechoic to a heterogenous pattern with highly reflective echoes in a fibrotic gland with parenchymal and ductal calcifications. Although characteristically seen as predominantly anechoic masses with acoustic enhancement and often slightly thickened walls, pseudocysts may exhibit atypical findings including multiple septations, internal echoes that may or may not layer dependently, and absence of transmission[33,34] (Figs. 11-19 and 11-20). Ultrasound can assist in selection of the optimal site for entering a pseudocyst to perform internal drainage by indicating the wall thickness and relation to nearby

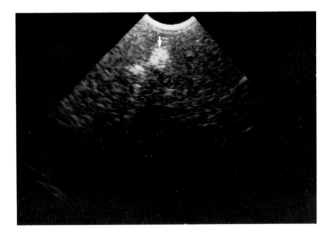

Fig. 11-17. Sclerosing hemangioma of the liver. A well-defined echodense lesion (arrow) is seen within the liver on this longitudinal scan. No acoustic shadowing is noted. (From Mittelstaedt CA, Staab EV, Drobnes WE et al: The intraoperative uses of real-time ultrasound. Radiographics 4:267, 1984.)

structures, and can help to distinguish inflammatory swelling from cyst.[7,15,18,30] A complicated pseudocyst, on the basis of ultrasound alone, may be impossible to distinguish from hematoma, abscess, or even cystic neoplasm.[34] At times, it is difficult to completely exclude surgically correctible lesions in the face of changes produced by inflammation. In these instances, ultrasound can help exclude cyst or abscess within areas of pancreatic or peripancreatic swellings, and dilated ducts in chronic pancreatitis.[15]

In a study of patients with pancreatic inflammatory disease evaluated in the OR, ultrasound was found helpful in 67 percent of operations, while assisting in the diagnosis in 8 percent, giving improved localization of the abnormality in relation to visible anatomic landmarks in 40 percent, and excluding significant pathology from an area suspected on basis of gross appearance in 19 percent.[7]

With chronic pancreatitis, irregular areas of increased sonic density are seen.[19] The gland is usually atrophied with greater sonic density than the normal gland and is associated with an irregularly dilated duct that has calcifications and posterior shadows.[22] In surgery for chronic pancreatitis, ultrasound helps to define structures and identify the site of the pancreatic calcifications or intraglandular cysts.[19]

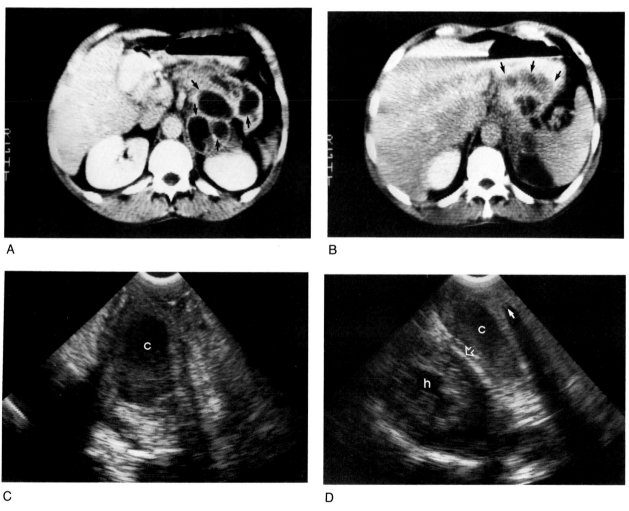

Fig. 11-19. Pancreatic pseudocyst. **(A)** Enhanced CT scan. A multiseptated pseudocyst (arrows) is seen within the pancreatic tail. **(B)** Enhanced CT scan, at a higher level that **(A)**. A poorly defined mass (arrows) is seen posterior to the stomach. **(C)** High transverse scan demonstrating a cystic mass *(c)* posterior to the stomach. This pseudocyst had developed since the CT scan in **(B)**. **(D)** Longitudinal scan showing the pseudocyst *(c)* inferior to the diaphragm (open arrow). A nasogastric tube within the stomach is casting an acoustic shadow (arrow). The OR ultrasound clearly defined the nature of the pancreatic mass that had developed since the earlier CT scan. (*h*, heart) (From Vincent LM, Mittelstaedt CA: Intraoperative abdominal ultrasound. p.95. In Sanders RC, Hill M (eds): Ultrasound Annual 1984. Raven Press, New York, 1984.)

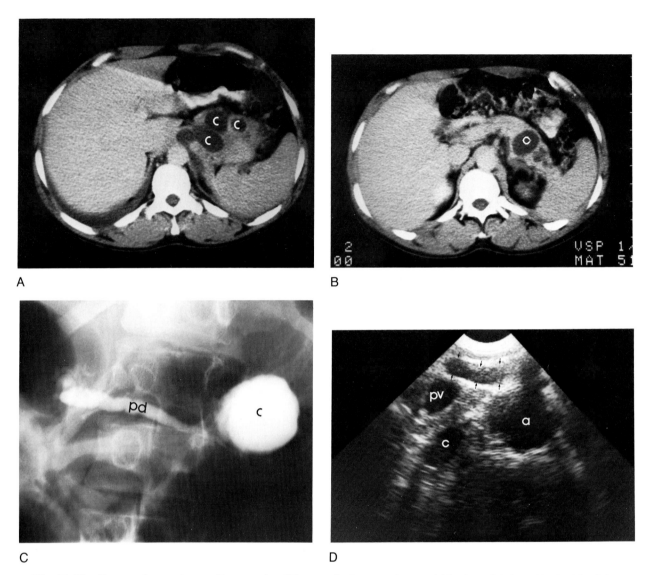

Fig. 11-20. Pancreatic pseudocyst. Preoperative CT scans display pseudocysts *(c)* in the tail **(A)** and body **(B)** of the pancreas. At ERCP **(C)**, the cyst *(c)* in the body was seen to fill with contrast with injection of the pancreatic duct *(pd)*. At surgery, the cysts in the tail were found but the cyst in the body could not be located. **(D)** Magnified transverse scan shows a dilated pancreatic duct (arrows) anterior to the aorta *(a)*, inferior vena cava *(c)* and main portal vein *(pv)*. *(Figure continues.)*

The ultrasound appearance of a pancreatic carcinoma is not specific but it has been found to provide diagnostic aid in 61 percent of operative procedures for tumor.[7,14] However, there are signs suggestive of malignancy that include pancreatic duct dilatation, stricture or invasion of the superior mesenteric vein, and common bile duct dilatation without biliary stones.[7,14] These may help establish the diagnosis of malignancy.[7,14] Many tumors have been shown to have a hypoechoic appearance with poorly defined margins without acoustic enhancement[7,14,19,22] (Fig. 11-21). Other investigators have reported a hyperechoic or isosonic pattern.[14] In cases in which tumor and inflammatory changes cannot be dis-

tinguished, ultrasound can be used to guide a needle biopsy of a pancreatic mass.[14,30] Also, ultrasound has been found useful in the identification of nonpalpable pancreatic masses.[35]

Ultrasound can be extremely helpful in evaluating the resectability of a lesion.[7,14,30] Tumor involvement of the superior mesenteric vessels and portal vein can be detected.[7,14,22,30] With tumor involvement, there is loss of movement with respiration, irregular vein wall, and loss of linearity of parenchymal/vein interface to complete occlusion.[19,22] Partial or complete occlusion of the portal vein with secondary thrombosis may be seen with distal pancreatic ductal dilatation.[19,22] With identification of

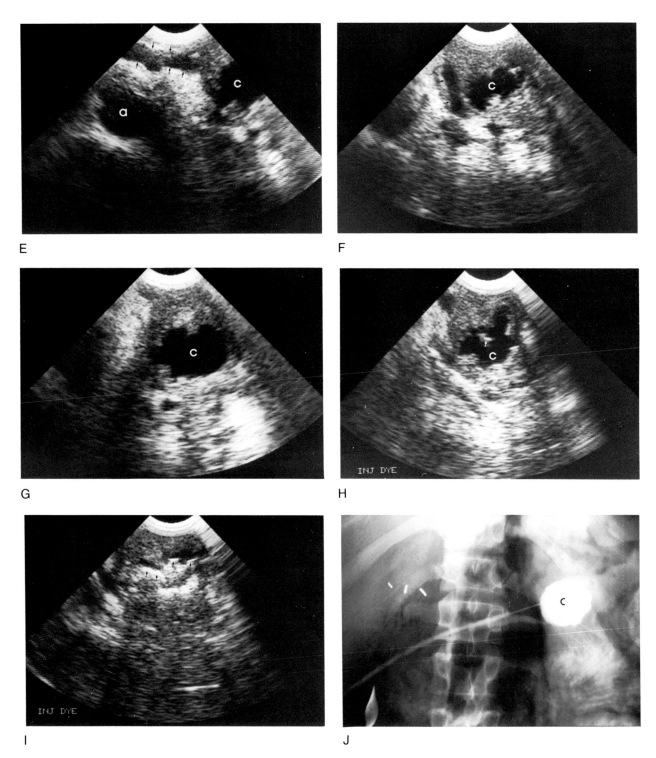

E

F

G

H

I

J

Fig. 11-20 *(Continued).* By angling to the left transversely **(E)**, the cyst *(c)* is seen as well as the duct (arrows). (*a,* aorta.) With slight change in the transducer position on **(F)**, the relationship of the duct (arrows) and cyst *(c)* are shown. (*a,* aorta.) **(G)** The cyst *(c)* has irregular borders and is anechoic. **(H)** With ultrasound visualization, a needle (arrows) was inserted into the cyst *(c).* **(I)** Without changing the transducer position, contrast was injected (arrows) into the cyst causing a reflective pattern. **(J)** Radiograph taken showing contrast injection within the cyst *(c).* It does not communicate with the other cysts so a second cyst drainage procedure was undertaken.

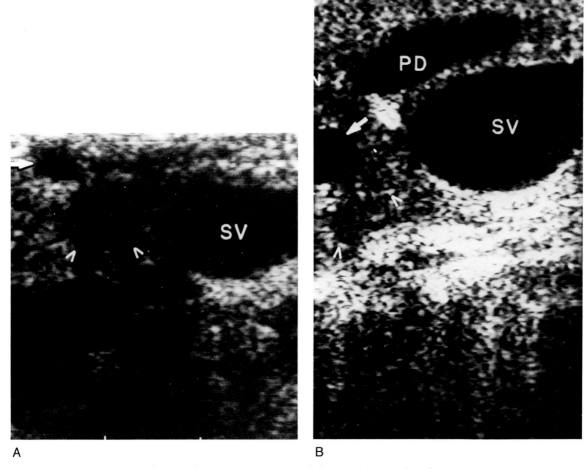

A   B

Fig. 11-21. Pancreatic carcinoma. **(A)** Transverse image (along the long axis) of the pancreas demonstrates an ill-defined hypoechoic mass 5 × 5 mm, a carcinoma, in the ampullary segment (arrowheads) of the pancreas abutting the gastroduodenal artery (arrow) and the confluence of the superior mesenteric and splenic veins *(SV)*. Demarcations at the bottom of the image are centimeters. **(B)** Transverse image (along long axis) of the pancreas demonstrates an ill-defined 1 cm hypoechoic adenocarcinoma (arrowheads) surrounding the common bile duct (arrow). The dilated pancreatic duct *(PD)* and the confluence of the superior mesenteric and splenic veins *(SV)* are also visible. (From Rifkin MD, Weiss SM: Intraoperative sonographic identification of nonpalpable pancreatic masses. J Ultrasound Med 3:409, 1984.)

portal vein infiltration by tumor, the surgeon can decide the feasibility of a pancreaticoduodenotomy or may choose a palliative bypass procedure.[22] Duct termination with tumor involvement has been described as having the presence of a shelf or complete blockage with intrinsic tumor invasion, or an abnormally proximally tapering duct due to external obstruction.[14]

Endocrine tumors can be particularly difficult to localize at surgery. Lobulations of the pancreas pose a problem in their diagnosis.[6] Because of its small size (most less than 2 cm and not visible from the surface of the gland) and 10 percent potential for multiplicity, the tumor is difficult to localize preoperatively and intraop-

eratively.[24,36,37] Ultrasound has been found to be useful in detection of these tumors and exclusion of tumors at sites considered to be suspicious on the basis of operative findings.[6,24] With accurate localization, a simple enucleation procedure may be performed.[24] Enucleation carries less morbidity and mortality than does pancreatic resection, especially if it is "blind."[24]

All endocrine tumors in one series were found to be hypoechoic, with adenomas being the most pronouncely hypoechoic[6,24,36,37] (Fig. 11-22). Therefore, in cases in which a mass is palpated and found to be hypoechoic at ultrasound, a tumor is suspected. Ultrasound is particularly important in helping to locate these islet cell tumors

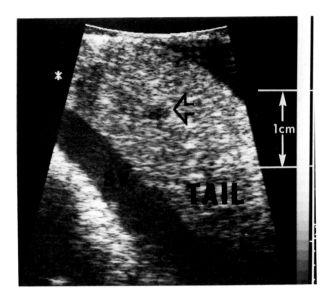

Fig. 11-22. Islet cell tumor. Insulinoma. Transverse high-frequency (10 MHz) image demonstrates a 0.4 cm hypoechoic mass (arrow) within the distal body of the pancreas. This was one of five similar-sized insulinomas in a patient with MEN-I syndrome. Four were identified sonographically. (*SV*, splenic vein.) (From Charboneau JW: Shallow body structures come into sharper focus. Reprinted with permission from Diagnostic Imaging 11:90, © 1984 by Miller Freeman Publications.)

of the pancreas because of the failure to find such lesions might necessitate "blind" resection of a part of the pancreas or performance of total gastrectomy.

Because radiography during pancreatic surgery is rarely applicable, ultrasound provides unique imaging information that may facilitate surgical therapy.[7] In evaluation of pancreatic tumors, ultrasound has been found to be helpful in 61 percent of cases, to assist in making the diagnosis in 39 percent, to assist in localization in 18 percent, and to aid in exclusion in 4 percent.[7]

Vascular

There have been recent reports of the use of ultrasound during arterial reconstructive surgery to supplement information from the preoperative arteriogram and to detect vascular defects immediately after restoration of blood flow.[4,38,39] Intimal flaps are the commonest defects observed; others include strictures or thrombi.[4,30,38,39] In most instances in which defects are seen, vessels are not reentered because the defects are considered too small or located in nonstrategic sites or both.[30,38]

When ultrasound and arteriography are compared, they are found to be equal in terms of sensitivity, speci-

ficity, efficiency, and predictability of a negative test.[39] In one series, the predictability of a positive test is 77.8 percent by ultrasound and 59.1 percent for arteriography.[39] In determining the usefulness in detecting vascular defects after extremity bypass graft reconstruction, the accuracy of ultrasound has been reported to be 94.4 percent and that of arteriography 83.3 percent.[40] Fewer needless reexplorations occur with ultrasound.

The greatest advantage of ultrasound is its ability to observe the active motion of the intimal flaps in cadence with arterial pulsations.[39] If a flap is seen a decision can be made whether to reexplore. However, ultrasound is oversensitive in detection of strictures, thrombi, and intimal flaps.[39] This modality is capable of recognizing lesions too small to be of clinical significance.[39]

There are limitations to the ultrasound evaluation of vessels.[22,38,39] Because the scan field is small, proper orientation may be difficult. Unlike arteriography, only the vessels exposed can be scanned by ultrasound; the arterial tree distal to the operative site cannot be viewed. However, the use of ultrasound can provide better information in instances in which the decision is now based solely on the clinical assessment and it may reduce the need for operative arteriography.

Other Applications

Because intraoperative ultrasound is still evolving, its applications have not been fully identified. Other applications might include the localization of foreign bodies for removal, and characterization of any unsuspected mass seen at surgery.[2-4]

CONCLUSION

Intraoperative ultrasound is as yet a new frontier; its applications are still being "staked out." Its impact is likely to become considerable because of the quality and quantity of new information available. Whether this modality will be used only under particular conditions or receive general adoption for ordinary use remains to be seen. While the advanges of this modality are many, its disadvantages will determine its future role.[1]

The scarcity of commercially available dedicated equipment is the biggest disadvantage; but, this is not likely to continue to be a major factor. For the time being, general purpose sector systems can be easily adapted for some but not necessarily all OR studies at the present time.

One of the general drawbacks to the procedure remains the general inexperience of the surgeon regarding ultrasound principles, technique, and interpretation. Ultrasound is one of the most "user-dependent" of all radiographic procedures.[1] Logistic problems will ultimately be a limiting factor precluding routine use if the surgeon remains entirely dependent on the sonologist; though some degree of collaborative effort between the sonologist and the surgeon will always be necessary. In many instances, it may be desirable for the surgeon to have "hands on" the transducer, especially in cases with limited access, confusing anatomy, or with guidance for needle localization.

Ultimately the development of picture archival and communication systems (PACS) may support the practicability of the routine use of OR ultrasound.[1] Most of the logistical obstacles may be eliminated with the examination by the surgeon in the operating room, while the sonologist monitors the study in his or her own department.

REFERENCES

1. Vincent LM, Mittelstaedt CA: Intraoperative abdominal ultrasound. p.95. In Saunders RC, Hill M (eds): Ultrasound Annual 1984. Raven Press, New York, 1984
2. Mittelstaedt CA, Herbst CA, Vincent LM et al: Follow-up: Intraoperative gallbladder ultrasound. Proceedings from the 28th Annual Convention of the American Institute of Ultrasound in Medicine, J Ultrasound Med 2:18, 1983
3. Mittelstaedt CA, Fried FA, Staab EV et al: Intraoperative renal real-time ultrasound. Proceedings from the 28th Annual Convention of the American Institute of Ultrasound in Medicine, J Ultrasound Med 2:19, 1983
4. Sigel B: Operative Ultrasonography, Lea and Febiger, Philadelphia, 1982
5. Sigel B, Coelho JCU, Machi J: Operative real-time B-mode ultrasound scanning. p. 201. In Sanders RC (ed): Ultrasound Annual 1982. Raven Press, New York, 1982
6. Sigel B, Duarte B, Machi J et al: Operative ultrasonography for endocrine tumor. Proceedings from the 28th Annual Convention of the American Institute of Ultrasound in Medicine, J Ultrasound Med 2:21, 1983
7. Sigel B, Machi J, Beitler JC et al: Appraisal of utility of operative ultrasound in pancreatic surgery. Proceedings from the 28th Annual Convention of the American Institute of Ultrasound in Medicine, J Ultrasound Med 2:20, 1983
8. Lytton B, Cook JH: Intraoperative Ultrasound. p. 340. In Resnick MI, Sanders RC (eds): Ultrasound in Urology. Williams & Wilkins Company, Baltimore, 1979
9. Cook JH, Lytton B: Intraoperative localization of renal calculi during neprolithotomy by ultrasound scanning. J Urol 117:543, 1977
10. Sigel B, Coelho JCU, Spigos DG et al: Real-time ultrasonography during biliary surgery. Radiology 137:531, 1980
11. Sigel B, Spigos DG, Donahue PE et al: Intraoperative visualization of biliary calculi. Current Surgery 36:158, 1979
12. Machi J, Sigel B, Spigos DG et al: Experimental assessment of imaging variables associated with operative ultrasonic and radiographic cholangiography. J Ultrasound Med 2:535, 1983
13. Sigel B, Coelho JCU, Sharifi R et al: Ultrasonic scanning during operation for renal calculi. J Urol 127:421, 1982
14. Sigel B, Coelho JCU, Nyhus LM et al: Detection of pancreatic tumors by ultrasound during surgery. Arch Surg 117:1058, 1982
15. Sigel B, Coelho JCU, Donahue PE et al: Ultrasonic assistance during surgery for pancreatic inflammatory disease. Arch Surg 117:712, 1982
16. Lane RJ, Coupland GAE: Ultrasonic indications to explore the common bile duct. Surgery 91:268, 1982
17. Sigel B, Coelho JCU, Nyhus LM et al: Comparison of cholangiography and ultrasonography in the operative screening of the common bile duct. World J Surg 6:440, 1982
18. Sigel B, Coelho JCU, Spigos DG et al: Ultrasonic imaging during biliary and pancreatic surgery. Am J Surg 141:84, 1981
19. Lane RJ, Glazer G: Intra-operative B-mode ultrasound scanning of the extra-hepatic biliary system and pancreas. Lancet 2:334, 1980
20. Plainfossé MC, Merran S: Work in progress: Intraoperative abdominal ultrasound. Radiology 147:829, 1983
21. Marshall FF, Smith NA, Murphy JB et al: A comparison of ultrasonography and radiography in the localization of renal calculi: Experimental and operative experience. J Urol 126:576, 1981
22. Lane RJ: Intraoperative B-mode scanning. J Clin Ultrasound 8:427, 1980
23. Mittelstaedt CA, Staab EV, Drobnes WE et al: The intraoperative uses of real-time ultrasound. Radiographics 4:267, 1984
24. Charboneau JW, James EM, Van Heerden JA et al: Intraoperative real-time ultrasonographic localization of pancreatic insulinomas: Initial experience. J Ultrasound Med 2:251, 1983
25. Thuroff JW, Alken P, Riedmiller H et al: Doppler and real-time ultrasound in renal stone surgery. Eur Urol 8:298, 1982
26. Marshall FF: Intraoperative localization of renal calculi. Urol Clin North Am 20:629, 1983
27. Stafford SJ, Jenkins JM, Staab EV et al: Ultrasonic detection of renal calculi: Accuracy tested in an in vitro porcine kidney model. J Clin Ultrasound 9:359, 1981
28. Rubin JM, Baglet DH, Lyon ES et al: Intraoperative real-time ultrasonic scanning for locating and recovering renal calculi. J Urol 130:434, 1983
29. Cook JH, Lytton B: The practical use of ultrasound as an adjunct to renal calculous surgery. Urol Clin North Am 8:319, 1981
30. Sigel B, Coelho JCU, Machi J et al: The application of real-time ultrasound imaging during surgical procedures. Surg Gynecol Obstet 157:33, 1983

31. Levine SB, Lerner HJ, Leifer ED et al: Intraoperative cholangiography. Ann Surg 198:692, 1983

32. Carroll BA: Gallstones: In vitro comparison of physical, radiographic and ultrasonic characteristics. AJR 131:223, 1978

33. Laing FC, Gooding GAW, Brown T et al: Atypical pseudocysts of the pancreas: An ultrasonographic evaluation. J Clin Ultrasound 7:27, 1979

34. Sarti DA, King W: The ultrasonic findings in inflammatory pancreatic disease. p.178. In Raymond HW, Zwiebel WJ (eds): Seminars in Ultrasound. Vol. 1. Grune and Stratton, New York, 1980

35. Rifkin MD, Weiss SM: Intraoperative sonographic identification of nonpalpable pancreatic masses. J Ultrasound Med 3:409, 1984

36. Lane RJ, Coupland GAE: Operative ultrasonic features of insulinomas. Am J Surg. 144:585, 1982

37. Sigel B, Duarte B, Coelho JCU et al: Localization of insulinomas of the pancreas at operation by real-time ultrasound scanning. Surg Gynecol Obstet 156:145, 1983

38. Sigel B, Coelho JCU, Flanigan P et al: Ultrasonic imaging during vascular surgery. Arch Surg 117:764, 1982

39. Sigel B, Flanigan P, Schuler JJ et al: Imaging ultrasound in the intraoperative diagnosis of vascular defects. J Ultrasound Med 2:337, 1983

40. Sigel B, Coelho JCU, Flanigan DP et al: Comparison of B-mode real time ultrasound scanning with arteriography in detecting vascular defects during surgery. Radiology 145:777, 1982

Index

Page numbers followed by *f* indicate figures; those followed by *t* indicate tables.